Reddy and Rajkumar's

Short Cases in
SURGERY

Including Orthopedics

Second Edition

Reddy and Rajkumar's

Short Cases in
SURGERY
Including Orthopedics

Second Edition

C M K REDDY

DSc (Hon), FRCS (Glas), FRCS, FRSH (Eng), FICS, FICA (USA)

General and Vascular Surgeon

Emeritus Professor of Surgery, The Tamil Nadu Dr MGR Medical University
Examiner to MBBS, MS, MCh (Vascular), National Board and FRCS (Ire)
Senior Consultant and Director of Continuing Medical Education Program, Apollo Hospitals
Surgeon–Director, Halsted Surgical Clinic, Institute of PG Education and Research
President, Indian Chapter, Royal College of Surgeons in Ireland
Visiting Professor and Member, Board of Directors, Sri Ramachandra Deemed University
Visiting Professor to Colorado University of Health Sciences, Denver, USA
Recipient of Dr BC Roy National Award, as Eminent Medical Teacher and
Lifetime Achievement Award by the Tamil Nadu Dr MGR Medical University

Formerly Honorary Professor of Surgery and Surgeon, Stanley Medical College and Hospital
Senate and Governing Council Member and Chairman, Board of Studies, TN Dr MGR Medical University
Chennai, TN

and

J S RAJKUMAR

MS DNB (Surg) FRCS (Eng), FRCS (Edin), FRCS (Glas), FRCS (Ire), FICS, FIMSA, FAIS, FRSM (Lon)

General, Laparoscopic Surgeon and Surgical Gastroenterologist

Chairman, Lifeline Multispeciality Hospitals, Chennai
Surgeon–Director, Rajaratnam Institute of Gastrointestinal Diseases
Visiting Professor, Rajah Muthiah Medical College, Chidambaram
Visiting Lecturer, Sri Ramachandra Medical College and Research Institute
Examiner to FRCS (Edin)
Chennai, TN

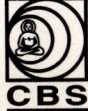

CBS

CBS Publishers & Distributors Pvt Ltd

New Delhi • Bengaluru • Chennai • Kochi • Pune

Hyderabad • Kolkata • Manipal • Mumbai • Nagpur • Patna

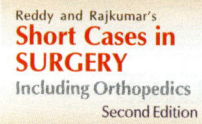

ISBN: 978-81-239-2260-7

Copyright © Authors and Publisher

Second Edition: 2013

First Edition: 2001

Published by Satish Kumar Jain for

CBS Publishers & Distributors Pvt Ltd

4819/XI Prahlad Street, 24 Ansari Road, Daryaganj, New Delhi 110 002, India.

Ph: 23289259, 23266861, 23266867   Fax: 011-23243014   Website: www.cbspd.com
e-mail: delhi@cbspd.com; cbspubs@airtelmail.in

Corporate Office: 204 FIE, Industrial Area, Patparganj, Delhi 110 092
Ph: 4934 4934   Fax: 4934 4935   e-mail: publishing@cbspd.com; publicity@cbspd.com

Branches

- **Bengaluru:** Seema House 2975, 17th Cross, K.R. Road, Banasankari 2nd Stage, Bengaluru 560 070, Karnataka
  Ph: +91-80-26771678/79   Fax: +91-80-26771680   e-mail: bangalore@cbspd.com
- **Chennai:** 20, West Park Road, Shenoy Nagar, Chennai 600 030, Tamil Nadu
  Ph: +91-44-26260666, 26208620   Fax: +91-44-42032115   e-mail: chennai@cbspd.com
- **Kochi:** 36/14 Kalluvilakam, Lissie Hospital Road, Kochi 682 018, Kerala
  Ph: +91-484-4059061-65   Fax: +91-484-4059065   e-mail: kochi@cbspd.com
- **Pune:** Bhuruk Prestige, Sr. No. 52/12/2+1+3/2 Narhe, Haveli (Near Katraj-Dehu Road Bypass), Pune 411 041, Maharashtra
  Ph: +91-20-64704058, 64704059, 32342277   Fax: +91-20-24300160   e-mail: pune@cbspd.com

Representatives

- **Hyderabad** 0-9885175004 • **Kolkata** 0-9831437309 • **Manipal** 0-9742022075
- **Mumbai** 0-9833017933 • **Nagpur** 0-9021734563 • **Patna** 0-9334159340

Printed and bound in India by Nutech Photolithographers.

to

---

our parents,

all our teachers
who taught us to sail the ocean of surgery

and

our wives,
Nirmala Reddy and Chitrakala Rajkumar,
who endured our discussions during
odd hours at night

Foreword

I am delighted to write this Foreword for the book, which impressed me, on perusal, as a very useful work for those pursuing higher learning in surgery.

Topics have been properly selected, the sentences have been carefully phrased and it is being released at a time when it is most needed by the postgraduate students of MS, National Board and Fellowship of the Royal colleges. While adhering to syntax, the matter has been compressed to convey maximal data in the space provided. Several color photos, line diagrams, algorithms and table forms added, should help in understanding the subject better, while breaking the tedium.

The accent on recent advances, gleaned from printed and on-line media as well as the addition of special topics such as chemotherapy, radiotherapy, nutrition, lasers, etc., will be particularly welcomed by exam-going postgraduates and practising surgeons.

Both the authors, whom I know well, have been doing excellent academic work for several decades: Prof CMK Reddy served as Honorary Professor at Stanley Medical College for 3 decades. Having been an examiner to MBBS, MS, MCh (Vascular), National Board and FRCS (Ire) for several years, he can judge the pulse of students with great precision. He has been acclaimed as one of the greatest teachers and his concise method of teaching has won appreciation from all corners.

Dr JS Rajkumar has an enormous academic foundation, with a brilliant career in Madras Medical College; a number of gold medals, including the coveted Johnstone medal, to his credit. He has proved himself to be a versatile surgeon, popular teacher and an asset to the medical community and I am happy that both these academicians have come together in this laudable project. The practice and perspective in surgery has evolved considerably over the last two decades and need less to say the authors have done well to combine the old with the new and package it into an enjoyable and purposeful reading.

I congratulate them for presenting this book to the young surgeons as a gift for the millennium.

Prof S Vittal

MS, FRCS (Ed), FICS, FIMSA, FAIS, FTASc

President, International College of Surgeons, Indian Section
Past President, Association of Surgeons of India, Founder President
Indian Association of Endocrine Surgeons, Visiting Professor
Madras Medical College, Chennai 600 031
Consultant Surgeon, Apollo Hospitals
Overseas Surgical Tutor, Royal College of Surgeons, Edinburgh, UK
Member, Editorial Board, *British Journal of Surgery*

Preface to the Second Edition

Prompted by the tremendous response from the medical students, especially postgraduates, we have ventured to bring out the second edition of our book *Short Cases in Surgery*. We also wanted to eliminate some deficiencies in the first edition of the book published in 2001, incidentally updating the previous chapters, since significant advances have taken place in virtually in every subject and every field of medicine. Chapters on surgical pathology, anesthesiology, radiology (diagnostic and interventional), endovascular surgery, portal hypertension, evaluation of an abdominal mass, minimal access surgery, medical audit including evidence-based medicine, medical ethics, stoma care general principles of orthopedics and common orthopedic problems, have been added.

There is no area in surgery without recent advances, hence meticulous updating of all the chapters was done, keeping an exam-going UG/PG surgical student in mind, so as not to overburden with information, which may be relevant only to students at superspeciality level in those areas. It is not easy to decide how much information to be given to a student but with our vast experience as teachers and examiners, we filtered the plethora of data available on every subject to the optimal level. Experienced consultants in various specialities of medicine have generously contributed in chapters of their interest and their involvement in shaping this book is highly appreciated.

Several clinical pictures, line diagrams and tables are added to make it student-friendly, so also 'jewels of gyan' to highlight important points for easy review and remembrance.

With countless medical advances, it seems virtually impossible to create a truly updated volume and when viewed through the lens of evidence-based medicine, some of the so-called standard treatment of yesterday, crumbles for want of solid scientific proof of their efficacy, giving way to newer methods of therapy. The rapid infiltration of modern technology into medicine has overshadowed to some extent the importance of delivering individualized care and ethical practice. Inherent lack of interest of the practitioners to read current medical literature, and attend continuing medical education courses and workshops has also contributed in a large measure to the suboptimal care to a patient and increased tendency for litigations.

These facts have been constantly kept in mind, while updating every chapter and we hope that the book would benefit junior surgeons in the examinations and later in practice.

The authors sincerely acknowledge the contributions made by several experts to reshape the book and by providing appropriate clinical pictures. Mr A Kumaaran, Techlogic, Coimbatore, who worked for several months to computerize all the material, to design attractive pagination, illustrations and giving finishing touches to the book, deserves special mention in this context.

We are grateful to the CBS Publishers & Distributors Pvt Ltd, New Delhi, for generously allowing sufficient time to us for editing the book to our full satisfaction and undertaking the job of printing and publishing the book. We also appreciate their plan for making the book available on-line, for the convenience of reference by surgical students in remote parts of the world.

CMK Reddy
JS Rajkumar

Acknowledgments

The authors gratefully acknowledge the contributions by the following senior consultants.

Dr V L Arul Selvan MD DM (Neuro) DNB (Medicine)
  Sr Consultant Neurologist, Apollo Hospitals, Chennai
Prof Arvind Krishnamurthy MS MCh (Surg Onco) DNB (Surg Onco) FICS FAIS
  Addl Professor and Sr Consultant Surgical Oncologist, Cancer Institute (WIA), Chennai
Dr V Balaji MS FRCS (Ed) FRCS (Eng)
  Sr Consultant Vascular Surgeon, Apollo Hospitals, Chennai
Prof G Balakrishnan MS MCh (Plast) FRCS (Eng) DSc
  Sr Consultant Plastic and Hand Surgeon, Right Hospital, Chennai
Prof N Deen Muhamed Ismail MS (Ortho) D Ortho
  Sr Consultant Orthopedic Surgeon, Madras Medical College, Chennai
Dr C M Kishore MS FRS
  Consultant General and Laparoscopic Surgeon, Halsted Surgical Clinic, Chennai
Dr S Krishnan BSc MD (Rad Therapy)
  Sr Consultant Radiation Oncologist, Head, Clinical Research, Dr Rai Memorial Medical Centre, Chennai
Dr Neha Kantawala MS FMAS FIAGES FALS
  Consultant General and Laparoscopic Surgeon, Lifeline Multispeciality Hospitals, Chennai
Dr K Raghavendran MD (Anes)
  Sr Consultant Anesthesiologist and Co-ordinator, Apollo Children's Hospitals, Chennai
Dr K R Reddy MS
  Sr Consultant General and Laparoscopic Surgeon, Laxmi Multispeciality Hospital, Kakinada
Prof Sandhya Sundaram MD DNB (Path) MNAMS
  Professor and Sr Consultant Pathologist, Sri Ramachandra Medical College and Research Institute, Chennai
Dr R Venkatasubramanian MS DNB (Surg) MNAMS MRCS FNB (MAS)
  Sr Consultant General and Laparoscopic Surgeon, Apollo Hospitals, Chennai
Dr A N Vivek MS (Ortho)
  Consultant Orthopedic Surgeon, Lifeline Multispeciality Hospitals, Chennai

Several consultants, who provided appropriate clinical photographs and those who worked for technical excellence of the final product deserve special mention.

Mr A Kumaaran and his team members, Dr N Suganthi (Coimbatore), Mr C Prabhu Ebenezer, Mr D Mohana Sundar, Mrs K Haritha, Mrs C Leeladevi, Dr J R Anirudh, Mr S Senthil Kumar, Ms Meena Kesan and many others, were of immense assistance in this regard.

Contents

Orthopedics

A Synopsis and Common Orthopedic Short Cases

01 Introduction

Please **do not skip this chapter!** The broad basics of clinical approach are dealt with in the following few pages, in order to equip you to answer several questions on the fundamentals of surgery, which are frequently posed by the examiners. The value of obtaining a comprehensive history and eliciting relevant physical findings should not be underestimated in clinical medicine and its role in providing expedient, cost-effective medicare.

It cannot be over-emphasized that many mistakes in clinical practice still occur, not because one is not aware of the latest information about the disease, but because the fundamental principles laid down for good clinical examination are overlooked.

Protocol of case writing (presentation)

Every student and clinician should be familiar with the standard protocol of case presentation or recording, so as not to miss any important aspect of a particular disease and should always aim for thoroughness in considering even remote possibilities of diagnoses, though common conditions deserve preference. It may be appropriate to remember two diagonally opposite aphorisms in this context: 'if you make a rare diagnosis, you may be rarely correct' and the other 'if you don't consider rare possibilities, they become still rarer!'

It is important that surgical students possess sufficient knowledge of certain basic subjects, such as embryology, applied anatomy including surface markings, physiology, pharmacology, pathology, basic anesthesia, definitions of common terms in clinical vocabulary and normal values of commonly performed laboratory investigations, as these figure during clinical discussions in examinations at all levels. No wonder, students are unsuccessful in the examination, though their diagnoses might be acceptable, if gross deficiency is identified in the areas mentioned above, that are necessary

for proper understanding of the science and craft of surgery.

This is the suggested foolproof scheme:

1) History
2) Physical examination
3) Provisional diagnosis
4) Differential diagnosis
5) Investigations
6) Clinical/Final diagnosis
7) Treatment
8) Prognostic evaluation
9) Follow-up of progress
10) Final outcome

1) History

Needless to say, this is a very important aspect of understanding the pathological sequence as well as the causal relations to various symptoms in a particular case. Patients cannot be tied down to an orderly sequence; freedom should be given to express in their own words and in their own style. Specific questions may be put whenever they seem to be straying away from relevance, or if any part of their history needs more details. Leading or suggestive questions, such as 'does the pain radiate to the left arm' or 'do antacids relieve your stomach pain' may save time, but may elicit thoughtless answers in the affirmative, from a 'not-so-alert' patient; instead it is preferable to ask 'where does your pain radiate' or 'what relieves your stomach pain'. Questions such as, 'what are you suffering from' (asking for the diagnosis), should also be avoided, unless the patient himself happens to be a doctor!

As a rule, history taking should not be stereotyped and has to be tailored to the individual patient, depending upon their level of intelligence and orientation. However some structured approach is necessary to avoid glaring omissions, particularly when the interrogator is relatively inexperienced. It may sound odd, but true that one has to mentally

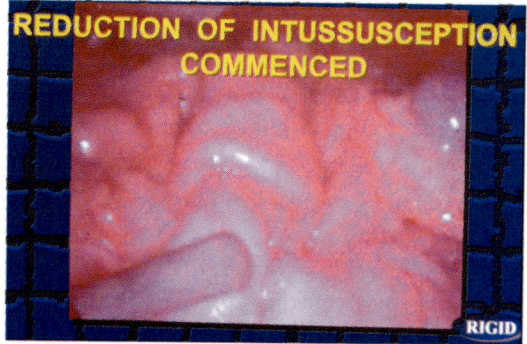

Fig. 1.1. Laparoscopic view of reduction of ileo-ileal intussusception (courtesy: Lifeline Hospitals, Chennai)

work out the differential diagnosis, based on the chief (presenting) complaints itself, so that no relevant history is omitted, either positive or negative. To illustrate this point, in a case of splenomegaly, unless one had worked out the various possibilities like portal hypertension, chronic malaria, tropical splenomegaly, blood dyscrasias, amyloidosis or autoimmune diseases, history taking can never be complete, since each of the conditions will require certain points to be elicited in the history.

By careful observation of the manner in which a patient narrates history, e.g. laying undue emphasis on unimportant matters, an experienced clinician can mostly identify a functional disorder mimicking an organic disease. In fact one of the important attributes for an efficient and popular physician is to be able to sort these out, at the time of the first visit itself, so that investigations in the wrong direction can be avoided.

Munchausen's syndrome is named after a laparotomophilic malingerer, who presented to several hospitals, at various times, with typical symptoms and signs of surgical diseases, luring them to carry out multiple laparotomies, for no organic illness, before the days of noninvasive imaging techniques. Unusual difficulty may be experienced in eliciting proper history in children, very aged, or those with a hearing defect, depressed cerebration, mental imbalance and language problems, requiring innovative techniques.

a) Personal data

Name: Knowing the name of the patient and addressing him or her by the name, during interrogation would bring the patient emotionally closer, since the dearest thing in the world for any one is his name.

Age: Not only should one ask for the age of a patient but should also correlate with the general appearance. It is not rare to find an uneducated rural patient unable to give his/her correct age.

Some diseases are peculiar to certain ages, e.g. congenital anomalies like cleft lip or palate, meningocele, sacrococcygeal teratoma or a club foot may be seen at birth, while conditions like thyroglossal cyst, polycystic kidney, branchial cyst may manifest later in life. True benign tumors are rare in children; if any mass has features of a benign tumor in a child, it is most probably a hamartoma (hamartia: defect or sin). Wilm's tumor (nephroblastoma) and neuroblastoma of suprarenal are found in infants, Burkitt's tumor in the preschool age (3-7 yrs), sarcomas in young adults and carcinomas in later life. In thyroid for example, differentiated carcinomas occur in younger ages (20-50), whereas anaplastic tumor occurs usually after 50. Stricture urethra and prostatitis are the common causes of urinary obstruction in young adults, whereas benign hypertrophy and carcinoma prostate are encountered in men over 50.

Gender: Diseases of genital tract/organs are different in either sex. Diseases of breast, thyroid, biliary tract, cervical rib and femoral hernia are more common in females, whereas carcinoma stomach, inguinal hernia, carcinoma lung are seen more in males. Certain x-linked diseases like hemophilia affect only males, but females may be carriers of these diseases.

Race and religion: Vascular diseases, colonic tumors are common in the West, Burkitt's lymphoma and keloids in Africa, bilharziasis in Arabian countries. In Jews and Muslims, who practice circumcision during childhood, carcinoma penis is extremely rare. Basal cell carcinoma is seen in white-skin races.

Occupation: Workers in aniline dye factories are more prone for carcinoma urinary bladder, those who work in asbestos factories run a high risk of developing pleural mesothelioma and people using rapid vibrating tools develop Raynaud's phenomenon of upper limbs. Conditions like 'student's elbow' and 'house maid's knee' are due to olecranon and prepatellar bursitis respectively.

Residence: Geographical distribution of certain diseases make it very important to record the place of permanent residence of the patient. Hydatid disease is common in the southern districts of TN, whereas dracunculosis is prevalent in western districts of AP (India), where step-wells are used for drinking purposes. Cat scratch fever (viral) is common in UK, bilharziasis in Egypt, malaria, filariasis, amebiasis and tuberculosis in the East Asia (tropics). Kangri cancer is seen in Kashmiris due to constant irritation by heat over the abdominal wall and cancer oral cavity is seen more in a population with a peculiar habit of smoking cigars with lighted ends inside the mouth (chutta cancer), prevalent in certain tobacco-growing coastal districts of AP (India).

Weight and height: Patient's weight has to be recorded with minimal clothing and height without any foot-wear. Any unusual value has to be taken into clinical discussion, like obesity, emaciation, gigantism, dwarfism etc. The fact that simple fluid retention could increase weight has to be remembered. Obesity, besides being a predisposing cause for many illnesses like hypothyroidism (relative), diabetes mellitus, hypertension, osteoarthrosis, dependent edema (benign) of legs, exertional

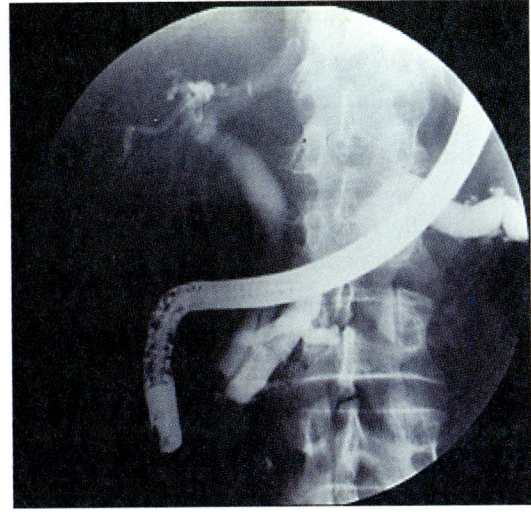

Fig. 1.3. Endoscopic retrograde cholangiopancreatogram (ERCP) showing dilated CBD and pancreatic ducts
(courtesy: Lifeline Hospitals, Chennai)

dyspnea, may give false high readings of blood pressure and make palpation difficult in groin hernia, abdominal masses or thyroid nodule etc. It may also pose problems during anesthesia, recovery following surgery and wound healing, considerably increasing the morbidity and mortality.

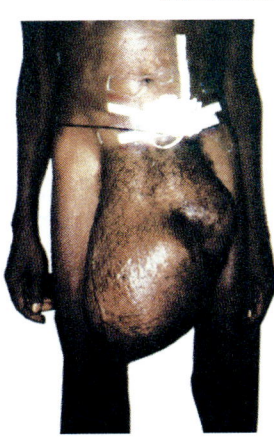

Fig. 1.2. Huge scrotal hernia (scrotal abdomen); note the evidence of creating pneumoperitoneum, through a cannula in the hypogastrium

(courtesy: Halsted Surgical Clinic, Chennai)

Body mass index (BMI)

The current practice is to measure the weight of an individual interpolated against the height, as body mass index.

(BMI: weight in KG/ height in M^2)
Under-weight: <18.5
Normal: 18.5 to 24.9
Over-weight: 25.0 to 29.9
Obese: 30.0 to 34.9 (Class I)
Very obese: 35.0 to 39.9 (Class II)
Morbid obesity: >40 (Class III)
Super obesity: >50 (Class IV)

b) Chief complaint(s)

If there are more than one, they should be mentioned in the chronological order. The patients often understate the duration or consider certain pre-existing disease as insignificant, hence it may be prudent to ask 'were you perfectly alright prior to this symptom?'

c) History of present illness

This is the most important of all, since occasionally there may not be any physical findings, as in peptic ulcer or ulcerative colitis, one has to depend largely on history, to proceed further. To avoid missing any important point, it is mentally divided into three parts:

i) to elaborate the chief complaint, in full detail

ii) to elaborate any other symptoms patient may be having, but not mentioned under chief complaint and last but not the least

iii) symptoms referable to general health of the patient, such as appetite, bowels, micturition, weight, cough, fever, sleep, etc. should be elicited in full detail, to clinch their causal relation to the main disease.

Though the present complaint may be of recent nature, if any symptoms patient had earlier, appear to be related, the history of present illness can start from that point onwards, to

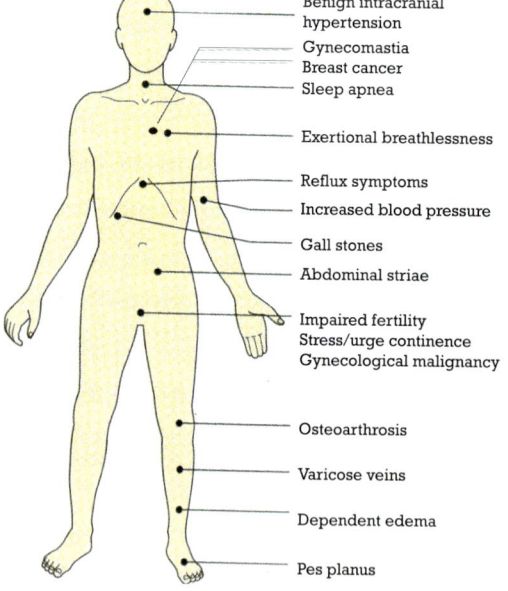
Fig. 1.4. Obesity-related diseases

narrate the sequence of events till date. For example, patient may come with acute epigastric pain, appearing like perforated peptic ulcer; if he gives history of acid-peptic disease for months or years earlier, with typical periodicity etc, one may start describing the present history from the time, he first experienced those symptoms. It is important to know the mode of onset (insidious or sudden), any precipitating factor like NSAIDs (for acute erosive gastritis), alcohol indulgence (in acute pancreatitis), or trauma, etc. If the patient is able to state precisely the date and time of onset of symptoms, it probably had an acute onset.

Specific food intolerance, such as fatty food (biliary pain), spicy food (acid-peptic disease) etc. has to be elicited. Though the earlier combination, 'fat, flatulent, fertile, female of forty' was considered high risk for gallstones, it is now realized that neither a 'slim, symptomless, sterile, man of sixty', nor a 'postpartum primi, who was a pre-pregnancy pill taker' is exempt. Next is to find out the progress of the disease, change in symptoms, rate of growth of a mass, any regression with/without treatment, and secondary manifestations, local, regional or systemic. If there has been ulceration over a mass, was it spontaneous or due to counter irritants applied over it. In a malignant breast mass, for instance, it is important to know if the overlying ulcer was due to tumor infiltration or due to external applications, as it would alter clinical staging and prognosis. If more than one area is involved, it is important to know where it originally started and which was subsequently involved, as in a case of oral cancer involving cheek and gum.

In cases of malignant tumor with skin ulceration, it is very pertinent to know if it started as an ulcer or as a subcutaneous swelling with intact skin that subsequently ulcerated, since in the former instance it might be an epithelioma or basal cell carcinoma, whereas in the latter case it is likely to be a

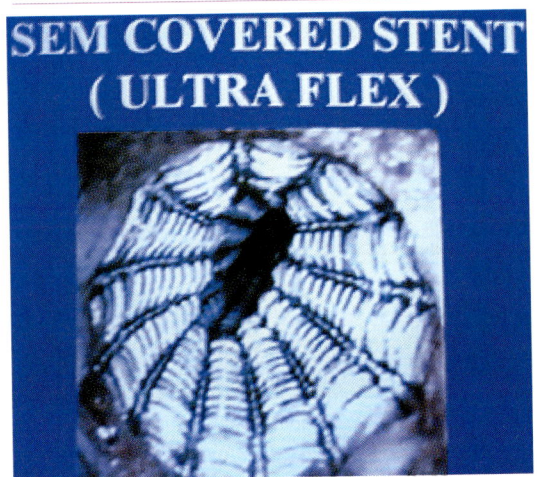

Fig. 1.5. Advanced carcinoma esophagus
Endoscopic placement of a covered self expandable
metal (SEM) stent which has memory, to retain original
shape
(courtesy: Lifeline Hospitals Chennai)

melanoma (arising from deeper layers of skin) or soft tissue sarcoma, infiltrating the skin. Local pain or fever at the onset of a swelling is generally in favor of an inflammatory lesion since neoplasms are neither painful, nor exhibit constitutional symptoms in initial stages.

Hematemesis is vomiting of frank blood, whereas if it is altered (coffee-ground), it is melenemesis, seen in slow bleeding disorders of upper GI tract. Occasionally bleeding from mouth and pharynx may confuse the picture, as also vomiting of swallowed blood from hemoptysis.

Melena is passing black tarry stools due to presence of altered blood and is an important symptom in ulcerating lesions of gastrointestinal tract, such as acid-peptic disease (APD), malignancy, inflammatory bowel diseases (IBD) etc. Generally, upper GI bleeding causes melena, but it may be from as low as distal colon. On the other hand, lesions of distal colon and anorectum produce frank (unaltered) bleeding per rectum (hematochezia), but it may be rarely seen in states of rapid transit from massive bleeding in the upper GI tract (proximal to

duodeno-jejunal junction). About 50-100ml of blood is required to alter the natural color of stools, whereas as little as 5-10ml, can give occult blood positivity.

Considerable weight loss generally indicates an organic disease. For example, if a child is 'incessantly' vomiting for several months, as reported by the mother, but not lost any weight, it is likely that he/she is suffering from some functional disorder. It may also be an important clue to distinguish a malignant lesion from a benign one, since weight loss is a usual phenomenon in cancers, for the following reasons:

1. Strategic location of the tumor obstructing food passages (esophageal carcinoma)

2. Actual loss of blood, electrolyte and protein-rich fluid from ulcerated tumors (colon carcinoma)

3. Humoral factors released such as tumor necrosis factor (TNF), which in turn raises serum levels of leptin (leptos: slender), a hormone which decreases food intake and increases energy loss, affecting bone marrow and GI tract

4. Competing with the host nutrition (only in disseminated tumors)

5. Psychological reasons (hence diagnosis should not be disclosed point blank, to the patient

Some negative aspects in the history may be equally important, e.g. thromboangiitis obliterans is not considered in a nonsmoker or adhesive small bowel obstruction without a previous history of laparotomy or peritonitis.

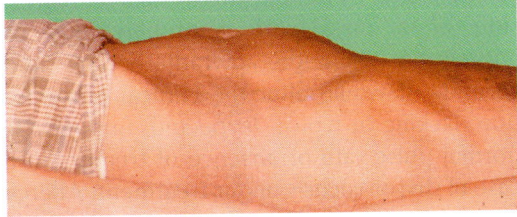

Fig. 1.6. Abdominal aortic aneurysm (AAA) pulsatile epigastric/umbilical mass better appreciated by tangential inspection
(courtesy: Halsted Surgical Clinic, Chennai)

d) Past history (medical/surgical)

All major illnesses suffered or previous surgical procedures undergone should be noted. History of typhoid fever will support a diagnosis of cholecystitis and history of pulmonary tuberculosis, may support the diagnosis of abdominal or genitourinary Koch's disease. Surgical incisions in line with ilioinguinal/iliohypogastric nerves could weaken the conjoint tendon and predispose to inguinal hernia (surgery on kidney, ureter, lumbar sympathectomy, appendectomy or surgery to expose iliac vessels, including renal transplantation). Local recurrence following excision of a mass generally suggests malignancy or a specific granuloma. Symptoms of acid-peptic disease appearing years after surgery for DU, might signal anastomotic ulcer or an ulcer diathesis. History of injury or immobilization of limb may predispose to deep vein thrombosis and its late sequel, postphlebitic syndrome. Childhood diseases like mumps (infertility), rheumatic fever (valvular disease of heart), bleeding tendencies (hemophilia or thrombocytopenic disorders), poliomyelitis (phantom hernia or club foot), etc. may also be important. Though delicate, history of exposure to sexually transmitted diseases (STD) has to be elicited, but it should be emphasized that the absence of such a history does not exclude the diagnosis of STD; nor does a positive history automatically establish the diagnosis.

e) Treatment history

It is important for two reasons: it may give a valuable clue to the diagnosis; such as regression of a mass with antituberculous or antimitotic chemotherapy/radiotherapy and secondly it would alter the clinical presentation, lacking in typical (expected) findings, as normal pulse rate or absence of tremors in a case of thyrotoxicosis under treatment. Allergy to drugs/certain foods/ adhesive tapes/iodised antiseptic external paints, etc. should be noted in bold, to avoid life-threatening misadventures.

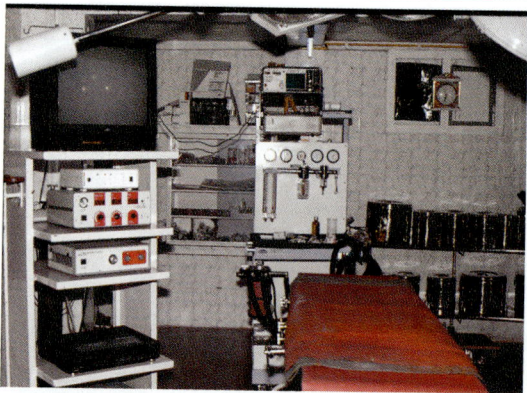

Fig. 1.7. Laparoscopic unit
(courtesy: Halsted Surgical Clinic, Chennai)

Even if there is history of a mass regressing with some treatment given by the family physician, one cannot exclude the possibility of malignancy or specific infection, as lymphoma may respond promptly to steroids, or a tuberculous granuloma may regress with streptomycin, kanamycin or ofloxacin given inadvertently as a general antibiotic.

Immunisation history may also be noted here. Therapy received for any chronic or concomitant illness, such as NSAIDs, steroids, thyroxine, antidiabetic, antihypertensive, antiplatelet, anticoagulant, psychotrophic agents, laxatives, contraceptives or diuretics etc. which might influence the selection of drugs to be given, has to be recorded. For example it may be disastrous to give IV calcium gluconate if the patient is receiving digitalis preparations. Similarly anti cholinergic agents or α-adrenergic agonists might precipitate acute urinary retention in a case of BPH.

f) Personal history

Diet, smoking, tobacco chewing, snuff or jarda, alcoholism have to be noted. The significance of smoking cigars with lighted ends inside the mouth, is already described. Marital status, number of children and whether she breast fed them, are all important, because carcinoma breast is more common in women with no or few children and if they were not breast-fed, due to uninterrupted estrogen influence on

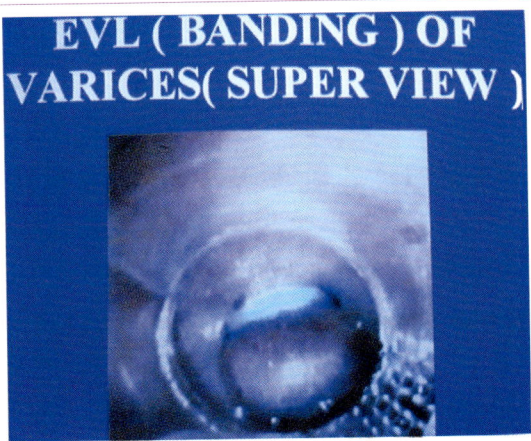

Fig. 1.8. Endoscopic esophageal variceal banding - the strangulated varix is seen
(courtesy: Lifeline Hospitals, Chennai)

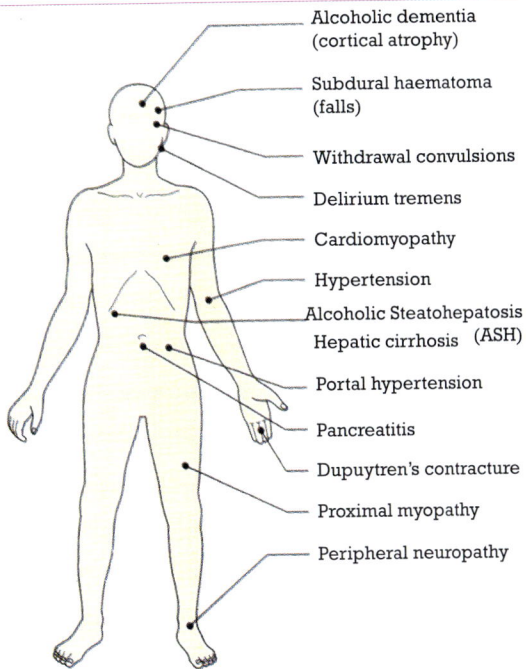

Fig. 1.9. Alcohol-related diseases

mammary tissue. Carcinoma cervix uteri is more common in multiparous women.

Menstrual and obstetric history is important, including regularity, nature and quantity of bleeding or other symptoms such as leukorrhea, metrorrhagia (or menostaxis), dysmenorrhea or dyspareunia. Number of pregnancies or miscarriages, whether they were delivered normally or by Cesarean section and for what indication and the present state of health of children should be ascertained. Menstrual status is also important in the management of carcinoma breast. Pain in the lower abdomen occurring exactly during intermenstrual period is due to minimal bleeding at the time of rupture of Graafian follicle, known as Mittelschmerz (mittel: middle; schmerz: pain) disease, which may be confused with appendicitis or salpingitis.

Severe abdominal pain with signs of internal hemorrhage in a young woman who missed a period, may point to ruptured ectopic (tubal) gestation. Surprisingly, some women would not have missed a period at all! A suprapubic mass, dipping into the pelvis in a woman of child bearing age, who has amenorrhea is, in all probability pregnancy unless proved otherwise (even if her husband had undergone sterilization operation!).

g) Family history: Some diseases run in families, like hemophilia, dyshormonogenic goitre, diabetes mellitus, primary hypertension, certain malignancies (breast, MEN syndromes, etc) are a few examples. To know if the parents of the patient had any major illness and if not alive, what was the probable cause of death, is important, so also the siblings and children of the patient.

It should be realized that a young patient may have reservations about disclosing history of smoking, drinking or exposure to STD in the presence of his parents or other elder members of the family. It is better to ask such questions in total privacy, taking the patient into confidence.

2) Physical examination

It is done under three headings: General, loco-regional and survey of other systems.

General

At the outset, patient's build, state of nourishment and hydration and whether in acute distress (pain, circulatory collapse or dyspnea) has to be noted along with the attitude taken by the patient. Problems, such as severe pain, external bleeding, upper airway obstruction, tension pneumothorax, acute cardiac tamponade or patient in a state of shock, should be given immediate attention for relief, before detailed history/ physical examination could be attempted or full cooperation of patient could be expected.

Physical examination should be done on a comfortable bed, in good day light (as far as possible), preferably completely stripped of clothes, covered only by an examination gown or sheet. While examining a child, it is better to have one of the parents by the side and if the patient is female, a female nurse/attendant should be by the side, to avoid misunderstanding later on (of course if the physician is a female, the reverse may be desirable).

A) Mental and intellectual state has to be assessed first, to know the reliability of history narrated by the patient. If there is any doubt, it is prudent to have an intelligent attendant to stand by for help. Five levels of mental faculties and consciousness may be noted:

I) Fully conscious and orientated to time and space

ii) Fully conscious but disorientated and incoherent

Faculty Measured	Response	Score
Eye Opening	Spontaneous	4
	To verbal command	3
	To pain	3
	No response	1
Motor response	To verbal command	6
	To localized pain	5
	Flexes and withdraws	4
	Flexes abnormally	3
	Extended abnormally	2
	No response	1
Verbal response	Oriented, converses	5
	Disoriented, converses	4
	Uses inappropriate words	3
	Make incomprehensible sounds	2
	No response	1

Table-1.1. Glasgow coma scale (GCS)
Grading:< 8points: severe injury
9-12 points: moderate injury
>12 points: minor injury

iii) Stuporous: Drowsy, but responds to questions and superficial stimuli

iv) Semicomatose: Responds only to deep/painful stimuli

v) Comatose: Deeply unconscious, not responding to even painful stimuli

Glasgow coma scale (GCS) is a reproducible way of evaluating the consciousness level, based on eye opening, verbal and best motor responses, often used to monitor patients with head injuries.

B) Attitude: Patients with peritonitis would like to lie still, whereas they would be tossing and curling about if it were a colic. A patient with cerebral irritation would lie still and resent light and one with hydrophobia would avoid looking at light or water. Attitude of the limb also may give a clue to the diagnosis, as in fracture neck of femur, with externally rotated leg without movement. Patients with serious unilateral lung disease, would not like to lie on the opposite side, as it would interfere with the normal excursions of the only functioning lung. Patients with limb ischemia prefer to drop the leg low, whereas those with venous

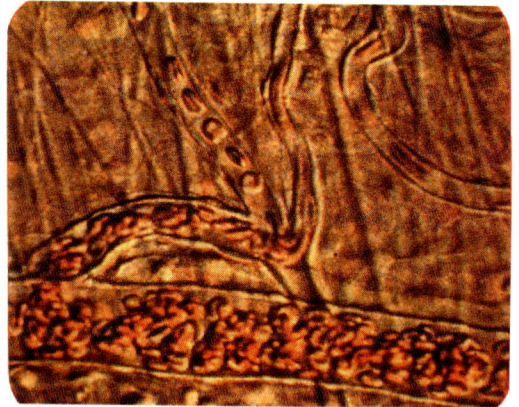

Fig. 1.10. High power magnification of capillary blood flow
(courtesy: Halsted Surgical Clinic, Chennai)

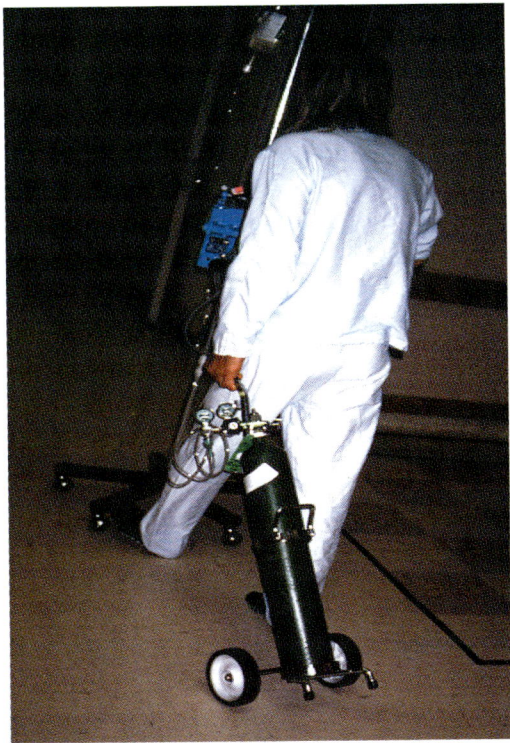

Fig. 1.11. Manpower problem?

An elderly patient carrying the oxygen equipment and IV fluids and stand (on wheels), all by himself to the Radiology department for investigations

(courtesy: Halsted Surgical Clinic, Chennai)

mask-like or expressionless face of Parkinsonism or hypothyroidism, Moon face of Cushing disease and adenoid facies in hypertrophied adenoids are a few examples. An experienced physician can study the face and decide if one has an organic disease, functional (psychosomatic) disease or is a malingerer, within a few moments of interview.

e)   Skin: Skin is the largest organ in the body and many internal diseases are expressed by cutaneous manifestations: Typical generalized pigmentation of Addison's disease or pigmentation and dermatitis of legs in congenital hemolytic anemias are almost diagnostic. Any generalized skin disease has to be noted, before color, cyanosis and jaundice are observed. Mycosis fungoides is the skin involvement in lymphoma (NHL), due to cutaneous response to T-cell lymphomatous infiltration, generally over nonexposed areas and may manifest years before obvious lymph nodal disease.

i)   Anemia: Pallor is indicative of severe anemia, but if it is confined to one limb it may indicate acute arterial occlusion (thromboembolic) or due to vasomotor instability seen in Raynaud's diease/phenomenon. Nail beds, lower conjunctiva, tongue and lips are the usual sites of observation. Intense distress or vasovagal shock may produce marked pallor of face. Koilonychia (spoon-shaped nails) may be associated with severe iron deficiency anemia.

insufficiency would keep it elevated for relief of discomfort. Similarly if there is a perianal abscess or prolapsed inflamed piles, they sit at the edge of chair or on one buttock and if one has a whitlow with digital abscess, he may keep it elevated to get relieved of the throbbing pain.

c)   Gait: Diseases of locomotor system would alter gait (see chapter on Gait)

d)   Facies: 'Face is the index of mind' and it can also give a clue to many diseases. Risus sardonicus of facial tetanus with trismus, Hippocratic face of generalised peritonitis with severe toxemia,

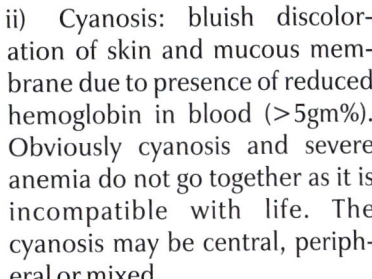
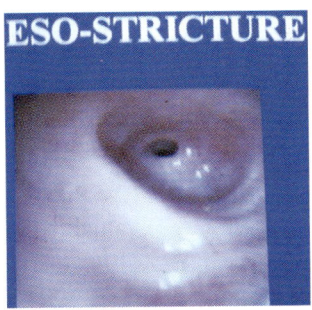

Fig. 1.12. Endoscopic view of a tight benign stricture of the lower esophagus
(courtesy: Lifeline Hospitals, Chennai)

ii)   Cyanosis: bluish discoloration of skin and mucous membrane due to presence of reduced hemoglobin in blood (>5gm%). Obviously cyanosis and severe anemia do not go together as it is incompatible with life. The cyanosis may be central, peripheral or mixed.

The central type is seen in cyanotic heart diseases, COPD, asphyxia, methemoglobinemia, sulphemoglobinemia and carboxyhemo-globinemia. The latter is seen in carbon monoxide poisoning and produces generalized cherry red discoloration of skin. Central cyanosis is seen over the tongue besides other areas like nail-bed, tip of nose, lips, palms and toes.

The peripheral type is due to excessive reduction of Hb in capillaries when blood flow is slowed down as in Raynaud's disease/ phenomenon, exposure to cold, ergotism, frost bite etc. It can be observed in all areas mentioned except the tongue.

The mixed type can occur in low cardiac output states, such as cardiogenic shock, acute pulmonary edema, congestive cardiac failure, where skin blood flow is diverted to vital organs, by differential vasoconstriction.

iii) Jaundice: yellowish discoloration of skin and mucous membranes due to increased circulating bile pigments, more than 2mg%. Elevated bilirubin levels between 1-2mg may not be clinically detected, hence known as chemical or preclinical jaundice. Areas observed are upper sclera, nailbed, under surface of tongue, ear lobule and tip of nose. The high elastin content of the sclera and its affinity for bilirubin, makes the yellow discoloration of the sclera, first to appear and last to disappear. Minimal jaundice may be easily missed when examined under artificial light. Severe anemia may go undetected in the presence of jaundice. In long standing cases, the color may turn green due to formation of biliverdin. In obstructive jaundice there is intense itching due to circulating bile salts, scratch marks being evident all over the body. In this, urine will be high colored but motion is pale or clay colored.

iv) Hair: Hair color and texture are racial characteristics and are genetically determined. Gender-based hair distribution and other secondary sexual characteristics start around puberty. Common baldness in men is an inherited character and it may be seen in some elderly women.

Patchy hair loss (alopecia) may be seen in certain skin disorders, as well as following burns, radiation, herpes zoster or over a sebaceous cyst. Metabolic causes of hair loss include hypothyroidism and severe iron deficiency anemia. It may be a conspicuous feature following anti-mitotic therapy for malignancies.

f) Clubbing of fingers: Due to hypertrophy of tissue in the base of nails, the angle between nail base and adjacent skin is obliterated and in extreme cases the terminal segment of fingers are bulbous, like the ends of a drumstick. It may be congenital, but acquired clubbing is seen in cyanotic heart diseases, chronic suppurative lung diseases or COPD. Minimal clubbing may also be seen in pulmonary tuberculosis, bronchogenic carcinoma, chronic inflammatory bowel diseases and polyposis coli. In hypertrophic pulmonary osteoarthropathy, besides clubbing there may be periosteal thickening of bones of forearm and leg.

Mechanism of clubbing: It is supposed to be due to hypoxia-induced A-V shunting and/or neovascularization of terminal phalanges of fingers.

g) Generalised edema (anasarca) or skin disorders have to be noted. Anasarca may be due to cardiac, renal, hepatic, nutritional or hormonal reasons. Unilateral edema of a limb is due to some local pathology, such as lymphatic/venous obstruction or soft tissue inflammation. If the edema is pitting, firm digital pressure over the skin for about 10 seconds, would produce a depression, lasting for about 30 seconds.

h) Evidence of generalised lymphadenopathy (lymphoma, tuberculosis, sarcoidosis or infectious mononucleosis etc.) has to be noted.

I) Pulse: (normal 70 to 80/min) This gives a valuable clue to several diseases and generally indicates the severity of illness. It may be recorded under the following sub-headings:

1) Rate: increased in fever, any toxemic conditions including active tuberculosis, hyperkinetic state of circulation (AVM, beriberi, PDA, Paget's disease of bone, anemia,

hyperthyroidism, aortic regurgitation etc. Anxiety states also produce tachycardia, but it comes down during sleep or tranquilization; hence sleeping pulse rate distinguishes functional from organic causes of tachycardia. Bradycardia is seen in athletes, hypothyroidism, complete heart block or in vasovagal episodes. During febrile episodes, usually there is about 8 beats/minute increase for every 1°F raise of body temperature (Meister's rule). Relative bradycardia is considered typical of typhoid fever.

2)   Rhythm: Regular or irregular; if the latter, it is either regularly irregular (sinus arrhythmia) or irregularly irregular (atrial fibrillation or multiple ectopics).

3)   Tension indicates blood pressure and is not an accurate way to assess arterial pressure; but with experience some approximation may be arrived.

4)   Volume indicates pulse pressure, in turn reflecting the cardiac stroke volume. Low volume pulse is seen in peripheral failure, low cardiac output as well as hypovolemic states. High volume pulse is seen in hyperdynamic circulatory states already mentioned and is typically appreciated with arm gradually elevated, while holding it around the mid-forearm. It is also known by several names: hyperkinetic, water-hammer, Corrigan's, collapsing pulse etc.

5)   Character of pulse: it may be hyperkinetic (already mentioned), pulsus alternans (left ventricular failure), pulsus paradoxus (cardiac tamponade), slow rising (aortic stenosis) etc. Delayed pulse may be seen in subclavian steal syndrome (radial) and coarctation of aorta (femorals).

6)   Condition of vessel wall, mostly for atherosclerosis, seen as diffuse thickening and beaded feeling in Monckeberg sclerosis. In elderly hypertensives, the brachial artery may be elongated, tortuous and appears to be dancing with each heart beat, known as locomotor brachii.

J)   Blood pressure: (normal 120-110 systolic and 90-70 diastolic. In patients over 50, the diastolic may remain unchanged but systolic may go up to some extent, but it is important that in any age, the brachial blood pressure above 130 (sys) and 90 (dia) respectively is considered abnormal.

Arterial blood pressure is generally recorded with a sphygmomanometer over the brachial artery in supine position. The sharp bruits heard over the brachial artery with a stethoscope, just distal to the cuff as it is being deflated, are known as Korotkoff sounds, which appear at systolic and disappear at diastolic pressure. Inflating the cuff of the apparatus well above the expected systolic pressure is important, since occasionally a silent zone may appear in between, giving a false low systolic reading.

In vascular cases it is better to record BP in both arms and if possible in both thighs (femorals). Normally systolic pressure in the right upper limb is higher than the left, by about 5-10mmHg, since the brachiocephalic trunk is in line with ascending aorta, whereas the left subclavian artery arises from the aorta at a right angle. The pressure recorded in the thigh (femoral) is higher by about 10-15 mmHg over brachial pressure, firstly because common iliac arteries are the terminal branches arising almost in line with aorta and secondly it needs greater force to compress the femoral artery surrounded by strong thigh muscles.

High systolic with normal diastolic pressure is in favor of a rigid aorta due to atherosclerosis. The significance of wide pulse pressure is already discussed. If the patient is a hypertensive on drug therapy, it is advisable to record brachial pressure in both supine and standing positions to see for any postural difference. In obese patients and those with sclerotic peripheral vessels, false high systolic pressures may be recorded, as more external pressure is required to compress the vessel, to obliterate blood flow.

k)   Respiration: This gives useful information leading to diagnosis but also valuable in

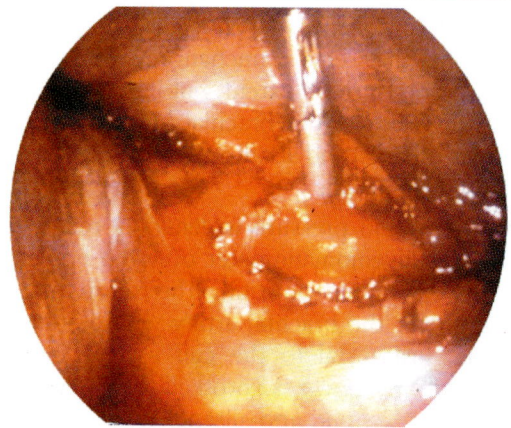

Fig. 1.13. Thoracoscopic Heller's cardiomyotomy. Bulging mucosa is seen, after dividing the muscularis (courtesy: Lifeline Hospitals, Chennai)

assessing patient in critical conditions or under anesthesia. Tachypnea is seen in fever, shock, metabolic acidosis (e.g. Kussmaul's breathing in diabetic ketosis), atelectasis of lung, hypocalcemic tetany, functional syndromes (hysteria etc). Bradypnea is seen normally in athletes, but may be due to cerebral compression. Gradual deepening with hyperventilation alternating with periods of apnea is termed as Cheyne-Stokes breathing and is considered as poor prognostic significance. In terminal stages of respiratory failure, increased excursions are attempted by bringing extrathoracic (accessory) muscles like sternocleidomastoid (SCM), strap and scalene muscles, into action, with the result the lower jaw is depressed during inspiration acquiring the name, jaw breathing. Indrawing of intercostal, subcostal and supraclavicular spaces during inspiration, indicates upper airway obstruction, so also stridor, as in laryngeal diphtheria or foreign body in tracheo-bronchial tree.

Respirations may be thoraco-abdominal (normal), purely thoracic as in generalised peritonitis or purely abdominal as in the rigid chest seen in ankylosing spondylitis. Normally during inspiration, abdominal wall moves forwards to accommodate the downward swing of the diaphragm and vice versa. In paradoxical respiration, part of the chest wall may move inwards during deep inspiration due to a flail chest. Likewise abdominal wall may move inwards during inspiration due to diaphragm moving upwards under increased negative thoracic pressure as in diaphragmatic palsy due to phrenic nerve lesion or eventration.

l) Temperature: Normal oral temperature is 98-99°F (Fahrenheit) or 37°C (Celsius or Centigrade) It is usually recorded from under surface of tongue, axilla or rectum. Temperature of mouth or rectum is about 1°C more than axillary temperature. The pattern of fever may give a clue to the nature of fever and three types are recognized clinically:

i) continuous: the temperature never touches normal at any time and the fluctuation is less than 1^{0} C.

ii) if the daily fluctuations exceed 2^{0} C, without touching normal during any part of the day, it is known as remittent fever and high remittance is termed hectic fever.

iii) if the fever is present only during some part of the day, touching normal in between, it is called intermittent and if the rise of temperature occurs once a day, it is called quotidian, once in two days, it is tertian and if it is once in three days, it is termed as quartan fever.

Most of the fevers show their peak toward evening because of exhaustion of the temperature regulatory system and other compensatory mechanisms by the end of the day.

Loco-regional examination

Naturally this is the most important aspect of the entire exercise and it is in this area that most of the 'heat' is generated between the examiner and the examinee. It may be recorded under the following sub-headings

(a) inspection
(b) palpation
(c) percussion
(d) auscultation
(e) measurements
(f) movements and

(g)   regional lymph nodes.

a)   Inspection: It is important to overcome the temptation of putting one's hands on a swelling, without proper inspection of the lesion and its surroundings. The aphorism 'one sees not what the mind knows not' is very apt in this context, because an uninformed observer misses many points, which an experienced physician can pick up by inspection.

b)   Palpation of a lesion would not only confirm several points noted by inspection, but adds more information, so that 'short-listing' the differential diagnoses is possible. Generally masses appear to be much larger by palpation, than realized by inspection. Clinching the anatomical plane of the lesion, so that the tissue of origin may be postulated, is an important, but often overlooked piece of information. It also identifies if a mass is likely to be benign or malignant and if it is resectable or not, both very useful in the management of the case.

There are two expressions for a hard mass, bony and stony hard. The physical feel of the mass may be the same, but by clinical examination, if the swelling appears to be arising from the bone, it should be termed bony hard, otherwise it may be called stony hard.

Fluctuation has to be elicited to know if a swelling is cystic or solid.

Rules for eliciting fluctuation

1.   Freely mobile swelling has to be fixed, to avoid total displacement of the mass (displacement enmasse), e.g. fibroadenoma breast or a testicular swelling

2.   It has to be elicited in two directions. A fleshy muscle may 'appear' fluctuant across but not in the longitudinal direction

3.   Fix the mass with four (passive) fingers (both thumbs and middle fingers) and apply pressure by alternate index (active) fingers. The impulse may be appreciated by the other index finger or the passive fingers.

4.   *Paget's test* may be done when the swelling

is too small (<2cm); if the swelling is soft in the center and firm in the periphery, it is likely to be a cystic swelling and vice versa.

5.   Very soft swellings such as a lipoma or Warthin's tumor of parotid, may give false sense of fluctuation (pseudofluctuation).

6.   Bilocular cystic swellings, if they are communicating, exhibit cross fluctuation. e.g. multiple meningoceles, hydrocele en-bisec or a psoas abscess above and below the inguinal ligament.

c)   Percussion: Left middle finger (pleximeter finger) is placed over the area and its middle phalanx is tapped with the tip of right middle or index finger (percussing finger), to observe the resonance over the mass. It is important to use only wrist movements but not elbow of the right hand, during percussion.

d)   Auscultation is least important, except over chest/abdomen, major vessels, hernia or a highly vascular lesion. An abnormal sound heard over chest, arising from heart and its entry/exit points is known as a *murmur*. Similar sound heard over a vessel distal to a stenotic segment or an arterio-venous malformation (AVM), creating turbulence of flow, is known as *bruit*. A soft sound heard over a highly vascularised soft tissue (enlarged hyperactive spleen, vascular sarcoma, placenta or lactating breast) is called a *souffle*. The sound heard over an AVM or a patent ductus arteriosus (PDA) is typically of machinery character.

Venous hum is an indistinct continuous low sound of musical character heard over a large

Jewels of Gyan - 01.1

To be examined in erect position
Conditions, such as varicose veins, groin hernia, Malgaigne bulging, communicating hydrocele, undescended testis, varicocele, lymph varix, breast mass, mobile kidney, engorged veins over anterior abdominal wall etc. require the patient to be examined both in erect as well as supine postures.

vein, usually internal jugular, in sitting position, disappearing on assuming recumbent posture. It may be normally present and is considered innocent, thought to be due torrential blood flow returning from brain and disappears on gentle jugular compression. It is also known as *'bruit de diable'* (devil's noise) and may also be heard over epigastrium in portal hypertension, with widespread collaterals.

Kenaway's sign: venous hum heard over an enlarged spleen in portal hypertension or Egyptian splenomegaly, which may also be heard in the epigastrium, more so on deep inspiration, due to the compression of the spleen, causing engorgement of splenic vein.

Auscultation is also used to identify friction rub of pleura, pericardium or peritoneum, locating the position of trachea in difficult cases, to assess the size of a hollow viscus by ausculto-percussion and to identify succussion splash over the chest (hydro-pneumothorax) or over the epigastrium (gastric stasis due to outlet obstruction).

e) Measurements (mensuration) and movements are usually important in orthopedics, as in fractures, dislocations, articular or extra-articular disorders. Recording abdominal girth serially may indicate the progress of distension in cases of intestinal obstruction, to help the surgeon make a decision either to continue nonoperative treatment or to proceed with laparotomy. Recording the range of respiratory excursions during each visit, should guide a physician as to the improvement or otherwise, in a case of ankylosing spondylitis. In case of a swelling, thought to be malignant, its size is needed for proper clinical TNM staging.

f) Regional lymph nodes: No examination of a surgical condition is complete without systematic inspection and palpation of regional lymph nodes, noting the following points: anatomical group, number, sizes, consistency, fixity to each other, to overlying skin. surrounding tissue and adjacent bone. Fixity to each other should not be confused with matting, typically

seen in tuberculous lymphadenitis, due to periadenitis. In the latter instance, nodes are flat, attached to each other, like a mat, grooves felt distinctly between them. Variable consistency due to caseation is diagnostic of tuberculous lymphadenitis, though rarely secondaries in cervical nodes from papillary carcinoma thyroid may undergo cystic degeneration. Secondary skin changes such as ulceration, fungation and sinus formation should be noted.

Survey of other systems

This should be done system-wise, in order of preference based on the provisional diagnosis as indicated:

a) Cardiovascular system & peripheral pulses
b) Respiratory system & chest
c) GI Tract & abdomen
d) GU System & external genitalia
e) Musculoskeletal system & extremities
f) CN System & cranium
g) Endocrine system & neck
h) PV and PR examination should never be omitted. It is true but hard to believe that polyp of rectum (in children) and carcinoma (in adults) have been missed by many a physician, for want of carrying out a simple digital examination of rectum in their offices, only to regret later.

i) Examination of groins and external genitalia: Groin is a colloquial term used to include inguinal, femoral regions and labia majora or root of scrotum and while describing the extent of a swelling, it is preferable to specify the particular anatomical area, rather than use such a collective expression.

j) Ocular fundus examination should be done, using an ophthalmoscope, as part of routine physical examination, in diabetics, hypertensives and those with visual, neurological or vascular diseases.

3) Provisional diagnosis

It is nothing but the most probable and first in the differential diagnosis; rest of the conditions are mentioned in the order of preference, under differential diagnosis. As far as possible one should try to fit in all the findings of a patient into a single diagnosis, rather than giving out more than one unconnected diseases. If such a case is given in the examination, where two conditions co-exist, general instructions are given to the examinee, to examine only one of them, ignoring the other, to avoid confusion at the time of discussion and management. However incidental diseases like lipoma, a scrotal hydrocele or a goitre should be mentioned in passing, under survey of systems, but if there is any element of doubt that they might be related, more detailed description is mandatory, to clinch their pathogenic significance in that particular case. For example, in a patient with pulmonary/renal tuberculosis having a scrotal hydrocele, the possibility of tuberculous epididymo-orchitis with secondary hydrocele cannot be overlooked. Likewise, a loin mass in a hypertensive, may be a congenital polycystic kidney, with secondary hypertension.

In giving out a provisional diagnosis, include anatomical, functional and pathological aspects of diagnosis adding any complications if already evident. For example in a goiter, one has to say, solitary nontoxic goitre, probably an adenoma of thyroid. In malignancies, generally accepted stage of disease has to be included, e.g. in carcinoma breast (4cm), with mobile ipsilateral axillary nodes without obvious dissemination, it should be stage-II (of Manchester) or T2-N1-MO (of TNM staging). Where there is no standard protocol of staging, TNM staging can be given with universal acceptance. It is to be noted that N in TNM staging refers only for regional nodes and not any node in the body. Any other node (than regional) should come under M (metastasis), as in a case of contralateral node involvement in carcinoma breast.

In ambiguous cases, a systematic approach, by some working classification of diseases, usually leads to 'narrowing down' the possibilities. These usually fall into one of the following categories:

a) congenital
b) traumatic
c) inflammatory, acute, subacute or chronic and nonspecific or specific
d) neoplastic, benign or malignant, latter primary or secondary
e) degenerative
f) metabolic
g) hormonal
h) toxic or poisonous
i) functional, psychosomatic or psychiatric
j) iatrogenic (iatros: physician)
k) idiopathic (idio: peculiar; pathos: disease)

4) Differential diagnosis

Any leading symptom or sign may be taken to work out the various conditions associated with those findings, in the order of preference or frequency of occurrence. All the findings in a given case should be remembered while considering the order of preference, for example if a patient has an epigastric mass and melena, ulcerating lesions of GI tract, like carcinoma stomach or colon must be considered first before including others like a hepatic neoplasm, lymphoma or a pancreatic tumor.

If amongst the various possibilities, no clue is available as to what should be given as provisional diagnosis, one can go by statistical data and put them in their order of frequency, so that the most common will be the provisional diagnosis; the rest constitute differential diagnosis. To illustrate this, in a solitary nodular goitre, without features of malignancy, adenoma thyroid may be given out as the provisional diagnosis, as it is the most common disease of the thyroid, presenting as a solitary nodule. This exception notwithstanding, it is inadvisable to propose a histological diagnosis, in a clinical context, e.g. better to label as soft tissue sarcoma rather than fibrosarcoma or liposarcoma.

5) Investigations

Routine investigations like hematology, urinalysis may be mentioned only in passing. Under special investigations, less expensive noninvasive investigations should be done before more expensive and invasive ones are considered, especially if the former studies do not give us the desired information to proceed with the management of the patient. Always look for the shortest route to clinch the diagnosis, rather than waste time and money in carrying out unimportant investigations. Microbiological, histopathological or cytological study to arrive at a conclusion, should be considered early in the diagnostic processs. Investigations which do not influence the diagnosis, management or prognostication are purely academic and should be avoided, to prevent unwanted escalation of cost of medicare in the long run.

Establishing tissue diagnosis is vital in many surgical diseases, which may be by biopsy (excision, wedge, edge, punch or needle) or cytology (aspiration or exfoliative). Fine needle aspiration cytology (FNAC), also known as aspiration biopsy cytology (ABC), introduced by Scandinavian pathologists, has become very popular clinching study over the last three decades, a simple, least invasive and 'reasonably' sensitive, with the main advantages of the report being available on the same day and high patient compliance. However, it needs a trained cytologist, to be able to accurately interpret the morphology of a single cell or a clump of few cells. Many still prefer wide-bore needle biopsy, whenever the size of lesion is over 2-3cm, not only to improve accuracy, but to be able to get sub-classification, level of differentiation and immunohistochemistry (IHC) in cases of tumors, to facilitate expedient management.

Whenever any single finding is materially altering the course of events, such as an enlarged lymph node in the opposite axilla or an SOL in the liver, in a case of stage I or II breast carcinoma, that fact should be established beyond any doubt, by tissue diagnosis, since it is disas-

trous to presume it as metastatic and label the patient as having an incurable disease, only to find later that it was non-malignant, denying the patient the benefit of curative therapy.

Without histological conformation, it is wise to refrain from carrying out radical or mutilative surgery for suspected malignancies. Having established the tissue diagnosis of malignancy, some more investigations are necessary for proper staging of the disease, before planning therapy. Needless to say, prudent selection of investigations would not only help to arrive at a diagnosis expediently, but saves a lot of time and expense to the patient, besides sparing them the distress of unnecessary or possibly risky investigations.

In this context, it is to be remembered that many investigations done for patients in some of the western countries are not considered to be cost-effective and done more to satisfy the legal requirements, invariably hiking the overall cost of medicare exorbitantly, whether it is the individual, the insurance company or the state, that bears the brunt. It is apt to recall Hutchinson's remark here, that 'the process of curing the illness should not be more grievous than enduring it'.

6) Clinical diagnosis

The diagnosis arrived after all the relevant investigations with or without tissue diagnosis is known as clinical diagnosis, based on which treatment may be planned. In certain abdominal emergencies, only a 'working diagnosis' as to the need for laparotomy, is possible, having eliminated non-surgical conditions, to a reasonable extent and such an approach, without insisting on a definitive diagnosis, is both logical and scientific.

In cases of malignancy, appropriate clinical staging has to follow diagnosis and if there is no standard staging available, internationally accepted

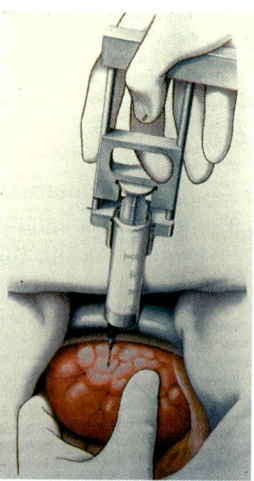

Fig. 1.14.
Cameco syringe for FNAC
(courtesy: Lifeline
Hospitals, Chennai)

TNM staging may be used. In case of carcinoma breast for example, both TNM and Manchester staging have to be described, as the former is more precise for comparison of results and the latter is useful for translating into treatment protocols. It should be realized that therapeutic strategies are decided only after final (patho-logical) staging has been arrived, after com-plete diagnostic and staging work up, such as chest skiagram, USG/CT/ MRI/PET-CT, biopsy, tumor markers/receptors, skeletal survey, node sampling, laparoscopy etc.

7) Treatment

It may be general or specific, which may be medical or surgical.

General treatment includes rest, alteration in personal habits like alcohol or smoking etc., adjustments in diet, nutritional supplements, tranquilization and anabolic steroids (when-ever needed).

Specific treatment: If the disease has an accepted medical therapy, it should be tried first, clearly outlining the dose and duration, monitoring not only the improvement (subjec-tive and objective) but also any expected or unexpected side effects of therapy that may require interruption of a particular drug.

Selection of antibiotic agent

Though it is ideal to decide after the microbial sensitivity data is available, in critical situations it is desirable to initiate empirical therapy

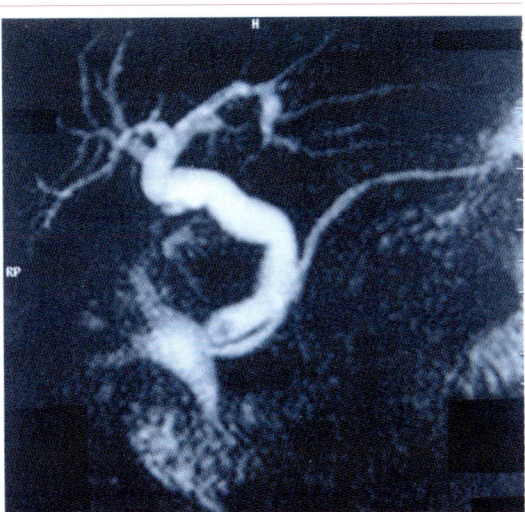

Fig.1.16. Magnetic resonance cholangio-pancreatogram (MRCP) showing a dilated CBD with a calculus in the lower end. It has largely replaced conventional ERCP (courtesy: Lifeline Hospitals, Chennai)

immediately, based on the following factors:

1. The source of infection and most likely organism involved, e.g. coliforms and anerobes in appendicitis, salmonella in cholecystitis, staphylococci in furuncle or carbuncle, streptococci in throat or tonsil infection and in burn wounds, initially Gram positive and later Gram negative organisms

2. Comorbidities, such as diabetes, renal insufficiency or immunosuppression

3. Severity of infection and potential to cause systemic manifestations (SIRS)

4. Distribution of the agent to the site of infection

Collection of material for culture and sensitivity studies should be done at the earliest opportunity, preferably before commencing antibiotic therapy. It is wise not to withdraw a particular antibiotic, if the patient shows clinical improvement, even if the report says 'not sensitive' to the agent already started, but an additional drug may be started based on the report, if warranted.

If surgical treatment is suggested, spell out the indications for the same in that particular

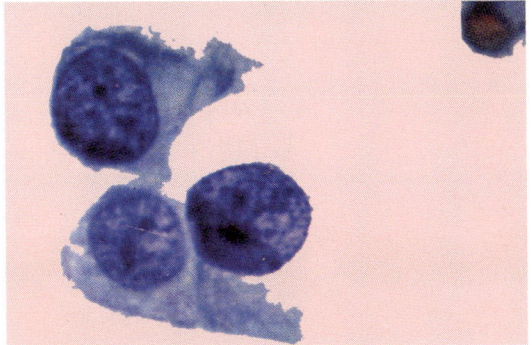

Fig. 1.15. Malignant cells seen in FNAC of breast mass (courtesy: Histo Lab, Chennai)

patient, before mentioning the name of the operation. Surgical management has to be dealt with under five headings:

1. preoperative evaluation and preparation
2. surgical procedure including the choice of anesthesia
3. immediate postoperative management
4. advice to be given at the time of discharge, including chemo/radiotherapy (CRT) for malignancies
5. anticipated late complications and their management

Whenever surgery is proposed for malignant disease, it should be defined if it is a curative or palliative procedure and what form of adjuvant treatment (radiotherapy, chemotherapy, immunotherapy, hormonal therapy etc) should follow and its timing in sequence. Turnbull technique of early control of vascular pedicle to minimize spread of cancer, may be employed in appropriate cases.

When preoperative radiotherapy &/or chemotherapy is given to 'down-stage' tumor, sometimes reducing a nonresectable tumor to a resectable one, it is known as neoadjuvant therapy. Tumors like desmoid and soft tissue sarcoma, once considered radio-resistant, are now with improved technique, being treated with neoadjuvant RT, to improve the prospects of surgical resections (see chapter 24, on Radiotherapy).

A palliative procedure should be aimed at relieving some troublesome symptom to improve the quality of life (without which it is debatable if one should only prolong the suffering in incurable malignancies) and should not cause undue morbidity (or mortality) to the patient. This should also help the patient return home early, to spend the 'remaining' days with family and children rather than with doctors and nurses in the hospital. *Hospice care* is also offered to terminally ill patients, not only to provide necessary physical and emotional support, but to give them the privilege of 'dying in dignity' (J M Zimmerman).

If a solitary secondary is detected in a patient with cancer, it is justifiable to resect it, with a curative intention, provided:

(a) the primary tumor is eminently curable,

(b) thorough investigation excludes any other site of spread

(c) the procedure can be performed without much of additional morbidity (or mortality), with the available expertise and infrastructure.

(d) excision of the secondary should extend survival of the patient, e.g. hepatic mets from colorectal, ovarian and pancreatic neuro endocrine tumors.

In the new millennium, it may be well to appreciate the current philosophy of treating malignancies, with limited resection, preserving the organ and to depend more on adjuvant forms of therapy. Procedures like breast conservative

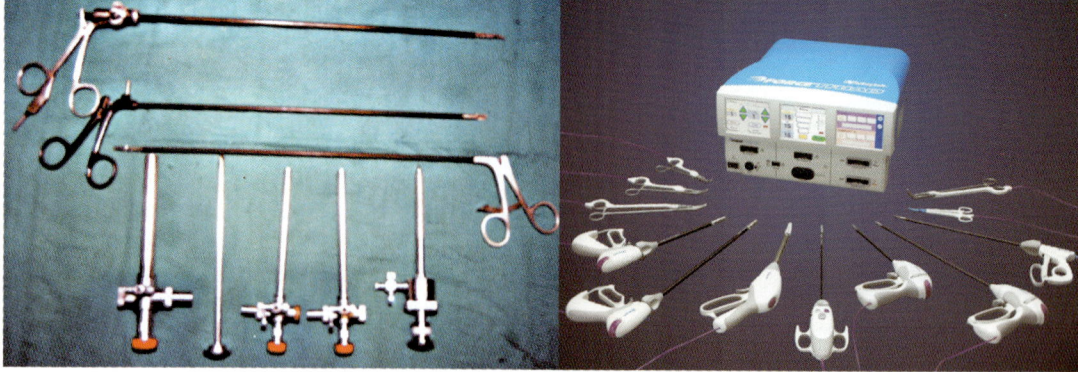

Fig. 1.17. Laparoscopic trocars, cannulae and hand instruments
(courtesy: Lifeline Hospitals, Chennai)

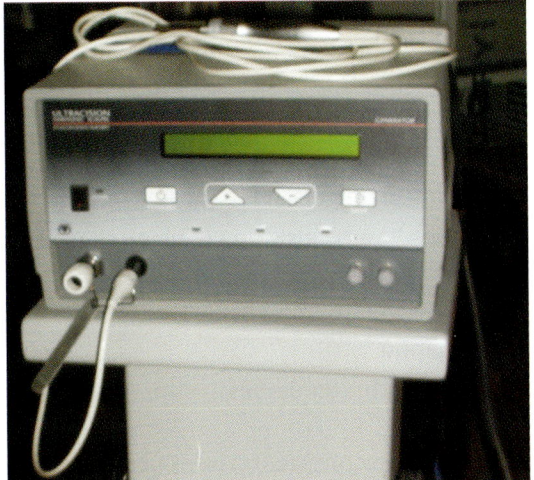

Fig. 1.18. Harmonic shears (ultrasonic scalpel)
High frequency ultrasonic oscillations coagulate and cut tissues
(courtesy: Halsted Surgical Clinic, Chennai)

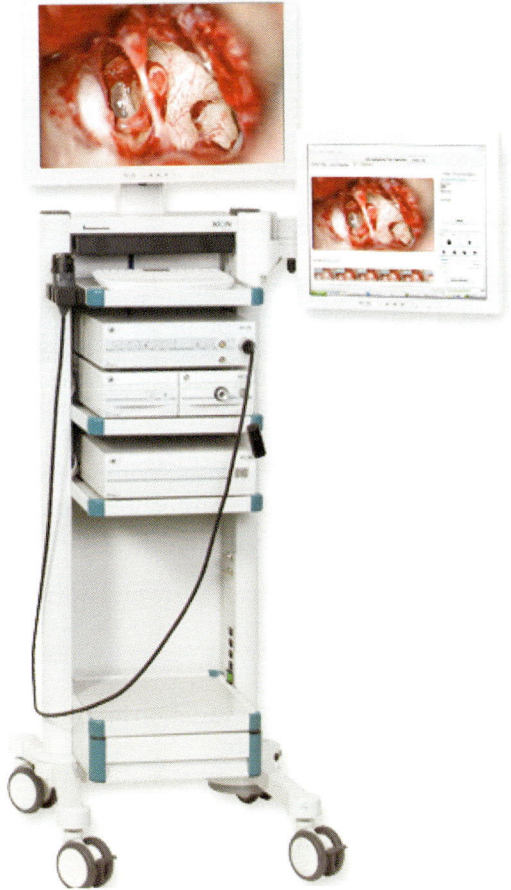

Fig. 1.19. Video-endoscopy unit
The images are magnified and findings can be documented

surgery for cancers, limb salvage procedures for bone sarcomas are gaining momentum and the 'fashion' of doing more and more extensive radical surgeries for cancers prevailed in the sixth and seventh decades of the last century have been outdated, fully realizing that malignancies are basically systemic diseases with local manifestations and any amount of local treatment is incomplete without some form of systemic approach. One recalls an anecdote stated in the late sixties by a pathologist, that a surgeon had performed such an extensive procedure for an advanced cancer that at the end of the operation, he was not sure which was the patient and which was the surgical specimen! Such surgical 'gymnastics' are rarely advocated in current practice.

Minimally invasive or key-hole surgery is the revolution of the decade, which has taken the entire world by storm and has come to stay; hence one should get familiarized with the indications and expected complications of these procedures, with a clear line drawn between surgery and adventurism in the operating rooms! As more and more innovative procedures are being evolved, it may not be an exaggeration to say that in the years to come, the role of a general surgeon may be largely limited to operating for the complications of endoscopic surgery.

In this era of evidence-based medicine, we are not expected to manage patients based on 'anecdotal' observation of a few cases nor such strategies are accepted in qualifying examination or court of law. (see chapter 100)

Scheme of examining a LUMP or MASS

A lump or swelling is a general term meaning any abnormal mass of tissue, but the term tumor indicates a neoplastic process and should not be used if the intention is not to mean it.

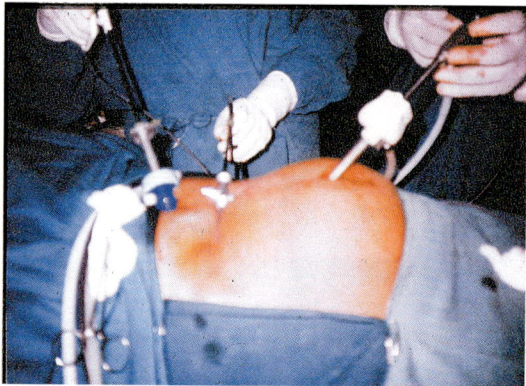

Fig. 1.20. Laparoscopic cholecystectomy in progress
(courtesy: Halsted Surgical Clinic, Chennai)

The information given in Chapter 1 has to be applied while examining a mass. Without risk of repetition, the general protocol is briefly summarized here.

History

Duration
Mode of onset
Pain
Starting point, progress or variation in size
Similar swellings elsewhere
Secondary changes
Pressure effects
Impairment of function
Constitutional symptoms
Bowels, micturition and menstruation
General health status
Previous treatment and its effect
Past history, including co-morbidities
Personal history
Family history

PHYSICAL EXAMINATION

1. General examination, including vital signs
2. Loco-regional examination
a) Inspection

Location, shape, edge, number, cough impulse movement with respiration, deglutition, protrusion of tongue and posture

pulsations, peristalsis, overlying skin and secondary changes

Pressure effect, trophic changes and deformity

b) Palpation

Local warmth, tenderness, size, shape and extent

Surface, edge, consistency, translucency, cough impulse, reducibility, compressibility, fluctuation, fluid thrill, pulsations, mobility, anatomic plane, surrounding structures

Underlying bone, movements of joint in the vicinity

c) Percussion
d) Auscultation
e) Regional lymph nodes
f) Measurements
g) Movements
h) Pressure effects

3. Vaginal and rectal examination

4. Survey of other systems in an order, with preference to those relevant to the condition

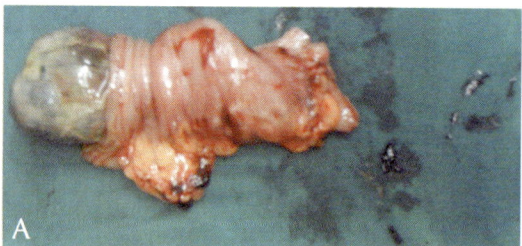
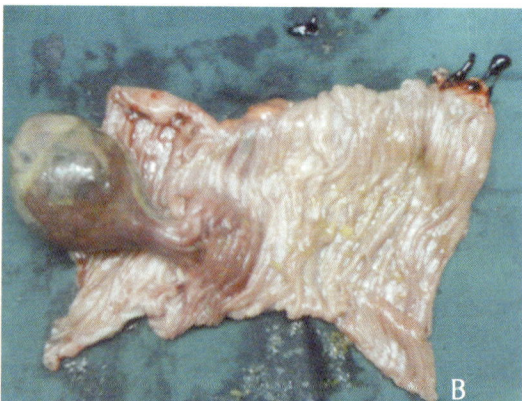

Fig. 1.21. A. Pedunculated adenoma of small bowel causing intussusception
B. Opened specimen showing the stalk of the tumor
(courtesy: Halsted Surgical Clinic, Chennai)

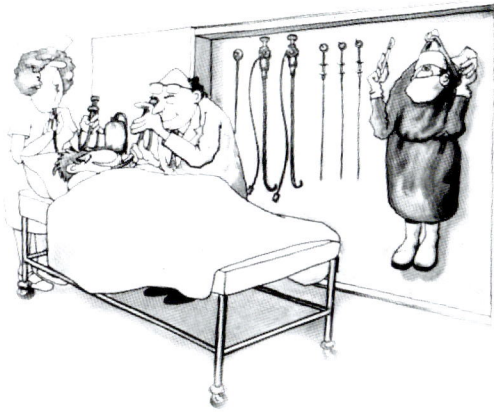

Fig. 1.22. With the advent of endoscopic surgery, is the general surgeon obsolete?
(courtesy: Lifeline Hospitals, Chennai)

Provisional diagnosis, differential diagnosis, investigations and final diagnosis.

The subjects of the final pathological diagnosis, prognostic evaluation, follow-up of progress, condition at discharge and final outcome shall be discussed under the appropriate chapters. In case of mortality, findings of an autopsy, if performed, should be recorded for retrospec-tion. In developed countries, the academic standard of any teaching hospital is judged by the percentage of autopsies done for hospital deaths. Some of them go to the extent of obtaining the consent for postmortem examination, at the time of entering into hospital for any illness, along with the permission for carrying out investiga-tions and treatment. However, most clinici-ans feel that such a 'blanket package' is undesirable, as it overlooks the emotional undercurrents of a patient who gets admitted for some minor illness.

The importance of skills of communication and clinical observation/ presentation cannot be overemphasized, as these forms the main basis on which a student is assessed in a qualifying examination at any level. Even in practice, mastering this art certainly makes one

Urogenital	Undescended testis
	Exstrophy of bladder
Increased peritoneal fluid	Ascites (tuberculosis, nutritional etc.)
	Presence of Ventriculoperitoneal shunt
	Peritoneal dialysis
Increased intra-abdominal pressure	Repair of gastroschisis/ exomphalos
	Severe ascites- liver failure, chylous etc
	Meconium ileus
Chronic respiratory disease	Cystic fibrosis
Connective tissue disorders	Ehlers-Danlos syndrome
	Hunter- Hurler syndrome
	Marfan syndrome
	Mucopolysaccharidosis
Miscellaneous	Developmental dysplasia of hip

Table 1.2 - Risk factors for development of hernia in children

Jewels of Gyan - 01.3

Some misnomers in medicine

Adenolymphoma	is not a lymphoma
Anemia	is not absence of blood (low Hb)
Cock's peculiar tumor	is not a tumor (infected sebaceous cyst)
Cystosarcoma phyllodes	is not a sarcoma
Daughter scoleces of hydatid	the nematode is a hermaphrodite
Enteroteratoma	is not a teratoma (it is an umbilical adenoma)
Essential hypertension	is never essential to any patient
Hematoma	is not a tumor (collection of lymph is not called lymphoma)
Malignant exophthalmos	is not a cancer
Malignant hydatid	is not a cancer, but a disseminated abdominal hydatid
Malignant hypertension	is not malignant
Malignant melanoma	all melanomas are malignant
Mycosis fungoides	is cutaneous lymphoma, not a fungal disease
Mycotic aneurysm	is not due to fungal infection (bacterial)
Physiological goiter	is pathological (due to physiological stress)
Pott's puffy tumor	is an infection, not a tumor
Pregnancy tumor	is a pyogenic granuloma
Pretibial myxedema	not seen in myxedema (only in treated cases of Graves' disease)
Rectum	means straight. In humans, it is anything but straight
Sternomastoid tumor	is considered birth injury not a tumor
Stethoscope	is not for seeing but for hearing

a popular and cost-effective clinician in the long run.

Jewels of Gyan - 01.4

DOs & DON'Ts during clinical discussion

ALWAYS	NEVER
Do noninvasive and less expensive investigations first	Say there is no differential diagnosis
Find a short route to establish the diagnosis	Propose radical or mutilative surgery for malignancy without tissue diagnosis
Discuss the medical treatment (if available), before proposing surgery	Do academic investigations, which do not influence the management
Do staging investigations after confirming the diagnosis of malignancy	Take undue risk to life of a patient while offering palliative therapy
Appropriate adjuvant therapy should follow surgery for cancers	Suggest radical surgery if your aim is only palliation

02 The Making of a Surgeon

Education is not filling a bucket, it is lighting a fire - W B Yeats

Surgical training has come a long way since the days of Kocher and Halsted.

The 'Making of a Surgeon' a monumental work by Ian Aird, written several decades ago, catalogued the trials and tribulations that every doctor had to go through before he completed his surgical training. The little book talked of the changes in personality, mindset, and habits that were required of a surgeon in training.

The 20th and early 21st century, had seen a tremendous growth in the field of surgery. Unfortunately, surgical training had not yet been standardized in most countries across the globe. In developed countries, there are stringent requirements that trainees perform a certain number of supervised surgeries, and demonstrate a stipulated number of skill sets, before they are allowed to operate on patients. Several training programs insist on vivisection (animal surgeries) but this is becoming more difficult, due to the intervention of the animal

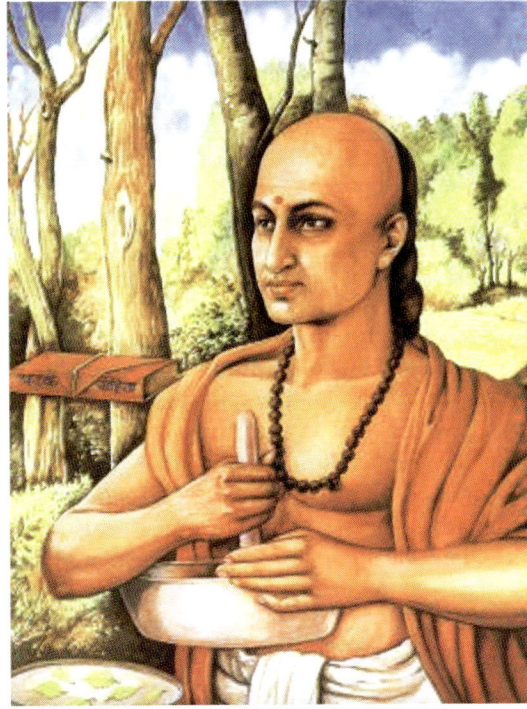

Fig. 02.02. Saint Charaka (300 BC)

rights activists all over the world. This has brought in the electronic simulators and virtual reality trainers, which are quite useful for predominantly two dimensional operations like laparoscopic surgeries. However, their main drawback is the lack of 'haptics' or the tactile feel of human flesh, which is quite crucial to the ultimate precision of good open surgery.

How does one monitor training? Ideally a surgical training program must not only be monitored carefully by the senior surgeon, but training should take place in a series of steps: initially didactic lectures to the surgical trainees done by teachers, followed by demonstration of the surgery by the surgical tutor known as the 'mentor'. After the initial tutoring and mentoring, the trainee must be able to operate under the careful supervision of one of the

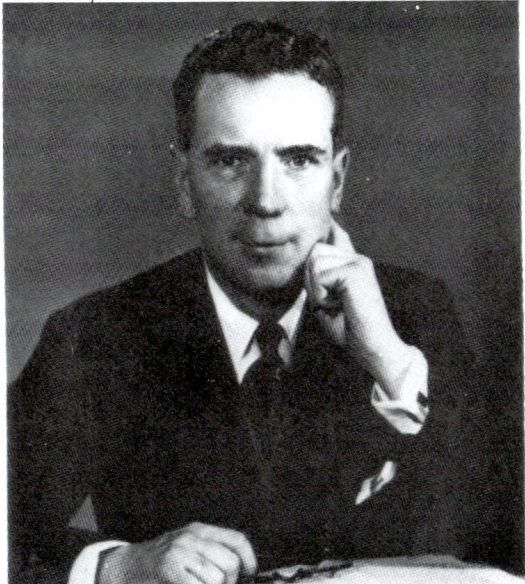

Fig. 02.01. Ian Aird (1905-62) - author of 'Making of a Surgeon'

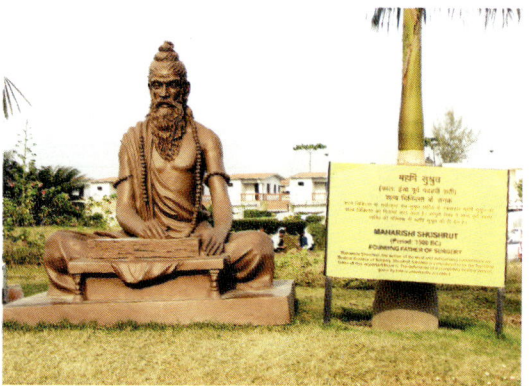

Fig. 02.03. Maharishi Sushruth (1500 BC) - statue at Patanjali Yogpeeth, Haridwar

mentors - a 'proctorship' program. This should be paralleled by courses and fellowships that result in credentialing (credere: to believe or trust), which means that the surgical trainee can be trusted to perform that particular procedure within known international standards. There is a constant tussle between the 'theoretical' surgeon who is looked at as too bookish on the one hand, and the "butcher" (or surgical technician) who is a raw cutter, with little interest or flare for the theoretical finesse of surgery.

The ideal surgeon is a judicious combination of the two, i.e., he should be well versed with the theory behind the operation, which includes the pathophysiological changes that will result, the anatomical basis of his approach etc. whilst having a high degree of manual dexterity to

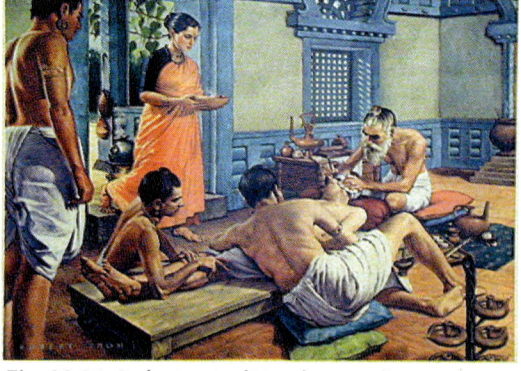

Fig. 02.04. Sushruta - traditional ayurvedic treatment - a tooth being extracted without anesthesia

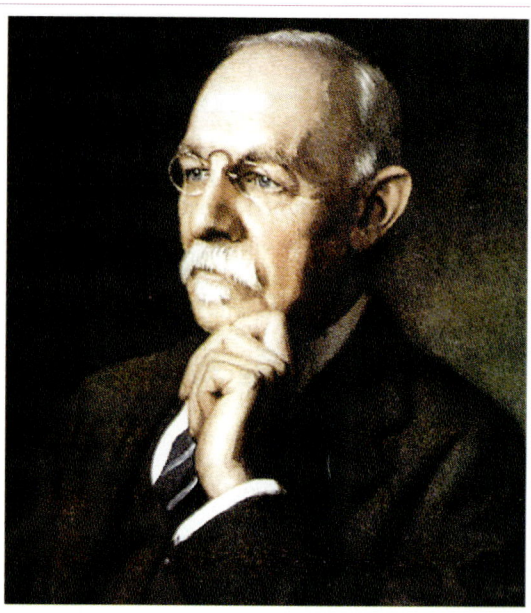

Fig. 02.05. William Stewart Halsted (1852-1922)

perform the operation as meticulously as possible. Primarily, every surgeon must realize that the surgical degree is only a passport into the exciting world of surgery, not a certificate of guarantee of technical excellence. Some countries think that it is only an entry point and tune their syllabi accordingly. At every stage of development, a surgeon must affiliate himself with courses, workshops, continuous medical education program etc. so that he is constantly abreast of techniques and changing technology. This has brought up the need for reassessment and recertification, done compulsorily at intervals in some countries like USA, UK, and Australia etc.

Surgical training, although started by Charaka and Sushruta, was brought to light into the western world by the likes of William Halsted, Theodor Kocher, Theodor Billroth and Harvey Cushing. It is interesting that Halsted, who was the fastest and flashiest surgeon when he was operating in New York, evolved to be a meticulous, painstakingly slow, and gentle handler of tissues in his later years in Baltimore at the Johns Hopkins Hospital. It is important that the surgeon thinks of the patient as a continuum starting from the point of surgery to the post operative period. This philosophy has been encapsulated in the early 20th century 'choose well, cut well and get well'.

'Change is the only permanent thing', goes an old adage. The surgical environment has always been one of constantly changing variables. As an evolving surgeon one must not only be aware of change, but be abreast of it. This means embracing changing trends and technological advances. One must always be aware of one's roots, and the tradition of modern surgery can directly be traced back to a few pioneering surgeons as mentioned above. Choosing one's operative procedure, and more importantly, the decision to operate, is vitally important to the surgical outcome. Indeed, it is said that good surgery is 25% dexterity and 75% decisiveness.

Charles Darwin, while proposing the theory of evolution said, "it is not the strongest species that survives nor the most intelligent, but the

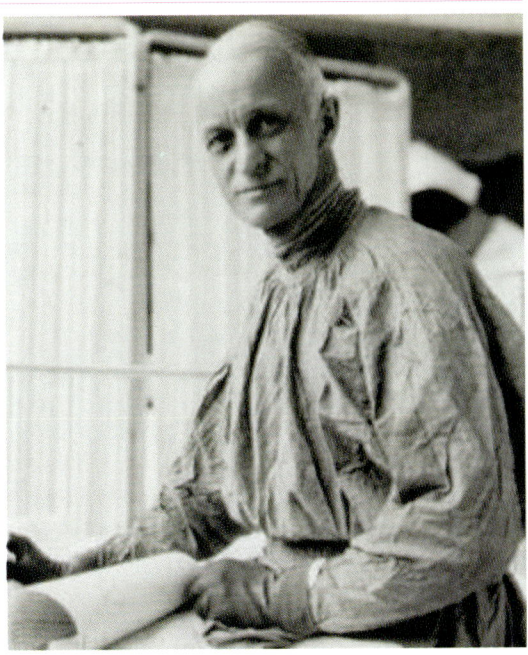

Fig. 02.07. Harvey Williams Cushing (1869-1939)

one most capable of adapting to the changed environment".

During the conduct of surgery, the focus of surgeon should always be on the ultimate clinical result, and every move that respects anatomy and every therapeutic maneuver that supports the patient's deranged physiology will contribute to that result. The legal sword of Damocles perched atop every capped head should ensure documentation of every step of the operation. In this respect, it may be well worth remembering Murphy's laws:

1. 'The more complex a procedure, the more likely it is to go wrong'. It's better to think of a simpler procedure that is equally effective, under the circumstances.

2. 'If there is even one single step in the entire operation that could go wrong, it will'. Don't underestimate the potential risk of any wrong step, however trivial it may appear to be. Depending on 'mother nature' to rectify our mistakes may be disastrous.

3. 'If we think everything is going on well, something obvious may have been overlooked'.

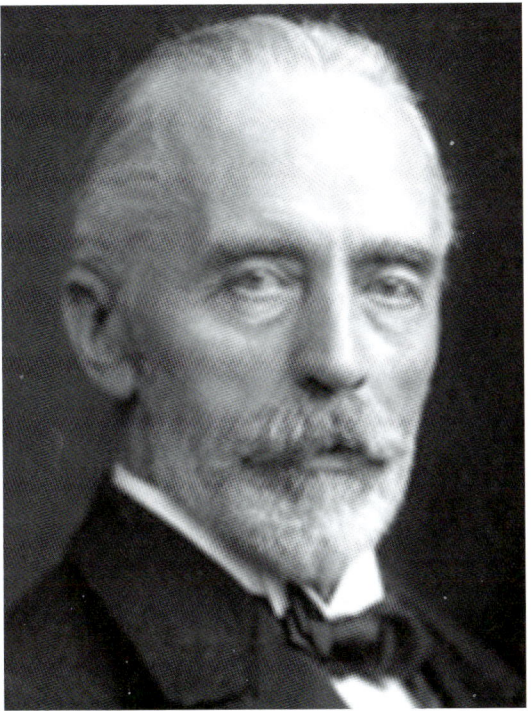

Fig. 02.06. Theodor Kocher (1841-1917)

A surgical operation is a combination of several small details and don't neglect any step or detail during a procedure. Interestingly, Murphy himself was an optimist!

A Chinese proverb: *One who leaves the luck out of his plans usually finds it.*

If one were to recount a few crucial advances that pushed forward the groundswell of surgical growth, they would be:

1. General anesthesia (Morton)
2. Surgical training bodies
3. Antisepsis and asepsis (Lord Lister)
4. Meticulous gentle tissue handling (Kocher and Halsted)
5. Antibiotics (Alexander Fleming)

1. General anesthesia

Ever since the first clinical demonstration of ether for general anesthesia by William Morton in 1846, it has gripped alike the fraternity of surgeons and patients and soon within a few decades, thousands of operations were being performed under ether or chloroform anesthesia. Simultaneously the accidental discovery of the local anesthetic effect of the coca seed, led to the use of cocaine as a local anesthetic, spearheaded by Halsted, (who, sadly later became addicted to it, while experimenting on himself). Thus the combined growth of local and general anesthesia provided a powerful shot in the arm to enhance the growing science and craft of surgery.

2. Surgical training bodies

Interestingly, the Royal College of Surgeons of Edinburgh offered comprehensive surgical training 500 years ago in which the trainees were taught only surgical procedures. A full 300 years later MBBS (Bachelor of Medicine and Bachelor of Surgery) course were started by the University of London. Thereafter, aspiring surgeons first became physicians and then acquired the further technical skills to become full-fledged surgeons. A point to note, that all of us are basically physicians. Though the physicians know when to operate, the surgeons, in addition, know how to do it.

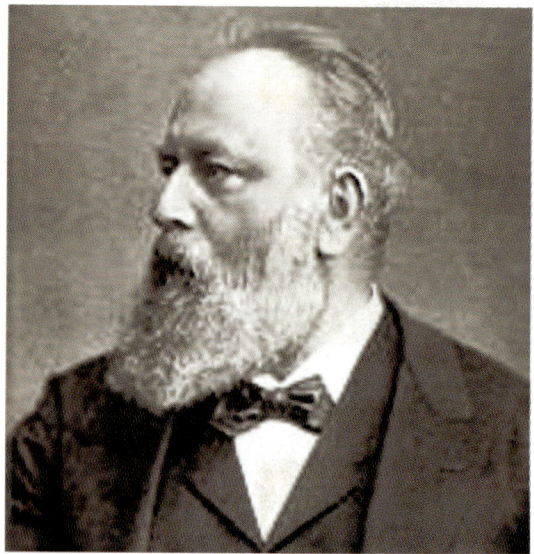

Fig. 02.08. Theodor Billroth (1829-94)

Halsted was the brain behind the residency training system in USA, by incorporating 3 essential components; the period of training was increased from 3 to 5 years, the trainees were made to work for the hospital, as part of learning and they were paid adequate stipend (sustenance allowance), so as not to depend on their parents.

3. Antisepsis and asepsis

Lord Joseph Lister's pathbreaking work gave a precedent for surgeons on both sides of the Atlantic to follow. Concepts of a clean surgical field evolved directly therefrom, meticulously propagated by Louis Pasteur, even before the advent of surgical gloves, preparation of skin with carbolic acid was carried on until it was replaced by less irritant and more effective agents like povidone iodine and cetrimide. The principles enunciated by Lister are very much relevant even today.

4. Tissue handling

Kocher in Europe brought down the mortality rate of thyroidectomies simply by gentle, atraumatic tissue handling and greatly reducing wound sepsis, then the leading cause of death. This also culminated in his receiving the Nobel prize in 1909 (the first surgeon, to be so honored).

Using newer technology in the operating room was second nature to the brilliant and charismatic Harvey Cushing who quickly deployed the newly invented Roentgenograph to make great strides in Neurosurgery (pneumo-encephalography, discography etc).

5. Antibiotics

Another significant factor that made a great

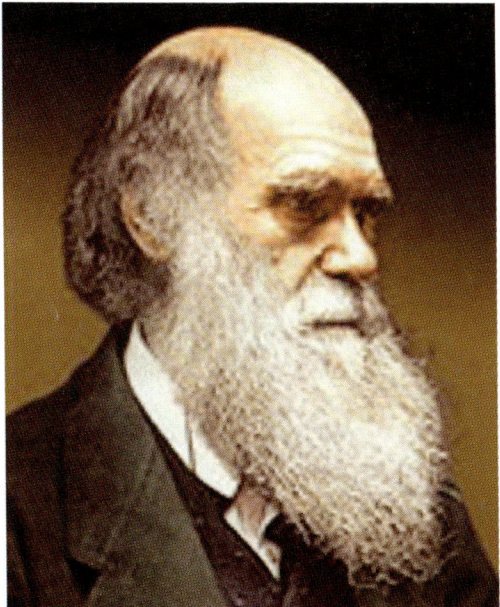

Fig. 02.09. Charles Darwin (1809-82)

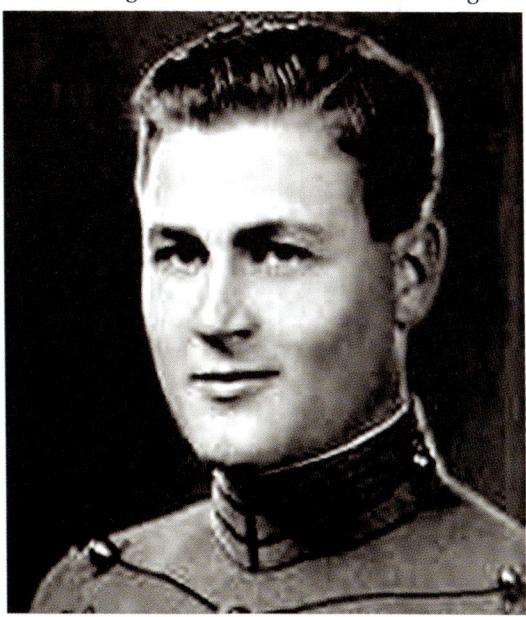

Fig. 02.10. Edward Murphy (1918-90)

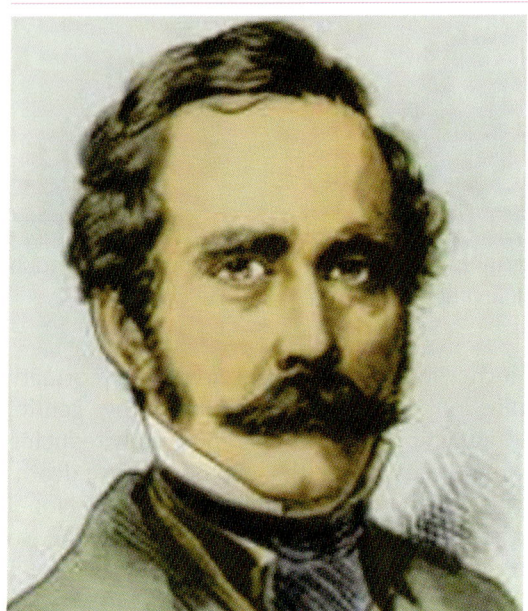

Fig. 02.11. William Thomas Green Morton (1819-68)

difference to surgical mortality and morbidity was the advent of antibiotics, when Alexander Fleming discovered penicillin from a mould in 1942. (see chapter 4 on Asepsis).

INFORMATION EXPLOSION

The huge technical and scientific explosions have made access to information a basic human right. This has resulted in profound changes in the surgical milieu, especially those of public perception. For example, the demand for safety and transparency has resulted in unearthing the sad statistic that of 234 million surgical operations performed every year across the globe, 7 million have debilitating complications leading to about 1 million deaths annually. Most alarming is the information that about 50% of these deaths are potentially preventable.

The UK Study called NCEPOD (National Commission on Enquiry of Perioperative Deaths) looked exclusively at the cause and prevention of perioperative deaths and found that about 50% of the human errors were related to overworked and fatigued staff, prompting a sea change in the NHS hours of work (where surgeons worked over 80 hours of week in the years gone by, now it is reduced to 40 hours).

This information access has permitted patients to participate actively in decision making and often times the final choice between, for example, a pancreatic resection and a bypass, rests on the patient's shoulders. It is good for every young surgeon to constantly recall the Latin phrase, Primum non nocere, which means above all, do no harm.

A combination of algorithms. protocols and guidelines are available for most diseases. These, used judiciously, will steer the confused surgical trainee across the rocky waters of rapid decision making.

ALGORITHM: a series of steps to deal with a problem, with multiple verticals.

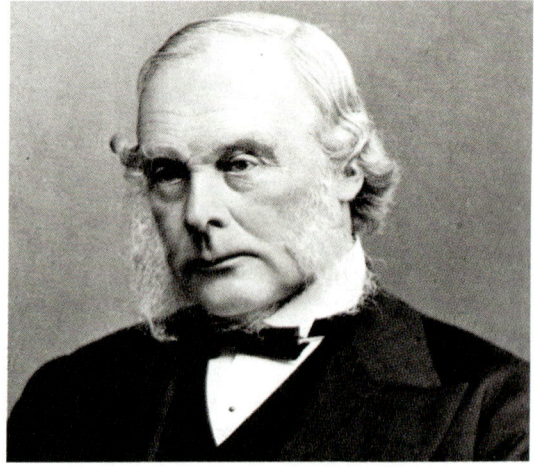

Fig. 02.12. Lord Joseph Lister (1827-1912)

PROTOCOLS: a formal pre planned sets of rules applicable within a practice or an institute.

GUIDELINES: best practice advisory recommendations.

Note: protocols are local and guidelines are global!

Despite the above preventive measures, adverse events will occur, and when they do, it should be properly documented, more to modify the system and prevent repetition, rather than to merely blame the operating surgeon! The action sequence checking (or checklist manifesto) is being widely introduced, with the objective of reducing errors maximally, as followed by the aircraft pilots, before takeoff.

The practical operative experience of the trainees has now been eroded by public pressure on health care systems to deliver consultant performed rather than consultant supervised procedures. This point is of significance in the training milieu, with a large number of private hospitals taking part in surgical education.

The three periods of surgical interaction for every trainee are preoperative, intra-operative and postoperative and the requirements and check lists in each part are herewith detailed:

PREOPERATIVE

In the early 20th century, the maxim, Choose well, cut well, get well was coined to envisage all the three aspects of the operation. These days, the preoperative period, is one of intense decision making for the surgeon and the patient. It is imperative that the surgeon in training participates in every aspect of this phase.

The concept of informed consent has now become paramount before surgery, and it implies that a complete understanding of the various negative aspects of the surgery has been given to the patient and kith and kin by the concerned surgical team. It is often difficult to decide how much to disclose to the patient, before any procedure, since mentioning some remote complication may cause undue anxiety and may even culminate in the refusal of the procedure. As a general rule 'all possible' complications need not to be discussed, but only those probable (>1%). Documentation of the same is vital in the current scenario of increased tendency for litigation.

Very often, there are a number of equally viable options that could be exercised in the treatment of a given patient. The most optimal one for that particular patient is chosen and a multidisciplinary approach is sometimes required, especially for tumor related surgeries, e.g. a planned rectosigmoid resection may be deferred based on a CT or MRI showing bulky disease, and referred instead for preoperative chemoradiation. Being part of such a multi-disciplinary process will serve to widen the perspective of young surgeons. Pertinent to this is Voltaire's immortal quip, The best is often the enemy of the good!

Preoperative information gathering should be

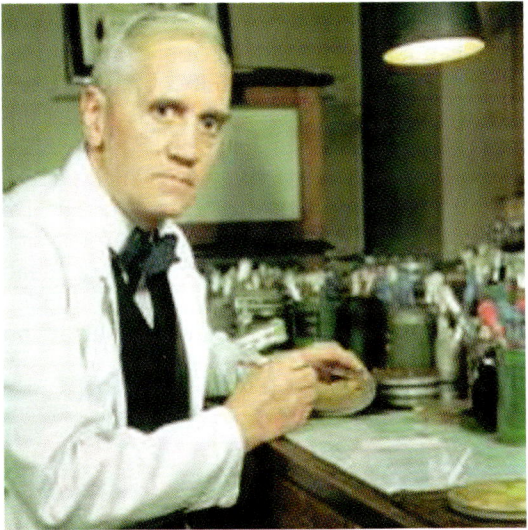

Fig. 02.13. Alexander Fleming (1881-1955)

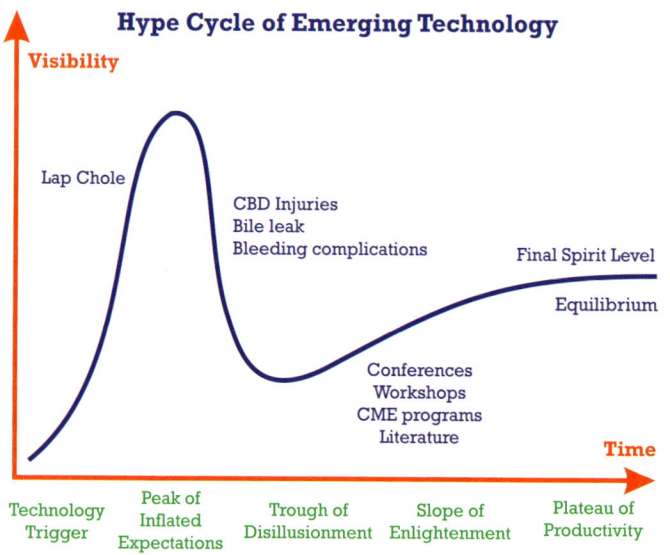

Hype Cycle of Emerging Technology

Visibility

Lap Chole

CBD Injuries
Bile leak
Bleeding complications

Final Spirit Level

Equilibrium

Conferences
Workshops
CME programs
Literature

Time

Technology Trigger | Peak of Inflated Expectations | Trough of Disillusionment | Slope of Enlightenment | Plateau of Productivity

Fig. 02.14. Gartner's Hype Cycle, taking laproscopic cholecystectomy as an example

done on the basis of a careful patient interrogation and analysis of tests. At this point, it is important to point out the value of medical statistics, which unfortunately remains a Cinderella specialty in medicine. Understanding the importance of prospective double blinded controlled clinical trials and the input they provide towards decision making, will lay a rock solid foundation to build the edifice of a

surgical career. See chapter 100 on Evidence-based medicine.

Reports of meta-analysis and a Cochrane trial analysis should be looked at as gospel truth and a discerning postgraduate should know all recommendations from these two sources regarding the surgical procedure.

New methods of treatments are constantly cropping up in the horizon. There will then follow a period of conflicting evidence confusing the picture. Although a postgraduate should be aware of what is new, he should not wildly embrace an unproven technique. Indeed, it is best to wait for approval of the technique by a third party who is unconnected with the hype surrounding the procedure. The apex court of evidence- based medicine still remains meta-analysis, but these trials will take a considerable period of time to appear in surgical literature. The above facts would most aptly apply, in recent times, to minimal access surgery. It is worthwhile to remember the Richardson curve that every new treatment modality seems to follow.

TRIAGE

One cannot concentrate on only one patient when faced with a multiplicity of patients and this happens sometimes in the accident and emergency department, especially during mass casualties. One needs to choose which patient would benefit most from treatment, e.g. if a single doctor is confronted by four sick patients, and if one of them is nearly dead (couldn't be helped) and one fairly well (need not be helped), then he should concentrate on

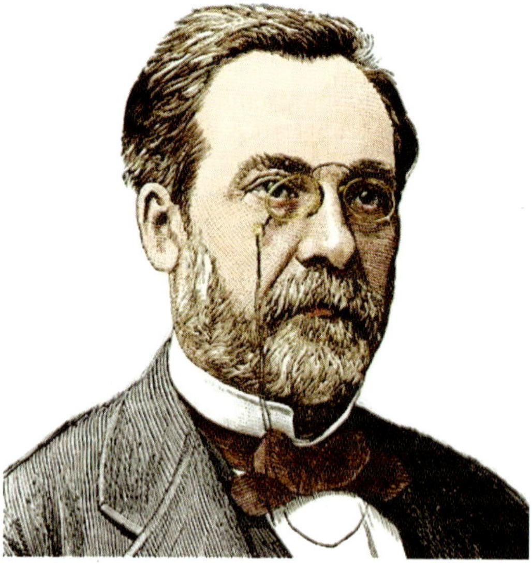

Fig. 02.15. Louis Pasteur (1822-1895)

Jewels of Gyan - 02.5

Meta-analysis

Comparison of differently structured clinical trials in order to elicit a statistically significant conclusion, i.e. comparing apples and oranges.

the other two patients who can be saved by emergency care.

CHANGING FEATURES

In some acute disease conditions, the clinical features may show rapid changes within a few hours. Hence the need for repeated examinations, as the trend of changing features will allow decision making about taking to the OR etc. If in doubt, it is best to defer decision by an hour or two provided the patient is stable, and be re-examined by the same observer, thoroughly thereafter.

GET HELP

The third eye phenomenon is defined as the extra input we receive by getting the help of another surgeon. One should never be too over-confident to seek help as the patient should always be the centre point of all surgical decisions, not the ego of individual surgeons.

TRAWLING

This means performing a huge battery of tests, hoping that one of them will hit upon the diagnosis. Although encouraged by corporate hospitals, this practice is a drain on the patient's purse and good clinical judgment will allow short listing of relevant investigations in each case and thereby expedient diagnosis.

CHECK IT OUT YOURSELF

Some investigations, like endosonography, Doppler, CT-angio, etc., are operator dependent. When in doubt, the junior surgeon is best advised to speak to the person who has performed the same, which will serve the clarify issues. This includes free interaction with the surgical pathologist as well.

RATIONALE FOR SURGERY

Before entering the OR, the surgeon should be sure about the rationale for the particular procedure in that specific patient. The chain of decision making should run through the surgeon's mind so that he is clear with the logic of choosing the operation.

INTRA-OPERATIVE

EXCEL EVERYDAY

Skill and commitment to surgical excellence do

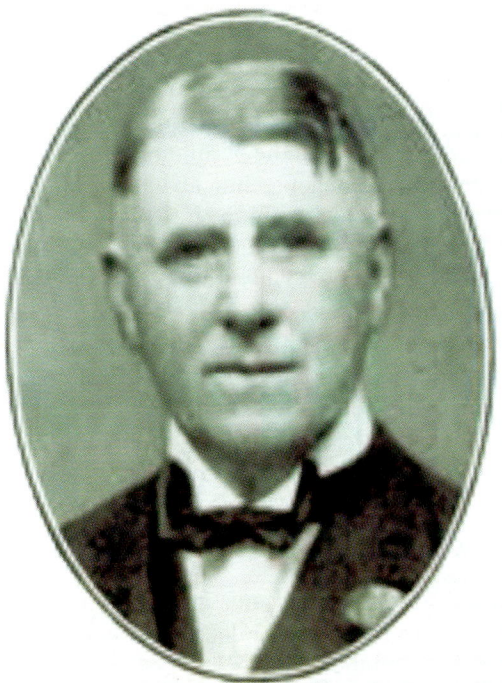

Fig. 02.16. Lord Berkley George Andrew Moynihan (1865-1936)

not appear by themselves when needed. They are carefully constructed, nurtured and converted into second nature. By force of repetitively striving for precision, surgical activity should become ingrained in a surgeon.

RIGHT CHOICE

The perfect operation can still be a failure if the patient selection has been faulty or if postoperative management is insufficient. A useful take home message here: The operation is over only when the patient goes home well.

SURGICAL TECHNIQUES

Alternative measures of learning surgical skills are now the recommended route. These can be in the form of conferences, workshops, virtual reality, animal labs etc. It is said that every surgical movement is played out in the cerebral cortex a microsecond before the hands start doing it. Lord Moynihan of Leeds was said to walk around theatres with a suture in his hand, using every spare minute to practice ambidexterous knot tying!

IMMITATE

It is useful to watch and copy experts, given that imitation is the highest form of flattery! When observing the senior surgeon at work, it is important to look at the peripheral aspect of the field and the smaller technical details as well, as excellence depends upon the trivia (Michaelangelo). At the end of the day, aggressive repetition of moves will result in skill, dexterity, precision and speed.

Watching well captured videos on surgical procedures is another method of training, in which the operative field is zoomed to understand the finer details, preferably with the comments by experienced surgical teachers. 2-way interactive live surgical workshops organized by acknowledged surgeons, have recently become as very popular with the junior surgeons and postgraduates to learn operative skills and decision makings in complex situations.

Complication rate is not necessarily lessened by the experience of a surgeon, but when it occurs, it is better accepted.

KNOW YOUR ANATOMY

The greatest of surgeons have always spent long and arduous hours in the anatomy dissection rooms. One must be completely familiar and comfortable with all aspects of anatomy and there is simply no substitute for this. The overall operating time and complication rate of a surgeon who has good command over anatomy is considerably less than his fellow surgeons.

Other basic sciences as applied to surgery, such as embryology, physiology, pathology, pharmacology, anesthesia etc. are no less important in the making of a comprehensive surgeon.

TISSUE DISSECTION

Remembering that every unnecessary grasp of tissue could revitalize cells and predispose to infection. Living tissues are capable of reacting to irritation or trauma (inflammation) and therefore should be handled with the utmost gentleness. A senior surgeon once commented that tissues should be handled as gingerly 'as

Jewels of Gyan – 02.6

Postoperative Fever – Commonest Causes

Day 0: Blood transfusion, drugs
Day 1: Atelectasis
Day 2: Wound infection
Day 3: UTI, central or peripheral line infection
Day 5: DVT or wound infection
Later: Abscess formation

the surgeon's own urethra'. Absolute hemostasis is a must while avoiding excessive strangulation or charring of tissue. Careful and symmetrical re-apposition of tissues will permit minimal scarring of the wound. The diathermy and employing drainage have to be as minimal as necessary, realizing their potential to cause tissue damage and infection.

ENGAGE BRAIN BEFORE KNIFE

Instead of rushing to start the operation, it is far better to move in a smooth and calm progression. As part of a checklist, one must ascertain that he is dealing with the correct patient, side, site, instrument and equipment. After reaching the target site, it is advisable to stop again. If faced with advanced infection or cancer, one should start at the periphery and work towards the centre of the disease process, in order to minimize spreading bacteria or malignant cells. If one is not sure of achieving the desired result, there is no harm in seeking senior assistance or backing off. Nowhere in medicine is it truer that discretion is the better part of valor.

EMERGENCY SITUATION

One should not lose focus on the primary objective of the surgery. If a lesser procedure within the reach of the surgeon can be safely done, then that option is quite acceptable, for e.g. if a junior surgeon opens up a patient with large gut obstruction, and is not confident of carrying a bowel resection, a proximal colostomy, simple and safe, will tide him over the crisis and achieves the desired result.

MISCONCEPTION

This is a cortical event, and a frequent cause of errors, especially in laparoscopic surgeries. Once the structure is identified, the cortex labels it so, not permitting a challenge of this assumption. Many a common bile duct has been crippled because it was labeled as a cystic duct. A safe and cautious surgeon is one who has a low threshold for generating a doubt and urge for verification. When in doubt, do not proceed before confirmation!

SWABS

It's best to use as few swabs and as large ones as possible to accomplish the given task. There should be equal panic whether the swab counts of the OR nurse are more or less than the numbered swabs on the board. Either is a signal to recheck the wound thoroughly. Having a radio-opaque thread built in the swabs is a certain way to exclude retained swabs, if the wound was already closed. A trapped swab in a wound is called a 'gossypoma' both because *Gossypium hirsutum* is the taxonomic name for cotton and probably also because of the unwanted gossip that ensues during surgery!

FIGHTING INFECTION

Reducing tissue revitalization is important, as this is a predisposing factor to infection. The oxygen tension in a wound is dependent on pO_2, blood pressure, hypovolemia and sympathomimetic effects including inadequate analgesia. Another factor is the prolonged exposure of the wound to the atmosphere with

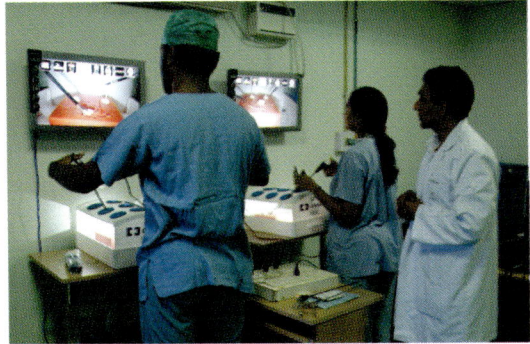

Fig. 02.17. Hands-on training in laparoscopic surgery on a virtual module

Jewels of Gyan - 02.7

What do you do as a surgeon, when the nurse says at the end of an operation, she is getting one pad excess?

Answer: Obviously the initial count was wrong. Then we do just the same as what we have to do when one pad is less.

its drying effect. Constantly keeping these factors in mind will ultimately reduce the incidence of infection.

Prophylactic antibiosis, as discussed, in the chapter 04 on Asepsis, should be given with the objective of maximum bactericidal levels while the skin is being incised by the knife.

POSTOPERATIVE CARE
MONITOR APPROPRIATELY

Operation notes should be followed by mention of what parameters need be monitored, for how long and how to react if changes occur, for eg., routine half hourly pulse, blood pressure and temperature monitoring is not necessary for a young healthy man undergoing a hernia procedure or an uneventful laparoscopic appendectomy.

OPERATIVE FINDINGS AND DRAINS

A full detailed record of the operative procedure is essential including special details like tourniquets, drains and tubes. A sketch of the incisions with attached drains etc., will elucidate matters considerably. When in doubt, it is better to label the T-tube and drain, to avoid inadvertent removal of the one for the other.

COUNSELING RELATIVES

It is extremely important to discuss especially with the relatives of a patient who has had a major procedure or a poor risk surgical candidate and apprise them of the exact situation. Sometimes it is better to delay breaking very bad news for a day or two in order to lessen the stress for the family.

DRUGS

The preoperative medication like antihypertensives, bronchodilators, thyroxin and anticonvulsants, should be restarted as soon as possible. Oral hypoglycemic agents and antiplatelet aggregation drugs are started more slowly to avoid possible hypoglycemia and post operative bleeding respectively. See chapter 101 on Anesthesia.

ABC

Throughout the postoperative period the vital function of airway, breathing and circulation need to be monitored. It is sad that this basic premise is often forgotten with disastrous results.

ANALGESIA

Whichever the analgesic protocol that is followed it is imperative that the patient is kept as pain-free as possible. Small repeated doses of pain killers are a good way to avoid the specter of respiratory depression. See chapter 85 on Postoperative Analgesia.

RESTLESSNESS

Apart from wound pain, the restless patient might be having an unemptied and distended bladder. Hypoxia is another important cause for the same, as is an uncomfortable position or pressure from the edge of the bed or some other apparatus.

Jewels of Gyan - 02.8

The 6 Ws of Postop Fever

Wind:	Atelectasis
Water:	UTI or IV line
Wound:	wound infection
Walking:	DVT
Wonder drugs:	Drug fever
Whereabouts not known:	Deep-seated abscess

ATELECTASIS AND DVT

As soon as a patient is awake he should be encouraged to take deep breaths, cough, and to start intensive spirometric exercises, keeping in mind that inadequate lung expansion postoperatively, is the commonest cause of fever in this period.

Every patient should also be persuaded to walk as soon and as early possible, since low molecular weight heparin and TED stockings do not guarantee immunity against DVT.

Lung complications and DVT are the commonest causes of postoperative death.

Modern medicine is a science but practicing it is an art
The fact the patient is going home well doesn't necessarily mean that we have done the right thing

03 Preoperative Preparation

This is as important as the operation itself, for several reasons. Ideally, the patient is admitted only a few hours before surgery (previous evening for operation next morning), since the incidence of wound infection is directly related to the number of preoperative hospitalization days. This is due to replacement of normal (relatively harmless) resident bacterial flora of the patient's skin by the hospital bacteria, which are more resistant to antibiotics. For minor surgery done under local anesthesia or 'day-care surgery', they are asked to report just an hour or two before, for general evaluation, premedication as well as for skin preparation.

They should be advised to abstain from alcohol, smoking or other forms tobacco abuse, for at least two weeks before an elective procedure and have strict control of diabetes and hypertension, for a few days prior to surgery. The high incidence of respiratory and cardiovascular complications in smokers and hepatic problems in alcoholics have to be impressed on the patient.

For elective surgery its is preferable to maintain good glycemic control, with glycosylated hemoglobin (HbA1c) levels under 7 (known as 'euglycemic clamp'). Perioperative control of sugar is preferably done by a titrating scale with soluble insulin, by round-the-clock blood/urine check, because of its labile nature, as a response to stress. Even on the day of surgery, since the patient is generally fasting, insulin may be administered after starting the intravenous line, just before the operation. Under normal circumstances, it is virtually not possible to induce hypoglycemia, while an intravenous glucose drip is on flow.

No effort should be spared to assess cardiac, pulmonary, renal, hepatic and cerebral functions preoperatively, whenever their dysfunction is identified/anticipated based on history and physical findings and it may be prudent to defer elective surgery, till clearance is obtained from the experts after supporting investigations. There is the additional risk of inducing renal insufficiency while operating on patients with obstructive jaundice.

In grossly obese patients, particularly with ventral hernia, it is advisable to make them lose weight before surgery, by postponing it for up to 2-3months if needed. Firstly it makes anesthesia and surgery more comfortable; secondly postoperative cardiopulmonary morbidity is considerably less and thirdly they may not be interested in doing so after surgery. Hence they should inculcate diet/exercise discipline prior to any elective operation, in their own interest. In patients with a history of bronchospastic disease, it is safe to 'cover' them with parenteral bronchodilators and corticosteroids, before induction of anesthesia.

Besides previous major illnesses or surgical procedures, history of allergy to drugs, bronchospastic or convulsive disorders, use of corticosteroids, thyroid dysfunction, cardiac/cerebral ischemia etc. which need attention during anesthesia, has to be recorded and passed on to the anesthesiologist, while taking instructions for premedication. Early in the morning is the best time to operate on children, obviating the need for starvation. It is equally ideal for adults, particularly major operations, leaving the entire day at the disposal of the recovery room staff, to monitor them, with seniors around. Sedation in the previous night may be needed as a 'routine', more so for apprehensive patients (not surgeons!). About six hours of starvation is advisable for adults before a major anesthetic, which may be reduced to three hours in children.

Even if the patient is on anticoagulant/antiplatelet agents, there is sufficient evidence that a surgical procedure may be performed safely, without risk of additional bleeding. However, most surgeons play safe by withdrawing them 3-5 days before the operation and restart a few days later. In more emergent situations, fresh frozen plama (FFP), or platelet-rich plasma (PRP) infusions are given perioperatively, to reduce risk of bleeding.

Special preparation is necessary in certain situations, such as gastric outlet obstruction or colon surgery, by gastric decompression and bowel lavage respectively, before surgery. Bowel preparation for colon surgery is mainly mechanical, earlier accomplished by repeated enemas, now largely replaced by an osmotic laxative, like mannitol or polyethylene glycol/electrolyte solution (Peglec). The main drawback of the earlier practice of giving intestinal antibiotics (bacteriological bowel prep), is staphylococcal superinfection, known as pseudomembranous enterocolitis. There has been however, a recent evidence-based trend to do away with preoperative colonic lavage altogether.

Euthyroid state is mandatory for surgery for thyrotoxicosis, to avoid a 'storm'. More elaborate perioperative medical preparation is required, under supervision of an endocrinologist, for surgery for a pheochromocytoma, Cushing's syndrome or Conn's disease. If the patient has intestinal obstruction, nasogastric aspiration and monitoring of fluid/electrolyte/acid-base balance may be very important. Anemia and hypoproteinemia are commonly seen in patients with liver disease, malignancies, gastrointestinal and nutritional disorders, requiring build up, if they need surgery, by appropriate blood component therapy.

DVT prophylaxis may be considered in high risk group using low molecular weight heparin (LMWH) starting before (or soon after) surgery and pressure-gradient elastic support to the legs and feet (see chapter 82). Surgery for orthopedic, neurological and vascular diseases and in obese patients, major chest/ abdominal/pelvic surgery, major amputations, advanced malignancy, congestive cardiac failure and those with thrombophilic state or previous history of DVT, is considered high risk and they have to be suitably covered by prophylaxis against major thromboembolic catastrophies.

Preoperative transfusion of blood components may be indicated only if the Hb is less than 8gm. Autologous transfusion (using patient's own blood), collected a week or two before surgery, is the safest but not very popular, except in some vascular cases. Each time, blood is drawn and an equal volume of a colloid solution, such as hydroxyethyl starch (HES) or polygelatin is infused, not only to restore volume but for reducing viscosity by hemodilution, beneficial for microcirculation. Another novel method, when more units of blood are required, is to start collecting blood from the patient 6weeks before surgery, at weekly intervals. The first unit collected is transfused back, before collecting two units on the second week and those two units are given back to him, to collect 3 units on the third week and so on, so that on the week before surgery six units of his own blood are available for intraoperative use. The principle of this procedure is to avoid administration of blood stored in the bank for too long, with the consequent loss of quality.

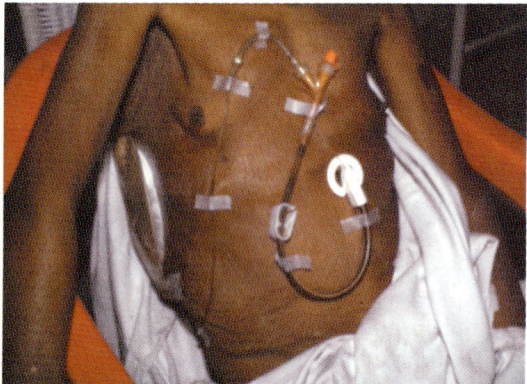

Fig. 3.1. Malignant obstructive jaundice
Note a percutaneous endoscopic gastrostomy (PEG) for feeding and a percutaneous transhepatic biliary drainage (PTBD) for decompression
(courtesy: Lifeline Hospitals, Chennai)

In addition to the problems of mismatching and infectious diseases, the patient must be guarded against post-transfusion reactions, which include transfusion-related acute lung injury (TRALI), cardiac overload and iron overload, which follow multiple transfusions. Preoperative blood transfusion is generally avoided since there is evidence that the immune system is affected by the donor blood due to the transfusion-related immune modulation (TRIM), which can lead to increased risk of infection and cancer recurrence, post-transfusion graft-versus-host disease (GVHD), when the donor immune system attacks the host's blood cells and microchimerism (when small amount of donor blood persists in the recipient's body, causing ongoing low grade GVHD).

Local skin preparation is done, to provide a surgically clean area, before the operation. Skin shaving should be done after a clean bath, not earlier than an hour before surgery, since if more time is allowed, colonization of hospital flora occurs in the serum exuding through microscopic cuts, created during shaving; in this respect, clipping is superior to shaving. The area may be gently scrubbed with chlorhexidine or povidone iodine and a sterile towel is wrapped in place, before transporting to operating room. Sometimes, all this is done in the ante-chamber of the operating room itself, while the patient is waiting following premedication. For bone surgery, a 24-hour skin preparation is required, especially if an implant is likely to be placed. If skin or bone grafting is planned, the donor area also requires similar preparation, as also the back, for spinal anesthesia.

The side of planned surgery should be marked to avoid the not too uncommon catastrophe of operating on the 'wrong' side. Verifying it from the patient on the operating table, who is under the influence of premedication is neither ethical nor legal and is best avoided.

In clean-contaminated cases, where a poten-tially unsterile hollow viscus, such as small bowel, vagina or urinary bladder, is being entered, prophylactic antibiotics are indicated. The most popular method described by Burke, consists of starting a high dose of a bactericidal agent (preferably a single drug) intravenously 30min. before making the incision, to continue through the operation and for about six hours later. It may be continued as necessary, if frank infection is encountered during surgery, further treatment being guided by the microbiological study of the pus. Postoperative wound dressings have attracted considerable attention ever since the experiment on medical students conducted by Billroth, wherein he concluded that an open wound is less likely to get infected than a closed one. There are enough defense mechanisms in the wound after 48hours to prevent entry of bacteria; hence clean wounds may be safely left open after 2 days. This also facilitates inspection of the wound by seniors, during their rounds, so that early signs of infection may be detected and appropriate action initiated. It is important to realize that in more than 95% of wound infections, the process starts during surgery (endogenous). No external dressing can prevent a smoldering wound infection from becoming clinically apparent, which is usually in 48-72hours. In fact, under the dressings, accumulated serum and sweat form a fertile anaerobic culture medium for bacterial growth and many pathogenic microbes can be identified, if a swab from the under surface of the dressings is cultured after 2-3 days !

The choice of anesthesia, is largely the prerogative of the expert, but preferences of the surgeon and the patient cannot be totally discarded. Whenever major anesthetic is necessary, the anesthesiologist should examine the patient in the previous evening, review all relevant laboratory reports, explain the patient the nature of anesthesia, general risks involved and for him/her in particular and postoperative precautions to be followed by the patient, such as limb movements, coughing/breathing exercises, early ambulation etc. In a situation, where significant risk is involved, it may not help to discuss the issue with the patient, but responsible attendants may be taken into confidence on probable risk/benefit equations, by the anesthesiologist/surgeon, generating candid interaction, before they are asked to sign as witness for an informed consent given by the patient. In critical situations, it is wise to get additional moral and legal protection by inviting a second opinion from a fellow consultant in the subject concerned, even if such request had not originated from the patient's side, more so if such desire had surfaced from them.

At this juncture, it should be realized that the majority of litigations following surgery are related to complications of anesthesia rather than surgery, though the surgeon, as the 'captain' of the team, cannot disown vicarious responsibility, for the ultimate unfavorable result. Improper communication seems to be the main reason for such 'heart burns' and it is very important to explain the therapeutic options with their score, to the patient/attendants, to involve them in decision-making to some extent, to keep them periodically appraised of the progress of a critically ill

patient and maintain some amount of 'transparency' in various steps being taken from time to time. This compassionate approach creates a cordial doctor-patient relationship in the long run, leaving very little scope for mistrust and confrontation.

Prevention of misadventures in surgical management

Concerned about the unacceptably high incidence of perioperative human errors leading to morbidity and mortality (totalling around 7 millions out of estimated 234 million operative procedures carried out globally every year), the World Health Organization (WHO) had designed a check-list (similar to that followed by aircraft pilots), calling it as Alliance for Patient Safety (2004) to prevent surgical misadventures.

The CHECK LIST divided into 3 steps, namely, before induction of anesthesia, before making the surgical incision and before the patient leaves the OR, mainly focuses on:

1. Identification of the patient, disease and the procedure
2. Well informed consent
3. Side and site to be operated

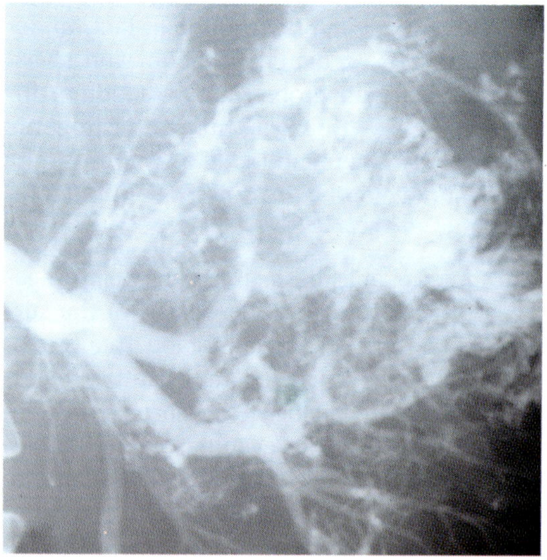

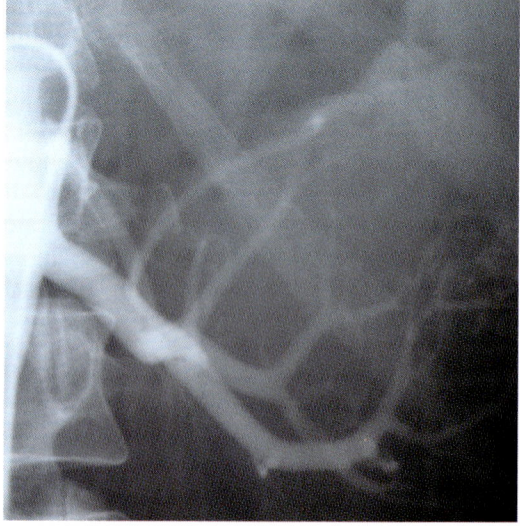

Fig. 3.2. Therapeutic embolization. Renal angiogram demonstrating a vascular renal cell carcinoma.

Fig. 3.3. Post-embolization angiogram
(courtesy: Halsted Surgical Clinic, Chennai)

4. Pre-anesthetic precautions

5. Preoperative precautions

6. Functioning of the equipments

7. Attention to co-morbidities

8. Areas where the surgical team might possibly err.

Every surgeon is earnestly urged to adopt these precautionary measures, to protect the clients against 'avoidable' complications and to live up to their expectations, as well as to steer away from litigations, when they submit themselves to us for a surgical operation with great confidence.

04 Asepsis and Sterilization

Asepsis has come a long way since Ignaz Semmelweiss (1818-65) in Vienna, drastically decreased the mortality from puerperal sepsis by washing his (ungloved) hands between successive vaginal examinations. Like all geniuses during their times, he was rewarded by being shut away in a lunatic asylum for the rest of his life. Later Robert Koch postulated that a particular microorganism could be considered responsible for an infection:

(1) when it is found in adequate numbers at the focus,

(2) it can be cultured in pure form and

(3) the lesions could be reproduced by injecting it into another host. Subsequently Lord Joseph Lister (father of antiseptic surgery) and Louis Pasteur introduced the concept of having a clean and sterile field during surgery, which has become an integral part of the surgeon's conduct in the operating room. Sterilization is the process wherein all microbes, including spore forms are destroyed, whereas disinfection implies destroying only the vegetative forms and not spores. Asepsis is prevention of

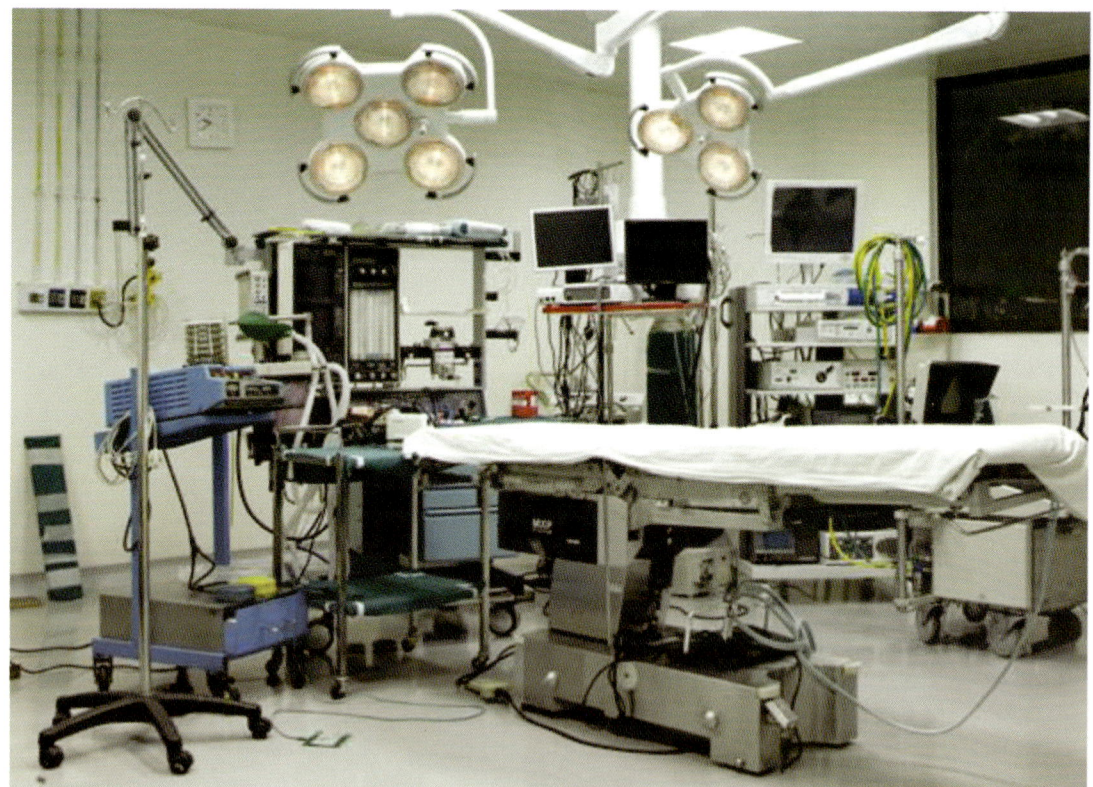

Fig. 4.1. Modern operation room set up
(courtesy: Lifeline Hospitals, Chennai)

William Stewart Halsted introduced rubber gloves for his scrub nurse, **Caroline Hampton** (who later become Mrs. Halsted), to protect her hands from the corrosives, such as mercuric chloride used to sterilize the instruments. One of Halsted's students, **Joseph Bloodgood**, introduced their routine use by the entire operating team.

microbial invasion into healthy tissues and antisepsis refers to treatment of infection, once the invasion occurred.

The introduction of surgeon's gloves by William Halsted, though totally unintentional, is another landmark in the subject of aseptic surgery, since any amount of scrubbing of hands will only make them 'surgically clean', but not sterile in its real sense. However adequate scrubbing up to elbows is equally important, if one realizes that over 25% of gloves examined following a 2-hour operation, show punctures, creating a serious breach in the 'sterile concept'. This is one of the facts driving the push for routine double gloving. Repeat scrubbing with brush, for a second operation in succession, is neither warranted nor without risk of ploughing the permanent skin flora to the surface; hence simple soap wash is all that is needed for subsequent operations, provided the person has not left the surgical arena in between. In the operating room, only those who are scrubbed and gloved are allowed to handle sterilized instruments used during surgery. If any sterile item has to be picked up by the 'circulating staff', it is done with the help of a long crocodile-toothed instrument, called Chietle's forceps, which is always kept immersed in antiseptic lotion and is returned to the lotion jar immediately after use. The very principle of wearing caps and face masks during surgery is under debate, it may turn out to be more of esthetic value rather than anything else and probably more helpful more in protecting the operating team from the patient, than the reverse!

On the skin, there are three types of bacterial flora,

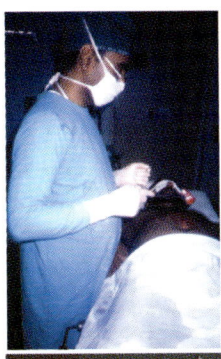
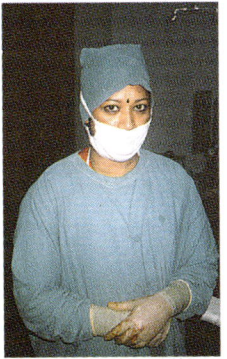
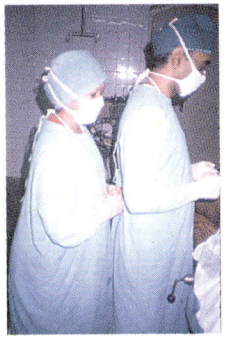

Fig. 4.2, 4.3 & 4.4. What not to do in the operating room

(a) transient,

(b) resident and

(c) permanent.

The transient flora are very labile, change within a few minutes of entering into a new environment and can be eliminated by simple soap wash. The resident flora are more difficult to alter; it may take 12-24hrs. of stay in an environment, to acquire the new flora and they are eliminated by a good five minutes hand scrub.

The permanent flora are situated in the roots of the hair follicles, sebaceous and sweat glands and are extremely difficult to get rid of, but reach surface along with sweat and sebaceous secretions; any amount of scrubbing during surgery cannot eliminate them, hence the obvious need to wear gloves. Minimally invasive surgery (MIS) has much less incidence of infection, compared to standard open surgery.

Some of the common mistakes committed in the operating room, breaching sterility are:

a) while preparing the skin to be incised, leaning on the table after wearing the operating gown: this contaminates the front of the surgeon's gown and then the main drapes, when the surgeon leans on to them during surgery. *Till the patient is completely draped, the surgeon should not touch the table.*

b) wearing the mask, exposing the nostrils, facilitating droplet infection of the surgical wound.

c) while shifting the assistant from the head to footside of the surgeon, his front (clean) should not come in contact with the back of the surgeon (potentially contaminated); instead he should roll over the back of the surgeon, with his back, taking a full circle.

Nosocomial Infection

(Nosos: disease; komeion: to take care of) syn: Hospital acquired infection

There are several situations and points of entry for the infecting organism into the patient, in the hospital:.

1. Surgical site infection (SSI) is the commonest. Main sources are:

a) Institution related (exogenous): hygienic conditions in the ward, operating room environment, sterilization of instruments, drapes and attire of the surgical team

b) Patient related (endogenous-95%): lack of personal hygiene, preoperative bath or harboring infection somewhere, too long preoperative stay in the hospital (acquiring hospital bacterial flora) and local hair clipping/shaving and its timing (ideally it should be done just before surgery)

Diabetes mellitus, obesity, anemia, hypopro-teinemia, vitamin deficiency, immune-compromised state, advanced malignancy, those in shock, on long term steroids or consume tobacco products or alcohol have higher incidence of SSI

c) Procedure/surgeon-related: rough tissue handling, inexpedient surgery (too long exposure of wound to the atmosphere and its drying effect), leaving dead space, mass ligatures, overuse of diathermy, inadvertent leaving foreign bodies, wound irrigation with toxic chemicals, inappropriate use of antibiotics, implants, suture materials and drains

2. Related to I.V cannula or indwelling catheters, such as urinary, central venous, jugular access for hemodialysis

3. Related to intubations: endotracheal, nasogastric

4. Procedure-related: lumbar/cistern

puncture, abdominal paracentesis or inter-costal chest tube, PTBD or PTC, joint aspiration, angiography, angioplasty etc

5. Patient-patient spread

a) keeping clean and infected patients in the same ward (not isolating grossly infected patients)

b) not employing routine hand wash (chlorhexidine+alcohol) before/after handling patients during ward rounds

c) improper management of hazardous hospital waste and sharps

6. Healthcare workers to patients:

a) employing HCW, carrying serious infection

b) not using protective attire - gloves, cap, face mask, shoe cover and apron, where appropriate

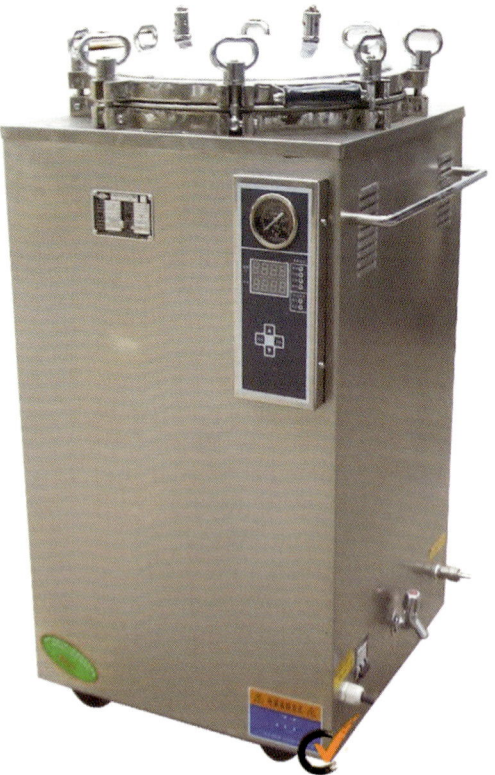

Fig. 4.5. Vertical type of autoclave

Methods of sterilization
a) Physical methods

I) Autoclaving: The principle that the boiling point of a solution can be raised by increasing the atmospheric pressure around it, is utilized in autoclaving as well as in pressure cookers. Water is boiled in a closed sturdy metal container, not allowing the steam to escape, raising the pressure inside the chamber to around 15lbs/sq.inch and elevating the boiling point to 125-135°C. At this temperature, all bacteria and spores are destroyed within 5-10minutes. Basically two techniques are employed in this process:

Pack method

Packed material to be autoclaved is kept in a separate central chamber, without coming into direct contact with the steam. A thermosensitive dye is used on a sticker (Signalock), to indicate if the required temperature is reached, ensuring adequate sterilization.

Caddy method

The instruments are kept in the central chamber, packed in metallic drums with vents to allow the steam to enter. After the required process is over, those vents are shut by some sliding device and the drums (also called bins or caddies) are removed and stored for use when necessary. Articles generally autoclaved: blunt instruments, linen, dressing material, gloves, diathermy cords etc.

ii) Boiling: Blunt instruments, rubber catheters etc. may simply be boiled for 30minutes, but this may not destroy spores.

iii) Gamma radiation: Using Cobalt-60 source, sharp objects such as blades, scissors and needles, suture materials, plastic material such as PVC catheters and drains etc. may be packed and sterilized effectively.

iv) Ultraviolet rays: This is generally used to sterilize operating rooms and laboratories, since they do not penetrate.

b) Chemical methods

Gluteraldehyde 2% (Cidex or Glutihyde) is used

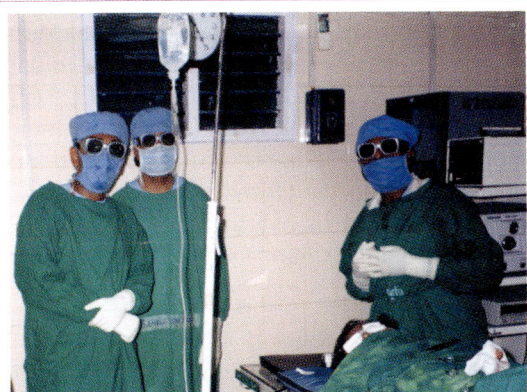

Fig. 4.6. Protective goggles, while operating on a patient with HIV infection
(courtesy: Lifeline Hospitals, Chennai)

for the endoscopes and endoscopic instruments; the vegetative forms are eliminated within 10-15minutes, but it may take several hours to destroy spores. Though the activated solution has a life of 2-4weeks, it is desirable to discard it daily, if grossly contaminated instruments have been immersed.

I) Ethylene oxide has been widely used to sterilize reusable materials intolerant of heat, its only drawback being explosive property, when mixed with air. Hence it is mixed in the sterilizing chamber with carbon dioxide, nitrogen and methyl bromide, exposure is maintained for 12hours at room temperature. It is toxic if inhaled and it should not be allowed to leak into working places; after the sterilization process, the room should be ventilated liberally for several hours.

ii) Chlorhexidine+cetrimide+alcohol complex (Savlon or Microshield): Solution containing 7.5% chlorhexidine gluconate, 15% cetrimide and 5% isopropyl alcohol is diluted and used for fast disinfection, since it requires only 2-5minutes of immersion.

iii) Tincture cetrimide, chlorhexidine or povidine iodine is used for surface disinfection for skin preparation of patient and hand scrub for operating team.

iv) Fumigation: This is used to disinfect operating, delivery rooms, laboratories or septic/isolation wards. Formalin or ethylene oxide vapour is generally used for this purpose. Initial dusting and cleaning of the equipments, such as anesthesia, suction or ventilating machines, monitors, overhead lights etc. should be done before filling up the closed room with fumes, kept for 6 hours or overnight. Contaminated linen and blankets may also be disinfected by this process.

v) plasma irradiation is a form of radiation sterlization, but without ionizing radiation. It utilizes an inert gas in plasma form.

Studies done regarding the use of laminar flow and other sophisticated methodology in the operating suits, such as disposable surgical attire, incise adhesive drapes, wound guards etc. have concluded that they did not contribute to superior results in terms of reducing surgical infections. After some minimum cleanliness and tidiness of the operating rooms, the most important factor that influenced the incidence of infections was surgical technique, such as gentle tissue handling, use of fine instruments and suture material, expedient surgery, leaving minimum dead space and foreign bodies, avoiding mass ligatures, anatomi-

cal restoration of tissue layers, good hemostasis, proper use of prophylactic antibiotics etc.

Erysipelas (meaning red skin) is spreading cuticular lymphangitis, usually due to Streptococcus pyogenes (β-hemolytic strain), but mixed infection is not uncommon. Poor personal hygiene, recurrent respiratory infections, immunosuppression, debilitating illness etc are the predisposing factors. The infection develops around a scratch or abrasion, rapidly spreading to the adjacent skin, associated with fever, toxemia and leukocytosis. It has a discrete margin and can spread to areas devoid of subcutaneous tissue, such as external ear or ala of the nose, whereas cellulitis (which is a speading inflammation of subcutaneous tissue planes), cannot spread to those areas (Milian's ear sign) and has diffuse borders.

Face, arms and legs are the most common sites, the involved skin turns pink, edematous and shiny with occasional blisters of serum and pus, associated with regional lymphadenopathy. Swabs taken from the punctured blisters provide the necessary microbial information and the choice of antibiotic. The florid infection responds promptly to antibiotics, such as penicillin, clindamycin or erythromycin, though it may take several weeks for the skin color to return to normal.

Clostridial infections
Tetanus

With world-wide distribution, it is caused by a spore-bearing Gm positive anaerobic bacillus, Clostridium tetani, the terminal spore giving a classical drumstick appearance. Though the incidence in the western world has come down, with vigorous campaigns for active immunization, it still causes significant morbidity and mortality in developing countries. It is found in manured soil, capable of invading any wound, more so with devitalized hypoxic tissue.

It produces two powerful exotoxins, tetanospasmin and tetanolysin. The former inhibits

Jewels of Gyan – 04.1

How do you sterilize/disinfect?

Foley's catheter	Gamma irradiation
Artery forceps, scissors etc.	Autoclave
Ureteric catheter	Ethylene oxide or gamma irradiation
Laparoscopic hand instruments	Plasma irradiation, gluteraldehyde
Electrical cords	Ethylene oxide, gamma irradiation
Pad, gauze	Autoclave

cholinesterase at the motor endplates, leading to excess of local acetylcholine and sustained state of tonic muscle spasm, not unlike that seen in strychnine poisoning. The toxin also travels along the nerve fibres to CNS, causing hyperexcitability of motor neurons in the spinal anterior horn cells, resulting in widespread spasm of skeletal muscles, in response to sensory input. Once the toxin gets fixed to nervous system, its action becomes irreversible and cannot be neutralized by antitoxin. Tetanolysin causes hemolysis and is a mild cardiotoxic, both are not considered clinically significant.

Incubation period may be 2 to 10days (average one week) and as in case of rabies, closer the wound is to CNS, earlier the symptoms appear and more serious the natural course of the disease. Rarely the infection may be dormant in the tissue, to manifest under suitable conditions, months or years later, called latent tetanus.

Symptoms and signs: Its manifestations are usually generalized, but may be confined to area of entry point, known as local tetanus, with minimal systemic features. Bacteria entering through the umbilical stump causes neonatal tetanus (tetanus neonatorum), in which difficulty in sucking may be the initial presentation, gradually becoming generalized tetanus.

Vague discomfort over the neck, lumbar region, abdomen and jaw are the initial symptoms, followed by muscles spasms and trismus. Dysphagia may be seen due to involvement of pharyngeal muscles and typical face of painful smile (risus sardonicus), caused by the spasm of the muscles of facial expression. There may be fever, tachycardia and leukocytosis as a response to infection, respiratory distress due to thoracic muscular spasm or generalized toxic convulsions, but the patient may remain mentally alert, till end. Other types

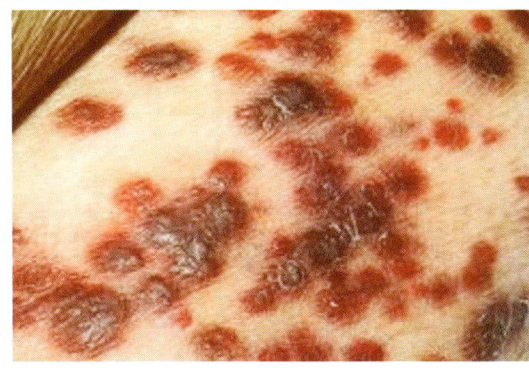
Fig. 4.8. Kaposi's sarcoma
(courtesy: Halsted Surgical Clinic, Chennai)

involving various regions are: cephalic tetanus (involving cranial nerves), bulbar tetanus (involving deglutition and respiration), otitis tetanus (following CSOM), postoperative (after surgery) or puerperal tetanus (after an abortion or delivery).

Diagnosis is made mostly by clinical features rather than laboratory support. Demonstration of bacilli in the wound is not diagnostic nor its absence excludes the disease. Opisthotonus and emprosthotonus are the terms used to describe backward and forward curvatures of spine due to the spasm of the muscles of spine. The bending of the body like a bow earned the disease the name, 'dhanurvatha'. Orthotonus refers to spastic fixation of the body and limbs in straight position. The muscle spasms may be so violent as to cause rupture of muscles/tendons or fractures.

Differential diagnosis: Dental sepsis, tonsillitis, seizure disorder, meningo-encephalitis, hypocalcemic tetany, strychnine poisoning, delirium tremens etc.

Treatment

Prevention by active immunization with adsorbed tetanus toxoid is ideal, the routine use of which (as triple antigen for children) has brought down the incidence to a large extent. Liberal wound

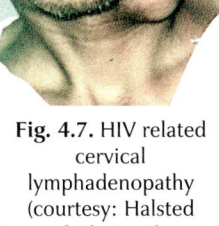
Fig. 4.7. HIV related cervical lymphadenopathy (courtesy: Halsted Surgical Clinic, Chennai)

Virus	Cancer	Etiological Probability
RNA Viruses		
HIV	NHL	
	Kaposi sarcoma	
	Hairy leukoplakia	
	Squamous cell Ca	
HCV	Liver Cancer	25%
	NHL ?	
DNA viruses		
HBV	Liver cancer	50%
HPV	Cervical cancer	100%
EBV	Burkitt lymphoma	>90%
	Hodgkin's lymphoma	>50%
	Nasopharyngeal Ca	100%
	Post-transplant lymphoma	>80
KSHV	Kaposi sarcoma	100%
HTLV 1	Adult T-cell leukemia	100% (Human Tlymphotropic virus)
Human Herpes Virus	Kaposi saricoma	
	Primary effusion lymphoma	
Bacteria		
Helicobacter pylori	Gastric carcinoma	30%
	MALT lymphoma	100% (Low grade NHL)
Parasites		
Schistosoma hematobium	Bladder SCC or adeno Ca	
S. mansoni	Liver Ca	
S. japanicum	Colon Ca	
	Splenic lymphoma	
	SCC of prostate?	
Distomiasis (liver fluke)		
Clonorchis sinensis	Cholangiocarcinoma	
Opisthorchis viverrini		
Plasmodium falciparum	Burkitt lymphoma	

Table-4.1. Infection as a cause of cancer

debridement and irrigation is helpful to reduce the bacterial load. The only way to counter the effects of toxins once infection has occurred is by giving hyperimmune tetanus antiglobulin, at the earliest. The immune response following tetanus infection is so poor that the patients recovered from it still need immunization. A booster dose of toxoid may be routinely given to the immunized patients undergoing surgery, if it had not been given during the previous six months and for an unimmunized patient with a dirty injury, both passive and active immunization are recommended.

Patients with clinical tetanus need skilled nursing care to prevent complications. They should be confined to a quiet room, to avoid external stimulation triggering muscle spasms, but the practice of isolating the patients in a remote ward is unnecessary, since the infection doesnot spread from patient to patient and it precludes close assessment of progress by senior consultants. The medical team must be sensitive to identify the usual problems of lack of mobility, such as pressure sores, venous thrombo-embolism, pulmonary and urinary infections. Rhabdomyolysis leading to 'crush-like' syndrome, affecting the renal functions, may be observed.

Tetanus immunoglobulin (TIG) 5000 to 10,000 units, is administered as soon as the diagnosis is made. If the patient is not allergic, high dose IV Penicillin G (10million units per day) is the antibiotic of choice, alternately doxycycline or clindamycin may be used. Liberal use of skeletal muscle relaxants, analgesics, anxiolytics, nutritional and ventilatory support are the main stay in the management. Tracheostomy may be needed if prolonged ventilatory support is anticipated. Attention to eye care, bladder and bowel function is also important. The value of high doses of magnesium in preventing muscle rigidity and seizures (lower doses are routinely used in eclampsia) is under evaluation. The overall mortality of tetanus is around 40%, hence the importance of prevention.

Gas gangrene (see chapter 17 on Gangrene)
VIRAL INFECTIONS

Both RNA and DNA viruses have been associated with human oncogenesis. Viruses are simple forms of life containing RNA or DNA genome wrapped in a viral capsid of protein and has the potential to replicate within living host cells. After invasion, the host cells turn into manufacturing units for viral particles. The infection may kill the host cell or may remain latent in the cell and can survive for long periods, predisposing to cancerous change in the host cell, known as insertional mutagenesis. Though the mechanism is not clearly understood, there is sufficient data in favor of viral oncogenesis ; all patients with the above mentioned cancers were found to be infected with the culprit virus and cancer cells contain the viral genome.

Human immune deficiency virus (HIV) and Surgeons

It is a retrovirus, containing reverse transcriptase, trasmitted most commonly by sexual encounter between the partners; other modes are: mother to fetus (vertical transmission), use of infected needles (in drug addicts), blood transfusion and between patient and health care workers (HCW), particularly surgeons. It is expected that 30% of those infected with HIV, will develop full-blown AIDS.

The patients with HIV infection develop opportunistic infections, such as tuberculosis (though most commonly M.tuberculosis, atypical mycobacteria like M.avium intracellulare are also encountered), oral/esophageal candidiasis, pneumocystis carini pneumonia, cryptosporidial diarrhea, cryptococcal meningitis, toxoplasmosis (SOL in brain) etc. They are also prone to secondary malignancies (they are called secondary because their origin is related to a known cause), such as NHL, Kaposi's sarcoma, hairy leukoplakia and squamous cell carcinoma. Surgery may be required in them for HIV-related conditions, such as intestinal obstruction, biopsy of a lymph node, a cerebral SOL etc. or diseases unrelated to HIV infection.

AIDS anal syndrome:

Warts, diarrhea, suppuration, ulceration, fissure and incontinence (in homosexuals).

Diagnosis

History should identify the high risk group for acquiring the infection. Detecting the disease in its early stages may be difficult, especially within the first few weeks, before the serological tests turn positive (window period of danger). The virus can be isolated from blood, semen, saliva, tears, urine and cervical secretions of infected patients. ELISA (enzyme-linked immunosorbant assay) and Western Blot tests only identify the antibodies, after the window period, but polymerase chain reaction (PCR) can detect the DNA of the antigen (the virus) itself, even during the window period, when antibody tests are negative (before sero-conversion). Three strains of virus, HIV-0, HIV-I, and HIV-II have been so far identified.

Prevention/protection

UNIVERSAL PRECAUTIONS FOR SURGERY ON HIV PATIENTS

Provide face mask to the patient
Allow minimum number of personnel in the operating room

Staff with abrasions or ulcers are not allowed

Wear shoe covers, water-proof sheets, gowns, gloves, eye protection to every one

During surgery

All the above + double gloves and protective goggles to the surgical team
Use of heavy duty face mask

Jewels of Gyan – 042

Tackling hair at operative site	
Clipping	Best
Shaving immediatly before	As good, standard
Shaving several hours before	Dangerous
No shaving or clipping	No difference to infection but dressing may be uncomfortable
Chemical depilation	Ideal but time consuming and expensive

Avoid jerky hand movements causing injuries by sharps or needle sticks
Transfer sharps through a kidney tray
Prefer scissors or diathermy to knife
Skin clips are preferred to sutures
Use instruments where possible instead of fingers

All the team members must wash their hands thoroughly at the end of procedure.

After the procedure, all instruments used should be immediately washed with soap and autoclaved or immersed in gluteraldehyde.

The aim of prevention should be to protect HCWs from getting infected not only from a known case, but also as a routine in all cases coming in contact during day to day professional activities, be it medical, surgical, obstetric or endoscopic. Beware of 5-Hs in practice, homosexuals, heroin addicts, highway drivers, healthcare workers (HCW) and hemophiliacs!

The healthcare workers are constantly at high risk, unless appropriate preventive protocols are strictly adhered to, while dealing with patients in general, realizing the high infectious potential of the disease during the window period (after acquiring infection and before sero-conversion) of any patient. This implies that unless tested by PCR, which detects the viral antigen, routine screening for HIV anti-bodies, is not 100% fool-proof, to identify the risk of carrying the disease, while performing a procedure or choosing a blood donor.

If any member of the surgical team has developed a skin breach, while operating on a known HIV patient, the wound should be allowed to bleed liberally and quickly washed with soap and 1% sodium hypochlorite solution. Prompt testing of a baseline ELISA is mandatory and combination drug therapy (post-exposure prophylaxis - PEP) with zidovudine, lamivudine and indinavir, is immediately commenced, under the guidance of a specialist. The test may be repeated every two weeks, for 3-6 months or

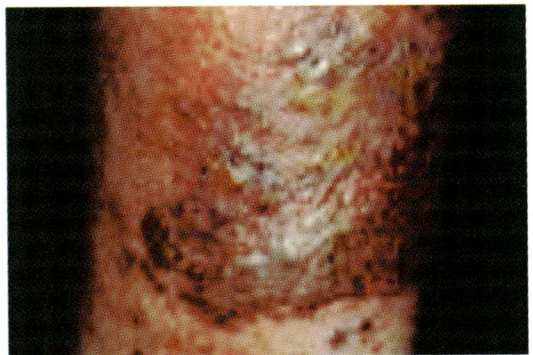

Fig. 4.9. Erysipelas of the arm

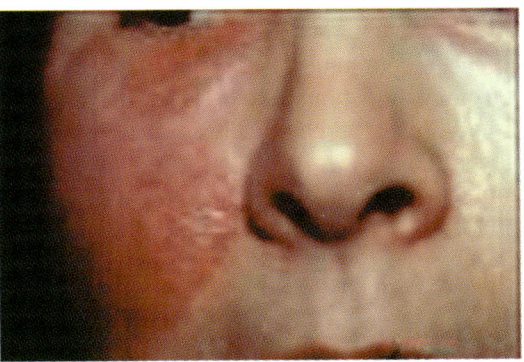

Fig. 4.10. Erysipelas of the face

till it turns positive, to decide further course of therapy, based on the merits of the situation.

HIV patients are usually monitored by the estimation of viral load, CD4 (cluster differentiation) and total lymphocyte count (TLC). Readings of <10,000 replications of the viral load, >500/cmm of CD4 and >1500/cmm of TLC, bear a favorable prognosis. With the advent of newer antiviral drugs, the outlook in the patients with HIV infection has greatly improved. Several thousands of patients have survived for over 15 years with a zero-virus count in the peripheral blood and it has now become a chronically manageable disease, though, as on date, neither a cure nor a preventive vaccine, is in sight.

Hepatitis B virus (HBV) and Surgeon

It is a hepadenovirus, with outer surface coat (HBsAg) and inner nucleocapsid core (HBcAg). The circulating form of the latter is HBeAg, a marker of viral replication and activity. It is transmitted by needle stick, blood transfusion, administration of sera, sexual or perinatal infection. Though not realized, this is more infective and dangerous than HIV, 1% developing fulminant hepatitis and 10% going into carrier state, cirrhosis and hepatocellular carcinoma, particularly when it is acquired in childhood. Health care workers are at great risk of infection, mostly surgeons, by injury of the hands by sharp instruments, while operating on infected patients. The average incubation period is 30-100days. Hepatitis-C, D (parenterally transmitted) and E (enterally transmitted), also have been recognized.

Diagnosis: HBsAg, Anti HBcAb, HBeAg

Prevention: 3-dose vaccine against HBV is available and is strongly recommended to all exposed to risk of infection. If suspected immediately after a needle puncture or sexual encounter, Hepatitis B immunoglobulin (HBIG) may be given.

Treatment: Interferon-2b has been extensively tried with some success, notwithstanding the long duration (1 year) and high cost of therapy. Recently, oral therapy with lamivudine, hepavirin (for six months) and a herbal *(Phyllanthus amarus*)* compound (for 30days), has shown promising results, in terms of reducing viral load and faster sero-conversion with the added advantage of being cheap and compliant.

Protecting patients from dangerous nosocomial infections, such as hepatitis-B or HIV, is a statutory requirement and it is equally important to protect the health care workers (HCW) against such hazards. Routine laboratory detection of these infections in all patients coming for surgical treatment is neither practical nor cost-effective and as such is not done. In the absence of such safe 'routines', it becomes imperative for the operating team, to observe standard precautions, such as avoiding needle/knife injuries to hands, wearing waterproof gowns and masks.

* discovered at Chennai

Hospital waste disposal

In the recent times, acute awareness of nosocomial infections or the hazards of solid/liquid/biological/chemical/radioactive waste generated in the hospital, disposed into regular municipal outlets, has necessitated certain measures to be followed to make the hospitals 'hazard-free' to the general public as well as to the HCWs in the campus. Environmentalists have given certain statutory guidelines to dispose all hazardous biomedical solid waste generated in clinical establishments, by incineration, autoclaving, hydroclaving, microwaving, wormiculture, ozonization, plasma torch technology, deep soil burial etc. The hospital washings and liquid effluents from toilets have to be suitably treated and disinfected by chlorination (1% sodium hypochlorite) or other chemicals, before being allowed into regular sewers. Sharps such as needles, blades etc. should be blunted or shredded and disinfected before disposal. Statistically, trying to recap the needle is the most common cause of accidental injury to the hands of HCWs, hence it should be avoided. For fear of unscrupulous recycling, all plastic items, made of polyvinyl chloride (PVC) should be deformed and disinfected, but never incinerated, since the noxious fumes generated, such as furons and dioxins (incriminated in certain endocrinopathies), may create atmospheric pollution. However newer plastic material, made of high or low density polyethylene (HDPE or LDPE) may be safely incinerated. The personnel handling such hazardous waste should be properly immunized, motivated, trained, supervised and physically protected by suitable gloves, masks, overshoes and goggles.

Segregation at the point of generation into different categories is essential, since it is not possible to do so later; furthermore, mixing a small fraction of bio-hazardous material (15%) with the rest makes the entire volume hazardous, thus increasing the cost of its disposal.

Since it is not practical to create and maintain a waste disposal facility for each medical establishment, including medical and dental offices, employing a common treatment facility has been found to be most appropriate, eco-friendly and cost effective, which is currently being adopted in all the cities and towns in the country, proactively monitored by the pollution control department of the state.

05 Sutures and Staples

Suturing is an integral part of any surgical procedure and with biotechnological advances, a variety of materials are made available to a surgeon, requiring judicious use at appropriate places, fully realizing their physical and biological properties.

An ideal suture material should possess the following features:
a) good tensile strength
b) minimal tissue reaction
c) good knotting property
d) should not harbour infection

e) should be easily available and affordable
They may be classified according to their physical characteristics as follows:

l) monofilament sutures: e.g. polyamide (nylon), polypropylene (prolene or vylene), polyester (terylene, dacron etc), polydiaxanone (PDS) and metallic sutures, clips and staples. The main disadvantage of monofilament material is that it has poor knotting property, requiring several knots to secure a ligature.

ii) mutlifilament or braided sutures: e.g. cat gut, polyglycolic acid (dexon), polyglactin

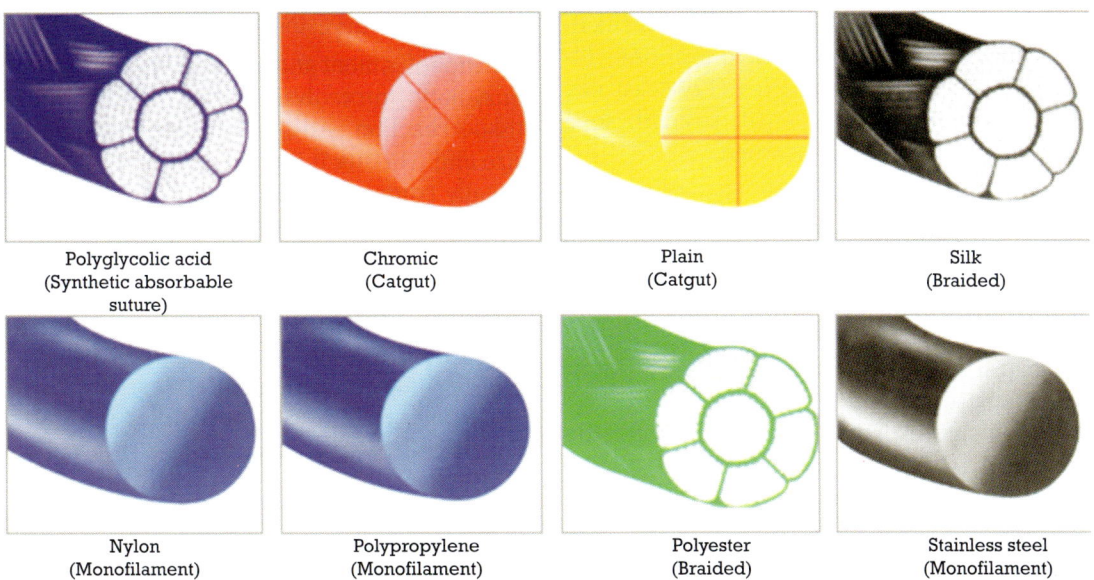

| Polyglycolic acid (Synthetic absorbable suture) | Chromic (Catgut) | Plain (Catgut) | Silk (Braided) |
| Nylon (Monofilament) | Polypropylene (Monofilament) | Polyester (Braided) | Stainless steel (Monofilament) |

Fig. 5.1. Cross section of suture materials

Classification	Monofilament	Multifilament
Absorbable	Surgical gut (Plain & Chromic) Poliglecaprone 25 (Monocryl) Polydiaxonone (PDS)	Polyglycolic acid (Dexon) Polyglactin 910 (Vicryl) Polyglactin (Vicryl) Coated Polyglactin (Vicryl) Rapide
Nonabsorbable	Polyamides (Nylon) Polypropelene (Prolene) Stainless steel (Ethisteel) Polyesters (Terylene & Decron)	Surgical Silk (Silk worm) Surgical Linen (Linum plant) Surgical Cotton (Cotton wool) Polyamide Braided (Sutupak) Polyester Braided (Mersilene)

Table-5.1

(vicryl), braided polyester (mersilene), silk (fibres of silk worm cocoon), cotton (hair of cotton seed), linen (fibres from plant linum) etc. The main drawback of braided material is it possesses 'interstitial spaces', where bacteria may lurk, perpetuating infection and exciting granulomatous reaction.

iii) glues (butyl cyanoacrylate or fibrin) and welding (cryo or laser)

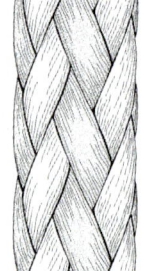

Fig. 5.3. Magnified view of braided suture material

They are also grouped according to their absorbable nature as follows:

i) absorbable sutures: e.g. catgut, plain (gets absorbed in 7 days), chromicized impregnated with chromium trioxide (3-4weeks), polyglycolic acid (4-8weeks), polyglactin (4-8weeks), polydioxanone (4-8weks), biodegradable staples (12weeks) etc. They lose much of their tensile strength, long before they are actually absorbed.

ii) nonabsorbable sutures: e.g. silk, polypropylene, polyester, silver, stainless steel, alloy metallic sutures, clips and staples.

iii) living tissue such as fascia lata, vas deferens etc. have been used in herniorrhaphy.

Biological sutures of historical interest, not in common use
Collagen sutures from tendo Achilles of cattle

(plain and chromic)
Cargile membrane from submucosa of cecum of ox
Fascia lata (bovine or human)
Kangaroo tendon

Natural absorbable sutures

Surgical gut is 99% collagen made from submucosa of sheep or beef intestine, taken from antimesenteric border. The more fibrous mesenteric border is used for making tennis gut. There is no clear information in the literature how the name of 'cat' is associated with it, except this collagen thread was supposed to have been used in a stringed musical instrument by name 'catchu' in yester years !

It is monofilament and absorbed by a process of enzymatic proteolysis, hence excites local tissue reaction. Absorption rate depends on size and whether it is plain or chromicized and usually completed within 60 to 120 days, but the effective tensile strength lasts only for 5 days for plain and 20 days for chronic gut. It is sterilized by gamma irradiation and kept supple by the liquid preservative. Allergic reaction to surgical gut may be due to iodine preservative earlier used or impurities such as mucopolysaccharides, not fully separated during the process of cleaning of the animal intestines.

Since it is derived from animal protein, its immunological and microbiological status is always unpredictable, with instances of catgut being incriminated in producing severe local reaction and postoperative infections, such as tetanus.

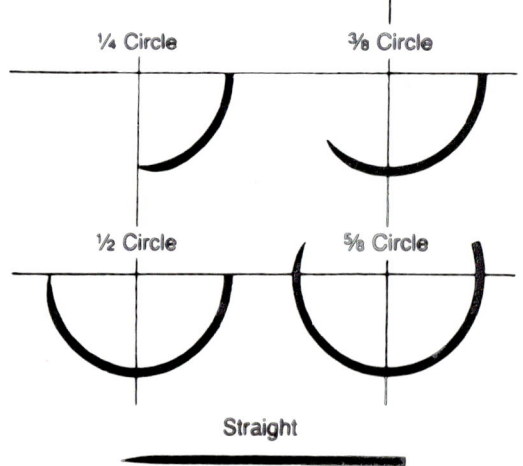

¼ Circle   ⅜ Circle

½ Circle   ⅝ Circle

Straight

Fig. 5.2. Different types of needles

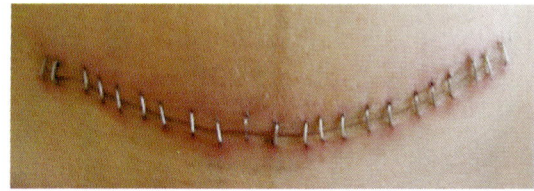

Fig. 5.4. Stapled skin closure after thyroidectomy
(courtesy: Laxmi Hospital, Kakinada)

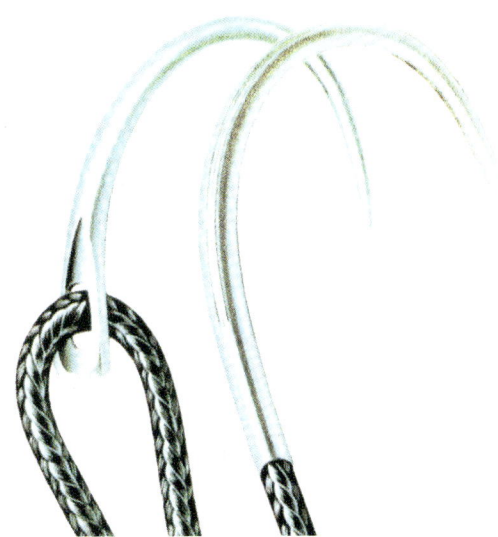

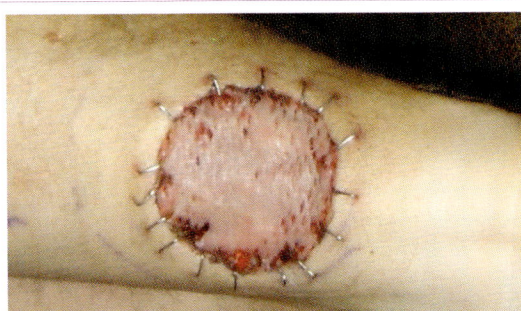

Fig. 5.7. Fixation of skin graft by staples

Fig. 5.5. Eyed and eyeless (atraumatic) needles

Synthetic absorbable sutures

There are many synthetic absorbable sutures available, manufactured from carbohydrates, eliminating allergic reactions. They may be monofilament (Monocryl and PDS) or braided (Vicryl). Their strength is twice that of surgical gut, with slower loss of tensile strength (30 days) and rate of absorbtion (by process of hydrolysis completed by 100 days), hence evoke minimal tissue reaction. They are sterilized by ethylene oxide, with over 5 years of shelf life and are considered to be superior to the surgical gut, practically meeting all the requirements of an ideal suture material, and suitable for all types of surgical procedures.

Coating: The Vicryl is coated with calcium stearate (for lubricating effect while the suture passes through tissues) and lactic acid (helps to retain tensile strength longer)

Vicryl Plus, coated with a broad spectrum antibacterial agent, triclosan, effective against common bacteria associated with surgical site infection (SSI).

Vicryl Rapide has been specially treated to lose the tensile strength in 10 days and totally absorbed within 40 days, particularly useful in areas with high cosmetic consideration or where its presence is required only for a short period, as in pediatric, dental, plastic and urologic (circumcision, urethroplasty etc) surgery.

Monocryl (Poliglecaprone-25) is composed of two co-polymers - glycolide and caprolactone, with loss of tensile strength in 14 days and complete absorption period of 120 days. It is the most flexible monofilament absorbable material, with excellent knotting properties.

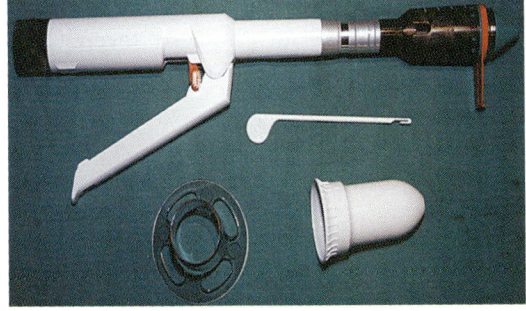

Fig. 5.6. A circular stapler gun for end-to-end anasto-
mosis(EEA) in hemorrhoid surgery
(courtesy: Lifeline Hospitals, Chennai)

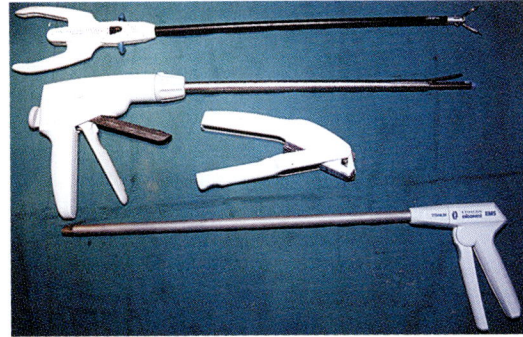

Fig. 5.8. External (skin) stapler and endoscopic staplers
(Endostapler)

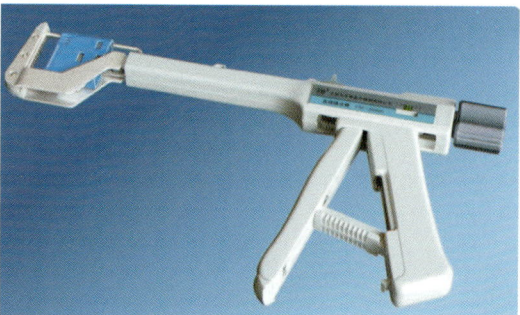

Fig. 5.9. Linear stapler (no knife)

PDS (Polydiaxanone) is a monofilament material, made by polymerizing para dioxanone molecules, to form a strong pliable filament. It loses tensile strength in 40 days and takes about 180 days for total absorption.

Nonabsorbable sutures

Silk: It is made from the fibres of silk worm cocoon, basically consists of keratin-like protein. After braiding to increase the strength, it is coated with wax, to reduce capillary action and friction while passings through tissues. Though the tissue reaction is very minimal, it gets encapsulated by fibrous tissue within 3 weeks.

Linen: it is made from the fibres from plant, linum, with similar properties as silk, but has a unique quality of gaining some tensile strength, when wet by tissue fluids.

Cotton: It is derived from the hair of cotton seed, with identitical properties of silk or linen, but weaker in comparison.

Polyamides (Nylon, it is so called because the formula was supposed to have been described

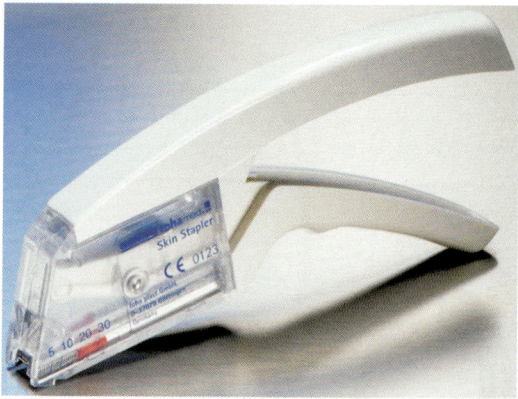

Fig. 5.11. Skin stapling device

simultaneously in New York and London). They lose approximately 25% of tensile strength in one year and are stiffer to handle than silk.

Polyesters (Terylene and Dacron and combination of both, Tevdec) are chemically extruded from a polymer and braided into sutures, with extremely high tensile strength, which is retained indefinitely. Hence it has become the suture of choice in cardiovascular surgery. Teflon or PTFE coating over the material makes them smooth and eliminate 'sawing' effect while drawing through tissues. Ethibond is a polyester suture with polybutylene coating, considered superior to Teflon or PTFE.

Polypropylene (Prolene): is a monofilament, chemically extruded from a purified and dyed polymer, with extremely high tensile strength, which is retained indefinitely. It has the property of expanding upto 30% before breaking, very useful in areas where 'give and

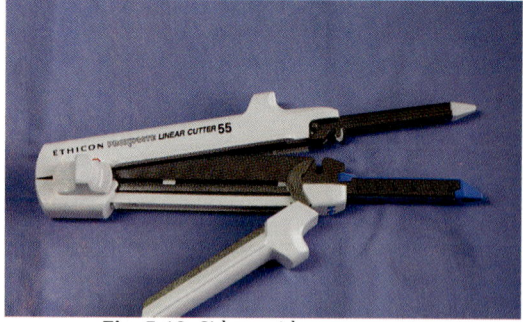

Fig. 5.10. Side-to-side anastomosis

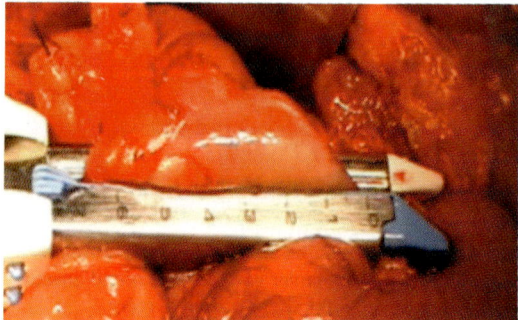

Fig. 5.12. Bowel transection using linear stapler

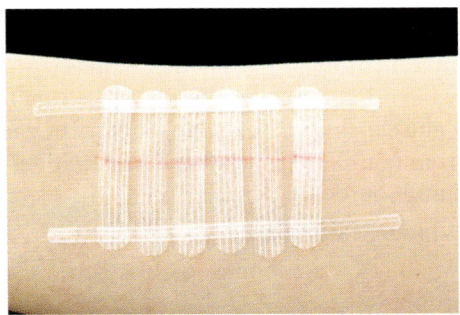

Fig. 5.13. Steri-strips closure of skin
Courtesy: Laxmi Hospital, Kakinada

take' is required due to local swelling or muscular activity. It is very inert, has very low friction coefficient and slides through tissue readily. It is sterilized by ethylene oxide and has become the most popular material currently used in many specialities. The drawbacks of polypropylene are the tendency to fracture on crushing and poor knotting property, requiring multiple throws for fixation.

Stainless steel: It had an enviable place, for its strength and inertness, before the advent of polypropylene. However, the drawbacks are, it cuts through the tissue if tied too tight, the barbs at the cut end of the wire may traumatize gloves and skin and its tendency to kink and fracture. It is still the material of choice to close sternotomy and orthopedic surgery, but in other areas such as Thiersch 'wiring' for rectal prolapse, it has been replaced by polypropylene.

Selection of suture material

It is based on the following factors

Degree of tissue tension anticipated

Rate of healing of tissues approximated

Presence of body fluids, such as bile, urine, intestinal juice, soaking the material

Presence of or potentiality for infection

Desirable tissue reaction and cosmesis

Handling comfort and knotting property

Cost and availability

Coating the fine suture materals with prostacycline is being tried currently, e.g. In microsurgical sutures, to discourage platelet aggregation and formation of microthrombi, over their intraluminal segments.

In atraumatic or eyeless suture, the suture material is firmly swaged to a needle, by special technology during manufacturing, so that no additional trauma occurs when the needle and suture are drawn through tissues. They are available with curved (held with needle holders) or straight (hand-held) needles, either round bodied or cutting. Suturing friable tissue, such as kidney or liver, anastomoses of bowel, blood vessel, nerve or ureter are ideally done using these sutures. Regular or eyed sutures are used only because of their low cost. Cutting needle should be used for suturing skin, breast tissue, cartilage, tough fascia or atherosclerotic artery, whereas for other tissues round-bodied needle is preferred.

Other special types of needles

a)   **reversed cutting,** where cutting edge is on the convexity of the needle, with less chance of suture cutting through while ligating, useful in areas like cornea, plastic surgery, etc.,

b)   **micro-tipped,** with very fine sharp tip used in microvascular surgery, vaso-vasostomy, etc.

c)   **taper-cut,** combination of cutting and round body, in which the distal sixteenth alone is cutting while the remaining is rounded, used in tough but vital structures, such as heart muscle.

d)   **CC (calcified coronary)** needle for cardiovascular use for atheromatous vessles

e)   **BV (blood vessel)** needle for fine vascular anastomosis

f)   **JB (Juergen Breuner)** needle, a specially designed round bodied, for GI surgery

g)   **Ethiguard needle:** Blunt tipped dolphin-nosed needle eliminating the risk of accidental puncture of surgeon's fingers, but specially designed to pass through tissues with ease. It is also very useful in operating on patients known to have bood borne infections, such as hepatitis and HIV and while handling friable organs, like liver, spleen and kidney.

Size of suture material

The diameter increases with the number starting with 1, but thinner than no.1, is graded as 0 and it becomes thinner with increasing number of '0's. For example no.3 suture is thicker than no.2, whereas no. 3-0 is is thinner than no. 2-0. Commonly used sizes range from no. 3 to 12-0, thinnest sutures being used in corneal and microvascular surgery, with the help of operating microscope.

Most of the sutures nowadays are supplied in presterilized, alcohol filled, sealed foils for ready use during surgery. The outer wrap is peeled apart, exposing the sterile inner foil, which should be picked up by the assisting personnel, by a sterile instrument and opened for use. Those materials not so supplied, such as nylon, cotton or linen may be autoclaved before use.

Staples in surgery

Michel's clips have long been used for skin closure, wherever cosmetic considerations prevailed, such as neck incisions. A straight or circular row of staples may be placed by firing a 'preloaded gun', for various types of intestinal surgery, coming very handy in difficult anatomical situations such as esophageal or low rectal anastomoses. But in other areas, it is debatable if the time saved by these devices is worth their cost, particularly in developing countries. Different types of 'guns' are manufactured, for end-to-end, end-to-side, lateral closures, endostapling of bowel, ligation and division of omentum, fascial and skin closure etc. improving handling comfort and enlarging applications.

Advantages: reduction in operating time, blood loss and tissue handling. 'B' type of stainless steel staples provide hemostasis, yet permit nutrition to pass through, to the cut edge of suture line, avoiding tissue hypoxia or impaired healing.

Disadvantages: cost, availability and requires training and expertise.

The endostaplers with 3 rows of staples on either side of knife, have revolutionized complex surgery like laparoscopic bariatric surgery.

Implants in surgery

Definition: it is an extraneous material surgically fixed into a patient, to serve the function of a muscle, fascia, bone, vessel etc. They may be from non-biological (synthetic) or biological (natural) sources.

Non-biological implants

1. **Stainless steel** bones plates, screws and arthroplasties.

2. **Tantalum titanium** coarse mesh for acetabular floor and fine mesh for hernial repair, as well as for bone plates and screws.

3. **Chrome-cobalt alloys:** bone plates, screws and arthroplasties.

Textile material

Dacron

1. **Woven tubes** - small interstices with minimal blood loss, poor penetration by fibrous tissue and poor fixation of pseudointima, are used for large blood vessel replacement.

2. **Knitted tubes** - large interstices; so preclottng is necessary, good fibrous tissue penetration and early pseudointima formation ; suitable for smaller vessel replacements.

3. **Sheets and felts** for attachment of heart valves and breast prostheses.

4 **Spun sutures.**

Polyethylene sheets for hernial repair

Teflon is used similar to dacron. Polytetrafluoroethylene (PTFE: Goretex) grafts are made from expanded teflon and are relatively non-porous. Velour prostheses are modified knitted grafts of dacron or teflon.

Biological implants

Biografts remain the first choice for aortocoronary bypass and vascular bypass below the groin. Biografts may be

1) autograft: from the same individual (commonest)

2) homograft: from another individual of the same species

    a)   isograft: genetically identical donor, such as monozygotic twin (rare)

b)   allograft: genetically not identical (second commonest)

3) heterograft: from a different species. One biological implant that is getting popular, is the porcine collagen mesh (Surgisis), which promotes tissue ingrowth in patients with infected meshes, after the inevitable mesh removal.

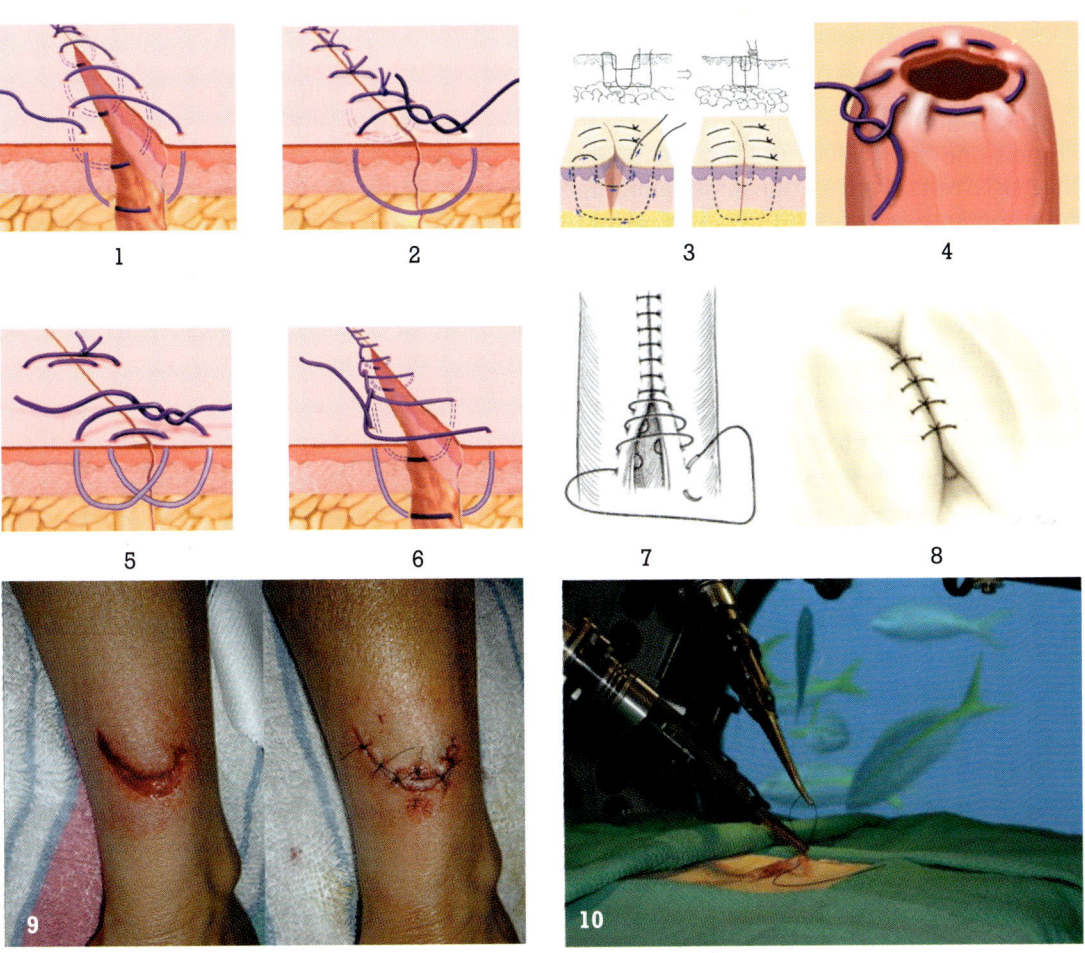

Fig. 5.14.
1. Simple running suture; 2. Simple interrupted suture; 3. Vertical mattress suture; 4. Purse-string suture
5. Far and near tension suture; 6. Running locking suture; 7. Connell full thickness inverting bowel suture
8. Lembert seromuscular bowel suture; 9. A laceration closed with simple interrupted sutures
10. Suturing by robotics.

Surgical pathology was born out of surgeon's curiosity, in fact early surgeons also took pleasure in looking into the microscope to diagnose disease conditions !!

The gross evaluation, careful handling of specimen and accurate interpretation is the cornerstone upon which the final pathologic diagnosis rests. Perhaps the most important requirement is a good communication between the surgeon and the pathologist in terms of provision of clinical information, representative biopsy and requirement of special laboratory procedures. Futhermore, to obtain maximum information, a surgeon must familiarize himself with various pathological techniques and their indications.

Diagnostic surgical techniques

There are two major types of specimens submitted for surgical pathology analysis, viz.

Biopsies and surgical resections.

Biopsies

Biopsy, by definition, is the removal of a piece of tissue for examination of histological architecture and cellular details. The different procedures include

1. Open biopsy - it refers to the tissue obtained during surgery. This may be incisional or excisional. *Incisional biopsy* entails the removal of a wedge of the lesion with adjacent normal margins while in *excisional biopsy* is, the entire lesion is excised with surrounding rim of normal tissue. Incisional biopsy is preferred in large lesions, keeping in mind the final incision for surgery. All small lesions should be excised in toto.

2. Core biopsy - which are obtained through the use of large-bore needles, sometimes under image guidance, such as ultrasound, CT scan or MRI. It involves the targeted removal of a needle core of tissue from the suspected site. Different types of needles are used depending on the site of lesion; however, Tru-cut needle is now the most preferred device.

3. Endoscopic biopsy - is probably the most commonly performed tissue sampling procedure. As the specimens are small, interpretation is difficult and multiple biopsies are desirable.

4. Cone biopsy - a cone biopsy is surgery to remove a cone-shaped piece of tissue from the cervix and cervical canal. Cone biopsy may be used to diagnose or treat a cervical condition and use of diathermy is.avoided to preserve tissue architecture, hence it is also called_cold conization.

5. Punch biopsy - a biopsy performed using a punch, an instrument for cutting and removing a disk of tissue. This is usually performed for cervix uterus, anorectal diseases, cheek, tongue, skin lesions etc.

Surgical resections

Surgical resection specimens are obtained by the therapeutic surgical removal of an entire diseased area or organ. These procedures are often intended as definitive surgical treatment of a disease in which the diagnosis is already known or strongly suspected. However, pathological analysis of these specimens is critically important in confirming the previous diagnosis, staging the extent of malignant disease, establishing whether or not the entire diseased area was removed, determination of the surgical margin, identifying the presence of unsuspected concurrent diseases, and providing information for postoperative treatment, such as adjuvant chemotherapy in the case of cancer.

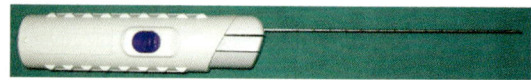

Fig. 6.1. Tru-cut (core) needle biopsy gun
(courtesy: Halsted Surgical Clinic, Chennai)

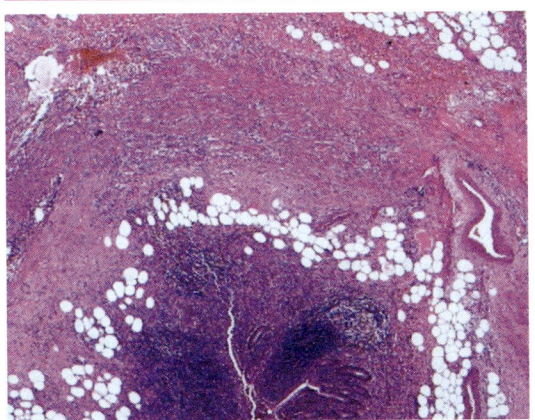

Fig. 6.2. HPE of acute appendicitis
(courtesy: Prof Sandhya Sundaram, Chennai)

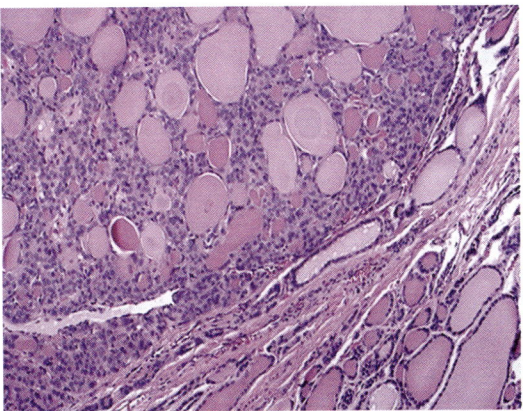

Fig. 6.3. HPE of colloid goiter
(courtesy: Prof Sandhya Sundaram, Chennai)

General principles of tissue sampling

The main objective of a tissue biopsy is to obtain a sample with well-preserved architecture and which is representative of the underlying pathologic process. Although there may be practical difficulties, certain guidelines should be followed irrespective of the nature of biopsy.

1. Large lesions require multiple biopsies to include focal changes within the entire lesion.

2. Biopsies should be avoided from the central necrotic area. A peripheral lesional area along with adjacent margin is likely to be more informative.

3. In cases where it is required to establish the presence of invasion, a whole thickness would help in accurate evaluation.

4. In lesions with thick capsules, it is important to ensure that the biopsy transgresses the capsule to include the actual lesion.

5. When electrocautery is used for biopsy, cautery-induced artifacts may obscure cellular details. In such cases biopsy should be larger and low setting coagulation mode should be used.

6. The tissue should be handled with minimal grasping irrespective of the instruments used to avoid crushing artifacts.

7. Many specimens are difficult or impossible to orientate once removed from the patient. Hence, orientation has to be performed by the surgeon at the time of excision using easily identifiable markers.

Possible techniques to orient include:

Sutures of varying lengths and number
Subdivision of the specimen in separate labeled containers
A diagram outlining the details should accompany the specimen
Orientation of small biopsies i.e. small intestinal biopsies can be accomplished by placing the base of the biopsy on a plastic mesh.
However, it is always preferable to discuss a complicated specimen with the pathologist in person.

Surgical pathology work flow

Specimen handling

Fixation: most specimens should be fixed as soon as they are removed, except in situations where more information is obtained by examination of fresh tissue. The usual fixative is 10% buffered formalin (never concentrated formalin), which is suitable for most samples. However some tissues fix better in alternative solutions e.g. testicular biopsies in Bouin's, gluteraldehyde for electron microscopic studies.

The precautions that need to be taken include Suitable sized containers with at least 8-10 times the volume of fixative to specimen

Specimen must be totally immersed in the fixative

Accurate labeling of the container

Minimal delay between obtaining the tissue and its arrival at the laboratory.

Fresh specimen (without fixative) to be sent if special procedures like smears, dabs, culture, enzyme histochemistry and molecular pathology are required.

Request form each specimen must be appropriately labeled with a complete and signed request form. The form must contain the details of patient identification, unit and consultant, date and nature of procedure, adequate clinical history, operative findings, previous reports if any and provisional diagnosis..Infectious specimen should be clearly labeled as it is left in fixative for longer time before cut up. Culture swabs should be taken before fixation.

Gross sampling - the type of specimen determines the method of grossing, therefore, contrary to practice by surgeons, they are best left uncut or unopened, provided they arrive at the pathology department the same day. Gross specimen, if considered to be of special interest should be photographed before being cut up.

Tissue processing - the aim of tissue processing is to embed the fixed tissue in a supporting medium that permits the subsequent cutting of histological sections without any distortion. Paraffin wax is the most satisfactory and widely used embedding medium. The processing steps are:

Dehydration - to remove the fixative and tissue fluids by treating with alcohol and acetone.

Clearing - of tissue by chemicals which are miscible with dehydrating agents and

Embedding medium, e.g. xylene or toluene. Embedding in paraffin wax

These are usually currently done by automatic tissue processor.

Cutting and staining - sections are cut on a microtome and mounted on glass slides before staining. Haematoxylin and eosin is routinely used as it provides excellent cellular and architectural details and enables the vast majority of histological diagnosis. In certain situations special stains are needed to identify specific components.

Surgical reports - although routine reports are made available within 3 working days, sometimes this may not be possible due to variety of reasons. Some tissues take longer time to fix, special treatment e.g. bone, deeper level cuts or additional sampling to study in detail. Special stains may be required before a firm pathological diagnosis is made. Finally, difficulties may be encountered with interpretation, which may require consultation and second opinion. For reporting tumors the AJCC (American Joint Committee on Cancer) guidelines are used.

Frozen sections

This technique involves freezing of fresh tissue and then sectioning it in a special cabinet, the cryostat. Tissue is frozen using solid CO_2 or liquid nitrogen .the ice acts as the embedding medium. The cut frozen sections are stained immediately with H&E stain for immediate reporting to surgeon. However this is an exacting technique and the interpretation is more difficult than regular paraffin sections..

Purpose of frozen section study

1. To establish the nature of suspect lesion [benign/ malignant]

2. To ensure disease free margins in resection of malignancies or benign disorders, e.g. Hirschsprung's disease.

3. To confirm whether the biopsy obtained in a difficult case contains sufficient material for a diagnosis to be established.

Guidelines for dispatch of frozen tissue material

Frozen specimens should be sent unfixed, i.e., not in formalin.

Should not be allowed to dry

To be sent wrapped in wet gauze piece

Although a definite diagnosis is possible in most cases, there are instances where it may have to be deferred until paraffin sections are examined. In such situations the surgeon may have to postpone definite surgical treatment or decide based on other criteria until the routine paraffin section report is available.

Frozen sections in patients undergoing elective surgeries, should always be booked with the pathology department prior to the operation.

Cytopathology

In terms of techniques used, cytology may be classified as

1. **Fine needle aspiration cytology** - FNAC is a simple and the most commonly used procedure. The patient should be adequately counseled about the procedure and consent obtained. FNAC is performed by using 20-23 gauge needle attached to a 10 ml syringe. The patient is positioned to allow the most optimal digital palpation of the mass. Larger needles may be used, but they carry a higher risk of complications, including tumor seedling. The skin overlying the mass is prepared; the mass is grasped with the left hand and held in a fixed and stable position. The mass is entered, and multiple passes are made without exiting the skin surface. Adequate negative pressure is maintained by traction on the syringe plunger. If a cyst is encountered, it should be completely evacuated, and fluid and capsule should be sent for cytology. A small drop of aspirated fluid is placed on a glass slide. A smear is made with the help of another slide. One of the smears is immediately placed in 95% ethyl alcohol for H&E /pap staining while other samples should be air dried for staining with May Grunwald, Giemsa or Lieshmann's stain.

Advantages of FNAC

Safe, cost effective and rapid reporting

Done as an out patient procedure

Acceptable rate of sensitivity and specificity

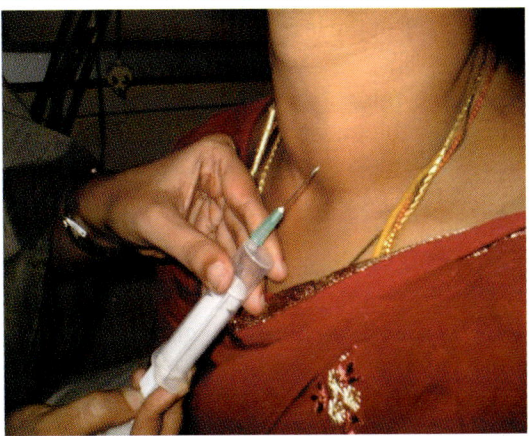

Fig. 6.4. FNAC of a thyroid lump
(courtesy: Prof Sandhya Sundaram, Chennai)

Readily repeatable

Disadvantages

Unsatisfactory aspirates

Diagnostic information limited

Interpretation bias

For diffuse lesions not reliable

Caution to be exercised in

FNAC of testicular masses

Pulsatile lesions

Malignant melanoma (primary site FNAC to be avoided)

Coagulation disorders

Other offshoots of cytology

Brush cytology - which is employed in endoscopic work. Brushings are obtained from

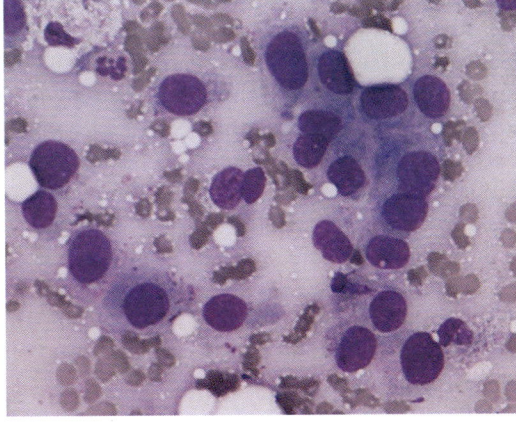

Fig. 6.5. Cytology of malignant cells in breast carcinoma
(MCG stain x400)

the surface of the lesions and transferred on to glass slides.

Imprint cytology - surgeons infrequently use imprint cytology, which entails the application of a sterile glass slide on the cut surface of the tissue. It is particularly useful in lymph node pathology.

Scrape cytology - where edge of one glass slide is used to scrape the surface of the tissue and then smeared on another glass slide. This consistently produces a better yield.

Squash cytology – in which a small bit of tissue sample is crushed between two slides. This is highly sensitive in detection of CNS tumors.

Irrespective of the technique used, a cytological diagnosis is made on the cellular characteristics and the degree of cohesion of cells. Though a highly useful first line investigation, the inherent disadvantages include unsatisfactory aspirates with limited diagnostic information.

Ancillary studies

Conventional H&E preparations give baseline information on the pathologic process, but with the advent of a variety of special techniques, additional information is possible.

Familiarity with the types of special studies is important, as it may throw further light on the prognosis of the disease.

These include

1. Special stains: these are stains other than H&E used to aid diagnosis in certain situations for e.g. periodic acid Schiff stain to diagnose fungal elements. They are not as specific for any particular tissue. Nonetheless, for many years, this panel of stains aids pathologists in diagnoses. A common stain is the mucicarmine stain which highlights mucin a bright pink on a background of yellow. The presence of mucin within a malignant tumor may indicate glandular differentiation suggesting that it is an adenocarcinoma.

2. Immunohistochemistry (IHC) refers to the process of detecting antigens (e.g. proteins) in cells of a tissue section by exploiting the principle of antibodies binding specifically to antigens in biological tissues. These stains became part of the pathologists' armamentarium during the 1980's, which has revolutionized the practice of diagnostic pathology as well as opened new insights into basic research. These stains are monoclonal antibodies and depending upon the tissue stained, it may clinch the diagnosis or narrow down the differential diagnosis.

Applications

To diagnose/confirm tumor of known or unknown histogenesis, e.g. C-Kit, PKC-theta, and CD34 for a GIST

As prognostic marker in cancers, e.g. Ki- 67 in brain tumors

To predict response to therapy, e.g. ER/PR in breast cancer

To identify infections, e.g. CMV/EBV viral infections.

3. Immunofluorescence & electron microscopy are particularly useful in renal, skin and soft tissue lesions.

4. Molecular pathology is an emerging discipline within pathology which is focused in the study and diagnosis of disease through the examination of molecules within organs, tissues or bodily fluids. It is a scientific discipline that encompasses the development of

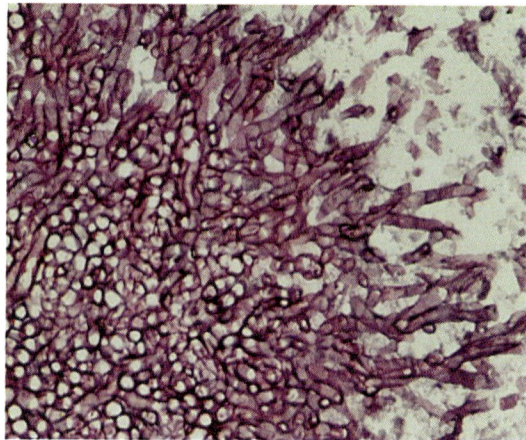

Fig. 6.6. Periodic Acid schiff stain showing fungal hyphae
(courtesy: Prof Sandhya Sundaram, Chennai)

molecular and genetic approaches to the diagnosis and classification of tumors using DNA or RNA. The common techniques include fluorescence in-situ hybridization (FISH), polymerase chain reaction (PCR), flow cytometry and DNA micro array etc.

A surgical pathology report once issued becomes a part of the patient's medical record used primarily for treatment and for follow up.

Therefore, through all this, the interaction between the surgeon and the pathologist is of prime importance, as it is for a common good- the patient well-being.

Specificity and sensitivity of FNAC

Specificity: low false positives
Sensitivity: low false negatives

They vary greatly due to diversity of tumor types and complexity of cytological patterns of individual lesions. It also depends on the tumor site and the experience of the cytopathologist interpreting the lesion.

In deeper organs, like lung, liver pancreas, kidneys, bone and soft tissues etc., the sensitivity may vary between 67-99% and specificity between 96-100%. Follicular neoplasm of the thyroid constitutes a gray zone and a diagnosis exclusively on cytology may not be feasible. Studies in literature have reported

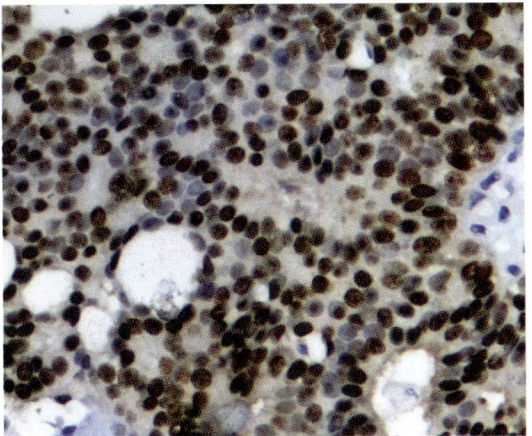

Fig. 6.7. Immunohistochemisry for estrogen receptor with nuclear positive breast cancer
(courtesy: Prof Sandhya Sundaram, Chennai)

Jewels of Gyan - 06.1

Sensitivity = low false negative
Specificity = low false positive

an increase in accuracy when a cytopathologist performs the FNAC and uses immediate assessment to guide specimen adequacy.

Specificity and sensitivity of core biopsy

Sensitivity of needle core biopsies in breast tissue is reported around 87% for free hand automated gun core biopsy while it is about 98% for image assisted biopsy techniques.

In a study on core biopsies for thyroid nodules, the sensitivity was found to be 61% and specificity of 100% for malignant lesions.

Reasons for false negatives in a needle biopsy

(1) technical or sampling errors, Technical difficulties (e.g. poor lesion or needle visualization, deeply located lesions, dense fibrotic tissue) cause inaccurate sampling but can be reduced by using modified standard practices.

(2) it is often due to a nonrepresentative sample performed without image guidance

(3) core-needle breast biopsies may miss areas of invasive cancer in specimens in which lesion is predominantly noninvasive

(4) failure to recognize or act on radiologic-histologic discordance, which is of critical importance in US-guided core needle biopsy.

(5) Lack of imaging follow-up after a benign biopsy result; even patients with concordant benign findings after US-guided core needle biopsy are directed to undergo follow-up imaging because there may be difficulty in the recognition of false negative findings.

(6) Small size of the specimen, crush artifact and destruction of the lesional area by hemorrhage or infarction.

Optimization of technique, radiologic-histologic correlation, and post biopsy follow-up are therefore mandatory.

Special fixatives for muscle, testis and kidney biopsies

Muscle: they are to be sent fresh. A part of it is used for enzyme histochemistry and other half is fixed in neutral buffered formalin.

Testis: Bouin's fluid is ideal however if not available neutral buffered formalin may be used for optimum results.

Kidney: the tissue to be divided into 3 parts:

1. Neutral buffered formalin or modified Bouin's fluid for routine studies

2. 2.5% gluteraldehyde for ultrastructural analysis by electron microscopy (EM).

3. Fresh tissue is required for immuno-fluorescence, specimen is wrapped in aluminum foil, placed in a cryotube and delivered to the laboratory on ice.

Multiple small specimens, such as gastro-intestinal biopsies, should be mounted on a piece of filter paper and labeled.

Lymph nodes may be sent fresh to facilitate other ancillary testing like flow cytometry etc. FNAC smears are to be fixed with methyl or ethyl alcohol spray.

Organ/tissue	Sensitivity	Specificity
Breast	73-95%	87-100%
Thyroid	88-99%	80-100%
Salivary gland	66-100%	96-99%
Lymph nodes	87-100%	88-99%

Table - 6.1. Diagnostic accuracy of FNAC of superficial organs

Jewels of Gyan - 06.2

Immunohistochemistry of some cancers

Lymphoma Basic Panel
Hodgkin's disease (HD)
Classical Hodgkin's disease	CD 15+	CD 30+	EBV Probe +
Nodular lymphocyte predominant HD	CD 45+	CD 20+	EMA $\pm$

Non-Hodgkin Lymphoma (NHL)
B-Cell	CD 45+	CD 20+	CD 3 –ve
T-Cell	CD 45+	CD 3 +	CD 20 –ve

Epithelial malignancies: EMA (Epithelial membrane antigen) positive
Pan cytokeratin positive site specific depending of CK-7 and CK-20 positivity
Melenoma: HMB45 positive
Neural tumors: S100 positive

An abscess is a collection of pus in a pathological space, lined by granulation tissue. An empyema is a collection in a physiological space, e.g. pleural cavity, anterior chamber of the eye and gallbladder.

The types of abscess are:

I.   acute pyogenic abscess
II. chronic nonspecific abscess or an antibiotic-induced granuloma (antibioma)
III. pyemic abscess
IV. abscess from infected cysts
V.   cold abscess

I.   ACUTE PYOGENIC ABSCESS

Pathology: This is the commonest type, of universal distribution. A suppurative lesion is one in which there is cell death and liquefaction, both tissue cells and those of exudates are killed by toxins of pyogenic organisms and liquefied by the action of proteolytic ferments released from the dead leukocytes. The resultant whitish-yellow alkaline fluid, or *pus*, containing living and dead bacteria, leukocytes and macro-phages, fills up the cavity along with cellular debris. *Cellulitis* is a spreading inflammation of tissue planes, which precedes suppuration. *Phlegmonous inflammation* (phlegma: a flame) is a particularly angry form of suppuration, which spreads rapidly along the lines of fascial planes. The wall of the abscess is lined by granulation tissue and phagocytic histiocytes, called *pyogenic membrane*, which eventually gets fibrosed, as the abscess resolves, with or without drainage. Occasionally an abscess may empty itself to the exterior or into an adjacent hollow viscus, e.g. lung abscess, opening into bronchial tree with spontaneous resolution.

Clinical features

The history of each abscess varies depending upon the source of infection (e.g. tooth infection or an infected prosthetic valve of heart), but the symptoms, such as throbbing pain (due to pulsations of vessels in the wall), fever (due to release of pyrogens), are characteristic. This disease truly exhibits all the four cardinal features of acute inflammation, stated by Celsus, *calor* (heat), *rubor* (redness), *dolor* (pain) and *tumor* (swelling) and the fifth, added by Galen, *functio laesa* (loss of function). A painful, warm, tender, cystic swelling, not confined to one anatomical plane, of a few days duration, associated with fever and limitation of neighboring joint movement, due to spasm of adjacent muscles, is almost always present. In cases treated with antibiotics or in the elderly debilitated, such local/systemic signs may be dull, unimpressive and confusing.

The pain is relieved to some extent by elevation, which reduces the amplitude of arterial pulsations, and aggravated by dependency; thus a patient with whitlow is typically seen with hand elevated above his head. The intensity of pain is related to tissue tension and therefore varies from place to place; an abscess

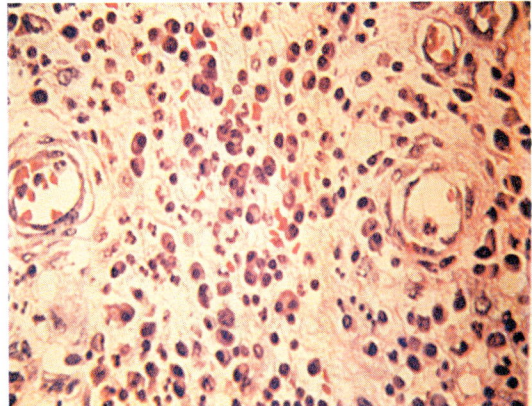

Fig. 7.1. Histology of pyogenic granulation tissue
(courtesy: Histo Lab, Chennai)

Jewels of Gyan - 07.1

A basic (but often forgotten!) adage
Cellulitis : Antibiotic
Abscess : Adequate drainage

in the pulp space or middle ear is more painful than one in the scrotal or abdominal wall. Fever in pyogenic abscess is of high remittent (hectic) type, more pronounced in children and may be absent in elderly. Features of abscesses in special areas, commonly seen in practice, are described later. An abscess can be differentiated from cellulitis by the circumscribed nature and fluctuation, though often both coexist; diagnostic needling is an expedient office procedure, to clinch the issue, in such cases.

Differential diagnosis

Degenerated sarcoma, leaking aneurysm, cold abscess, infected cyst, hematoma, hidradenitis suppurativa etc.

Investigations

a) Polymorphonuclear leukocytosis, with a shift of *Arneth index* to left (more immature cells seen) often provides a vital clue to the underlying acute suppurative process.

b) Toxic stippling of leukocytes may also be seen in severe cases.

c) *Imaging* by skiagraphy/USG/CT/MRI are resorted to delineate a deep-seated abscess and to chalk out the shortest route for its drainage.

d) *Needling* is an expedient and foolproof method of diagnosing an abscess; besides providing material for bacteriology, it has the virtue of being a clinchng office procedure. For deep-seated abscess, USG/CT-guided or laparoscopic aspiration may be necessary.

In a breast abscess, often it may be curative.

Treament

Adequate drainage, breaking into all the loculations, should be done under cover of appropriate antibiotics. *Hilton's method* of drainage consists of making a skin incision over the swelling and pushing a blunt instrument, such as a sinus forceps, deep into the cavity and opening it parallel to the axis of deeper neurovascular structures (especially useful in the neck). Straight incisions have a tendency to close by the tissue elasticity; hence either a cruciate or circular (excising a disc) incision is preferred; the latter is also known as *deroofing* the cavity. While draining an abscess in the depth, the shortest route is the best and it is advisable to introduce a drain (penrose, finger stall of a glove, corrugated rubber or plastic etc.), to come out at a dependent point, if necessary by making a counter stab incision for the purpose.

In areas such as parotid, breast, ischiorectal, or any deep seated location, fluctuation as an indication of ripening, may not be readily appreciated and there is no need to wait for it before proceeding with drainage.

Effective antibiotics should be continued till total resolution of adjacent cellulitis takes place. However, it should be realized that liberal drainage of the cavity and subsequent wound care, is more important than antibiotic administration. Daily wound lavages with normal saline or diluted hydrogen peroxide, reduce the bacterial count and clear any debris gradually, acting complementary to other forms of therapy.

Complications

1. Injury to overlying/underlying vessels and nerves, during drainage

2. Secondary hemorrhage, as severe hemoptysis developing in a lung abscess (pseudoaneurysms of Rasmussen, found in the wall)

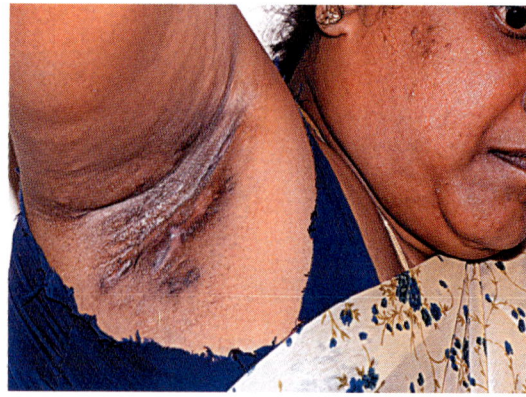

Fig. 7.2. Hidradenitis suppurativa of the axilla (courtesy: Lifeline Hospitals, Chennai)

3. Bacteremia, toxemia, septicemia and pyemia with metastatic abscesses

4. Sinus formation: it is interesting to know that a surgically drained abscess heals well, whereas if the abscess is allowed to spontaneously open to the exterior, by necrosing the overlying skin, it may form a persistent sinus, taking much longer to heal or may never heal. Such a complication is seen most in perianal suppuration.

5. Fistula: if the abscess is the result of a diseased hollow viscus, simple drainage may form a fistula

6. Chronicity: goes into chronic state, under the influence of antibiotics and NSAIDs.

7. Sympathetic effusion of the adjacent joint

8. Ankylosis: when it heals by fibrosis, restriction of movements of a muscle, tendon or joint may take place.

9. Thromboembolism: if the abscess is located near a major vein, thromboembolism may occur. Infection may also spread along venous channels and lead to thrombosis of veins at a distance, as seen from the perinasal/perioral facial sepsis tracking down into pterygoid plexus of veins and from there spreading intracranially to cavernous sinus, causing thrombosis. In the preantibiotic era, this zone in the face was known as *dangerous area*.

10. Intestinal adhesions/obstruction: may occur in undrained intraperitoneal absces-ses

11. Spread to neighboring structures: as in a mastoid/middle ear infection producing an intracranial abscess or a liver abscess opening into pleural/pericardial space.

12. Hidden abscesses: such as pelvic or subphrenic spaces, may cause complex clinical syndromes of declining health, until a high index of suspicion by an alert clinician leads to its discovery. The popular adage, 'pus somewhere, but pus nowhere, pus under the diaphragm', has to be remembered here. Absence of specific complaints, except general feeling of ill health, malaise, anorexia etc. earned the name, 'not doing well' syndrome, to these occult abscesses.

Abscesses in special areas

a)   palmar abscess: as the skin and subcutaneous tissues of the dorsum are loose, the swelling is seen more dorsally, even if the abscess is on the palmar aspect. Drainage may be done by incisions along the creases or via the interdigital spaces, meticulously avoiding injury to digital nerves and vessels.

b)   pulp abscess: as the blood vessels to distal phalanx travel through limited spaces, separated by septae, accumulation of pus under tension may endanger vascularity, leading to necrosis of the distal digit.

c)   parotid abscess: is located under a tough parotidomasseteric fascia; hence fluctuation develops very late and should not be waited for, to institute drainage.

d)   abscess of solid viscera, such as brain, lung, liver, spleen and kidney.

e)   pelvic abscess : develops as a complication of pyogenic peritonitis of any etiology, pus collecting in the rectovaginal (Douglas) or rectovesical pouch, which are the most

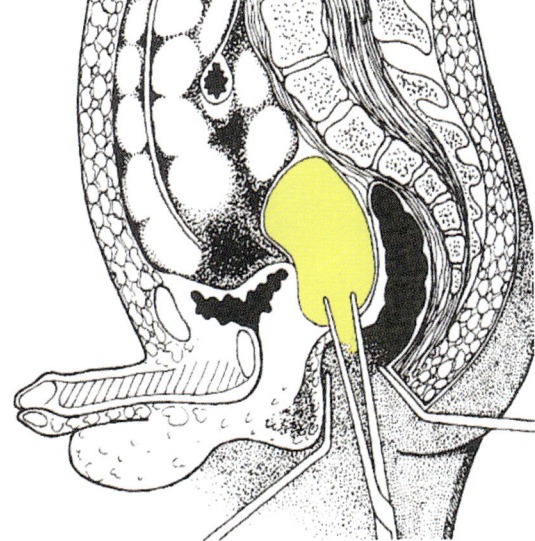

Fig. 7.3. Transrectal drainage of pelvic abscess in male

dependent peritoneal spaces in the erect posture. Besides general features, symptoms of irritation of rectum (mucous diarrhea or tenesmus) and bladder (frequency and strangury) predominate. After confirmation by digital (PV/PR) examination, USG/CT and needling, it may be drained through the posterior fornix of vagina (in women) or anterior wall of rectum (in men). More extensive collections, with loops of bowel expected to be involved, should be drained by anterior (laparotomy) approach.

f) subphrenic abscess: is a more complex subject with at least six anatomical spaces, where pus may collect. They are:

i) *right anterior intraperitoneal* bounded by right lobe of liver (below and behind), diaphragm (above), coronary and right triangular ligaments (behind), rib cage and diaphragm (lateral) and falciform ligament (medial).

ii) *right posterior intraperitoneal* (hepatorenal pouch of Morison) bounded by right lobe of liver (anterior), right kidney and rib cage (posterior), right triangular ligament (above), rib cage and diaphragm (lateral) and hepatic flexure of colon (below). This is the most dependent of all peritoneal spaces, in the supine position.

Iii) *right extraperitoneal* in relation to the upper pole of right kidney (laterally placed), same as perinephric abscess and a space related to bare area of liver (in paramedian location).

iv) *left anterior intraperitoneal* bounded by left lobe of liver, gastrohepatic omentum and stomach (posterior), rib cage and diaphragm (anterior), left triangular ligament (above), falciform ligament (on the right) and gastrosplenic ligament and diaphragm (lateral).

v) *left posterior intraperitoneal* (lesser sac or omental bursa) bounded by left lobe of liver, gastrohepatic omentum and stomach (anterior), left triangular ligament (above), rib cage and spleen (lateral), folds of gastrocolic omentum below and left kidney and pancreas (posterior). It communicates with right posterior space, through epiploic foramen (of Winslow). Collection of fluid in this space occurs in pancreatic pseudocyst.

vi) *left extraperitoneal* in relation to the left kidney, as in left perinephric abscess.

g) perinephric abscess may develop from the spread of infection from the kidney, renal pelvis, appendix, pancreas and rarely hematogenous. It may also come from ruptured liver abscess, due to the intimate relationship of the right kidney to the bare area of liver, so also as a

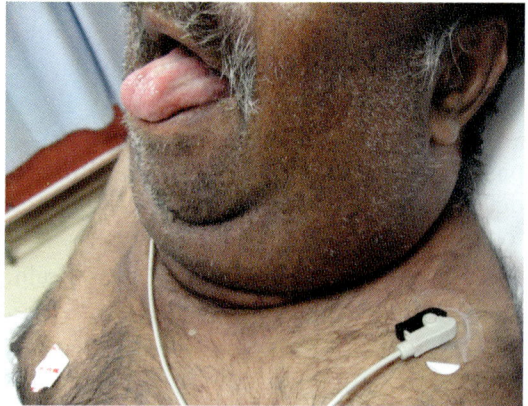

Fig. 7.4. Ludwig's angina
(courtesy: Laxmi Hospital, Kakinada)

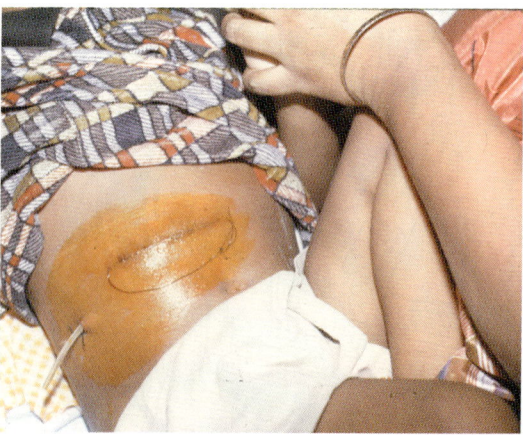

Fig. 7.5. Pig-tail catheter draining right subphrenic abscess
(courtesy: Lifeline Hospitals, Chennai)

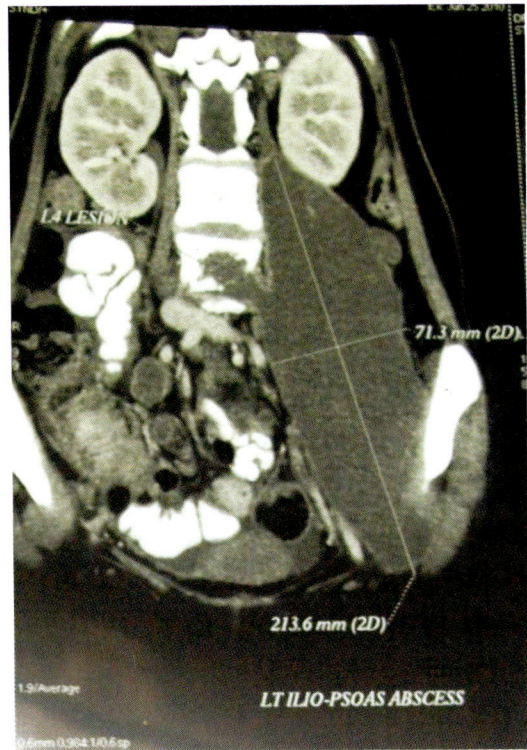

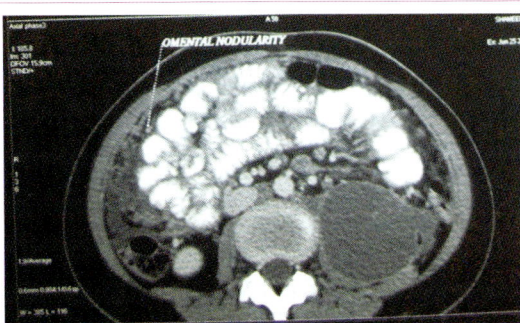

Fig. 7.6 & 7. large tuberculous psoas absess (cold)
(courtesy: Halsted Surgical Clinic, Chennai)

sequel of colonic diverticulitis or malignancy. Though rare, tuberculous cold abscess, from caseated renal cortical granuloma, diseased retroperitoneal lymph nodes or vertebra, is another pos ility.

In classical pyogenic abscess, high fever, severe pain, tenderness, local warmth and fullness over the loin (renal angle) are present. Scoliosis may be seen due to spasm of paraspinal muscles on the affected side. Pus cells in the urine may be conspicuously absent, unless the primary focus is in renal pelvis (pyelonephritis). The psoas shadow may be obscured and there may be restricted mobility of the diaphragm on that side. After confirming the diagnosis by USG/CT scan, liberal drainage of the pockets of pus through a loin incision has to be carried out, under cover of higher antibiotics (or anti-tuberculous therapy). Preliminary diagnostic needling may be done under USG guide, but its curative role is limited. The source of infection has to be treated on its merits, to prevent recurrence.

h) Appendicular abscess: An abscess may form in relation to an inflamed appendix, if the acute infection is not properly treated nor timely surgery performed. It may be a natural course of suppuration in cases of an appendicular mass and may occur in various locations, depending upon the position of appendix, such as retrocecal, retroileal, preileal, paracolic or pelvic. Clinically it is identified when high fever and leukocytosis are associated with a tender mass in the right iliac fossa, during 'resolution' of acute appendicitis, under conservative treatment.

After confirming the presence of an abscess by USG/CT, appropriate surgical drainage and antimicrobial therapy based on bacteriological study, generally cures the condition. Any attempt to remove the appendix at the time of drainage of an abscess may be associated with risk of bowel injury and fistula formation and is unwarranted. The need for 'interval' appendectomy, however has to be evaluated few weeks after the resolution of infection.

I) psoas abscess: Development of an abscess within the psoas sheath may be acute (nonspecific) or chronic (usually tuberculous). The pathogenesis of acute abscess is from secondary infection of a hematoma, formed following some injury. In tuberculous retroperitoneal lymphadenitis or spondylitis, caseous material tracks down under the psoas sheath, into the groin, presenting as a bilocular mass, often exhibiting cross fluctuation. Local pain, presence of a mass and persistent psoas

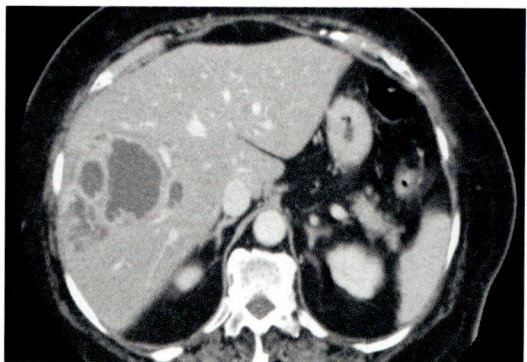

Fig. 7.8. CT scan showing multiple liver abscesses

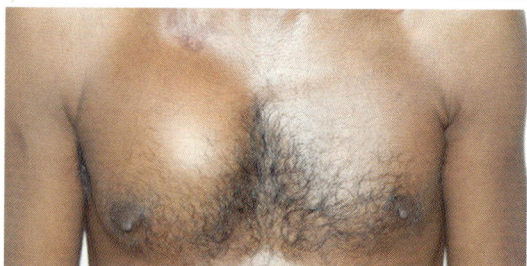

Fig. 7.9. Retromammary abscess in a HIV patient
(courtesy: Lifeline Hospitals, Chennai)

spasm, with hip joint flexed and medially rotated, are the typical features. The diagnosis may be confirmed by USG/CT scan and treated by drainage through a muscle-splitting extraperitoneal approach, under cover of higher antibiotics or anti-tuberculous therapy, as the case may be, followed by physiotherapy to restore hip movements.

There is increased incidence of tuberculous psoas abscesses in the era of HIV. Retroperitoneoscopic drainage is a recent innovation in the management of this disease. (see chapter 18).

J) *Bezold's abscess:* is a complication of middle ear suppuration, pus tracking along the sternocleidomastoid (SCM) muscle and surfacing in the neck. Pus may also collect in relation to posterior belly of digastric (*Citelli's abscess*) or root of zygoma (*Luc's abscess*).

II. CHRONIC NONSPECIFIC ABSCESS (SYN: ANTIBIOMA)

This results from inadvertent administration of antibiotics for an abscess, without drainage, allowing it to become chronic, and is commonly encountered in the breast. The wall gets fibrosed, the contents may be sterile and inspissated and external signs of inflammation may be lacking. The cutaneous lymphedema with peud'orange appearance, hard consistency, lack of intrinsic mobility and regional lymphadenopathy make it clinically indistinguishable from malignancy. History of acute onset of pain/ swelling, treated by antibiotics is

suggestive of a chronic abscess, confirmed by USG and needling.

Treatment

Smaller abscesses may be excised (*abscessectomy*), whereas larger ones are *deroofed* (subtotal excision) and curetted, sending the material for histopathology. Simple drainage often results in a nonhealing sinus, in view of the organized abscess wall.

III. PYEMIC ABSCESS is a complication commonly seen in children convalescing from serious infections, such as typhoid fever, measles or chicken pox or those in immune-compromised states. Pyemic emboli get lodged in various parts of the body, developing into abscesses, without much local/ systemic signs of inflammation. After identifying any focus of sepsis, as a source of emboli, each abscess is treated on its merits, by drainage under cover of appropriate antibiotics, with good results.

IV. INFECTED CYSTS, such as sebaceous, lymph or dermoid cysts, may mimic abscesses, with minimal external features, depending upon the thickness of the sac. Local pain, tenderness, warmth and loss of free mobility are usually seen, which may be confirmed by needling. In a sebaceous cyst, with suppuration, the doughy consistency becomes soft and cystic and discharge of a bead of pus may be seen at the punctum. The pus with infected sebaceous material should be drained initially by an incision, to allow the inflammation to resolve. The cyst may not reform, if the lining membrane is totally destroyed due to infection; otherwise elective excision of the cyst may be planned, after a few weeks.

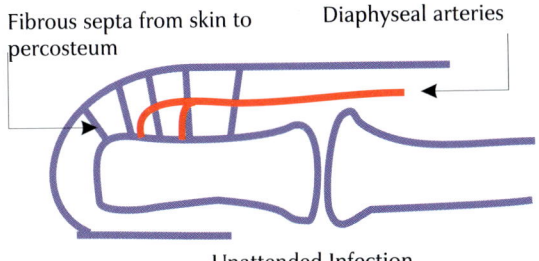

Fibrous septa from skin to percosteum

Diaphyseal arteries

Unattended Infection
↓
arterial thrombosis
↓
Ischemic Necrosis & Osteomyelitis

Fig. 7.10. Pathogenesis of osteomyelitis in digital infection
(courtesy - Halsted Surgical Clinic, Chennai)

V.   COLD ABSCESS: is described under tuber-culous lymphadenitis. (see chapter 42)

WOUND DRAINAGE

Indications

1. Presence of pus in the depth of the wound
2. Uncontrolled diffuse wound bleeding (oozing)
3. Anticipated sepsis in a contaminated wound
4. Anticipated intestinal, biliary or urinary leak
5. Anticipated lymph collection (e.g. lymph nodal dissection.
6. To maintain negative pressure in a closed space (e.g. to promote wound healing and in pleural cavity)
7. to create a controlled fistula (e.g. duodenum or CBD)

Types

1. Simple drain
    a. Corrugated rubber or plastic
    b. Penrose
    c. 'Cigarette' (with a gauze 'wick')
2. Tube
3. Suction or vacuum
4. Sump
5. Water-seal (to maintain negative pressure)

Drawbacks of employing a drain

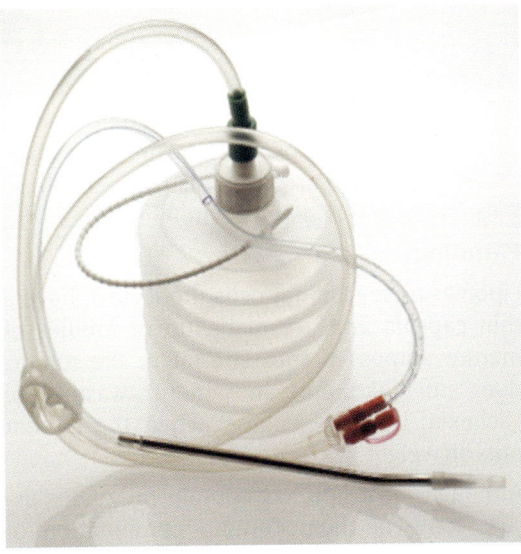

Fig. 7.11. Ambulant wound suction unit (Redivac)
(courtesy - Halsted Surgical Clinic, Chennai)

1. stiff drains may cause local pain and discomfort
2. being a foreign body, interferes with local defence mechanisms
3. forms a portal for entry of microorganisms
4. erosion into adjacent vessel or viscus
5. peritoneal adhesions, especially those in the lower abdomen
6. some drains may restrict ambulation
7. the idea of draining tends to make the surgeon less meticulous about hemostasis
8. the drain may be inadvertently retained in the wound
9. may result in a persistent sinus (e.g. tuberculous cold abscess)
10. a hernia may develop through the track created.

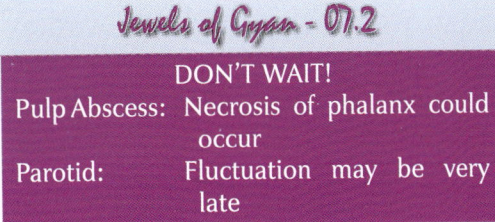

Jewels of Gyan - 07.2

DON'T WAIT!

Pulp Abscess: Necrosis of phalanx could occur

Parotid: Fluctuation may be very late

Definition: Benign tumor composed of mature adipose tissue. Due to its ubiquitous occurrence, it is often known as the *universal or ubiquitous tumor*.

Pathology

Lipomas arise from fat cells (lipocytes), have a thin capsule and are made up of lobules of mature adipose tissue. The fat in the tumor, does not take part in general wasting of cachexia, but may enlarge when the patient puts on weight.

Although most lipomas contain only fatty tissue, some of them contain combination of other tissues, e.g. fibrolipoma, angiolipoma, (renal pelvis), gangliolipoma (Dercum's disease, adiposis dolorosa) which are often painful and multiple, myelolipoma (adrenal), chondrolipoma etc. Lipoma differs biochemically from normal fat by the high levels of lipoproteins, lipase and contains increased precursor cells.

Locations of lipoma

a) *Subcutaneous lipoma*: Commonest variety, higher incidence in the back and neck, usually flat, but can be globular or rarely pedunculated. The following are its characteristics

i) Skin over the swelling will be normal but may be stretched if the tumor is large.

ii) Swelling not warm or tender.

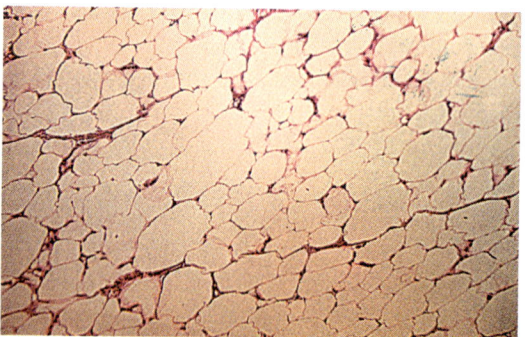

Fig. 8.1. Histology of lipoma
(courtesy: Histo Lab, Chennai)

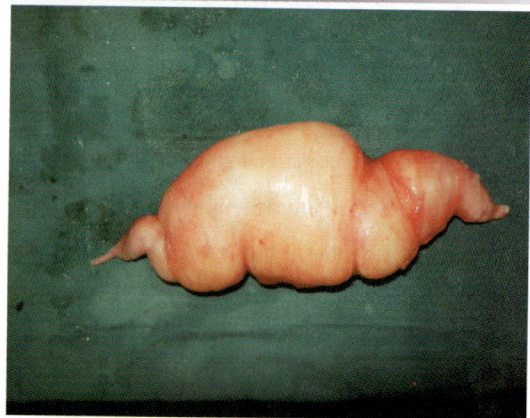

Fig. 8.2. Neurolipoma excised from forearm
(courtesy: Halsted Surgical Clinic, Chennai)

iii) Soft in consistency, no fluctuation but occasionally a sense of fluctuation (pseudofluctuation), may be appreciated.

iv) Transillumination is negative (rarely positive, because of translucent fat)

v) Surface is smooth, and lobulated, edge is soft and slips away from the examining finger (sign of slipping): this sign differentiates a lipoma from the yielding edge of a sebaceous cyst.

vi) The skin can be freely moved over it, but if the lipoma is moved or the skin held taut, dimples appear on the skin, at the site of attachment of the fibrous bands from the capsule of the lipoma.

Vii) The lipoma is always mobile over the deeper structures (if not, suspect the onset of

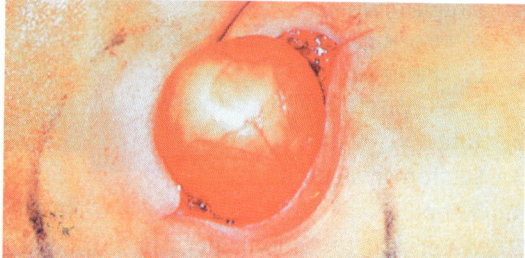

Fig. 8.3. Enucleation of a subcutaneous lipoma
(courtesy: Lifeline Hospitals, Chennai)

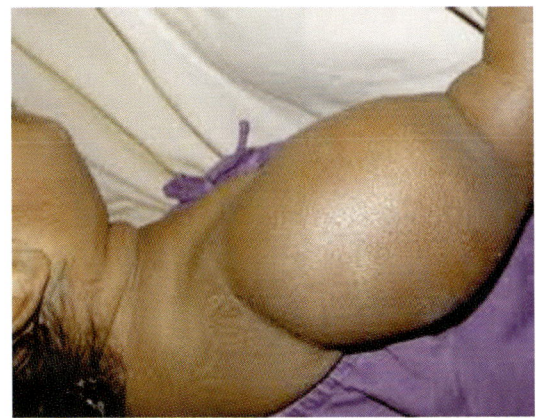

Fig. 8.4. Lipoma arm
(courtesy: Halsted Surgical Clinic, Chennai)

sarcomatous change or rarely infection).

b) *Subfascial lipoma*: in the scalp, palm or sole, lipomas may appear under the aponeurotic layer, where it is impossible to differentiate from a fibromatous tumor arising from these fasciae or dermoid cyst (in the scalp), hence this is best treated by excision. One peculiarity of any benign tumor in this plane is its movements become restricted on putting the underlying muscle to contraction, giving an impression that it is either arising from or fixed to the muscle, leading to an erroneous impression that the swelling in question might be malignant. In fact, it is because of limitation of 'moving space' within the fascia, when the muscle firms up.

c) *Intermuscular lipoma*: Lipoma occuring between the muscles has the following features:

i.   difficult to differentiate from a soft tissue sar

ii. has higher risk of malignant transformation into a liposarcoma.

iii. the presence of the lipoma mechanically interferes with muscle movements.

iv. As in a subfascial location, there may be restriction of intrinsic movements when the surrounding muscle groups are made to contract.

Early excision is indicated, for all the above reasons.

d) *Submucous lipoma*: may occur in the intestines, or in the bronchi. In the former situation, it acts as the apex of an intussusception, and in the latter, can cause partial bronchial obstruction. It may *assume* a polypoid shape, either sessile or pedunculated.

e) *Subserous lipoma*: is found in relation to the pleura or peritoneum, and may reach large sizes. A useful diagnostic aid is a CT scan which shows the capsulated, lobulated tumor, with pathognomonic low Hounsfield density.

f) *Subsynovial and intra-articular lipomas:* They occur in relation to joints. Bursae, synovial cysts (like Baker's cyst) or tumors/degeneration of cartilage are the differential diagnoses, in this situation.

Lipoma arborescens is regarded as hyperplasia, rather than a neoplasm, seen in association with osteoarthrosis of knee (rarely elbow), in which fat-filled pedunculated villi hang into the fluid-filled joint space. They may get detached and form loose bodies in the joint.

g) *Subperiosteal and intraglandular lipomas* are rare, e.g. in the pancreas or breast. Renal pelvis angiolipoma is a rare condition and sometimes found in association with multiple neuroectodermal diseases, such as Bournville's disease (phakomatoses, a hereditary syndrome, associated with disseminated hamartomas of eye, skin and brain).

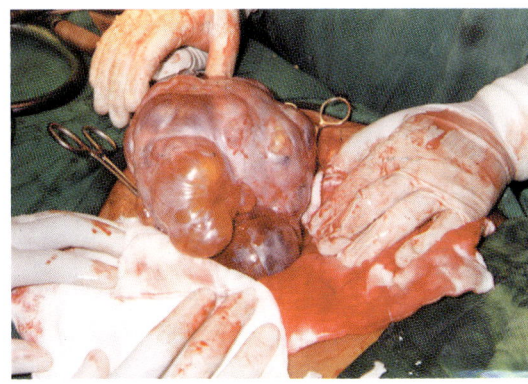

Fig. 8.5. Retroperitoneal lipoma being excised
(courtesy: Lifeline Hospitals, Chennai)

h) *Retroperitoneal lipoma* is rarely detected clinically, till it turns sarcomatous. However with the liberal use of USG/CT more of these are currently being discovered.

i) *Extradural lipoma* is also rare, seen in relation to spina bifida or other neural canal defects.

Lipomatosis is hamartomatous disease, with multiple mixed lipomas, distributed throughout the body, often painless and harmless. *Dercum's disease* is a variant, with multiple painful *ganglioliomas* (adiposis dolorosa). Excision is done only if any one of them is symptomatic or shows unusual growth and sometimes for a biopsy to reassure patient. At times these fatty lesions tend to increase in size, if the patient puts on weight.

Symmetrical lipomatosis (Madelung's disease, lipoma annularis colli) is an even deposition of fat in the neck It is not encapsulated and does not slip at the edge of the lesion. Higher incidence of this is seen in alcoholics, diabetics and in those with chronic liver disease.

Similar deposition of fat, known as diffuse lipoma, is commonly seen in axilla and spermatic cord.

Singawald syndrome: bilateral fibrolipomas over the sacroiliac joints, seen in elderly indi-

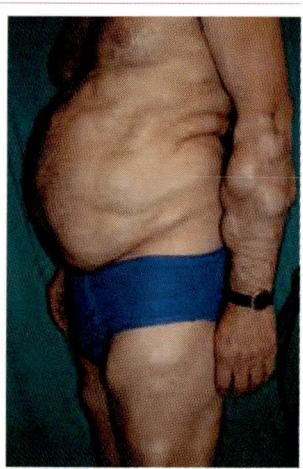

Fig. 8.7. Multiple lipomata
(courtesy: Lifeline Hospitals, Chennai)

viduals, without much clinical significance.

Differential diagnosis

Sebaceous cyst, dermoid cyst, neurofibroma and other soft tissue benign tumors. Lipoma may sometimes contain combination of tissue, e.g. angiolipoma, neurolipoma, fibrolipoma etc.

Complications of lipoma

1. Cosmetic problems

2. Pressure effects on subjacent nerves or vessels, especially axillary lipomas compressing the cords of the brachial plexus, but such an occurance is rare.

3. Trauma, leading to hemorrhage or fat necrosis, producing variability of consistency, often confusing with sarcomatous change.

4. Malignant transformation to liposarcoma is a rare, often disputed complication, more observed in the retroperitoneum, back, buttocks and thighs. This may be probably because benign tumors go undetected in these locations for a long time, allowing them to turn sarcomatous.

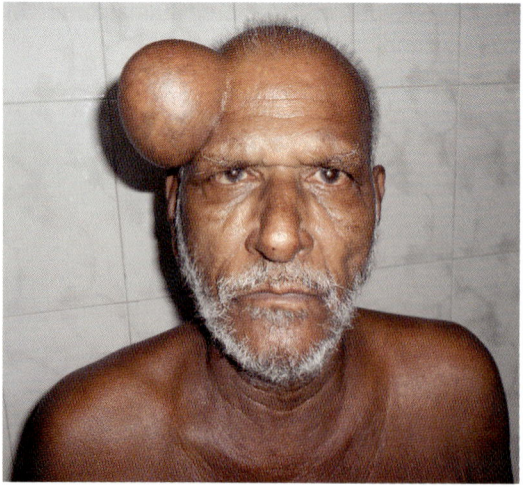

Fig. 8.6. Large lipoma, right temple
(courtesy: Halsted Surgical Clinic, Chennai)

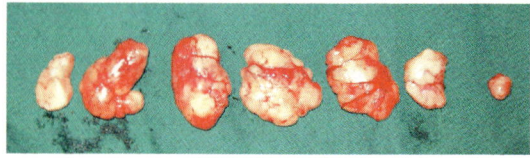

Fig. 8.8. Multiple lipomatosis.
Seven tumors excised from both forearms
(courtesy: Halsted Surgical Clinic, Chennai)

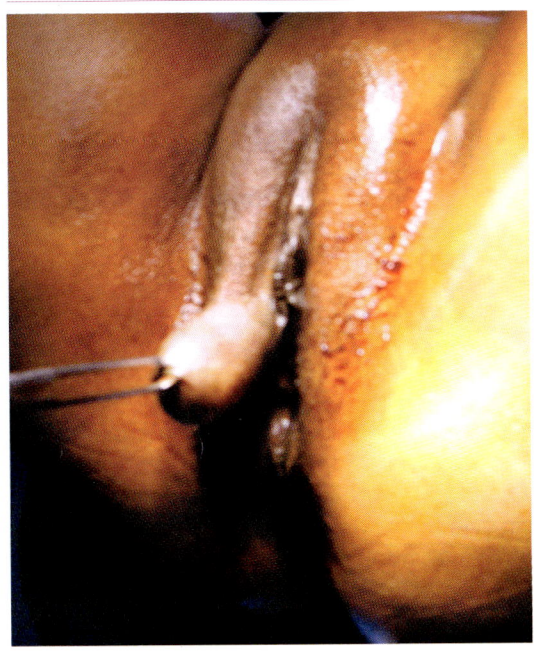

Fig. 8.9. A pedunculated lipoma of right labium majora (courtesy: Halsted Surgical Clinic, Chennai)

Features of malignancy in a lipoma: Recent spurt in growth, local pain, fixity, variable consistency, warmth, engorged veins in the vicinity, skin changes and secondaries to lungs and bones, but lymphatic spread is rare.

5.   Infection and abscess formation

6.   Saponification (soap formation), usually follows trauma.

7.   Myxomatous degeneration

8.   Calcification (dystrophic) in longstanding cases, especially following trauma/ necrosis

Treatment

Excision is ideal, wherever the location may be; an incision is made along the *Langer's lines*, avoiding crossing a joint line, the capsule is opened and the tumor is shelled out, carefully removing 'pseudopodia-like' extentions, known as *intracapsular* extraction (as done for a fibroadenoma, in contrast to the *extracapsular* excision of a sebaceous cyst).

If *sarcomatous* change is suspected, tissue diagnosis by a wide-bore needle or wedge biopsy should be done, before a *wide* (3-dimensional) *excision* can be planned. It is moderately radio/chemosensitive, these modalities are employed as post-excision adjuvant or preoperative neoadjuvant therapy, in an attempt to down-stage the disease. In advanced, nonresectable tumors, they may be employed for palliation.

Hibernoma is a variant of lipoma, rarely seen in man, situated in the interscapular region, axilla and thigh. It is believed to arise from brown fat similar to that seen in the hibernating gland of animals *(embryonic brown lipoblasts)*.

Recent advances: Where cosmesis is essential, such as over the face, an alternative method of treatment is by *liposuction* through a tiny incision. The fat tissue within the capsule is completely sucked out; but this procedure has a higher incidence of recurrence than by standard excision.

Introduction

The skin (cutis) and its derivatives constitute the integumentary system. It is the largest organ of the body, forming the external covering, consisting of two main layers: the epidermis and the dermis(corium).

The epidermal derivatives of skin include hair and hair follicles, sweat glands, sebaceous glands, nails and mammary glands.

Sweat glands are of two types:

I) *eccrine*, whose function is to secrete watery fluid on to the surface, to regulate body temperature; they respond to emotional stress,and are distributed all over, but more concentrated in axillae, palms, soles and forehead.

ii) *apocrine* (apo: from; krino: separate), in which cytoplasm of apical or free ends of the secreting cell forms part of secretions. They are larger, confined to axillae, areola of breast and urogenital area (breast is a modified apocrine gland), similar to scent glands in animals, by which they recognize their mates. In man they are odorless, but due to the action of bacteria, often acquire unpleasant smell.

The sebaceous glands belong to *holocrine* type, in which secreting cells themselves disintegrate into fatty material and extruded along with accumulated secretions. Most of the other exocrine glands in the body belong to the *merocrine* variety, wherein the secreting cells remain intact throughout the secretory process, only the secretions are drained out through the ducts.

Sebaceous glands of various sizes are distributed almost over the entire body, more concentrated over the scalp, face, neck, scrotum and upper back; these areas forming the common sites for the retention cyst. There are no sebaceous glands in the palms, soles and dorsa of feet, hence these cysts cannot occur in these locations. Most of them are associated with hair follicles, except in areas like vermilion of lips (Fordyce's spots), areola of women (Montgomery's tubercles), internal fold of prepuce (Tyson's glands), eye lids (Meibomian's glands) and labia minora.

SEBACEOUS CYST (syn: wen, epidermal cyst, pilar cyst)

It is an acquired retention cyst of sebaceous gland and contains sebaceous material, keratin and its breakdown products, within a squamous epithelial wall. The sebum, a yellowish pultaceous material, is responsible for the offensive odour when the cyst is opened. Occasionally a cheesy substance comes out of the punctum, which may contain a minute worm, Demodex folliculorum (hair follicle mite).

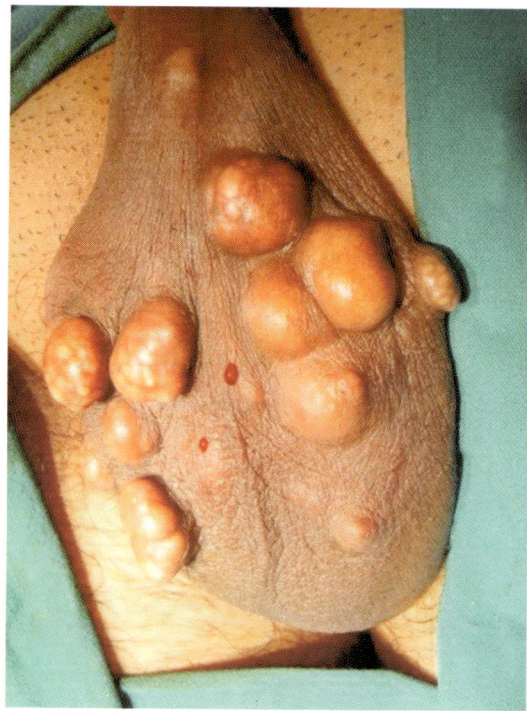

Fig. 9.1. Multiple sebaceous cysts of scrotum (courtesy: Prof T Gunasagaran, Chennai)

Pathology

If the sebaceous duct is blocked, the gland becomes distended with its own secretions and forms a cyst. It is in the *intradermal* (intracuticular) plane, though much of the swelling may be located in the subcutaneous fat. At the summit a black spot, the keratin filled orifice of the duct, known as *punctum*, is seen in most of the cases. Its intradermal location, compressing the adjacent roots of hair follicles, is responsible for absence of hair over the cyst, in contrast to subcutaneous swellings like lipoma or dermoid cyst, over which normal hair distribution is seen. The material, sometimes slowly extruded through the orifice gets hardened, becoming a *sebaceous horn*. Rarely the cyst may discharge its contents completely and regress or disappear spontaneously, a welcome event indeed.

Clinical features: It occurs in all ages, though rare before adolescence and presents as a hemi-

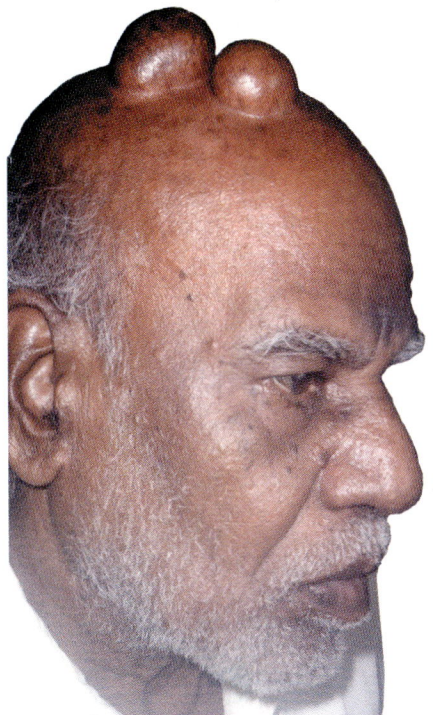

Fig.9.2. Sebaceous cysts, scalp
(courtesy: Halsted Surgical Clinic, Chennai)

spherical, nontender, intradermal, cystic swelling of varying size in the common regions indicated, with the typical punctum over its summit. It should be realized that the punctum is seen in only 50% of cases, but when present, it is pathognomonic. Thinned out skin with loss of hair over the swelling is typical. Often multiple, they are situated in intradermal plane, moving freely over the underlying fat and muscles, with the classical *sign of moulding*, attributable to the doughy consistency of the contents. It is not transilluminant and there is no regional lymphadenopathy.

Differential diagnosis

Lipoma, dermoid cyst (see table - 9.1), neurofibroma, preauricular cyst and chronic abscess.

Investigations

There are no specific investigations to diagnose this condition; if infection is suspected, aspiration bacteriology may be useful. FNAC is indicated, if malignancy within the cyst is suspected by recent spurt of growth, variable consistency and regional lymphadenopathy.

Treatment

Total *extracapsular* excision of the cyst, by an elliptical incision, either by standard dissection or by avulsion of the sac, is curative. Recurrence may be expected, even if a small portion of the sac is left behind. In the scrotum, multiple cysts may be treated by partial or subtotal excision of scrotum.

Reasons for employing elliptical incision

a) The cyst is intradermal, adherent to the skin, more at the summit
b) The punctum has to be excised, along with the cyst
c) The elliptical piece of skin to be removed, which is attached to the cyst, is used to apply traction on the cyst, to facilitate dissection.
d) Excision of redundant skin helps closure without laxity or dead space.

Complications

I. *Infection* is the commonest complication,

which produces minimal local or systemic signs, because of the thick sac covering it. Some warmth, tenderness and regional lymphadeno-pathy may be seen. By preliminary diagnostic needling, the infected (foul smelling) material is drained by an incision, under cover of antibiot-ics and allowed to heal by daily dressings fol-lowing hydrogen peroxide irrigations. The cyst may not reform if the lining membrane is com-pletely destroyed; otherwise elective excision of the cyst may be planned after total resolution of inflammation.

ii. *Cock's peculiar tumor* is the sequel of rup-ture of infected sebaceous cyst, resulting in ulceration and granuloma formation, closely mimicking fungating SCC. After excluding malignancy by a wedge/edge biopsy and con-trolling infection, total excision has to be done. It is not a tumor as the name implies.

iii. *Sebaceous horn*, described above, may be excised along with the underlying cyst.

iv. Sebaceous *adenoma* and *carcinoma* may rarely supervene, the latter is either BCC or SCC. Adenoma is treated by simple excision,

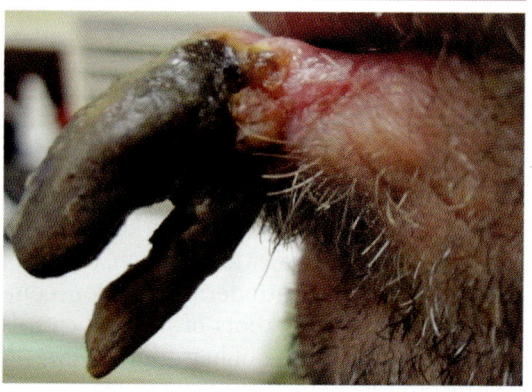
Fig. 9.3. Giant cutaneous horn on the lower lip

whereas carcinoma is treated on the merits of the tissue diagnosis, as described under those diseases.

Other malignancies which can rarely occur in a sebaceous cyst are Bowen's disease, mycosis fungoides and melanoma.

v. *Recurrence* is seen, if the cyst has been inad-vertently opened and part of the sac was left behind, during excision.

Multiple sebaceous cysts of scrotal skin (see chapter 28 on Scrotum).

	Features	Sebaceous cyst	Dermoid cyst
1	Location	Anywhere except palms & soles	Embryological lines of fusion (congenital type)
2	H/O trauma	Absent	Present (in implantation type)
3	Punctum	Usually present	Absent
4	Anatomic plane	Intracutaneous	Subcutaneous or subfascial
5	Hair over the swelling	Lost	Normal
6	Underlying bone	Normal	May be eroded
7	Incidence of infection	High	Minimal

Table-9.1. Differences between sebaceous and dermoid cyst

10 Dermoid Cyst

It is a cyst developed from entrapped ecto-derm. They may be classified as

(1) congenital (sequestration),
(2) acquired or traumatic (implantation),
(3) tubulo-dermoid and
(4) teratomatous types.

1. Congenital (sequestration) type is formed by inclusion of ectodermal cells, during devel-opment, at the embryonic lines of fusion. The common sites are:

a) in the midline, in the root of nose, neck, sublingual, mediastinal, retroperitoneal, presacral, postanal locations
b) external angular, at the outer canthus of the eye
c) postauricular, behind the ear
d) at the other lines of fusion of skull bones

Pathology

The cyst is lined by mature stratified squamous epithelium, with hair follicles, sebaceous and sweat elements. It contains white pultaceous (doughy) material, a mixture of keratin (not sebum of sebaceous cyst) and desquamated epithelial debris. Sometimes, it may get buried deep to the subjacent mesodermal elements, particularly in the head, to get situated in subperiosteal plane or causing a defect in the underlying skull bones with intracranial extention, the total lesion taking a dumb-bell shape. Infection, ulceration and malignancy (SCC or BCC) are rare complications.

Clinical features

Manifesting either at birth or in early child-hood, presents as a slow-growing painless, rounded (or oval), cystic swelling in the loca-tions mentioned. It generally remains small in the subcutaneous plane, but may grow to large size in deeper locations, such as under the tongue, mediastinum, retroperitoneum or infront of the sacrum. The intracranial compo-nent may produce compression of brain and focal fits.

On examination a cystic (or doughy) swelling in the subcutaneous plane, usually tethered to the underlying skull bone, without transil-lumination. A false feeling of a defect of the underlying bone, is often present, due to periosteal reaction around the base, without actual bony erosion. If there is an intracranial component, a detailed neurological evaluation is necessary.

Differential diagnosis

1. Sebaceous cyst: intracutaneous plane, punctum present, sparse hair over the swelling

2. Lipoma: flat, soft, lobular, with slipping edges. There will no bony erosion.

3. Meningocele: seen at birth, in relation to spine and cranium, compressible, with cough (cry) impulse and is brilliantly transilluminant. They may be multiple with cross fluctuation.

Investigations

Skiagram of the skull for bony defect and if pres-

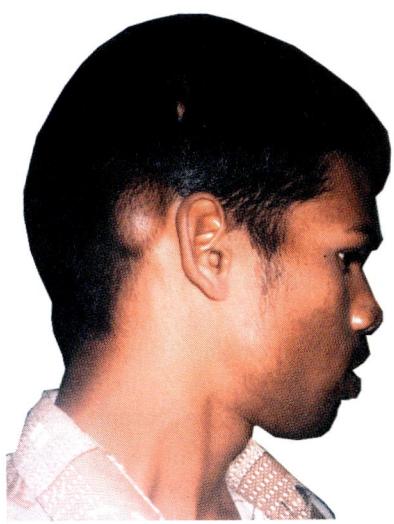

Fig. 10.1. Post-auricular dermoid
(courtesy: Halsted Surgical Clinic, Chennai)

ent, a CT scan to detect any intracranial extension, should be done, when the cyst is over the scalp. CT may also be useful in other locations, to define its anatomic relations.

Treatment

Total excision of the cyst, is the definitive treatment. Neurosurgical help may be required, to deal with the intracranial part, when present.

SUBLINGUAL DERMOID

This is a sequestration dermoid cyst in the floor of mouth, due to entrapped surface ectoderm at the level of the first branchial arch and is typically a midline swelling, either supra or inframylohyoid, but may rarely be paramedian.

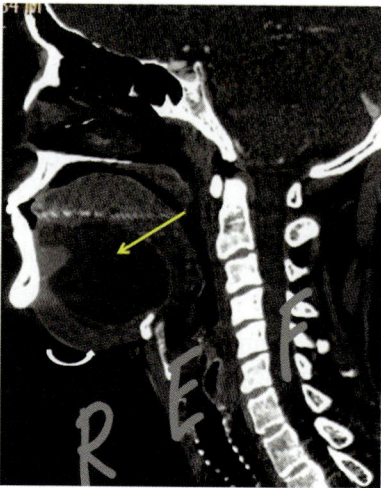

Fig. 10.2. CT showing sublingual dermoid
(courtesy: Halsted Surgical Clinic, Chennai)

Pathology

It contains cheesy, sebaceous material secreted by the ectodermal glands. It is lined by a thin squamous epithelium, containing, hair follicles, sweat and sebaceous glands with their secretions.

Clinical features

It occurs in the 2nd decade of life and presents

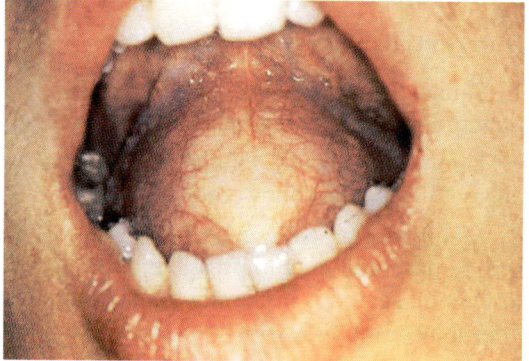

Fig. 10.3. Sublingual dermoid
(courtesy: Halsted Surgical Clinic, Chennai)

as a painless swelling in the floor of the mouth, below the point of chin. Pain is indicative of infection or hemorrhage. A slow-growing, rounded, tensely cystic swelling with a smooth surface, fluctuation and negative transillumination, it may be supramylohyoid, found in the floor of the mouth, covered by mucous membrane or inframylohyoid (cervical) type presenting in the submental region, producing a 'double chin' appearance. It is freely mobile and bidigitally palpable with some mechanical restriction of the movements of tongue, depending upon the size. Lymph nodes are involved only if there is secondary infection or rarely malignant change in the cyst.

Differential diagnosis

When it is inframylohyoid

1. Thyroglossal cyst: it moves up with deglutition and tongue protrusion

2. Submental lymphadenopathy: primary septic focus present, other nodes may be involved and usually not bidigitally palpable

When it is supramylohyoid

1. Ranula: thin-walled, brilliantly transilluminant, in a more superficial plane

2. Hamartoma and benign tumors of tongue: they are attached to tongue

Rarely, when it presents laterally submandibular/sublingual sialadenopathy: bidigitally palpable, firm or cause of ductal obstruction, such as a calculus may be present.

submandibular/submental lymphadenopathy and plunging ranula (see above).

Investigations

Only routine baseline investigations and those

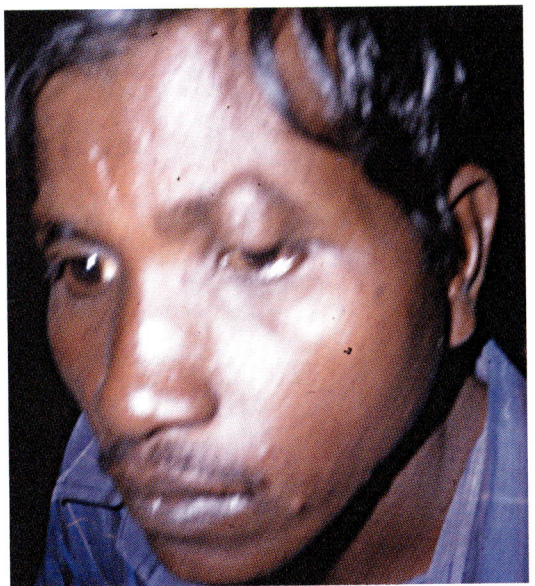

Fig. 10.4. Implantation dermoid of the upper eye lid
(courtesy: Lifeline Hospitals, Chennai)

for lymph nodal diseases, such as tuberculosis, lymphoma, nonspecific lymphadenitis. When in doubt, needle aspiration may be done, to clinch the cystic nature or to diagnose secondary infection. US/CT scan may be helpful to delineate the mass, before surgery.

Treatment

Excision of the cyst, either through the floor of the mouth (supramylohyoid) or through the neck (inframylohyoid). In large midline lesions, where profuse bleeding is anticipated, preliminary bilateral external carotid control, would be desirable (or one side, if it is laterally placed).

Complications

Infection and malignancy (SCC). Needle aspiration would confirm infection, besides providing material for bacteriology. USG and guided biopsy are useful, if malignancy in the cyst is suspected, by its rapid growth, variable consistency and regional lymphadenopathy and treated as SCC elsewhere, after confirmation.

Complications of surgery may be injury to submandibular ducts and lingual or hypo-glossal nerves.

2. Acquired or traumatic (implantation) dermoid cyst

This follows punctured or penetrating injuries, when a tiny bit of skin is driven into the depth and gets implanted, hence commonly seen in parts of body vulnerable for injury, such as hands, feet and digits, in those exposed to such risk, like gardeners, tailors and house-wives.

Clinical features

An indolent, tensely cystic swelling, usually <2cm in size, in the locations indicated above, in an adult, is typical. Often the history of trauma may not be forthcoming, but on careful inspection, a 'tell-tale' scar of bygone injury may be seen.

Differential diagnosis

Ganglion, sebaceous cyst, soft tissue benign tumor, nodules of rheumatoid arthritis or gout, fungal granuloma etc.

Treatment

Excision of the entire cyst, under regional anesthesia, is curative.

3. **Tubulo-dermoid** is an epidermal cyst, developed from an unobliterated remnant of an ectodermal duct or tube; e.g. thyroglossal cyst, postanal dermoid (which may be a teratomatous type) and ependymal cyst in the brain (from neurectoderm).

4. **Teratomatous dermoid** develops from the totipotent cells, with dominant ectodermal elements. They contain derivatives of all three germinal layers and tissue not indigenous to the site (see under hamartoma), such as cartilage, bone, teeth, hair etc.

Common locations are ovary, testis, mediastinum, retroperitoneum, presacral and postanal regions. They are treated by appropriate surgery, in view of a high tendency for malignant transformation.

Tumor markers like β-hCG help to diagnose and follow up trophoblastic tumors.

CORN (syn: tyloma)

Definition: Localized cutaneous hyper-keratosis. There is an increased piling up of keratin, although the basal layer of the epidermis is normal, hence this is not a neoplasm but a form of hyperplastic response of epidermis, to repeated external pressure.

Etiology

Increase in weight, ill fitting footwear, and bony abnormalities like genu valgus, causing abnormal pressure at one point. If the area subjected to such pressure is small, a corn is formed, whereas if it is over a larger area, it results in a callosity.

Pathology

It is a cone shaped thickening of stratum corneum with the base upward and the apex in the subdermal tissue. There is a soft central core and a hard periphery. Pain is often felt, due to pressure on the subjacent sensory nerve terminals.

Differential diagnosis

Callosity and common plantar wart

Treatment

1. Losing weight and footwear correction.
2. Soft shoes or pads at the corn site.
3. Keratolytic topical agents like 40% salicylic acid (corn cap) etc.

If these measures do not help, excision is indicated under local anesthesia, of the entire lesion, with its apex. Culprit bony prominence if present, may have to be excised, for permanent cure. Whereever possible, after excision of a corn, the skin may be primarily closed, leaving the sutures for at least three weeks. This allows wound to heal by primary intention, thereby minimizing the scar. Postoperatively, the other measures indicated above have to be continued, to prevent recurrence.

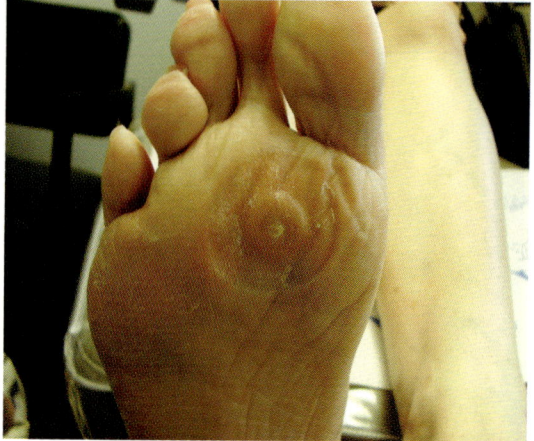

Fig. 11.1. Corn foot

CALLOSITY (syn: heloma)

Definition: A superficial, painless and circumscribed thickened white patch of hyper-keratosis, usually seen over the skin of sole or palm.

Etiology

Constant pressure subjected to an area of skin (small area produces a corn, whereas a larger area of pressure results in a callosity).

Pathology

A central parakeratotic (or orthokeratotic) horny plug situated within a funnel-shaped epidermal defect. Thickening and hypertrophy of the strata granulosum, corneum and basale. The retepegs are atrophic in this condition.

Differential diagnosis

Corn, adventitious bursa

Treatment

No specific treatment is required, except hand care (manicuring) and change of foot-wear, where indicated. Keratolytic agents like 40% salicylic acid (corn cap) are helpful to discourage recurrences following trimming.

12 Papilloma

Papilloma is a common benign tumor of skin, either sessile or pedunculated. It consists of a central axis of connective tissue, blood vessels and lymphatics.

Common sites

1. from the epidermis
2. from mucous membrane
a. squamous cell - in tongue, cheek, lip, larynx or esophagus
b. transitional cell - in the renal pelvis, ureter or urinary bladder
c. from the wall of a duct - in the breast
d. From the wall of a cyst - in the ovary or thyroid

Pathology

The central axis contains connective tissue, blood vessels and lymphatics. The surface varies according to the tumor site. It may be nearly roughened or composed of innumerable, delicate, villous processes, as in the case of renal, vesical or anal papilloma, where it behaves like a malignant tumor, as secondary growths arise by implantation of exfoliated cells. Furthermore, malignant change in transitional cell papillomas is well documented.

PAPILLOMA OF SKIN

A *cutaneous papilloma* is derived from either the squamous or basal layers. The squamous cell papillomas include the following types.

1. *Congenital or* nevus verrucosus: It may be single or multiple and appears either at birth or in early life. It is a warty growth, brownish in colour and may have large, horny excrescences.

2. *Infective papilloma* or verruca vulgaris. This common papilloma probably due to the human papillomavirus (HPV) infection. It may be single or multiple; a spontaneous regression is well known. It is usually seen in children or

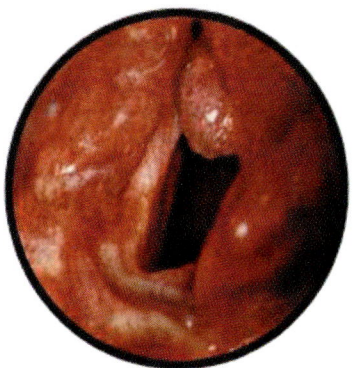

Fig. 12.1. Papilloma of the larynx
(courtesy:Prof. Ravi Ramalingam, Chennai)

adolescents affecting the fingers, palms and soles. When occurring in the plantar aspect, it is often difficult to differentiate it from a corn.

3. *Soft papilloma*, which often occurs in the eyelids of infected people.

4. *Keratin horn* is seen in old people and is associated with excessive keratin production.

5. *Basal cell papilloma* (syn: seborrheic keratoses, senile wart) see next chapter.

6. Acrochordons are small skin tags of fleshy papillomas, usualy seen over eyelids, neck, axillae and groins.

Mucosal papillomas: These are mucosal

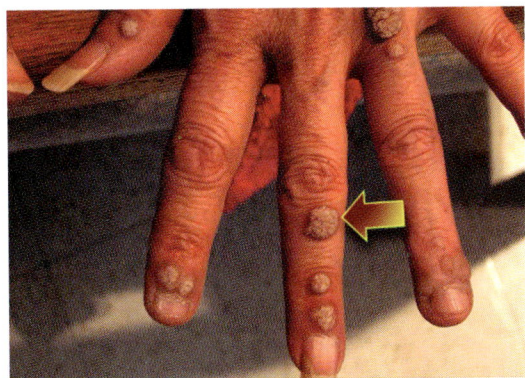

Fig.12.2. Multiple warts of fingers
(Courtesy: Lifeline Hospitals, Chennai)

exophytic growths usually less than 1.5cm diameter, resembling cutaneous warts. They are made up of numerous slender papillae having fibrovascular cores covered by keratinised stratified squamous epithelium superficial ulcer and infection is sometimes superimposed and even active epithelial hyperplasia is occasionally seen. However, dysplastic changes and malignant transformation are very rare.

Differential diagnosis

Corn, callosity, hemangioma, lipoma etc.

Investigations

Since it a surface lesion, no specific investigation is needed for the diagnosis

Treatment

Excision including the base is curative

5-FU ointment is found to effective to treat multiple cutaneous lesions

10% podophyllin application may be used for infective papillomata

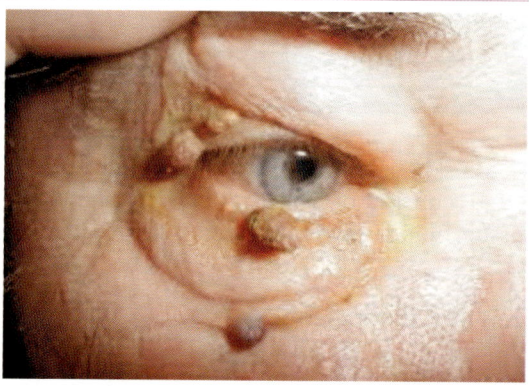

Fig. 12.3. Acrochordons of eyelids
(courtesy: Laxmi Hospital, Kakinada)

For plantar warts, the following measures may be useful.

a) Change of socks to the cotton variety.
b) Formaldehyde application to the wart
c) Silver nitrate application
d) Curettage, cryosurgery or excision to be carried out if the above measures fail.

13 Seborrheic Keratosis

(syn: senile wart, basal cell papilloma, verruca senilis) osis: abnormal

I t is a benign lesion, frequently pigmented and multiple. It affects the trunks, face, arms of persons in middle or old age.

Etiology

Seborrheic warts are common in caucasians (Caucasus: a mountain range in the Soviet Union) and often accepted as part of the ageing process, but uncommon in Indians. In women, they may occur at the time of menopause. There is little tendency for spontaneous regression or malignant change. Exposure to ultraviolet rays may play a role in the etiology. There may be a familial trait with an autosomal dominant mode of inheritance. A mutation of a gene coding for a growth factor receptor (GFR-3) has been associated with this diseases. Genetic predisposition may explain its occurrence as a manifestation along with visceral malignancies. Sometimes seborrheic keratosis may occur in patients who are on estrogen therapy.

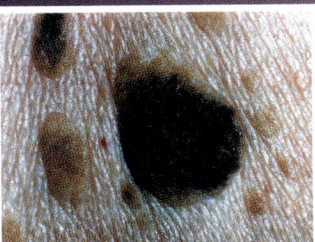

Fig. 13.2. Seborrheic keratosis
(courtesy: Lifeline Hospitals, Chennai)

Pathology

Arising from keratinocytes, the base of the lesion is at the superficial surface of the dermis and its outer surface is formed by thin, orthokeratotic epidermis, with an accumulation of immature epidermal cells in between, nourished by elongated and branched dermal papillae. Malignant transformation has been reported, in patients predisposed to it; however, considering the frequency of this lesion, this is a rare occurrence. The soft greasy surface is responsible for its descriptive name (sebum: tallow; rhoia: flow).

Clinical features

A verrucous plaque is seen, stuck on the epidermis, varying from yellow to black in color, ovoid to circular in shape and measures from 1 mm. to several centimeters. Sometimes the occurrence of seborrheic warts may be preceded by an inflammatory dermatoses.

Differential diagnosis

1. The superficial type has to be differentiated from simple and malignant lentigo.

2. The domed, pigmented variety may resemble a melanoma. Multiplicity of these lesions and the age of occurrence may give a clue to the diagnosis. If doubt persists, excision biopsy is recommended.

Investigation

Edge or excision biopsy is the only specific investigation.

Treatment

Seborrheic warts are removed with a sharp curette leaving a flat surface, which epithelialize within a week. Laser/cryosurgery are also successful in treating these lesions.

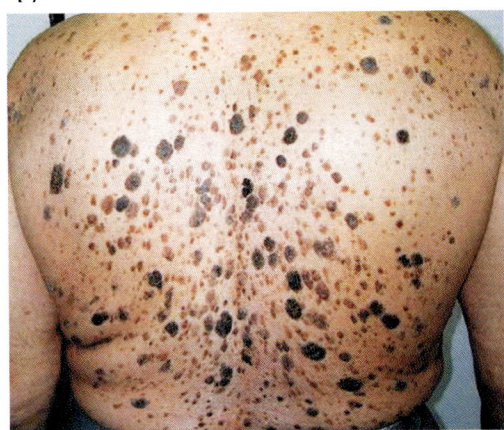

Fig.13.1. Seborrheic keratosis
(courtesy: Halsted Surgical Clinic, Chennai)

14 Pyogenic Granuloma

Definition: It is an exuberant growth of granulation tissue occurring at a site of chronic sepsis, usually in the distal extremities. This lesion looks like a hemangioma but has a typical history.

Common sites

It is most commonly seen on the face, fingers and toes, but can occur wherever there is a breach of epithelium and smoldering infection.

Pathology

Chronic infection in a wound causes excessive proliferation of capillary loops which grow from the base of the granulation tissue, protruding above the surface, which looks pale red, friable and soft. For reasons not clear, this often occurs during pregnancy, hence is sometimes termed as *pregnancy tumor*.

Clinical features

Typically there will be history of injury. The surface is covered by granulation tissue, (proud flesh) which bleeds easily with seropurulent discharge, depending on the nature of underlying infection. The growth is rapid and it often doubles its size in a few days, but never becomes very large. The lesions are generally painless, but they may be slightly tender, soft in consistency and partially compressible.

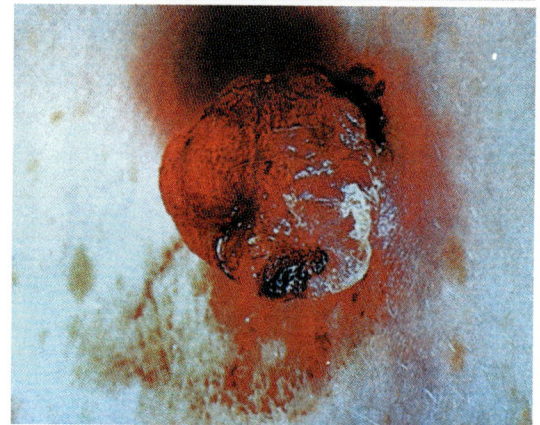
Fig. 14.2. Pyogenic granuloma of skin
(courtesy: Lifeline Hospitals, Chennai)

Regional lymph nodes are usually enlarged, sometimes undergoing suppuration with abscess formation.

Differential diagnosis

Infected hemangioma, specific granuloma such as tuberculous or mycotic, foreign body granuloma, chronic osteomyelitis, malignant skin tumors etc.

Investigations

Routine studies including bacteriological study (Gram stain and culture) of the discharge etc. X-ray of the underlying bone may be useful.

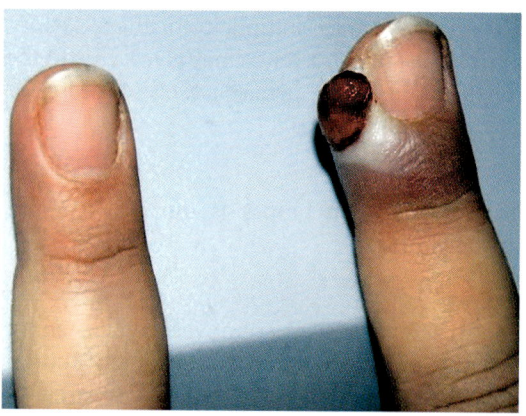
Fig. 14.1. Pyogenic granuloma, finger
(courtesy - Laxmi Hospital, Kakinada)

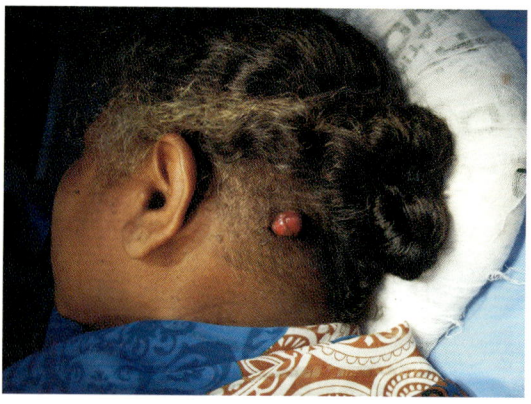
Fig. 14.3. Pyogenic granuloma
(courtesy: Halsted Surgical Clinic, Chennai)

Treatment

Apart from appropriate antibiotics to control infection, the excessive granulation tissue is chemically cauterized by silver nitrate solution or copper sulphate crystals. As an alternative, electrocautery or cryocautery may also be used. If the lesion is persistent, it may be excised by an elliptical incision and sent for histopathology. By themselves, lymph nodes may not need additional treatment, unless suppurated, when drainage is necessary by adequate incision.

INGROWN TOENAIL (syn: unguis incarnatus onychocryptosis- *onyx:* nail; *kryptos:* hidden) is a pyogenic granuloma commonly affecting the big toenail. It is a painful condition in which the nail grows laterally so that it cuts into one or both sides of the paronychium or nail bed. It should not be confused with a similar nail disorder, onychocyrtosis or convex nail (*kyrtos:* convex). Though the overt infection may resolve with aggressive medical treatment, the disease smolders with a great tendency to recur.

Causes:

1. Bad nail-care, including cutting the nail too short, rounded off at the tip or peeled off at the edges instead of being cut straight across

2. Ill-fitting shoes, as those that are too narrow or too short can cause bunching of the toes in the developmental stages of the foot (frequently in those under 21), causing the nail to curl and dig into the skin

3. Trauma to the nail plate or toe, which can occur by stubbing the toenail, dropping things on the toe or going through the end of the shoes (as during sports or other vigorous activity), can cause the flesh to become injured, the nail to grow irregularly and press into the flesh. Injury to the nail can cause it to grow abnormally, making it wider or thicker than normal or even bulged or crooked.

4. Predisposition, such as abnormally shaped nail beds, nail deformities caused by diseases,

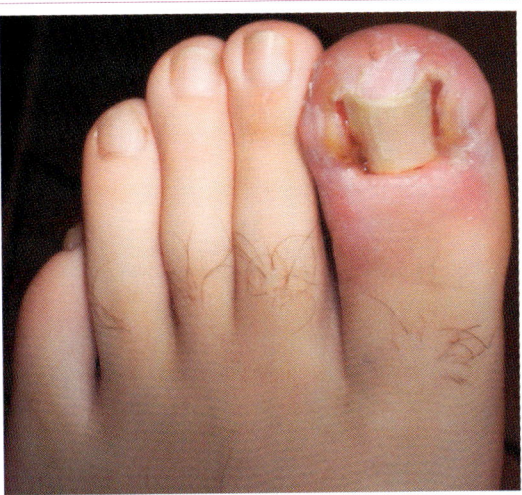

Fig. 14.4. Ingrown toenail
(courtesy: Halsted Surgical Clinic, Chennai)

or a genetic susceptibility

5. Ingrown toenails may be the result of a bacterial or fungal infections, appropriately treatable.

Prevention: Injuries to the toes can be prevented by wearing properly fitting shoes, especially when working or playing. Maintaining good hygiene, avoiding too much moisture and trimming the nails square flush with the tip of toe are some of the measures to prevent nail infection. Early identification, in the stage of initial inflammation, rather than delaying till a suppurating granuloma has developed, may be able to avoid surgery.

Treatment

Conservative: Treatment of ingrown toenail ranges from the use of antibiotics, soaking the afflicted area to surgery. The appropriate method is dictated by the severity of the condition. In nearly all cases, drainage of blood or watery discharge should mean a trip to the doctor, usually a podiatrist, a specialist trained explicitly to treat these conditions. In early stages, strapping the toe, to widen the angle between the nail and nail bed with a 'Band-aid' may be helpful. Most surgeons agree that trying to outwait the condition is nearly always fruitless, as well as agonizing, but it can be done

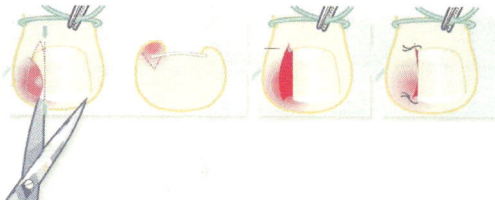

Fig. 14.5. Wedge resection for ingrown toenail

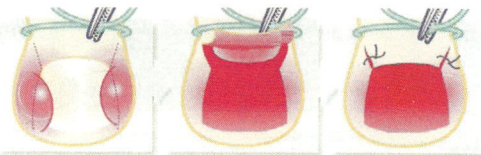

Fig. 14.6. Total nail removal for bilateral disease (courtesy - Halsted Surgical Clinic, Chennai)

as long as the condition is not too severe and if the individual has a high pain threshold. It has to be adequately covered by antibiotics and antimycotics to treat the associated soft tissue infection.

Vandenbos (nail-sparing) procedure

Unlike other procedures used to treat ingrown toenails, no part of the nail is removed, but involves excision of soft tissue of paronichium. An incision is made proximally from the base of the nail about 5 mm (leaving the nail bed intact) then extended towards the side of the toe in an elliptical sweep to end up under the tip of the nail about 3-4 mm in from the edge. It is important that all the skin at the edge of the nail be removed. The excision must be adequate often leaving a soft tissue deficiency measuring about 1x3cm. Based on microbiological studies, appropriate antibiotic or antimycotic agents have to be used along with daily dressings for a few days. This is suitable for early cases of ingrown toe nail and has high incidence of recurrence.

Wedge resection (standard operation) syn: Lateral onychoplasty

Removal of the offending piece of nail is a more popular and satisfying procedure. Under digital block anesthesia, an onychotomy in which the nail along the edge that is growing into the skin, about 3mm broad entire length of nail is cut away (ablated), the offending piece of nail is avulsed including a wedge of adjacent soft tissue and any lurking infection is liberally drained. Using a sharp curette or blade of knife, the entire root of nail segment (nail matrix or onychogenic tissue) is scraped and touched with phenol, to prevent regrowth of nail. A few nonabsorbable skin sutures are placed to reduce the raw area. This is done as an 'office' procedure and takes approximately 20 minutes, with a total healing time of about 2 weeks. Light dressings, an oral or topical antibiotic or a special soak may be used for about a week following surgery.

Rare procedures: Zadek's operation: In difficult or recurrent cases of ingrown toenail with persistent problem, total avulsion of nail may be resorted to, which is rarely required. This procedure, besides requiring more experience for a total removal of the nail matrix, has the disadvantage of long healing time and recovery time(> 2 months).

Still rarer and more formidable alternative is the Syme procedure, consisting of total nail matrix removal, skin flap transfer with or without partial osteotomy of the distal phalanx. Fotunately the cure rate with the standard operation is so high, these procedures are rarely needed, if ever.

15 Ulcer

Definition: A breach in continuity of skin or epithelium, due to molecular death of tissue. The latter half of the statement is added to exclude acute traumatic conditions. Loss of partial thickness of epithelium is called *erosion*, often seen in GI tract and cervix uteri. Common ulcers encountered in the clinical practice (and in examinations) will be discussed in detail here.

Healing of ulcer

This is accomplished by four natural mechanisms:

1. Growth of epithelium from the edges, at a rate of about 1mm per day, mostly depends of local tissue vascularity and absence of overt infection

2. Contraction of the ulcer base, a characteristic feature of newly laid collagen, which contributes over 75% of healing and varies from area to area, depending upon the laxity and suppleness of the skin and subcutaneous tissue

3. Centripetal pull by the myofibroblasts, attaching themselves to the epitheilial edge as well as to the base of the ulcer

4. In the absence of the above factors, it may heal by granulation tissue, with the formation of a thin pseudoepithelium, resulting in an unstable scar, with a high tendency to break down for trivial reasons.

Clinical examination

Inspection

1) Site: venous (gaiter area), arterial (tips of toes or fingers), pressure or decubitus ulcers (over the heels, sacrum etc).

2) Floor of the ulcer is visible, whereas the base can be felt only by palpation. It may be red (healthy granulation tissue), yellow necrotic tissue (spreading ulcer), pale (tuberculous), wash-leather (gummatous), blackish (mela-noma), irregular, bleeding to touch (malignant). What is seen between the floor and margin is the edge of an ulcer and the margin is the junction of ulcer with the adjacent normal epithelium.

3) Discharge: serous (healing or tuberculous), purulent (spreading), greenish (pseudomonas infection), sanguine (malignancy).

4) Edge: sloping (healing), punched out (trophic or gummatous), undermined (tuberculous), raised (BCC) and raised/everted (SCC)

5) Surrounding skin: pigmented (venous), dark, thin and shiny (ischemic), edematous (spreading ulcer), adjacent scar (Marjolin's ulcer).

Palpation

1) edge
2) base
3) mobility
4) friability or bleeding to touch
5) adjacent bony thickening
6) surrounding skin
7) probing for an associated sinus

Regional nodes, peripheral pulses, neurological deficit, venous varicosities, movements of the neighboring joint(s) have to be noted.

Systemic examination for cardiovascular, neurological, pulmonary disorders, splenomegaly (blood dyscrasias), syphilitic stigmata, has to be done.

Clinical classification: they are healing, spreading, callous (or indolent) and trophic

a) *Healing ulcer* shows healthy granulation tissue in its floor, with bluish sloping edge and minimal serous discharge, without adjacent cellulitis.

Traumatic ulcer, also known as footballer's ulcer, commonly seen over the feet, is a typical example of a healing ulcer.

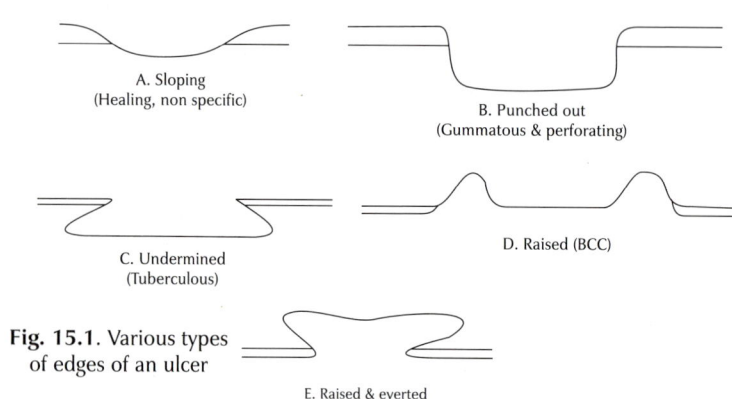

A. Sloping
(Healing, non specific)

B. Punched out
(Gummatous & perforating)

C. Undermined
(Tuberculous)

D. Raised (BCC)

Fig. 15.1. Various types of edges of an ulcer

E. Raised & everted
(SCC)

graded according to the neuropathy and trophic changes of soft tissue and bones:

1st degree: minimal sensory changes

2nd degree: severe anesthesia and sensory changes, without trophic ulcer

3rd degree: trophic ulceration without overt infection

4th degree: trophic ulcers, infection and deformities

b) *Spreading ulcer* shows unhealthy slough, without granulation tissue in the floor, purulent or offensive discharge, with cellulitis around but no sign of epithelialization. Its size increases, with gradual loss of more and more epithelium.

c) *Callous* (indolent) *ulcer* has a whitish floor, due to pale unhealthy granulation tissue, neither has a tendency to heal nor to spread with time.

d) *Trophic ulcer* (trophikos: nourishment) is due to lack of either nutrition (ischemic) or sensory innervation, to an area, usually feet and hands, which are vulnerable for injury. (vide infra)

Special types of ulcers

1) *Diabetic ulcer* (see also under gangrene)

Diabetic foot is a complex subject, which is

5th degree: severe neuropathic (Charcot's) arthropathy

Vibration sense is tested to detect early neuropathy in the extremities (*biothesiometry*) and pressures are recorded to identify points of maximal pressure distribution in the sole of the foot (*podobarometry*), for 'custom-making' of microcellular rubber (MCR) shoes, in high risk patients. MCR shoes may be sufficient in 1st & 2nd degrees, but for 3rd degree and above, moulded insoles, using sophisticated technology may be necessary, available only in a few centres in India.

2) *Ischemic ulcer:* is due to ischemic necrosis of the skin, usually at the tips of toes or fingers, which may be acute or chronic. This has been described in detail in chapters 77 and 79.

Certain special types of ischemic ulcers are described here:

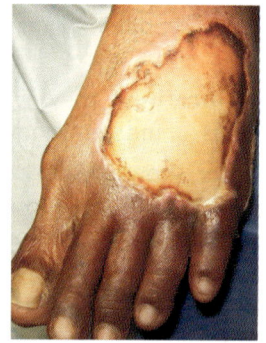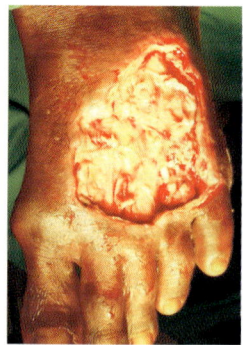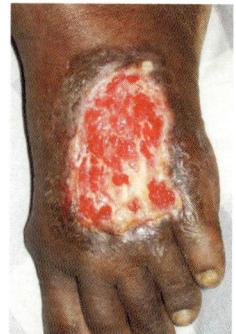

Fig. 15.2. Traumatic ulcer dorsum of the foot 1.Before slough excision 2.After slough excision 3.Ulcer ready for skin graft (courtesy: Halsted Surgical Clinic, Chennai)

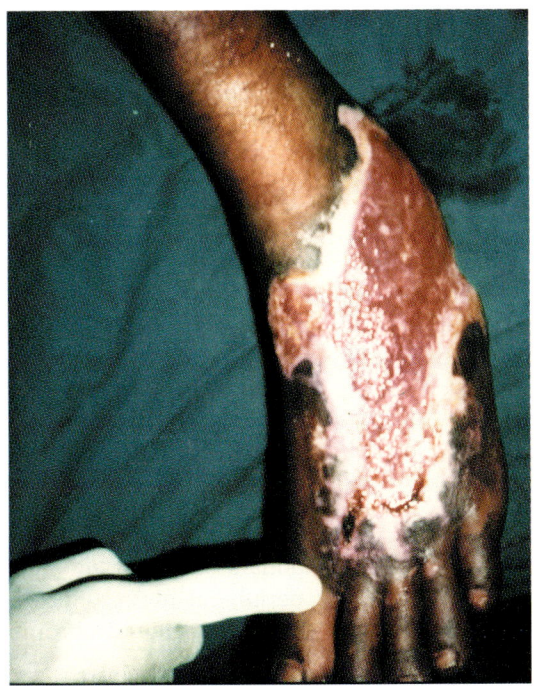

Fig. 15.3. Ulcer resulting from diabetic foot infection
(courtesy: Halsted Surgical Clinic, Chennai)

a) Pressure sores (syn: decubitus ulcer, bed sore), are the commonest and clinically significant type under this category; earlier considered to be neuropathic in nature,they are actually due to ischemia of skin and subcutaneous tissue as a result of prolonged pressure against bony prominences, in debilitated, bed-ridden or comatose patients. Pressure sores are predisposed by abrasive injury, anemia, malnutriton and moisture. Common sites are over sacrum, ischial tuberosity, greater trochanter, heels, malleoli, elbows, occiput and scapula. It should be identified early in vulnerable patients, by erythema, blistering or induration, so that preventive measures may be intensified. The disease may be divided into 4 stages:

Stage-I: early erythema, induration and tenderness

Stage-II: blistering, skin break-

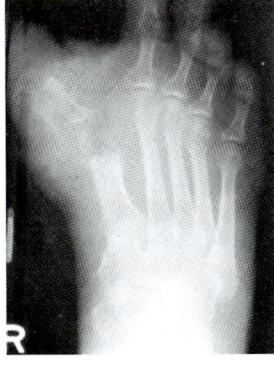

Fig. 15.4. diabetic infection with osteomyelitis
(courtesy: Halsted Surgical Clinic, Chennai)

down limited to dermis, local swelling

Stage-III:ulcer/crater formation into subcutaneous tissues with slough or eschar

Stage-IV:necrosis extending beyond fascia, into the ligaments and bones (osteomyelitis)

Prevention

Turning the patient frequently and powdering the back after drying are generally helpful. Using excess cotton or foam rubber padding over the pressure points and alternating air/water mattress (Alfabed), which periodically redistributes the pressure points, are routinely used while nursing aged, debilitated, less mobile patients, particularly in an ICU set up. Ultraviolet/infra-red rays to the area also improve regional blood flow to the base of ulcer.

Other situations of pressure necrosis and ulceration are:

(a)   cuffed endotracheal intubation and

(b)   Sengstaken-Blakemore tube for esophageal tamponade. As a routine precaution, these tubes, when required to be retained for longer periods, should be periodically deflated (once every six hours) for a few minutes and reinflated, to avoid continuous pressure leading to mucosal sloughing and ulceration.

Treatment of decubitus ulcer

It is a troublesome complication that needs to be prevented by aggressive paranoid measures. Contrary to general belief, lack of mobility in bed even for 1 or 2 days may be enough to show prodromal features of skin necrosis. Lack of protective reflexes for changing posture on occasions of persistent pressure in comatose or debilitated patients is the main factor. Though conventionally it is termed an ulcer, deeper tissue up to the bone are often involved, making spontaneous healing difficult. It should be realized that development of a decubitus ulcer is an indication of poor quality of nursing care provided to the patient.

Specific treatment

a) for superficial ulcers, off-loading the pressure points, immediate debridement and local care, to allow it to heal either by epithelialization or secondary intention

b) for deep ulcers (besides above indicated measures):

Antibiotic impregnated wet dressings

Desloughing agents

Appropriate systemic antibiotics

Nutritional support

Agents to promote growth of granulation tissue

Platelet-derived growth factor (RhPDGF) and epidermal growth factor (RhEGF) may be helpful to promote granulation tissue and epithelialization respectively

Local infrared therapy or wound vacuum therapy may reduce the wound healing time

Suitable reconstructive procedure, either by primary closure, skin grafting or flap closure, when the wound is clean and dry with healthy granulation tissue.

b) *Martorell's ulcer* is seen in diabetic, hypertensive men over 50, due to sudden ischemia, probably thromboembolic, a patch of necrosis develops on the outer aspect of calf, leaving a deep, nonhealing ulcer.

c) *Bazin's ulcer,* seen only in women, is considered to be due to obliteration of perforating branches of posterior tibial and peroneal arteries of leg, associated with *erythrocyanosis frigida*, a condition in which skin of leg becomes hypersensitive to the changes in external temperature.

d) *Cryopathic ulcers* are due to exposure to extreme degree of cold, two such conditions are commonly seen in people living in snowy zones, namely chilblains (or perniosis) and frost bite. Acute ischemic blisters, ulcers, pregangrene or gangrene may occur in these conditions, depending upon the temperature level and duration of exposure, usually in the legs and feet, due to vasoconstriction and arteriolar thrombosis affecting cutaneous microcirculation.

3) *Trophic ulcer* (syn: neurogenic ulcer, ischemic ulcer, perforating ulcer): This ulcer occurs in response to repeated pressure in a small area which is devoid of sensory innervation or adequate blood supply. They are not true ulcers by definition, since an ulcer is only skin deep, whereas in trophic ulcer, deeper tissue, like fat, fascia etc. are also deficient, hence the name perforating is more appropriate for this ulcer.

Predisposing conditions

The common conditions associated with this type of ulcers are: peripheral nerve injuries, Hansen's disease, diabetes mellitus, chronic arterial occlusion, syringomyelia etc.

Etiopathogenesis

Commonest type of trophic ulcer is a *pressure* (bed) *sore* (vide supra). Initially a callosity is formed due to constant pressure, later leading to necrosis of the fatty tissue between the bone and the skin. Ulceration and suppuration then occur and the entire process is painless because of lack of afferent nerves. The term trophic ulcer was coined earlier because of the misconception that the nerves carry a trophic substance to the skin and the ulcer develops due to denervation. It is now known however that the pressure is the primary factor involved and absence of sensory innervation is secondary, which results in poor inflammatory response to injury, because the *axon reflex*, that triggers tissue reaction, is mediated through the afferent nerves. When there is no inflammation, there is no repair, leading to nonhealing callous ulcer, burrowing up to the bone. As the area of pressure against a bony prominence, such as sacrum or head of metatarsal, is well demarcated, these ulcers have a sharp punched out edge.

Sites: Pressure points on the skin are all vulner-

Feature	Ischemic Ulcer	Neuropathic Ulcer
Location	Digital tips	Pressure points in the sole
Pain and tenderness	Present	Absent
Black eschar	Present	Absent
Local temperature	Cold	Normal
Peripheral pulses	Absent	Normal
Sensory deficit	Absent	Present

Table-15.1: Differences between ischemic and neuropathic ulcers

able sites for trophic ulcers. Thus for ambulatory patients, the heel, the ball of the foot and the plantar aspect of the big toe are affected. For patients who are supine and in bed, the sacral and tendo Achilles areas are involved.

Treatment

a) The primary cause of the trophic ulcer should be dealt with. Further pressure is prevented by periodically turning the patient over and caring for the skin and other precautions mentioned under pressure ulcer. In the sole of foot, prevention is possible by the use of MCR shoes to redistribute the pressure points. The MCR shoes are made to order, to suit the individual foot, after mapping the pressure points, by podobarometry.

b) Desloughing and debridement are carried out.

c) The ulcer is then covered by a variety of reconstructive methods using rotation or myocutaneous flaps. As the area is denervated further recurrence should be prevented by paranoid caution.

4) *Venous ulcer*: is probably the commonest ulcer of the leg, caused by chronic ambulatory venous hypertension. Its pathological sequelae are described in chapter 82.

5) *Tropical ulcer*: This is a specific type of nonhealing ulcer found in the tropics, due to infection by *Vincent's organisms (Bacillus fusiformis and Borrelia vincentii)*, notorious for its indolence. Microbes gain entry through a crack or abrasion, excite a painful local reaction with regional lymphadenopathy, initial pustular lesions soon break down forming undermined ulcers, mimicking tuberculosis, with serosanguineous discharge. When heals, usually after several months, a parchment-like pigmented scar is left. It is also known as *phagedenic* (phagos: eat) ulcer.

Treatment

Ideally this disease process should be picked up at an early stage, before inflammatory necrosis has occurred. Early institution of appropriate antibiotic therapy is all that is necessary. For a chronic nonhealing tropical ulcer, at least three weeks of broad spectrum antibiotics (cephalosporins, nitroimidazoles, fluoroquinolones etc.) should be attempted, followed by split skin grafting, if there is no attempt for epithelialization.

6) *Tuberculous ulcer*

Cutaneous manifestation of tuberculosis is known as *lupus vulgaris*, which may be acquired through a close contact suffering with the disease. Another mode of formation is by breakdown of a cold abscess leading to a painful nonhealing ulcer. Typically it has an undermined edge, with thin serous discharge and red angry-looking floor, often associated with a sinus leading to some underlying structure, such as lymph node or bone, where the disease had originated. In the tongue, pharynx, larynx and urinary bladder, they tend to be multiple and superficial. Tuberculous ulcers often heal with much fibrosis and disfigurement. A rare and unimportant variant of this, caused by Mycobacterium ulcerans, with similar features is known as *Bairnsdale ulcer*. For investigations and treatment, see chapter 18.

7) *Syphilitic ulcer*: Ulcers may be seen in every stage of syphilis, *Hunterian chancre* in

primary, snail-track or *serpigenous ulcers* of mucocutaneous junctions in secondary and *gummatous ulcers* in tertiary stages, the last variety is of some relevance to surgeon. Gummatous ulcers occur commonly on the anterolateral aspect of the leg as a result of granulomatous lesion, starts as a subcutaneous nodule, later undergoes central necrosis and ulceration, which is painless, with punched out edges, floor covered with typical wet wash-leather slough, without regional lymphadeno-pathy. It has to be differentiated from a tropical ulcer; history, involvement of other systems, specially CNS and serological tests for syphilis (STS) clinch the diagnosis. A healed lesion may leave a circular paper-thin scar, with pigmenta-tion around. For detailed investigations and treatment, see chapter 54 (tongue).

8) *Pyogenic ulcer*: Children with poor hygiene often have recurrent ulcers due to pyogenic staphylo/streptococcal infection, in the leg and foot. The heightened antibody response to superficial streptococcal infection on the legs (impetigo) may result in conditions such as glomerulonephritis and rheumatic arthri-tis/carditis. Local care, appropriate antibiotics on a long term basis and improvement of hygiene are necessary for total control of dis-ease.

9) *Neoplastic ulcers*: are either primary skin cancers such as SCC, BCC and melanoma or

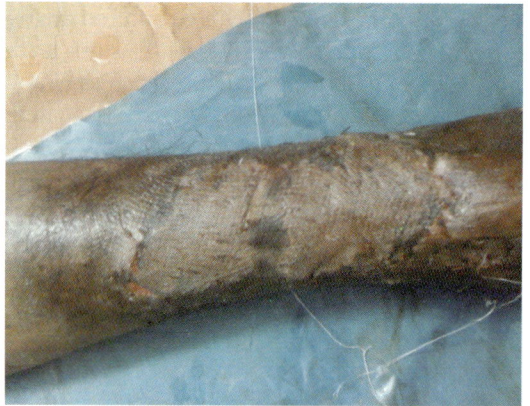

Fig. 15.5. Split skin graft placed over an ulcer
(courtesy: Laxmi Hospital, Kakinada)

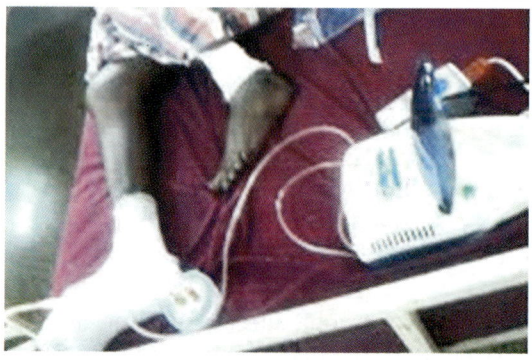

Fig. 15.6. The apparatus for vacuum therapy to the intractable ulcers
(courtesy: Laxmi Hospital, Kakinada)

those originating from the scars of burns or venous ulcers (Marjolin's ulcers) and from meta-static deposits in the skin (Sister Joseph's nod-ules) - refer appropriate chapters.

Ulcers in herpes simplex (HSV), cytomega-lovirus (CMV) and human immune deficiency virus (HIV), have been described in the chapter 53 (Mouth).

Aphthous (dyspeptic) ulcer - see chapter 53

Dental ulcer - see chapter 54

Solitary rectal ulcer - see chapter 75

Arterial ulcer - see chapter 77

Venous ulcer - see chapter 82

Recent advances

Enhancing skin wound healing by direct delivery of intracellular ATP

1. To circumvent the problem of poor blood supply, highly furogenic lipid granules (ATP visicles) at 100 to 200 nm size, are used to encapsulate magnesium adenosine triphos-phate (Mg-ATP). When these vesicles come in contact with cell membrane, they fuse and deliver their contents into the cytosol. After successful studies on mice, it is being studied on humans, to see its reproducibility in terms of promoting ulcer healing.

2. Recombinant human platelet-derived growth factor - rhPDGF (Plermin) and recombi-nant human epidermal growth factor rhEGF (Regen-D)) have been found to promote granulation tissue and epithelialization respectively in various types of nonhealing

	Agent	Composition	Function	Commercial Names
1.	Debriding agents			
	Hydrogen peroxide	H_2O_2	Bubbles and releases nasent O_2, debredes particles in depth and crevices	
	Edinburgh solution of lime	Hypochlorite	Debriding action	EUSOL
2.	Polymeric films	Polyurethane	Allows water vapor permeation	Opsite, Tagaderm
3.	Hydrocolloids	Hydrophilic colloid particles	Impermeable to fluids & bacteria	Duoderm, Intrasite
4.	Alginates	Seaweed polymer, that forms a gel when it absorbs fluid	Absorbs exudates, non-adherent	Algisorb Sorbsan
5.	Medicated Gauze	Soframycin Zinc oxide Neomycin Bacitracin	Topical antibiotic	Sofratulle
6.	Platelet-derived growth factor (RhPDGF)	Acts through tyrosinekinase receptor	Stimulates angiogenesis	Plermin
7.	Epithelial growth factor (RhEGF)	acts through tyrosinekinase receptor	Stimulates epithelialization	Regen-D

Table-15.2. Some of the local wound care modalities currently practiced

ulcers and have gained wide acceptance in the recent times in clinical practice. However the high cost precludes their routine use in all types of ulcers.

3. The use of continuous suction to create a vacuum over a healing wound. The constant negative pressure seems to hasten closure of the wound.

4. Stem cells, hailed as the holy grail of medicine, are now used to culture keratino-cyte sheets used to cover ulcers as an autograft

5. Magnetotherapy and resonance therapy are also being tried to hasten healing of intractable ulcers.

DERMAL COVER

Whenever possible, primary skin closure, by mobilizing the lateral flaps if necessary, is the simplest and most preferred method of closing gaps of skin generated out of excision of a lesion, such as a sebaceous cyst, hemangioma, breast malignancy etc. However, large non-healing ulcers, skin loss due to trauma, burns or extensive surgery, which are incapable of epithelialization, require skin cover, by grafting or transplantation.

Indications

Injuries: avulsion, degloving, crushing etc

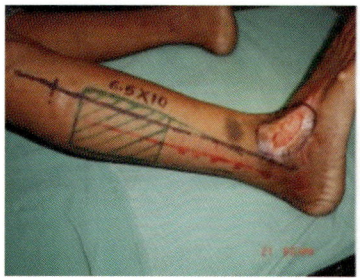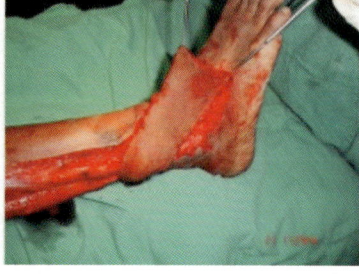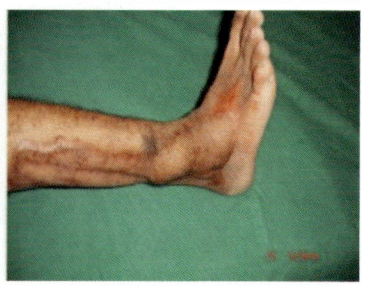

Fig. 15.7. Peroneal perforator based calf flap rotated to cover a non-healing ulcer over dorsum of foot
(courtesy: Prof G Balakrishnan, Chennai)

Postoperative: wide excision of large tumors, post-burn escharectomy, guillotine amputation etc.

Diseases causing skin loss: venous ulcers, decubitus ulcers, diabetic ulcers, necrotizing fasciitis, Fournier's gangrene, cancrum oris etc

Reconstructive procedures: excision of cheek, tongue, filarial penis, urethral or vaginal reconstruction

Types of skin grafts

Classification depending upon the thickness of dermis and the technique

Free grafts: the graft is totally detached from the donor site and laid over the recipient area

Split thickness (Thiersch) graft this is the most common type of skin graft, consisting of epidermis and part of dermis, harvested by using a Da Silva, Humby's or Watson's knife or Brown's pneumatic dermatome. The donor site has the potential for complete re-surfacing within 2 weeks, grown from the residual skin adnexae, ready to donate fresh layer of skin if necessary for grafing.

The front of thigh is the most preferred donor area, for its technical convenience and concealed location. Where immediate skin cover is required for early recovery, split thickness skin graft is the first preference. Depending upon the thickness of the split skin graft being harvested, which may be programmed in the dermatome, it is further

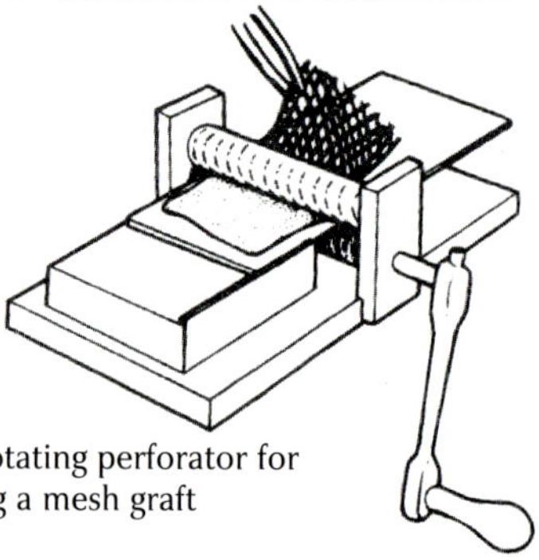

Fig. 15.11. Rotating perforator for creating a mesh graft

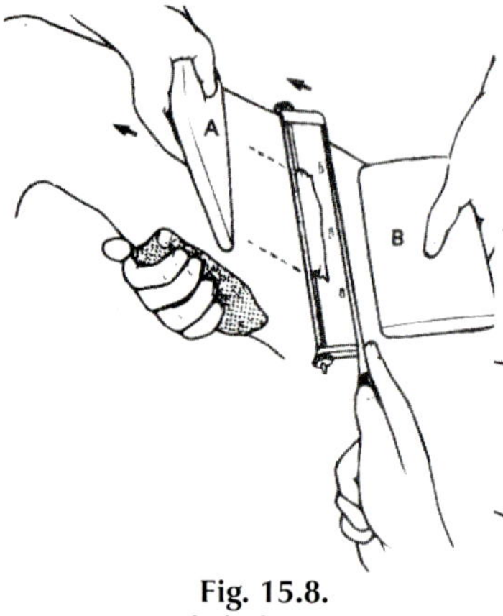

Fig. 15.8.
Humby's dermatome

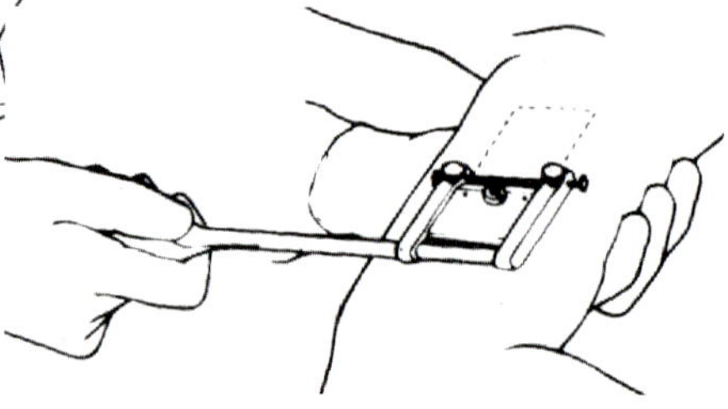

Fig. 15.9. Da Silva dermatome

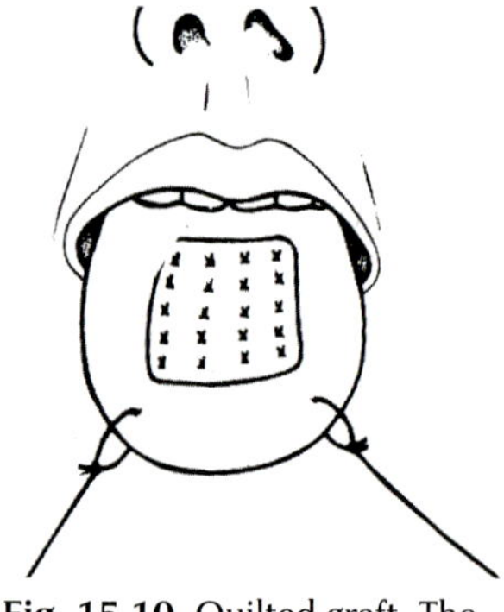

Fig. 15.10. Quilted graft. The graft is fixed over the tongue with multiple sutures

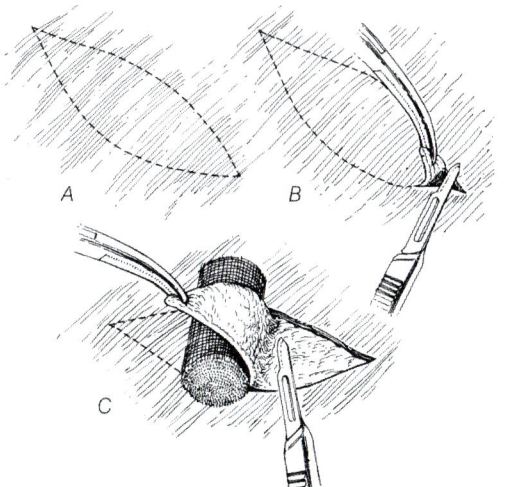

Fig. 15.12. Technic of harvesting full thickness skin graft

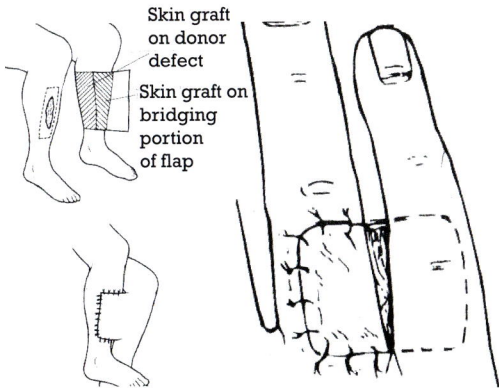

Fig. 15.14. Cross leg and cross finger flaps

divided into 3 categories, thin (10 microns), medium (15 microns) and thick (20 microns). For split skin graft, it may take about 72 hours for the neovascularization to develop and accordingly first wound inspection may be done after 72-96 hours.

The intermediary gaps, thus created by the 'button-holes', get covered in due course by the growth of epithelium from the edges of the grafted skin.

Mesh graft: Converting the skin sheet into a mesh by making multiple stab wounds (or by mechanical devices) is useful to cover larger area with the graft and allow tissue fluid and lymph to escape, facilitating better graft take.

Pinch graft: Small circular pinches or 'postage stamps' of skin are sometimes employed to cover uneven raw surfaces. Quilted graft is used over a mobile structure like tongue or other highly vascular areas, with high possibility of bleeding beneath the graft. The graft is immobilized by multiple anchoring stitches, to ensure better fixity.

Full thickness (Wolfe) graft consists of entire skin devoid of subcutaneous fat, harvested manually by using a scalpel. Lax skin over the neck, groin or abdominal wall is the preferred donor site, so that the resultant defect may be primarily closed.

Composite graft contains multiple compo-

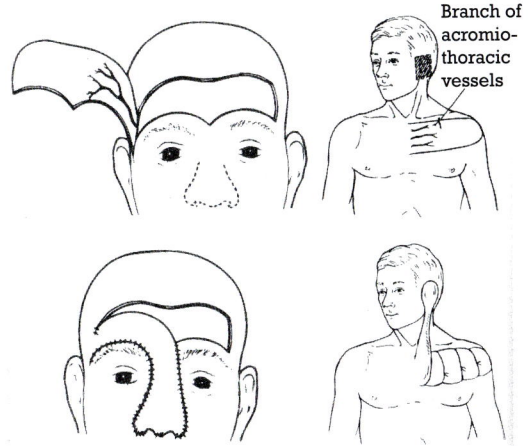

Fig. 15.13. Forehead and deltopectoral flaps
(courtesy: Prof R M Kirk, London)

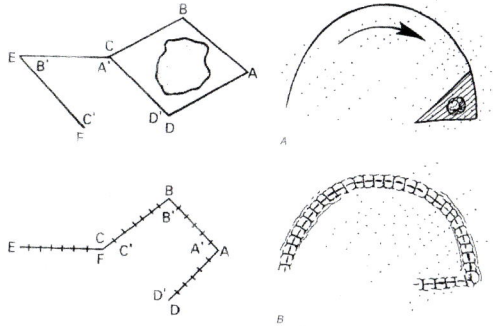

Fig. 15.15. Rhomboid and rotation flaps
(courtesy: Prof R M Kirk, London)

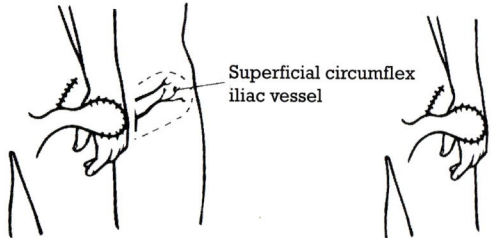

Superficial circumflex iliac vessel

Fig. 15.16. Groin flap based on superficial circumflex iliac vessels

nents, such as bone (fibula, radius, iliac crest, rib etc), cartilage, muscle, fat etc.

The neovascularization of the full thickness skin graft may take about 7 days, hence for clean cases, first inspection of the wound may be carried out around that time. However, in not-so-clean cases or where infection is suspected (fever, wound discharge etc), earlier inspection of the graft is desirable.

Pedicled flaps are used in areas of impaired vascularity of the ulcer bed, exposed bone, cartilage, tendons etc. They are two types, namely *random flap*, where there is no definite vascular base (flap nourished by dermal and subdermal plexus) and *axial flap* in which definite blood supply is provided by native vascular tree, oriented longitudinally in the flap.

E.g. Cross leg or cross finger flaps forehead flap based of superficial temporal artery, Narayanan flap for cheek reconstruction, median forehead flap based on supratrochlear vessels for nasal

reconstruction etc. deltopectoral (DP) flap for the defects of neck and face, rotation of advancement flaps e.g. following excision of pilonidal disease (Limberg flap) or for a pressure sore over the sacral area.

Myocutaneous flaps: the principle that blood supply to the skin overlying a muscle is derived from the muscular branches is employed.

E.g. Latissimus dorsi (LD) flap or transverse rectus abdominis myocutaneous (TRAM) flap for breast reconstruction.

Sternomastoid myocutaneous flap for cheek reconstruction.

Microvascular free flap transfer is the latest and most sophisticated technique, wherein a part of the body, such as a muscle, bone, finger or toe is transferred and fixed in an another part, by anastomosing the arteries and veins, using operating microscope, to the vessels in the recipient area.

E.g. 'Chinese' forearm flap based on radial artery, fibular flap based on peroneal artery, thumb reconstruction using a toe etc.

Classification depending upon the source of the skin

Autograft: from the same person (commonest)

Homograft is from the same species, which may be:

Allograft: from an individual genetically not identical (next common)

Isograft or syngenic graft: from an individual

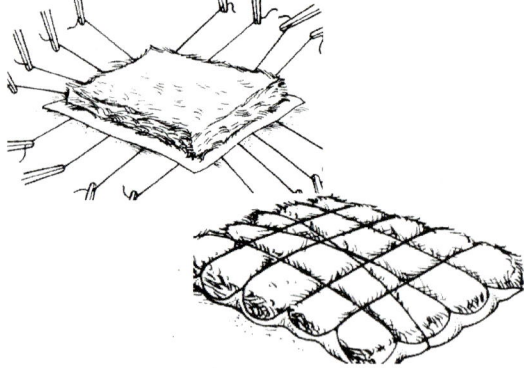

Fig. 15.17. Method of fixing the skin graft to edges of the wound over a gauze pad

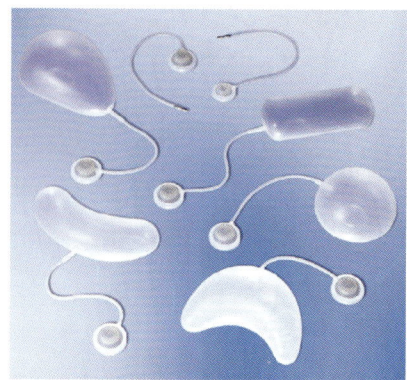

Fig. 15.18. Different types of tissue expanders

genetically identical (e.g. uniovular twin)

Xenograft or heterograft: from another species, e.g. pig, chimpanzee etc.

Skin substitutes: these are useful for temporary skin cover, when the skin defect is very large and donor area is insufficient, e.g. collagen sheets (collagen peptide bound to nylon or silicone - Biobrane), amniotic membrane etc.

Tissue expanders are used to expand the available skin over a period of weeks or months, to be utilized for the future reconstruction or covering a skin defect, e.g. scalp, breast etc.

Causes of failure of the 'take' of a skin graft

1. Infection is the commonest cause for graft failure. Presence of frank sepsis, especially with β-hemolytic streptococci, may be a contra-indication for skin grafting

2. poor vascularity of the ulcer bed or over an exposed bone, including arterial insufficiency. One novel technique adopted when the graft has to be placed over an exposed bone, is to make multiple drill holes in the cortex (under strict aseptic conditions) and allowing the marrow to sprout out and provide granulation tissue cover to the bone, within a few days (Fig. 17.8).

3. anemia

4. hypoproteinemia

5. hypovitaminosis, especially water soluble vitamins (B and C)

6. local tissue edema due to any reason, including venous insufficiency

7. lack of adequate immobilization. During the first 48 hours, there is a growth of delicate vascular and connective tissue elements into the graft from the ulcer bed and if the graft is not kept absolutely immobile, the sheering effect will disrupt the neovasculature and adversely affect the survival. If the graft is placed in the vicinity of a joint, total immobilization with a plaster of Paris (PoP) splint is essential for a few days and first inspection of the wound should be carried out only after 72-96 hours

8. thickness of the graft. Since the survival of the graft during the first 2-3 days is by the diffusion of the nutrients from the ulcer surface through the layers on the graft, thinner it is, better the chances of survival

9. immune compromised states

Recent advances: Use of cultured autologous keratinocytes, derived from pinches of patient's full thickness skin from some other area, overcomes the problem of shortage of donor skin. The removed skin bits are minced, trypsinized to separate the epithelial cells from the dermal layers and cultured in standard growth media. After achieving a multilayered epithelial tissue, containing stratum basale and stratum corneum, the microthin sheets are carefully transferred on to the large raw areas (usually for post-burn defects), allowed to get fixed and grow further, to provide skin cover.

Feature	Split Thickness	Full Thickness
Harvesting	By mechanical gadgets	Manual
Thickness	10-20 microns	Full thick skin
Layers of skin	Epidermis+part of dermis	Epidermis+dermis
Donor site	Heals spontaneously	Requires skin cover
Wound contraction	Occurs	Very minimal
Aim	Rapid skin cover	Cosmesis
Chances of graft survival	Excellent	Fair
First wound inspection	72-96 hours	7 days (in clean cases)
Pigmentation	Abnormal	Normal
Resistance to injury	Weak	Good
Usually done by	Every surgeon	Plastic surgeon

Table-15.3. Differences between Split skin graft and Full thickness skin graft

16 Sinus and Fistula

Sinus: hollow or a bay; Fistula: pipe or tube

Definition: A **SINUS** is an abnormal blind tract leading from the exterior, lined by granulation tissue or epithelium. Although sometimes there may be an abscess cavity in the depth connected to the sinus, there is no viscus or epithelial surface leading to it. The rider 'lined by epithelium or granulation tissue' is added to exclude the acute traumatic condition.

A **FISTULA** is an abnormal track lined by granulation tissue or epithelium, connecting two hollow viscera or one to the exterior, known respectively as internal or external fistula.

Local causes of a persistent sinus or fistula see fig.16.1

i)   presence of a foreign body (e.g. suture material, necrotic tissue like a sequestrum or synthetic mesh used for hernioplasty).

ii)   presence of specific disease (e.g. tuberculosis, amebiasis, Crohn's disease or actinomycosis).

iii) malignancy or chemo/radiation.

iv)   epithelialisation or dense fibrosis of the track, occurs in the course of several weeks of nonhealing.

v)   presence of an abscess in the depth that communicates with the track (Zimmerman's abscess) and inadequate drainage.

vi)   distal obstruction to the natural passage (e.g. stricture of the bowel/urethra distal to the site of fistula).

vii) recurrent trauma or movement (e.g. nonhealing of a fistula-in-ano attributed to continuous sphincteric action).

Etiology

i)   *Congenital*: preauricular, branchial, tracheo-esophageal, recto-vaginal, recto-urethral etc

ii)   *Inflammatory*: apical infection of tooth, Crohn's disease, perianal, urethral (watering can perineum), tuberculous, amebiasis, actinomycosis etc.

iii) *Neoplastic*: Carcinoma of colon causing fistula on the abdominal wall or anorectum leading to multiple perineal fistula etc.

iv)   *Iatrogenic*: (iatros: physician) this may be inadvertent or deliberate (or therapeutic).

a)   inadvertent: cricopharyngeal, duodenal, biliary, pancreatic, ileal, cecal etc

b)   therapeutic: A-V fistula for hemodialysis, gastrostomy, choledochostomy, gastrojejunostomy, ileotransverse colostomy, biliary-enteric bypass, suprapubic cystostomy etc.

Systemic causes may be general debility, immune suppression, diabetes, anemia hypoprotenemia, avitaminosis etc.

History

i)   presence since birth or early childhood is in support of a congenital type

ii)   history of tuberculosis or its contact

iii) history of surgery, 'draining' a cold abscess or appendectomy in typhlitis of Crohn's or amebiasis, flank drainage for peritonitis due to duodenal/ileal perforation

iv)   history of passing 'rice grains' or bone chips is in favour of chronic nonspecific osteomyelitis with a sequestrum

v)   if it follows abdominal surgery, nature, quantity of drainage and if it is increasing or decreasing, is important. High output fistula is one which drains more than 500 ml or 10ml/kg body weight per day

vi)   passing flatus/stools via naturalis, will ensure absence of significant distal bowel obstruction

vii) passing gas/feces per urethra indicates entero-vesical fistula

viii) incontinence (dribbling) of urine, following pelvic surgery or difficult labor, without normal voiding is vesico-vaginal fistula (VVF), whereas if the patient is also voiding normally in between, it is likely to be uretero-vaginal fistula (UVF), other ureter normally draining into the bladder.

ix) if any treatment has been given, its nature and effect may give a clue to the diagnosis

General survey

Chest, spine, ribs etc, should be examined for tuberculous affection, especially in a cold abscess presenting with a sinus. In recurrent fistula-in-ano, abdominal examination along with proctosigmoidoscopic/colonoscopic examination is important (chapter 74)

Local examination

1. *Site*: diagnosis is often made by its location alone:

a) preauricular sinus situated at the root of the helix or on the tragus, due to failure of fusion of tubercles of the ear.

b) pilonidal sinus may be in the natal cleft (at the level of the first piece of coccyx), in the interdigital cleft or at the umbilicus (chapter 26).

c) branchial fistula: in front of the lower third of anterior border of SCM, can present later in life although congenital (its relation to tonsillar disease is described in chapter 90)

d) multiple sinuses in the neck with lymph node enlargement, are commonly due to tuberculosis although rarely due to actinomycosis.

e) a sinus situated directly over a bone and fixed to it, is almost always due to osteomyelitis.

f) located in the anterior perineum, discharging urine, is urethral fistula, which may be multiple (watering-can perineum)

g) perianal location is classically a fistula-in-ano, though anterior ones may be confused with urethral and posterior with pilonidal disease.

h) in Dracunculosis (guinea worm infestation), it is located around the ankle/foot, (parts coming in contact with water), due to its hydrophilic property.

2. *Number*: some diseases like tuberculosis, Crohn's disease, actinomycosis, ulcerative colitis and malignancy produce multiple fistulae, while most other sinuses/fistulae are single.

3. *Opening*: if the sinus/fistula opening shows granulation tissue it usually indicates a foreign body, such as a nonabsorbable suture material or an implant in the depth. The margin is blue and undermined in tuberculosis and blue diffusely all around in Crohn's disease.

4. *Discharge*: it may be urine, feces, saliva or bile, depending upon the viscus it communicates with. In actinomycosis, yellowish clumps of ray fungus, 'sulphur granules' and in osteomyelitis rice grains or bone chips are characteristic. It may be purulent in nonspecific disease or if foreign body is present, usually associated with an abscess at the inner end. In dracunculosis, sinus in the leg may discharge larvae and bits of the nematode or occasionally the worm itself may stick out through the opening.

5. *Surrounding skin*: a scar in the surrounding region with openings indicates chronic tuberculous lesion, (*scrofuloderma*), so also a scar over a bone could indicate bone surgery resulting in a sequestrum. Skin excoriation or digestion indicates pancreatic or intestinal juices, rich in proteolytic enzymes.

6. *Tenderness*: if present, it is in favor of an inflammatory lesion like osteomyelitis.

7. *Mobility*: if the sinus is fixed to the underlying bone, the diagnosis of osteomyelitis is very likely. Fixity to subjacent lymph node is suggestive of tuberculosis or malignancy.

8. *Regional lymph nodes*: they may be nonspecific or specific, such as tuberculosis or malignancy.

9. *Probing*: it should be done by gentle force, with a blunt malleable probe, taking extreme care not to create a false passage, which may convert a sinus into a fistula. The depth of the

sinus, presence of a foreign body and commu-nication with a hollow viscus are made out by this examination. In perianal sinuses, it has to be done under direct vision by a bivalved rectal speculum, generally before surgery.

Investigations

I) Besides routine investigations, examina-tion of discharge for bacteria/fungi to identify the underlying organism, such as M.tuberculo-sis, Entameba histolytica, Nocardia madurae or Actinomyces israelii. If the discharge is col-lected in a test tube filled with water and shaken, 'sulphur granules' can be made out at the bottom, pathognomonic of actinomycosis. Under the microscope, these granules show Gram positive filaments and Gram negative clubs (which are only tissue debris and not spores).

ii) Immunologic studies for tuberculosis (Mantoux, IgA/IgM/IgG, PCR)

iii) X-ray:

(a) Plain skiagram may show a radio-opaque foreign body or sequestrum (dead bone appears more dense, as it has more mineral content than normal bone).

(b) Contrast study: *Sinogram* or *fistulogram* is done by injecting a contrast material, such as iothalamate meglumine (Conray) or sodium diatrizoate (Urographin) into the sinus/fistula, through a polythene catheter introduced and mouth closed water-tight, by a purse-string suture tied around, to prevent back-spill; skiagrams (two views) will indicate its entire course and relation to important structures in the vicinity, the presence of abscess cavity in the depth, the ramifications of the tract etc. providing information useful during surgery.

iv) CT and MRI scan: These sophisticated investigations are useful in identifying an abscess in relation to a sinus or a fistula, espe-cially in the chest, abdomen or pelvis. An MRI also gives an excellent definition of the multiple tracts of a fistula.

v) Biopsy: This is very crucial in intractable cases, to establish the diagnosis, once and for all. If there is no mass at the surface, the sinus track may be gently dilated and curetted, col-lecting the lining granulation tissue for histopathology.

Treatment

The definitive treatment of a sinus/fistula, natu-rally depends upon the cause. Chemotherapy for tuberculosis, Madura mycosis or actino-mycosis will generally make the sinus heal, whereas if it is secondary to a foreign body or a sequestrum, it should be removed surgically. All side tracks should also be removed and any abscess cavity present liberally drained. In cases of duodenal/ jejunal fistula, liberal appli-cation of zinc oxide/calamine (Siloderm) around the mouth would prevent skin excoria-tion due to activated proteolytic enzymes.

In high output fistula, it may be convenient to apply an 'ostomy' bag over it, not only to avoid frequent need for dressings, but also to mea-sure the quantity, helpful in assessing the prog-ress. A fistula requires surgery more often than a sinus. Excision of a perianal fistula and its ram-

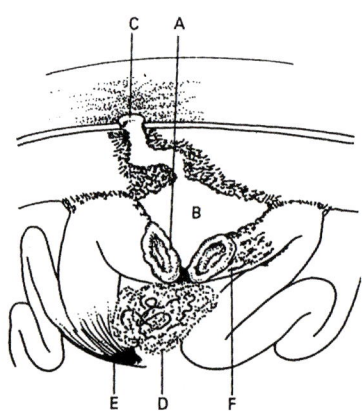

Fig. 16.1. Causes of nonhealing of an intestinal fistula
a) total disruption of the anastomosis
b) abcsess in relation to the track
c) epithelialization of the track
d) foreign body
e) distal bowel obstruction
f) specific pathology (TB, Crohn's, actinomycosis or malignancy)
        (courtesy: Laxmi Hospital, Kakinada)

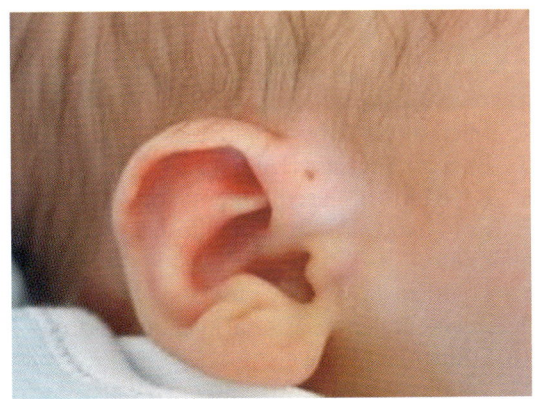

Fig. 16.2. Preauricular sinus
(courtesy: Dr B S Madhusudanan, Chennai)

ifications (*fistulectomy*) or complete laying open (*fistulotomy*) may be curative, however, if specific disease like amebiasis, tuberculosis or Crohn's disease underlies the fistula, appropriate therapy should be combined for total cure.

In a situation where excisional surgery would compromise vital physiology, such as a high fistula-in-ano, injection of tissue adhesive glue (cyanoacrylate) into the track, to cause obliteration, is a recent advance in its management.

Sinuses in special areas

Preauricular sinus

The auricle develops from the fusion of six tubercles grouped around the external auditory osteum. Failure of fusion of these tubercles leads to the formation of either a cyst (dermoid) or a sinus, located just in front of the helix of the ear. Rarely, the track passes through the cartilage, to open into the inner aspect of the external ear.
Differential diagnosis: Tuberculous sinus from the preauricular lymphadenitis or Infected sebaceous cyst

Treatment: Careful excision of the entire cyst or sinus, by preliminary injection of a dye (methylene blue) into the track, to ensure total removal, sometimes including a bit of pinna cartilage.

Median mental sinus: This is a rare congenital condition seen in children, as a sinus adherent to jaw in the midline submental region, due to improper fusion of both halves of Meckel's cartilage, destined to form the mandible. After excluding dental sepsis as the cause of the sinus by an x-ray, total excision is the treatment.

Submental (dental) sinus: is due to an apical infection of the lower incisor teeth, leading to an abscess, breaks through the mandibular table and tracks between the two mentalis muscles, to open in the submental region (often in the midline), repeatedly discharging pus. Typically the sinus is fixed to the jaw and on suspicion, a dental x-ray would confirm the 'root' cause, which has to be dealt appropriately. The culprit tooth may have to be extracted as a last resort, for permanent cure of the disease, by eliminating the source of infection.

Watering-can perineum (multiple urethral fistulae)

Commonly arising following a rupture or drainage of periurethral abscess, under the background of a stricture, urine leaks through multiple openings resembling a watering-can. The fistulae heal, if the stricture is adequately treated, either by dilatation or endoscopic internal urethrotomy. Rarely urethroplasty (reconstruction of urethra) using perineal skin flap or buccal mucosa, may be required.

Pilonidal sinus: see chapter 26
Perianal sinus: see chapter 74

Thyroglossal sinus: see chapter 88

Branchial sinus: see chapter 90

17 Gangrene

Definition: GANGRENE is macroscopic death of tissue, with superadded putre-faction. This commonly occurs in parts accessible to microbes, such as limbs, appendix, bowel or gall bladder, whereas if bacteria cannot readily invade, it results in *infarction*, as in brain, heart, spleen, kidney or testis.

Ulcer or gangrene?

If there is a black patch over a toe due to ischemia, should it be called as an ischemic ulcer or gangrene, since both are due to death of tissue (necrosis)? By definition, ulcer is only skin deep, hence if on examination, only skin appears to be involved, it is an ulcer. If deeper tissues are also involved, it should be labeled as gangrene.

Causes of gangrene

a. Vascular causes are the commonest, to produce gangrene of extremity

1. Senile endarteritis obliterans
2. Thrombosis of an atherosclerotic artery
3. Embolism, from the heart (in atrial fibrillation, bacterial endocarditis, myocardial infarction etc), atheromatous plaques and aneurysm

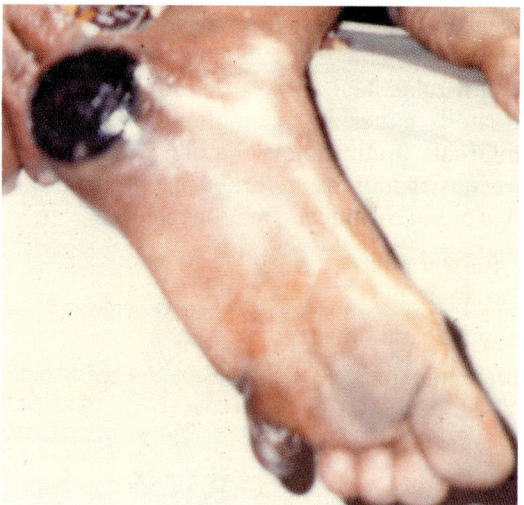

Fig. 17.1. Gangrene of heel and little toe (TAO) (courtesy: Halsted Surgical Clinic, Chennai)

4. Microangiopathy of diabetes
5. Buerger's disease (TAO)
6. Raynaud's disease/phenomenon
7. Cold exposure: frost bite, trench foot, chilblains etc.
8. Ergotism (St. Antony's foot)
9. Accidental intra-arterial injection of drugs
10. Strangulated bowel
11. Venous gangrene
12. Syphilitic gangrene, due to endarteritis

b. Infective

Furuncle (boil), *carbuncle, cancrum oris, gas gangrene, Meleney's gangrene* of abdominal wall, *synergestic* (Fournier's) *gangrene* of the scrotum, *necrotizing fasciitis, diabetic gangrene* etc.

c. Traumatic, may be direct or indirect

Direct: Crush injury, pressure sores and constriction gangrene of strangulated bowel

Indirect: Gangrene from injury to vessels as in supracondylar fracture of humerus or femur

d. Physical: Burns, scalds, frostbite, irradiation and electricity

e. Chemical: Acid or alkali burns

f. Neurological syringomyelia, tabes dorsalis, peripheral nerve lesions

Features of gangrene

Arterial pulsations, venous filling and capillary response to pressure, are absent. The part is cold and discolored, without sensations or functions. It may be of dry or moist types.

DRY GANGRENE

This occurs in ischemia of slow onset, with intact venous flow, such as atherosclerosis or thrombo-angiitis obliterans (TAO). The tissues are dessicated, dry and shrivelled, blackish from disintegration of hemoglobin and greasy to touch (*mummified*). A definite *line of demarcation* is seen, between the dead and viable tissue.

MOIST (WET) GANGRENE

This occurs as a result of sudden arterial and venous occlusion as in acute arterial occlusion, due to thromboembolism, strangulation of bowel or due to aggressive infection, as in diabetes mellitus. Bacterial invasion and putrefaction invariably occur, the affected part becomes swollen and discolored due to cellulitis and the epidermis may be raised with blebs. Crepitus may be felt due to infection by gas-forming organisms. The rapid spread of infection and tissue necrosis overrun local defenses, prevent formation of a line of demarcation and results in toxemia or septicemia, with a threat of losing both limb and life, unless promptly intervened.

Differential diagnosis

I)   Ischemic ulcer: This has to be differentiated from gangrene. It develops almost always at the tips of toes or fingers and is only 'skin-deep'; if deeper tissues are dead, it becomes a gangrene.

ii)   Trophic ulcer: see under ulcer (chapter 15)

iii)   Spreading cellulitis due to non-clostridial gas-forming organisms, such as pyogenic cocci and bacteroides, may mimic gas gangrene in many respects, especially if it follows trauma.

Investigations

Routine blood, urine studies, including sugar, lipid profile and VDRL, a chest x-ray, an electrocardiogram etc.

Specific: largely depend upon the type of gangrene.

X-ray of the part for calcification of vessels, gas bubbles in the depth and any bony involvement or fractures

Segmental blood pressure recordings, ankle/brachial or toe/ankle index

Doppler/Duplex recording of arteries/veins of the part (see chapters 77 & 82)

Angiogram, if direct arterial surgery is contemplated

Discharge from the ulcer for Gram stain and culture

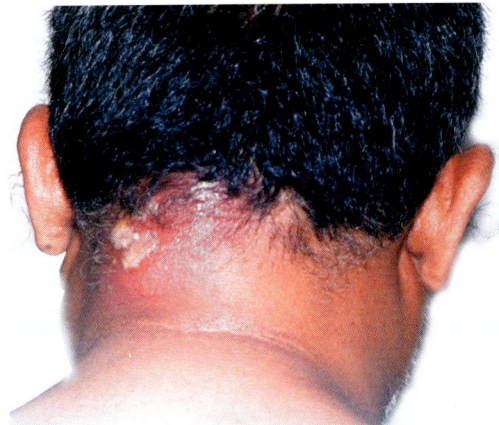

Fig. 17.2. Carbuncle of the nape of neck (courtesy: Lifeline Hospitals, Chennai)

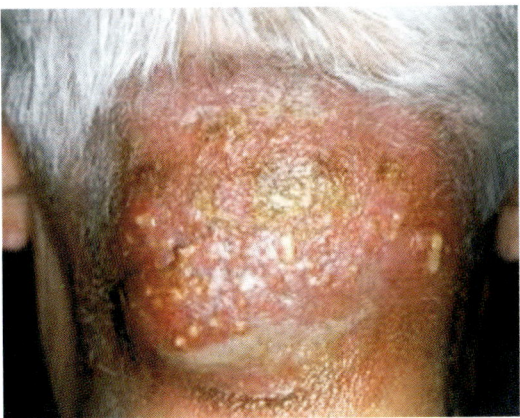

Fig. 17.3. carbuncle, nape of neck (courtesy: Laxmi Hospital, Kakinada)

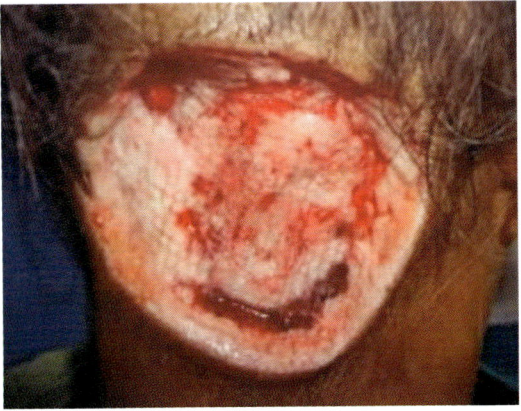

Fig. 17.4. Debrided carbuncle (courtesy: Laxmi Hospital, Kakinada)

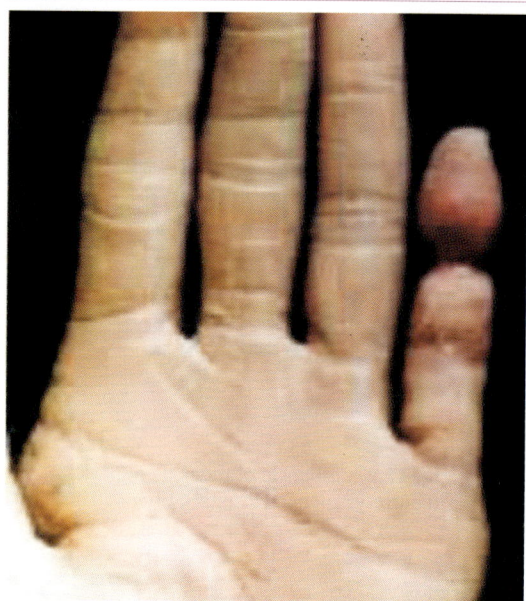

Fig. 17.5. Ainhum of little finger

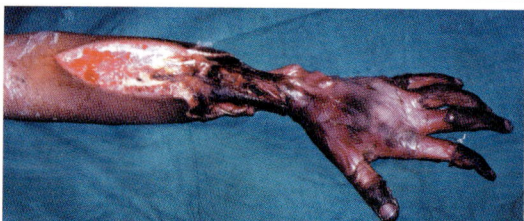

Fig.17.6. Extensive gangrene of the hand and the forearm due to high voltage electrical burn (courtesy: Halsted Surgical Clinic, Chennai)

Treatment

General: Diabetes, dyslipidemia, cardiac arrhythmia and anemia have to be attended to, if present. Appropriate antibiotics for infection, including gas gangrene, should be started. Associated arterial insufficiency has to be treated on its merits, as described in chapter 77.

Local: The limb is kept dry and the skin protected from pressure. Minor surgical procedures like excision of dead tissue (debridement) or draining an abscess, may be done as necessary. A life saving guillotine amputaion may be required for a badly crushed limb or rapidly spreading gangrene, either clostridial or otherwise.

SPECIFIC TYPES OF GANGRENE

(I) **BOIL or FURUNCLE** (furnace: heat): It is an infective gangrene, caused by Staphylococcal infection of hair follicle or sebaceous gland, with perifolliculitis. Initially the infection causes suppuration and central necrosis which drains out after a few days, through the necrosed overlying skin. Rarely, it may resolve without suppuration (blind boil). Diabetics are more prone for this disease, especially in summer season, due to excessive sweating.

Clinical features: A painful indurated swelling develops, gradually spreading to the surrounding tissues. In areas like external ear or nostril, where the skin is attached to the underlying cartilage, tension builds up in the lesion, causing extreme pain. Acute regional lymphadenitis may be present.

Stye (syn: hardeolum) is boil over the eye lid in

	Feature	Diabetic	Atherosclerotic
1	Age	Young	Elderly
2	Type of gangrene	Moist	Dry
3	H/o claudication	Absent	Present
4	Location	Any where	Mostly toes
5	Peripheral pulses	Well felt	Absent
6	Pathology	Microangiopathy	Macroangiopathy
7	Neuropathy	Often associated	No association
8	Arterial surgery	Not possible	May be possible
9	Sympathectomy	No effect	May help under 50
10	Level of amputation	Limited	Minimum is below-knee

Table – 17.1: Differences between diabetic and atherosclerotic angiopathy

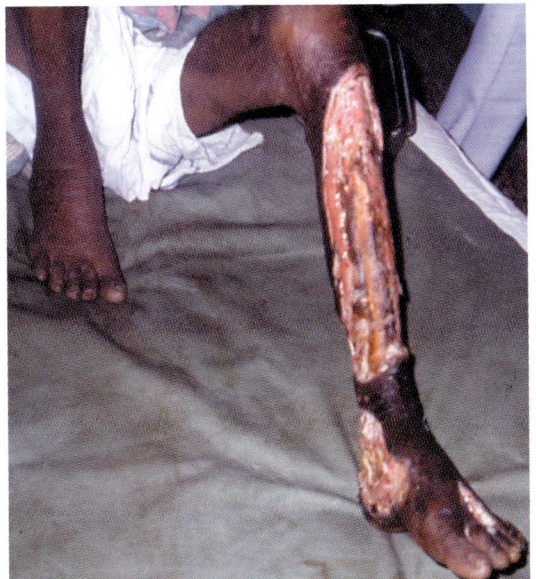

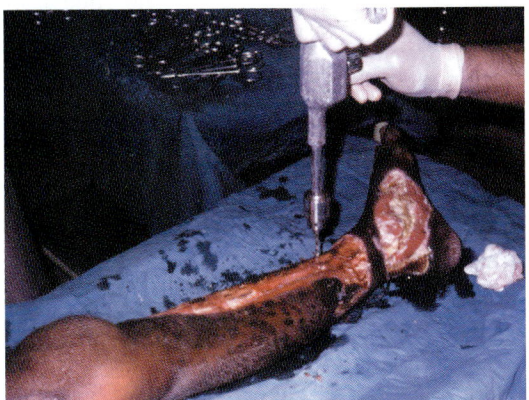

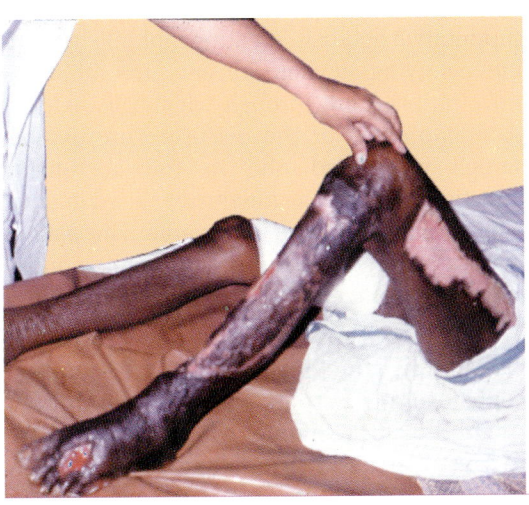

Fig. 17.7. Extensive necrotizing diabetic infection of leg and foot, exposing the medial surface of the tibia
17.8. Result of daily liberal debridement; drill holes are being made into the exposed bone to allow growth of granulation tissue from the marrow
17.9. Final result following skin grafting
(courtesy: Halsted Surgical Clinic, Chennai)

relation to the eyelash follicle.

Dangerous boil: Boil (or any infection) over the face (the so-called dangerous area), may cause intracranial spread of infection into cavernous sinus, via anterior facial vein and ophthalmic veins, with serious consequences; hence should be aggressively treated.

Treatment: Under cover of appropriate antibiotics, extraction of the overlying hair allows drainage of the cavity and application of local heat, leads to resolution. Rarely it may need drainage by a surgical incision.

Hidradenitis suppurativa (apocrinitis): Recurrent multiple boils usually seen in the axillae and sometimes groins, leading to recurrent multiple abscesses, with considerable scarring from the healed lesions. Common the ages of 10 to 30, with female preponderance (3:1), can be very troublesome to eradicate.

Under cover of appropriate antibiotics, selected by the sensitivity study, the abscesses have to be laid open, but recurrence is the rule. As a last resort, the entire skin bearing the disease may have to be excised and defect primarily sutured or covered with skin graft,

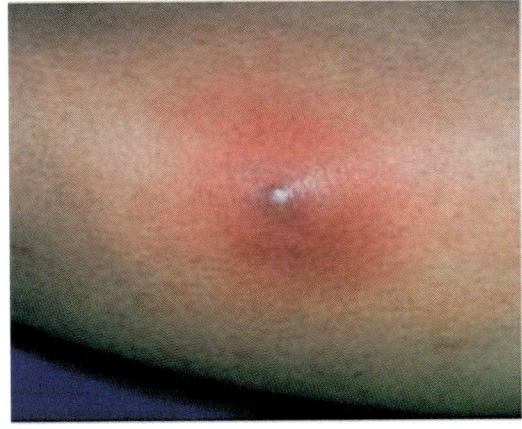

Fig.17.10. Boil or Furuncle

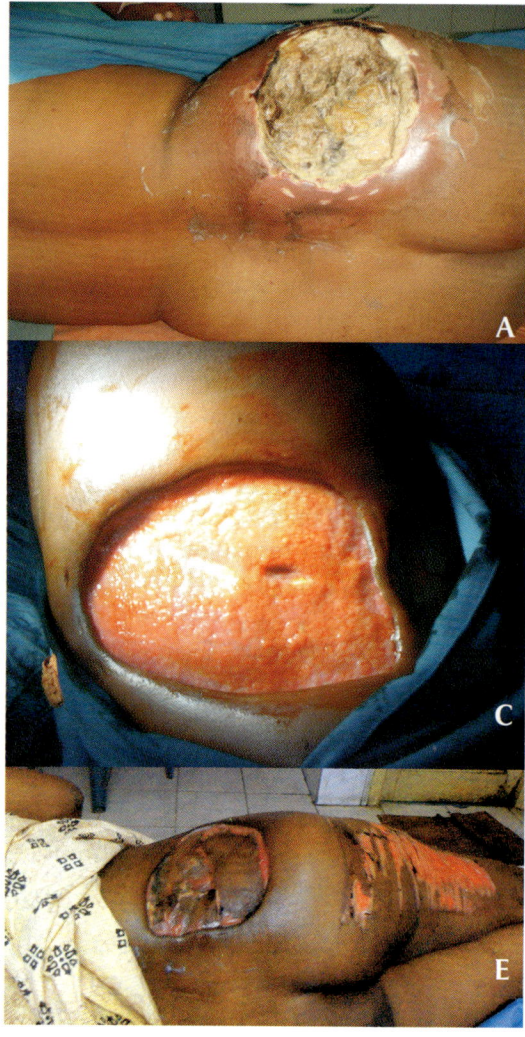

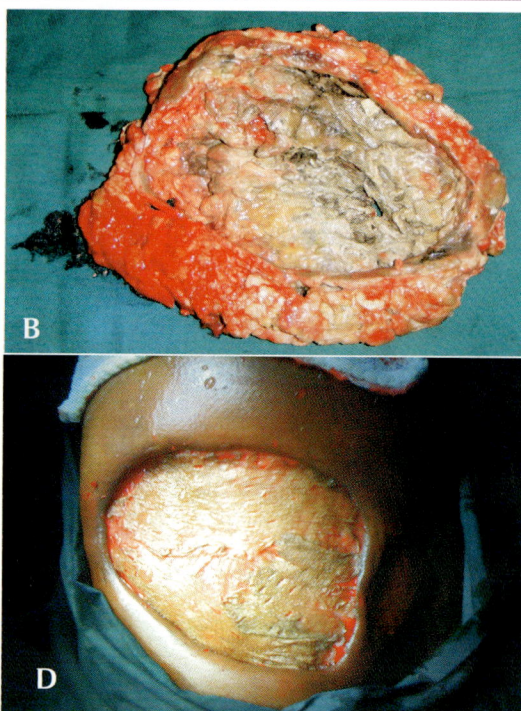

Fig. 17.11.
A. Necrotizing fasciitis of gluteal region following an intramuscular injection
B. Excised necrotic tissue
C. Meticulous daily debridement resulting in a healthy granulating ulcer
D. Split thickness skin graft applied over the ulcer
E. Final result after total 'take' of the graft
(courtesy: Halsted Surgical Clinic, Chennai)

with gratifying result. Anti-perspirant drugs (such as propranolol) and sprays may be of help in reducing recurrences.

(ii) CARBUNCLE (means charcoal and it was thought to resemble smoldering coal): It is an infective gangrene of skin and subcutaneous tissue, usually caused by Staphylococcus aureus. It is uncommon under 40, seen often in diabetic male patients and those with poor immunity, common sites being over the back of neck (nape) and chest, where the skin is thick and less vascular.

The skin becomes painful and red, with subcutaneous induration, which goes on to supputative necrosis, creating multiple holes in the overlying devitalized skin, resembling a sieve (cribriform), through which pus exudes, pathognomonic of the disease. Considerable slough is formed due to the necrotizing infection and if not aggressively treated in time, may spread, involving larger area. The patient may become very toxic and glycemic control may be difficult, endangering life.

Treatment: Appropriate antibiotics such as cloxacillin, flucloxacillin, 3rd generation cephalosporins, strict glycemic control by round-the-clock soluble insulin therapy, have to be instituted immediately, but early

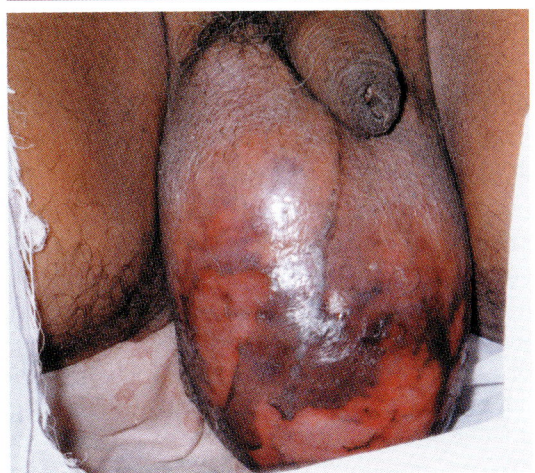

Fig. 17.12. Fournier's gangrene of scrotum
(courtesy: Lifeline Hospitals, Chennai)

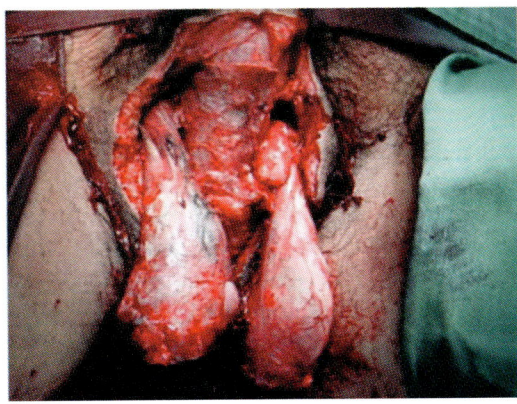

Fig. 17.13. Fournier's gangrene of scrotum. Both testes
exposed following excision of skin
(courtesy: Lifeline Hospitals, Chennai)

deroofing and slough excision by a cruciate incision, using minimal analgesia, could be life saving. If methycillin-resistant staphylococcus aureus (MRSA) is suspected, higher antibiotics like vancomycin or meropenum, may have to be used. Once the infection is contained, the wound granulates and contracts with amazing speed, rarely requiring skin cover by grafting. Use of infrared therapy may be helpful to promote granulation tissue.

Renal carbuncle: It is also common in diabetics, following debilitating illness and those with immune-compromized state, initialy starts as an abscess in the renal parenchyma, usually due to hematogenous infection by Staphylococcus or coliform bacteria from a focus of sepsis elsewhere. It may also follow from secondary infection of a hematoma due to a blunt injury to the kidney.

Local signs of inflammation, resembling perinephric abscess and usual constitutional symptoms may be present and gradually a part of the renal parenchyma is replaced by capsulated necrotic mass. An SOL may be reported in relation to the kidney by ultrasonography or CT scan, mimicking malignancy. Under cover of high antibiotics, image-guided percutaneous needle aspiration may be attempted, failing which, open surgery to excise the slough and drain the pus, is required.

(iii) CANCRUM ORIS (syn: Necrotizing stomatitis) is a severe form of stomatitis, leading to infective gangrene, occurring in malnourished, immune-compromised children, typically following an attack of typhoid, gastroenteritis, diphtheria, measles, whooping cough or worm infestation. Dental sepsis is often blamed, since the presence of erupted teeth appears necessary for the onset of the disease and it starts from the gingivae. It is caused by opportunistic bacteria such as Vincent's organisms (Borrelia vincentii and Fusobacterium fusiforme), starts as ulceration over the cheek and lips, goes on to deeper

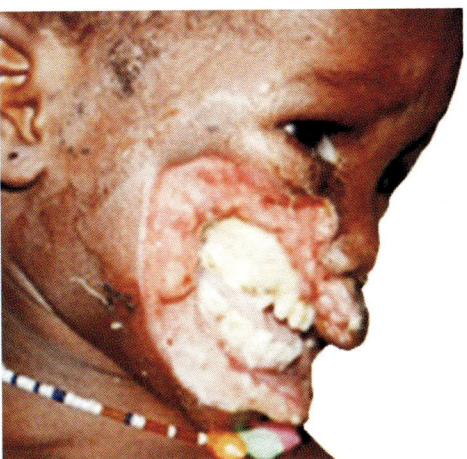

Fig. 17.14. Cancrum oris

planes, causing necrosis of all the layers of those structures, including the underlying bone, leaving a wide defect. As a result, the patient's nutrition is further worsened, which may lead to fatal outcome. In view of the impaired tissue response, local signs of inflammation may be minimal, but systemic complications such as septicemia, SIRS or MODS may supervene. In course of natural healing, considerable scarring and disfigurement may result, restricting the jaw movements.

Treatment: Nutrition has to be improved either by nasogastric or parenteral feeding. Infection has to be aggressively controlled by appropriate antibiotics, including high dose penicillin, cephalosporins and metronidazole and gentle excision of slough has to be carried out. Ultimate defect may need reconstructive cosmetic surgery, often requiring pedicled tube skin grafting, when the condition improves. Rarely a wedge resection of mandible may be needed (Esmarch's operation), for ankylosis of temporomandibular joint. The overall prognosis of this condition is poor.

(iv) DIABETIC GANGRENE is a multifactorial variety of infective gangrene:

a) *microangiopathy*, leading to tissue hypoxia

b) *neuropathy*, dampens inflammation

c) increased but unutilized tissue glucose, due to lack of insulin, the so called 'poverty amongst plenty', nourishing invading microbes

d) *immunosuppression*, occurring in diabetes, reducing local tissue resistance and phagocytic activity.

e) *Macroangiopathy* due to hastened atherosclerosis in diabetics is another factor, significantly influencing the outcome. Though microangiopathy is ubiquitous in diabetes, there appears to be no actual vasoocclusive disease of the small vessels, contrary to the earlier belief. Hence they should not be denied the benefit of arterial reconstruction, if associated macroangiopathy exists. Angiopathy is related more to its duration rather than the severity of diabetes, hence it was rarely seen in IDDM in the pre-insulin era, as the survival was not long enough.

Callosities and trophic ulcers develop on the sole, whereby infection gains entry into deeper planes, involving fascia, tendons and bone.

The differences between diabetic and atherosclerotic gangrene are given in table 17.1, but it should be realized that both being common disorders, they may coexist, with overlapping features.

Investigations

Routine blood and urine examination. X-ray of the foot to rule out osteomyelitis.

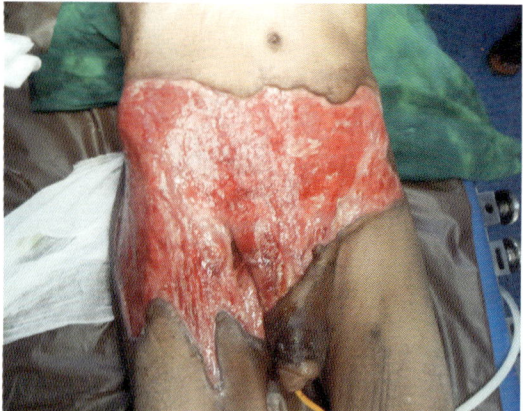

Fig. 17.15. Meleney's gangrene of the abdominal wall, after slough excision and control of infection

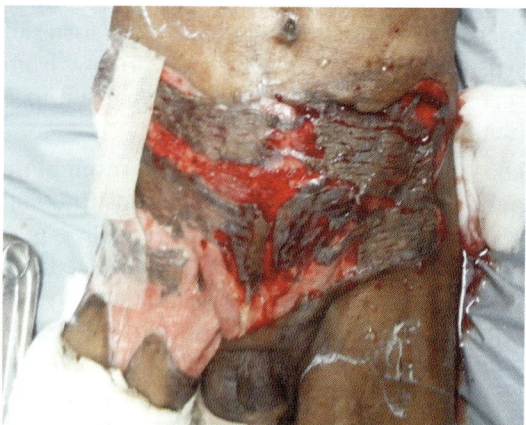

Fig. 17.16. Meleney's gangrene of the abdominal wall, after split skin graft applied

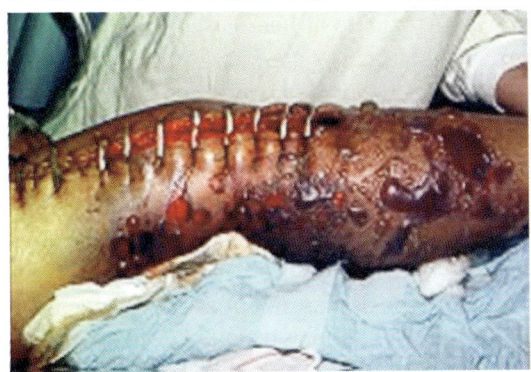

Fig. 17.17. Gas gangrene, lower limb
(courtesy: Mohan Nursing Home, Chennai)

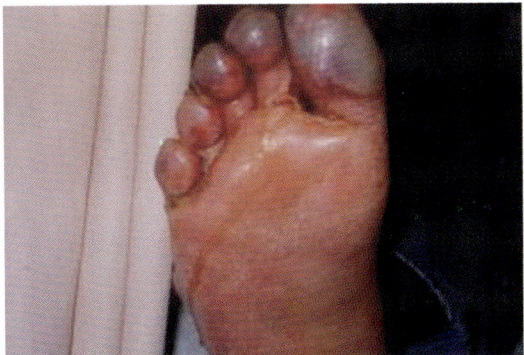

Fig. 17.19. Frostbite

Treatment

In view of its *labile* nature, due to infection or stress, the diabetes mellitus must be brought under control by *soluble insulin*, given round-the-clock, under plasma/urine sugar monitoring. Thorough wound debridement should be done to allow it to granulate, because it is a race between the infection and the patient. The key word in the management of diabetic infection is *aggressiveness* in excising the devitalized tissue and laying open pockets of pus, every day while carrying out wound dressings. Experience has shown that if the vascularity is adequate, even apparently hopeless necrotizing infections may be brought under control by this approach, salvaging the limbs. If arterial insufficiency is coexistent, loss of limb may be inevitable, unless it is simultaneously investigated and treated on its merits. Use of myocutaneous flaps (e.g. medial head of gastrocnemius may be rotated into the sole) or other reconstructive procedures may be needed to give cover to nonhealing diabetic ulcers. If not treated aggressively and adequately, the patient has to 'pay through his foot' and may ultimately leave hospital without it.

(v) TRAUMATIC GANGRENE

This may be due to crushing (direct), injury to blood supply (indirect) or protracted pressure, bed sores being a common example of the latter.

Extensive hopeless crush injuries of extremities are best treated by early amputation, at an appropriate level. Cut injuries or dismembered fingers/limbs are often salvaged by microvascular reconstruction, provided the severed parts are brought 'clean and cold', within a few hours following injury, to institutions having necessary infrastructure and expertise. (see

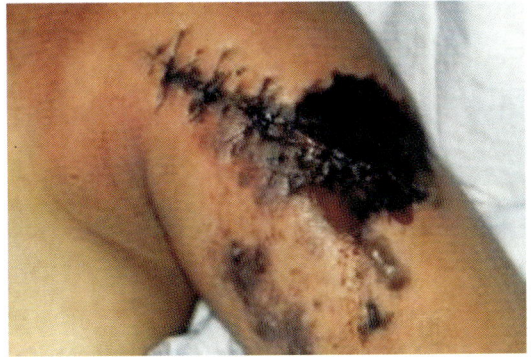

Fig. 17.18. Gas gangrene, deltoid region
(courtesy: Halsted Surgical Clinic, Chennai)

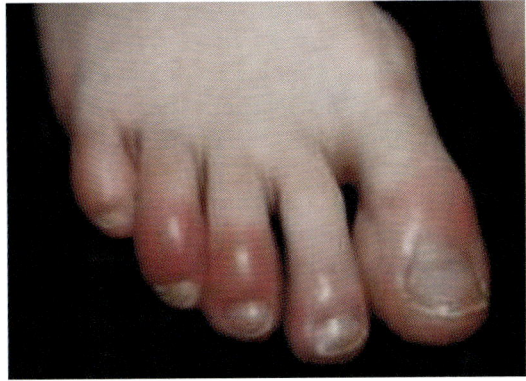

Fig. 17.20. Chilblains

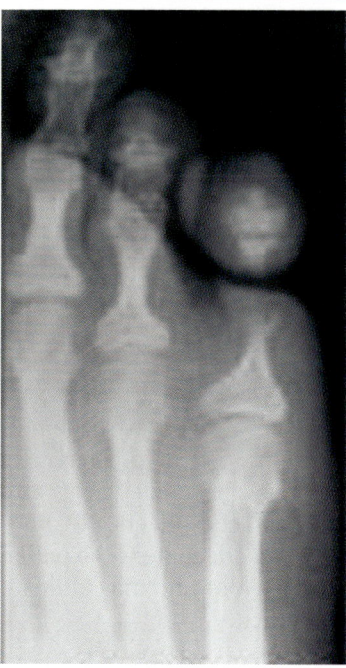

Fig. 17.21. Ainhum - X- ray of foot

chapter 77 on microvascular surgery)

Expanding hematoma, absent peripheral pulses and cold extremity indicate major vascular injury. If it is associated with a fracture in that region, vascular repair should be done only after stabilizing the bone by internal/external fixation. Either trimming and direct anastomosis or vein grafting should be done (see chapter 77).

(vi) GAS GANGRENE is a type of necrotizing soft tissue infection, with high propensity for wide spread tissue destruction, exotoxemia and high mortality, caused by *Clostridium welchii* (perfringens), *C. novyi* (edematiens), *C. septicum* and *C. histolyticum*. These anaerobic organisms are commensals of the gastrointestinal tract and form a source of potential infection in bowel necrosis including gallbladder and appendix, perineal surgery, septic abortion and ischemic muscle injury. The exotoxins produced by them are:

(1) lecithinase, also known as alfa toxin (hemolysis, toxemia and dermonecrosis),

(2) beta toxin (toxic necrosis),

(3) proteinase (breaks down collagen) and

(4) hyaluronidase, also known as invasin or spreading factor (breaks down hyaluronic acid, a cement substance of tissues); all resposible for toxemia and rapid invasion, more in the longitudinal (along muscle bundles) than transverse direction, to occur.

The gas in the tissues, not necessarily specific of Clostridial infection, is usually due to anaerobic and rarely aerobic bacterial metabolism, resulting in the production of insoluble gases such as hydrogen, nitrogen and methane.

Clinical features

When typical local pain, skin necrosis, discoloration, blistering, crepitus and tachycardia are present in a patient injured in a road accident, the diagnosis is easy, but in subtle cases, much myonecrosis may occur before clinical recognition. Later on, signs of toxemia, such as irritability, dyspnea, tachycardia out of proportion to fever, may develop. They may also foam in internal organs such liver (foaming liver). A plain skiagram and CT scan may be very helpful in identifying the extent of disease, by showing slivers of gas. Bacteriology of the tissue fluid may clinch the invader, Gram positive rods (Clostridia) or cocci (strepto or staphylococci).

Treatment

Broad spectrum antibiotics, including high doses of crystalline penicillin should be given immediately on suspicion: alternately clinda-

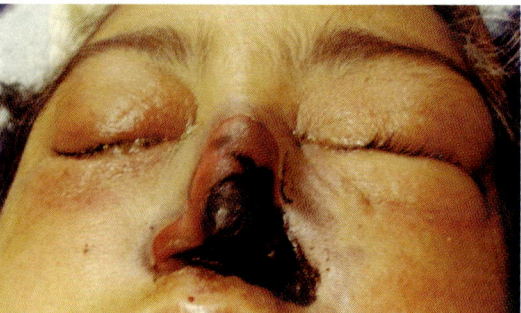

Fig. 17.22. Severe necrotizing diabetic infection with gangrene of nose and cellulitis of face

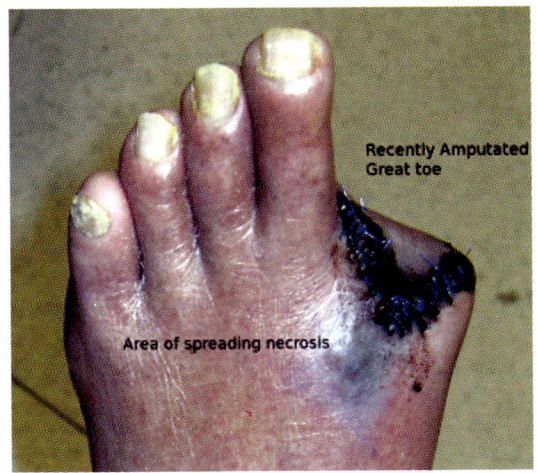

Fig. 17.23. Reuslt of premature amputation for a toe gangrene due to fem-pop occlusion, before revascularization

mycin and metronidazole may be used. *Polyvalent antiserum* (22500 i.u) against all the three strains (C.welchii 9000; C.edematiens 9000 and C.septicum 4500i.u) may be given both as prophylaxis and therapy for established cases, but its role in the latter is doubtful. Liberal surgical debridement is often lifesaving; this may amount to a guillotine amputation in extensive cases with severe toxemia. Role of hyperbaric oxygen therapy, given at 300% atmospheric pressure, in a specialized chamber, is controversial, besides it is cumbersome and not possible in all centres. Though it

has been shown to improve results in Clostridial infections, it has no effect in non-Clostridial infections, besides its complications such as pneumothorax, eardrum injury, air embolism, neurotoxicity, visual defects, tendency for seizures etc. Other supportive measures including blood transfusion, have to be employed. Overall mortality in this disease is around 25%.

(vii) IDIOPATHIC SYNERGISTIC GANGRENE of scrotum (syn: Fournier's gangrene) is an acute ischemic necrosis of the scrotal skin, due to synergistic action of staphylococcus aureus and microaerophilic streptococci (either hemolytic or nonhemolytic), causing obliterative arteritis of dartos and skin. The onset is sudden, without any heralding systemic signs, the entire scrotal skin turning black 'overnight'. Rarely it may be a disturbing complication following surgery for inguinal hernia, circumcision or scrotal hydrocele. Toxemia sets in slowly, with suppuration occurring under the dead skin, which pours out when the overlying skin is incised. Similar, but more morbid lesions may occur following surgery on the abdominal wall, groin and perineum, known as *Meleney's progressive synergistic gangrene*, or spontaneously in any part of the body, known as *necrotizing fasciitis*, with extensive involvement of skin, subcutaneous tissue, fascia and muscles.

The common type of necrotizing fasciitis (type-I) is polymicrobial (anaerobes, coliforms and streptococci. The rarer type-II is monomicro-

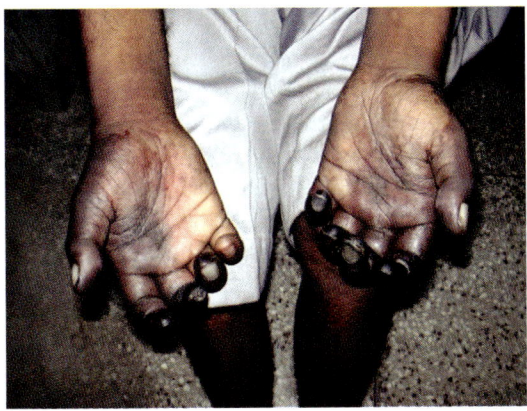

Fig. 17.24. Bilateral symmetrical digital gangrene due to autoimmune vasculitis
(courtesy: Halsted Surgical Clinic, Chennai)

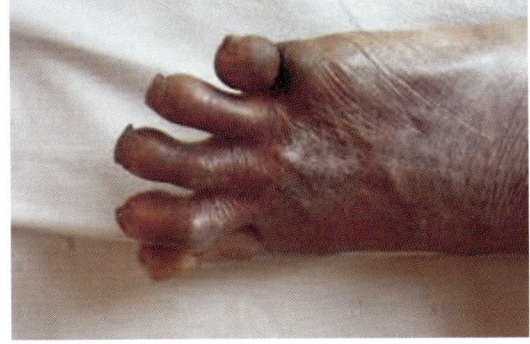

Fig.17.25. Ainhum of little toe
(courtesy: Halsted Surgical Clinic, Chennai)

Feature	Dry gangrene	Moist gangrene
Onset	Slow	Sudden
Etiology	Gradual occlusion of artery	Sudden occlusion of artery & vein
Spread	Slow	Fast
Line of demarcation	Present	Absent
Appearance	Dry & mummified	Turgid & swollen
Adjacent cellulitis	Minimal	Severe
Constitutional symptoms	Minimal	Present
Infection	Minimal	Gross
Treatment	Elective	Emergency
Threat to life	Minimal	Considerable

Table - 17.2. Differences between dry and moist (wet) gangrene

bial, usually by group-A, β-hemolytic strepto-cocci.

Treatment

Not much different from that of gas gangrene; liberal slough excision and irrigation with diluted hydrogen peroxide solution should be done, under cover of wide spectrum antibiotics, selected by microbiological studies. Other supportive therapy, such as macro and micro-nutrients, anabolic steroids, blood transfusions etc are necessary. After excision of necrosed skin in scrotal gangrene, the testes hang by the spermatic cords without any support, but the lax scrotal skin contracts so fast, that providing skin cover by surgery is rarely necessary. *In general Fournier's gangrene carries a much better prognosis than the other types of necrotizing soft tissue infections.* In atypical cases of such necrotizing infections, rarely underlying specific diseases, such as fungal or tuberculous

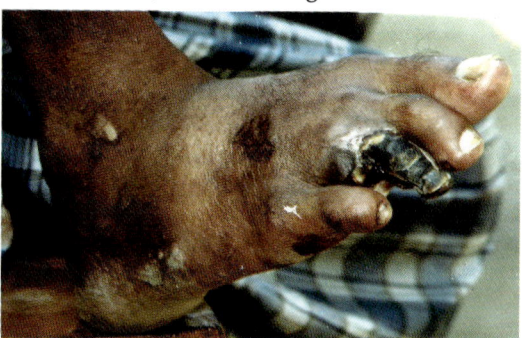

Fig. 17.26. Toe gangrene due to Buerger's disease (courtesy: Halsted Surgical Clinic, Chennai)

infection may be responsible for 'resistance' to conventional therapy.

Gangrene due to arterial occlusion (see under limb ischemia, chapters 77 & 79)

Drugs, such as ergot alkaloids taken for migraine can affect the ear, nose, fingers and toes. Repeated unintentional ingestion of ergot leaves by those living in forests, produced pedal ischemia, known as *St. Antony's fire. Infiltration of a local anesthetic mixed with adrenaline for digital or penile blocks, may produce severe vasoconstriction, leading to disastrous tissue necrosis.* Similar ischemic accidents of spinal cord have been reported following addition of adrenaline to the spinal anesthetic agents, with an aim of prolonging their effect.

Acidental intra-arterial injection of drugs: described in chapter 79

Ainhum (syn: dactylolysis spontanea)

This affects mostly African males, who walked bare-footed in their childhood. A fissure appears at the level of the inter-phalangeal joint of a toe, usually the 5th, which becomes a fibrous band, encircling the digit, causing necrosis. The treatment is either by a relaxing incision, 'Z' plasty or later amputation, which happens spontaneously as the disease progresses. The etiology of this disease is unknown.

VENOUS GANGRENE described in chapter 82

Physical causes of gangrene

Exposure to cold

Local pathological response to exposure to cold

include frost nip, frost bite, which may be superficial or deep, trench foot and chilblains.

In *frost nip*, there is cutaneous blanching, sensory impairment and while rewarming, painful hyperemia and with only loss of epidermis, is evident.

In *superficial frost bite*, there is patchy full thickness skin loss, with a slow tendency for reepithelialization within weeks.

In *deep frost bite*, more extensive tissue loss due to spasm and microthrombosis of blood vessels, the extent is often difficult to assess, leading to development of dry gangrene, with a line of demarcation.

The is due to more prolonged exposure to nonfreezing temperatures, muscular inactivity and illfitting shoes. There is sensory loss, producing a feeling of walking on cotton wool. Erythema and superficial necrosis of skin may be present, associated with constitutional symptoms like fever, malaise and weight loss. Initial anesthesia may be replaced by hyperalgesia. When it heals, it leaves thin pigmented skin, with wasting of fat and muscles and joint stiffness. This condition may rarely occur in the upper limb in shipwreck survivors.

Chilblains (syn: perniosis, erythema pernio) are multiple localized swellings due to recurrent cold injury, mimicking Raynaud's phenomenon, often with intractable itching and pain. The disease starts in childhood, with familial tendency and female preponderance. The nodules are infiltrated by round cells, which may ulcerate, discharging serous fluid. A variant of this, known as *Bazin's disease* is seen in adolescent women, due to cold sensitivity of over exposed areas.

Treatment

Besides routine investigations, ankle/toe index and TcO_2 estimation are useful in assessing the magnitude of ischemia. The affected part should be warmed veryslowly, to room temperature. Anticoagulant, antiplatelet and rheological agents are beneficial given early, to improve microcirculation, so also intra-arterial vasodilators and sympathetic blockade, to relieve vasospasm. Amputation should be delayed, keeping the probability of viable deeper tissues, till a definite line of demarcation develops.

Exposure to heat

Thermal and electrical burns may cause extensive necrosis of the soft tissue, depending upon the degree and duration of exposure.

CHEMICAL GANGRENE

They are due to chemical burns caused by strong acids or alkalis and are often the result of industrial accidents, assaults or inadvertent use of undiluted solvents and drain cleaners. The gangrene is due to direct effect on tissue, besides secondary vascular damage. Some chemicals, such as phenol, hydrofluoric acid may produce severe systemic effects from their absorption and may prove fatal. Overzealous attempts to neutralize the offending agent, may add thermal burns, due to the heat generated during the chemical reaction, further complicating the matter.

18 Abdominal Tuberculosis

(syn: Koch's abdomen)

ABDOMINAL TUBERCULOSIS is mostly a gut-borne infection, the other source being genital tract in females. Since *pasteurization* of milk has become a mandatory requirement in the dairy industry, bovine (dysgonic - no affinity to glycerol) species of Mycobacterium tuberculosis has been replaced by human (eugonic - affinity to glycerol) strains. Pre-existing open pulmonary infection is the rule, bacilli gaining entry into the gut through swallowed sputum. Consumption of raw (unprotected) milk, as a source of infection, is still possible, mostly in the rural population.

Microbiology

Mycobacterium tuberculosis (human) and M. bovis (bovine) are acid and alcohol fast, aerobic non-motile, non-capsulated and non-sporing bacilli. Diagnosis may be confirmed by culture (Lowenstein Jensen or Dorsett's egg media) or guinea pig inoculation, approximately taking 2 and 6 weeks respectively. The infection may be prevented by BCG (Bacilli Calmettee Guerine) vaccination. The other Mycobacteria relevant to man are, M.leprae, M.smegmae and M.ulcerans and M.avium (the last one is seen in HIV infected patients, causing intestinal obstruction).

Pathology

The typical histological unit is known as *tubercle* (from which the disease gets its name) consisting of a central area of caseation necrosis surrounded by epithelioid cells and giant cells, further surrounded by round cells and finally by fibrosis. The *Langhan* type of giant cells (true foreign body giant cells) are large oval or spindle shaped cells with fragments of nuclei situated in either pole with engulfed bacteria, which are typical but not pathognomonic of tuberculosis.

For purposes of understanding the pathology, abdominal tuberculosis may be divided into four types: *intestinal, lymph nodal, peritoneal and solid organs;* however in most of the patients, combinations of these various types may be present, in a way facilitating the diagnosis, since such a combination is rarely seen in other abdominal conditions. Other abdominal viscera commonly affected by tuberculosis are: female genital tract, duodenojejunal flexure, kidney, urinary bladder, colon, rectum, stomach, spleen and esophagus, in that order.

Each type is further subdivided into
Intestinal: *ulcerating* and *hyperplastic,* both may lead to *cicatrization* and intestinal obstruction, with or without treatment.

Lymph nodal: *hyperplastic* and *caseating,* latter leading to *cold abscesses* tracking down to various fascial planes, including psoas sheath.

Peritoneal: *exudative* (common), *plastic* (dry type) also known as *peritonitis sicca, loculating* (combination of the above two) and *purulent* types; the latter may be due to secondary infection, usually from salpingitis in women.

Solid organ: splenic, hepatic, genitourinary and others

INTESTINAL TUBERCULOSIS

The lymphoid tissue in Payer's patches are initially infected, but it differs from typhoid in that it does not remain confined to them, but spreads circumferentially, resulting in *girdle ulcers*. The edges of these ulcers are ragged, irregular and undermined, with tubercles covering the floor. The bowel wall is thickened, with serosal congestion and usually associated with enlargement of regional nodes. It can affect any part of bowel but commonest site is ileocecal junction or terminal ileum, because this region of bowel is rich in lymphoid tissue and food stays there much longer than in other segments of bowel.

Fibrosis, typical of the tuberculous process, makes the perforation of ulcers rare, in striking contrast to typhoid ulcers. Besides mural cicatrization, kinking due to adhesions may also be a cause for bowel obstruction. With strictures producing incomplete obstruction, over the background of enteritis, patients may have the typical alternating diarrhea and constipation or features of malabsorption. Bowel proximal to obstruction may be enormously dilated, loops visible through the anterior abdominal wall, in emaciated patients. If multiple segments are involved, bowel in between may dilate, producing typical sacculation and due to narrowing of terminal ileum, almost resembling Crohn's disease, a *string sign* may be seen in barium meal pictures. Emptiness of right iliac fossa may be noted (as in intussusception) due to pulled up cecum (signe de Dance).

Differential diagnosis

Appendicular mass, carcinoma cecum, lymphoma of bowel and Crohn's disease (regional enteritis) are the common conditions to be considered; amebic granuloma, unascended (pelvic) kidney, tumor of an abdominal testis, intussusception and worm colic are uncommon, while actinomycosis is very rare in India.

PERITONEAL TUBERCULOSIS

It may have an acute presentation, but is more often insidious. The origin of infection is either from the gut, lymph nodes, Fallopian tubes and rarely hematogenous, as in the miliary type.

The ascitic form is the most common; gradual, uniform abdominal distension brings the patient to the doctor. As the fluid enters the processus vaginalis, congenital hydrocele may appear in a male child and increased intra-abdominal pressure may predispose to an umbilical hernia. Besides ascites, a transverse mobile mass is felt in the upper abdomen, due to *rolled up omentum*, floating in the exudate.

The fibrous (plastic) type or peritonitis sicca produces wide spread adhesions, resulting in subacute or acute intestinal obstruction or a

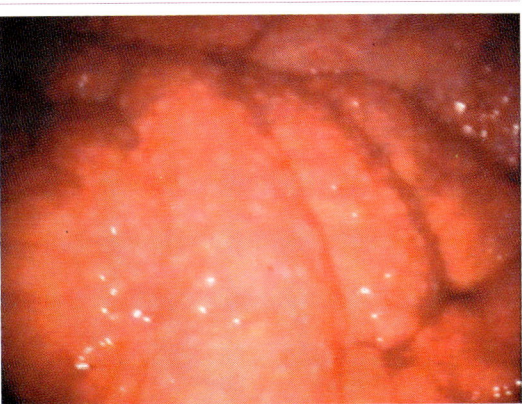

Fig.18.1. Laparoscopic view of abdominal tuberculosis showing military nodules over the bowel (courtesy: Lifeline Hospitals, Chennai)

blind loop syndrome due to grossly sacculated segments of small bowel.

When the above two types co-exist, a loculated or encysted type of peritonitis may result. Depending upon its location, a pancreatic pseudocyst, mesenteric, ovarian cyst or a huge hydronephrosis have to be differentiated from it. If omentum and loops of bowel surround and get adherent to a loculation, it is known as *abdominal cocoon*.

Purulent type is rare, usually secondary to tuberculous pyosalpinx, but may be due to a ruptured cold abscess from caseated nodes. The pus may open into adjacent bowel or find its way out near the umbilicus or both, rarely resulting in a fecal fistula.

TUBERCULOUS MESENTERIC LYMPH-ADENITIS

It is caused by spread of infection from Peyer's patches; often several nodes enlarge, mimicking a lymphoma or metastatic carcinoma. The presence of ascites is strongly against the former. Calcification of nodes in a skiagram is neither pathognomonic nor any indication of 'dead' infection. Rarely acute lymphadentitis may occur, mimicking intestinal obstruction, acute appendicitis or filarial lymphangitis. Caseated nodes may form a cold abscess within the leaves of mesentery called '*pseudocyst*' of *mesentery*.

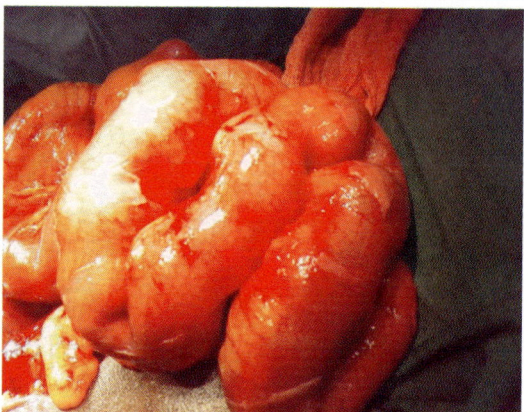

Fig. 18.2. Abdominal cocoon in tuberculosis

Psoas abcess

This results from caseation of retroperitoneal nodes or involvement of vertebral body. Commonly affected vertebra are T12 and L1 because:

1. junction of the fixed and mobile parts of the spine

2. proximity of cisterna chyli

The pus may track down into the psoas sheath, presenting as a mass in the iliac fossa and another in the femoral region. Typical psoas spasm leading to hip flexion and cross fluctuation between the two swellings, make the diagnosis easy.

It is treated by open or retroperitoneoscopic drainage of the abscess, under cover of anti-tuberculous therapy.

Enlarged matted lymph nodes sometimes produce external compression of small bowel resulting in intestinal obstruction; such a condition is known as *tabes mesenterica*. Fixed loop of duodenojejunal junction at the ligament of Treitz is a favourite site for such external compression by the nodes.

Investigations

Apart from routine studies, including ESR, Mantoux, stools for occult blood, chest and KUB film, barium study, analysis of aspirated ascitic fluid, ultrasonogram, laparoscopy or laparotomy may be needed to clinch the diagnosis. Study of immunoglobulins (IgA, IgG & IgM, for antibodies) and polymerase chain reaction (PCR), for Mycobacterial antigen, may give the additional diagnostic support, if tissue for diagnosis cannot be obtained.

Barium meal findings: *Sacculation* of small bowel, hurried transit time, string sign (of Kantor), ileocecal angle becoming obtuse, by *pulled up cecum* due to fibrosis, may be present. Unless judiciously used, a study with thick barium may precipitate frank intestinal obstruction. In a case of subacute/incomplete occlusion of the lumen, a very thin barium or a water soluble contrast, meglumine diatrizoate (Gastrografin) should be a safer option.

ASCITES
Mechanism of ascites

It is the result of balanced effects of plasma and peritoneal colloid osmotic pressures and hydrostatic pressures, which exchanges fluid and proteins between the intravascular compartment (capillary bed) and peritoneal fluid, the so called third compartment. Protein-rich fluid enters the peritoneal space when capillary permeability is increased, as in peritonitis of disseminated peritoneal malig-nancy (carcinomatosis peritonei).

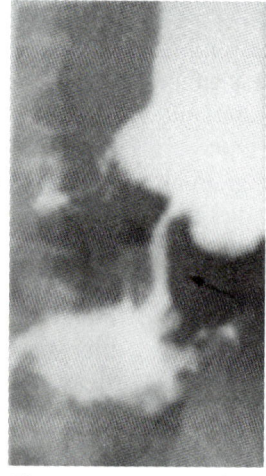

Fig. 18.3. Barium meal picture showing ileal stricture in tuberculosis

Other situations of increased capillary pressure are, generalized water/sodium retention, congestive cardiac failure, constrictive pericarditis or inferior vena caval obstruction. Local (intra-abdominal) raise of capillary pressure may occur in portal hypertension, including Budd-Chiari syndrome. Capillary oncotic pressure is lowered in hypoproteinemia, due to reduced protein intake, impaired absorption, abnormal losses or defective protein synthesis (as in cirrhosis).

Transudate	Exudate	Extravasation type
Hepatic *	Tuberculosis *	Pancreatic ascites
Nutritional	Malignancy *	Chylous
Cardiac	Pyogenic (nonspecific)	
Renal		
Myxedema etc		

* Most common causes

Table – 18.1 Causes of ascites

Feature	Transudate	Exudate
Appearance	Clear	Thick or Cloudy
Sp. Gravity	<1015	>1018
Proteins	<2.5 gm%	>3 gm%
Serum-ascitic fluid albumin gradient	>1.1	<1.1
LDH fluid/serum ratio	<0.6	>0.6
Glucose fluid/serum ratio	<0.8	>0.8
Fluid cholesterol	<45mg%	>45mg%
Cell count	Minimal	More

Table – 18.2 Differences between transudate and exudate

Tissue diagnosis of tuberculosis may be established by the following:
a) upper GI endoscopy
b) lower GI endoscopy
c) excision biopsy of an abnormal external lymph node, if present
d) guided needle biopsy of internal lymph nodes
e) peritoneal biopsy using Cope's needle
f) laparoscopy/laparotomy

SOLID ORGAN TUBERCULOSIS

The commonest in this type is genitourinary tuberculosis, which is almost always secondary to pulmonary infection.

Genital: Male: epididymo-orchitis is the commonest, due to retrograde spread from the prostatic urethra, via the vas deferens (see chapter 29)

Female: The tubo-ovarian involvement occurs first, uterus (endometritis) being affected only in a later stage.

Urinary: In the order of frequency, the kidney, urinary bladder and the ureter are involved.

Other solid organs involved are liver, spleen and pancreas, wherein this etiology has to be

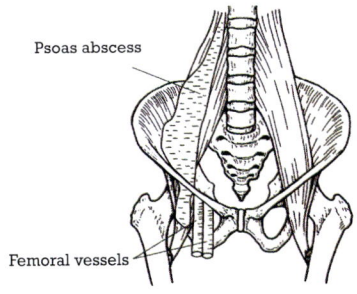

Psoas abscess

Femoral vessels

Fig. 18.4. Scheme of right psoas abscess tracking into the groin

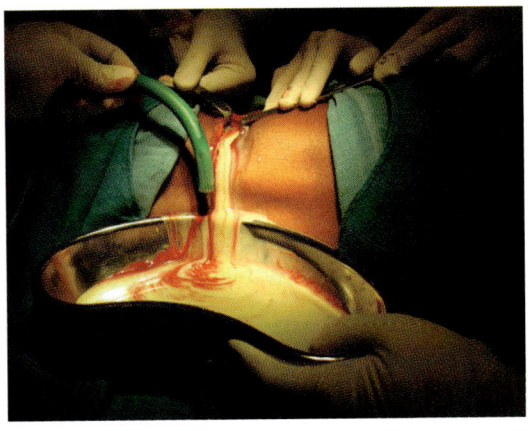

Fig. 18.5. Drainage of psoas abscess

119

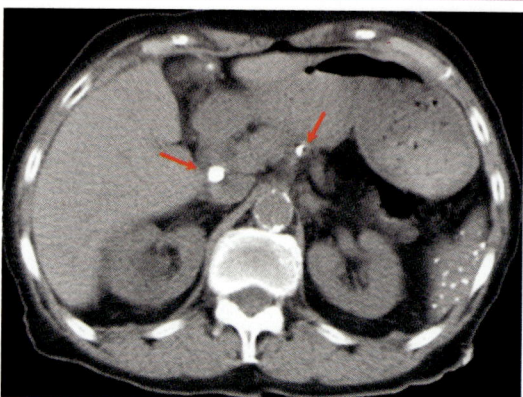

Fig. 18.6. CT scan of the abdomen showing calcified tuberculous lesions in the spleen and lymph nodes (courtesy: Halsted Surgical Clinic, Chennai)

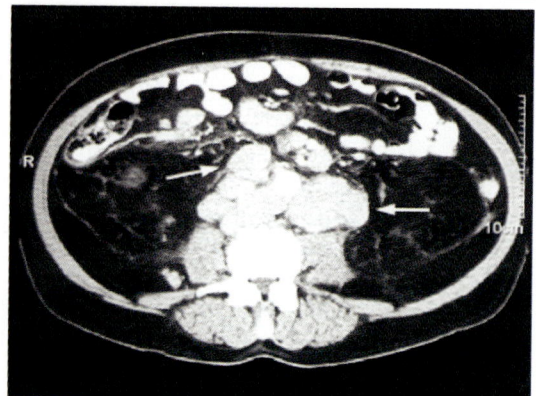

Fig. 18.7. CT scan of abdomen showing multiple paraaortic lymph nodes in tuberculosis (courtesy: Halsted Surgical Clinic, Chennai)

considered when an abscess is encountered in these situations.

Treatment

Abdominal tuberculosis is primarily treated with multi-drug chemotherapeutic regime for 6-12 months, depending upon the clinical response, as judged by patient's subjective improvement, weight gain, resolution of any mass present and erythrocyte sedimentation rate (ESR). Completion of standard course of medical therapy is mandatory, even if surgery is done, for total cure.

Chemotherapy for tuberculosis: The earlier classification as first and second line drugs is not followed any longer, grouping as bactericidal and bacteriostatic, may be more practical. They are given as combination therapy for 6-12 months, as necessary. Hepatic tuberculosis, although rare, may confuse the issue and the second line non-hepatotoxic drugs may have to be used, e.g. ofloxacin, cycloserin or kanamycin.

Bactericidal agents

a) *Streptomycin* (Sm): 0.5-2.0gm/IM/day. It is neurotoxic, particularly eighth nerve is commonly affected.

b) *Rifampicin* (Rmp): 300-600mg/day, in single dose, on empty stomach in the morning and patient should be cautioned that the urine will be colored deep orange, for a few hours follow-

ing taking the drug. Hepatotoxic, hence periodic enzyme monitoring is necessary, during treatment. Cutaneous flushing and pruritus may also be seen.

c) *Isoniazide* (INH): 300-600mg/day, in single dose, usually first drug to start and last drug to stop. Peripheral neuropathy is a well known dose dependent toxicity of the drug, countered by pyridoxine (vit.B6), which is given along with INH, to prevent neurotoxicity.

d) *Pyrazinamide* (Pzm): 30mg/kg/day, generally not used alone for fear of developing resistance. Hepatotoxicity and hyperuricemia are the known side effects.

Bacteriostatic agents

e) *Para-amino salicylic acid* (PAS): 5-10gm/day, may cause gastrointestinal disturbances.

f) *Ethambutol* (Emb): 400-1200mg/day, optic neuritis, to be monitored by color vision and visual fields.

g) *Thiacetazone* (Tzn): cutaneous , liver and bone marrow toxicity can occur.

h) *Cycloserine* (Cys): CNS toxicity and convulsions, preveted by concomitant administration of pyridoxine (vit.B6).

l) *Ethionamide* (Etm): useful against atypical strains, it may cause gastrointestinal disturbances

j)   *Prothionamide* (Pto)

k)   *Terizidone* (Trd)

l)   *Levofloxacin (Lfx)*

m)   *Moxifloxacin (Mfx)*

Other drugs like *kanamycin* (Kmc), *amikacin* (Am), *ciprofloxacin* (Cipro), *ofloxacin* (Ofx) etc. also have antituberculous property.

Current recommendation of WHO: 4 drugs (Rmp+INH+Pzm+Emb) daily for 2 months, followed by 2 drugs (Rmp+INH) daily for 4 months.

Modified regime of Tuberculosis Research Centre (India), which is proved to be equally effective, is to administer the same drugs, but only thrice a week, under strict supervision, for six months. This has an advantage in the cost, compliance and side effects.

Indications for surgical intervention

i)   intestinal obstruction (commonest)
ii)   cold abscesses
iii)   not responding to adequate chemotherapy or uncertainty of diagnosis
iv)   coexisting malignancy suspected

Principles of surgery: Limited resection of involved bowel or enteroplasty (stricturo-plasty), as necessary, for intestinal obstruction. Ileocecal resection and end-to-end ileo-ascending colic anastomosis is the standard procedure for ileocecal disease. Blind bypass sometimes may be necessary if multiple adherent loops, densely plastered, prevent thorough exploration. Being a benign condition, with near normal life expectancy, resection of obstructing bowel segment (or a mass), is pref-erable to bypass, to avoid blind loop syndrome and to exclude associated malignancy. Draining the cold abscesses, often multiple, curetting the caseous material and closing the cavity primarily may be done by laparoscopy/laparotomy. Psoas abscess may be drained extraperi-toneally, through a suprainguinal muscle-splitting incision.

Tuberculosis co-existing with malignancy is not an uncommon occurrence, favourite sites being the lungs (bronchogenic carcinoma), lymph nodes and cecum (lymphoma). This should be kept in mind whenever the patient is not responding to anti-tuberculous chemother-apy as expected, or shows deterioration during therapy.

Recent advances

1)   Adenosine deaminase (ADA) is an enzyme secreted by lymphocytes on contact with myco-bacterium tuberculosis. Estimation of this enzyme is a sensitive indicator of tuberculosis of serous cavities (pleural, pericardial or peritoneal); there is a small false positivity in lymphomas, due to dedifferentiation of lym-phocytes. However ascites is a rare feature of lymphomas.

2)   For solid organ tuberculosis, PCR may be done even on a paraffin-fixed slide. This is espe-cially important in cases of granulomatous hep-atitis, wherein this helps to differentiate Koch's disease from a chronic viral pathology.

3)   As in ovarian malignancy, high levels of CA-125 may also be found in peritoneal tuberculo-sis; hence this marker should be used with cau-tion while evaluating a female patient with ascites.

19 Basal Cell Carcinoma (BCC)

(syn: rodent ulcer, tear cancer)

Definition: This is a locally invasive carcinoma of the basal surface of the epidermis and occasionally from outer root sheath of hair follicles, which arises probably from pleuripotent cells.

Etiology

Exposure to sunlight, especially in fair-skinned people (e.g. Caucasians resident in tropical countries) and those suffering from xeroderma pigmentosa (inadequate repair of DNA after sunlight induced injury).

Arsenic (earlier used in skin ointments) usage predisposes to BCC.

Highest prevalence is in Australia, due to actinic exposure. The *ozone layer* in the atmosphere filters the solar actinic rays to a large extent, so that their deleterious effects on humans are minimized, but as the ozone layer is becoming thinner and interrupted in recent times, people exposed to sun light for protracted periods of time are becoming more vulnerable.

Pathology

Six clinical types are commonly described:

i) Nodulo-ulcerative type: (commonest) with typical rolled and beaded (pearly)edge and the floor showing scabs over some areas.
ii) Pigmented BCC (dark brown color mimicking a melanoma).
iii) Field fire type: Advancing edge but healing center, destroying large areas rapidly.
iv) Morpheic type: (rarest) appearing as red raised plaques or streaks.
v) *Fibroepithelioma*
vi) *Superficial* BCC

In the scalp, this tumor is known as epithelioma adenoides cysticum or *turban tumor*.

BCC cannot occur in mucosal areas which do not have pilosabaceous adnexa, such as lips, tongue, cervix uteri etc.

Histology

Cells in island patterns, extending down from the epidermis. Peripheral cells in the islands have a *palisade* arrangement. No cell nests, keratinization or prickle cells (see SCC), but stromal cells, chronic inflammatory cells and fibrovascular tissue are present. They are hyperchromatic small cells, with oval nuclei and little cytoplasm. It may be differentiated type (keratotic or sebaceous BCC) or most aggressive undifferentiated (solid) type.

Spread: Primarily by local invasion, lymphatic and hematogenous spread are very rare, but described. Characteristically it burrows into the deeper tissues or bone, hence the name, *rodent ulcer*.

Symptoms

A nodule or ulcer, classically above a line (*Ohngren's line*) joining the angle of the mouth to the lobule of the ear (90%). Itching or bleeding may occur. Multiple lesions occur especially in the basal cell nevus (Gorlin's) syndrome. The common site in the face where tears roll down, earns the name 'tear cancer'.

Signs

Nodule is the initial presentation, which under-

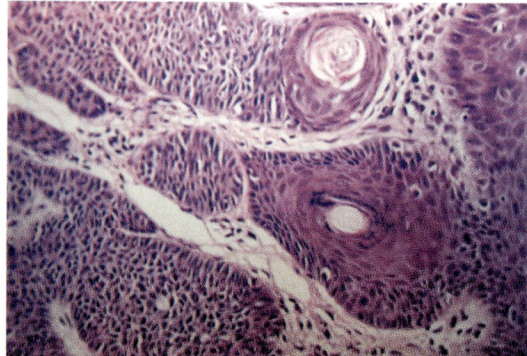

Fig. 19.1. Histology of BCC, showing typical palisading (courtesy: Lifeline Hospitals, Chennai)

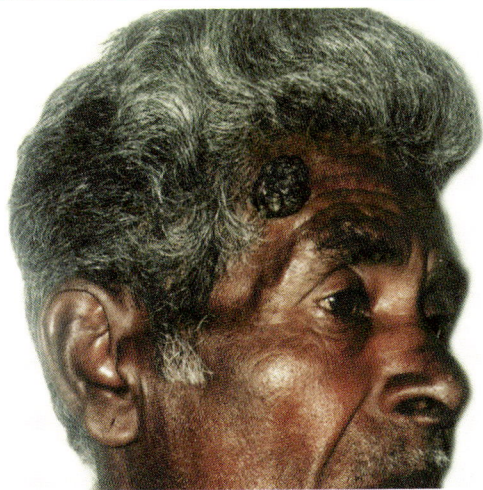

Fig. 19.2. Basal cell carcinoma, forehead
(courtesy: Dr A.V Tanuja, Chennai)

goes central necrosis resulting in an ulcer. As the growth spreads, the ulcer margin becomes irregular and as it erodes deeper tissues, the edge becomes more raised, but never everted, in contrast to SCC. The floor is covered with fibrin crust and the base is the underlying normal tissue. Some rodent ulcers may appear cystic, due to central tumor necrosis. As a rule, regional nodes are not enlarged.

Differential diagnosis

SCC, seborrheic keratoses, keratoacanthoma, amelanotic melanoma and infected hemang.ioma.

Investigations

X-ray of the region for bony erosion and edge biopsy to establish diagnosis are the specific investigations necessary. A chest x-ray and an abdominal ultrasonogram may be done as a routine, for proper staging of the disease.

Treatment

1. Surgery is the treatment of choice, with a cure rate of over 90%. Excision with a margin of about 5mm is recommended in all dimensions, for total clearance, special attention to be given to the depth, to avoid late recurrence. Skin closure after excision may be by primary suturing, skin graft (full thickness with a proper color match, for cosmetic reasons) or a rotation flap.

Indications

(i)   when radiotherapy is contraindicated,

(ii) for recurrence or

(iii) for new lesion adjacent to radiated site

(iv) more extensive resection with tissue reconstruction, may be necessary for advanced lesions sometimes following down-staging by neo-adjuvant RT.

2.   90% of BCC will be cured by RT as well. Fractionated doses, over a few weeks decreases scarring and necrosis. Lesions not amenable to RT are those very close or attached to adjacent cartilage or bone.In elderly patients, with a low risk of a second malignancy, RT is ideally indicated.

3.   Nd:YAG or carbondioxide laser (unfocused beam) may be used for small lesions.

4.   Cryotherapy with liquid nitrogen at -196°C is useful for elderly patients.

5.   5-Fluorouracil cream as a topical treatment is useful for small flat nodules, but recurrence is frequent, probably due to residual disease in the depth.

CYLINDROMA (syn: Turban tumor)

It is considered to be a peculiar benign variant of BCC or trichoepithelioma, may be inherited as autosomal dominant trait, generally seen over scalp and face. It may be single or more commonly multiple, arranged in translucent cylinders, forming an extensive turban-like swelling over the scalp, with little tendency for ulceration. The condition has to be differentiated from multiple sebaceous

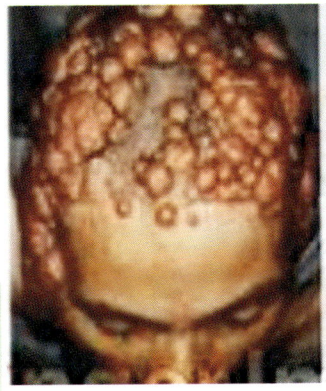

Fig. 19.3. Turban tumor
(courtesy: Halsted Surgical Clinic, Chennai)

cysts or eccrine spiradenoma. It is less aggressive than the standard BCC and carries better prognosis, if adequately excised and the resultant defect covered by a free skin graft or a flap. Smaller lesions may be excised using laser. Occasionally malignant transformation may occur (malignant cylindroma) and has to be managed like BCC.

(syn: epithelioma, epidermoid carcinoma)

Definition: SQUAMOUS CELL CARCINOMA (SCC) of the skin arises from the prickle cell layer of the epidermis.

Etiopathogenesis

1. SCC is usually seen in fair-skined persons who had excessive exposure to sun light, during childhood.

2. more common in males.

3. it is the cumulative life time exposure to ultraviolet rays (from sunlight), that determines the development of SCC.

4. there is an increased incidence of SCC in persons, treated with PUVA (psoralen-UVA was used to treat psoriasis). In sunlight induced cancers, ultraviolet-B rays are more carcinogenic.

5. patients on immuno-suppresive therapy after organ transplantation or patients infected with HIV have a higher incidence of SCC. In these patients the ratio of BCC to SCC is altered, suggesting that the normal immune system may control SCC, mediated through T-cells.

6. chronic inflammation, ulceration, sinus or scar tissue may predispose to SCC(Marjolin's ulcer).

7. exposure to ionising radiation can result in the development of SCC, several years later.

8. topical agents used to chronic skin conditions can some times be carcinogenic and cause SCC.

9. industrial exposure to chemicals is a major risk factor for SCC.

a) in cotton spinning mills, contact with cotton oil was found to cause SCC.

b) scrotal malignancies in chimney sweepers (described by Sir Percival Pott) due to prolonged contact with carcinogenic soot.

c) some industries dealing with paraffin tar, shell oil and creosote oil have an high inci-

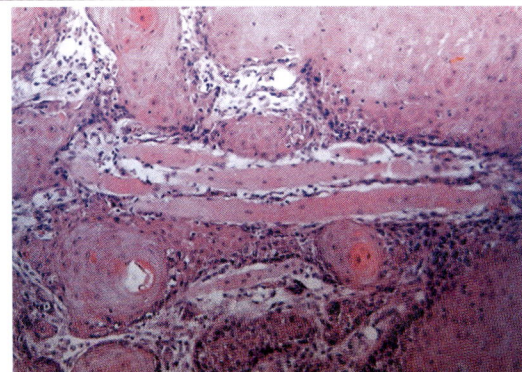

Fig. 20.1. Histology of SCC, showing keratin pearls (courtesy: Lifeline Hospitals, Chennai)

dence of SCC in their workers.

10. heavy alcohol and tobacco abusers may develop SCC of mucocutaneos junctions especillay in the buccal area.

11. Kangri cancer (Kangri: glowing coal): in some northern states of India (Kashmir), people employ a basket of hot charcoal, called kangri, under the clothes over the anterior abdominal wall for purposes of warmth. Due to chronic thermal irritation they develop SCC of abdominal wall. The warming appliance is also known as Kairo in Japan and Kang in China.

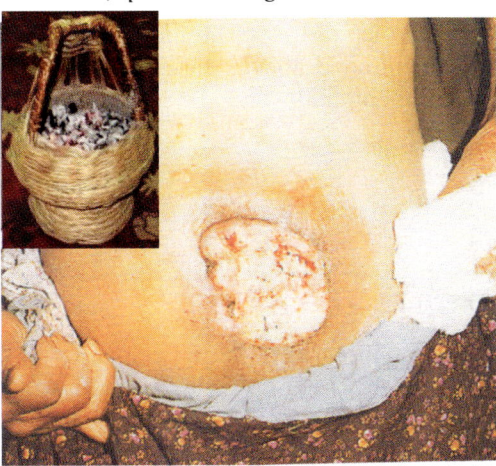

Fig. 20.2. Kangri cancer common in Kashmir (India). Inset shows the Kangri with burning coal. (courtesy ; Laxmi Hospital, Kakinada)

12. Chutta cancer: in tobacco growing areas the workers have a peculiar habit of smoking cigar (chutta) with lighted end inside the mouth, leading to SCC of oral cavity.

13. very rarely SCC may develop from a BCC, which is known as basi-squamous carcinoma

14. conditions such as sebaceous or branchial cyst may predispose to SCC

Other factors may be responsible for development of SCC in specific locations, such as chronic cervicitis and erosion (for uterine cervix), chronic bronchitis, asbestos, nickel, chromium, inorganic arsenic etc. (for bronchus). (see also under lips, tongue, cheek, penis for details).

15. There is accumulating evidence that suggests a causative role of the human papillomavirus (HPV), especially in SCC larynx, penis and cervix uteri.

Sites

Any part of the body covered by stratified squamous epithelium may be the site for an SCC, eg: skin, mouth, penis, esophagus, anus, ectocervix uteri etc. It can also occur at other sites, such as gallbladder or urothelium, as a result of squamous metaplasia of columnar and transitional epithelium respectively, usually due to chronic irritation by a calculus.

Precancerous diseases: Besides various diseases mentioned above, these are some precancerous conditions:

1. Bowen's disease
2. Senile keratosis
3. Lupus vulgaris
4. Xeroderma pigmentosum
5. Actinic kerotosis
6. Leukoplakia
7. Burn scar, chronic venous ulcer or balano-posthitis

Pathology

Macroscopically two types are described:

1. Ulcerative type (commoner): Epithelial malignancy generally starts as an ulcer, whereas tumor arising from the the depth (e.g. STS), presents as a mass, with intact skin, which may later ulcerate, an important point of difference in the history.

2. proliferative type

Microsco pes

i) carcinoma-in-situ (intraepithelial or preinvasive carcinoma)

There is an increased, irregular cellular proliferation of the prickle cell layer, atypical mitotic activity, cellular pleomorphism and other features of dysplasia with intact basement membrane.

ii) invasive carcinoma

In this, groups of malignant cells from the main mass of origin bud off to invade the basement membrane, deeper connective tissue and muscle. This is accompanied by the fibrous desmoplastic response, which may be dense

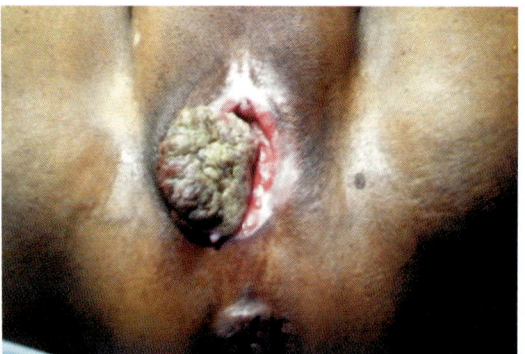

Fig. 20.3. Polypoid squamous cell carcinoma of vulva (courtesy Laxmi Hospital, Kakinada)

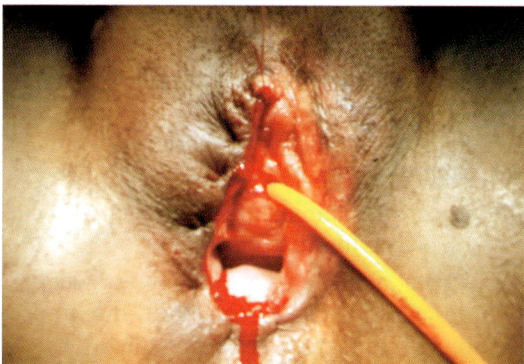

Fig. 20.4. After wide local excision (courtesy Laxmi Hospital, Kakinada)

and acellular as in scirrhous type or loose and avascular in other types.

Cell-mediated immunity is involved in checking the growth and spread of SCC, as seen by the presence of lymphocytes in abundance around tumors of low grade malignancy and during the earlier stages of cancerous change. After surface ulceration, a more acute type of neutrophilic response occurs secondary to bacterial inflammation.

Degree of differentiation

SCC, as other malignancies, vary considerably in the degree of differentiation of tumor cells.

Well differentiated tumors manifest epithelial pearls (keratin pearls, horn pearls or cell nests), which are groups of cells producing a central whorl of keratin, surrounded by prickle cells and a barely recognizable stratum granulosum. They carry better prognosis.

Poorly differentiated SCC shows no obvious keratin but only groups of prickle cells with high mitotic figures. It may be said that the lesser the attempt at prickle cell formation and keratin production, the more anaplastic the tumor and worse the prognosis.

Broder's grading: depending upon the degree of differentiation, four grades have been described:

Grade I: < 25% undifferentiated tumor cells.

Grade II: 25 to 50% undifferentiated cells.

Grade III: 50 to 75% undifferentiated cells.

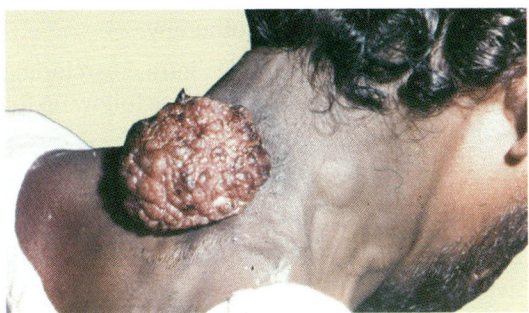

Fig. 20.5. Typical cauliflower-like SCC of the nape of neck
(courtesy: Prof T Gunasagaran, Chennai)

Grade IV: >75% undifferentiated cells.

The higher the grade, faster the growth and spread, hence worse the prognosis.

Variants of SCC

a)   Papillary (transitional cell) carcinoma

Some SCC of Nasopharynx and bronchi have a papillary structure and are composed of transitional type of epithelium, however, the term transitional cell is better avoided.

b)   Verrucous carcinoma

SCC some times forms a slow-growing papillomatous mass, well differentiated, late to metastasize, such variety occurs on the sole of the foot or cheek, masquerading as a simple wart but burrowing into deeper tissue. It is also called epithelioma cuniculatum.

c)   Spindle cell carcinoma

Occasionally the cells of a SCC are fusifom or spindle shaped, which is so highly undifferentiated, that it may be impossible to distinguish this from a sarcoma or an amelanotic melanoma.

d)   Marjolin's ulcer: described later

Spread

1.   local spread by continuity and contiguity.

2.   lymph spread is the commonest, occurs by embolism and permeation. The nodal involvement varies with site of the primary lesion occurring late in tumors of the hand or from a scar of a chronic ulcer, but early in cancers of the foot, face and neck.

3.   blood spread occurs rare and late, if any.

Clinical features

Symptoms

1.   the primary lesion often manifests as a red indurated papule that appears denovo superadded to an actinic keratosis. It expands rapidly producing an ulcer, which may bleed to touch (bleeding ulcerating nodule is seen more commonly in SCC than in BCC).

2.   painless initially, becomes painful as it invades deeper structures.

3. enlarged lymph nodes may sometimes be the presenting symptom, before primary tumor is noticed (occult primary SCC, common in nasopharynx and laryngopharynx).

Signs

1. typically an ulcerated mass, commonly seen over the face, neck, back and the dorsum of the hand.

2. not warm, usually not tender

3. irregular shape

4. raised and everted edges

5. floor is covered by necrotic tumor, and sero-sanguineous discharge. In advanced cases, deeper structures, such as muscle, tendon, cartilage, bone etc. may be exposed. While describing the floor of a malignant ulcer, the word 'granulation tissue' should never be used, since such tissue is seen only in chronic inflammatory condition.

6. base is indurated, which is one of the pathognomonic signs of epithelioma.

7. in early stage, it can be moved with the skin, over the underlying structures, but later on with tumor invasion, it becomes fixed to them.

8. involvement of regional lymph nodes is a very important clinical sign of SCC; it may be due to three reasons:

    a) metastatic,
    b) secondary infection
    c) sinus histiocytosis, due to immune response to the tumor. Thus, it should never be assumed that palpable lymph nodes are always due to malignant spread.

Differential diagnosis

1. keratoacanthoma
2. seborrheic keratosis
3. pyogenic granuloma
4. Amelanotic melanoma
5. spindle cell STS
6. fungal granuloma
7. tuberculous ulcer

Investigations

Among the specific investigations, establishing tissue diagnosis by biopsy and proper staging of the disease, by imaging methods, are most important.

Biopsy: Either edge, punch, incisional or excisional biopsy should be performed depending upon the size and site of the tumor. Needle biopsy (fine or wide bore) is used for deeper lesions and nonulcerated lymph nodes. In a very small skin SCC, an excision biopsy with adequate margins may be both diagnostic and therapeutic.

Having made the tissue diagnosis, even if there are no obvious secondaries, staging investigations are necessary, before planning treatment.

Treatment

a) Treatment of primary tumor

i) Surgery: Wide excision of lesion should be done with a margin of 1 cm of normal tissue all around. In case of tumor involving finger, toe or penis, amputation may be indicated. In the limbs, amputation may be required, if a functionally useful limb cannot be offered to the patient after adequate clearance. However, mutilative surgery like a major amputation should not be done, unless there is a reasonable chance for cure.

Indications for surgery

1. large, but mobile lesions

2. well differentiated tumors, since they are less chemo/radiosensitive

3. radiotherapy is inadequate.

4. recurrence after radiotherapy

Moh's microsurgery (vide infra, carcinoma penis) may also be done, but close follow up for recurrence is mandatory.

ii) Radiotherapy: indicated when

1. there is contraindication for surgery.

2. the growth is small or too large and extensive

3. genital mutilation is undesirable in a young man with carcinoma penis

4. as a complement to chemotherapy in

patients with anal carcinoma

5. the tumor is poorly differentiated

6. to down-stage an advanced disease, making it resectable, as in carcinoma cervix (neoadjuvant therapy)

Contraindications

1. verrucous carcinoma
2. tumor has involved underlying bone or is too close to the eyes
3. Recurrence following radiotherapy

iii) Chemotherapy

1. It is used as adjuvant or neoadjuvant form.

2. as palliative therapy for advanced or disseminated tumor

Drugs used are: bleomycin, cis-platinum, 5-FU, taxanes etc.

Newer modalities of treatment of early tumors, under evaluation
1. Laser radiation (photodynamic therapy)
2. Local immunotherapy
3. Interferon

b) Treatment of metastatic lymph nodes (see under lymph nodes, chapter 42)

1. there is no place for prophylactic lymph node excision, they are removed enbloc, only when they are clinically involved.

2. secondary nodes are not as radio-sensitive as the primary SCC.

3. possibility of their enlargement due to secondary infection should be excluded by a 2-week course of appropriate antibiotics, before considering them as metastatic.

4. if the nodes can be removed enbloc with the primary tumor, it may be done at the same time, but if two separate incisions have to be made, the node excision is done after 4-6weeks following primary surgery (see under penile carcinoma, chapter 33).

5. even if the primary tumor is treated by radiation, mobile secondary nodes may be excised.

6. involvement of regional lymph nodes, reduces the survival rate considerably.

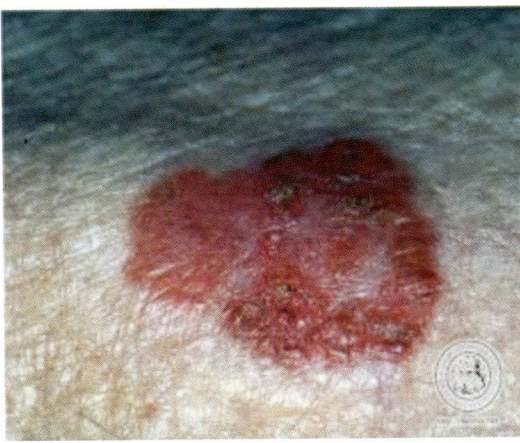

Fig. 20.6. Bowen's disease
(courtesy: Dr A V Tanuja, Chennai)

7. fixed nonresectable nodes may be irradiated for palliation.

8. the role of FNAC of lymph nodes is limited, since negative report has no value.

Calcifying epithelioma (of Malherbe) is nothing but a mummified epidermal cyst with calcification and not an SCC. It is mentioned here merely because of the inappropriate nomenclature.

BOWEN'S DISEASE (syn: precancerous dermatosis, intra-epidermal SCC)

It is the most characteristic form of carcinoma-in-situ of the skin, but unlike in other sites, it rarely becomes invasive. It is often treated for considerable period of time, as 'eczema', by patients and doctors alike!

Presentation

Crusted patches, which are flat and pink in color in areas of the skin exposed to actinic radiation but may occur on non-exposed areas as well, removal of which reveals a bleeding surface.

Clinical features

A non-elevated scaly lesion which progressively enlarges with clearly demarcated margins. If ulceration occurs, malignant change (SCC) should be considered; an edge biopsy clinches the diagnosis. It is commonly seen over the trunk in a middle age person.

Pathology

Immunosuppression, chronic solar exposure, use of arsenic compounds and HPV-16 infection are incriminated in the etiology. Atypical squamous cell proliferation of the skin, which may be of variable thickness, histologically mimicking Paget's disease of the breast or a melanoma; sometimes associated with cancers in the respiratory, gastrointestinal or genitourinary systems.

The lesion may be considered as SCC-in-situ, with a tendency for lateral spread and carries a high risk (upto 50%) of developing invasive skin cancer, more so in genital disease, over a period of 6-7 years. Immunosuppression, chronic solar exposure, use of arsenic compounds, HPV-16 infection etc have been incriminated in the etiology, common site being the trunk in a middle-aged patient.

Differential diagnosis

Actinic dermatitis, eczema, psorisis, morpheic disease (BCC), Paget's disease and SCC.

Investigations

Exfoliative cytology or edge biopsy

Treatment

Early Bowen's lesion is easily treated by cryotherapy or vaporization with CO_2 laser. Radiotherapy has a limited role, so also chemo-

therapy, either systemic or topical.

Excisional surgery, with 5mm margin, is the treatment of choice; a lesion of the prepuce is best treated by circumcision and if it is on the glans in a young man, brachytherapy with radium mould is recommended, as for an early SCC.

Topical application of 5-FU or Imiquimod (an immune response modifier) is found to be effective. Moh's micrographic surgery may be useful in poorly demarcated lesions or in areas where tissue-sparing is vital.

Marjolin's ulcer (Scar cancer)

Definition: This is an SCC arising in a chronic ulcer or a scar. Chronic venous ulcer and burn scars are the commonest predisposing conditions, but it may take several years for this change to occur, though it may be shorter in postburn scarring.

Pathology

This is a well differentiated SCC, resulting from chronic inflammatory response in an ulcerated scar tissue, which turns neoplastic. The fibrosis of the underlying scar obliterates blood/lymph channels and disrupts sensory nerve endings. The above facts largely influence the biological behavior of this malignant ulcer.

1. The lesions are typically very slow growing owing to the lack of blood supply.

2. Lymphatic spread is rare and if any, occurs

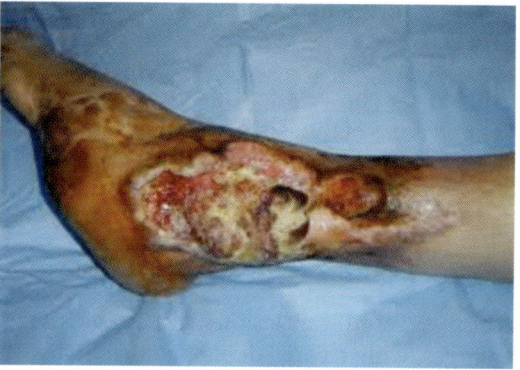

Fig. 20.7. Marjolin's ulcer developed in a chronic venous ulcer
(courtesy: Halsted Surgical Clinic, Chennai)

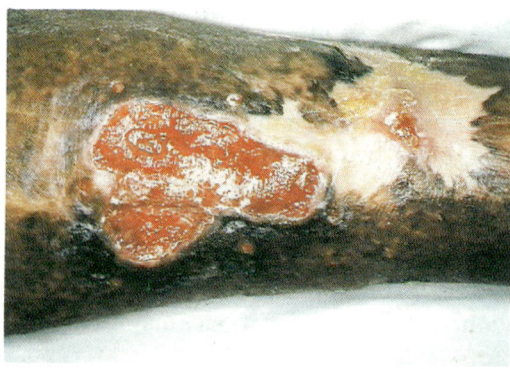

Fig. 20.8. Marjolin's ulcer developed in burn scar
(courtesy: Halsted Surgical Clinic, Chennai)

late, because of obliterated lymphatics.

3. These are usually painless because of the impaired sensations.

Differential diagnosis

Other chronic ulcers such as tuberculous, gummatous and tropical ulcers.

Investigations

If malignancy is suspected in a chronic ulcer, a four-quadrant edge biopsy, should be done to clinch the issue. Once tissue diagnosis is established, investigations to stage the disease may be done.

Treatment

Surgery

Definitive treatment is by wide excision of the lesion with at least 2.5cm margin all around (as for SCC), followed by appropriate skin reconstruction. Involved regional lymph nodes should be dealt as in SCC, after excluding secondary infection by a course of broad spectrum antibiotics. In head and neck regions (postburn), however a margin of 1cm is acceptable because of the less aggressive nature of the malignancy.

Radiotherapy

In contrast to SCC elsewhere, it is not very radiosensitive, due to extensive fibrosis and poor vascularity. For the same reason, there is no role for chemotherapy; however these modalities may be useful to down-stage/palliate the disease in locally extensive or disseminated disease.

Recent advances

In a highly undifferentiated tumor, detection of antikeratin antibodies, will identify the tumor as SCC (keratinocyte origin).

Jewels of Gyan - 20.1

Points to know about Marjolin's ulcer ('scar cancer')

1. Rare
2. Slow growth
3. No pain
4. Late nodal spread
5. Fibrosis of base
6. Not radio or chemosensitive
7. Adequate surgery offers good prognosis

21 Pigmented Nevus

(syn: mole, benign melanoma or freckle)

They may be congenital or acquired, though this division appears to be arbitrary.

The *congenital* moles are *hamartomatous (hamartia: defect or sin)* lesions arising from melanoblasts and melanocytes.

Origin

Although an earlier theory, that epithelial cell rests penetrate into the dermis and produce pigments in deeper layers, still exists, the neurectodermal theory has earned wider acceptance in recent times. In early embryonic life, neurectodermal cells with common cytochemical property (APUD), from the neural crest migrate all over the body along with peripheral nerves and some get incorporated in the basal layer of epidermis. The black pigment is melanin, synthesized from an aminoacid phenylalanine > dehydroxyphenylalanine (DOPA) > melanin, hence histochemically they are all DOPA positive, but some may lack the pigment (amelanotic type).

CONGENITAL HAIRY NEVUS

A warty epidermis with hair growth, which may be elevated from the surface due to infection of

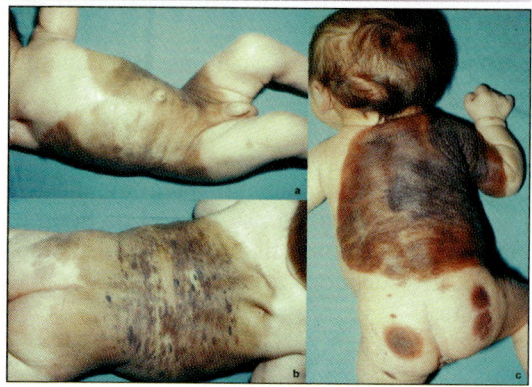

Fig. 21.2. Congenital giant hairy nevi

subjacent sebaceous elements. An extensive type, known as *giant hairy nevus*, is seen in infants, often with bathing-trunk distribution, which creates a major cosmetic problem, besides its malignant potential. There is also a non-hairy counterpart, with smooth surface.

The *acquired* moles are classified based on the layer of origin and the progression of the lesion:

1. DEEP DERMAL OR 'BLUE NEVUS'

They arise in the deep dermis, due to overlying layers of epidermis, they appear bluish, commonly seen on the face, limbs or buttocks in children (Mongolian spot), almost never becomes malignant.

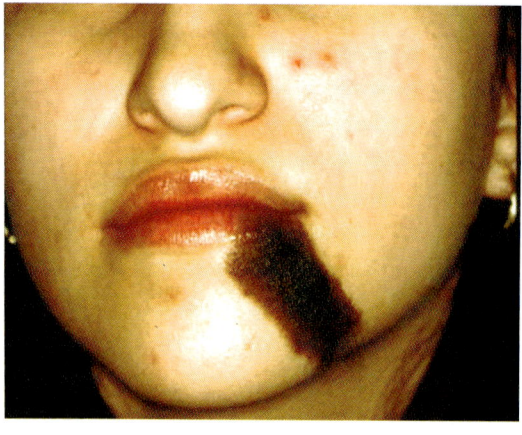

Fig.21.1. Congenital hairy nevus

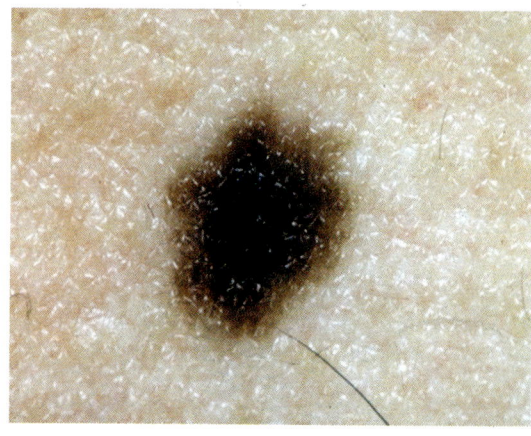

Fig.21.3. Junctional nevus

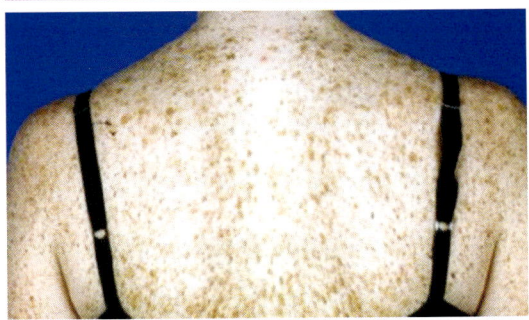

Fig. 21.4. Lentiginous freckles
courtesy Halsted Surgical Clnic, Chennai

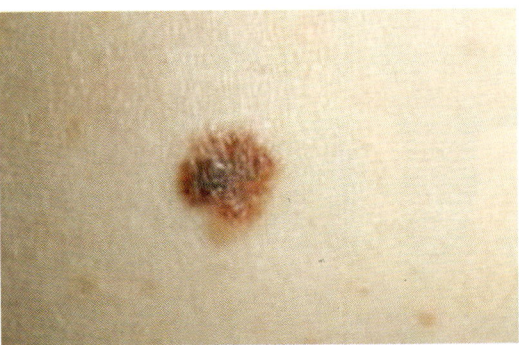

Fig. 21.5. Compound nevus

2. JUNCTIONAL NEVUS

This lesion occurs at the basal or junctional layer of the epidermis and is essentially made of immature cells, with a very high incidence of malignancy. They commonly occur in the palms, soles, digits and genitalia. Microscopically, the cells have clear cytoplasm and dark nuclei, with melanin granules.

3. COMPOUND NEVUS

When both the above components are present, it is called compound. Though the intradermal component is stable and benign, the junctional component is the one that turns malignant.

4. LENTIGO (syn: Hutchison's freckle, senile benign melanoma)

This is a large area of dark pigmention occuring on the head and neck area of elderly people. Nodular changes and malignant transformation

may occur, but they carry better prognosis compared to other types of melanoma.

Early ominous features may be ABCDE: **a**symmetry, **b**order irregularity, **c**olor variegation, **d**iameter (>6mm in typical locations) and **e**levation above skin surface.

Clinical features

Nevi are commonly seen in children and adolescents, yet some may appear in later life, probably due to associated pigmentation under hormonal influence (α-melanocyte stimulating hormone α-MSH, derived from cleaved ACTH of adenohypophysis) and over 95% of them are multiple. Those located over genitals, palms and soles have the highest malignant potential.

Treatment

Most nevi pursue an uneventful course, grow very slowly for a time, remain quiescent for long and gradually atrophy, hence rarely require active treatment.

Excision is the preferred option, especially if

Jewels of Gyan - 21.1

When a mole is no longer a 'mole'

Rapid increase in size
Irregularity of the edge
Itching or discharge
Ulceration, crusting or hemorrhage
Increase in density of pigmentation
Regional lymphadenopathy
Nodule formation
Satellite nodules/pigmentation around the lesion

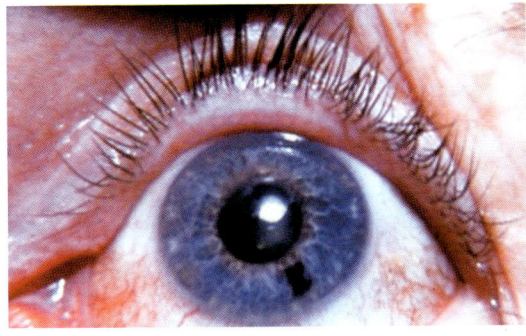

Fig.21.6. Pigmented nevus of iris

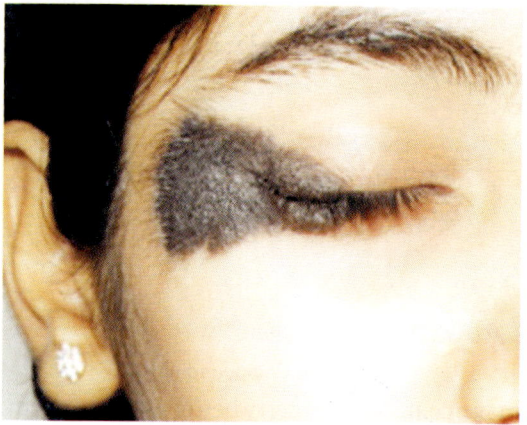 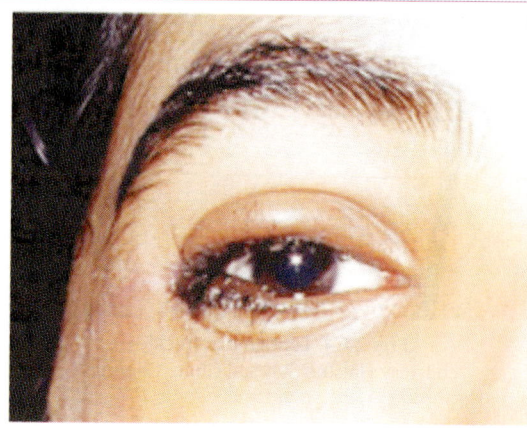

Fig. 21.7 and 8. Congenital hairy nevus, excision and skin grafting done
(courtesy: Dr B S Madhusudanan, Chennai)

a)   a junctional nevus is suspected
b)   repeated trauma may occur
c)   cosmetic considerations exist
d)   there are any features to suggest the onset
of malignancy (vide supra)

The excision should have a 5 mm margin of macroscopically normal skin, with the exception of moles present at birth, where the margin may be less. The lesion should be subjected to histopathology as a routine in all cases.

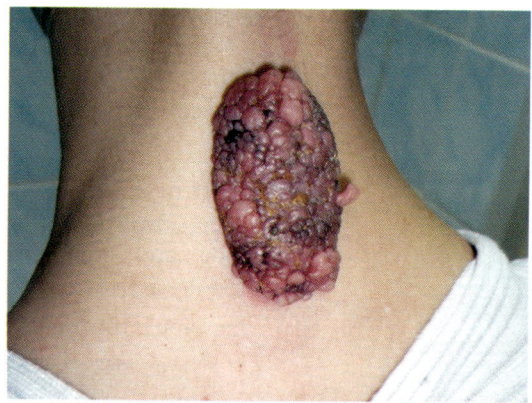

Fig. 21.9. Congenital nevus over the nape of neck
(courtesy: Laxmi Hospital, Kakinada)

22 Malignant Melanoma

The term MALIGNANT MELANOMA, used as a force of habit, is probably superfluous, as all melanomas are malignant. They arise either in a preexisting junctional/compound nevus (90%) or denovo (10%), the cell of origin is the melanoblast of the epidermal junction. A small proportion of melanomas (<5%) do not produce melanin pigment and are known as *amelanotic* melanomas.

Types of melanomas

1. Superficial spreading
2. Lentigo maligna
3. Nodular
4. Site specific melanomas
   a) Melanomas in giant hairy nevus
   b) Acral lentiginous (volar, plantar, subungual, mucosal, anorectal, conjunctival, ocular and genital)
5. Amelanotic type

Etiology

Sunlight, especially ultraviolet-B rays on the skin of Caucasians (more in Australians), blacks are rarely affected, except the acral lentiginous type in palms and soles. The role of trauma and pregnancy is debatable. This tumor is unknown before puberty. About 50% of malanomas arise from a preexisting mole

Features of malignancy in a benign mole: recent increase in size, itching , crusting , bleeding, ulceration, irregular border, appearance of satellite nodules/pigmentation or enlargement of regional nodes.

1) Superficial spreading melanoma (SSM) is the commonest (70%) variety, seen over the back, chest and legs, presents as an elevated, pigmented plaque with irregular surface/border and varying colors.

2) Lentigo maligna melanoma (LMM) also known as melanotic freckle of Hutchinson, occurs in patients over 60. It is the least virulent variety and presents as a large pigmented patch which slowly enlarges over a few years. Increased thickness and appearance of nodules help to differentiate this from its benign counterpart.

3) Nodular melanoma (NM) is a highly malignant type which affects younger individuals (mean age 45). It presents as a raised, brownish-black lesion with a sharp edge, which ulcerates early and bleeds easily and its vertical growth is rapid compared to lateral spread.

4) Acral lentiginous melanoma (ALM) is seen in blacks and usually in the palms, soles and under the nails.

5) Amelanotic melanoma This type is the most malignant, with de-differentiation, the melanocytes lose the melanin producing property. The lesion is pink instead of black, nodular, resembles SCC, DOPA reaction negative and carries worst prognosis.

Pathology and growth pattern

The two patterns of growth exhibited by melanoma are horizontal (radial) and vertical, corresponding to the two types of cells. The less malignant (lentigo maligna and superficial spreading) types have predominantly horizontal growth, by advancing cells known as 'surround' cells, with large hyperchromatic nuclei, multiple nucleoli and are different from the

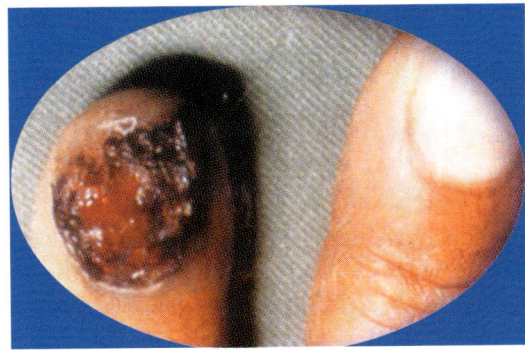

Fig. 22.1. Acral lentiginous melanoma, nail bed (courtesy: Lifeline Hospitals, Chennai)

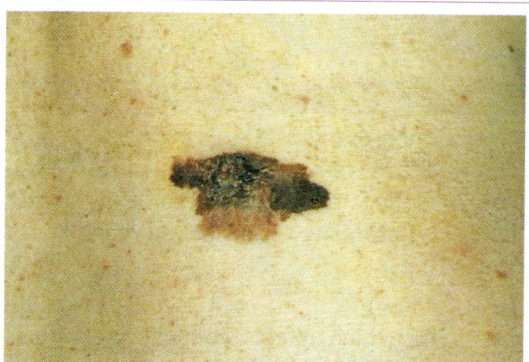

Fig. 22.2. Superficial spreading melanoma

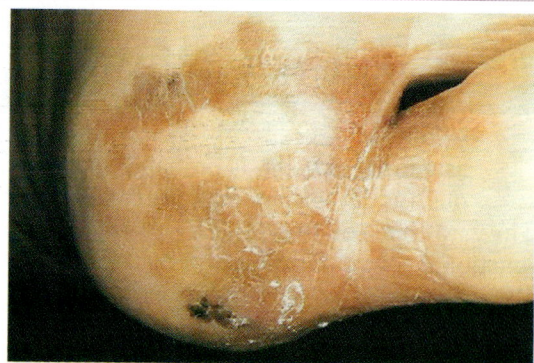

Fig. 22.4. Acral lentiginous melanoma

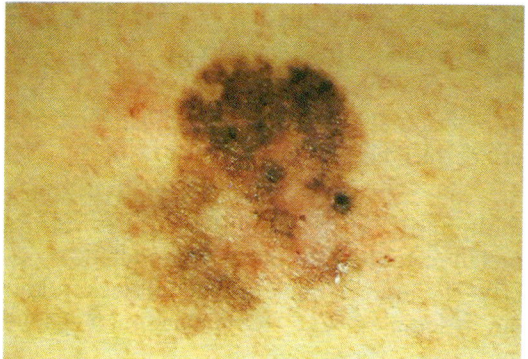

Fig. 22.3. Lentigo maligna melanoma

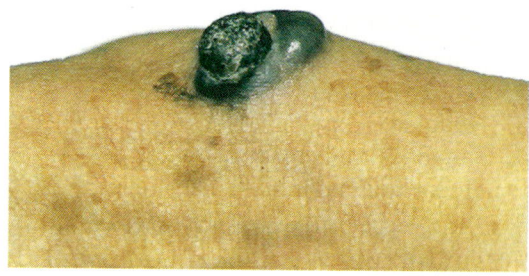

Fig. 22.5. Nodular melanoma

cells within the tumor. These *surround* cells are more typical in the superficial spreading melanoma than in lentigo maligna and are rarely seen in nodular type, with very little lateral growth, but exhibit vertical expansion.

The main type of malignant cell is the *nodule cell* in the central part of the melanoma, which is spindle shaped, with coarsely clumped nuclear material and fine granules in the cytoplasm. Some of the nodule cells have an epithelioid appearance, whereas others spindle appearance, the latter being more active. Hence it may be stated that the biological behavior of melanoma depends upon the type of cell playing dominant role. Identification of a histochemical tumor marker, DOPA, a precursor of melanin, in the tumor cells, by the so called *DOPA reaction* is very valuable, to the pathologist, in doubtful cases, to clinch the diagnosis of melanoma. Poorly differentiated tumors are DOPA negative, hence carry worse prognosis.

Histological features of malignancy

1, increase in junctional activity
2. increase in nuclear cytoplasmic ratio
3. increase in cell size
4. cytoplasm is filled with fine melanin granules
5. vacuolated cells in the epidermal layers
6. tumor cell clumps in the sub-epidermal lymphatics
7. lymphocytic invasion

Pathological staging

A) Clark's levels of invasion

Level 1: all tumor cells are above the basement membrane of the epidermis-dermis junction

Level 2: extension into papillary dermis

Level 3: extension into papillary reticular junction

Level 4: extension into reticular dermis

Level 5: subdermal fat involved, this indicates worsening prognosis with vertical spread.

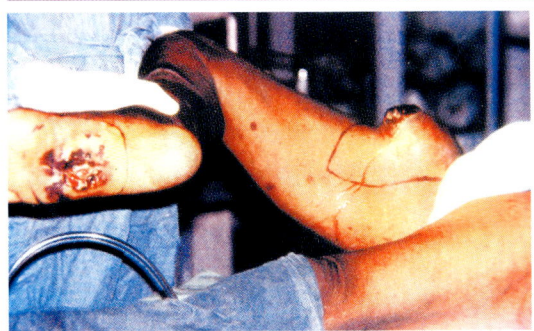

Fig. 22.6. Melanoma sole with inguinal nodes
(courtesy: Lifeline Hospitals, Chennai)

B) Breslow's staging

A more accurate way is to measure the exact tumor thickness with micro-calipers,(optical micrometer) which appears to correlate with prognosis in early lesions, but in developing countries, neither early tumors are seen often nor micro-calipers freely available !

Stage I: <0.75mm (best prognosis)

Stage II: 0.76 to 1.50mm

Stage III: 1.51 to 3.00mm

Stage IV: >3.00mm

Clark vs Breslow comparison

CLARK level1   : Breslow Stage 1

CLARK levels 2 & 3 : Breslow Stage II

CLARK levels 4 & 5 : Breslow Stage III & IV.

Clinical staging

Stage I: only the primary lesion

Stage II A: lesion + satellite nodules

Stage II B: lesion + satellite nodules +
              regional nodes

Stage III: distant metastases

Spread

Contiguous spread: Melanoma cells grow radially from the periphery causing a 'halo' sign; deep fascia acts as a strong barrier against deeper invasion.

Lymphatic spread: Commonest mode, both by *embolism* and *permeation* of lymphatics.

Satellite nodules, (within 2cm of the macroscopic edge of the primary tumor), and *in-transit* nodules, appearing more towards the direction of lymphatics, interspersed between the primary tumor and regional nodes, occur due to lymphatic permeation. Nodules develop along the course of lymphatics (e.g. in leg and thigh from foot), called 'intransit' metastatic nodules. Lymphatic spread is not seen in melanoma of the choroid plexus, since CNS has no lymphatics but seen very early in mucosal melanoma, such as anal canal, due not only to rich in lymphatics, but to constant movements, propelling the lymph.

Hematogenous: Liver spread is favored by melanoma, as also lungs, bones and brain; the small bowel serosa and the mesentery are also unusually targeted for metastases by this tumor. Eye lesions can metastasize to the liver many years after enucleation (beware of enlarged liver in a patient with glass eye!).

Symptoms

Whenever a 'benign' mole shows the features indicated above, melanoma should be suspected. Weight loss, dyspnea, melanuria and hepatomegaly et.c. indicate metastatic disease.

Signs

Common sites: Palms, soles, extremities and mucocutaneous junctions. The BANS acronym is useful to remember forlocations of poor prognosis, i.e. **b**ack, **a**xillae, **n**eck and **s**oles.

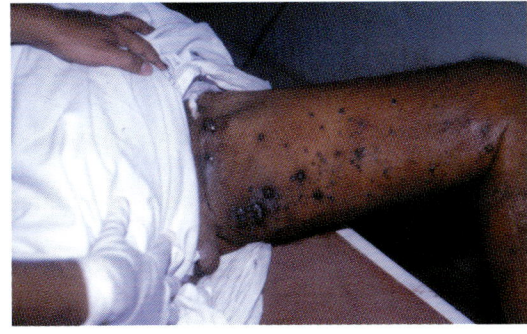

Fig. 22.7. Melanoma with intransit metastatic nodules
(courtesy: Dr K Sreekanth, Hyderabad)

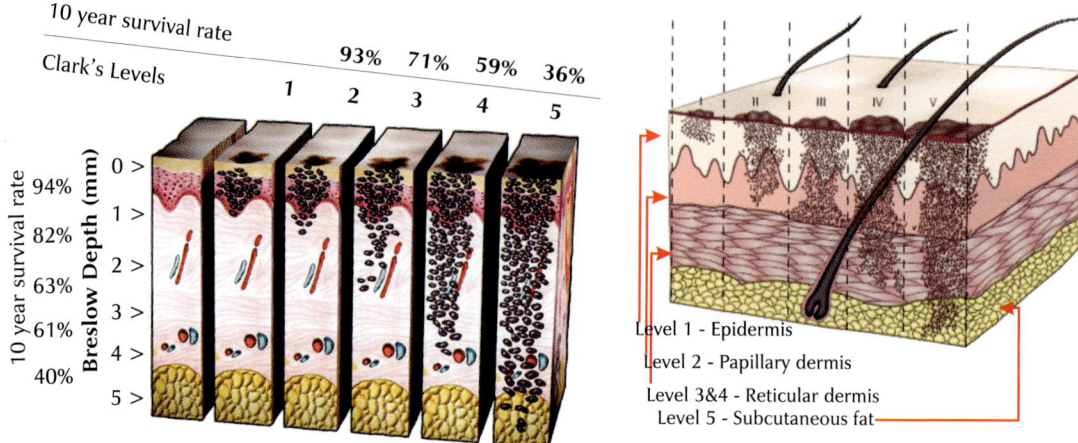

Fig. 22.8. Clark vs Breslow comparison

Fig. 22.9. Clark 's levels of melanoma invasion

Color: Varying degrees of pigmentation, from brown to black, darker the pigmentation, more the malignancy, except in the virulent amelanotic melanoma, which is pink and fleshy like an SCC.

No warmth or tenderness.

Surface: Crusting, ulceration, bleeding often seen.

Consistency: Firm to hard, with the same being felt in the satellite nodules.

Mobility: Easily mobile on deeper structures, but fixed to skin.

Lymph nodes: Often enlarged, with satellite nodules between them and primary lesion (intransit deposits).

Systemic spread: General examination to rule out hepatic, pulmonary and cerebral metastases.

Differential diagnosis

1. Pigmented basal cell carcinoma - site of the lesion, pearly edge
2. Kerato acanthoma - uniform, often sponta-neously disappears
3. Pyogenic granuloma - granulation tissue is uniform, no nodularity or pigmentation
4. Pigmented squamous papilloma.

Spontaneous regression: has been occasionally reported in the SSM and LMM, probably due to immune attack against the tumor, mounted by the T- lymphocytes.

Investigations

Edge or wedge biopsy, including junction of normal skin should be done at the earliest

Chest X-ray, USG of liver and liver function tests are mandatory in all cases, others such as CT brain, skeletal survey only if indicated.

Lymphangiography and lymphoscintigraphy are of limited value and not routinely done.

Melanuria is seen in disseminated tumors, where the urine is dark-stained or turns dark on standing for a few minutes.

Treatment

Surgery

Excision biopsy with a margin of 1 cm of healthy skin, for most small melanomas and 3 cm for larger ones, is usually adequate. All corners of the excised specimen, properly identified and labeled, should be examined histologically, to ascertain the adequacy of clearance.

The principles of melanoma surgery:
1) Radial clearance in all directions is manda-tory.
2) The deep fascia is preserved if possible, because of its 'barrier effect' for the invasion by the tumor.
3) Incisional biopsy is only used for very large

lesions, and is avoided as far as possible.

4) Involvement of the deep dermis (reticular), should dictate a clearance of 3cm all around and 5cm towards the direction of lymphatics.

5) Amputation of the phalanx (if distal) or digit (if proximal), is done for subungual melanoma.

6) Choroid melanoma requires enucleation of the eye and has a high predilection for liver metastasis

7) Anorectal melanomas are treated by abdomino-perineal resection (APR), as they are always distal to the pectinate line (anoderm). The tumor is aggressive, carrying a poor prognosis, with <10% 5-year survival.

Primary closurure of the wound after excision of melanoma should follow the basic principles of skin cover, such as closure without tension, split skin grafting (from the contralateral limb) or rotation flap closure. Split skin is preferred to full thickness, because it facilitates early detection of local recurrence under the graft.

Radiotherapy

Only useful to palliate an advanced primary tumor, reduce pain of bone metastases or to arrest the growth of cerebral secondaries.

Chemotherapy

Regional: For distal extremity melanoma, with satellite deposits or recurrent disease, isolated limb perfusion technique has been tried, with some benefit. Phenylalanine mustard (Melphalan) is the drug infused into the femoral artery and recovered from the femoral vein. Besides considerable blood loss, intimal damage with subsequent thrombosis of vessels is a common complication of this procedure.

Systemic: Phenylalanine mustard, vindesine, dacarbazine(DTIC), 5-FU, methotrexate have all been used, with only palliative effect.

Immunotherapy

Spontaneous regression of malignant melanomas has been well documented and is proof that the T-lymphocyte system responds to the presence of the malignant melanocytes and sometimes causes disappearance of the tumor. For this reason, this tumor has been the main target for the researchers, to study the benefits of immunotherapy. The logic that an accelerated immune response may restrain tumor growth is used in immunotherapy. Also, since the tumor and the metastases are mostly superficial, follow up of progress is easy.

Intralesional BCG (bacilli Calmette-Guerin vaccine for tuberculosis) has a beneficial effect in reducing the size of thick melanomas and sometimes causes regression. Systemic BCG or polyvalent bacterial vaccine, Corynebacterium parvum, Bordetella pertussis, levamisole (Vermisol), thymic hormone (thymosin), tinocordin (Immu-Mod), arabinoxylan, g-interferon and interleukin-2 are the drugs, under trial. *Allogenic human melanoma vaccine*, prepared from several different human melanoma cell lines (Can Vax), to prevent recurrence or progression of disseminated melanoma, is now available.

Treatment of metastases

A. Lymphatic secondaries

When there is no enlargement, prophylatic regional lymph node dissection does not improve survival and should only be used if the primary lesion is within 10cm of a major nodal group e.g. melanoma in the groin or axilla. A relative indication is a thick melanoma (Breslow-III or IV, within 15cm of a major nodal group)

In obvious clinical or lymphangiographic involvement, block dissection is the treatment of choice. Mono-bloc procedure (lesion+nodes) is preferred, by a single incision, if the primary and secondaries are in close proximity. Otherwise 3-4 weeks interval is recommended. If any doubt about nodal involvement exists, an FNAC is employed, but it should be realized that a negative report has limited value, as anywhere else. A positive correlation between node involvement and tumor thickness is generally seen.

Sentinel node concept

This was initially described by Cabanas, for penile carcinoma, popularized by Morton for melanoma, but also useful in breast. when regional nodes are not clinically palpable. It is based on two principles, 1. existence of orderly and predictable pattern of drainage, 2. first lymph node as effective filter Intradermal injection of radioactive agent or isosulfan blue is given around the primary tumor, the first lymph node that picks up the isotope is identified by hand-held gamma probe or by blue color, which is removed for histopathology. This gives an accurate indication of micrometastases to the nodal field. (See chapter 95)

Endolymphatic therapy

Radioactive isotopes of iodine or phosphorus are injected subdermally along with lipiodol, which is taken up by the nodes. The lymp nodes are monitored over four weeks, if they regress, the patient may be closely observed, otherwise block dissection is indicated.

B. Hematogenous secondaries

Palliation is the only of aim, in such lesions, e.g. skeletal or cerebral radiotherapy, reserving surgery for problems like intestinal obstruction. Chemotherapy with agents like dacarbazine (DTIC), isolated perfusion of hyperthermic limb, immunotherapy etc. have been attempted.

Melanoma and pregnancy

Since melanocyte-stimulating hormone (MSH) is markedly elevated during pregnancy (the reason for darkening of the areolae during first trimester of first pregnancy), the effect of pregnancy on the growth of melanoma is of some concern, but not conclusively proved. However, many workers feel, that a 'safe gap' of two years, should be recommended before allowing pregnancy, in a patient treated for melanoma. The tumor has the potential to spread to placenta and fetus.

Recent advances: Promising effects of the use of Interferon-alfa (IFN) and a monoclonal antibody, ipilimumab in disseminated melanoma is under evaluation.

Feature	SCC	BCC	Melanoma
Incidence	Commonest	Common	Uncommon
Origin	Prickle cell layer	Basal cell layer	Melanoblast
Site	Trunk, limbs, oral cavity	Face	Head, neck, digits, eye, palms and soles
Appearance	Ulcerated, cauliflower	Nodular, ulcerative	Nodular ulcerative
Ulcer margin	Everted	Rolled out, beaded	Irregular
Indiration of base	+ + + +	+ +	+
Scabbing	Never forms	Occurs	Never
Pigmentation	Absent	May be present	Mostly present (90%)
Spread	Lymphatics	No lymphatic spread	All modalities
DOPA reaction	No	No	Mostly
IHC expression	Cytokeratin	None	S100
Prognosis	Good	Very Good	Bad

Table - 22.1. Differences between squamous cell Ca, basal cell Ca and melanoma

23 Tumor Growth and Staging

Understanding tumor growth has helped the modern surgeon adopt effective strategies to tackle neoplasia. Synthesis of DNA occurs in a relatively short interval in the 'cell cycle' the pattern of which was revealed by radioactive-labelled thymidine. Tumor growth in relation to DNA synthesis in the cell cycle is called tumor kinetics. The cycle passes through the following phases:

G0: some cells have division capacity but are temporarily removed from the cycle; when suitably stimulated they move to G1.

G1: Apparent metabolic rest.

S: Synthetic period (of DNA)

G2: Premitotic period.

M: Mitosis (cell division)

A normal cell divides only to replace a lost cell (total cell number is constant). A cancer cell divides and adds to existing cells (total cell number is continually increasing). Tumor growth is the outcome of three combined parameters and is expressed as tumor doubling time (TDT), i.e. the time taken for a given amount of tumor tissue to double its volume, which may range from 4 to 500 days. Leukemia and lymphoma have the shortest TDT, followed by sarcoma, with carcinoma having the longest TDT.

1. Growth fraction (Gf) = the ratio of actively dividing cells to resting cells.

2. Cell cycle time (Tc) = (for human cells) 40-80 hours.

3. Cell loss coefficient = the ratio of cells lost to cells produced. It is 100% for normal tissues (zero growth) and 95-99% in cancer. In tumors, reduction in cell population may be due to exfoliation by friction (skin and gastrointestinal tract), central necrosis, biologically inadequate cells, metastases (washed away) and destruction by host defences or to the presence of resting cells.

A cancer may therefore be viewed not as a mass of very rapidly dividing cells but as tissue with cells dividing at an approximately normal rate but failing to lose cells in the normal fashion and therefore gradually increasing in size. TDT is constant for any tumor, i.e. a cancer that can double its size in 2 days will have quadrupled its size in 4 days and be eight times its original volume in 6 days (such proportional increase in size with unit time is termed exponential growth). The human body contains approximately 5×10^{13} cells; a tumor is clinically detectable when it reaches 10^9 cells = 1 gm = 1cm in size and when it reaches 10^{12} = 1 kg the patient is near death. A tumor is therefore clinically detectable and treatable during the last 10 to14 of its 35-odd doubling times, in other words in only the later third of its existence!

TUMOR STAGING

A single mutated cancer cell starts to grow locally to form a tumor composed of malignant and stromal cells, which spreads to adjacent and distant organs via lymphatic and blood vessels. The cancer growth pattern depends on the cell of origin and type of mutation(s); it can therefore progress slowly or rapidly in a very short time. Staging procedures are examinations and tests performed to define the extent of cancer within the body and they focus on the size of the tumor, lymph node involvement, and distant metastases. In the majority of malignancies, treatment is tailored to tumor stage in order to obtain best outcome in terms of survival and treatment-related toxicity. The aim of staging is therefore to avoid under- and overtreatment. It is important that the staging investigations should follow, after having made the tissue diagnosis of a cancer, before planning therapy.

Clinical staging

Over time, different staging systems and staging classifications have evolved and even today they are being fine-tuned with new outcome data. The most commonly used staging system is the TNM system (Table 23.1), which is based on 3 variables: tumor size (T0-T4), extent of lymph node involvement (N0-N3), and presence of distant metastases (M0-M1). Recent trend is to combine histologic grading, which is equally relevant to determine the overall outlook and rename it as TNMG staging. Though in most types of cancer TNM staging is used, different staging systems are used for central nervous system cancers, lymphomas (Ann Arbor staging classification), leukemias, multiple myeloma, and gynecological cancers (International Federation of Gynecology and Obstetrics/FIGO).

In breast, Manchester staging (stages I, II, III & IV) is also employed to understand the treatment protocol, since it becomes too complicated to interpolate the combinations and permutations of TNM staging against various forms of therapy by the clinician.

In colo-rectal cancers, Dukes' staging is also popular, to identify the depth of tumor invasion, the loco-regional and distant spread.

Pathological staging

The pathological classification (post-surgical or pTNM) is based on the evidence acquired before treatment, supplemented or modified by the additional evidence acquired from surgery and from pathological examination.

The pathological classification can be determined in the primary tumor

pTX: primary tumor cannot be assessed
pT0: no histological evidence of primary tumor
pTis: carcinoma-in-situ
pT1-pT4: according to this size and/or local extension of primary tumor.

Regional lymph nodes

pNX: regional lymph nodes cannot be assessed histologically

pN0: no regional lymph node metastases

pN1-pN3: increasing involvement of lymph nodes.

Primary tumor (T)	
Tx	Primary tumor cannot be evaluated
T0	No evidence of primary tumor
Tis	Carcinoma-in-situ
T1-t4	Size and/or extent of the primary tumor
T1: <2cm; T2: 2-5cm; T3: 5-10cm; T4: >10cm	
Regional lymph nodes (N). Involvement of any nodes other than regional is considered metastasis	
Nx	Regional lymph nodes cannot be evaluated
N0	No regional lymph node involvement
N1, n2, n3	Involvement of regional lymoh nodes (number and/or extent of spread)
Distant metastasis (M)	
Mx	Distant metastasis cannot be evaluated
M0	No distant metastasis
M1	Distant metastasis
Histological grading (Broder)	
G1	Well differentiated (>75% differentiated cells)
G2	Moderately differentiated (50-75% differentiated cells)
G3	Poorly differentiated (25-50% differentiated cells)
G4	Undifferentiated (<25% differentiated cells)

Table-23.1 TNMG staging

	FEATURE	BENIGN	MALIGNANT
1	Number	May be multiple	Usually single
2	Growth	Slow	Rapid
3	Precancerous conditions	Absent	May be seen
4	Outline	Circumscribed	Irregular
5	Dilated veins over the skin	Absent	May be present
6	Secondary changes of skin	Absent	May be noted
7	Tissue planes	Confined to a plane	Don't respect planes
8	Pressure effects	Late	Early
9	Local warmth	Absent	May be present
10	Fixity	Absent	Present (may be late)
11	Intrinsic mobility	Present	Absent
12	Consistency	Uniform	Variable
13	Regional or distant spread	Absent	May be present
14	Cut surface	Becomes convex	Flat or concave
15	Encasing capsule	Usually present	Absent
16	Standard treatment	Simple excision	Wide (3-dimensional) excision
17	Tumor markers	Absent (unless functional)	May be present
18	Histology	Resembles native tissue	Usually dedifferentiated
19	Prognosis	Excellent	Variable (usually bad)

Table - 23.2. Differences between benign and malignant tumors

24 Radiotherapy (RT)

Use of ionizing radiation for therapeutic purposes is known as radiotherapy (RT). Ionizing radiations damage both neoplastic and normal tissues, by breaking the DNA strands. As it affects actively dividing cells, normal tissues are less vulnerable for damage and rapidly recover while neoplastic tissues do not, resulting in the therapeutic benefit. A radiation dose is defined as the energy absorbed per unit of mass and is expressed in rads or in Grays (1 Gray = 1joule/Kg =100 rads). RT is used mainly for malignancies and rarely for benign conditions (e.g. thyrotoxicosis and some skin conditions); it may be as radical (curative), palliative, adjuvant or neo-adjuvant therapy.

Radiation can be considered as packets (quanta) of energy in the form of photons (e.g. x-rays, ultraviolet light) or particles (e.g. protons, neutrons, and electrons). As these packets of energy penetrate into tissue, they produce ionizations either directly or indirectly in biologically important molecules. The subatomic collisions caused by the particle types of radiation can induce direct biologic damage within cells, which is termed *direct ionization*. X-rays, on the other hand, transfer their energy to chemical intermediates within tissue, and it is these intermediates that produce the actual biologic damage. This is called *indirect ionization*. Thus, particulate radiation is direct and x-radiation indirect.

TUMOR RESPONSE

Radiocurability refers to the eradication of tumor at the primary or regional site and reflects a direct effect of the irradiation, which may not parallel the patients' ultimate outcome. *Radiosensitivity* expresses tumor response to irradiation. No significant correlation exists between radiosensitivity and radiocurability. Thus, a tumor may be fairly radiosensitive yet incurable and vice versa.

Tumor response to irradiation is not necessarily a good measure of radiosensitivity. Most tumors contain a proportion of rapidly proliferating tumor cells and inflammatory cells that show an early response to irradiation.

The response of a tumor to irradiation will depend on the programmed lifetime of terminally differentiated cells within the tumor, the proliferation kinetics of the malignant clonogens, and the removal rate of dead cells. In general, local control for rapidly regressing tumors will be slightly higher than that for slowly regressing tumors. Despite this observation, reduction in total dose on the basis of tumor response is not warranted.

The interpretation of slow tumor regression is somewhat more complex. Slow regression can be due to slow tumor proliferation and cell loss kinetics. It also may indicate a mass of residual stroma without viable tumor cells, as is commonly seen in Hodgkin's disease, pituitary adenomas, and choroidal melanomas. Finally, slow regression may be due to persistent tumor. The issue is clouded further by the fact that a small proportion of most tumor types will regress slowly even though the majority may regress quickly.

In view of the heterogeneity of tumor response, obtaining early post-irradiation biopsies of a slowly regressing tumor often is unnecessary and sometimes is misleading because of the impossibility of distinguishing sterilized but still living tumor cells from those that have retained their reproductive integrity. Since early post-irradiation biopsies are associated with considerable risk of tissue necrosis, the advisable approach usually is to avoid performing such biopsies if a tumor continues to regress; often, they are not indicated sooner than three months after therapy.

Radiation oncologists are much like surgeons in that they attempt to cure disease by local eradication of a tumor. This concept represents

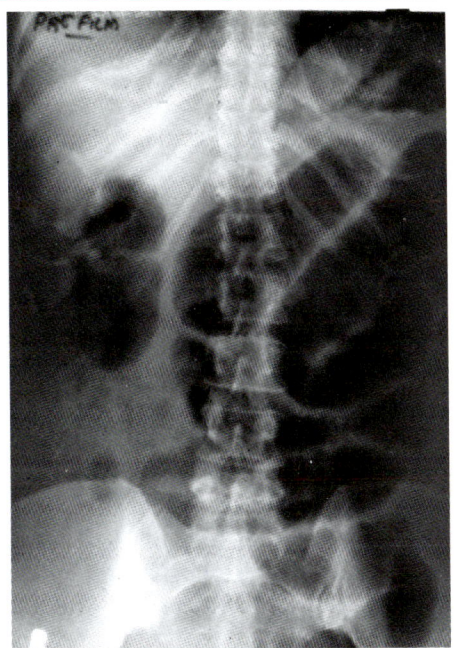

Fig. 24.1. Radiation enteropathy with bowel
obstruction
(courtesy: Lifeline Hospitals, Chennai)

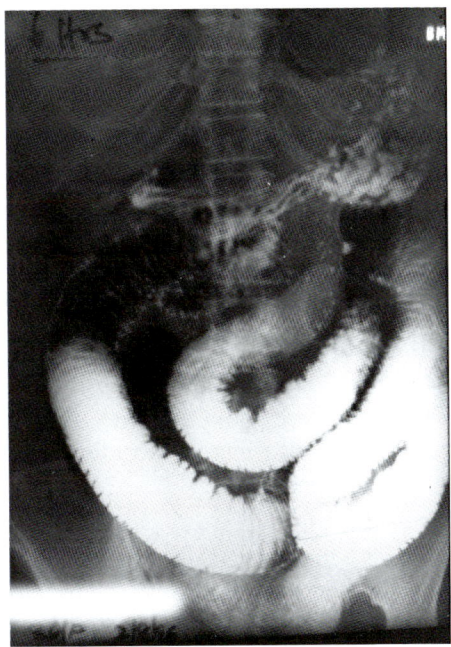

Fig. 24.2. Barium meal picture of radiation enteropathy
showing loss of mucosal markings
(courtesy: Lifeline Hospitals, Chennai)

local control, implying that the tumor will never return to the treated area; on providing local control, a higher probability of cure would be expected. Oncologists tend to evaluate therapies in terms of response rates.

A *complete response* is defined as the absence of clinically detectable tumor, whereas a *partial response* is defined as a greater than 50% reduction in tumor mass. Radiation oncologists tend to place less emphasis on response rates than do their peers in other oncologic specialties, as a complete response does not necessarily translate into a clinical cure and a partial response most likely will translate into a complete failure.

Development of computer graphics has led to progress in the form of treatment planning advances. In particular, 3-dimensional treatment planning systems and intensity-modulated radiotherapy (IMRT) techniques have significantly improved the ability to localize radiation dose to difficult locations and unusual shapes. These "conformal" treatment planning tools allow for more effective treatment of tumors while offering better and precise protection adjacent normal tissues.

Cancer response to RT

1) *Type of cell:* highly radiosensitive (e.g. Burkitt's lymphoma, Wilms' tumor and seminoma) or moderately sensitive (e.g. BCC, SCC, transitional cell carcinoma and osteogenic sarcoma). STS, and recurrent tumors following previous RT are generally radio-resistant. Note, that while seminoma needs 2000r, Hodgkin's disease requires 4000r. and SCC, breast/rectal carcinoma need 6000r.

2) *Differentiation* of cells: Radiosensitivity is directly proportional to reproductive activity and inversely proportional to the degree of cell differentiation. Thus, germinal cells and spermatogonia are very sensitive, while neurones are resistant (except medulloblastoma). Anaplastic cancers are generally radiosensitive and 'melt' quickly, only to regrow equally fast.

3) *Blood supply:* Hypoxic cells are radio-resistant, e.g. in large rapidly growing cancers, those in association with syphilis or post-inflammatory scarring, following therapeutic embolisation (to reduce vascularity) etc. Hyperbaric oxygen therapy increases the radiosensitivity of cancer, as do nitroimidazole derivatives, such as misonidazole and they are known as radio-sensitizers.

4) *Localisation:* The more localised the cancers, the easier their control (e.g. BCC, carcinoma of the cervix) and the better the results (provided they are radiosensitive), debulking (cytoreduction) also increases radiosensitivity of the tumor.

Assessment of tumor

Radiation is administered after the extent of the cancer has been accurately assessed by surface anatomy, examination under anesthesia, radiography, preoperative insertion of radiopaque markers around the target and computerized simulators. Radiation dose depends on age, condition of patient, type of cancer and the target volume (the larger the tumor load, the greater the number of radiation fractions required). Deep-seated cancers are most often treated by multiple convergent beams or by rotational therapy.

Total body radiation

In the era of total body radiation followed by bone marrow transplant (BMT) rescue, it is important for the clinician to be aware of the side effects.

Immediate effects

1. Very high dosage (>5000r. single exposure) produces *cerebral syndrome* (nausea, vomiting, tremors, convulsions and death).

2. Moderate dosage (800-5000r. single exposure) produces *gastrointestinal syndrome* (nausea, vomiting, diarrhea, dehydration and death).

3. Low dosage (<800r. single exposure) produces *hematological sydrome*.

(mild nausea and vomiting but mainly bone marrow aplasia with pancytopenia manifested by infection and bleeding tendencies.

Late effects

1. Premature ageing (progeria)
2. Cataract
3. Infertility
4. Fetal abnormalities
5. Malignant disease
6. Genetic effect

Local effect of radiation on the skin (in chronological order)

1. Erythema followed by pigmentation.
2. Fibrinoid necrosis with endarteritis and radionecrotic ulcer (painful, indolent, with clean-cut edge and sloughing floor)
3. Fibrosis with absent hair follicles and accessory glands (delayed healing following injury). Skin becomes atrophic with telangiectasia.

Types of RT

A) External beam therapy

1. Conventional x-ray therapy (ortho-voltage 10-500 KV) either superficial or deep.

2. Mega voltage (1.2 - 40 MV) from:

a) Y sources ^{60}Co, ^{137}CS teletherapy.

b) X-ray sources from linear accelerator giving sharper, deeper but more extensive radiation.

c) Particle beam (electrons) from linear accelerator.

d) Betatrons (circular electron accelerators)

e) Cyclotrons and synchrotrons producing heavy particles, e.g. neutrons.

Note: (a) and (b) are electromagnetic radiations while (c), (d) and (e) are particle radiations.

B) **Brachytherapy** (brachys: short; tele: at a distance)

In this technique, radioactive sources are inserted within or close to the cancer tissue.

1. Intracavitary

Used mainly in gynecology for treatment of carcinoma of cervix and corpus uterus, radium, ^{137}Cs, ^{90}Y (bladder carcinoma) and

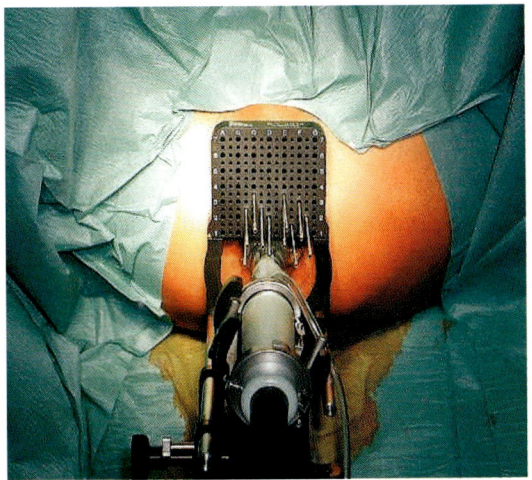

Fig. 24.3. Brachytherapy for carcinoma anal canal

^{198}Au, colloid (in malignant effusion- ascites or pleural) are used. One method involves insertion of a special applicator (under anesthesia) and is left in for 24hours, which may have to be repeated as necessary. The cathetron technique involves inserting a shielded ^{60}Co source holder under general anesthesia after-loading it mechanically from another room.

2. Interstitial

It involves application of moulds under general anesthesia (e.g. radium and ^{137}Cs needles, ^{192}Ir, ^{192}Ta and ^{90}Y wires; ^{198}Au grains; and radon seeds). Used in tongue and bladder carcinoma and also following surgery (unresectable tumor) of parotid, apical lung cancers, STS and for breast conservation.

C) Sytemic radiotherapy

This works like 'target-guided missiles', using radioisotopes, such as ^{131}I (for thyrotoxicosis and thyroid carcinoma), ^{32}P(for polycythemia rubra vera) etc. When systemically administered, these isotopes emitting radiation energy, are taken up preferentially by malignant cells in much higher concentrations than by normal cells.

Clinical applications

i) Radical radiotherapy (alone), with the aim of cure, e.g. SCC (skin, oral cavity, larynx and cervix uteri.

ii) Planned combination of surgery with radio-therapy, e.g. seminoma (with improved 5 year survival of from 50% to 80%) and carcinoma of pharynx.

iii) Radiotherapy may be preoperative as neoadjuvant form (e.g. hypernephroma and rectal carcinoma), or more commonly post operative (e.g. breast carcinoma).

iv) Planned combination of cytotoxic therapy with radiotherapy, as sandwich form (e.g. late stage malignant lymphoma and tumors of head and neck).

v) Palliative radiotherapy, e.g. in bronchogenic carcinoma to control profuse hemoptysis, bone pain, pressure effects such as dysphagia, dyspnea and superior vena caval obstruction; in breast carcinoma to control bone pain (due to metastasis); in advanced cervical carcinoma to control bleeding and for retrobulbar deposits causing proptosis

SUMMARY

Many advances in radiation oncology have occurred since the discovery of x-rays in 1895. Initially, radiation oncology was largely empirical and based mainly on clinical observations. Modern radiobiology provides a rationale for both normal tissue and tumor response to irradiation.

These responses are based on 4-'R's of radiobiology:

1. reoxygenation of hypoxic cells
2. repair of sublethal damage
3. repopulation of cells between fractions
4. reassortment of cells to more sensitive phases of the cell cycle.

Since cell killing is a random process, no single dose of radiation will guarantee a cure. Radiation oncologists attempt to provide the highest probability of tumor control while minimizing the risk of serious complications and are in constant search for ways to increase the tumor response and improve patient care.

Today, advances in all aspects of oncology have led to a realistic possibility of cure of more than 50% of newly diagnosed cases of cancer. Researchers hope that future advances will continue to improve benefits of radiation oncology and cancer care for all.

Morbidities related to Radiotherapy

1. Immediate effects (within 6-8 weeks)

Fatigue, lassitude, anorexia, nausea and emesis

Skin reactions: more in neck, axilla and inguinal folds (more so with combined chemo+- radiotherapy-CRT).

Bowel symptoms may occur with abdominal or pelvic irradiation

Hematological toxicities and infections may occur in about 10 to20%, especially after CRT

2. Late effects

Apical and para-mediastinal fibrosis

With mantle/neck radiation: Lhermitte phenomenon (electric-like shock wave spreading down the body when the patient flexes the neck, commonly seen in multiple sclerosis and other cord lesions)

Occasional pericarditis and/or effusion

Gonadal dysfunction or infertility, especially with CRT

Development of secondary (metachronous) neoplasms upto 10%, after about 20 years of treatment

Hypothyroidism

Cardiac dysfunction, coronorary artery disease, if left heart received >25gy.

Pulmonary fibrosis in up to 10% after CRT.

Intensity modulated RT (IMRT)

It is a type of 3-dimensional radiation therapy that uses computer-generated images to match radiation to the size and shape of a tumor. In IMRT, thousands of tiny radiation beams (or beamlets) enter the body from many angles and intersect the tumor. Since the intensity of each beamlet can be controlled, the radiation dose can wrap around normal tissue, create concave shapes and turn corners. The aim is to deliver a higher radiation dose to a tumor with less damage to nearby healthy tissue. IMRT may be used, for example, to treat a tumor that surrounds the spinal cord and spare the cord itself.

During treatment, the radiation intensity of each beamlet is controlled, and the beam shape changes hundreds of times during each treatment, by employing a device called a multileaf collimator, which adjusts the size and shape of the computer-determined radiation beams. As a result, the radiation dose bends around important healthy tissues in a way that is impossible with other techniques. Because of the complexity of these motions, physicians use special high-speed computers, treatment-planning software, diagnostic imaging and patient-positioning devices to plan treatments and control the radiation dose during therapy.

For IMRT to be effective, the anatomical position of the tumor and surrounding healthy tissues must be accurately defined. Conventional CT, PET-CT or MRI provide the necessary 3-D anatomical information. Surgeon plays a key role by keeping markers during surgery and

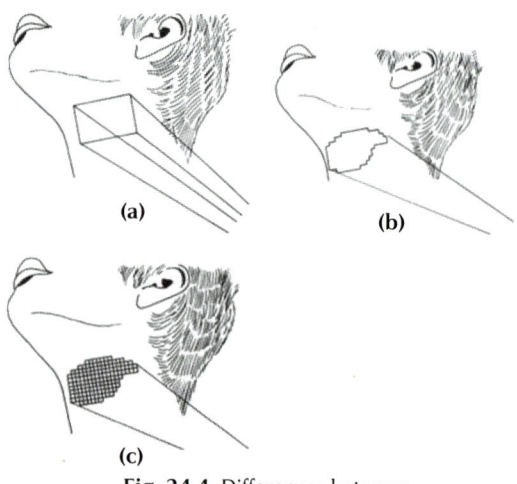

Fig. 24.4. Differences between
(a) conventional radiotherapy (RT)
(b) conformal radiotherapy (CFRT) without intensity modulation
(c) CFRT with intensity modulation (IMRT)

working closely with oncologist to define the treatment area. It's also important to accurately position and immobilize the patient during treatment. Another innovation is image-guided RT (IGRT), in which entire radiation dose calculation is done under CT image guidance.

Stereotactic radiosurgery and RT

Stereotactic radiosurgery (SRS) and radiotherapy (SRT) represent an increasingly important option in treatment of central nervous system diseases. Both SRS and SRT are flourishing, non invasive techniques of precise high precision RT for localized benign and malignant lesions in intracranial and extracranial sites, called stereotactic body radiotherapy (SBRT).

The rationale is to give a highly precise dose of irradiation to the target volume with little radiation to surrounding normal tissues. It may allow dose escalation without increasing radiation related morbidity and/or has a potential to decrease RT induced morbidity.

To achieve their goals, SRS and SRT, certain prerequisites have to be fulfilled: - high resolution 3-D images, accurate immobilization, relative lack of internal organ motion and external fiducial reference markers to align the treatment machine so that the lesion is accurately targeted. The choice between SRS and SRT depends on many factors, such as target volume, presence or absence of organ or tissues at risk, close to PTV and the indication for treatment.

Current recommendations

SRS

1. Arteriovenous malformations

2. Brain metastasis

3. Functional radiosurgery (e.g. for trigeminal neuralgia)

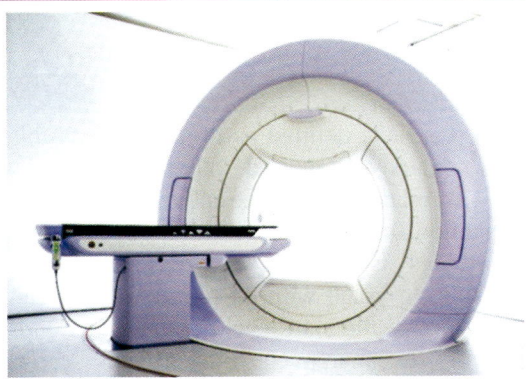

Fig. 24.5. Stereotactic radiotherapy unit (courtesy: Dr S Krishnan, Chennai)

SRT

1. Pituitary Adenoma
2. Craniopharyngiomas
3. Meningiomas
4. Acoustic neuromas
5. Gliomas

Complications (3-10%) dependent on normal brain tissue\volume adjacent to nidus irradiated. Majority occur within 3 years of therapy.

Headaches and dizziness due to cerebral edema, radio necrosis, convulsive disorder, infarct and hemiparesis or cyst formation

Rarely mortality (< 0.2%) may occur from fatal internal bleeding

Recent advances in RT

1. Administration of chemical and physical radiosensitizing procedures such as hyperbaric oxygen, hyperthermia (lethal to malignant cells) and imidazole group of drugs (metronidazole, misonidazole etc).

2. Use of particle radiation, e.g. fast neutrons, protons and negative pimesons (O_2 independent).

25 Scar Hypertrophy and Keloid

A scar is defined as the residual visible mark of a wound. When the intensity and duration of the active phase of scar formation are increased, it undergoes hypertrophy. This is marked by proliferation of fibroblastic tissue without blood vessels, elevated above the skin level but never extends beyond the margin of the original scar(as against keloid, which overshoots it). It may spontaneously regress in some cases and in any event does not continue to grow beyond 3 to 6 months.

Etiology

1. Increased skin tension at the time of closure
2. Chronic hypoxia
3. Healing by secondary intention
4. An autoimmune mechanism
5. Racial and familial, occurring more in negroes and orientals
6. Altered collagen kinetics (decreased collagenolysis) and ground substance alteration

Clinical features

1. Common in younger individuals
2. Scars crossing the natural skin creases or Langer's lines are more vulnerable for hypertrophy.
3. Never spreads onto the surrounding normal skin
4. No claw-like processes
5. No itching nor increased vascularity
6. May regress after 6 months
7. If excised, recurrence is uncommon

Differential diagnosis

Keloid: This is irregular growth beyond the original scar with itching and hyper vascularity. It continues to grow even after 6 months and secondary smouldering infection in the crevices producing local inflammation and pain, is very common. Presternal and deltoid regions as well as the pinna of the ears are its favourite sites.

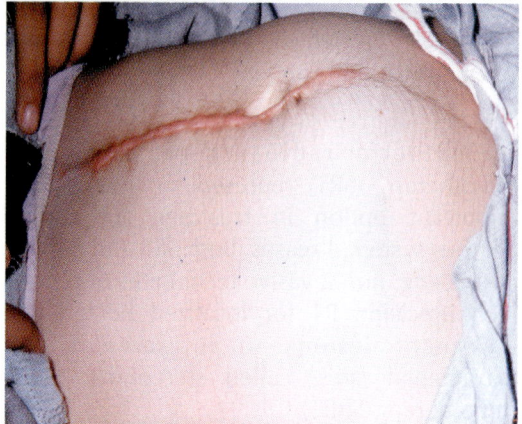

Fig. 25.1. Scar hypertrophy, abdominal wall (courtesy: Lifeline Hospitals, Chennai)

Recurrence with greater vigor following excision is the rule.

Management

Prevention, by avoiding some of the factors mentioned above is the best. Infection, persistent suture material or granulation tissue are dealt with immediately. Injections of depo-steroids, into the scar, are helpful to discourage further growth. Application of constant pressure by elastic compression reduces fibroblastic activity; this is particularly useful for post-burn scars. This also helps to reduce lymphedema of the area. Prolonged use of the silicone gel sheet, supported by external pressure is also found to prevent and resolve scar hypertrophy.

Surgery

The principle of surgery is excision of the hypertrophic scar and reconstruction of the skin with minimal tension, by direct suturing or 'Z' or 'V-Y' plasty, ideally done after about 6 months, allowing for spontaneous regression. Advancement or rotation flaps and skin grafting may be rarely necessary. Laser surgery, a recent introduction, appears to score over earlier methods of treatment.

KELOID (kele: tumor; eidos: form) is considered a form of cellular fibroma, due to an overgrowth of a scar or may arise denovo, in vulnerable individuals. Colored races are more prone for this troublesome disease (Negro women often invoke them as decorations), but other races also exhibit individual susceptibility. It may develop in healed burns, surgical wounds, cuts, needle punctures, vaccination/tattoo marks, scratches etc. or without any provocation, presternal region and ear lobules being the favourite sites. Multiparous women are the commonest victims of keloid and it differs from simple hypetrophy of scar by the lesion extending well beyond the original scar and its potential to develop without a predisposing injury or scar. It has been suggested that in many instances, it may be an exaggerated proliferative reaction to a foreign body, such as dislocated hair, cotton/wool fibers, keratin debris etc. (Glucksmann). The altered collagen kinetics seen in scar hypertrophy, appears to be exaggerated in this disease and the amount of collagen is about 20 times compared to normal scar.

They present as irregular elevations from the surface, freely mobile over the underlying fat, with thin skin cover and uneven surface forming deep crevices, which harbour infection.

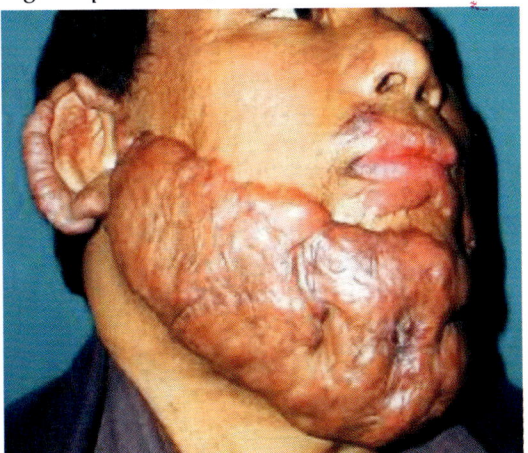

Fig. 25.2. Extensive keloid, neck, face and ear from burn wound
(courtesy: Halsted Surgical Clinic, Chennai)

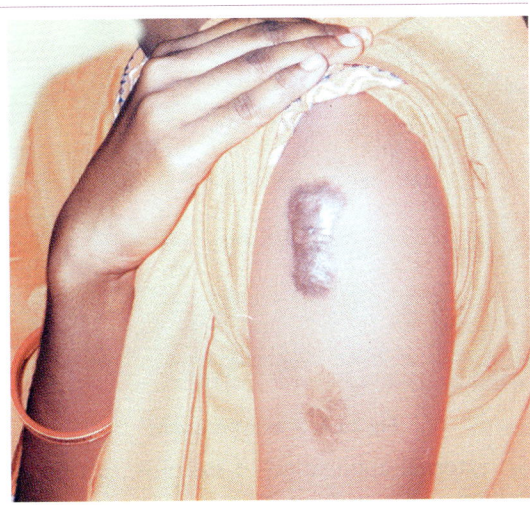

Fig. 25.3. Keloid of vaccination scar, deltoid region
(courtesy: Halsted Surgical Clinic, Chennai)

Over the presternal region, they may be typically butterfly-shaped and grow to enormous size. Itching and pain are usually present, sometimes associated with cellulitis, purulent discharge and regional lymphadenopathy, due to often associated infection. They contain a significant number of mast cells as compared to normal skin or scar, explaining the severe itching over the lesion, relieved to some extent by oral or topical antihistaminic therapy.

Management: No specific investigations are necessary for the diagnosis. As they recur with greater vigour following excision, aptly called 'plastic surgeon's nightmare', surgery alone of any kind should be avoided. The therapeutic options are:

1. intra-lesional injection of deposteroid or the socalled 'supersteroids' like clobetasol or triamcinolone (Kenacort) and hyaluranidase (Hyalase). Skin atrophy and development of telangiectasia may be seen following this therapy.
2. excision followed by injection of steroids into the wound margins.
3. superficial radiotherapy
4. excision followed by superficial radiotherapy after 48-72 hours.
5. Laser excision

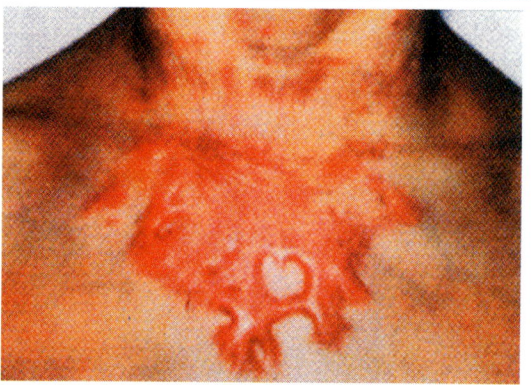

Fig 25.4. Scar hypertrophy

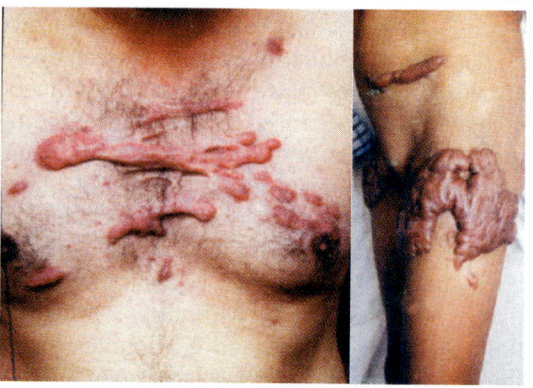

Fig 25.5. Keloids of presternal region & thigh

6. external application of steroids, to relieve itching

7. Early use of pressure garments and silicone sheeting has been found to be effective, by increasing the activity of collagenase due to local warmth produced.

The more common areas for keloids: earlobe, presternal, deltoid and upper back.

Less common areas: eyelids, genitalia, palms, soles and across joints.

	Feature	Hypertrophic scar	Keloid
1	Incidence	More common	Less common
2	Racial predilection	No	Afro-caribbean race
3	Familial tendency	Absent	Present
4	Occurance	Soon after injury	Months/years later
5	Location	Flexor surfaces	Ear lobe, anterior chest wall and deltoid region
6	Amount of collagen	6-7 times normal	20 times normal
7	Skin color	More in fair-skinned individuals	More in dark-skinned
8	Extent of lesion	Confined to scar	Extends beyond the scar
9	Pathology	Hypertrophy of mature fibroblasts	Proliferation of immature fibroblasts
10	Pruritus	No	Severe (due to presence of mast cells)
11	Regression	Spontaneous within a few months	No
12	Recurrence after excision	No	Notorious

Table-25.1. Differences between scar hypertrophy and keloid

26 Pilonidal Disease

(pilo: hair; nidus: nucleus/nest)

(syn: pilliferous cyst, jeep driver's disease, coccygeal sinus)

Most commonly located in the natal cleft with male preponderance, has both congenital and acquired etiological factors, though the latter has more following.

Congenital type (the veracity of this is being questioned) seen in children and in young women, whereas the acquired type, more common, seen in adult males having dense hair, with rough texture.

Etiology

Congenital sinuses in this region may be due to the patency of the tail end of the neural canal or a complication of post anal dermoid cyst; these are not true pilonidal diseases.

Acquired (virtually all the cases)

1. The disease affects predominantly obese men with thick black, straight hair and deep natal cleft

2. Movement of buttocks causes broken hair to be driven into the skin cracks in the cleft.

3. Usage of toilet paper may sweep perianal hair into the cracks

4. The embedded hair within the skin sets up chronic infection resulting in an abscess or a sinus. If there is no infection, it can result in granulomatous reaction and cyst formation.

5. Interdigital pilonidal sinus is an occupational disease of hair dressers and sheep shearers, who clip wool from the animal.

6. Recurrence is possible even after adequate excision, probably due to the same etiological factors operating.

7. This was so common in drivers during the second world war that it was popularly known as 'jeep driver's disease'

8. A strong point in favor of acquired hypothesis is that if the tuft of hair within the sinus is examined carefully, their heads are inside with the roots sticking outside. Furthermore, in barbers the hair present in the sinuses is not their own, but belong to the customers !

Other sites for pilonidal sinuses are

(1) In hair dressers, a small black spot or a palpable lump (barber's nodule) may be seen in the interdigital clefts of right hand, which may get infected, forming a sinus.

(2) umbilicus

(3) axilla

(4) over the scalp following sutured lacerations

(5) clitoris

Pathology

Uncomplicated pilonidal cyst may go unnoticed, patient usually presenting with an infected cyst or a sinus discharging pus, following its rupture. The track of the sinus is notorious for its ramifications, leading to the formation of more than one external opening (sinuses). The track is usually lined by granulation tissue, though stratified squamous epithelium may be seen at its mouth. In about 25% of cases, no hair is found in the lesions.

Microscopically it has an appearance of a sinus tract lined by inflammatory tissue with foreign body (giant cell) granuloma, in which tufts of

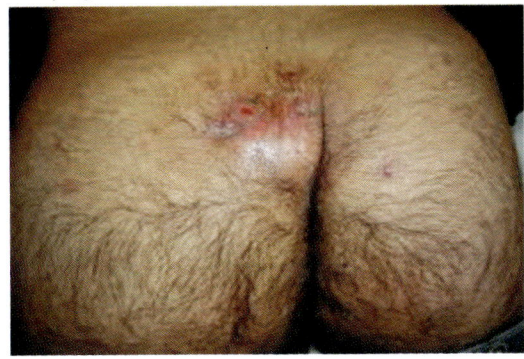

Fig. 26.1. Pilonidal abscess
(courtesy: Dr C J Reddy, Gudur)

153

hair are embedded. Contents: hair, granulation tissue and epithelial debris fill the cavity. Typically the roots of the hair are projecting outside, a point in favor of the acquired theory.

Complications

1. Recurrent abscess formation
2. Complications related to any focus of chronic sepsis, like cellulitis, pyemic abscesses, reactive arthritis/fibrositis, amyloidosis, etc.
3. Superadded malignancy (SCC)
4) Osteomyelitis of sacrum/coccyx

Clinical features

With male/female ratio of 4:1, the disease usually manifests during third decade. A recurrent painful swelling or sinus usually containing a tuft of hair, with purulent discharge in the post-coccygeal region is rather unmistakable. Despite its chronicity, neither the general condition nor the normal activities of the patient is affected. This condition rarely occurs in blondes, as their hair is thin and soft. The primary sinus may have multiple openings even up to six, situated in the mid line.

Differential diagnosis

1. Infected sebaceous/dermoid cyst
2. Perianal suppurative conditions
3) Hidradenitis suppurativa
4) Osteomyelitis of the sacrum/coccyx
5) Tuberculosis of sacro-coccygeal joint

Investigations

A sinogram may be done to identify the ramificatons and their relationship to the underlying bony structures, but is not routinely required. Though expensive, MRI is the most reliable investigation, to understand the topography of the lesion. Other investigations like an x-ray chest/ sacro-coccygeal region, Mantoux test, bacteriological study of the discharge, immunological tests for tuberculosis or biopsy of the curetted material in the sinus tract, may be performed as necessary.

Treatment

Surgery is the only definitive treatment; drug therapy is used only to control infection and relieve pain in acute cases.

1) Incision and drainage of an abscess may have to be done, as a preliminary step to control overt sepsis, before definitive surgery is planned.

2) Several operations have been described for pilonidal disease:

i) 'Fistulotomy' (laying open the sinus) may be done, to lay open the entire tract and to remove the hair and inflammatory debris. This marsupialises the pathological cavity.

ii) Excision of tract with saucerisation (like for a fistula-in-ano) is a safe procedure but the process of secondary healing of the deep cavity might take several weeks, leaving a painful scar. Needless to say, this is preferred if there is residual infection in the depth. Secondary suturing may be done after a week or so, to minimize healing time and the resultant scar.

iii) Excision of tract and primary closure of the wound, retaining the sutures for 2-3 weeks is the most popular procedure, since the wound heals by primary intention, resulting in minimal scarring. Preliminary injection of a dye, such as methylene blue, to ensure excision of all ramifications and meticulous hemostasis, with the help of diathermy are essential prerequisites for this operation. Prophylactic antibiotics are indicated in view of the proximity to the anus. Perioperative attention to local hygiene and depilation of unwanted hair in that region are necessary for optimal results.

Whenever injection of dye is done into the track for identification, excess material should be rinsed out thoroughly with normal saline, leaving only the lining of the track colored. Otherwise, if the track is entered during surgical dissection, the spilt dye stains the entire wound, misleading the extent of excision needed.

iv) In extensive disease, use of myocutaneous flap or other reconstructive procedures may be necessary, e.g. Limberg flap.

v) Excessive transverse stretch of the healed

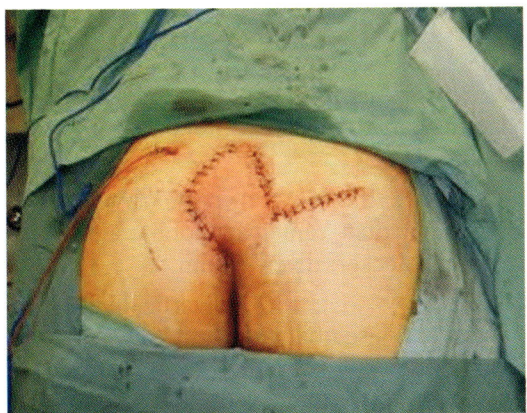

Fig. 26.2. Limberg flap cover for pilonidal surgery
(courtesy: Laxmi Hospital, Kakinada)

wound, may lead to break down and reinfection, which can be prevented by closing the vertical deep wound transversely (Karydakis procedure).

Postoperative care and precautions

1) if the wound is left open, daily dressings following sitz baths are necessary.

2) if suturing is done, they should be retained for minimum two weeks.

3) patient should not sit on buttocks for about 2-3 weeks , following primary closure.

4) observing proper local hygiene, and periodic depilation or clipping are useful, in preventing recurrence.

5) losing weight certainly benefits obese patients in the long run.

Causes of recurrence

1) Operative: one of the ramifications has been left behind, during surgery

2) Postoperative: repeat of original process, new hair driven into the skin cracks.

27 Umbilicus

Embryology: The umbilical cord is the connecting stalk, covered by ectoderm, that anchors the caudal end of the embryo to the trophoblast (placenta). The midgut develops from the central part of the yolk sac. It communicates with the rest of the yolk sac through the vitellointestinal duct. The umbilical cord consists of:

I)   allantois, which later becomes urachus

ii)   omphalomesenteric or vitellointestinal duct

iii) umbilical veins(two)

right - disappears early

left - carries oxygenated blood from the placenta to the fetus, to the left branch of portal vein and into the IVC through the ductus venosus. This is thought to be the route by which neonatal umbilical sepsis spreads to portal vein, causing thrombosis and its consequences in later life, such as cavernous malformation of portal vein and prehepatic (presinusoidal) portal hypertension.

iv)   umbilical arteries (two) arising from the internal iliac (hypogastric) arteries of the fetus, carrying reduced blood to the placenta.

v)   Wharton's jelly, a soft homogeneous mucoid material, with thin interlacing collagen fibers, providing a 'solid state' to the umbilical cord.

Developmental anomalies of the umbilicus

I)   vitellointestinal duct anomalies

ii)   urachal abnormalities

iii) others

i)   Vitellointestinal duct abnormalities

Patency of vitellointestinal duct to a variable extent, can give rise to several clinical conditions. A cyst or a tumor may also form at the mouth of the opening of the vitellointestinal duct.

a)   If the entire duct is patent, it gives rise to a vitellointestinal (ileo-umbilical) fistula, dis-charging small bowel contents through the umbilicus.

b)   If only the enteric part of the vitellointestinal duct remains unobliterated, it is known as Meckel's diverticulum.

Meckel's diverticulum: (diverticulum means a wayside house of ill fame and it lives upto its reputation)

It is a true diverticulum, present in about 2% of population, usually 2 inches long, located at about 2 feet from the ileocecal junction and 2% of them produce complications (only 2% of students seem to know this!). It may contain ectopic gastric or pancreatic tissue, conferring it the potential to ulcerate, bleed or perforate; other complications of the diverticulum are, diverticulitis, intussusception and gangrene.

c)   Sometimes a fibrous cord, representing the obliterated remains of the vitellointestinal duct, runs from the diverticulum to the anterior abdominal wall, when it may act as a fulcrum for a volvulus and if it lies free, it may cause interloop knotting of bowel or adhesive intestinal obstruction.

d)   If only the parietal end of the vitellointestinal duct is patent, a blind sinus discharging mucus is the result. Sometimes a protuber-

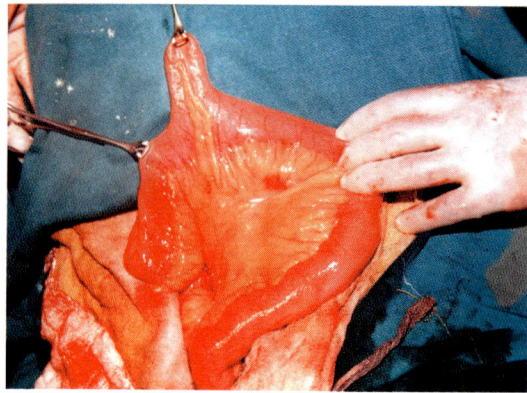

Fig. 27.1. Meckel's diverticulum
(courtesy: Lifeline Hospitals, Chennai)

ant, granular epithelial mass is seen, known as a *raspberry tumor* or *umbilical adenoma*.

e) If the central portion of the vitellointestinal duct remains patent with the obliteration of its both (enteric and parietal) ends, sequestration of secreted mucus occurs, with the formation of a cyst, known as *enterocystoma*, usually hanging from its attachment to bowel.

Clinical features

The problems related to Meckel's diverticulum are rarely diagnosed preoperatively. Recurrent periumbilical pain in a young patient, should alert the clinician to consider such a possibility. As indicated above, depending upon the pathology, the picture ranges from simple intestinal colic, local/ diffuse peritonitis, passing

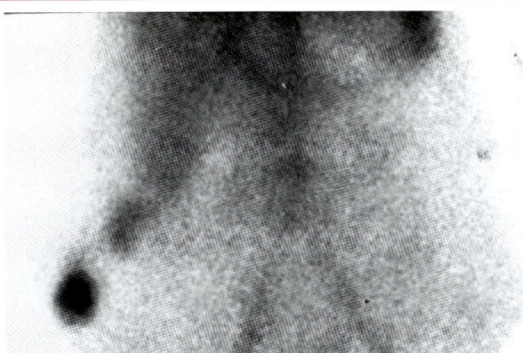

Fig. 27.3. ^{99m}Tc scintiscan showing Meckel's diverticulum
(courtesy: Lifeline Hospitals, Chennai)

altered blood or red current jelly stools, to frank intestinal obstruction. When the Meckel's diverticulum forms a content of an inguinal hernia, it is called Littre's hernia.

Differential diagnosis

Acute/recurrent appendicitis, mesenteric lymphadenitis, worm colic, necrotizing enteritis, congenital bands, jejunal diverticulitis, Crohn's disease etc. The conditions commonly responsible for fecal discharge from the umbilicus are

(1) congenital - vitellointestinal anomalies
(2) infective - tuberculosis
(3) neoplastic - carcinoma.

Treatment

Treatment of vitellointestinal duct disease naturally would depend upon the type of anomaly and clinical presentation. Generally, these anomalies are treated by excision of the entire vitellointestinal tract, with (in case of a Meckel's diverticulum), a 'V' resection of the involved antimesenteric part of the ileum. If peritonitis, hemorrhage, intussusception or intestinal obstruction is present, urgent laparotomy/laparoscopy is imperative, with appropriate pre and postoperative treatment.

Incidentally discovered Meckel's diverticulum, during the course of laparotomy/laparoscopy for other purposes, should be resected, to prevent complications, unless contraindicated by overt sepsis, multiple injuries or malignancy,

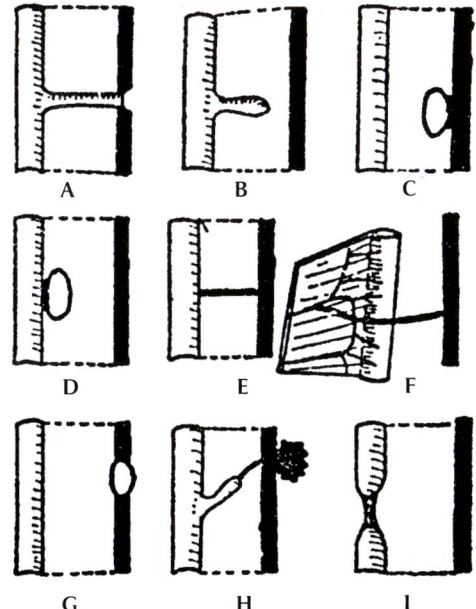

Fig. 27.2. Anomalies of vitellointestinal duct
a) Entero-cutaneous (umbilical) fistula
b) Meckel's diverticulum
c) Subumbilical (properitoneal) cyst
d) Paraileal cyst or enterocystoma
e) Fibrous band
f) Fibro-vascular band
g) Parietal cyst
h) Raspberry tumor
i) Ileal stenosis/atresia

where additional morbidity may not be justified.

(ii) Urachal abnormalities

Embryology

The urachus is the duct through which the allantois communicates with the fundus of the urinary bladder and contributes to its formation. It gets obliterated later to become the median umbilical ligament, running from the vesical fundus to the umbilicus in the properitoneal plane of the anterior abdominal wall. Abnormalities of a patent urachus cause vesico-parietal disease, which is parallel to the enteroparietal disease, caused by vitello-intestinal duct abnormalities. The following are the types described:

1. Complete patency of the urachus resulting in a fistula between the urinary bladder and the umbilicus, which may manifest even in middle or older ages.

2. The umbilical and the vesical parts of the urachus are obliterated, leaving behind only a secreting mid portion, resulting in a urachal cyst, located in properitoneal plane of the infraumbilical anterior abdominal wall.

3. Sometimes the umbilical end remains patent giving rise to a urachal sinus discharging small amounts of mucus which may become mucopus, by superadded infection.

4. Only the vesical end remains patent, forming a congenital vesical diverticulum.

Investigations

An ultrasound scan will reveal a urachal cyst in the properitoneal plane, whereas a cystogram or a sinogram will reveal a complete fistula, sinus or diverticulum.

Treatment: The only definitive treatment is surgery and once the patent portion of the urachal sac is excised, recurrence is very rare.

Differential diagnosis of umbilical mass

1. Umbilical or paraumbilical hernia (see chapter 45)
2. Inflammatory conditions

a. Umbilical granuloma
b. Pilonidal sinus
c. Omphalitis with abscess: it is often seen in obese individuals with deeply placed umbilicus; pain, discharge and tenderness are the main features. Sometimes, the infection spreads and a painful cystic swelling is found at the umbilicus (umbilical abscess). Chronic omphalitis may be associated with umbilical calculus (umbolith). vide infra

Treatment

Antibiotics followed by omphalectomy.

3. Neoplastic conditions

i) Benign 'tumors', peculiar to this region are (both of them are not true neo-plasms):

a) *Umbilical adenoma* (syn: raspberry tumor):A partially unobliterated vitellointe-stinal duct accounts for this lump, which is not a tumor. The mucosa of the terminal part of the vitellointestinal duct prolapses through the umbilicus and gives rise to a tumor-like swelling, discharging mucus and bleeding after trivial injury. If features of intestinal obstruction are present, intra-abdominal vitellointestinal anomaly has to be considered.

Treatment

The definitive treatment is omphalectomy and complete excision of vitellointestinal remnants, including Meckel's diverticulum, if necessary by laparotomy.

b) Endometrioma (syn: umbilical endometriosis): This is due to spillage and implantation of endometrial tissue in the wound after any operation involving opening the uterus (hysterotomy). It is also not a true neoplasm, and presents as a bluish, painful, tensely cystic swelling around the umbilicus, in women around 30-40years. This may ulcerate and discharge blood during menstrual periods (known as vicarious menstruation, often seen in naso-pharyngeal endometriosis with recurrent epistaxis). Increased pain/swelling during menstruation is pathognomonic of this condition. In those who had premature surgical menopause by hysterectomy, cyclical exacerbation is still noted, if ovaries were not removed.

Treatment

Omphalectomy along with excision of the endometriotic nodule.

ii) Malignant tumors

(a) Primary malignant tumors of the umbilicus or anterior abdominal wall, are quite rare, usually it is a malignant fibrous histiocytoma or a fibrosarcoma. The clinical features are as described for soft tissue sarcomas anywhere. Blood-borne metastasis may occur, to lungs and bones and if lymphatics are involved, to groins and axillae, because of the watershed zone of the umbilicus. Desmoid tumor is another primary tumor in this region, with low malignant potential (chapter 37).

Investigations and treatment: as for STS or desmoid tumor.

(b) Secondaries (Sister Joseph's nodules)

This is the commonest tumor presenting at the umbilicus and is indicative of advanced intra-abdominal malignancy, the usual sources being the GI tract, ovary, rarely the breast. Inner quadrant breast tumor spreads via lymphatics of rectus sheath, the falciform ligament into the liver, umbilicus being involved by retrograde embolization. Ulceration, secondary infection and bleeding are not uncommon from these

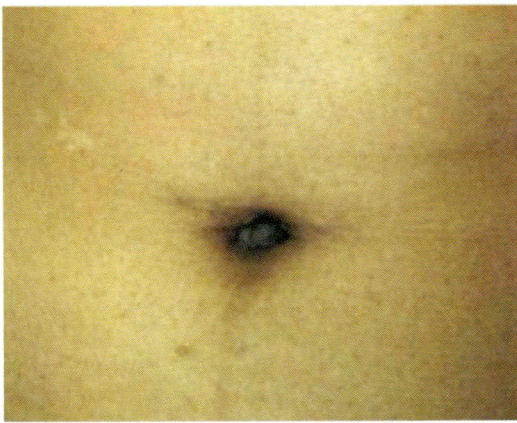

Fig. 27.4. Umbilical endometrioma
(courtesy: Halsted Surgical Clinic, Chennai)

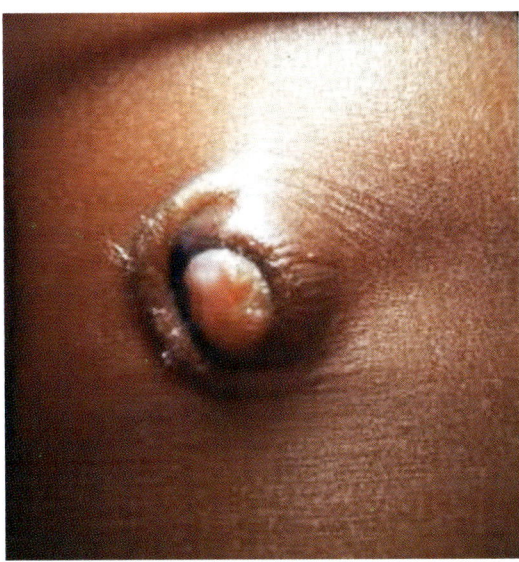

Fig. **27.5**. Umbilical granuloma
('Raspberry tumor')
(courtesy: Dr C J Reddy, Gudur)

lesions. Rarely, if the gut malignancy lies immediately deep to the umbilicus, contiguous infiltration of the umbilicus may lead to fungation or fecal fistula.

UMBILICAL GRANULOMA

Definition: Excess granulation tissue at the stump of the severed umbilical cord, resulting in pyogenic granuloma, which prevents epithelialization.

Treatment

1) appropriate antibiotics to control infection.
2) chemical cautery (silver nitrate or copper sulphate).
3) cryocautery (using a cryoprobe).
4) electrical cautery under local anesthesia.

If this persists despite repeated destruction, one must suspect the possibility of an umbilical adenoma or a sinus/fistula.

Chronic omphalitis with abscess

Although true omphalitis occurs in infants after the umbilical cord is severed, it is also seen in adults especially obese individuals, due to embryonal duct remnant. It is necessary at laparotomy to ascertain that no associated abnormalites like Meckel's diverticulum are present which should then be dealt with accordingly.

Pilonidal sinus of umbilicus

Sometimes encountered in the umbilicus, characterised by a purulent discharge, it presents as a lump with a small tuft of hair in the sinus, often seen in obese hairy men, with improper local hygiene.

Treatment

i)   excision of the sinus, if small
ii) omphalectomy, if large and either primary closure or marsupialization.

Umbilical hernia is described in chapter 45.

Umbilical calculus

(syn: umbolith)

(a rare cause of an umbilical nodule)

Capillary suction effect of a deep umbilicus may sometimes draw in desquamated cells from the skin, hair and clothing, which get fixed together to form an umbolith or an umbilical calculus. Although small concretions are usually asymptomatic, when they coalesce, a large calculus may be formed, giving rise to persistent infection and an umbilical abscess.

Treatment

Extraction of calculus and omphalectomy if there is a persistent umbilical abscess.

28 Scrotum

Scrotal skin is a very common site for sebaceous cysts (chapter 9) and synergistic infective gangrene of Fournier (chapter 17)

SPERMATOCELE

This is a cyst developed from the sperm-conducting apparatus of the epididymis, presenting as a painless, rounded, cystic mass on the postero-superior aspect of the head of the epididymis. The size rarely exceeds 2cm, but when it does, it may be mistaken for a third testicle ! It is unilocular and transilluminant, containing thin, opalescent fluid with spermatozoa, resembling rice water.

Management

Scrotal USG and needling/analysis of fluid are confirmatory. If it is small and otherwise asymptomatic, it may be left alone. Larger and troublesome ones are excised, if they reaccumulate

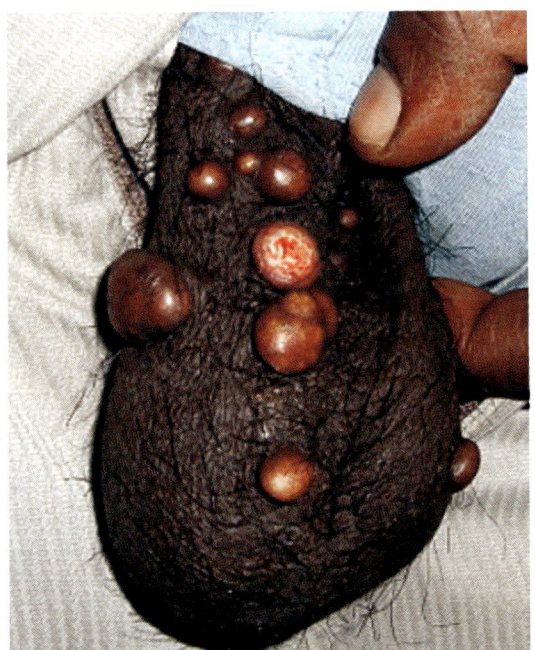

Fig. 28.1. Multiple sebaceous cysts, scrotum
(courtesy: Dr C M Kishore, Chennai)

after aspiration. In the young, surgery is preferably done under magnification, carefully avoiding damage to the seminal conduits with subsequent blockage.

ACUTE EPIDIDYMO-ORCHITIS

When the inflammation is confined to epididymis, it is epididymitis and when the body of the testis is also involved, it is called epididymo-orchitis.

Causes

a) retrograde spread from the urinary tract (urethra, prostate, seminal visicles or vas), in men with bladder outflow obstruction or following prostatic surgery. Sexually transmitted gonococcal/chlamydial infection is another common cause.
b) instrumentation of urethra, such as indwelling catheterization or cystoscopy
c) filariasis
d) mumps orchitis

Clinical features

Acute pain and swelling of the epididymis and testis, associated with fever/chills is the usual mode of presentation. Tenderness, edema and redness of the hemiscrotum are typically seen. It has to be differentiated from torsion (vide infra) or a hematocele. Elevation of the scrotum relieves pain in this condition, whereas it aggravates the symptoms in torsion of testis (Prehn's sign)

Investigations

Routine blood counts, blood smear for microfilaria and if necessary, USG/Doppler study of scrotum

Treatment

Treat the cause, with antibiotics (doxycycline is specific for chlamydial infection), antifilarial drugs, NSAIDs etc

Natural course: It may resolve, suppurate to form an abscess or sinus or go into chronicity, leading to infertility due to testicular atrophy or conduit block.

CHRONIC EPIDIDYMO-ORCHITIS

The common causes are:

1) filariasis (see chapter 41)
2) tuberculosis
3) nonspecific, which may be due to:
    a) UTI/prostatitis,
    b) urethral instrumentation/transurethral surgery,
    c) indwelling urethral catheter
    d) urethral stricture
4) syphilis of testis with epididymal extension.

CHRONIC NONSPECIFIC EPIDIDYMO-ORCHITIS

In most cases, a chronic urinary infection with seminal vesiculitis, prostatitis and urethritis predisposes to epididymitis.

In a clinical context, it may be stated that:

1) epididymis is involved first: tuberculosis or nonspecific

2) testis is involved first: syphilitic or lepromatous orchitis

3) if both are involved simultaneously: filariasis

Treatment

Any cause of chronic UTI or urethral obs-

truction, like a stricture should be identified and treated. Rigorous broad spectrum antibiotics are tried for 4-6 weeks, surgery in the form of epididymectomy or orchidectomy is advised as a last resort.

TUBERCULOUS EPIDIDYMO-ORCHITIS

This is a common cause of chronic epididymo-orchitis in the west, but in tropical countries, the incidence of filarial disease outnumbers tuberculosis.

Pathogenesis

Retrograde infection from infected seminal vesicles, as part of urinary tuberculosis, affects the globus minor initially. If the globus major is primarily involved, the source is probably hematogenous.

Clinical features

Slightly tender and indurated nodule of the epididymis is the first sign. Other nodules soon appear and eventually a firm painless, craggy mass is felt behind the testis. Beading of vas deferens, due to multiple tubercles, testifying to the source of infection, is pathognomonic of this disease. In a third of the patients a small secondary hydrocele is present. The body (mediastinum) of the testis usually remains uninvolved till late stages of infection. A fluctuant subcutaneous swelling may appear (cold abscess), which may open through the skin, forming a sinus, typically on the posterior aspect of scrotum, in contrast to a gummatous ulcer, located anteriorly due to the primary involvement of testis.

Swollen tender seminal vesicles may be felt by digital examination of rectum, as irregular induration, just above the prostate. The presence of urinary tuberculosis (approximaly over 2/3rd of the cases) corroborates the diagnosis. They may also seek medical help for infertility, due to conduit block leading to azoospermia, if the disease is bilateral.

Investigations

Despite plenty of pus cells present in urine, routine microbiology is usually reported as

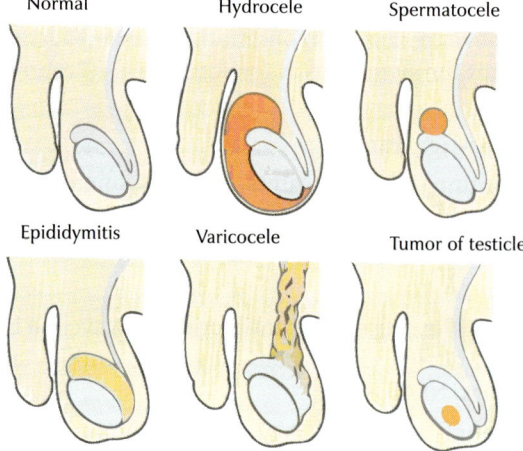

Normal   Hydrocele   Spermatocele

Epididymitis   Varicocele   Tumor of testicle

Fig. 28.2. Common scrotal conditions

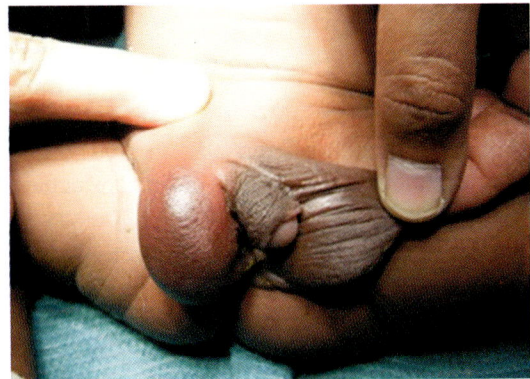

Fig. 28.3. Torsion of right testis

sterile (sterile pyuria), it may specifically be examined for AFB, supported by an USG, intravenous urogram (IVU), a cystoscopic evaluation and biopsy, to establish the diagnosis.

Chest x-ray, ESR and immunological tests such as Mantoux, IgM/IgG, PCR etc.

Special culture of urine and semen may be useful, but rarely needed for the diagnosis.

Histopathology of the granulation tissue obtained by curetting the sinus often clinches the diagnosis.

Treatment

Anti-tuberculous chemotherapy with 4-drug regime should be started immediately on confirming the diagnosis, which may be less effective in genital than in urinary tuberculosis, but sufficient in the majority of patients. If it does not resolve in 12 weeks of adequate therapy, epididymectomy (common) or orchidectomy (rare) may be needed for cure.

TORSION OF TESTIS

Torsion of the spermatic cord or testicle is an important condition peculiar to prepubertal males, because if it is not promptly diagnosed and intervened, loss of the testis is inevitable.

Predisposing factors

The normal anchorage of the testis, which prevents rotation about its axis, may be disturbed in the following conditions:

1) Inversion of the testis (commonest predis-posing cause).

2) High investment of the tunica vaginalis, which causes the testis to hang within the tunica like a clapper in a bell.

3) Where the body of the testis is separated from the epididymis by a long mesorchium, torsion of the body can occur without involving the cord.

4) Undescended testis

5) Trauma which could be straining, lifting heavy weights or coitus.

6) Ambient temperature: the torsion is much commoner in the colder months.

7) A well developed cremaster

It is well known that testicular torsion usually occurs in the direction away from the median septum i.e., clockwise on the right and anti-clockwise on the left. This corresponds to the insertion of the cremaster fibres into the cord and sudden spasm of a well developed muscle is accepted as the final triggering factor. The torsion may be intravaginal (within the tunica) or extravaginal; the former is more common than the latter.

Clinical features

Commonly seen in the peri-pubertal period (between 10-20), the symptoms vary with the degree of torsion. Sudden agonising pain in the groin and lower abdomen followed by vomiting

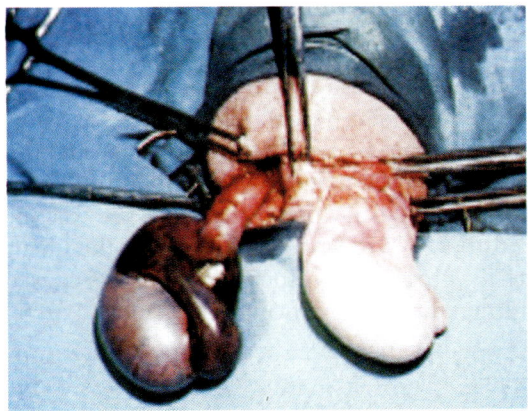

Fig. 28.4. Necrosed testis following torsion. Orchidopexy of the opposite testis being carried out

is the common presentation. Nausea and vomiting are very common. In incompletely descended testicles it is difficult to differentiate this condition from a strangulated inguinal hernia. Acute attacks of scrotal pains, spontaneously relieved within a few hours, is diagnostic of recurrent torsion, which requires careful evaluation and early 'prophylactic' orchidopexy.

Local examination

The hemiscrotum is swollen and tender, with edema of the scrotal skin being present, often making it difficult to differentiate it from an acute epididymo-orchitis. Elevation of the scrotum relieves pain in the latter (by reducing the edema) but aggravates the pain in torsion, by increasing the venous congestion (Prehn's sign). The testis can sometimes be made out lying in the horizontal position. Presence of the horizontal lie of the contralateral testis would clinch the diagnosis of torsion testis (Angell's sign). High scrotal tender testis may also been seen (Deming sign). Fever and leukocytosis are conspicuously absent.

Differential diagnosis

a) in the scrotum: acute epididymo-orchitis and acute traumatic hematocele

b) in the inguinal canal: acute epididymo-orchitis, funiculitis and strangulated inguinal hernia

1) Acute epididymo-orchitis: This is unusual under the age of 25 and systemic symptoms frequently precede the scrotal pain (it is vice versa in torsion testis). Vomiting is rare and relief of pain by scrotal elevation is an important diagnostic point in this condition. Except for fever/leukocytosis, it cannot be distinguished from torsion of a canalicular (inguinal) testis. Presence of associated funiculitis causes further diagnostic difficulties.

2) Acute traumatic hematocele: history of injury, followed by a tensely cystic swelling in the hemiscrotum, without constitutional symptoms; ecchymosis of the skin may be seen and

aspiration with a wide bore needle would draw frank/altered blood, which, along with an USG may clinch the diagnosis. If the fluid reaccumulates even after aspiration, indicating continued bleeding from the injured testis, scrotal exploration should be done, to evacuate the clots and evaluate/repair testicular injury.

3) Strangulated inguinal hernia (in torsion of canalicular testis): There is no certain way to distinguish between the two, but it is not very crucial, since both of them require urgent surgery. When there is a doubt about the diagnosis, immediate exploration is warranted, before bowel/ testis undergoes necrosis.

Recent advances

A Doppler ultrasound study is a useful method of differentiation as there will be no flow in torsion testis in contrast to high flow in acute epididymo-orchitis. Another method is by doing an urgent ^{99m}Tc perfusion scan, which shows no uptake by ischemic testis. Needless to say, these tests are useful only if they can be done expediently, without losing precious time.

Treatment

Manual external de-torsion has been attempted in the first hour but only by a few surgeons, most preferring immediate surgery. The principle mentioned earlier, clockwise on the right and anti-clockwise on the left should be taken into account and gentle untwisting attempted. If pain increases, while doing so, it should be abandoned in favour of immediate exploration.

Even if de-torsion is successful (rarely!), surgical fixation of the both testes (orchidopexy) should be performed as soon as possible. In all other cases immediate surgical exploration is the treatment of choice. If the testis is found viable, it must be fixed, to prevent recurrence. This can be done either by excision of a portion of the tunica vaginalis or by simple eversion as in a hydrocele (Lord's plication), producing adhesions between the testis and scrotal wall. The color, pulsations of the vessels in the cord and

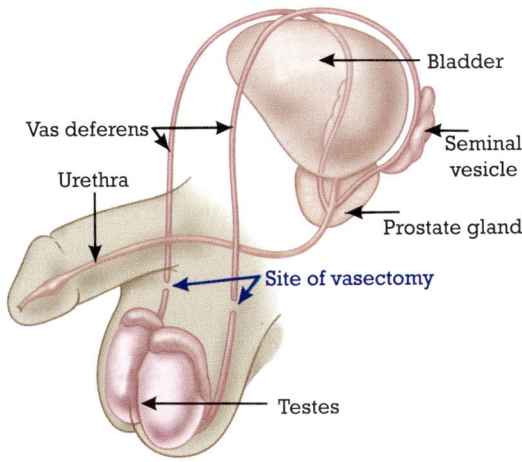

Fig. 28.5. Scheme of vasectomy

bleeding from a fine needle puncture of the testis are useful in establishing viability. Intraoperative Doppler may also be used for the same purpose. A totally infarcted testicle is best removed.

The contralateral testis should be fixed at the same time, as most often the predisposing factors are bilateral and the only remaining testis should be preserved at any cost.

Prognosis

If testicular fixation can be performed within 6 hours of the 'attack', the prognosis is excellent, otherwise almost always the testis is damaged beyond salvage. Procrastination in this situation may be disastrous.

Sympathetic orchidopathia: Following necrosis of testis due to torsion, the opposite (normal) testis also undergoes inflammatory changes, leading to late dysfunction. Some autoimmune

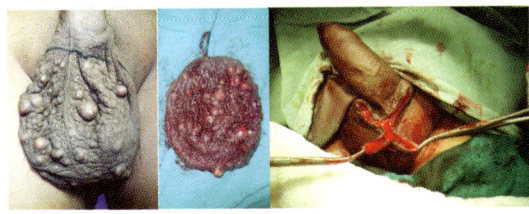

Fig. 28.6. A. Multiple sabaceous cysts of scrotum **B.** excised anterior scrotum, **C.** scrotal reconstruction (courtesy: Laxmi Hospital, Kakinada)

process is believed to be responsible for such an affliction, akin to sympathetic ophthalmia. This catastrophe may possibly be averted by early orchidectomy for torsion.

Filarial scrotum - see chapter 41

Tumors of testis: see chapter 32

Male sterilization

Vasectomy is the most common method of permanent male sterilization, with the advantage of being an out-patient procedure, requiring only local anesthesia. The principle is to surgically interrupt both vasa deferentia in the root of scrotum, to prevent spermatozoa from the testes from mixing up with the rest of seminal fluid, thereby turning the individual infertile. In view of its physical, emotional and social consequences, adequate counseling of both partners is essential, including the prospects of reversal and the facility to store (cryo-preservation) the semen in a bank, to be used if a future contingency arises.

Indications for vasectomy

1. Birth control for family planning
2. Medical contraindications to further pregnancy for the wife
3. Economic factors
4. As an adjunct to prostatectomy to prevent retrograde epididymo-orchitis (not considered essential nowadays)
5. Eugenic reasons: where offspring is undesirable due to high risk of genetic transmission of an incurable hereditary disease

Standard procedure: It is generally done under local anesthesia, supplemented by some sedation, if the patient is apprehensive. Two tiny incisions on either side (or one in midline) of scrotum are made, the vasa are delivered, divided and both the ends tied with fine chromic catgut. About 1-2 cm of the vas may be excised to minimize the chance of recanalization as well as to protect against litigations, by sending the bits for histopathology. The small incisions may be closed with some absorbable material and the patient discharged immediately, to resume

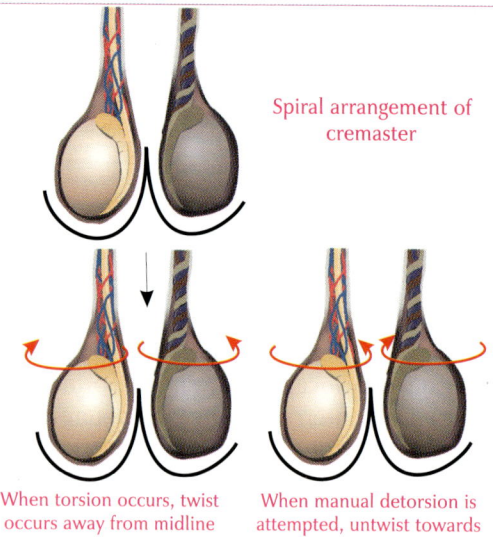

Spiral arrangement of cremaster

When torsion occurs, twist occurs away from midline

When manual detorsion is attempted, untwist towards midline

Fig. 28.7. Scheme of testicular torsion

normal activities within a day or two.

No-scalpel vasectomy: By using a sharp mosquito clamp, the skin is punctured, the vas carefully grasped, delivered and cut. The skin wound is so small that no sutures are required.

Fascial interposition of both cut ends is employed by some surgeons to discourage recanalization. Clips (VasClip), Endoluminal devices (Intra-Vas device) and injected plugs (Medical-grade polyurethane MPU or Medical-grade silicone rubber MSR) are also used by some to occlude the vas, but these are not very popular.

Outlook: Sexual intercourse may be resumed after a week, but with precautions against pregnancy, for a few ejaculations, 'washing off' the entire distal seminal conduit from spermatozoa. It is advisable for the couple to adopt other methods of contraception, till the semen analysis done after about 10 ejaculations confirms azospermia (incidentally proving the technical accuracy of the operation). Irrigating the prostatic side of vas with spermicidal agents (e.g. euflavine) may be done to achieve instant sterilization.

Complications: Hematoma, wound infection are common to any surgery

post-vasectomy pain: It is considered to be due to the pressure on the epididymis by the testicular secretions, with an incidence of about 3-5%, appearing months or years after surgery. It may get exaggerated during intercourse or physical exertion and needs only reassurance and symptomatic therapy.

Sperm granuloma: A small tender nodule may develop at the proximal (testicular side) stump of vas, due to the local reaction of the accumulated spermatozoa. This may also account for some cases of post-vasectomy pain.

Sterilization failure: The incidence of failure is about 1 in 2000 vasectomies (tubectomy has a much higher failure rate, 1 in 300). Spontaneous recanalization of vasa deferentia has been documented, accounting for the failure.

Psychological impact: Majority of men have no significant emotional problems, a few may develop 'sterility-complex' from which they

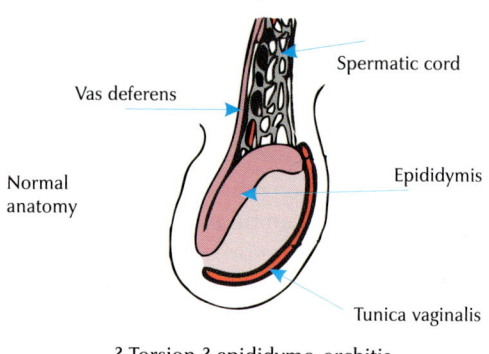

Normal anatomy

Vas deferens

Spermatic cord

Epididymis

Tunica vaginalis

? Torsion ? epididymo-orchitis

Check other side
If horizontal lie

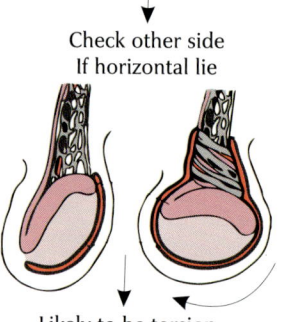

Likely to be torsion
(Get a doppler if available)

Fig. 28.8. Angell's sign in torsion

generally get over. There is reported marginal increase in libido, probably due to the lack of fear of conception, following vasectomy. The incidence of loss of libido is very rare, more related to the emotional than the physical effects of surgery and may be helped by appropriate counselling.

Vasectomy reversal

The reversal operation, vaso-vasostomy may be necessary if there is a need for another child, but its success depends on several factors, such as technique of vasectomy (closer it is to epididymis, inferior the results), interval between the operations (shorter the better), development of autoimmune reaction (antisperm antibodies) and production of abnormal sperms (poikilo or asthenospermia). These factors influence the ultimate fertility rate (functional success), though technically the conduit may have been restored (anatomical success).

The introduction of microsurgery (doing 2-layer anastomosis under an operating microscope, without using a stent), has improved the prospects of anatomical success of the operation.

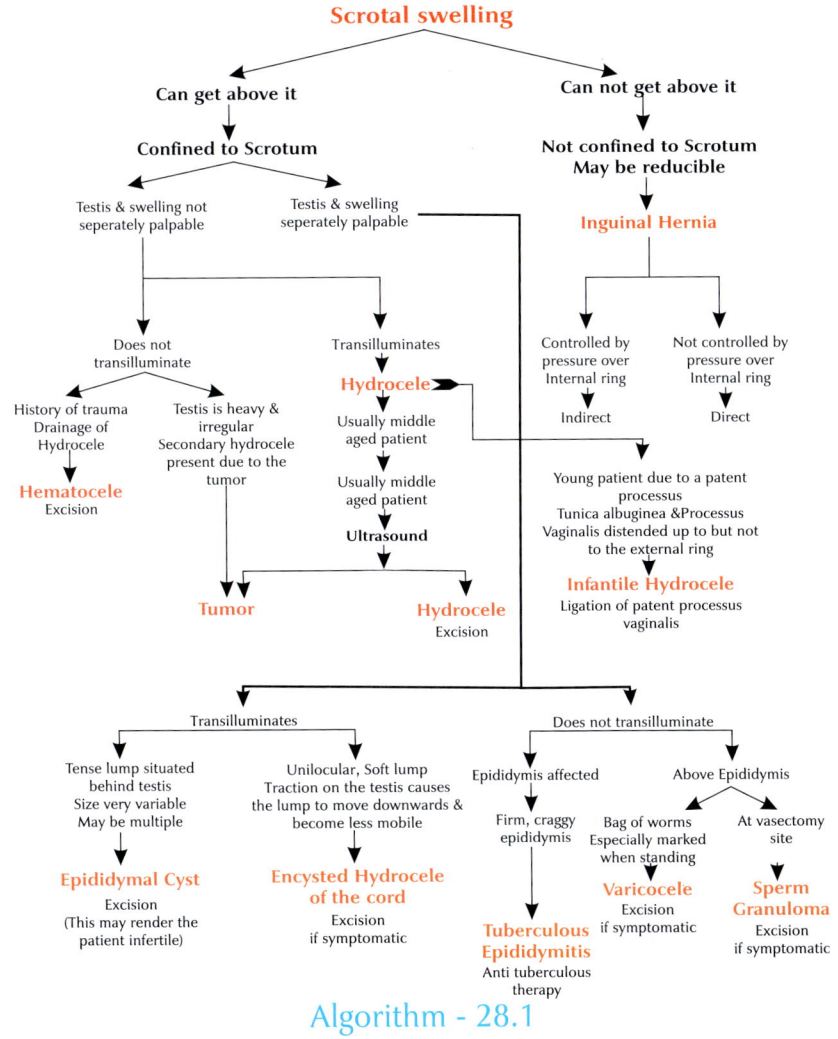

Algorithm - 28.1

29 Hydrocele

HYDROCELE is an abnormal collection of serous fluid within a sac, contributed by the processus vaginalis.

Etiologic classification

1) *Primary* or *idiopathic:* this occurs in the absence of any identifiable disease in the testis or epididymis. Although the etiology in the primary variety is not clear, its prevalence in areas endemic to filariasis and the finding of high titres of anti-microfilarial antibodies, in the hydrocele fluid, support filarial origin more in the tropics.

2) *Secondary:* when it is secondary to a known disease of the testis or epididymis, which may be: traumatic, inflammatory or neoplastic. Obstruction to testicular lymphatics as in filariasis or damage to them during certain operations like varicocele excision, vasectomy or inguinal herniorrhaphy, may also lead to secondary hydrocele.

Inflammations may be acute or chronic and nonspecific or specific

Neoplasms causing hydrocele are always malignant, either primary or secondary

Topographic classification

Depending upon the location of the fluid, there are several varieties of hydrocele.

1) **Vaginal hydrocele:** This is the commonest variety, where the collection of fluid in the tunica vaginalis and is confined to scrotum.

2) **Infantile hydrocele:** Collection of fluid in the tunica, extending onto the spermatic cord,

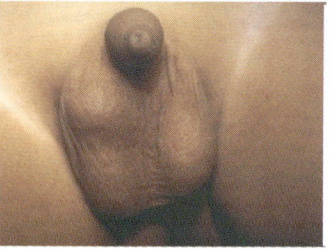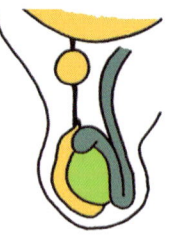

Fig. 29.1. Encysted hydrocele of the cord

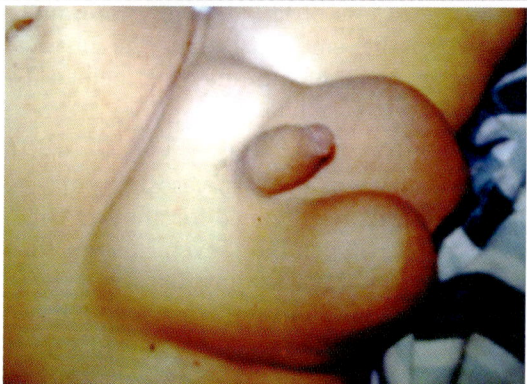

Fig. 29.2. Bilateral infantile hydroceles
(courtesy: Dr C M Kishore, Chennai

upto the internal ring, where the processus is obliterated, assuming a retort shape.

3) **Congenital or communicating hydrocele:** entire processus vaginalis is patent, freely communicating with the peritoneal cavity. The fluid trickles into the scrotal sac, while the child is up and playing about, and empties itself during sleep.

4) **Encysted hydrocele** of the cord: The processus gets obliterated in the inguinal canal as well as just above the testis, fluid getting sequestrated in between. It can be felt separate from the testis, but gets pulled down, on applying downward traction on the testis (traction sign).

5) **Hydrocele of canal of Nuck** is a similar encystation of fluid, in relation to the round ligament (ligamentum teres) in the inguinal canal, in females. Contrary to the encysted hydrocele in males, it is located mostly in the inguinal canal.

6) **Funicular hydrocele:** proximal part of the processus is patent, communicating with the peritoneal cavity, but closed distally, above the testis.

7) **Bilocular hydrocele** (syn: hydrocele enbissac): It starts off as infantile type, but due to increased pressure within, the inguinal compo-

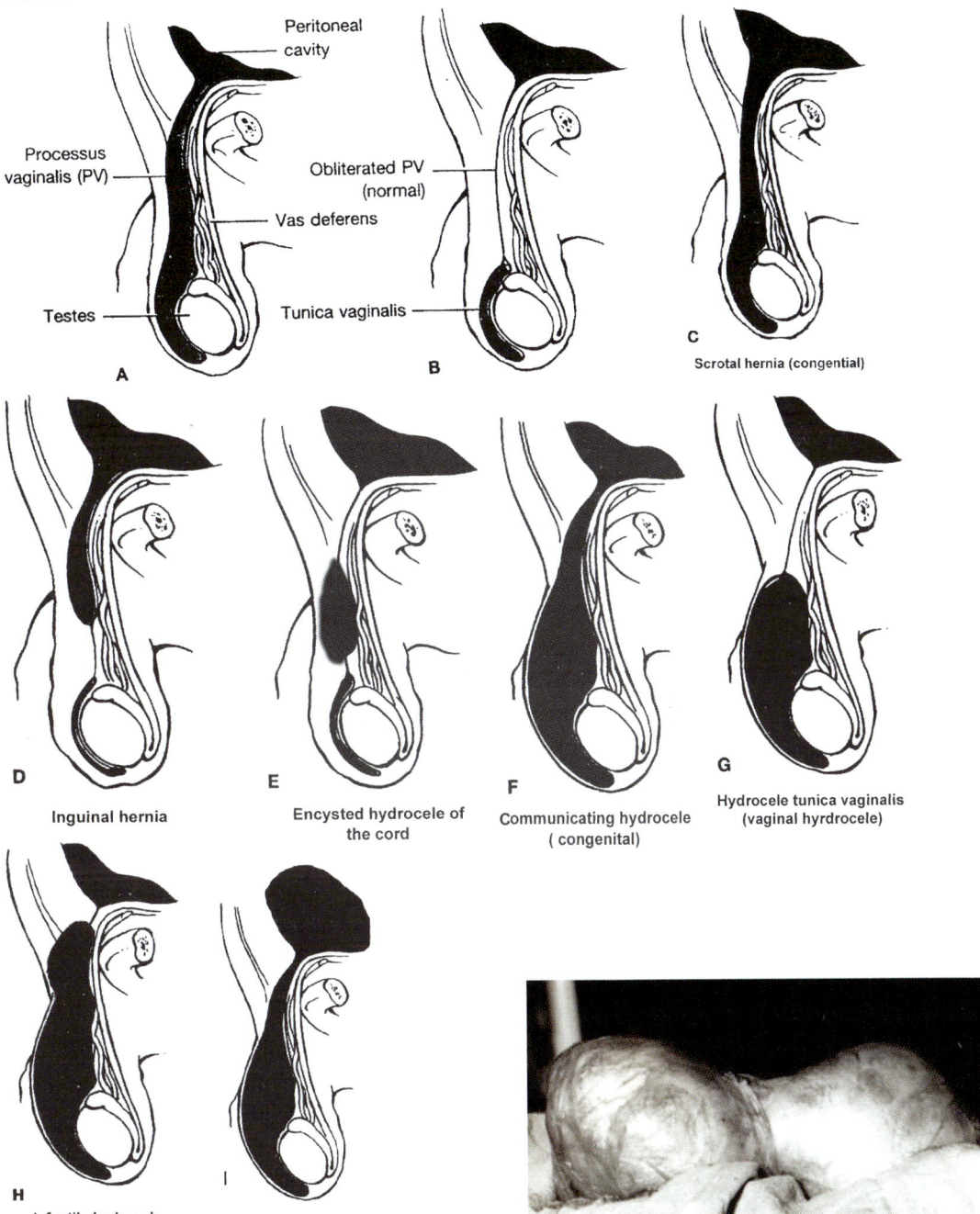

Peritoneal cavity

Processus vaginalis (PV)

Obliterated PV (normal)

Vas deferens

Testes

Tunica vaginalis

A

B

C
Scrotal hernia (congential)

D
Inguinal hernia

E
Encysted hydrocele of the cord

F
Communicating hydrocele (congenital)

G
Hydrocele tunica vaginalis (vaginal hyrdrocele)

H
Infantile hydrocele

I
Bilocular hydrocele

Fig. 29.3. Types of hernia and hydrocele
A. Normal Inguino-scrotal anatomy in the fetus
B In mature infant; **C** to **I.** Abnormalities caused by persistence of a portion or whole of the processus vaginalis

Fig. 29.4. Bilocular hydrocele delivered before emptying

nent dissects its way into extraperitoneal plane, expanding to form another locule inside. Besides a retort shaped inguino-scrotal swelling, another cystic mass is felt in the iliac fossa, exhibiting cross fluctuation.

8) **Hydrocele of hernial sac** is due to sequestration of fluid in the hernial sac, unable to return into the peritoneal cavity, due to an omental plug occluding the neck of the sac.

9) **Diffuse hydrocele of the cord:** this is actually a lymph varix of the cord, usually due to lymphatic obstruction and not a true hydrocele.

10) **Gibbon's hernia** is a large hernia producing secondary hydrocele, due to compression of venous and lymphatic channels.

Pathology

The collection of fluid may take place, due either to defective resorption (as in primary) or to increased secretion (as in secondary); the fluid has the characteristics of an exudate (sp. Gr >1018 and proteins >3gm%), in the latter. Initially the fluid is thin, straw colored, containing sodium chloride, carbonates, proteins and some fibrinogen, but does not coagulate spontaneously. With the passage of time, it may look 'oily' due to the presence of cholesterol crystals.

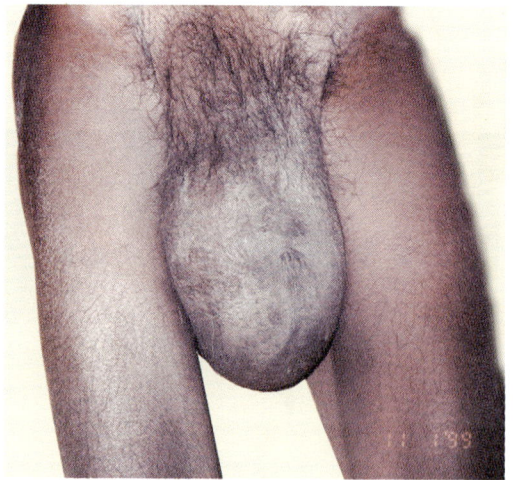

Fig. 29.5. Large bilateral vaginal hydrocele with buried penis
(courtesy: Halsted Surgical Clinic, Chennai)

Occasionally, small fibrin covered loose bodies may be seen, formed from precipitated salts. Rarely spermatozoa may find their way into hydrocele fluid, probably by transmigration from the epididymis.

Over a period of time, both fluid and sac get thickened, due to repeated trauma and/or sterile inflammation. In long standing cases, the wall may become so thick with deposition of calcareous plaques on the tunica, that it may feel cartilaginous and not be translucent. Fibrinous adhesions (synechia) may form within, converting it into a multiloculated sac. The hydatid of Morgagni may be considerably elongated, the significance of which is not clear. Left untreated, the congenital and funicular types may allow herniation of omentum/ viscera, with enlargement of the neck of the sac.

Clinical features

Insidious painless scrotal swelling is the commonest presentation of an uncomplicated hydrocele, producing physical and esthetic difficulties. In the congenital type, the typical history from the mother is that, the swelling disappears at night, only to appear towards the end of the day, as the child plays around. History of trauma or acute or chronic pain, is present in secondary types.

Signs

The findings depend upon the type of hydrocele. In the vaginal type, which is the commonest of all, a vertically oval, cystic, nontender, transilluminant swelling, is found in one or both sides of scrotum, depending upon whether it is unilateral or bilateral. The swelling is confined to the scrotum (can get above it), with the dartos and skin freely moving over it. Sometimes a gentle hour-glass constriction is

Jewels of Gyan - 29.1

Negative Transillumination

The reasons for negative transillumination in a hydrocele may be simplified as:

thick skin, thick sac and thick fluid.

	Feature	Vaginal hydrocele	Inguino-scrotal hernia
1	Situation	Scrotal	Inguino-scrotal
2	Shape	Oval	Pyriform
3	Reducibility	Absent	Present
4	Cough impulse	Present	Absent
5	Consistency	Cystic	Elastic or doughy
6	Transillumination	Positive (usually)	Negative
7	Resonance	Absent	May be present (enterocele)
8	Testis	Not felt separate	Felt separate

Table-29.1: Differences between a vaginal hydrocele and inguino-scrotal hernia

seen in the primary type, due to tension of fluid, bringing out the real shape of tunica. Other point of difference is, in primary type, the testis can never be felt within the hydrocele, whereas due to laxity of fluid in some secondary types, it feels like a balloon partly filled with water and the testis can be felt. To avoid the posteriorly placed testis coming in the way, transillumi-nation must be always carried out side-to-side and not antero-posteriorly.

It should be realised that there are certain types of hydroceles, where one cannot get above the swelling, such as congenital (communicating), infantile, bilocular hydrocele and encysted hydrocele of the cord. A 'pseudo impulse' may be felt in these types, due to displacement of

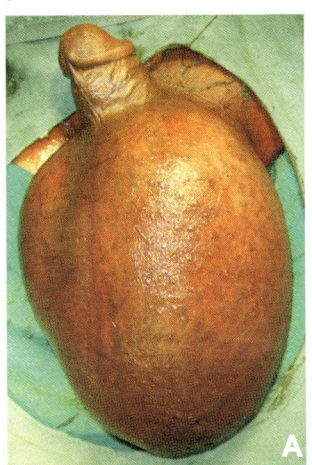 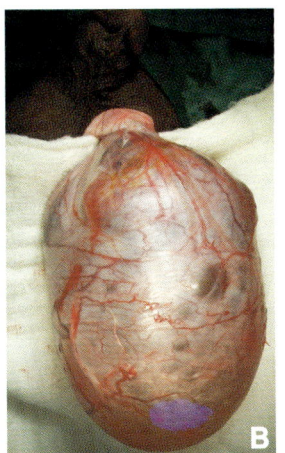 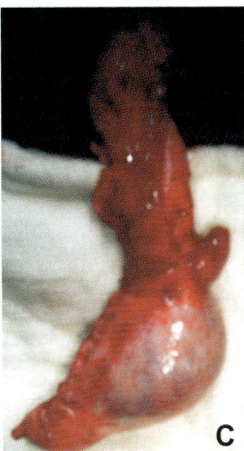

Fig. 29.6. Subtotal excision and eversion of tunica
A. Large left vaginal hydrocele; B. Hydrocele sac delivered from scrotum; C. Testis and spermatic cord after the procedure

Jewels of Gyan - 29.2

Hernia of a hydrocele
Localized thinning of tunica leading to a pseudopodium-like projection, usually seen when fluid is under tension and the sac is thick.

Hydrocele of a hernia
Fluid sequestration in a loculus of an indirect inguinal hermia, resembling a hydrocele. This is seen in long standing cases with adhesions within the sac.
This is more often seen in a ventral hernia.

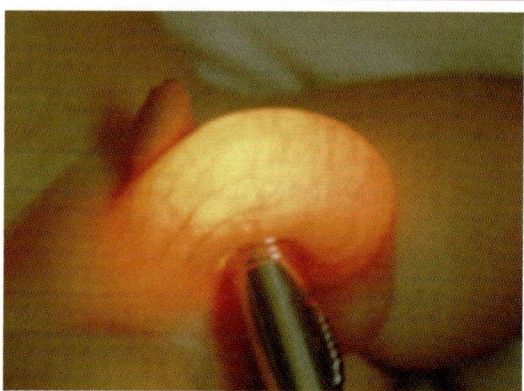

Fig. 29.7. Eliciting transillumination in a hydrocele
(courtesy: Laxmi Hospital, Kakinada)

fluid out of the inguinal canal into the scrotal part of the sac, during coughing.

Being common conditions, differences between vaginal hydrocele and inguino-scrotal hernia are of great clinical significance (Table - 29.1).

Differential diagnosis

1) inguinoscrotal hernia
2) causes of secondary hydrocele, such as inflammations and neoplasms
3) spermatocele
4) filarial scrotum; A hydrocele is a mere collection of fluid in the sac, whereas in filarial scrotum, all the components of scrotum (skin, subcutaneous tissue, testis, epididymis, spermatic cord etc) are involved; there may also be a secondary hydrocele.
5) complications, such as hematocele or chylocele.

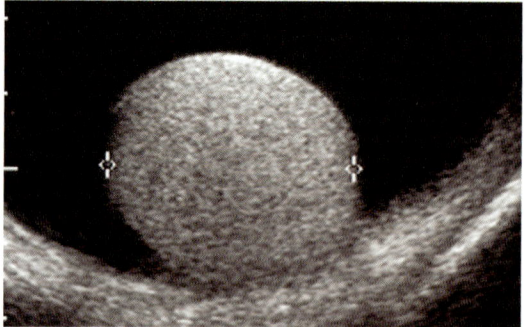

Fig. 29.8. Ultrasonography of the testis in hydrocele
(courtesy: Laxmi Hospital, Kakinada)

Investigations

No specific investigations are needed to diagnose a hydrocele but only to exclude conditions producing secondary hydrocele, such as filariasis, tuberculosis and tumors.

a) night blood smear for microfilaria: see chapter 41, on filariasis.

Treatment

Definitive treatment for a hydrocele is surgery; essentially the sac is excised &/or everted, after draining the fluid and excluding obvious diseases of the testis and epididymis. Simple aspiration should be avoided, for fear of introducing infection and injury to testis. A diagnostic tap may be done, if infection or chylocele is suspected. Rarely judicious use of aseptic aspiration (therapeutic) may be indicated to gain time for surgery, if someone is heading for his wedding or a major sports event, where such a burden is undesirable.

Surgery: There are three types of operations for the vaginal hydrocele.

1) **Lord's plication** is done when there is minimal fluid and a thin sac. The sac is incised along with skin and dartos, fluid let out, testis lifted up to evert the sac and few plication sutures are placed, before returning the testis into its hemiscrotum. A separate incision may be needed to plicate opposite sac, if necessary. This operation can be conveniently done under local anesthesia as a 'day care' procedure.

2) **Jaboulay's operation** is the commonest procedure done for a moderate vaginal hydrocele, which involves delivering the entire sac, by a paramedian scrotal incision and performing eversion of the tunica vaginalis; the fluid secreted by the (everted) sac, gets absorbed by subcutaneous lymphatics. Even if there is minimal fluid on the opposite side, it is advisable to carry out the same, through a septal window, which may be closed with a figure of '8' stitch after returning the testis to its habitat.

3) **Subtotal excision** of sac *with or without eversion is done for large hydrocele, wherein*

either a small rim of sac is retained, just enough for snug eversion or thick sac is excised as close to the testis as possible and a locking catgut stitch is run all-round the testis for hemostasis. The latter procedure is necessary for a highly thickened sac, which has a feel of a coconut shell.

In view of high incidence of a granuloma and sinus formation, nonabsorbable suture materials are not used in scrotal surgery (except for skin, which may be removed later or for microsurgery on epididymis/vas, where 5-0 or 6-0 polypropylene is used).

Hydrocele communicating with peritoneal cavity, such as congenital or funicular types, should be treated as a hernia (herniotomy), by inguinal incision. The tunica should be 'routinely' everted, by delivering the testis into the wound, to prevent a vaginal hydrocele developing later. The sac of an encysted hydrocele of the cord may be either excised in toto or everted by wrapping around the cord, after partial excision. Infantile and bilocular hydroceles are treated in a similar fashion, through an inguino-scrotal incision, carefully protecting cord structures, particularly venous plexus and the vas.

Management of secondary hydrocele is done on the merits of the underlying disease, following relevant investigations.

When to suspect a tumor? Recent onset with recognizable growth of the scrotal swelling, which feels uneven and heavy, with variable consistency and loss of testicular sensation. There may be cord thickening and enlargement of para-aortic lymph nodes. An USG of the scrotum/abdomen and tumor markers, like α-fetoprotein (AFP), carcino-embryonic antigen

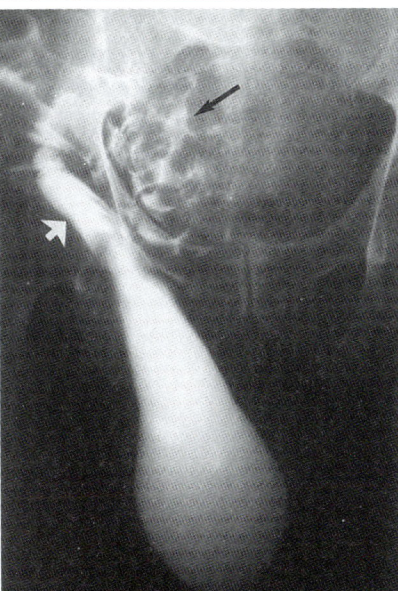

Fig. 29.9. Contrast study of a congenital hydrocele demonstrating communication with the peritoneal cavity
(courtesy: Laxmi Hospital, Kakinada)

(CEA) and β-human chorionic gonadotropins (β-hCG), are helpful in suspected patients. Examination of aspirated hydrocele fluid is of little help.

What to do? If there is high suspicion by these tests and if the patient is elderly, it may be expedient to proceed with high (inguinal) orchidectomy and plan further treatment based on the pathology report. In young men however, scrotal exploration and if necessary inspection of bivalved testis *(Chevassu maneuver)*, with preliminary application of a non-crushing vascular clamp on the cord, is mandatory before committing to orchidectomy. A frozen section report would be very handy for the surgeon in such situations, to eliminate even a remote chance of removing the testis for a benign disease. Preoperative ultrasound-guided needle biopsy is advocated by some, but without universal approval, since it may open up new pathways of lymphatics from the scrotal skin, towards the inguinal nodes. Furthermore, a negative report cannot override a strong clinical conviction.

Complications of hydrocele

1. infection
2. trauma and hemorrhage, leading to hematocele
3. herniation
4. rupture
5. physical/esthetic disability
6. defective spermatogenesis
7. calcification of sac
8. masking an underlying testicular disease (malignancy). Of these, first is most common and last is the most dangerous.

1) Infected hydrocele: Systemic and local symptoms should alert the clinician, confirmed by local warmth and tenderness, in making a diagnosis of infection. Immediate aspiration of fluid should be done through a wide bore needle and sent for microbiology (Gram stain and culture), before starting appropriate antibiotics. If treated early, minimal infection may resolve, but if the fluid is frankly purulent, it should be drained under local anesthesia, by adequate incision. In any event, standard surgery for hydrocele must not be done in the presence of infection, as it may lead to a nonhealing sinus and eventually to orchidectomy.

Sometimes following gross infection, the hydrocele may not reform (a welcome sequel?), which is attributable to the severe damage to the secreting epithelium and adhesions (synechia) which develop between tunica vaginalis and albuginea. Of course, it is not to say that introducing infection is one way of treating a hydrocele! In cases of infected hematocele in elderly, after identifying by aspiration, prior to making the incision in the operating room, it is prudent to proceed with 'clean' orchidectomy, without opening the sac and spilling the contents into the wound. Whenever infected fluid is encountered on one side, surgery for the contralateral hydrocele should be deferred.

2) it is vulnerable for repeated trauma, resulting in a hematocele, with high risk of infection.

3) Herniation is felt like a soft 'pseudopodium' over the hydrocele with thick sac, due to defect in the outer layers of the sac, through which the inner layers herniate. By itself, it does not need treatment.

4) Rupture of the sac may rarely occur with extravasated fluid getting absorbed and the hydrocele disappearing, but only to recur soon.

5) Physical disability may produce a typical broad gait in large hydroceles.

6) Defective spermatogenesis due to increased local warmth appears logical; this has not been borne out by concrete evidence, so also 'pressure atrophy' of testis, in long standing cases.

7) Masking an underlying testicular neoplasm may be a serious problem related to scrotal hydrocele. In suspicious cases, an USG of the scrotum and tumor markers should be done, to exclude an SOL in the testis.

Complications of surgery for hydrocele

i) scrotal hematoma: if it is of considerable size, it should be immediately evacuated by reopening the wound in the operating room and resutured.

ii) infection is usually related to collection of lymph/blood in the wound. Aggressive treatment with high antibiotics and liberal drainage is necessary, lest the testis may undergo avascular necrosis.

iii) persistent sinus is the result of deep-seated infection or a foreign body, such as a suture material, but rarely a specific disease like tuberculosis may be responsible. Simple curetting, to retrieve a suture is generally curative, the granulation tissue obtained may be sent for histopathology, to exclude specific disease.

iv) Fournier's gangrene is a rare complication (see chapter 17).

30 Undescended Testis

Definition: This term is used when there is an arrest of testicular descent in any part of the normal pathway. The incidence goes up to 20%, in premature babies, under 1.0 kg birth weight, but there is no higher incidence than average population, once the conception goes beyond 32 weeks. At birth, undescended testis is seen in about 4% of 'normal' infants but most of them descend; only <1% failing to reach scrotum, by the end of one year, out of which one half may remain undescended permanently. This condition was first described by Hunter (1786).

Embryology

The testes are formed in the abdomen from the mesenchymal cells derived from the yolk sac, known as genital folds in the retroperitoneum. Gubernaculum testis(of Hunter) is a fibromuscular cord that runs from the lower pole of the testis to the floor of the scrotum (gubernaculum meaning one that governs), traversing the inguinal canal. This explains the 'U' bend seen at that origin of vas difference at the tail of epididymis (globus minor) It has several points of distal attachments, called the tails of Lockwood, going to supra-inguinal, pubic, perineal and femoral areas. This guides the testis into the scrotum by 'railroad' technique. If any of the other tails become more operative, the testis might reach ectopic sites. It may also get arrested while descending in its normal pathway, resulting in abdominal, canalicular (within the inguinal canal), external inguinal and high scrotal testis.

Processus vaginalis is a fold of peritoneum drawn with the testis during its descent, its fundus becoming the tunica vaginalis, while the rest obliterates after complete testicular descent, forming the vaginal ligament. It may remain unobliterated in states of incomplete descent, predisposing to the development of an indirect inguinal hernia. If this is imperfectly obliterated, it may reopen in later life due to increased abdominal pressure for any reason, to manifest an indirect inguinal hernia.

The descent of gonads is under the influence of gonadotrophic hormones, besides the effect of increased intra-abdominal pressure of the fetus in the last trimester and the role played by the gubernaculum. While normal children secrete no gonadotrophic hormones in urine, they are significantly present in cryptorchid boys and disappear following orchidopexy. This explains why administration of these hormones seldom help otherwise healthy children, to promote descent. Most important single peptide, calcitonin gene-related peptide (CGRP) responsible for testicular descent, has been identified.

The placement of testis outside the abdomen is essential for normal spermatogenesis, as high intra-abdominal temperature is detrimental to the process. Whether imperfect descent is responsible for underdevelopment of testis or the reverse, is debatable, most believe, both are

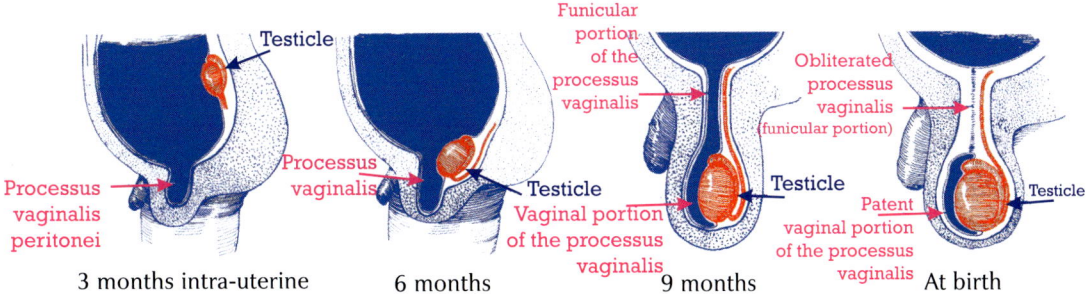

Fig. 30.1. Stages of normal descent of testis

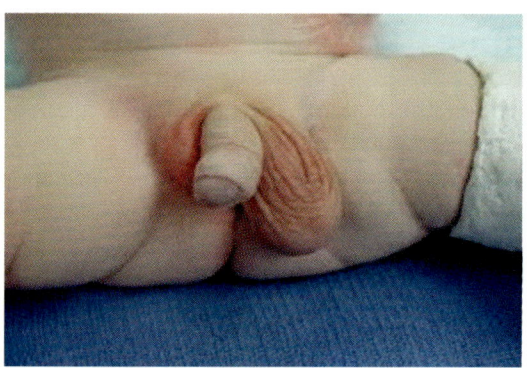

Fig. 30.2. Undescended right testis
(note right half of scrotum has not developed)

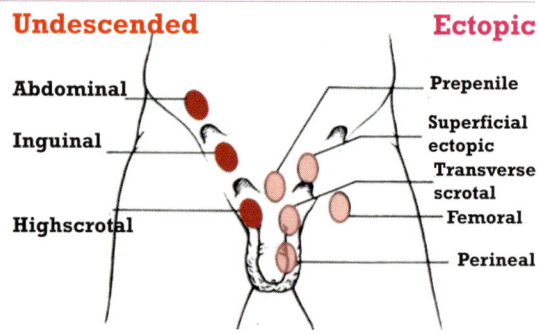

Fig. 30.3. Various positions of undescended and ectopic testis

possible, yet another attractive suggestion, that both may be related to a common etiological factor, cannot be ignored. It is also understood that the process of spermatogenesis is initiated in infancy, to attain its finale by puberty. Hence it is necessary that the testis should be brought down into the scrotum (orchidopexy), as early as possible, ideally around 2, in any case not later than 4 years.

Spermatogenesis gets totally arrested beyond recovery by about 12 years, if the testis remains undescended. The hormonal functions however, are unaltered by its placement, provided it is not grossly hypoplastic. The right testis descends later and remains at a slightly higher level in the scrotum than the left. Being a 'junior', all anomalies related to the development and the descent of the testis, are more common on the right side.

Diseases associated with testicular descent and development:

(i) Abnormal placement of tesis: unde-scended/maldescended/ectopic testis

(ii) Imperfect obliteration of processus vaginalis: communicating (congenital) hydrocele, indirect inguinal hernia

(iii) Imperfect fixation in scrotum &/or long mesorchium: torsion

(iv) Testicular development: hypoplasia/aplasia/agenesis

(v) Tumor: usually seminoma or embryonal carcinoma of testis

(vi) Trauma: particularly the canalicular type, is vulnerable for injuries

Certain terms used

Maldescent is generally used whenever the testis is not in its normal place. If it is arrested within the path of normal descent, it is known as undescended and if it has deviated from the normal path, it is termed ectopic.

Cryptorchism simply means the testis cannot be externally appreciated by inspection (or palpation) and is usually used synonymous with abdominal testis. If one testis fails to develop (patient has only one testis) it is known as monorchism and if both testes fail to develop, it is anorchism.

Types of undescended testes: As already indicated it may be

a) intra-abdominal: most often it lies intraperitoneally, just deep to the internal ring.

b) canalicular (inguinal): here, it may or may not be palpable, sometimes plunging in and out of the abdominal cavity through the internal ring, simulating cough impulse.

c) in the superficial inguinal pouch (of Denis Browne): when it has to be differentiated from retractile testis.

d) high scrotal, just outside the external ring: this also can mimic a retractile type.

Pathology

Spermatogenesis is markedly depressed or absent, due to raised temperature, when the testis is situated at sites other than scrotum, which affects the seminiferous apparatus. Fortunately, the androgen producing interstitial (Leydig) cells of the testis are unaffected, hence normal hormonal functions and secondary sexual development are seen.

Malignancy

Undescended testis has higher incidence of malignancy, such potential is seen wherever the testis may be placed, other than its normal location. However, it is highest in abdominal testis (incidence reaching equal to ovarian malignancy) and lowest in inguinal and high scrotal positions. Higher temperature, impaired growth may be readily blamed for such tendency, but whatever the factor responsible for its maldescence in the first place, might well be oncogenic, as seen by the fact that in cryptorchids, normally placed opposite testis also carrys an increased risk of malignancy.

Torsion: Long mesorchium, separating the testis from epididymis or imperfect external fixation, may lead to intravaginal or extra-vaginal torsion, respectively.

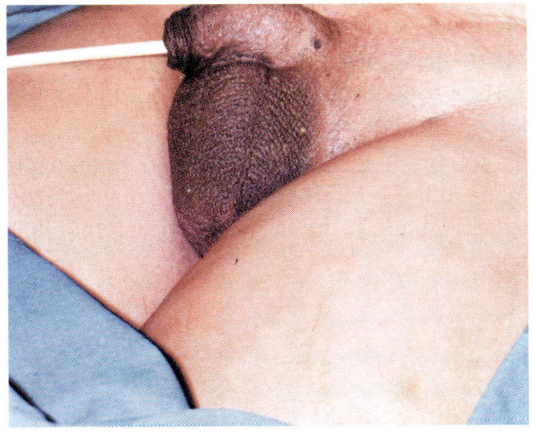

Fig. 30.4 Left undescended testis (hemiscrotum is hypoplastic) (courtesy: Lifeline Hospitals, Chennai)

Jewels of Gyan - 30.1

The complications of undescended testis may be remembered as TESTIS

Trauma

Epididymo-orchitis confusing abdominal pain

Sterility

Torsion

Inguinal hernia

Seminoma testis.

Clinical features

Symptoms

Usually the boy is brought by parents, with one or no testicle in the scrotum. Other rarer presentations are:

(i) an adult seeking medical advice for the same
(ii) inguinal hernia
(iii) torsion
(iv) infertility
(v) malignancy (usually seminoma), producing a pelvic tumor, causing diagnostic difficulties
(vi) ambiguous genitalia syndrome.

It is also vulnerable for trauma and other diseases, like epididymo-orchitis, which affect the fully descended testis.

Signs

It is important to differentiate this condition from a retractile testis, since the latter rarely requires active treatment. Well formed scrotal sac is in favour of retractile testis, whereas in unilateral undescended testis, one hemiscrotum is hypoplastic. Examination should also be done in standing position, to appreciate the extent of descence and associated indirect hernia. Squatting on a chair and increased abdominal pressure by Valsalva maneuver, are very helpful in pushing a retractile testis out of inguinal canal (Orr). If the testis is not felt in its normal location, careful examination of the inguinal canal, perineum, root of penis, femoral region and hypogastrium as well as for enlarged para-aortic nodes, must be performed.

Investigations

An USG of abdomen is the first choice, not only to locate the testis, but to assess its size, presence of paraaortic nodes and to detect associated urological anomalies. Karyotyping, semen analysis, tumor markers and study of hormonal profile may be necessary in appropriate cases.

Differential diagnosis

(i)   retractile testis

(ii) testicular agenesis or gross hypoplasia

(iii) testicular atrophy, following injury or infections

(iv) ectopic testis

(v)   torsion or epididymo-orchitis of an abdominal testis, may be confused as 'acute abdomen'.

(vi) intersex or ambiguous genitalia syndrome

Treatment

As already indicated, gonadotropic hormones have a very limited role, except in established deficiency states. Surgery to restore the scrotal location is the definitive treatment. The fundamental question, whether a testis should be retained or removed, in a given patient, is answered by considering the following factors:

(i)   spermatogenesis

(ii) hormonal functions

(iii) malignant potential

(iv) esthetic considerations

For a boy under 12, there is no question of orchidectomy, testes should be restored to scrotum, at the earliest. In adults with bilateral cryptorchism, even if both testes are expected to have lost their spermatogenetic function, at least one (better developed one, usually the left) has to be retained for hormonal functions. Emasculation is a more serious complication than infertility and the surgeon should not be a party to create such a psychosomatic disaster, hence bilateral orchidectomy should never be performed. Besides esthesis, placement of tes-

tis in scrotum also facilitates early detection of malignancy, if it occurs later on.

Orchidopexy: Ideally done around 2, but in any event, not later than 4years, either in one sitting or occasionally in stages. This has three essential surgical steps, mobilization of cord structures, scrotal fixation of testis and dealing with associated hernia, if present. First successful orchidopexy was done by Beven (1899).

(I) Mobilization: The coverings and contents of the spermatic cord, have to be carefully dissected. The vessels may be comfortably mobilized up to as high as the lower pole of the kidney, by extraperitoneal digital separation. If necessary, the medial crus of the internal ring (including the inferior epigastric artery), may be divided, to reduce the lateral convexity of their course. Dividing the peritoneal process (hernial sac) that accompanies the cord, would provide additional release.

(ii) Scrotal fixation (orchidopexy): In order to prevent retraction, several procedures have been described.

a) Subdartos (extradartos) pouch is the most popular, where in, a space is created between the skin and dartos, at the bottom of scrotum, to house the testis.

b) Keetley-Torek operation: a staged procedure, where the testis is initially implanted in the thigh, allowing the cord structures to elongate, subsequently brought down and fixed in the scrotum, at a second stage.

c) Ombredanne's procedure: an opening is made in the scrotal septum, through which the testis is made to lie in the contralateral compartment.

d) Ladd and Gross operation: the testis is fixed to the bottom of the scrotum by a nonabsorbable stitch.

e) Denis Browne procedure: in addition to the above (d), it is anchored to the upper medial thigh, with an elastic band, to permit postoperative mobility of the child.

f) Microvascular technique: This is a sophisticated surgery done for short vascular pedicle, which involves anastomosing the testicular vessels to inferior epigastric or pudendal vessels, restoring circulation, in a testis brought down into scrotum.

g) Laparoscopic staged approach: This is now becoming popular in cryptorchid infants, to locate the testis and to divide the spermatic (testicular) vessels in the retroperitoneum, so that the testis can be brought down into the scrotum, at a second stage. It is also useful to deal with the abdominal testis, in adults.

h) Orchido-celiopexy (intrabdominal fixation of testis), when it can not be brought down into the scrotum, is mentioned only to be condemned.

(Iii) For associated indirect hernia, simple herniotomy would suffice, repair of posterior wall (herniorrhaphy) may be considered, on the merits of local anatomy.

Orchidectomy: The indications have been already discussed, in general it may be said that prevention/early detection of malignancy form the main aim of this procedure, overriding other considerations.

Ectopic testis

As detailed, depending upon the activity of the tails of Lockwood, testis may be placed in abnormal locations, away from the normal path. The common types are:

a) suprainguinal: in the superficial inguinal or subinguinal pouch of Denis Browne (between Scarpa's fascia and external oblique aponerurosis)

b) pubic: at the root of penis

c) perineal: located in the anterior perianal region

d) femoral: near the fossa ovalis in the femoral triangle.

The most important aspect about ectopic testis is that the cord structures are not short, the scrotum is well developed and the processus vaginalis is usually not patent, facilitating comfortable orchidopexy. Defective spermatogenesis and malignant predilection are also

Jewels of Gyan - 30.2

Not all cryptorchids are invariably sterile

As Sir Astley Cooper was teaching a batch of students that sterility was the rule, one of the students, who was a cryptorchid, rushed out to commit suicide. Sadly a postmortem on his testis showed viable sperms. Medicine being a science of probabilities, only thumb rules apply and dogmatism may be risky.

31 Varicocele

Definition: Dilated elongated, tortuous veins of the pampiniform (pampinus: tendril) plexus of the spermatic cord.

Veins of the spermatic cord consist of:

a) those draining the testis and epididymis.

b) those accompanying the vas deferens.

c) cremasteric veins

In the scrotum, the veins of the pampiniform plexus are about 15-20 in number. As they pass proximally in the inguinal canal, they number 4-8 and coalesce further to enter the deep inguinal ring. Intra-abdominally, there are often two veins, called testicular (spermatic) veins. The right testicular vein enters the IVC, just below right renal vein (rarely into the renal vein itself) at about the level of L-2 and the left one into the left renal vein at a right angle. There are no valves in this system, except at their termination.

Etiology

1. Idiopathic: failure of the valve at the caval/renal vein entry

2. Sagging testis in a pendulous scrotum

3. Secondary to renal carcinoma of the left kidney or left renal vein thrombosis.

4. An SOL in the inguinal canal or retro-peritoneum, compressing the gonadal veins

Why is left sided varicocele more common?

i) The left testicular vein drains into the renal vein at a right angle.

ii) The loaded, mobile sigmoid colon may press upon the left testicular vein, impeding venous flow.

iii) The left suprarenal vein drains into the left renal vein, whereas the right, directly into the IVC. Catecholamines from the adrenal medulla on the left, bathing the area may cause incompetence of the valve.

iv) Left renal vein passes between the aorta and superior mesenteric artery and is prone for compression (nut cracker effect).

v) The left testis is normally placed at a lower level than the right, increasing the length and hydrostatic pressure o f the venous plexus.

vi) In 16%, the left testicular artery arches over the left testicular vein, and may compress it (Nathan and Hale).

VARICOCELE AND SPERMATOGENESIS

Scrotal temperature is about 2-3° C lower than the abdominal, which is essential for normal spermatogenesis. Because of reflux and stasis of blood in the scrotal veins, varicocele raises the temperature in the scrotum, which is detrimental to the process, more so if it is bilateral (Barfield). However, occasional normal fertility in men with bilateral varicoceles remains unexplained.

Another factor proposed is the reflux of adrenal hormones (catecholamines and steroids) into the testicular veins.

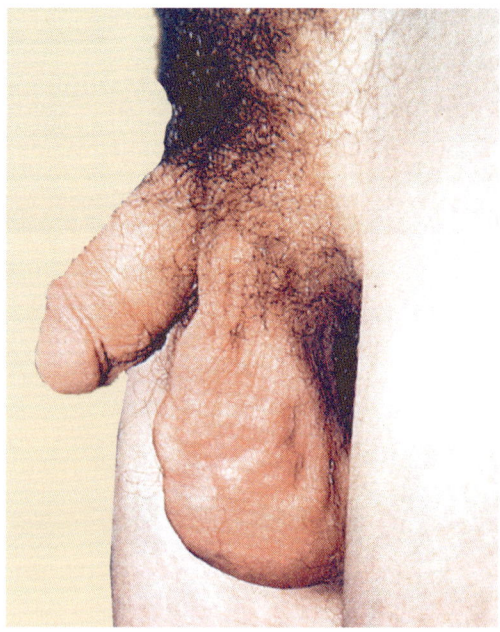

Fig. 31.1. Varicocele (bag of worms) (courtesy: Lifeline Hospitals, Chennai)

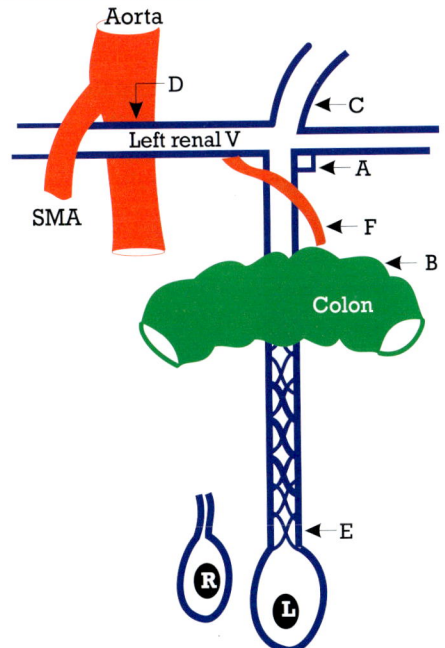

Fig. 31.2., Why varicocele is more common on the left
A. Left testicular vein joins renal vein at 90°
B. Mobile loaded sigmoid colon
C. Left suprarenal vein enters renal vein at the same level
D. Left renal vein may be compressed by SMA
E. Left testis is at a lower level
F. Left testicular artery crosses and compresses the testicular vein (16%)

Clinical features

The classical sufferer is a tall, young man with a pendulous scrotum.

Symptoms

i) often asymptomatic, detected by routine scrotal examination

ii) vague dragging discomfort in the scrotum is the most frequent complaint

iii) patients with bilateral varicoceles may present with subfertility or infertility.

Signs

The patient should be examined in standing position also.

Inspection: Dilated and enlarged veins may be obvious.There may be visible impulse on coughing and the ipsilateral testis may be atrophic in long standing cases.

Palpation: Typical feel of 'bag of worms', is unmistakable, which disappears in the supine position. Impulse (thrill) on coughing or by Valsalva maneuver is better palpated than seen.

If the veins are occluded by compressing the superficial inguinal ring with the thumb, the impulse/thrill will disappear and when the patient is made to stand up, they may be seen to rapidly fill up from below.

Bow sign: the patient is asked to bend forwards; while palpating the scrotal venous plexus between fingers, there will be a drop in their tension, as the abdominal viscera fall away from posterior abdominal wall, where the spermatic veins are located.

Investigations

i) If indicated, semen analysis for the sperm count/motility, to exclude oligo or asthenospermia.

ii) Ultrasound to show anechoic, multiple tortuous channels along the cord suggestive of varicocele. Abdominal study would detect any SOL, if present.

iii) Doppler flow study will confirm the presence of varicocele and reflux into the scrotal veins, disappearing on compressing the external ring.

iv) CT scan &/or IVU to rule out renal or retroperitoneal disease causing a secondary varicocele.

v) Thermography to detect raise in local temperature is rarely required.

vi) Appearance of unilateral varicocele, especially on the right (uncommon) side should alert the possibility of an SOL in the course of the testicular vein. On the left, the possibility of RCC permeating into renal vein has to be remembered. Recent development of a varicocele in an elderly, warrants investigation for a secondary type.

Differential diagnosis

Lymph varix, hydrocele, inguinal hernia, and diffuse lipoma of cord.

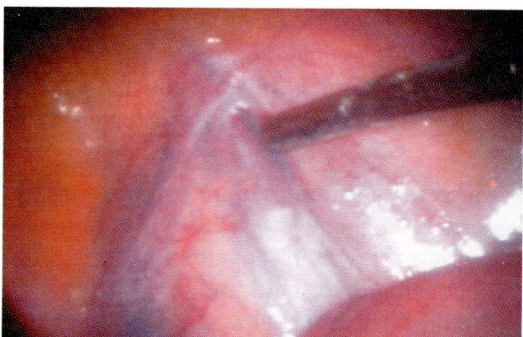

Fig. 31.3. Laparoscopic view of internal inguinal ring showing the spermatic veins and vas deferens (courtesy: Lifeline Hospitals, Chennai)

Treatment

Conservative: If the symptoms are not severe and there is no effect of spermatogenesis, reassurance and advice to wear supportive underclothing, may suffice.

Operative: Indications for surgery are bilateral varicocele with subfertility or persistent pain and discomfort. Among all the surgically correctable causes of male infertility, surgery for varicocele gives the best results. If properly selected and done, the improvement in seminal parameters are seen immediately, reaching its peak by 3-6 months.

(i) Scrotal approach: the pampiniform plexus can be exposed bilaterally through high scrotal incisions, but bleeding is often troublesome and can sometimes be complicated by a scrotal hematoma. Furthermore, a high recurrence rate and the likelihood of injury to testicular artery, make it a less preferred approach.

(ii) Classical (inguinal) approach: it is through an inguinal incision, similar to that of hernia. The cord structures are dissected out and the pampiniform plexus is isolated, ligated and divided, except 1 or 2 veins. The ends are tied together in order to lift up the testicles. This procedure is sometimes combined with an eversion of the tunica vaginalis in order to prevent a secondary hydrocele. Alternately in the inguinal canal, at the deep ring, the veins of spermatic cord confluence to form one or two veins, which are ligated without disturbing the posterior inguinal wall.

(iii) Paloma (suprainguinal) operation: the testicular veins are approached above the deep inguinal ring through a transverse incision made 3cm above the mid inguinal point. The muscles of the anterior abdominal wall are split in grid iron fasion and the peritoneum and extraperitoneal fat are pushed medially. The spermatic veins are seen on the posterior abdominal wall, lateral to the external iliac artery and are ligated.

(iv) Laparoscopic (retroperitoneal) method: the spermatic veins may be comfortably accessed laparoscopically, where the peritoneum overlying the posterior abdominal wall is incised, bringing the veins into vision. They are individually clipped and divided. Large tributaries are sometimes seen coursing along the vas and in the anterior abdominal wall, they should be either clipped or electrocoagulated, to prevent reflux into scrotal veins. The angle formed by the spermatic veins and vas deferens is the landmark for the external iliac vessels and this imaginary space is called triangle of doom, because application of unipolar diathermy in close proximity to the iliac vein may predispose to thromboembolic complications.

(v) Microsurgical ligation is becoming more popular, claiming best results. Through a small inguinal incision, the spermatic cord and testis are carefully delivered. Placing the cord under an operating microscope, the spermatic veins are clipped, preserving the arterial and lymphatic structures.

32 Testicular Tumors

Nearly 99% of testicular tumors are malignant, commonly presenting between the ages of 25 and 35. Earlier they all carried a dismal prognosis, but the advent of chemotherapy and monitoring by tumor markers have dramatically shifted their position to potentially curable malignancies.

Predisposing factors

Maternal hormones

It appears that a high level of circulating maternal gonadotrophins causes testicular hyperstimulation in utero itself, causing a series of changes that ultimately result in a testicular tumor at a later age. The proof is the high incidence of testicular cancers in dizygotic twins, in whom the circulating levels of hormones are very high, compared to monozygotic twins (interestingly the incidence of breast cancer is also high in dizygotics). This may also be a factor to explain high incidence of tumors in cryptorchids (see below). Klinefelter's syndrome (44-XXY) is also known to predispose to the development of seminoma.

Undescended testicles

Nearly 10% of testicular tumors occur in maldescended testicles. A cryptorchid has 30% higher risk of developing testicular malignancy compared to the normal; the contralateral normally descended testis is also not spared, suggesting a common factor in these patients. It is possible that a high levels of circulating gonadotrophins in bilateral cryptorchism is an initiating factor. Orchidopexy done after 6 years does not seem to significantly reduce the risk of testicular tumors. Even in cases who have had an orchidopexy between 2 and 6 years, dysplastic changes in the testicles are frequently seen. Thus it is believed that early orchidopexy considerably reduces, but does not totally eliminate the risk of subsequent testicular cancer.

In some cases bilateral dysgenetic testicles due to abnormality of chromosomal patterns, contribute to the development of cancer. Controversial predisposing factors in a recent large study include trauma and exposure to sexually trans iseases.

Classification of testicular tumors

According to the Great Britain Testicular Tumor Panel:

1) Seminoma (40%)
2) Teratoma (30%)
   Teratoma differentiated
   Malignant teratoma intermediate (teratocarcinoma)
   Malignant teratoma anaplastic (embryonal carcinoma)
   Malignant teratoma trophoblastic (choriocarcinoma)
3) Combined seminoma and teratoma (15%)
4) Interstitial tumors (1%)
5) Lymphoma (7%)
6) Secondary malignancy and others (7%)

WHO classification of testicular tumors: germinal tumors (98%) and non-germinal tumors, the latter arising from the non-germinal stroma of the testis and almost always benign. Germ cell tumors are subclassified into non-seminomatous germ cell tumors (NSGCT) and seminomas. Under the NSGCT:

* teratocarcinoma
* embryonal carcinoma

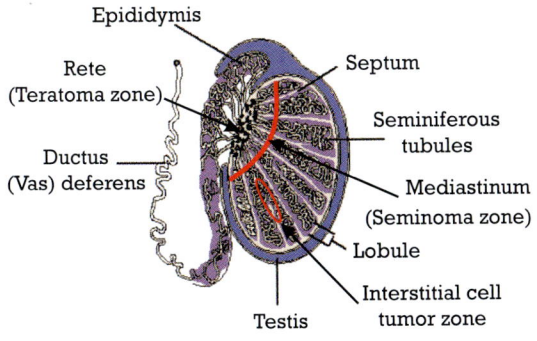

Fig. 32.1. Cross section of testis

| GROUP | Markers | | | Media-stinal spread | NPVM | % Pts | 5-Year Survival (%) |
	αFP (ng/ml)	β-hCG (ng/ml)	LDH (X N)				
NSGCT							
Good	<1,000 and	<1000 and	<1.5	no	no	58	90
Intermediate	<10,000 or	<10000 or	1.5-10	no	no	28	80
Poor	>10,000 or	>10000 or	10	yes	yes	14	50
Seminoma							
Good					no	90	90
Intermediate					yes	10	80

N: Upper limit of laboratory normal
NPVM: Non-pulmonary visceral metastases
Pts: Patients
Table-32.1. Prognostic evaluation of testicular tumors (IGCCCG)

* mature teratoma
* choriocarcinoma
* yolk sac tumor

A new (1997) classification of the International Germ Cell Cancer Collaborative Group (IGCCCG), is a prognostic indicator for germ cell tumors, which incorporates AFP, β-hCG, LDH, presence of mediastinal primaries and non-pulmonary visceral metastases (NPVM), for NSGCT. The seminomas are also divided into good and intermediate types based on the non-pulmonary visceral metastases. See table

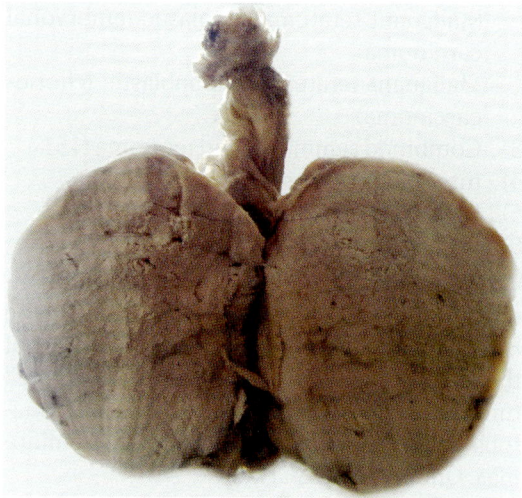

Fig. 32.2. Seminoma of testis (note homogenous fish flesh appearance, no necrosis or hemorrhage)

32.1.

Pathology

1) Seminoma

This is the commonest testicular tumor in an adult, with a peak incidence of 30-40 and a slightly higher incidence on the right side. It starts in the mediastinum testis and compresses the surrounding testicular tissue as it grows. Macroscopic appearance shows a homogeneous, pinkish and lobulated cut surface, without areas of hemorrhage or necrosis. It does not usually penetrate the tunica albuginea. Only the spermatocytic pattern makes small areas of cystic necrosis or hemorrhage. Microscopically there are of three types:

a) Typical seminoma

In this variety there are sheets of uniform seminoma cells divided into lobules by fibrous septa. The 'seminoma cell' is large and round and has a clear cytoplasm, a well demarcated cell membrane and a large central hyperchromatic nucleus with one or two prominent nucleoli. Tumor giant cells may be present and mitosis are infrequent. The septa between the lobules are infiltrated with lymphocytes, which represent the host immune response, more the lymphocytes along the septa, the better the prognosis.

b) Anaplastic seminoma

Feature	Seminoma	Teratoma
Cell of origin	Seminiferous tubules	Totipotent cells
Area	Mediastinum testis	Rete testis
Age	30-40	20-30
Incidence	More common	Less common
Shape of testis	Retained	Distorted
Consistency	Firm	Soft, cystic or firm
Spread	Lymphatic	Blood
Tumor markers	αFP	βhCG
Cut surface	Smooth & fleshy	Variegated, cystic
Radiosensitivity	Good	Fair
Prognosis	Excellent	Fair

Table-32.2. Differences between seminoma and teratoma

In this variety there is greater cellular and nuclear irregularity and tumor giant cells are frequently found. These are much larger than the seminoma cells with abundant mitotic figures.

c) Spermatocytic seminoma

This consists of three types of cells, namely

  i)   small cells with a narrow rim of eosinophillic cytoplasm resembling secondaries to metasites

  ii) medium sized cells with eosinophillic cytoplasm and

  iii) scattered giant cells

Seminoma spreads mainly by lymphatics, very rarely by blood stream. This tumor is never seen in children.

2) Teratoma

Teratomas of the testis arise from the totipotent cells in the rete testis, hence they may develop tissues derived from ectoderm, entoderm and mesoderm, occurring in younger ages compared to seminoma (25-35 years). Testicular tumors in infancy are always teratomas.

Macroscopically the homogenous lymph node-like appearance of the seminoma is absent. Multiple areas of cystic degeneration, hemorrhage and necrosis are seen in the cut section.

Mesoder-mal differentiation into cartilage may be seen.

Microscopically there are four varieties.

a) Teratoma differentiated (TD)

This has got two variants, the cystic teratoma (dermoid) and the solid mature teratoma. The cystic teratoma is nothing but a dermoid of the testis, similar to the dermoid cyst of the ovary. It has pultaceous material with a surrounding capsule. Extraneous tissue, such as hair, tooth, cartilage and muscle tissue can be made out. Like dermoid elsewhere, the prognosis is excellent.

Mature solid teratomas are composed of a mixed collection of differentiated cells like muscle, cartilage, squamous epithelium or intestinal wall. The stroma unlike the dermoid is a fibrous one. In adults, solid teratomas contain some elements of immature tissue and consequently may metastasize, testifying there malignant potential.

b) Malignant teratoma intermediate (MTI) syn: teratocarcinoma

It is the combination of embryonal carcinoma and teratoma. Here elements of immature tissue like primitive neurectoderm etc. are seen and sometimes the malignant foci reproduce the pattern of trophoblastic tissue or embryonal carcinoma.

c) Malignant teratoma anaplastic (MTA) syn: embryonal carcinoma, yolk sac tumor

These cells are truly pluri-potential and a complete spectrum of histological tissue may be reproduced, belonging to any of the germ cell layers. There are two types of embryonal carcinoma, the adult and the infantile variety. In the adult variety, a small tumor is seen in which the cells grow in alveolar, glandular tubular or papillary patterns. The neoplastic cells have an epithelial appearance and have hyperchromatic nuclei and prominent nucleoli. Tumor giant cells and mitotic figures are frequent and lymphocytes are hardly ever found. In the infantile form, which is the commonest type in infant and children, the individual tumor cells are quite metaplastic and contain vacuoles and granules of AFP.

d) Malignant teratoma trophoblastic (MTT) syn: choriocarcinoma

This is an aggressive testicular tumor in which the histologic hallmark is the presence of two types of cells viz. the cytotrophoblast and the syncytiotrophoblast. This is a rare tumor and often the primary is quite small. The lesion may sometimes present as a clot within the testis in the middle of which bits of grey tumor are made out. Microscopically the syncytiotropoblastic cell is large with many irregular hypochromatic nuclei and an abundant eosinophillic spatulated cytoplasm. Cytotrophoblast cells are regular and polygonal with a distinct cell border and a single fairly uniform nucleus. The syncytium cells form a cap and cytotrophoblasts grow in cords (cord and cap appearance). β-hCG is secreted in large quantities in this tumor, with early positive Aschheim-Zondek's (frog) test and sometimes producing gynecomastia or feminization. It is an aggressive tumor which

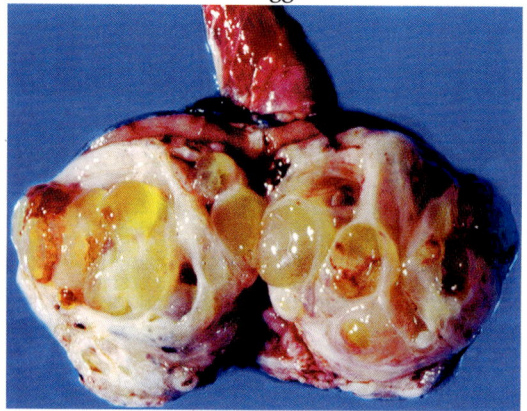

Fig. 32.3. Teratoma of testis (note multiple areas of cystic changes, necrosis, and hemorrhage)

rapidly spreads by all modalities, with very few surviving beyond one year.

3) Interstitial tumors

These occur at an early age and arise from the Leydig or Sertoli cells.

a) Leydig cell or prepubertal tumor

These are masculinizing and are often called pre-pubertal as they arise at that time. An excessive output of androgens causes extreme muscular development and sexual precocity. This results in a so-called infant Hercules appearance. Clinically the picture is the same as that of an adrenocortical virilizing tumor but a swelling of the testis is often palpable. Sometimes the contralateral testis may also hypertrophy in this condition. Removal of the testis results in complete suppression of the condition.

Histologically, the Leydig cells are large round cells with granular eosinophilic cytoplasm and a round central nucleus and with cytoplasmic inclusions made up of lipid granules and rod shaped crystalloids of Reinke. There are sheets of cells separated by a fibrous stroma.

b) Sertoli cell or postpubertal tumor

Rarer than Leydig cell tumor, often occurring post pubertally and marked by an excessive feminising hormone output. This causes gynecomastia, loss of libido and impotence. A high level of β-hCG is also noticed. Aschheim-Zondek test is positive. Histologically, regular tall columnar cells with vacuolated cytoplasm are seen.

Both these tumors are benign, dissemination almost never occurs and high orchidectomy is curative.

Clinical features of testicular tumors

There are four main clinical types or groups
1) typical,
2) metastatic,
3) atypical
4) hurricane type

1. Typical

Painless swelling of the testis is the commonest symptom. Only when the testis becomes twice or thrice the normal size does a sense of heaviness supervene. It is only in about 30% of the cases that pain is felt at all, which is of dull aching or dragging type. The normal sickening sensation felt around the umbilicus, on gentle squeezing the testis (testicular sensation), is classically lost in testicular tumors. In 10% of cases there is history of trauma on the affected side, which probably brings the swelling to attention.

2. Metastatic

The patient may present with para-aortic nodal enlargement, with insignificant scrotal findings. This is commonly seen in seminoma, which spreads mainly by lymphatics and may be associated with lumbar or abdominal pain. Rarely celiac and portal lymph nodes may cause obstructive jaundice. Chest pain, hemoptysis, dyspnea or cough may occur due to pulmonary metastasis, often seen in hematogenous dissemination from teratoma. Mediastinal or supraclavicular nodal involvement may also occur. Careful examination with high index of suspicion and appropriate investigations (imaging and tumor markers) generally provide the diagnosis.

3. Atypical

Acute presentation as 'epididymo-orchitis', with pain and swelling due to hemorrhage within the tumor, may be misleading. Lack of fever, leukocytosis and anticipated response to antibiotics and NSAIDs, should arise the suspicion of tumor. Slow growing tumors, such as well differentiated solid teratoma, may take as long as 2-3 years, to become clinically appreciable.

4. Hurricane type

Between the presentation of the testicular tumor and metastasis is only a matter of a few weeks and the patient rapidly succumbs. Hormonal manifestations patient may present with gynecomastia as in post-pubertal tumors or with virilization as in prepubertal tumors.

Physical examination

Local examination

The testis is enlarged by a smooth swelling (seminoma), a bosselated or irregular swelling (teratoma). The consistency is firm and regular in seminoma, but may be cystic in some areas in the case of a teratoma. The epididymis is initially normal, but as the disease progresses it may be involved. In a small percentage of patients a secondary hydrocele may be made out. Feeling heavy to lifting and loss of testicular sensation are pathognomonic features of a testicular tumor, occuring early in the course of the disease.

The spermatic cord remains normal initially but cremasteric hypertrophy secondary to the weight of the testis may cause it to become thicker, with increased testicular vascularity being a contributory factor. The vas deferens is almost never involved by a primary testicular tumor. Rectal examination should be performed, to detect any abnormalities of prostate and seminal vesicles.

General examination

All the sites of secondary spread should be evaluated

contralateral testis

abdomen, especially above the umbilicus

inguinal and iliac nodes may be involved, if scrotal skin is infiltrated or rarely by retrograde spread from the abdomen.

hepatomegaly
left supraclavicular fossa
edema of the lower limbs secondary to IVC obstruction
ureteric obstruction causing hydronephrosis.
Gynecomastia as a hormonal sequel

Differential diagnosis

i) Thick, calcified sac of long standing hydrocele

ii) An organized hematocele

Sometimes a history of trauma is not forthcoming and it is impossible to differentiate an organised clot between the layers of tunica vaginalis from a tumor. An USG and tumor markers may provide clues, but if they are equivocal, a high orchidectomy (in elderly) or scrotal exploration by Chevassu maneuver (in young) is recommended.

iii) Chronic epididymo-orchitis, either nonspecific or specific, such as tuberculous

This is a painful, tender, craggy epididymis in tuberculosis, with no loss of testicular sensation, but with history of fever and lymph node enlargement.

Staging

I   tumor confined to the testis
II   subdiaphragmatic node involvement
     A   < 2cm
     B   2 to 5 cm
     C   >5 cm
III supradiaphragmatic lymph node spread
IV   pulmonary, hepatic or other systemic spread

It is now agreed upon that tumor grading and markers should also figure in the staging along with nodal or visceral metastases, as they have a significant cumulative effect on survival.

Investigations

USG: An ultrasound scan of the scrotum to confirm the diagnosis, to evaluate the contralateral testis, ultrasound of abdomen to pick up para-aortic or iliac lymph nodes.

Radiograph of the chest is done to exclude metastasis.

Recently, PET-CT has replaced the above, as a single comprehensive study.

Tumor markers

I)   β-hCG for choriocarcinoma, AFP and LDH for the other teratomas

ii) placental alkaline phosphatase (PLAP) for seminoma

Needle biopsy and trans-scrotal orchidectomy are not recommended as they open up new lymphatic pathways, with increased risk of local recurrence and inguinal nodal metastases.

CT imaging of the thorax, abdomen and pelvis will complete the staging investigations in a confirmed germcell tumor.

IVU will detect compression of ureter by enlarged para-aortic nodes and also help to locate the kidney, which has to be shielded during radiation.

Lymphangiography may demonstrate secondary deposits in para-aortic lymph nodes and also helps to localize and outline the involved glands which can be progressively observed for shrinkage during therapy, but this imaging modality has been replaced by CT or MRI.

Contralateral testicular biopsy: Approximately 2% of those with germcell tumors will develop a second primary in the contralateral testicle. A precursor to this is the presence of carcinoma-in-situ(CIS), also known as testicular intra-epithelial neoplasia (TIN). Irregular coarse echogenic pattern and microcalcification in the ultrasound, may indicate CIS. However there is now increasing tendency to identify through a core needle biopsy of the contralateral testis either at the time of initial surgery on the testicle or more often at the end of the treatment programme. If CIS is found on the contralateral testicle, the role of giving a low dose RT to the testis, to obviate emasculation and sterility from orchidectomy, is being evaluated.

Treatment

A high or inguinal orchidectomy is the first step in the management of testicular tumors. Subsequent management is based on the staging, histological type and tumor markers.

Inguinal orchidectomy

Through an inguinal incision the inguinal canal is opened and the spermatic cord is brought out. It is clamped and divided at the level of the deep ring. Applying gentle traction on the cord, the testis is delivered into the wound and removed together. Excision of part of scrotum (hemiscrotectomy), is not recommended as a routine unless an inadvertent incisional biopsy was done earlier or the tumor had invaded the scrotal skin. Scrotal exploration and Chevassu maneuver: see under hydrocele (chapter 29).

Subsequent treatment of testicular tumors, depends upon the histology and the tumor load on hand, a summary of total therapy may be outlined here.

Seminoma

Stage I: High orchidectomy (HO) + RT

Stage II: HO + RT (+ chemotherapy with BEP- 3 cycles, if initial disease is >10cm)

Stage III: HO + 2 cycles of chemo (+ RPLND, if residual disease is >3cm), or otherwise, complete chemotherapy

Non-seminomatous tumors

Stage I: HO + surveillance (or RPLND, if the histology is aggressive or if tunica albuginea is breached)

Stage II: HO + chemotherapy. RPLND or salvage chemotherapy for high volume residual tumors

Stage III: HO + RPLND + Chemotherapy with cis-platinum, VP-16, Ifosfamide and bleomycin

Retroperitoneal lymph node dissection (RPLND)

It is more popular in the United States, but used in rest of the world only for management of residual masses after adequate chemo/ radiotherapy for NSGCTs. After a CT scan localization, through a long midline incision, retroperitoneum is completely exposed by incising the paracolic gutters and colonic mobilization. All enlarged lymph nodes and perivascular tissue, are removed. The disadvantages of the operation are its extensive nature and retrograde ejaculation and infertility, if both the L-1 sympathetic ganglia are damaged, during bilateral dissection.

Currently minimally invasive (laparoscopic) procedure has largely replaced the standard open surgery.

Management of residual masses

RPLND should be used to excise all masses >1cm, but in upto 50% of these patients they may not contain tumor, but only necrotic and fibrous tissue. More sensitive imaging methods, such as PET scan (positron emission transaxial tomography) will improve the selection criteria, sparing many of them from needless surgery, especially in teratomas (TD) containing differentiated or mature elements .

Mitramycin (or plicamycin), an antibiotic with antimitotic property, produced by streptomyces plicatus, is an RNA synthesis inhibitor, found to be useful against testicular tumors.

Long term toxicity

Although fertility is affected by chemotherapy, in course of time it returns to normal in those who had normal spermatogenesis prior to treatment. However, if it is very crucial, it may be safer to store the patient's semen in a sperm bank, for later use. Renal impairment, systemic hypertension, dyslipidemias and carcinogenesis are some of the well recocognized long term sequelae of chemotherapy. Bleomycin causes pulmonary fibrosis and Raynaud's phenomenon. Cis-platinum causes oto and nephrotoxicity, peripheral neuropathy and it persists in tissues in significant levels, long after the therapy is completed, which may be carcinogenic. Etoposide is known to cause leukemia. Overall it has been shown that among the long term survivors of testicular tumors, there is increased risk of developing acute leukemia, NHL, melanoma, malignancies of thyroid and GI tract.

Lymphoma of testis is usually NHL and is treated accordingly, with multimodality therapy (see chapter 42 on Lymph nodes).

33 Penis

Embryology: The genital tubercle in the embryo undergoes elongation and becomes the phallus. During this period, the urethral folds are pulled forward to form the walls of the urethral groove, both of them close over the urethral plate in the midline, to form the urethra. The most distal portion of the urethra, fossa navicularis, is formed later as invagination of ectoderm from the tip of the glans inwards to form a cord that subsequently canalizes.

Anatomy

The penis has three parts, the glans, the shaft and the root. It is composed of three columns of cavernous tissue, covered by fascia and skin, two dorsal, called corpora cavernosa, which expand at the base, inferior to the perineal membrane (called the bulb) and one ventral column, the corpus spongiosum, which houses the urethra. A tough covering encases the corpora cavernosa, known as Buck's fascia, which offers considerable resistance to the spread of malignancy into the cavernous tissue. Two tapering crura at the base are attached to the ischiopubic rami on either side. The entire glans is formed from the expanded spongiosum and is conical in shape, separated from the shaft by a circular (coronal) sulcus. The body of the penis is attached in the midline, to the front

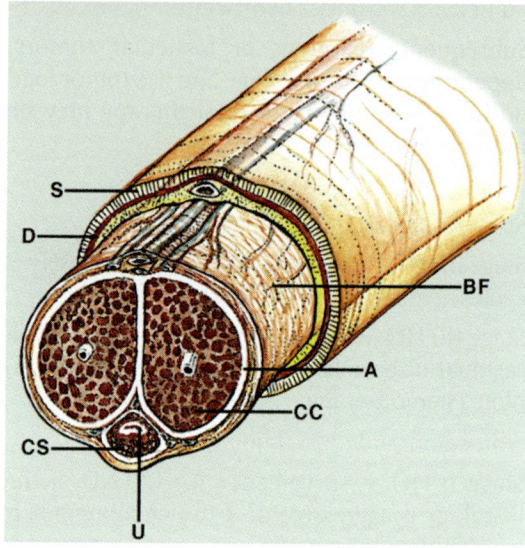

Fig. 33.2. Shaft cross section shows skin (S), dartos (D), fibroadipose tissue (yellow), Buck's fascia (BF) with numerous vessels and nerves, tunica albuginea (A) and corpora cavernosa (CC). Ventrally, the urethra (U) is surrounded by corpus spongiosum (CS) and tunica albuginea (white).

of the symphysis pubis, by a suspensory ligament.

Blood supply to the penis comes from the internal pudendal, through six arteries, two dorsal ones under the skin, two deep arteries in the substance of corpora cavernosa and two arteries of the bulb running within the corpora spongiosum, on either side of urethra. For functional reasons the arterioles directly open into cavernous tissue to produce turgidity on

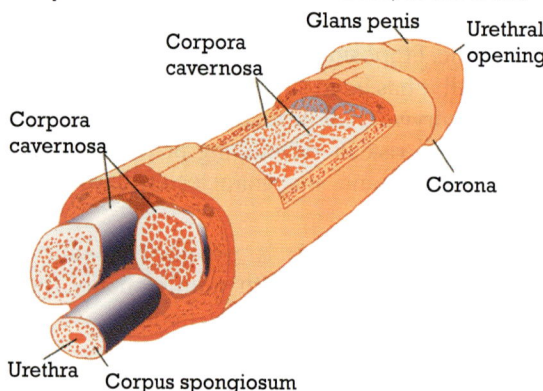

Fig. 33.1. Cross sections through the anterior part of the urethra

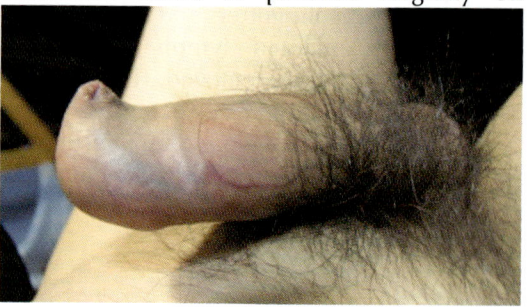

Fig. 33.3. Pinhole phimosis

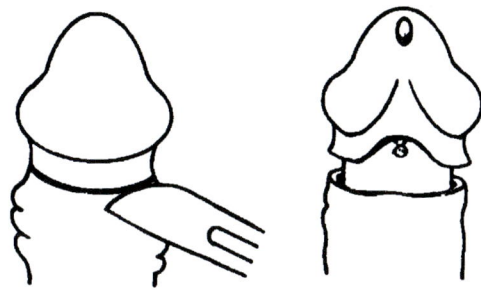

Fig. 33.4. Steps of circumcision Blandy's method

demand. The corkscrew configuration of the vessels permit elongation during erection.

Venous drainage by the same number of veins, but the dorsal ones lie antero-posterior instead of side by side, draining into long saphenous and prostatic plexus. Rest of the veins drain into pudendal veins.

Lymphatics from the penile skin drain into superficial inguinal nodes, whereas those from the body and glans drain into deep inguinal and external iliac groups. This explains the occasional involvement of external iliac nodes, skipping the inguinal nodes, by carcinoma penis.

Sentinel node concept - discribed later

PHIMOSIS

Definition: It is a condition in which the orifice of the prepuce is too small to permit free retraction over the glans penis.

In children under 6, the prepuce is normally adherent to the glans and retraction of the prepuce might be difficult. Although this gives a false impression of phimosis the external meatus is clearly seen and the prepuce is gently separated from the glans by releasing the adhesions by a blunt probe, under general anesthesia, enabling retraction over the glans.

Etiology

Congenital: In these cases the orifice is narrowed since birth and there is often a history of ballooning of the prepuce, followed by a thin stream of urine.

Acquired

Inflammatory: Long standing balanoposthitis

(inflammation of the glans and prepuce), especially in diabetes may lead to phimosis due to contraction of healed prepucial cracks. In course of time, adhesions develop between the glans and foreskin, complicating the matter further. Balanitis xerotica obliterans may also cause the same.

Traumatic: Occasionally vigorous trauma to the prepuce may cause prepucial fibrosis resulting in narrowing of the opening the prepuce.

Neoplastic: Underlying cancer of the penis may lead to this condition, and it must be suspected in an older patient, more so if he is a non- diabetic.

Clinical features

Difficulty in micturition is the main symptom, with the complaint of prepucial ballooning with a thin stream of urine.

In older patients, the symptoms of recurrent balanitis (edema, redness, pain and discharge per prepucial orifice), may be seen.

Back pressure effects of obstruction may cause residual urine in the bladder, bilateral hydroureters and hydronephrosis.

Rarely patients with minimal phimosis may present with paraphimosis, when the foreskin is stuck behind the glans penis. (vide infra).

In children, other congenital diseases such as pinhole meatus, urethral stricture or valves, should be looked for.

Complications

1. Balanoposthitis

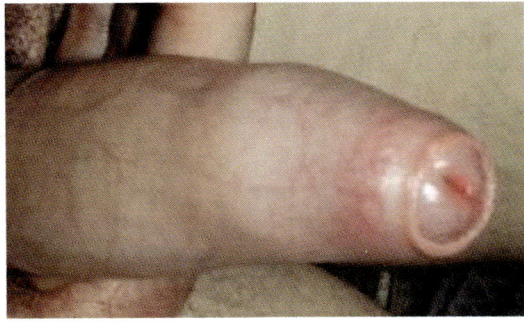

Fig. 33.5. Minimal phimosis with a risk of paraphimosis

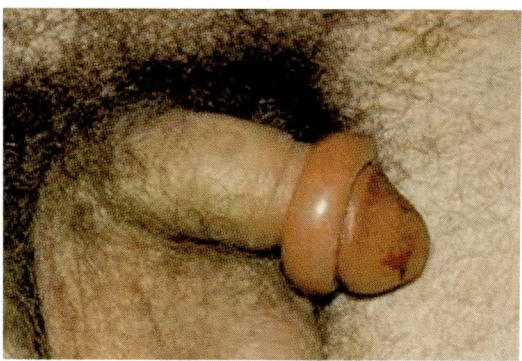

Fig. 33.6. Paraphimosis
(courtesy Laxmi Hospital, Kakinada)

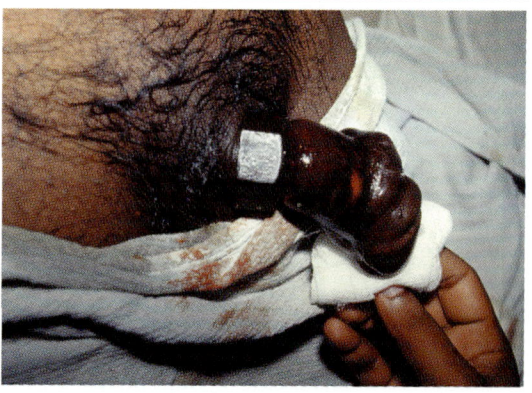

Fig. 33.7. Stangulating metallic ring, with impending gangrene of penis
(courtesy: Lifeline Hospitals, Chennai)

2. prepucial concretions due to inspissated smegma under the prepuce
3. acquired meatal stricture
4. obstructive uropathy, with effects on bladder, ureters and pelvicalyceal systems
5. paraphimosis
6. carcinoma due to prolonged contact of the carcinogenic smegma with glans penis.

Treatment

The definitive treatment is circumcision but a dorsal slit may sometimes be made as a first step, if extensive inflammation is present. This, along with antibiotics, allows the edema and inflammation to resolve within a few days, when circumcision may be performed. General anesthesia is preferred in children, but in adults a penile block, with 1-2% lignocaine (*without adrenaline*), is practised widely. It should be remembered that in hypospadias, neither a phimosis can manifest nor circumcision is advisable, since the prepucial skin may be required for urethroplasty later on.

Surgery: Circumcision (Blandy's method): A dorsal slit is made initially, the prepuce everted and cleaned, before it is cut circumferentially at two levels for outer and inner layers of the skin, ensuring some redundancy of prepuce to

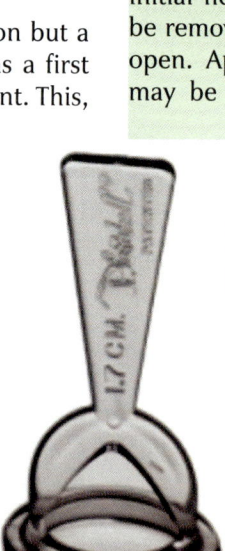

Fig. 33.8. Hollister plastibell for neonatal circumcision

accommodate penile erection, without the suture line getting too close to the coronal sulcus. The frenulum, considered to be the sexually sensitive area, should not be damaged and if it is found to be too short, it may be lengthened by 'V-Y' frenuloplasty. Fine absorbable sutures are used to approximate the skin edges, initial hemostatic compression dressings may be removed after 24-48 hours and wound left open. Appropriate antibiotics and analgesics may be used, but routine administration of estrogens, advocated by some, with an aim of preventing penile erection in the postoperative period is unwarranted, as the pain sensations originating from the stretched suture line, during the initial phase of erection will cause reflex inhibition of further tumescence.

Neonatal circumcision is practiced in developed countries and by certain races (jews), using a plastic bell (*Hollister plastibell or Gomco clamp*), the excess foreskin is crushed and excised, without the need for suturing. Besides improving local hygiene, it has brought down the incidence of penile carcinoma to a large extent. However if it is done in grown up children, as a religious ritual, it does confer some

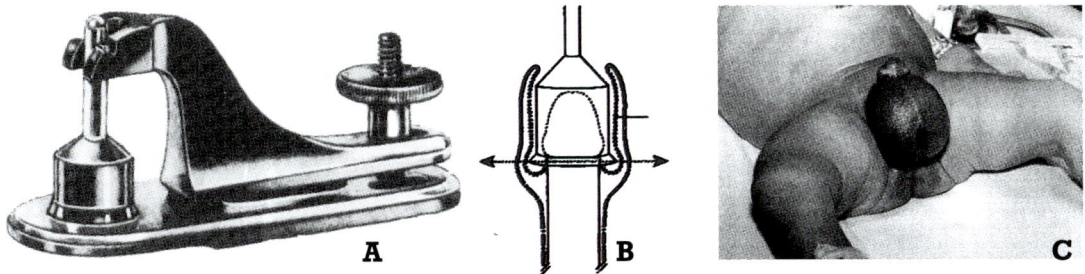

Fig. 33.9. A. Gomco clamp for neonatal circumcision
B. The clamp in place before the screw is tightened
C. A rare complication of bell circumcision - Fournier gangrene of scrotum

protection against malignancy, but does not eliminate the risk altogether.

PARAPHIMOSIS

Definition: Inability of the retracted prepuce to return to its normal position.

Etiology

Minimal phimosis is the common predisposing condition, which may be congenital or acquired due to chronic inflammation, leading to contracture of prepuce. Obviously tight phimosis does not produce this complication, since the prepuce cannot be retracted at all.

Pathology

The constricting band of phimotic prepuce around the coronal sulcus causes obstruction to the venous and lymphatic return from the glans penis, which sets up a vicious cycle of more constriction and more edema. In neglected cases arterial occlusion may supervene, leading to gangrene of the glans penis. The urethra is usually not involved and micturition is normal.

Clinical features

The patient presents with severe pain and swelling of the glans penis. The glans is edematous, congested with tight prepucial constriction around the sulcus. The shaft of penis is usually normal. Dusky hue of the swollen glans is an ominous sign of imminent necrosis, warranting urgent intervention.

Treatment

1. Application of ice cap and gentle manual compression may help to reduce the swelling.

2. Diluted hyaluronidase (Hyalase) in normal saline is injected into the swollen glans and prepuce, to tide over the situation, by facilitating absorption of the edema fluid and restoration of normal position of prepuce. Multiple punctures may also be made to drain the fluid out of the edematous prepuce and reduce its size.

3. If the above methods prove unsuccessful, the strangulating skin ring has to be released

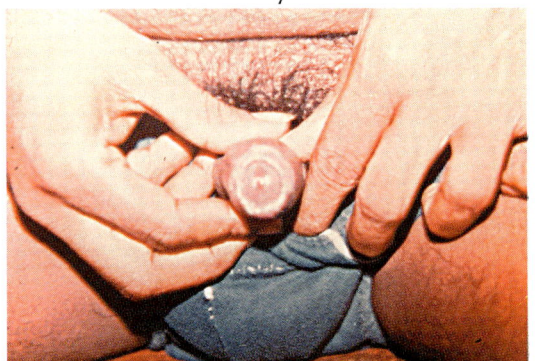

Fig. 33.10. Chronic balanoposthitis
(courtesy: Prof T Gunasagaran, Chennai)

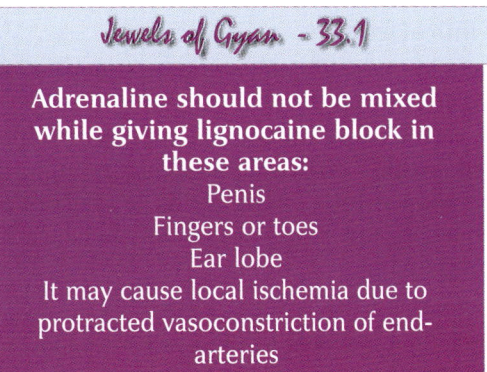

Jewels of Gyan - 33.1

Adrenaline should not be mixed while giving lignocaine block in these areas:
Penis
Fingers or toes
Ear lobe
It may cause local ischemia due to protracted vasoconstriction of end-arteries

immediately, under either local (in adults), or general anesthesia (in children). The surgical options are to cut the constricting band and reduce the prepuce, followed by standard circumcision either immediately or a few days later, allowing the edema to subside. A dorsal slit of the prepuce alone is another alternative.

Important precautions

(a) If it is planned to do under penile block anesthesia, adrenaline should never be added to lignocaine, for fear of inducing severe/protracted vasoconstriction and acute ischemia of glans penis.

(b) Monopolar diathermy should never be used to achieve hemostasis during surgery on penis, as it may thrombose the cavernous tissue at the base, by the current passing through it.

BALANOPOSTHITIS

Definition: Inflammation of the glans penis and prepuce. As they are very closely opposed, they are almost always involved together.

Causes

1. Most frequently it is due to retained secretions underneath prepuce with superadded bacterial or fungal infection, particularly when phimosis is present.
2. Skin conditions such as lichen planus and psoriasis.
3. Fixed drug allergy (FDA), especially to sulpha, affecting skin of the penis.
4. This is a very common manifestation in diabetics; sometimes this brings a latent diabetes to surface.
5. Antibiotic induced candidiasis.

Clinical features

In mild cases, the only symptoms may be itching and discharge from the foreskin.

In severe cases, the glans and prepuce appear red, with seropurulent exudate. Chronic balanoposthitis may lead to secondary phimosis and is a well known precancerous condition.

Investigations

Excluding diabetes mellitus is very important.

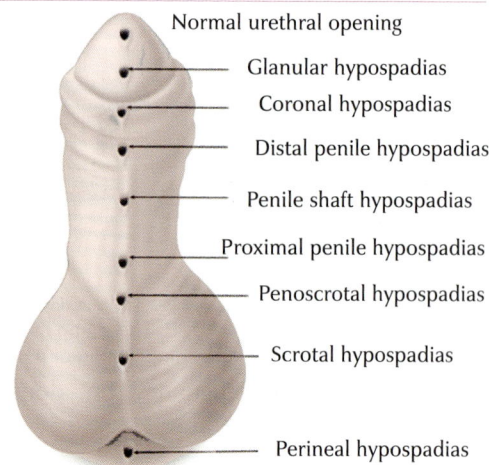

Fig. 33.11. Types of *hypospadias*

Other studies, such as serology for syphilis, microbiology for fungi and biopsy may be necessary in appropriate cases.

Treatment

Local hygiene and antimicrobial agents and if necessary a dorsal slit, followed by formal circumcision later on, should be performed.

HYPOSPADIAS

It is a condition where the urethra is not fully formed and the external meatus is located on the ventral aspect of the penis, proximal to the site of the normal opening.

Embryology

This is the commonest congenital anomaly of

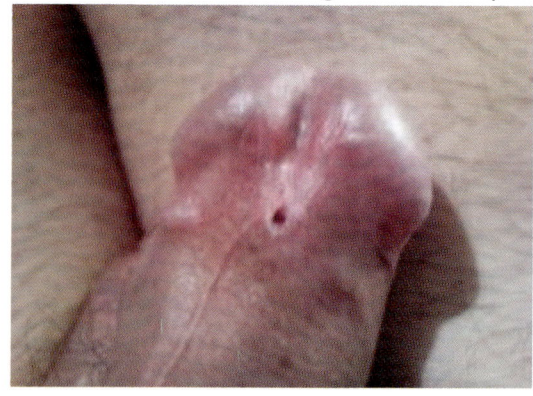

Fig. 33.12. Coronal hypospadias
(courtesy: Laxmi Hospital, Kakinada)

the male urethra, occurring in 3 out of 1000 male children. The penis/clitoris is developed from the genital tubercle, which shows a ventral groove developing into urethra in males and the labia minora in females (urogenital folds). Failure of the ventral urethral groove to close, for a variable distance so that the external urethral orifice recedes, results in hypospadias, either glandular, coronal, penile, penoscrotal or perineal, depending upon the site of the orifice. The urethra and its surrounding corpus spongiosum are not formed distal to the external orifice; the tissue beyond the orifice becomes a fibrous band, which produces a ventral bending of penis during erection, known as *chordee*. This fibrous band should be excised preliminary to reconstruction of the urethra, to achieve a full functional result.

Etiology

It may be familial or a result of hormone (estrogen and progesterone) therapy in early pregnancy.

Classification

According to the position of the abnormal meatus, it may be

1.   glandular - meatus located at the under surface of the glans, instead of the tip
2.   coronal - meatus located under the coronal sulcus
3.   penile - meatus located on the ventral aspect of the shaft
4.   penoscrotal - meatus located at the junction of penis and scrotum
5.   perineal - this is the most severe type, often

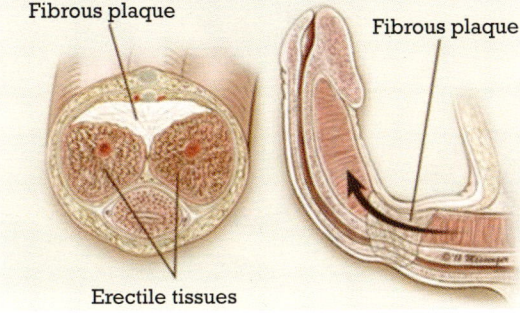

Fig. 33.13. Fibrous plaque in Peyronie's disease

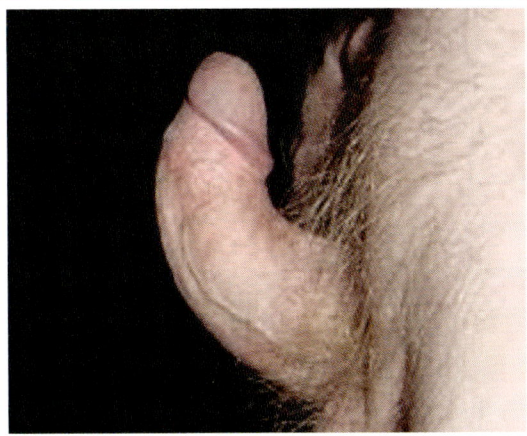

Fig. 33.14. Peyronie's disease

associated with maldescended testis and ambiguous genitalia. The scrotal sac is split (due to nonfusion) and the urethral meatus is located in between.

Pathology

This defect is associated with

1.   chordee, appreciated during erection, as explained above.
1.   external meatal stricture
2.   hypoplastic penis
3.   absence of prepuce on the ventral aspect, known as 'hooded prepuce'; hence it is impossible to have a combination of hypospadias and phimosis.

Complications

1.   obstructive uropathy and urinary tract infections

2.   chordee (a painful ventral bending of penis during erection, interfering with sexual intercourse).

3.   infertility, may be due to the failure of spermatogenesis, from associated abnormal development of testes or failure of intravaginal deposition of semen

4.   ambiguous genitalia and difficulty in sex differentiation (in the perineal type).

Specific investigations

1.   an IVU, to exclude other urological abnormalities.

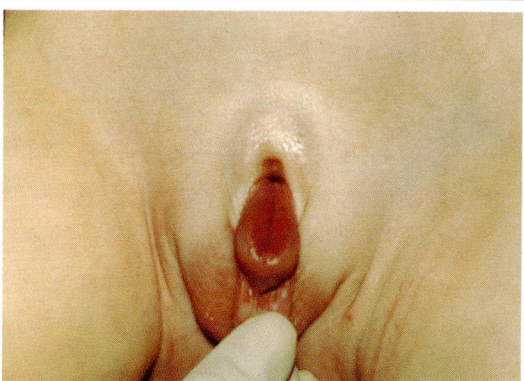

Fig. 33.15. Epispadias

2. Cystourethroscopy to exclude other ure-thral/vesical anomalies, but not mandatory in all cases.

3. karyotyping to identify the sex and any chromosomal abnormalities, in doubtful cases.

Treatment is only by corrective surgery, before preschool age, to avoid psychological problems. *Circumcision should not be done* in these boys and the precious skin should be saved for future urethroplasty. The glandular type may be left alone or may just need meatoplasty, if there is a stricture. Innumerable methods of repair have been described for the other types of hypospadias and the subject falls into a common ground covered by the urologist, pediatric surgeon and plastic surgeon, not to speak of a good general surgeon with special interest.

The main principles of surgery are:
(1) meatal dilatation
(2) correction of chordee
(3) ventral transposition of the prepuce and
(4) urethroplasty

Usually the first three are done at one sitting, at about 2-3 years of age and the fourth after a year or so, most often combined with urinary diversion, either perineal or suprapubic, for a few weeks. There is a growing tendency to carry out total reconstruction in a single stage, claiming satisfactory results, with obvious advantages. The major objection for one-stage repair was the fear of incomplete correction of chordee, but that is totally eliminated by the advent of artificial erection techniques, utilized during the procedure. This is done by injecting saline into the corpora cavernosa, using a fine needle, after application of a soft tourniquet at the root of the penis.

Urethroplasty

Preliminary urinary diversion either by perineal urethrostomy or suprapubic cystostomy is done. Denis-Browne method is the simplest, which consists of making a 'U' shaped incision starting on either side of the tip of the glans penis, going around the ectopic meatus. Mobilized lateral flaps of the central skin strip are sutured, creating a skin tunnel, starting from the abnormal meatus to the tip of the glans, in two fine layers, over which the lateral edges of skin is sutured in the midline, to cover the neo-urethra. A dorsal midline slit is sometimes made over the skin, to release tension on the main sutures. The success of this procedure lies in gentle tissue handling, proper mobilization of flaps, using fine suture materail and approximation of edges without tension.

Devine-Horton's operation is a one-stage urethroplasty, using a flip-flap technique, which utilizes a full thickness graft of the prepuce to form the tube and Byars' rotation flaps to cover it. Number of techniques described for reconstruction of hypospadias testify to their uncertain results, mostly due to the inherent healing problems in that region.

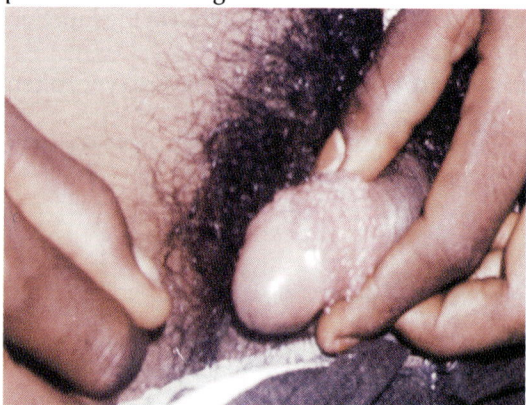

Fig. 33.16. Condylomata acuminata
(courtesy: Halsted Surgical Clinic, Chennai)

The urinary diverting catheter may be removed in 3-4 weeks, after ascertaining the complete healing of neo-urethral suture line, as it is notorious for poor healing and fistula formation.

EPISPADIAS

This is an anomaly in both sexes, where the urethral meatus is located on the dorsum of the penis/clitoris and is much rarer compared to hypospadias. According to the location of the ectopic meatus, it is called glandular, penile, penopubic and total epispadias, the last three being usually associated with urinary incontinence. The total type is associated with ectopia vesicae (exstrophy of the bladder).

Treatment is by surgery, using Denis-Browne technique, done around the age of 3.

PEYRONIE'S DISEASE

(Syn: induratio penis plastica)

In this condition, fibrous plaques of varying size are formed over tunica albuginea of one or both corpora cavernosa, usually on the dorsal aspect, causing bending of penis during erection.

Etiology: is unknown: trauma, vasculitis or collagen disorder have been incriminated, as in Dupuytren's contracture of the hand, which may occasionally coexist.

Clinical features

Occurs over 40, they present with painful erection with bending or feeling hard plaques on the penis, with impaired erection. On palpation, flat hard uneven plaques are felt over the dorsal aspect of shaft of penis. No local signs of inflammation or regional lymphadenopathy are seen. Spontaneous regression may occur in half of the patients, over a period of several years.

Treatment

It is empirical and symptomatic. Administration of drugs like para-aminobenzoic acid (PABA), antioxidants, such as vitamin A, E, b-carotene etc. local infiltration of hydrocortisone have all been tried with variable success. More aggressive treatment with excision followed by either tunica vaginalis graft or implantation of penile prosthesis has wider acceptance. Nesbitt's procedure of placing a nonabsorbable suture on the other side of cavernosa, to restore balance during erection is only of historical interest.

CONDYLOMATA ACUMINATA (syn: genital warts) are sexually transmitted, caused by human papillomavirus (HPV), developing into exophytic warty lesions around the frenulum, coronal sulcus, glans and also in the urethral meatus. They occur in places subjected to trauma during intercourse, in the female causing epithelial changes in the cervix, predisposing to carcinoma.

Other sexually transmitted diseases (STD), such as candidiasis, trichomoniasis, syphilis and gonorrhea, have to be excluded. Their association with HIV infection should also be borne in mind.

Treatment

Topical applications of 25% podopyllin in spirit, avoiding contact with adjacent skin and rinsed off. They may be excised using diathermy, cryo or laser and to eliminate moisture, which perpetuates the infection, circumcision may be helpful.

Ram-horn penis is described in chapter 42.

PRIAPISM

This is persistent painful erection of penis, the congestion being limited to corpora cavernosa.

Causes

1. Coagulopathy seen in blood dyscrasias
2. use of sildenafil, tadalafil or vardenafil
3. intracavernous injection of vasodilators, such as papaverine
4. prolonged sexual activity
5. autonomic neuropathy (rare)
6. venous compression due to malignancy (rare)
7. trauma leading to an AV fistula (rare)

Investigations to identify underlying cause, may include duplex imaging and coagulation profile.

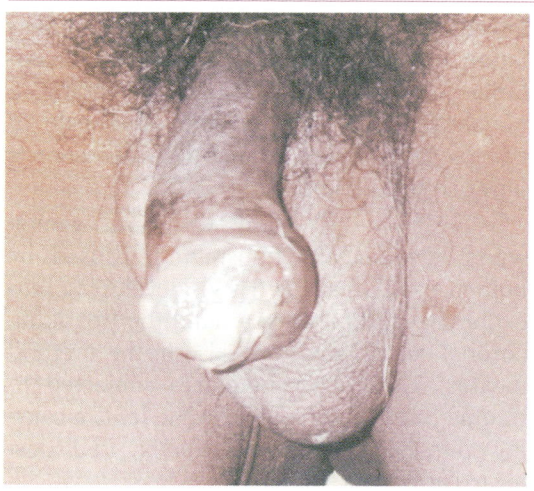

Fig. 33.17. Carcinoma penis
(courtesy: Halsted Surgical Clinic, Chennai)

Treatment

It requires care in a specialized centre; having excluded any predisposing disease, symptomatic therapy with analgesics, aspiration of stagnated blood in cavernous spaces, injection of vasoconstrictors, such as metara-minol, dopamine or adrenaline into both the carpora cavernosa, may be attempted. Surgery, to achieve detumescence, may be necessary by anastomosing carpora cavernosa with spongiosa, under cover of anticoagulation therapy. The overall prognosis in terms of symptomatic relief and functional restoration is not bright. Therapeutic embolization of internal pudendal artery, to shut-off the AVF, between the artery and cavernous tissue is also being attempted.

CARCINOMA PENIS

This is a common malignancy, accounting for upto 10% of all cancers in uncircumcised male population in Asian countries.

Predisposing factors

1. Age, usually after 5th decade, though rarely seen in younger ages
2. Phimosis
3. Local hygiene
4. Socio-economic status
5. Occupational

Circumcision: Carcinoma penis is almost unheard of in races like the Jews, who practice neonatal circumcision. A slightly higher incidence occurs in Muslims who undergo circumcision at around school-going age, but still much lower compared to the uncircumcised male population. About half of the patients with carcinoma penis are found to have phimosis, the chronic irritative effect of smegma within the prepucial sac possibly being the causative factor. The smegma is degraded by Mycobacterium smegmae to carcinogenic hydrocarbons and sterols.

Occupation: A higher incidence is noted in workers exposed to asbestos and paint.

Virus etiology: Two groups of viruses have been implicated, the herpes simplex type II and the human papilloma virus. A 3-8 fold increase in carcinoma cervix in the sexual partners of patients with carcinoma penis has been documented. *The Pincus' latent cancer theory* implicates a crossover of chronic, carcinogenic viral stimulation between patients with cancer penis and cancer cervix.

Premalignant lesions

1. Chronic balanitis
2. Leukoplakia
3. Bowen's disease
4. Erythroplasia of Queyrat (Paget's disease)
5. Genital warts

Pathology

Gross: Carcinoma penis usually begins as a small nodule or papillary lesion or an ulcerative lesion of the glans, prepuce or coronal sulcus. Origin from the skin of the shaft is rare. The lesion is ulcerated, with secondary infection in upto 90% of the cases. Foul smelling (characteristic) discharge and inflammatory induration of the deeper tissues may simulate tumor infiltration. Untreated, the tumor grows progressively producing distortion and destruction of the penis. It should be realized that SCC (or epithelioma) always starts as an ulcer, but if it is arising from the inner layer of prepuce or the glans in a patient with phimosis, initially only a hard nodule may be appreciated, till it erodes through the external layer. In late neglected cases, entire glans and part of the shaft may be destroyed by the infiltrating tumor.

Morphologic types

1. exophytic
2. scirrhous
3. ulcerative

Exophytic and scirrhous lesions are usually better differentiated with a more favorable prognosis compared to the ulcerative lesion, which unfortunately happens to be the commonest type. In the papillary type, the tumor grows towards the surface and fungates, only later producing an indurated base; thus the infiltrating and ulcerative lesions have a worse prognosis compared to the papillary and exophytic types.

Histological patterns of growth

1. Intra epithelial
2. Leukoplakia
3. Verrucous
4. Compact
5. Plexiform (highest degree of anaplasia occurs in this type)
6. Buschke-Lowenstein tumor, is a variant of condyloma acuminatum.

Buck's fascia, the tough fascia encasing the corpora cavernosa, acts as a temporary barrier against tumor invasion. Urethral involvement is also rare for some reason.

Carcinoma of the penis is similar to SCC occurring elsewhere and is usually moderate to well differentiated type. The cells involve the adjacent tissue, form keratinizing walls with central degeneration and form epithelial pearls or cell nests. However despite the inherently vascular nature of this organ, the malignant cells have a predilection to involve the lymphatics and the embolise to the regional lymphnodes and vascular dissemination is distinctly uncommon.

Spread: Metastases to the regional inguinal, femoral and illiac nodes is the commonest route of dissemination. Distant metastasis to the lung , liver, bone or brain is rare, more so, without regional nodal spread. *The commonest cause of death in advanced disease, is erosion of femoral vessels by the metastatic inguinal nodes, resulting in exsanguinating hemorrhage.*

Symptoms

1. Foul smelling discharge, bleeding
2. Exophytic growth
3. Mass or ulceration with inguinal nodal enlargement
4. Urinary retention or urethral fistula due to corporal involvement (rare)
5. Autoamputation of penis

Signs

1. Assess the primary; size, site, involvement of corpora, involvement of urethral meatus. If phimosis present, dorsal slit under local anesthesia, may be needed, for proper inspection
2. Involvement of shaft and root of penis and scrotum
3. Palpation of inguinal/iliac lymph nodes
4. Rectal and bimanual examination to assess if pelvic spread is present

Early diagnosis of this disease can be made only by a high index of suspicion in all ulcerating lesions of the penis. The inordinate delay in seeking medical advice is striking; the average period from the onset of ulcer to consulting a surgeon is around six months, even among the 'civilized' population.

Differential diagnosis

1. erythroplasia of Queyrat (Paget's disease of penis): reddened papular lesion on the glans, without ulceration
2. chronic balanoposthitis: signs of inflammation of prepuce and glans
3. granuloma inguinale: history of contact, large granulomatous, contiguous lesion, ripe pomegranate appearance
4. condyloma acuminatum: warty superficial lesion, around coronal sulcus
5. Buschke-Lowenstein tumor (syn: giant condyloma acuminatum) giant hypertrophic warty lesion, sometimes replacing glans, by destruction

6. herpes simplex: multiple circinate (scalloped) ulcers

7. syphilis, primary and tertiary: hard painless button-like chancre, with shotty nodes or gummatous punched out ulcer with washleather slough

8. fungal granuloma: clinically indistinguishable from other granulomas, often it is diagnosed by biopsy

9. tuberculous ulcer: undermined edges, evidence of tuberculosis elsewhere

Investigations

1. Baseline investigations (anemia and leukocytosis may occur as a part of chronic illness)

2. Rarely, azotemia secondary to urethral obstruction

3. Upto 20% of patients with carcinoma penis have hypercalcemia probably due to release of a parathormone-like substance produced by the tumor and its metastases (paraneoplastic syndrome)

Specific investigations

1. Biopsy: an edge biopsy is done, for diagnosis and grading of differentiation, however certain the clinical diagnosis might appear.

Radiology of chest and bones may provide evidence of metastasis as also a radio-nucleide scan.

IVU is only indicated if there is suspicion of ureteric obstruction secondary to retroperitoneal lymphadenopathy.

Lymphangiogram: The role of penile lymphangiography, to detect nodal secondaries, is not well established as the distinction bet-ween inflammatory and metastatic lesions is difficult, particularly in the inguinal/iliac region. A CT scan of abdomen and pelvis is indicated only if large nodes are present in the inguinal region, the lesion is high grade or if bimanual examination shows a lateral pelvic mass.

Staging: Jackson's and TNM, the first being the most popular one.

Jackson's staging: is convenient and widely used in practice for planning RT and surgery.

Stage I (A)   Tumor confined to prepuce or glans penis

Stage II(B)   Tumor invading shaft of penis (Buck's fascia)

Stage III(C) Inguinal nodes present, mobile and resectable

Stage IV(D) Tumor that invades penile nerves or scrotum, fixed/nonresectable lymph nodes and distant metastases.

TNM staging

Primary tumor (T)

Tx Primary tumor cannot be assessed
To No evidence of primary tumor

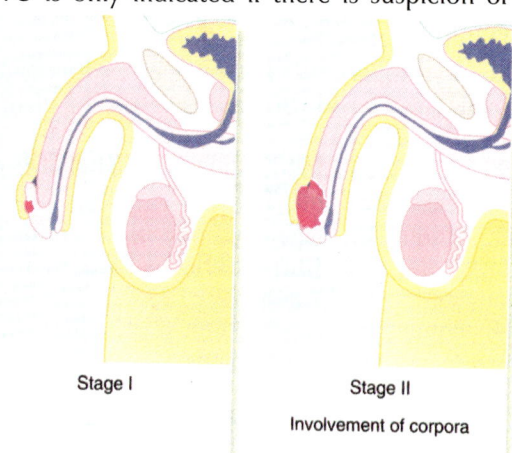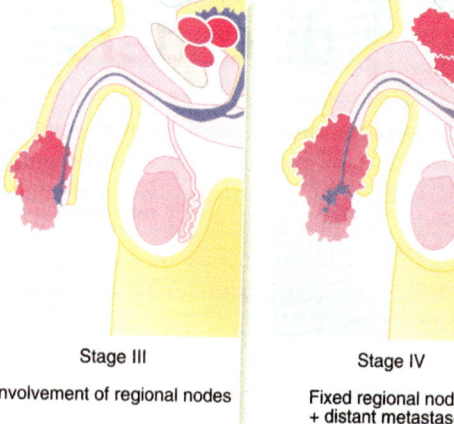

Stage I	Stage II	Stage III	Stage IV
	Involvement of corpora	Involvement of regional nodes	Fixed regional nodes + distant metastases

Fig. 33.18. Clinical stages of carcinoma penis

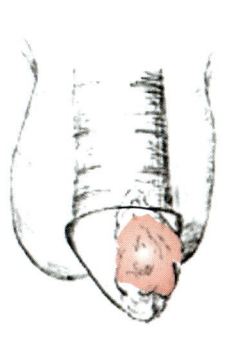 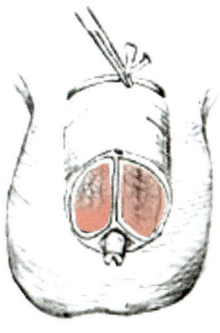 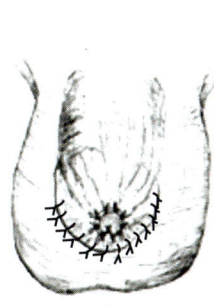 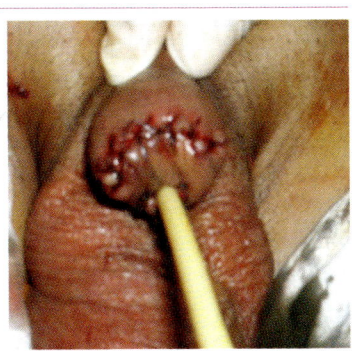

Fig. 33.19. Steps of partial amputation of penis

Ts Carcinoma-in-situ

T1 Tumor invades subepithelial connective tissue

T2 Tumor invades corpus spongiosum or cavernosum

T3 Tumor invades urethra or prostate

T4 Tumor invades other adjacent structures

Regional lymph nodes (N): The presence of nodal metastases halves the patients survival

Nx   Regional lymph nodes cannot be assessed

No   No regional lymph nodes metastasis

N1   Metastasis in single, superficial inguinal lymph nodes

N2   Metastasis in multiple, or bilateral superficial inguinal lymph nodes

N3   Unilateral or bilateral fixed deep inguinal or pelvic nodes

Distant metastases (M)

Mx   Presence of distant metastasis can not be assessed

Mo   No distant metastasis

M1   Distant metastasis present

Treatment

1. treatment of primary
2. treatment of regional lymphatics and lymphnodes
3. treatment of systemic metastases

Surgery

1. Circumcision may be sufficient, if only the prepuce is involved, but the recurrence rate is unacceptably high, upto 50%. It is curative for carcinoma-in-situ.

2. Wide local excision may be done, if a small lesion is situated over the glans in a young man, resulting raw area being covered by skin advanced from the shaft of penis. This is generally followed by brachytherapy, using isotope mould, to 'sterilize' the base.

The above two may be considered as conservative surgery.

3. Partial amputation of the penis; If the glans and distal shaft are involved and the lesion appears to be superficial; partial amputation with a 2.5cm margin proximal to the tumor gives the best result. A frozen section of the proximal margin may be obtained if possible, to confirm a tumor free margin. As a general rule, partial amputation is possible, if there is about 5cm gap from the tumor induration to the root of penis; 2.5cm clearance and 2.5cm stump. Some surgeons feel that once corpora cavernosa are involved, technically entire shaft is involved, hence nothing less than total amputation should be done.

In the absence of inguinal metastases the 5-year survival is upto 80%. The residual stump is usually adequate for upright micturition and sexual function.

4. Total amputation of penis with perineal urethrostomy, is done, when partial preservation cannot be done, by the criteria mentioned. If the lesion involves the proximal shaft or the specimen of partial amputation reveals tumor at the resected margin (preferably by frozen section), total amputation is the curative option. If the base of penis is involved and wide

elliptical incision around the root of penis is required for adequate clearance, the resultant large skin defect may be covered by advancement of anterior scrotal skin, on to the pubic symphysis or anterior abdominal wall.

For more locally advanced, low grade tumors with extension into the scrotum and perineum or with fixed large inguinal nodes, adventurous procedures, such as hemipelvectomy or hemicorporectomy with chemotherapy have been suggested in selected cases, but the role of such mutilation is doubtful and limited to very few cancer centres in the world. Low potential of the tumor for distant spread is the main attraction for such procedures.

Moh's micrographic surgery

This is a method of surgically removing skin cancers by excising the tissue in thin layers. Although more time consuming than other tissue sparing techniques it is ideally suited for the small distally located carcinoma. After excision, the area is allowed to heal by secondary intention. Meatal stenosis can sometimes form a problem following the surgery. This technique seems to provide cure rate equivalent to partial penectomy, leaving patients with more esthetic and functional residue.

Laser surgery

This is used to treat early disease (upto T2 lesion)

The CO_2 or the Nd: YAG laser are used and the lesion is fulgurated or excised respectively. The problem is that the depth of destruction due to laser is often difficult to assess, some times leading to stricture urethra due to uncontrolled tissue destruction. Since the tumor tissue is vaporized, histological documentation will not be available.

Radiation therapy (RT)

The advantage is that penile structure and function are retained. The main indications are:

1. Small, superficial, noninvasive lesion and the glans, in the young

2. As initial form of therapy, when surgery is refused

3. After failure of a course of topical 5-FU in the treatment of carcinoma-in-situ.

Problems related to RT

1. SCCs are typically radiosensitive but the

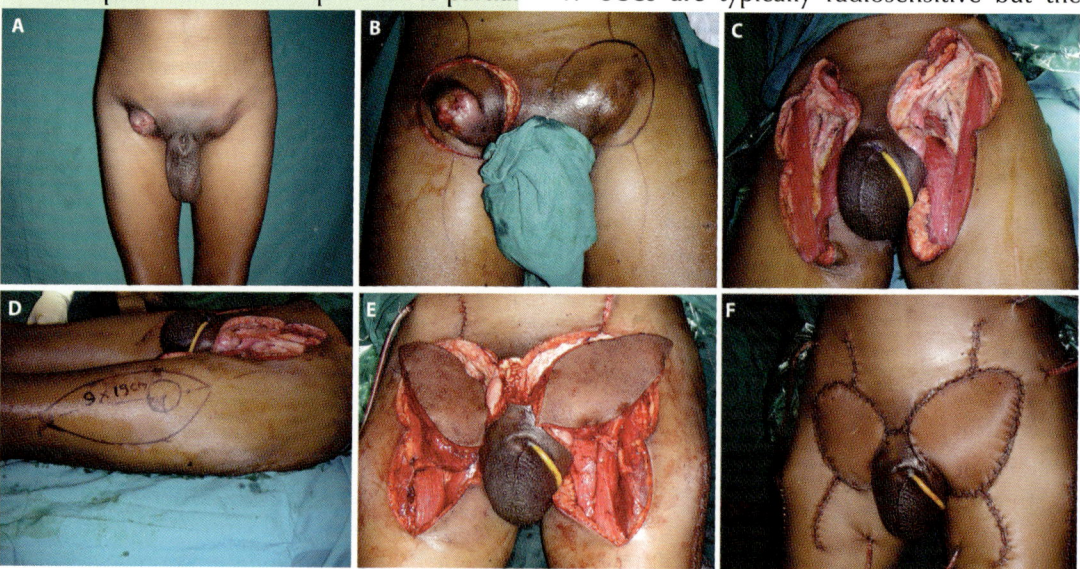

Fig. 33.20. Bilateral advanced inguinal lymphadenopathy, following amputation of penis
A. Inguinal masses fixed to skin **B**. Wide excision of the masses
C. Resultant skin defect **D**. Thigh rotation flaps marked **E**. Composite flaps to cover the defects **F**. Final result.
(courtesy: Dr B S Madhusudanan, Chennai

dose of radiation required to sterilise deeply infiltrating tumors may result in uretheral stricture, meatal stenosis or fistula. Any of these complications may require subsequent amputation of penis.

2. As expected, well differentiated tumors are less radio-sensitive than the anaplastic type.

3. In the presence of infection (which is the rule in this disease), the effect of radiotherapy is less than desirable.

4. The treatment schedule runs on for several weeks followed by several months of morbidity.

5. Careful longterm follow up is necessary to detect recurrence.

6. Recurrent malignancy is sometimes mistaken for an ulcerated post- irradiation scar

7. Radiation testicular damage

Types of delivery systems used:

1) external beam,
2) radium mould or
3) interstitial implants

The external beam therapy is ideal for radiation to lesions superficial to the fascia lata with negative nodes by histopathology.

RT for nodal disease

In patients with fixed, ulcerated and nonresectable inguinal nodes, RT may offer significant palliation, but secondary nodes are not as radiosensitive as the primary SCC, especially if they are the seat of secondary infection and surrounded by fat, which shields the tumor cells. It must also be realised that clinical evaluation of the groin becomes difficult after irradiation.

Chemotherapy: Mainly used as an adjuvant after lymphadenectomy in the high risk group (bilateral ilioinguinal nodes and less differentiated tumors) and for disseminated disease. Taxanes, bleomycin, cis-platinum, 5-FU and vincristine are used in various combinations.

Reconstructive surgery following amputation of penis:

Following partial penectomy, a microvascular procedure with a radial forearm flap provides for a phallic reconstruction with exogenous

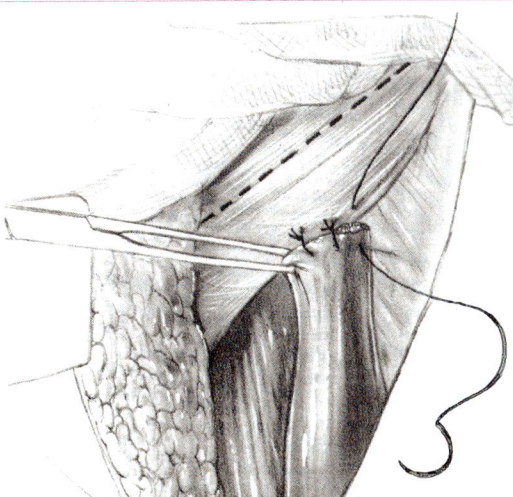

Fig. 33.21. Fixing the detached sartorius muscle over the femoral vessels

sensations, as some cutaneous nerves are also sutured. Similar procedures have been attempted following total penile amputation, using gracilis or rectus abdominis myocutaneous flaps and prosthetic stenting, but nothing can replace the natural anatomy and physiology of corpora, hence the unsatisfactory results.

Management of regional lymph nodes

The nodal presentation can vary from non-palpable nodes to fixed bilateral ilioinguinal lymphadenopathy. About 25% of patients have contralateral metastases even if the nodes are clinically palpable on one side. In patients with clinically positive inguinal nodes but without iliac nodes, ilioinguinal node excision has been shown to be superior to inguinal excision alone, which is supported by the observation that if the corpora cavernosa is involved (breaking through the Buck's fascia), lymphatic drainage can take place directly to iliac group, bypassing the inguinal, but this lacks universal approval.

Anatomy of inguinal nodes

They are broadly classified as superficial and deep groups. The superficial nodes, totally around 20, are located in a 'T' manner, vertically, along the long saphenous vein and horizontally, along the inguinal ligament, the latter further subdivided into medial and lateral groups. The efferent lymphatics from these groups pass through the cribriform fascia covering fossa ovalis (the fascia earns its name by the multiple perforations made by these channels).

The deep nodes are placed along the medial aspect of femoral vein, the highest of these is located in the femoral canal, called the node of Cloquet, which forms the junction between inguinal and iliac groups of nodes.

Lymphadenectomy: Nodal block dissection is performed only in the presence of clinically palpable inguinal nodes, having offered curative therapy to the primary lesion. It should be realized that 50% of palpable inguinal nodes are due to secondary infection and not metastasis and about 25% of impalpable nodes may show micro-metastases. A two-week course of appropriate antibiotics should be given, after eliminating the primary focus of sepsis, before presuming their involvement. It is important to identify patients, who are most likely to harbour subclinical nodal metastases, such as with poorly differentiated carcinomas or lesions that invade the basement membrane of the prepuce.

Sentinel node concept: see chapters 22 and 95 (melanoma and breast).

Bilateral lymphadenectomy should be considered in patients presenting with unilateral clinical adenopathy in T3-4 primary tumors, because of well established anatomic cross over of lymphatics, but the contralateral dissection however may be limited to inguinal nodes.

Timing of surgery for nodes: Excision of suspected metastatic nodes is done about 4weeks after resection of primary tumor, for the following reasons:

(1) high risk of wound infection and flap necrosis, if done synchronously and
(2) residual/spilt tumor cells in the surgical field, would be picked up by lymphatics, to reach and get filtered by the regional nodes,

within a few weeks.

Role of preoperative lymph node biopsy: There is some disagreement on this issue, whether it is useful or misleading, as 25% false negative results have been reported with FNAC. Excision biopsy is unwarranted before the main operation, as a negative reading in any case may be unreliable. Many prefer to proceed with nodal block dissection, if they do not regress with antibiotics or if they actually enlarge under observation. If biopsy of the *sentinel node* (most medial of the superficial horizontal group) is negative for tumor, the metastasis to illio-inguinal nodes is unlikely to have occurred.

Complications of nodal block dissection

1) wound collection of lymph and lymphorrhea this may be prevented to some extent by clamping and ligating the distal margin of the fat/fascia to be resected, in which afferent lymphatics travel. Suction drainage (Redivac or Hemovac) for a few days, quickly obliterating the dead space, also minimizes this problem.

2) flap necrosis is very common due to undermining and devascularization. It is advisable to avoid acute angles in the incision, the apex of which invariably necroses. An ideal incision is either a straight or a semilunar incision in this regard. Infection will necessarily supervene this complication.

3) wound infection can lead to disastrous consequences such as flap necrosis, lymphorrhea or secondary hemorrhage. This is largely

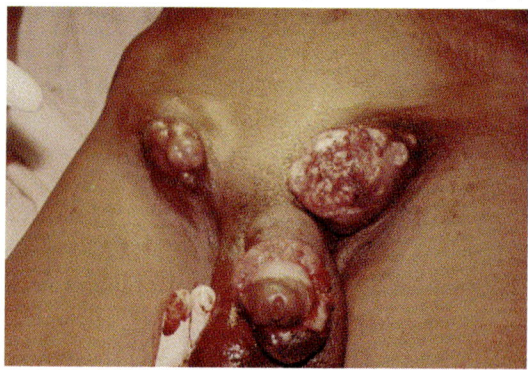

Fig. 33.22. Advanced carcinoma penis with fungating inguinal secondaries

dependent on several factors, including techniques of asepsis and surgery and can be prevented only to a small extent by prophylactic antibiotics. Once it develops, adequate antibiotic cover is necessary, guided by bacteriological information.

4) secondary hemorrhage: this also follows sloughing of overlying skin, precariously exposing the femoral vessels, leading to a catastrophe. This may be prevented by sliding the sartorius muscle medially to cover and protect the vessels and fixing it to the adjacent tissue, at the time of surgery.

5) lymphedema of the leg due to damage to the lymphatics, usually transient but may become permanent and troublesome. Elevation, elastic support and antiedema therapy alleviate this, but may have to be given for an indefinite period of time, depending upon the response. Scrotal edema also may occur, which lasts longer and more troublesome, in patients undergone bilateral surgery (see chapter 43).

6) lymphorrhea: occasionally the volume of lymph lost may be so high as to cause nutritional and fluid disturbances, especially in the neck, if the thoracic duct (on the left) or right mediastinal trunk is severed. If the output is high (>500ml/day), injection of sclerosant agents, such as polidocanol (3% as foam), bleomycin or tetracycline into the wound and/or parenteral octreotide (100mcgm I.M, t.i.d for 5 days) are found to be effective, to reduce the lymph leak, before surgical intervention is considered. The octreotide, however is more effective when given early, i.e., from 2nd or 3rd postoperative day. Topical application of collagen type I (Collerate RX) and

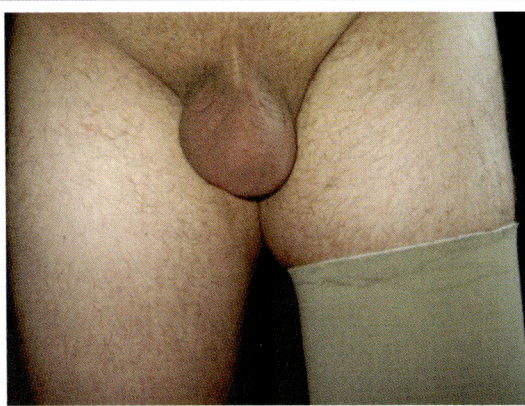

Fig. 33.23. Total amputation of penis with perineal urethrostomy (not visible)

gelatin matrix-thrombin tissue sealant (Floseal) are also found to be very useful in treating lymphorrhea following flap necrosis and wound breakdown.

Orchidectomy or not?

The proponents argue that following total amputation of penis, it is advisable to suppress sexual drive by bilateral orchidectomy. It also eliminates the obstructing scrotum, during voiding through a perineal stoma, but the consensus is against such a 'sadistic' approach. After all, there are many men who have the sexual desire but are impotent and they find their own means of quenching the sexual thirst. Moreover, trying to induce impotence, one should not risk creating emasculation and its psychosomatic consequences. Manual lifting of the scrotum, during micturition, to avoid 'dash and splash', is not such an inconvenient job that orchidectomy should be resorted to! This also prevents another problem, ammonia-induced dermatitis due to constant irritation of the scrotal skin with urine.

34 Cancer Chemotherapy

Drug treatment of cancer may be one of the following:

1. Cytotoxic antimitotic drugs.
2. Endocrine therapy
3. Immnunotherapy
4. Retinoids
5. Interferon
6. Systemic (metabolic) radiotherapy (radio-nucleides)
7. Supportive therapy (e.g. nutrition, antibiotics, analgesics, antiemetic (prokinetic) agents, tranquillizers, anabolic steroids etc.)

Cytotoxic therapy is defined as the use of drugs to halt the progression of cancer. They may be used for both primary and metastatic cancer and are lethal to both cancer and normal cells (unlike antimicrobial agents which are either bacteriostatic or bactericidal).

Cytotoxic therapy aims to bring about cure or prolong survival and has been partially achieved in hematological and childhood cancers. Cure by cytotoxics alone has been reported in acute lymphatic leukemia (children), Hodgkin's disease, Burkitt's lymphoma, Wilms' tumor, Ewing's sarcoma and rhabdomyosarcoma. Prolonged survival is made possible in acute leukemia (adults), lymphocytic lymphomas, multiple myeloma and neuroblastoma, but in adult solid tumors the picture is less encouraging. Cure has only been seen in relatively uncommon cancers, e.g. choriocarcinoma and seminoma. Prolonged survival has been claimed in ovarian and breast cancers.

Cytotoxics are given either as adjuvant 'prophylactic' chemotherapy over a prolonged period of time for patients presumably 'cured' (by surgery and/orradiotherapy) to address the subclinical (micro) metastases, e.g. early breast carcinoma, or as an aggressive multimodal therapy for certain disseminated cancers (e.g. childhood cancers which are relatively anaplastic and rapidly growing with high growth fraction); hence, a combination of radical chemotherapy, surgery and radiotherapy is employed. Such carefully designed multimodal protocols (to treat other solid cancers in adults) are becoming more popular throughout the world, with an aim of preserving the organs, while achieving 'cure'.

Classification of cytotoxic agents

This is according to their chemical structure and mechanism of action:

1. Polyfunctional alkylating agents: interfere with cross-linkage of DNA, e.g. nitrogen mustards (mustine), cyclophosphamide, chlorambucil, melphalan (phenyl alanine mustard), thiotepa (tetra ethyl thio phospharamide), busulphan, piposulfan etc.

2. Antimetabolites: interfere with nucleic acid synthesis because they are analogues of normal metablites and act by substrate competition, e.g. folic acid antagonist (methotrexate), purine antogonist (6-mercaptopurine), pyrimidine antagonist (cytosine arabinoside), halogenated pyrimidine (5- fluorouracil), glutamine antagonist (azaserine) etc.

3. Mitotic spindle inhibitors: cause mitotic arrest, e.g. colchicine and vinca alkaloids (vinblastine and vincristine).

Plant alkaloids form a broad group (including cocaine, morphine, quinine, atropine and vinca alkaloids).

4. Antitumor antibiotics: they bind with DNA to block RNA production, e.g. adriamycin, daunorubiucin, mithramycin, actinomycin-D, mitomycin-C, bleomycin etc.

5. Antiproliferative enzymes (L-aspara-ginase) act on protein synthesis.

6. Nitrosoureas: they affect DNA cross-linkage (CCNU, BCNU).

7. Inorganic platinium compounds (cis-platinum).

8. Miscellaneous group (procarbazine, hydroxyurea).

Malignant cells may develop primary (natural) or seconday (acquired) drug resitance (the latter is due to adaptation &/or mutation).

Toxicity occurs as a result of damage to rapidly dividing normal tissues.

1. Bone marrow: anemia, hemorrhage and infection (most drugs).

2. Gastrointestinal tract: stomatitis, vomiting, diarrheas (most drugs).

3. Lymphoreticular: Immunosuppression and infection (most drugs).

4. Hair follicles: epilation or alopecia (cyclophosphamide, vincristine and adriamycin).

5. Lung: fibrosis (chlorambucil and bleomycin) dose related.

6. Urinary bladder: cystitis and sterile hematuria (cyclophosphamide).

Hepato/nephrotoxicity: (methotrexate).

7. Skin: impaired wound healing, vesiculation and edema (most drugs).

8. Cardiotoxicity (daunorubicin and adriamycin) dose related.

9. Fetus: teratogenesis and abortion.

10. Local tissue damage if extravasated.

Careful choice of cytotoxic combinations, strict observance of total doses (many effects are dose related) and serial blood counts with symptomatic control (antiemetics, adequate hydration etc.) will minimize toxicity. Antiplatelet agents and NSAIDs have to be meticulously avoided while on chemotherapy, in view of the additional risk of causing thrombocytopenia and/or GI bleeding.

Contraindications

Use of an ineffective agent, availability of another superior approach, heavy tumor load, as in advanced disease (fatal toxicity is likely), pre-existing bone marrrow depression or active infection and when there are no means of assessing the progress of treatment.

Methods of cytotoxic use

1) Single agent continuous therapy

A constant blood level of a single cytotoxic drug is maintained until unacceptable toxicity, drug resistance or cure results.

2) Combination therapy

a) Continuous

This uses a number of drugs with various actions continuously; the cancer mass reduces only at the expense of simultaneous normal tissue toxicity which necessitates a rest phase for recovery during which time the cancer will repopulate.

b) Pulsing combination therapy

This is the most widely used treatment. Treatment is split into short intervals each of which is referred to as a pulse.

Its advantages are:

1. Maximal exploitation of the differential in recovery times between normal and malignant tissues.

2. Relative lack of toxicity allows therapy to continue indefinitely, increasing chance of cure.

3. Allows higher doses of individual drugs to be given so that a larger proportion of cancer cells are killed.

4. Recovery of normal tissues in between treatment pulses includes the restoration of the immune system which has further tumoricidal action against small cancer cell populations.

c) Sequential therapy

When combination chemotherapy is given in sequence, it is called sequential therapy. In Hodgkin's disease Stages IIIB and IV, 70-80% remission may be expected following the MOPP schedule:

Mustine HCl (nitrogen mustard) 6mg/m^2 (IV.) on day 1 and 8

Oncovin (vincristine) 1.4mg/m^2 (IV.) on day 1 and 8

Procarbazine 100mg/m^2 (oral) on day 1 to14

Prednisolone 40mg/m^2 (oral) on day 1 to 14

Six cycles (monthly) are usually given (with 2 weeks rest between the end of one course and the beginning of the next).

Administration of cytotoxic therapy

Systemic (oral and i.v)

More toxic but drug can reach micrometastases.

Local

Similar in effect to the other local methods of treatment (i.e. surgery and RT), which includes:

Regional cytotoxic therapy

Arterial infusion

1. Malignant melanoma (recurrent) - phenylalanine mustard.

2. Head and neck tumors - through the external carotid artery with methotrexate followed by antidote folinic acid (citrovorum factor) for rapid neutralization.

3. Liver secondaries - through the hepatic artery during laparotomy with 5- fluorouracil.

Extracorporeal limb perfusion: The main artery and vein to the tumor-bearing area are cannulated to maintain artificial circulation. The cytotoxic agent is given through the artery and retrieved from the vein, minimizing the systemic effects of the drug. Limb temperature can be raised (by immersing the limb in a water bath or covering it with hot towels), to cause vasodilation for increased rate of cytotoxic perfussion (hyperthermia, in itself may be lethal to cancer cells). This cumbersome method is sometimes used in malignant melanoma or soft tissue sarcoma of the limb.

Intracavitary

1. Pleural effusion due to secondary deposits or complicated malignancy of the breast and bronchus may lead to dyspnea and may be treated with instillation of cylophosphamide or thiotepa causing pleurodesis and fibrosis.

2. In ascites thiotepa or cyclophosphamide instilation is used with three objectives control of ascites, control of advanced primary disease and as adjuvant therapy at the time or resection for primary gastric, rectal and ovarian cancers.

Intrathecal

E.g. subarachnoid methotrexate injection in acute lymphatic leukemia since most cytotoxics cannot cross blood-brain barrier.

Topical

Creams and ointments, e.g. 5% 5-fluorouracil for skin carcinoma. It causes intense local reaction and is inferior to other means.

Targeted drug delivery concept

Also known as Smart Drug delivery is a method of delivering medication in a manner that increases concentration in the target tissue, such as solid cancers, with minimal systemic effect. This improves efficacy while reducing side effects. This requires the drug to be carried by delivery vehicles, such as liposomes, polymeric micelles, lipoproteins, nanoparticles, dendrimers etc. An ideal drug delivery vehicle must be non-toxic, biocompatible, non-immunogenic and biodegradable and most commonly used liposomes fulfill all the criteria mentioned. Stem cell therapy may also be considered as a type of targeted therapy, since it acts on particular tissue, with altered anatomy and impaired function, promoting cell regeneration.

In oncology it has many applications:

Breast cancer: Trastuzumab (Herceptin)
Lung cancer (non-smallcell): Gefitinib (Iressa)
Colon cancer: Cetuximab (Erbitux)
Bevaizumab (Avastin)
Lymphoma (NHL): Rituximab (MabThera)
Ca pancreas: Gemcitabine, Folfirinox, Erlotinib

GIST: Imitinib (Veenat), Sunitinib (Sutent) Prodrug therapy concept

This is a novel concept, antibody-directed enzyme prodrug therapy (ADEPT), the pretargeted antibody is conjugated to an enzyme that is capable of activating a subsequently administered inactive form of a drug (prodrug) in tumor tissue, exerting maximum effect in required areas. This eliminates systemic side effects of the chemotherapy to a large extent and may be very useful in patients who cannot tolerate standard forms of chemotherapy.

A number of enzymes have been used in preclinical trials of ADEPT, including lactamase (which can activate prodrug forms of doxorubicin and paclitaxel), cytosine deaminase (which can activate a prodrug form of 5-fluorouracil), and carboxypeptidase G2 (which can be used to produce nitrogen mustards).

Capecitabine (Xeloda), prodrug for 5-fluorouracil (5-FU) is in currently wide clinical use in advanced breast, colon and other GI malignancies.

VENOUS ACCESS DEVICES (VAD)

Treatment of cancer patient need safe and repeated access to the venous system to obtain blood samples, deliver IV fluids, cytotoxic drugs, antibiotics, and blood products; Most of the times peripheral device will be adequate, but occasionally the treatment plan requires

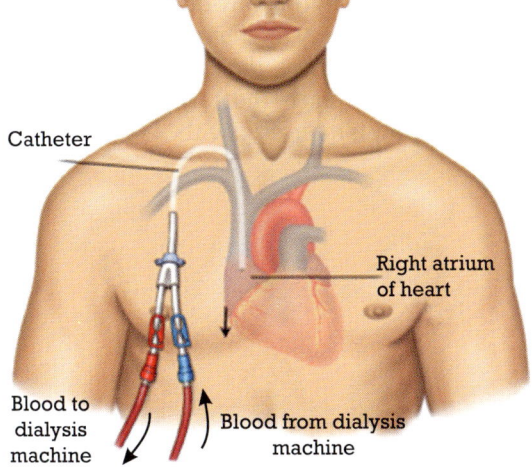

Fig. 34.1. Trans-jugular placement of central venous catheter (short term)

Catheter

Right atrium of heart

Blood to dialysis machine

Blood from dialysis machine

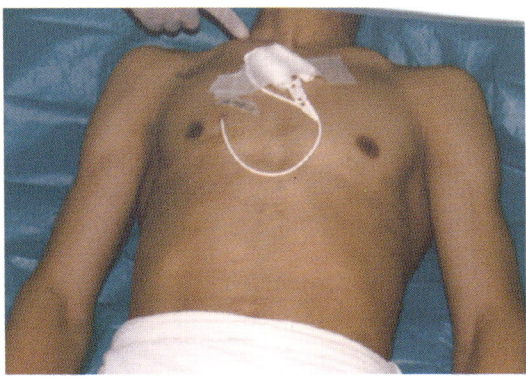

Fig. 34.2. Trans-jugular placement of catheter (short term)

central access device. This may be short or long term, depending on the diagnosis, duration of treatment and the treatment plan.

Any type of venous access needs care and maintenance to ensure optimal and safe function, and to prevent complications.

The quality of life of patients has improved dramatically in the past decade with development of access technology. Venous access devices are divided into two main categories: peripheral and central.

1) Non-tunneled central venous catheters, which are two types:

    A) Short term subclavian and jugular catheters

    B) Peripherally inserted central catheters

2) Tunneled central venous catheters

3) Implanted ports

Procedure of port implantation

Implantation in the operation theater under general or local anesthesia.

The common veins used are subclavian, internal/external jugular, and cephalic vein, the catheter will be advanced to the superior vena cava (Fig. 34.1 and 34.3).

In case of superior vena cava syndrome, obstruction of subclavian vein or tumor blockage; the saphenous or femoral vein access may be used to advance the catheter into the inferior vena cava.

The body of the port is usually placed in subcutaneous plane, about ½ inch under the skin over a bony area for stabilization.

The proximal end of the catheter is connected subcutaneously to the body of the port, which is implanted in the infraclavicular fossa over the pectoralis major fascia and sutured to the fascia layer.

Incision should not cross the diaphragm of the port since repeated access may cause stress to the suture line

Complications due to VAD

Immediate

1. Pneumothorax
2. Air embolism
3. Accidental arterial puncture and hematoma formation
4. Cardiac arrhythmias
5. Brachial plexus injury

Late complications

1. Infection
2. Catheter occlusion
3. Damaged catheter/fracture
4. Extravasation

The VAD has become an integral part of oncological management and there are many complications associated with it, which compromise the safety of the patient. The awareness of these complications and their prevention, early detection and treatment will ultimately increase the safety and patient's quality of life.

Implantable Venous Port

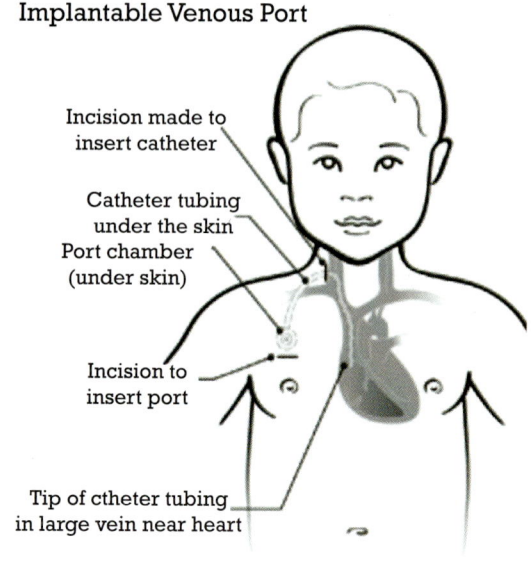

Incision made to insert catheter

Catheter tubing under the skin
Port chamber (under skin)

Incision to insert port

Tip of ctheter tubing in large vein near heart

Fig. 34.3. Trans-jugular placement of catheter with an implantable port (long term)

Caution: Preoperative therapeutic embolization is done for some vascular tumor, such as liver and kidney, to reduce vascularity during surgery. But it should not be done, if subsequent surgery is not being planned for some reason, since by making the tissue hypoxic, it disables the only other two options, namely radiotherapy or chemotherapy open to the patient. Further, the chemotherapeutic agent may not reach the target tissue, if its arterial supply is interfered with.

35 Spina Bifida

Definition: Also known as neural arch deformity or spinal dysraphism, this is a congenital defect in the posterior bony wall of the spinal canal due to failure of fusion in varying degrees of the laminae of the vertebrae. It may be very minimal, without external bulge, known as *spina bifida occulta* or may be more complicated, wherein either the meninges, spinal cord or its central canal may herniate, forming a cystic swelling over the spine (*spina bifida cystica*), commonly seen in the lumbosacral region. *Myelodysplasia* is the name given to anomalies of spinal column, associated with neurological deficit.

Embryology

The vertebral bodies develop segmentally around the notochord. Each vertebra is formed by the fusion of three components, the centrum and two lateral neural arches. The margins of the dorsal neural groove fuse, to form the neural tube, which becomes the central canal of the spinal cord. Failure of the arches to fuse in the midline results in spina bifida. The defect may be unilateral with one half of the spine developed or bilateral with absent arch. Varying grades of failure of the above process of fusion results in spina bifida occulta, meningocele, meningomyelocele and syringomyelocele. Folic acid deficiency during pregnancy is directly incriminated for the development of neural canal defects.

Pathology

This occurs due to both genetic and environmental factors. Differential growth of the spinal cord with vertebral canal occurs from the 10th week of gestation and goes on to puberty, which influences the clinical presentation. Congenital hydrocephalus may conceivably be an etiological factor for cystic spina bifida.

SPINA BIFIDA OCCULTA: This commonest type of defect usually occurs at the L-5 level and is mostly asymptomatic, without protrusion of intraspinal contents, and detected by routine palpation or a skiagram of lumbar spine. Symptomatic cases may be associated with a median bony spur, splitting the spinal cord in the midline (*diastematomyelia*).

The skin over the spinal segment is connected to the theca by a fibrous band called *membrana reuniens*. As the spine outgrows the cord, by differential growth, the membrana reuniens pulls on the nerve roots and causes neurological defects involving the feet and bladder, in childhood. Sometimes the symptoms may be due to a space occupying lesion (SOL), such as lipoma, developed in relation to the spinal theca and not the membrana reuniens.

Investigations

An x-ray spine would give the initial clue, further evaluation may be done by a CT/MR imag-

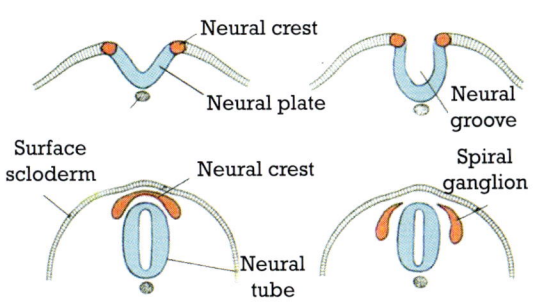

Fig. 35.1. Development of spine and spinal cord

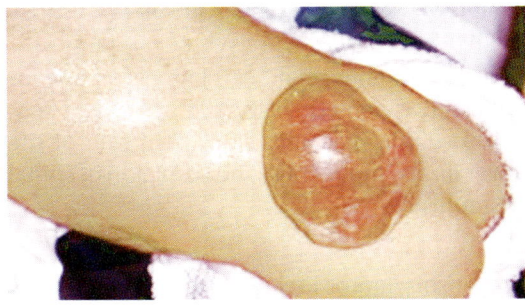

Fig. 35.2. Spina bifida with lumbar meningocele (courtesy - Dr R Jagadeeshan, Dublin)

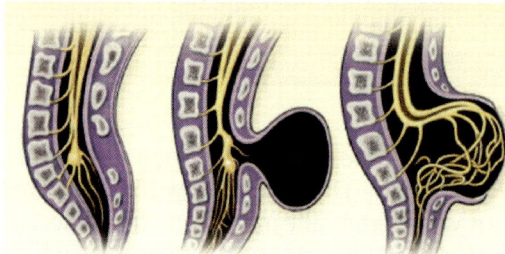

Spina bifida occulta   Meningocele   Myelomeningocele

Fig. 35.3. Schematic representation of spina bifida

ing. Detailed neurological recording is essential both for medical and legal purposes.

SPINA BIFIDA CYSTICA: This is also commonly seen in the lumbosacral region, associated with a cystic mass in the midline, often with congenital hydrocephalus. In 15% of cases, the cyst contains only dura and arachnoid, (*meningocele*). The skin overlying the mass is thin and atrophic. In the remaining, either a portion of the spinal cord and nerve roots also herniate (*meningomyelocele*) or the central canal of the spinal cord also comes in (*syringomyelocele*). In severe cases, the spinal cord itself may form a flat, vascular discoid mass at the site of the defect, devoid of any coverings (*myelocele*). The mass contains vascularised arachnoid, neural tissue containing mature neurons, ependymal lined cavities, spinal ganglia and roots.

On the midline or close to it, a luxuriant pony tail pattern of lesion has been described. Often a subcutaneous pigmented lipoma (nevolipoma) can be seen in the midline, which is almost always connected to the membrana reuniens, in the midline.

Orthopedic abnormalities: Talipes of one or both feet, asymmetry in the size of feet and legs, due to diminished muscle bulk in one of the lower limbs, should raise the suspicion of spinal dysraphism.

Neurological abnormalities

a) sensory/motor loss depends upon the level of involvement of the cord, higher the level more wide spread the deficit. This usually mani-

fests as weakness of one or both legs at birth or early infancy, with abnormal gait, may be made out at childhood. Alteration of deep tendon reflexes and an extensor plantar reflex are sometimes found.

b) sphincter dysfunction: with involvement of the autonomic nerves supplying the bladder, sphincter function may progressively deteriorate and often cause death due to uncontrolled dribbling and urinary infection.

c) meningitis: the meningeal presentation occurs in children with more overt dysraphism and may be fatal, in a few weeks after birth.

Diagnosis

1) After clinical examination, an x-ray of the entire spine should be taken, to look for the following defects:

    a) midline bony spur
    b) nerve/disc space
    c) malformed vertebral bodies
    d) hemivertebrae
    e) fused and malformed laminae
    f) widened spinal canal
    g) abnormal curvatures in the spine

2) CT/MRI myelography: should be done if the cutaneous stigmata and the radiological abnor-

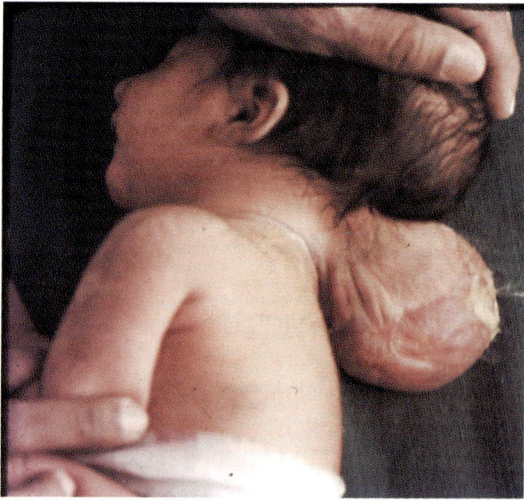

Fig. 35.4. Meningomyelocele in an infant
(courtesy: Prof R Narayanan, Chennai)

malities (described above) are found in conjunction with the diagnosis of spinal dysraphism, even if there is no obvious neurological deficit. Besides helping to decide about the need for surgery, they provide a 'road map' to the neurosurgeon, during the operation.

Screening

1. The α-fetoprotein (AFP) estimation in amniotic fluid and maternal serum is useful for early detection (when the neural defect is open, there is a leak of AFP from the spinal compartment into the amniotic fluid).

2. Maternal genomic screening and use of sophisticated antenatal ultrasonography, combined with maternal AFP, give a very high yield in the pick up of neural arch abnormalities, forming an indication for medical termination of pregna TP).

Treatment

1) Spina bifida occulta: operation is only indicated if the patient is persistently symptomatic:

a. a tuft of hair, a tail or a lipoma may cause cosmetic problem; these lesions are excised

b. if there are neurological symptoms due to the membrana reuniens, it has to be excised in its entirety.

c. orthopedic, urological or neurological symptoms may not be due to the membrana alone, but due to extra or intradural lipomas causing cord compression. After an MRI, such lesions should be excised. In diastematomyelia, decompression of the dorsal protrusion has to be performed, after CT myelography.

MENINGOCELE: This is the commonest and relatively harmless type among this group, wherein the meningeal protrusion through the neural arch defect contain only CSF, giving rise to a cystic swelling. The duramater may stop at the margin of the defect, with only arachnoid layer protruding; the overlying skin is intact, but atretic. Meningocele commonly occurs in the lumbosacral region, the occipital part of the skull or the root of nose, latter two are categorized under cranium bifida. Rarely, more than one defect may be present.

Anterior sacral meningocele is a much rarer condition, situated in the sacral hollow. Persistent low backache is the main symptom, the cystic mass felt by rectal examination. Increased sacral concavity, without destruction, seen on lateral skiagram is typical (scimitar sign), but diagnosis is clinched by a CT scan. Spina bifida cystica is often associated with congenital hydrocephalus, and may be causing it, which should be realized while planning treatment, as a preliminary shunt to decompress the ventricles might be required in such children, to stall any impact on higher intellectual functions.

Clinical features

1. present since birth
2. cystic, fluctuant swelling.
3. highly translucent
4. compressible.
5. expansive impulse when the child cries or coughs
6. overlying skin is normal and free.
7. edge of the bony defect can be felt all around
8. usually neurological manifestations are absent.
9. there could be associated hydrocephalus (Arnold-Chiari malformation).
10. if more than one present, cross fluctuation will be appreciated

Treatment

Meningocele: After allowing time for any skin ulceration/infection to resolve, reconstructive neurosurgery should be done, to excise the redundant skin and meninges, effecting primary repair, when the child is expected to lead a normal life.

Surgery for other types of spina bifida cystica such as meningomyelocele, syringomyelocele or meningoencephalocele, however, is more complex and often unsatisfactory. After excising the skin and meninges, the neural structures should be restored to their normal position. If an SOL, like an extradural lipoma is present, it should be carefully excised.

Myocutaneous flaps may be necessary to close defect following excision of a meningocele.

Unless aggressively treated, meningeal infection may kill the child within a few weeks of life, but if the child survives to lifelong disability, the emotional and socioeconomic impact on the parents is immeasurable.

Feature	Meningocele	Meningomyelocele
Contents	Membranes	Membranes and nerve roots
Transillumination	Brilliant	Partially transilluminant
Consistency	Cystic	Solid elements inside
External furrow	Absent	Present due to adherence of nerve roots to skin
Neurological defect	Absent	Present
Trophic ulcers	Absent	Present
Foot deformities	Absent	May be present
Prognosis after surgery	Good	Residual neurological defects

Table-35.1. Differences between meningocele and meningomyelocele

36 Neurofibroma

This is a benign tumor arising from the connective tissue of the nerve sheath. It is often considered a developmental disorder or a hamartoma rather than a true neoplasm with a familial predilection.

There are two common types of nerve tumors, with significant differences in clinical presentation and management:

1) neurilemmoma or Schwann cell tumor (Schwannoma), arising from perineurium is probably a true neoplasm

2) neurofibroma, arising from the endoneurium.

Types of neurofibroma

1. Solitary neurofibroma
2. Generalized neurofibromatoses
3. Plexiform neurofibromatoses
4. Elephantiasis neurofibromatosa
5. Cutaneous neurofibromatoses
6. Neurofibroma as part of a phakomatosis (phako: a freckle)

SOLITARY NEUROFIBROMA

Usually found in the extremities, in relation to peripheral (median or ulnar) nerves, though cranial nerves are not exempt (acoustic neuroma of 8th cranial nerve).

Pathology

Encapsulated, rounded swelling adjacent to a nerve. Some sensory/motor deficit may be pres-

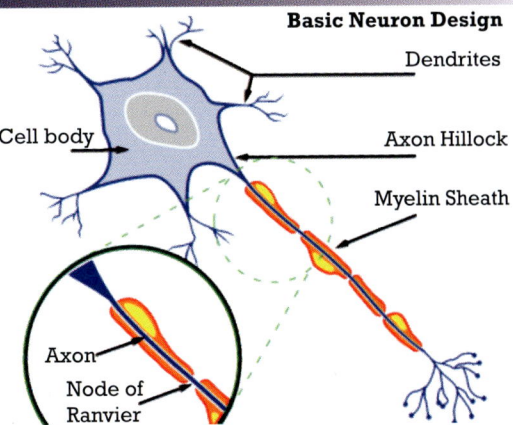

Basic Neuron Design

Fig. 36.1. Parts of a neuron

ent. Long slender cells with elongated nuclei are typically arranged in a palisade manner.

Clinical features

Swelling is the main feature with paresthesia or pain secondary to pressure. A firm swelling on the skin and subcutaneous tissue, in relation to a nerve, with restricted mobility along its axis and with a sensory/ motor deficit, in its distribution. Solitary neurofibroma also occurs, in relation to eighth cranial nerve at the cerebellopontine angle, called acoustic neuroma and in the dorsal nerve roots of the spinal cord, partly inside and partly outside the spinal canal, called a dumb-bell tumor.

Complications

1. Malignant change
2. Loss of sensation or motor power
3. Cystic degeneration

Differential diagnosis

1. other benign subcutaneous swellings, such as lipoma, myxoma, fibroma, hamartoma etc
2. when cystic degeneration occurs: any subcutaneous cyst, such as a sebaceous or lymph cyst

	Features	Schwannoma	Neurofibroma
1.	Origin	Arising from perineurium	Arising from endoneurium
2.	Location	Eccentric	Central
3.	Shape	Globular or ovoid in shape	Spindle shape
4.	Treatment	Can be excised separate from the nerve	Can be excised, but sometimes axonal damage occurs

Table-36.1. Differences between a Schwannoma and a neurofibroma

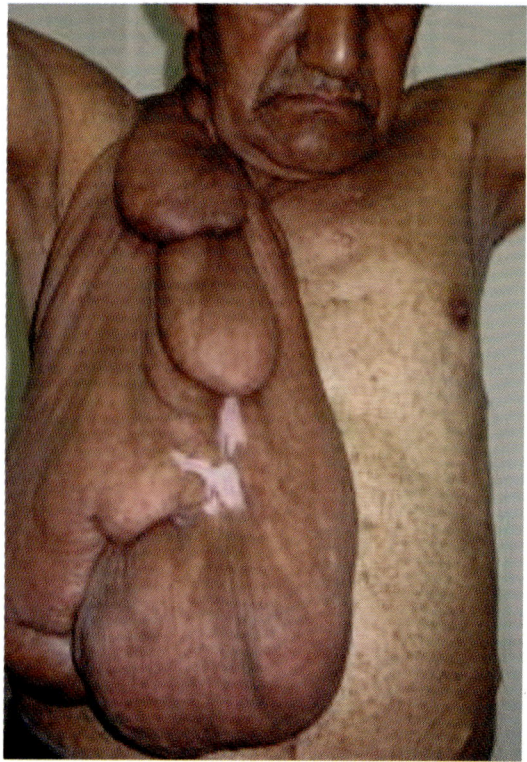

Fig. 36.2. Pachydermatocele
(courtesy: Laxmi Hospital, Kakinada)

Treatment

1. Excision of the neurofibroma without injury to the nerve is the ideal treatment, failing which, the entire tumor with the nerve is resected and neural ends are restored by either direct end to end anastomosis or interposition nerve graft.

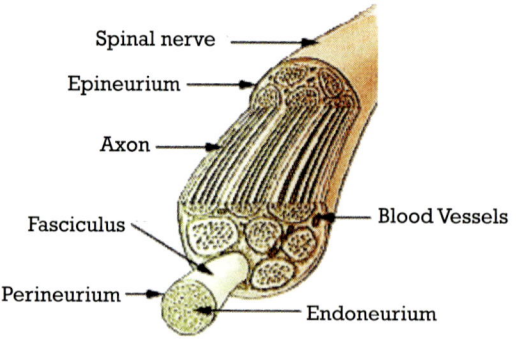

Fig. 36.3. Nerve fibre

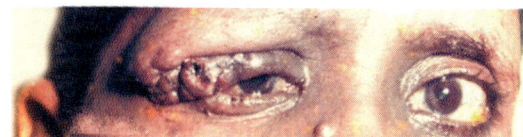

Fig. 36.4. Plexiform neurofibroma of face involving trigeminal nerve branches
(courtesy: Prof T Gunasagaran, Chennai)

GENERALIZED NEUROFIBROMATOSIS (NF)

NF - type 1 (von Recklinghausen's disease)

This is an autosomal dominant disease in which multiple subcutaneous neurofibromas are present, sometimes accompanied by neurofibromas of the cranial and spinal nerve, when it is called central neurofibromatosis (NF - type 2).

Clinical features

1. multiple subcutaneous nodules
2. café-au-lait spots (big nevus)
3. ocular manifestations like ptosis, exophthalmos, Lisch nodules of the iris and optic nerve lesion.
4. spine deformities like kyphoscoliosis
5. diaphyseal changes resulting in bowing of tibia and fibula
6. tendency for fractures leading to congenital pseudoarthrosis.

There is a generalised endoneurial developmental abnormality, in which not only cranial, peripheral and spinal neurofibromas, but other tumors involving neuroectoderm are present; e.g. pheochromocytoma from the adrenal medulla or multiple fibroepithelial tags. Neurofibromas of the spinal canal emerge through the intervertebral foramina, to acquire dumb-bell shape. Often, pigmented patches of the skin

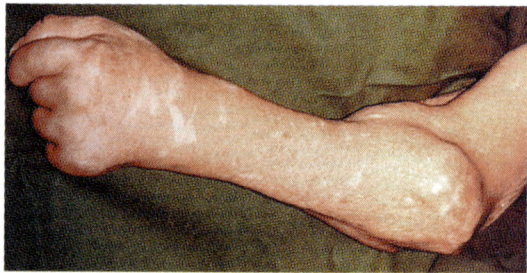

Fig. 36.5. Plexiform neurofibroma, forearm
(courtesy: Halsted Surgical Clinic, Chennai)

occur in these patients, known as café-au-lait patches (coffee and milk), because the neurectoderm is the common tissue of origin for the melanocytes and nerve tissue. Skeletal deformities like kyphoscoliosis may be present. If pheochromocytoma is associated, it needs primary attention.

The main component of NF-type 2 is (sometimes bilateral) acoustic neuromas, causing disturbabces in vestibular and cochlear functions of the VIII cranial nerve.

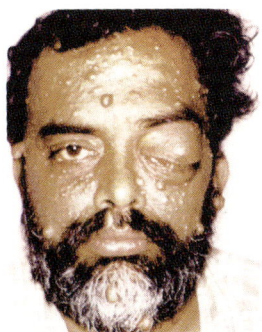

Fig. 36.6. Multiple neurofibromatosis on the face with left upper eyelid involvement

Complications

Same as for solitary neurofibroma

Treatment

Excision of all the lumps is impossible. When one of the tumors is painful, too large, or causing pressure symptoms on the underlying nerve, it may be excised. The other indication for excision is the possibility of a malignant change, but partial excision of a benign lesion is also believed to increase the tendency for sarcomatous transformation.

PLEXIFORM NEUROFIBROMATOSIS (syn: pachydermatocele)

This rare condition affects the branches of the trigeminal nerve. An excessive neural tissue overgrowth occurs in the subcutaneous planes and results in huge, edematous folds of subcutaneous tissue. Rarely it is seen in the limbs and the scalp. On examination, a large swelling, hanging in several pendulous folds in the affected region is made out, with a thickened nerve sometimes being palpated under the main swelling. Pigmentation of the affected area may also occur. Sarcomatous changes

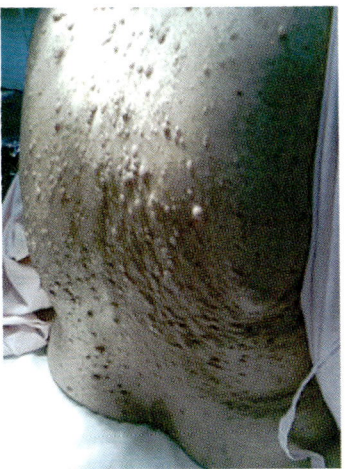

Fig. 36.7. Multiple neurofibromatosis (von Reclinghausen's disease)

have been described in this condition, more so following partial excision.

ELEPHANTIASIS NEUROFIBROMATOSA

This is a severe form of pachydermatocele, which involves the lower limb. It is called so because the affected skin becomes thickened, coarse and dry, resembling the hide of an elephant. This has to be differentiated from elephantiasis due to filariasis or lymphatic occlusion after radiotherapy or surgery.

CUTANEOUS NEUROFIBROMATOSIS

There are multiple neurofibromas, either sessile or pedunculated, with a prominent distribution over the chest, abdomen or scalp. The nodules are usually small, painful and discrete, without much appreciable growth. This is a hamartomatous lesion, to be differentiated from multiple lipomata.

Treatment

Reassurance and watchful expectancy is recommended, but when large, they may be excised for cosmetic reasons, as well as to allay the apprehensions of the patient by establishing tissue diagnosis.

NEUROFIBROMAS IN SPECIAL SITUATIONS

1. ACOUSTIC NEUROMA: This grows from the VIII nerve at the internal auditory meatus(cerebello-pontine angle). Early clinical features are deafness, tinnitus, headache and vertigo. Later with the involvement of the 5th, 6th and 7th cranial nerves, anesthesia occurs over the ophthalmic branch of the trigeminal nerve (eyelids and forehead). Facial muscle weakness often follows; when cerebellar pressure occurs, features of cerebellar palsy with increased intracranial tension occur.

Treatment

Excision through the posterior fossa approach

2. DUMB-BELL shaped neurofibroma occurs, as mentioned earlier, in the spinal canal, tumor partially located outside and partly inside, with the 'isthmus' in the neural canal, producing both root pain and peripheral symptoms, related to the nerve. It is treated by excision through laminectomy

3. STUMP NEUROMA: This occurs as a painful swelling at the amputation stump, usually due to proliferating nerve fibres from the cut end of the nerve. It is commonly seen arising from the sciatic nerve, after an above knee amputation. Apart from symptoms of pain (local and phantom-limb) and numbness, there may be severe discomfort when a prosthesis is fitted on the amputation stump. To minimize this local reaction, any major nerve should not be crushed or ligated but divided with a sharp scalpel, at the highest point possible.

Treatment

Excision of the neuroma after exploration.

PHANTOM-LIMB PAIN

Following major amputation, due to the impulses originating from the divided stump of the sensory nerves, patient often experiences the presence of the dismembered limb and also pain in relation to that region. The patient needs reassurance that the problem is innocuous and short-lived. The delusion is generally controlled with counseling and symptomatic treatment and does not warrant active intervention. Empirical use of calcitonin infusion is found to be helpful in some cases. Occasionally it may become chronic and intractable, requiring specialized psychotherapy.

4. SCAR NEUROMA: Sometimes, after any chest or abdominal surgery, a painful, nodular

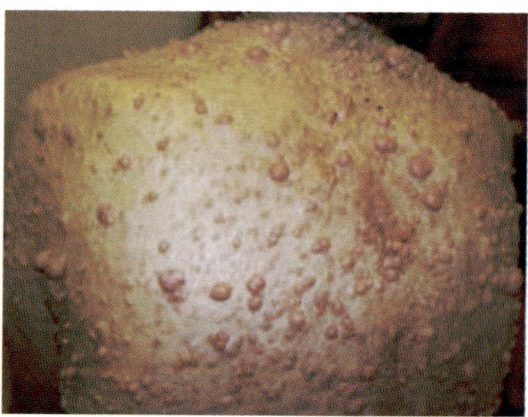

Fig. 36.8. Multiple neurofibromatosis (von Reclinghausen's disease) (courtesy: Dr C M Kishore, Chennai)

swelling may be seen or palpated at the site of the scar. This is due to a neuroma arising from the cut ends of the cutaneous nerve. The patient complains of pain and paresthesia over the scar, radiating along the distribution of the nerve. Saphenous nerve (during stripping of vein) and ilioinguinal nerve (during repair) may be similarly involved.

Treatment

A deposteroid injection sometimes prevents progression of this lesion, but if it is persistent, scar revision with excision of the neural nodules, is the only alternative.

Recent advances

The genetic background of neurofibromatosis is now well established. A transmissible lesion over the long arm of chromosome-17 (17q) causes faulty encoding of a protein, *neurofibromin*, responsible for the neuroectodermal differentiation. This also accounts for other tumors in these patients, such as Wilm's tumor, B-cell lymphoma, malignant Schwannoma and other types of STS.

NF- type 2 is considered to be the result of mutation of *merlin*, also known as *schwannomin* in chromosome 22q, which accounts for about 10% of cases of NF.

37 Desmoid Tumor

(syn: recurrent fibroid of Paget, musculo-aponeurotic fibromatosis)

Definition: (desmos: a band) This is a myofibroblastic tumor of low malignant potential which arises commonly from the musculo-aponeurotic layers of abdominal wall and behaves as a locally infiltrative tumor. Extra-abdominal sites are also common and occasional intra-abdomnal sites may occur.

Etiology

1. Congenital: In association with colonic polyposis, sebaceous cysts and frontal osteomas (Gardner's syndrome), typically intra-abdominal lesions (mesenteric) are seen. They occur in about 20% of patients with Gardner's syndrome and 10% of those with familial adenomatous polyposis coli (FAPC).

2. Traumatic: Some cases have been reported in assciation with trauma. It is very common in multiparous women, where recurrent stretching of the parietes may be an initiating factor.

Pathology

This is a non-encapsulated, non-metastasizing, slow growing and locally invasive tumor, arising from the fibroblasts of deep fascia and aponeurotic structures, with a distinct female preponderance (9:1). Microscopically, it is composed of uniform fibrocytes and fibroblasts with 1-3 oval small nuclei and associated with collagenization. Scattered dilated blood vessels, microhemorrhages and focal small round cell aggregates are seen. True fibromas are virtually nonexistent and desmoid is the only tumor, that comes close to the pathological description of a fibroma. Next to carcinoma, desmoid is the leading cause of death in FAPC, due to mesenteric fibrosis and bowel ishemia.

Myxomatous and frank sarcomatous changes have been described and should be suspected if rapid growth occurs, especially with areas of softening (indicating avascular necrosis), producing variable consistency.

Hormone sensitivity: The desmoid tumor may express hormone receptors (ER & PR) and may be hormone sensitive. This also explains the relationship of the use of oral contraceptives to the development of desmoid tumor and the benefits of tamoxifen therapy in this disease.

Clinical features

The commonest site is the anterior abdominal wall, but these have been reported elsewhere, such as aponeurosis-dense areas like palms, soles, supraclavicular and deltoid regions. A well-defined firm mass is seen, with an irregular surface and fixed to the fascia/aponeurosis in the region. By the Carnett's head or leg raising test, there is no change in the size of the swelling, but the intrinsic mobility becomes restricted, indicating its parietal plane of origin.

Differential diagnosis

Other soft tissue tumors, such as lipoma, neurofibroma, sarcoma etc. irreducible ventral hernia and hematoma of rectus sheath.

Investigations

The only specific investigation is the biopsy, which is best done at a site to be included in the

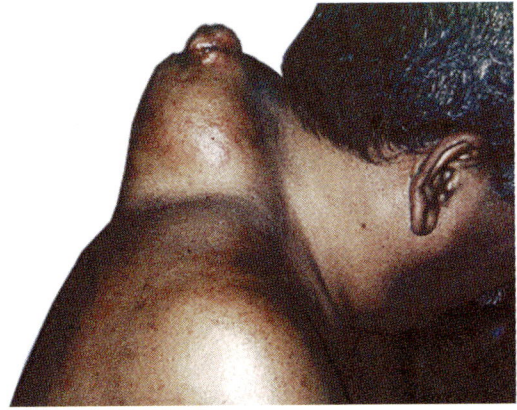

Fig. 37.1. Recurrent desmoid tumor, nape (courtesy: Halsted Surgical Clinic, Chennai)

future elliptical incision. FNAC is of limited value, but the sensitivity of a wide-bore (Tru-cut) needle, almost matches that of open wedge biopsy.

Chest x-ray and USG of abdomen should always be performed, because a slow growing soft tissue sarcoma can mimic a desmoid tumor. CT/MRI may be useful, to define the relation to the adjacent neurovascular structures as well as other vital organs.

Treatment

In view of its great potential for local recurrence, wide excision is always the first choice. It is only moderately radiosensitive and totally insensitive to chemotherapy. As recurrence is the rule if an adequate margin is not adhered to, excision of at least 2.5cm of normal aponeurosis all around is essential. After such a wide excision, it may be necessary to repair the defect with polypropylene (prolene) or polytetrafluoroethylene (PTFE) mesh. With improved techniques, radiotherapy is being offered as an effective alternative, particularly in areas, such as neck, axilla or femoral region, where adequate clearance is virtually impossible or as neoadjuvant therapy, to down-stage the tumor before surgery. It is also used as adjuvant therapy after surgery. Chemotherapy is of no value in the management of desmoid tumor, but high dose tamoxifen and prostaglandin inhibitors (NSAIDs) are being tried with some success.

38 Soft Tissue Sarcoma

Definition: SOFT TISSUE SARCOMAS (STS) are malignant tumors arising in the extra-skeletal connective tissues of the body (sarcos: flesh), developed from the mesenchymal derivatives, such as fibrous tissue, fat, skeletal/smooth muscle, lymph/blood vessel and synovium.

Etiology

1. Sarcomas affecting radiation fields have been described after irradiation for breast cancer and Hodgkin's lymphoma. These are most commonly fibrosarcomas and osteosarcomas, but it may take as long as a decade for this develoment to occur.

2. Lymphangiosarcoma may occur in the lymphedematous arm following axillary dissection for breast cancer (Stewart Treves syndrome).

3. Patients with von Recklinghausen's disease have a tendency (15%) to develop neurofibrosarcomas.

4. Patients with Gardner's syndrome may develop desmoid tumors or fibrosarcomas within the abdominal cavity.

5. Contrasts like thorotrast and polyvinyl chloride used earlier for angiograms have been associated with angiosarcomas of the liver and biliary tract.

6. There is no direct genetic predisposition to the development of soft tissue sarcomas, except 3 & 4 above.

7. Desmoid tumors of the abdominal wall occur following Cesarean section in some women.

8. Immunosuppression: Kaposi's sarcoma occurring in HIV/AIDS patients

9. Li-Fraumeni syndrome consisting of STS, breast carcinoma, melanoma etc

10. Many a time patients with an STS, give history of injury to that region; probably it helps to draw the attention of the patient to the swelling.

Pathology

1. Site: Because of their connective tissue origin, STS may occur anywhere in the body, however, about 50% are found in the lower extremity at or above the knee. An additional 20% are found in the trunk.

2. Histological types: The pathological classification of these tumors is based on the primitive cell of their origin.

Both benign and malignant tumors may arise from connective tissue and the pathological differentiation between them is crucial. Reactive lesions such as proliferative fasciitis and myositis ossificans, may sometimes grossly resemble sarcomas. Furthermore, some tumors of soft tissues appear histologically benign but exhibit aggressive biological behavior, to locally invade and metastasize. Examples are:

a. desmoid tumor

b. dermatofibrosarcoma protuberans (DFP)

c. well differentiated liposarcomas

Spread: Blood-borne pulmonary/skeletal metastasis and local invasion by contiguity occurs. Nodal spread through lymphatics is rare, but possible.

Common histological types

   i. Malignant fibrous histiocytoma (MFH) and fibrosarcoma - 65%
   ii. Liposarcoma - 20%
   iii. Rhabdomyosarcoma -10%
   iv. Leiomyosarcoma, synovial sarcoma, angiosarcoma, malignant Schwannoma etc. 5%

3. Grading: Histological grading is most widely accepted as the most important indicator of the biological nature of STS. They are categorized into low, intermediate and high grade tumors, based on number of mitotic figures,

Tissue of origin	Sarcoma
Mesenchymal (fibrous) tissue	Malignant fibrous histiocytoma (MFH) most common
Adipose (fat) tissue)	Liposarcoma
Synovial tissue	Synovial sarcoma
Blood vessels	Angiosarcoma
Lymph vessels	Lymphangiosarcoma
*Lymph node	Hodgkin's disease NHL, including Burkitt's lymphoma
Smooth muscle	Leiomyosarcoma (GIST etc)
Striated muscle	Rhabdomyosarcoma
Neural tissue	Malignant Schwannoma Neurofibrosarcoma
Uncertain	Epitheloid sarcoma
*not generally included under STS	

Table-38.1. Various types of soft tissue sarcomas

nuclear pleomorphism, degree of cellularity, stroma, vascularity and necrotic degeneration; the last is considered most important.

Clinical features

The typical presentation of an STS is a painless mass. As these arise in soft, pliable tissues, they may remain asymptomatic until they grow beyond the anatomic plane of origin. Pain is generally a late feature, attributable to hemor-

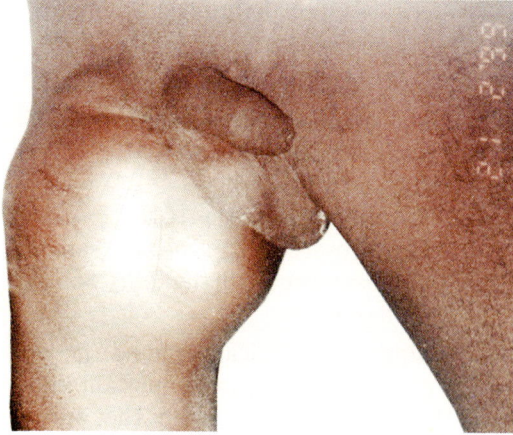

Fig. 38.1. Soft tissue sarcoma, right thigh (courtesy: Halsted Surgical Clinic, Chennai)

rhage/necrosis within or compression of adjacent structures, especially nerves. Hence a STS situated in fleshy areas such as retroperitoneum, buttocks and thighs, may reach large proportions before clinical detection. Fixity, variable consistency, local warmth and engorged veins over the mass go in favour of STS.

There is no single reliable physical sign to differentiate between benign and malignant soft tissue tumors. Neither the duration nor the rate of growth are helpful, making biopsy mandatory, with the only exception of a small soft tissue lump (<3cm), that persists unchanged for several years, which may be followed up without excision.

History

Comprehensive medical history needs to be elicited, with specific attention to family disorders, such as Gardner's syndrome, neurofibromatosis etc, site of origin, rate of growth, secondary skin changes, local pain, features of neurovascular pressure and evidence of regional/distant metastasis. History of previous biopsy/surgery, nature of treatment given and the response should be noted.

Physical examination

Besides location, size, shape, extent, consistency and intrinsic mobility, the following points have to be noted:
1. fixity to superficial and deep structures.
2. relationship to prior biopsy/surgery site, if done
3. functional status of the body part or extremity
4. concurrent medical disease.
5. pressure effects on nerves and blood vessels, and involvement of joint capsules especially for extremity sarcomas.
6. Involvement of viscera, such as GIT, and urinary tracts for trunk lesions and neurovascular structures of the head and neck for lesions in that area.

In a clinical context, having made a broad diag

nosis of STS, it is not always possible to give out the tissue type, but certain clues may be useful. If a preexisting lipoma, neurofibroma, fibroadenoma (breast), fibromyoma (uterus) or hemangioma is known, it becomes easy. Synovial sarcoma should be considered, if it is in the vicinity of a joint. In the absence of any lead, MFH/fibrosarcoma, being statistically most common, should be the best bet. (It is safe, and recommended, to merely propose the diagnosis of STS, unless pressed by the examiner).

Differential diagnosis

1. Hematoma - history of trauma or surgery
2. Chronic abscess-very difficult to distinguish even at surgery; USG/CTscan may show pus or antibioma
3. Myositis ossificans - history of injury and fracture, without progressive growth, biopsy negative.
4. Hemangioma - long standing history, typical bluish color, consistency and compressibility
5. Lymphangioma - long standing history and soft compressible, transilluminant mass, sometimgs difficult to distinguish from lymphangiosarcoma.
6. Lipoma - long duration, soft consistency, lobulation, slipping edge and free intrinsic mobility
7. Ganglion - typical site, mobility, size and plane of the swelling
8. Benign peripheral nerve tumor - well circumscribed mass, mobility restricted along axis of a nerve
9. Nodular fasciitis - painful tender, multiple, but often made out only at biopsy
10. Fibromatosis - possible to identify only by histology
11. Metastatic tumor - multiple typical sites, primary may be obvious and biopsy shows cell of origin
12. Lymphoma - nodular swelling in typical locations, other regions may be involved

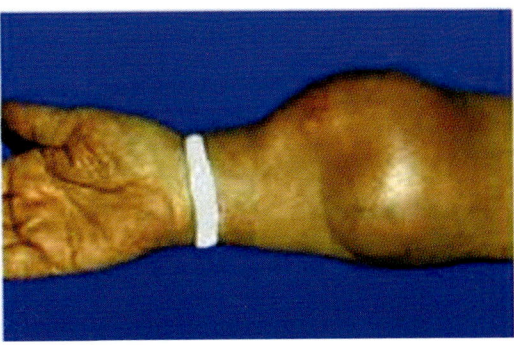

Fig. 38.2. Soft tissue sarcoma, forearm
(courtesy: Halsted Surgical Clinic, Chennai)

13. Bone sarcoma - Sometimes it is impossible to distinguish a sarcoma arising from the bone from periosteal or extraperiosteal tumors. An important point of difference is that the bone is usually expanded on all sides in the former, whereas in an extra-osseous tumor, infiltrating into the bone, bony thickening is seen only on that side.

14. Malignant melanoma or SCC - may be confused, if the tumor had come out through the skin and fungated. If the initial lesion was un ulcer, it indicates an epithelial tumor, on the other hand, if it was a subcutaneous or deep-seated mass, which later ulcerated, STS has to be considered.

Investigations

Radiology

1) X-rays
2) CT
3) MRI
4) Isotope (^{99m}Tc) bone scan

1. X-Rays: Routine: In STS, if bone erosion is suspected, plain x-ray is useful, and as good as an isotope bone scan. The sensitivity and specificity of an x-ray of pathologically confirmed periosteal invasion by STS is nearly 100%. About 80% of metastases in STS are seen in the lungs, pleura or mediastinum and are detectable by a plain chest skiagram.

2. CT Scan: Contrast enhanced CT allows visualization of major vascular, gastrointestinal and genitourinary structures providing important

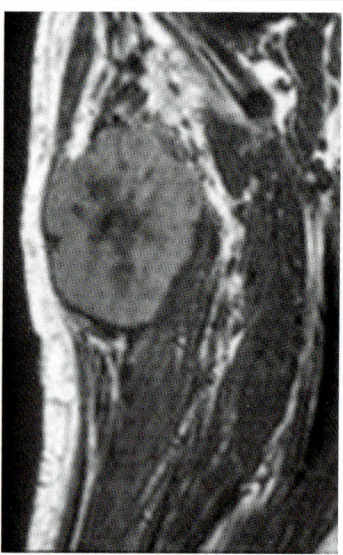

Fig. 38.3. CT scan of
STS thigh proved to be hemangiopericytoma

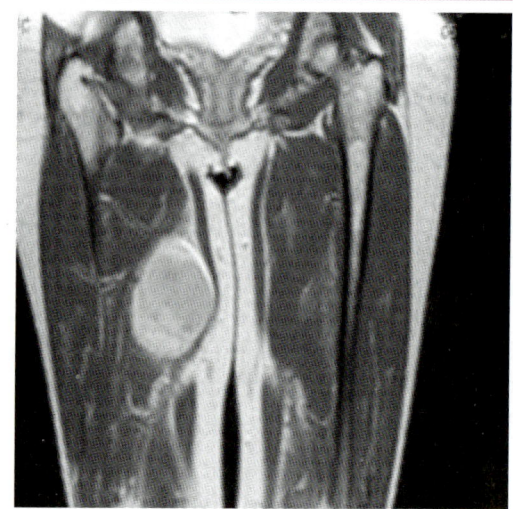

Fig. 38.4. CT scan showing STS of right thigh

information to plan treatment. It is ideal for intraabdominal and retroperitoneal lesions. Multi-slice (helical) CT of the chest is invaluable in detecting small lesions in the lung and the mediastinum.

Disadvantages of CT scan

a) tumors of muscle origin (most common) may be difficult to differentiate from surrounding normal muscular tissues.

b) only the transaxial views are obtained

3. MRI: Is the most useful single modality for evaluation of soft tissue sarcomas.

a) It offers better delineation between the tumor and surrounding tissue.
b) It allows both coronal and sagittal views (vis-a-vis CT Scan).
c) Specific muscle compartments may be easily outlined and this information is useful for surgical planning, especially compartmental excision.
d) Especially for extremity lesions, MRI is the investigation of choice.

The only disadvantage of an MRI is the high cost, thrice that of a CT scan.

Isotope bone scan: not routinely used for the evaluation of soft tissue sarcomas.

Angiography: If vascular resection and reconstruction is anticipated, an angiogram gives a very useful 'road map' to the surgeon. It is also helpful, while planning intra-arterial chemotherapy for unresectable tumors.

Biopsy: Many benign lesions may mimic sarcomas and a biopsy is mandatory.

Objectives of biopsy

1. to determine whether the lesion is benign or malignant and the type

2. to grade the tumor

3. to obtain all these data with minimal tumor disruption and spillage into the normal surrounding tissues.

Types of biopsy

(a) incisional or wedge biopsy
(b) excisional biopsy
(c) punch biopsy
(d) needle biopsy

(a) Incisional biopsy is simple to perform under local anesthesia and is the procedure of choice for most STS

Principles

The incision for biopsy should be placed directly over the summit of the tumor, in such a way that it is conveniently included at the time of definitive resection. Careful dissection without too much of elevation of skin flaps is necessary to minimize tumor spillage and hematoma formation.

i. Atleast a 1cc block of tissue should be obtained.

ii. Hemostasis must be meticulous.

iii. Drains are usually avoided

iv. For extremity masses, the biopsy incision should be oriented longitudinally, to facilitate subsequent incision and excision of a muscle group.

v. For truncal lesions, the incision should be placed parallel to the underlying muscle fibres.

b) Excisional biopsy may be done for small superficial masses. However, STS typically have a pseudocapsule of compressed normal tissue at the periphery of the lesion, with multiple prongs of tumor ('pseudopodia') invading through it, into the surrounding tissue, which may result in local recurrence. Therefore excision biopsy should be restricted to small (<3cm) superficial lesions only.

(c) Punch biopsy may be done for small superficial ulceroproliferative lesions, under local anesthesia.

(d) Needle biopsy is very useful in the setting of suspected metastatic or locally recurrent sarcoma as well as for an unresectable intrathoracic or intraabdominal STS. As tumor grading is equally crucial, many pathologists prefer a wide bore (tru-cut) needle, for proper sampling, rather than FNAC.

If a larger sample is required, the tumor may either be approached by standard open method or by minimally invasive (laparoscopic/thoracoscopic) technique.

Tumor markers by immunohistochemistry:

Some of these are useful in arriving at a specific diagnosis:

S-100 protein	for cartilage & soft tissue
Myoglobin	for striated muscle
Desmin	for muscle
Neurofilaments	for nerve
Vimentin	for mesoderm
Glial fibrils	for glial stroma

TNMG staging

T:	Tumor (primary)
T1:	<2cm
T2:	2-5cm
T3:	5-10cm
T4:	>10cm diameter
N:	Nodes (regional)
N0:	not involved
N1:	involved (proved) mobile
N3:	fixed nodes
M:	Metastases (distant)
MX:	not identified
M0:	none
M1:	present (proved)
G:	Grade (histological)
G1:	low
G2:	intermediate
G3:	high grade

AJCC staging scheme (American Joint Cancer Committee)

Stage I - IA:	G1 T1 N0 M0
IB:	G1 T2 N0 M0
Stage II - IIA:	G2 T1 N0 M0
IIB:	G2 T2 N0 M0
Stage III - IIIA:	G3 T1 N0 M0
IIIB:	G3 T2 N0 M0
Stage IV - IVA:	G2/3 T3/4 N1/2 M0
IVB:	G2/3 T3/4 N1/2 M1

Prognostic factors - see table 38.2

Treatment

As far as possible conservative surgery sparing

	Feature	Favourable	Unfavourable
1	Size	Small (<5cm)	Large (>5cm)
2	Site	Superficial	Deep
3	Histologic grade	Low	High

Table-38.2. Prognostic factors in an STS

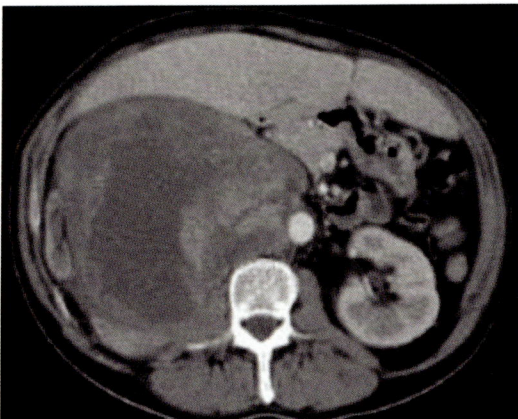

Fig. 38.5. CT Scan showing a large retroperitoneal liomyosarcoma, right side
(courtesy: Lifeline Hospitals, Chennai)

the affected limb and using a multi-modality approach is the accepted and preferred treatment for most of the STS.

Local treatment - objectives:

1. The complete eradication of local disease
2. Prevention of local recurrence
3. Prevention of distant spread
4. Preservation of tissue and function of limb/organ

Surgery

The extent of surgery is determined by the size, depth and anatomic relationships of the tumor, with the prime objective being to achieve negative surgical margins, regardless of the extent of the procedure.

1. Enucleation: Excision of a STS by dissection within the pseudocapsule or 'shelling out' should never be done as the sole treatment, since it is against the standard principles of cancer surgery.

2. Limited margin excision or local excision: This type of surgery is also associated with a local recurrence rate over 50%, but is sometimes resorted to in patients with tumor in close proximity to vital organs, bones or major neurovascular structures.

3. Wide excision: which is resection of a sarcoma along non-anatomic planes, with three dimensional clearance. With a recurrence rate of 25%, this is considered adequate for low grade tumors, when combined with adjuvant radiotherapy.

4. Radical resection: involves removal of all tissue in the anatomic compartment occupied by the tumor, including the origin and insertion of the entire group of muscles (compartmental excision) and a fascial plane, at least one uninvolved anatomic structure away from the tumor. Excellent result, similar to that seen with amputation may be achieved by this approach.

5. Amputation of limb: should be resorted to when a functionally useful limb cannot be achieved by wide local excision plus radio/chemotherapy because of extensive circumferential involvement of the limb. However, such mutilative procedures are justified only if cure of the disease is reasonably expected. Earlier, complete eradication of the tumor often required amputation including a joint proximal to the tumor; fortunately, because of early diagnosis and development of limb-preserving strategies over the years, nowadays it is required only in about 10% of cases.

6. Limb sparing surgery: In the last two decades, major advances have been made in the excision of skeletal and STS. For example a STS arising around the knee joint is best tackled by resection of the ends of the femur and tibia along with the knee, filling the gap by a tailor-made knee prosthesis, by the use of a preoperative MRI template of the joint. If necessary, vascular reconstruction is performed and tissue flaps are used to cover the main defect. When properly planned and executed, this approach seems to closely match the longterm results of amputations.

Treatment of regional nodes

These are involved in about 5% of STS, commonly seen in

(a) epitheloid sarcoma (48%),
(b) synovial sarcoma (17%) and
(c) embryonal rhabdomyosarcoma (12%) and

generally denote poor prognosis, as by then distant micro-metastases are expected to have occurred. Therefore elective regio-nal lymph node dissection is not warranted in STS; suspicious nodes should only be biopsied, as their involvement may influence in favour of palliative therapy.

(d) malignant fibrous histiocytoma

Principles of radical surgery for STS

1. As wide an excision as possible should be chosen

2. An elliptical skin incision should be used, encompassing all previous incision and drainage tracts

3. Thick subcutaneous skin flaps are raised to allow wide resections around the tumor

4. Early detection of structures that are to be preserved such as neurovascular bundles or bone

5. A wide margin of normal tissue around the tumor should be removed

6. The line of dissection should be carefully palpated and visualized through out the procedure

7. The actual tumor should not be entered or even visualized during the procedure.

Radiation therapy (RT): Although radiation therapy has been used by some as the sole therapy, the doses needed are sometimes unacceptably high; as such it is being used either as:

(a) preop. neoadjuvant therapy, to down-stage the tumor,

(b) postop. adjuvant therapy or

(c) palliative therapy in non-resectable tumors.

Advantages of preoperative RT

1. Eradication of tumor cells and preventing implantation in the wound

2. Tumor cells are better oxygenated preoperatively and are more radiosensitive, with downstaging of the tumor, before surgery.

Disadvantages

1. Compromise of wound healing

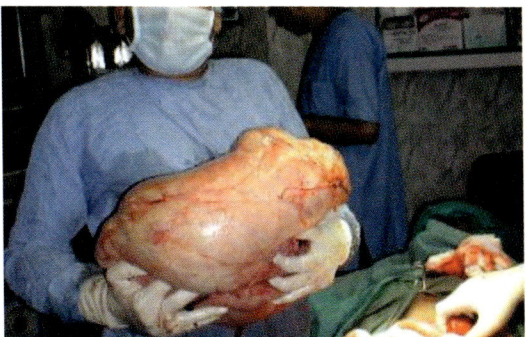

Fig. 38.6. A large retropertoneal sarcoma (20 Kg) occupying the entire abdomen, excised (courtesy: Dr. R.K. Mishra, New Delhi)

2. Incomplete tumor responses potentially resulting in a positive resection margin in an area that cannot be further irradiated

Postoperative RT

In the multimodality treatment for STS, this is routinely employed. Radiotherapy is most commonly given in the postoperative period.

Advantages

1. No interference with wound healing
2. The tumor bed can be marked with radio-opaque clips, at the time of surgery
3. Radiation treatment of minimal residual tumor, is more effective than treatment of bulky tumors.

Brachytherapy

Intra-operative or postoperative brachytherapy refers to the application of radioactive sources within or close to the tumor. Common isotopes used are: Iodine[125] seeds and Iridium[192] wires. Its main advantage is that high dosage of radiation can be delivered to the tumor bed, sparing adjacent normal tissue, whereas wound complications may be the main drawback.

Intraoperative RT (IORT) involves the use of a single high dose of electron beam or orthovoltage therapy at the time of surgery, delivered directly to the tumor bed, through open wound/abdomen/ thorax.

Chemotherapy: Most of the patients with metastatic disease in the lung have high grade sarcomas, requiring adjuvant systemic combination chemotherapy, with doxorubicin being the single most effective agent.

Chemotherapeutic regimes

1. CYVADIC: cyclophosphamide, vincristine, adriamycin & dacarbazine.

2. ACV: adriamycin, cyclophosphamide & vincristine

3. Nowadays, once the diagnosis of STS is made, preoperative (neoadjuvant) chemotherapy is given followed by planning for limbsparing surgery and postoperative RT. This regime of chemotherapy, surgery and RT being used successively, known as sequential multimodality therapy, has become standard in the management of STS.

Intra-arterial infusion therapy: This is possible if there is a single feeding artery to the entire area of tumor, usually in the limbs. Preoperative intra-arterial infusion of doxorubicin with or without synchronous radiation therapy has been advocated, in very large tumors for preoperative shrinkage, which is reported to be more effective than systemic therapy.

DERMATOFIBROSARCOMA PROTUBERANS (DFSP)

It is an intradermal sarcoma of low grade malignancy, rarely metastasizing, but with high tendency for local recurrence, involving mainly the trunk and extremities. It forms about 2-5% of STS and rarely conversion into frank sarcoma with a property to distant spread may occur (2-5%).

The disease has been linked with chromosomal translocation (17-22) and may occur in association with Gardner's syndrome. The translocation fuses collagen gene with platelet-derived growth factor (PDGF) gene, expressing as fibroblast, containing receptors for growth factor, turning into a neoplasm. The tumor is CD34 positive and its biological behavior has some semblance to a desmoid tumor.

Clinical features

it is a slow growing painless protruding hard

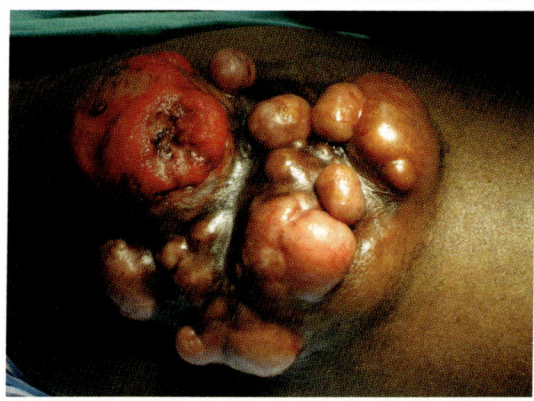

Fig. 38.7. Dermatofibrosarcoma protuberans of thigh

nodular mass, freely moving over the subcutaneous tissue, without regional lymphadenopathy. There may be surface ulceration more due to stretching of epidermis rather than tumor infiltration.

Treatment

It is not very chemo or radiosensitive, hence wide excisional surgery is the best option, but recurrences have to be anticipated. Mohs microsurgery has been found to be appropriate in some cases, which show deeper infiltration. A newer chemotherapeutic agent, imatinib mesylate has shown some promising results in recurrent or non-resectable tumors and appears to be more specific if the tumor is positive for gene translocation.

RETROPERITONEAL SARCOMAS

Sarcomas of the retroperitoneum are a subset of STS; by their anatomic location, making access difficult, the conventional methods of management discussed above are hard to apply. As 1/3 of retroperitoneal tumors are sarcomas, the potential benefit of establishing tissue diagnosis prior to definitive therapy is obvious.

Biopsy

A CT-guided (needle) or laparoscopic biopsy are very useful and eliminate the need for an open (laparotomy) biopsy, in this situation.

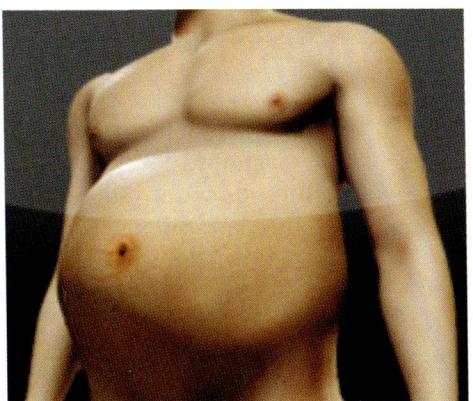

Fig. 38.8. Huge retroperitoneal sarcoma, occupying most of the abdomen

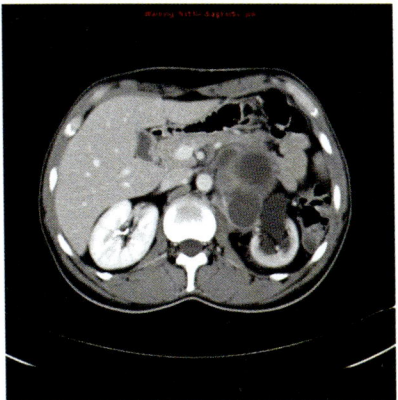

Fig. 38.9. Retroperitoneal sarcoma, compressing the left ureter causing hydronephrosis

Surgery

It forms the main stay of treatment but most retroperitoneal sarcomas are quite large at the time of detection, averaging >20cm in size, and with extensive local invasion. Consequently, it is uncommon for these tumors to be resected with negative microscopic margins and a true 'cancer clearance' is rarely accomplished.

Adjuvant chemotherapy

This gives some advantage by conferring a 'shoulder' on the survival curve, but it is over-compensated sometimes by drug toxicity.

Intraoperative radiotherapy (IORT) has been used with the objective of providing higher dose of radiotherapy to the target tissue with reduced risk of unwanted radiation to adjacent normal viscera. Although it gives a better control of local tumor, it has not influenced the long term survival rates.

Follow up and recurrence

Local recurrence is not uncommon because of the size and nature of these lesions, inspite of the ideal combination of therapy, given in the best institutions. Reoperation either for cure (rarely) or debulking (often), is being increasingly recommended, supported by chemo/radiotherapy, depending upon the merits of the situation. For distant dissemination, with little hope of curing the disease, some palliative systemic therapy, which can be tolerated (physically and financially), may be offered, fully realizing the score.

Special features of an STS

Most of them arise de novo

More common in extremities

Most common STS in adults is MFH

Most common STS in children is rhabdomyosarcoma

Most of them spread by blood stream to lung except retroperitoneal sarcoma goes to liver

MRI is the imaging modality of choice

Adequate surgery is the preferred treatment

Neoadjuvant or adjuvant radio/chemotherapy may be beneficial.

Jewels of Gyan - 38.1

STS

Plan incision of biopsy to be included in definitive procedure
Capsule like covering often present (beware!)
Surgery bulwark of therapy
Other modalities: only adjuvant to surgery

This involves stimulation of host immune mechanisms against cancer cells. The high incidence of cancers in kidney transplants and immune-deficient states together with the rare phenomenon of spontaneous tumor regression indicate the value of immune defences. Tumors differ antigenically from their hosts, this antigen difference is evident from the host's ability for allogenic inhibition (tumor cells lacking host antigen will not be allowed to grow when they are in the company of normal cells) and immunological surveillance to restrain tumor growth. Host immunoglobulins act either as:

1. antagonists to agents enhancing tumor growth.
2. unblocking antibodies that reverse the enhancement
3. beneficial cytotoxics that activate the complement system.

Cell-mediated immunity against a specific tumor antigen (type IV) as well as antibody-dependent cell-mediated (killer) cytotoxicity (type II) may be demonstrated in cancer patients.

Clinical uses

Usually employed after completion of other standard modalities of therapy, as it can only kill a small fraction of malignant cells. Immunotherapy may be specific or nonspecific.

Specific

Stimulation of the host immune response can be:

1. Active: Autologous tumor, e.g. patient's own tumor cells as well as transfer factor.
2. Passive: Use of antiserum specific to a particular antigen, e.g. antilymphocyte serum (ALS) in leukemia.

Nonspecific

Stimulation of general immune mechanisms by injecting BCG into melanoma nodules (leads to regression) or intrapleural injection of BCG folowing pneumonectomy (for lung cancer). Corynebacterium parvum, levamisole, tenocordin, arabinoxylan, retinoids and interferon are the other known nonspecific boosting agents.

Retinoids

They are nontoxic chemical modifications of preformed vitamin A (alcohol retinol). Vitamin A deficiency results in squamous metaplasia, which can be reverted after vitamin replenishment to actively secreting columnar epithelium. Therefore, retinoids prevent squamous metaplasia and their role in differentiation may be used in cancer prevention and preneoplastic conditions. (vitamin A is inferior to retinoids as it may be hepatotoxic). Clinical regression is noticed in actinic keratosis, BCC and malignant melanoma after topical therapy. Specific retinoid cytoplasmic receptors as well as immunostimulation may explain their mode of action. Further clinical studies are needed in this direction.

Interferon

Interferon (IF) is a protein, which was initially identified for its antiviral effects. If the inducing agent is a virus or double-stranded inducer, it is called Type 1 IF. Type II IF is produced if the immune-competent cells are stimulated by unrelated substances. It has three actions.

1. Binds to a surface receptor in the target cell and sets in motion a series of secondary messengers culminating in a change in the cells' general metabolic state (such changes inhibit virus replication using the genetic machinery of the host cell).
2. Complex inhibitory effect on cell growth and division.
3. Profound effect on the immune system (acting as a lymphocyte hormone)

According to heterogeneity, there are three families of IF:

a) (predominantly produced by leucocytes),
b) (produced by fibroblasts) and
c) (produced by antigen/mitogen-stimulated lymphocytes).

Including subtypes, there is a total of 14 different molecular species of IFs. Clinically, use of IF in myeloma, breast cancer and NHL, results in objective regression of these tumors.

It can cause some side effects (dose related) including anorexia, weight loss and central nervous system toxicity (metabolic encephalopathy). Other tumors, such as melanoma, renal cell carcinoma, lung cancer and Kaposi's sarcoma, respond to IF at a low rate (less than 20%). This anticancer potential of IF could possibly be utilized in adjuvant therapy in the early stages of solid tumors as well as in advanced disease.

Recent advances

1. The use of monoclonal antibodies, to deliver cytotoxics or radiation to their target tumors, is a new form of *passive immunotherapy*.

2. Enhanced immunity autologous tumoricidal cells (EIAT) are autologous stem cells harvested from the patient, cultured to boost their number and reinjected, to achieve a greater cell kill.

3. Tumor regression is noted following the use of antibodies prepared from the tumor itself, by a special process and may hold the key for future cancer cure.

It has been found that if antibodies were primed with cancer stem cells, they were capable of targeting cancer cells and conferring anti tumor immunity. The process of making a vaccine against cancer is seen at the end of the pipeline.

40 Endocrine Therapy for Malignancies

Hormones are defined as chemical mediators secreted by cells to affect ' target cells' at a distance (*endocrine*), as in most hormones; to stimulate nearby cells to secrete other hormones (*paracrine*), e.g. glucagon from α-cells of the islets of (Langerhans) pancreas stimulating β-cells to secrete insulin; or to act as neuro-transmittors (*neurocrine*). Each hormone binds to a protein (*receptor*), situated on the cell membrane or within the cell (cytosol), with a high affinity and specificity.

Hormone–receptor complex

Situated at the cell mebrane, this complex activates adenyl cyclase enzyme, leading to the production of adenosine monophosphate (AMP) as a second messenger which in turn stimulates intracellular metabolic events. Such a mechanism can be seen in catecholamines and peptide hormones, i.e., glucagons, LH, FSH , ACTH, while protein hormones, i.e., growth hormone, insulin and prolactin, activate membrane receptors by production of a second messenger other than AMP (probably a peptide).

Steroid hormones

All sex hormones being steroid in nature, diffuse through the cell membrane to bind to specific cytoplasmic receptor proteins, which then undergo a change in conformation and translocated to the cell nucleus, acting on the genome to induce transcription (RNA synthesis). Some target cells possess more than one receptor type, e.g. thyroid hormone acts via multiple receptor sites on the cell membrane, in the mitochondria, within the nucleus and in the cytoplasm. The receptor assay is of considerable clinical importance, permitting, for example, the development of specific hormone inhibitors.

Therapeutic manipulation of endocrine environment is carried out either by:

1) ablative therapy (surgical removal or radiation destruction of a particular endocrine organ) or

2) additive therapy, where exogenous natural or synthetic hormones or antihormones are administered, e.g. medical castration.

Endocrine therapy (unlike cytotoxic) is never curative - *eventually all hormone-sensitive tumors will become resistant*, and offers only a form of palliation in advanced endocrine-sensitive cancers (in less than 30% of cases) with successful control lasting for a maximum of 2-3 years.

Estrogen receptors (ER)

A) These provide a method of predicting the hormonal sensitivity of breast cancer. About a third of breast cancers have no detectable or significant receptor activity and must be spared from ineffective endocrine therapy (better treated by cytotoxic therapy). The remaining two-thirds, mainly in postmenopausal patients, must be considered for endocrine therapy with a 50% chance of response. Tumors with high receptor levels are more likely to respond. As samples of metastatic disease may be difficult to obtain for assay, receptor analysis of the primary should be done. There may be some quantitative differences in the receptor concentration in primary tumor and their later metastases, but it will not significantly alter the receptor status. *Tumors are labeled 'ER positive' if they contain >10 femto mol/mg of cytosol protein, 'borderline' if between 3 and 10 and 'negative' if they contain <3.*

Androgen and progesterone receptors (AR & PR) have also been discovered; the latter are present in a proportion of ER positive tumors, which respond to hormonal treatment better (90%), than those possessing ER alone (50%). PR are rarely found in tumors without ER, but when present, it materially improves the prognosis, since it responds well to endocrine therapy.

Estrogens

It has many anticancer actions: direct action on breast and prostatic tissue; pituitary-mediated effect as antiprolactin in breast carcinoma and antiinterstitial cell stimulating hormone in prostatic carcinoma; immune stimulation in both breast and prostatic carcinoma; increases testosterone-binding globulin; thus decreasing free testosterone in prostatic carcinoma. The preparations include (with oral daily doses):

Ethinylestradiol 0.1- 0.5mg t.i.d; stilbestrol 1-5mg t.i.d; trianisil chloroethylene (TACE) 12-24mg.

Fosfestrol tetrasodium (Honvan)

Usually inert, but under the action of acid phosphatase of prostatic carcinoma, free stilbestrol will be liberated and leads to rapid relief of sacral and pelvic pain following injection (250-500mg I.V/day), in patients with metastases to these areas (thus it may be diagnostic as well as therapeutic).

Androgens

Testosterone propionate 100mg thrice weekly (I.M), found effective in breast and renal cell carcinoma; but it may lead to hirsutism, hoarseness (in women), increased libido and baldness (in men). They may also exhibit anabolic effect, useful in cancer cachexia.

Progestogens

Medroxyprogesterone acetate (Provera) is useful in breast, renal cell, endometrial and ovarian carcinoma.

Antiprolactins

CB-154, L-Dopa and CG-603; used in advanced breast cancer. Bromocriptin or cibergolin are used against prolactinoma of pituitary.

Aminoglutethimide (Orimeten): A steroidogenesis enzyme blocker, it inhibits estrogen synthesis by blocking desmolase, which mediates the first step in the conversion of cholesterol to androgens in the adrenal glands (medical adrenalectomy), and aromatase, which mediates the conversion of endogenous androgens to estrogens peripherally. Clinically 250mg t.i.d with hydrocortisone 20mg b.i.d (to prevent a reflex rise in ACTH, which might overcome the adrenal block) is used in postmenopausal or oophorectomized women with metastatic breast cancers (especially ER positive), producing remission in 30%, with results comparable to those of surgical adrenalectomy.

Antiestrogens

Inhibit estrogen by blocking receptor sites in target organs in estrogen-dependent tumors. Orally active, they have minimal side effects like mild estrogenicity and possible prolactin inhibition. They are:

Tamoxifen citrate 10-20mg b.i.d. (may cause thrombocytopenia) - very popular drug in breast carcinoma.

Letrozole 2.5mg daily (causes arthralgia and osteoporosis)

Nafoxiden 60-90mg t.i.d. (causes dry skin, photophobia and cataract)

Clomiphene citrate 50mg b.i.d (causes hypergonadotrophinism)

Glucocorticoids

Complications such as hypercalcemia (due to bone metastases, immobolisation with osteoporosis precipitated by estrogen therapy), cerebral edema, autoimmune hemolytic anemia, general depression and anorexia are all treated with prednisolone. However, prolonged glucocorticoid therapy may cause many side effects:

Suppression/atrophy of adrenal glands

Na^+ and H_2O retention and K^+ depletion,

Weight gain and risk of heart failure

Hypertension

Susceptibility to infection

Cushinoid appearance with moon face and buffalo hump

Gastrointestinal tract problems (dyspepsia, acid-peptic disorders and perforation)

Osteoporosis

Hyperglycemia and diabetes

Psychosis with euphoria

Skin changes, problems in wound healing

Cataract

Myopathy.

Clinical uses

Breast carcinoma

Only 30% respond to hormonal manipulation. Prediction of the response depends on

a) laboratory tests (positive ER, tumor culture with different hormones and hormonal assay

b) clinical features (older age group and those with a long disease-free interval between primary treatment and appearance of first recurrence, show a better response;

c) postmenopausal status is favorable.

Early breast carcinoma

Treated by surgery + RT. One of the systemic forms of therapy is also given, sparing the other for recurrence.

Advanced breast carcinoma

1. Debulking or palliative surgery.

2. Palliative RT: in bone and skin metastases.

3. Premenopausal (within 3 years of menopause): Ovarian ablation and tamoxifen.

4. Postmenopausal (beyond 3 years of menopause): Antiestrogens (tamoxifen) or prednisolone in hepatic and lung infiltration. The antiestrogen is the drug of choice in soft tissue and pulmonary involvement. Relapse after ovarian ablation was treated earlier by secondary (major) endocrine ablation (MEA). However, such an endocrine 'mutilation' (adrenalectomy or hypophysectomy) has now been given up, and largely replaced by pharmacological agents, such as aromatase inhibitors, antiestrogens, corticosteroids, etc.

Cytotoxic therapy is classically indicated in endocrine failure or is used initially if the tumor is found to be hormone insensitive (e.g. ER negative) and in fairly aggressive diseases like fulminating carcinomatosis lymphangiosa. Either single or, usually, intermittent combination therapy is used (cyclophosphamide, methotrexate and 5-FU). Immunotherapy (by nonspecific stimulation of immune defense mechanism) and neutron therapy are under trial.

However, the current consensus favors cytotoxics in early and advanced breast cancer. In male breast carcinoma, bilateral orchidectomy is effective in two-thirds of cases. It appears to offer better tumor-control than oophorectomy in women. If relapse occurs, steroids and tamoxifen therapy is better than further endocrine ablative therapy.

Prostatic carcinoma

90% are hormone dependent, Flutamide and lutinizing hormone releasing hormone (LHRH) agonists (Gosereline) are the drugs of choice, with or without orchidectomy. Corticosteroids and aromatase inhibitors are also used to achieve 'medical adrenalectomy', especially in advanced cancers. Thromboembolism is a complication seen either due to tumor infiltration or to estrogen therapy. Bone metastases are controlled with megavoltage radiotherapy and obstructive uropathy is managed with transurethral resection of prostate (TURP) or radical retropubic prostatectomy.

Cancers of ovary, uterus (endometrial) and kidney (adenocarcinoma)

These organs are the embryological derivatives of the urogenital ridge and those cancers are treated with progestogens.

Thyroid carcinoma

Only papillary carcinoma is known to be hormone (TSH) dependent. Suppressive dose of thyroxine (0.3mg/day) is given to prevent the growth of the residual primary tumor and its metastases after total thyroidectomy. Other

41 Filariasis

This HELMINTHIASIS, caused by the nematodes, *Wuchereria bancrofti* or *Brugia malayi*, is widely prevalent in South India, directly proportional to the availability of breeding places for the mosquito vector, *Culex fatigans*.

Life cycle

The microfilaria in the peripheral blood of man (*definitive host*) are taken up by the female mosquitoes during their blood-meal. In the mosquito (*intermediate host*) they undergo further development and re-enter man, through the proboscis sheath of the mosquito. Unlike the malarial parasite, direct inoculation does not occur; the larvae are deposited on the surface of the skin, close to the puncture wound. They then penetrate the skin, probably due to the warmth, and reside in lymphatic channels. Sexual maturity of the worms then occurs and after fertilization, the microfilaria enter the blood stream.

Examination of night blood smear: Most of the pathological effects of filariasis are due to the adult worm. The migration of microfilaria into peripheral circulation during the patient's sleep hours, is typical; hence examination is generally done on a blood smear collected around midnight, for maximum yield. This is thought to be due to some vasomotor changes occurring during sleep, sending 'signals' to the parasite. If there is any shift of circardian sleep rhythm, such as night security personnel, their blood should be examined when they habitually sleep. The yield of this test may be enhanced by a 'provocative' dose of diethyl carbamazine (DEC), 300mg, given orally in the previous evening.

Pathogenesis of 'surgical filariasis'

i) Mechanical blockage of lymphatics by worms (adults)

ii) Release of toxic products by the parasite

iii) Superadded bacterial infection by strepto/staphylococci, causing lymphangitis

iv) Progressive lymphatic fibrosis, leading to further blockage

The main pathological manifestations may be

1. inflammatory: epididymo-orchitis, funiculitis, lymphangitis, lymphadenitis

2. lymphatic obstruction: lymph varix, lymphadenovarix, lymph vesicles, lymph scrotum, lymphedema of limbs

3. rupture: chyluria, chylocele, chylous ascites, chylothorax

4. continuing obstruction: elephantiasis of scrotum, leg/foot, forearm/hand, breast or vulva, 'ram-horn' penis

1. Inflammatory

a) Filarial fever: chills and rigors, more at night associated with signs of inflammation of target organs such as spermatic cord, epididymis, scrotal skin etc.

b) Lymphangitis and lymphadenitis: streaks of red inflamed lymphatics may be seen, along with painful lymph node enlargement. Retroperitoneal lymphangitis can mimic 'acute abdomen' with severe constitutional symptoms. The genital examination clinches the diagnosis, as the cord and scrotum are red and tender. Similarly, enlarged, painful, warm/tender lymph nodes with periodic fever and peripheral blood showing microfilariae, is the picture of acute or subacute filarial lymphadenitis.

c) Funiculitis and epididymo-orchitis: they both are actually parts of one continuous process, wherein inflammation of the cord structures (funiculitis) leads on to the involvement of the globus major of the epididymis , with obliteration of the sulcus between the testis and the epididymis. Thus, involvement of the upper pole of the epididymis is typical of filariasis, whereas in tuberculosis, the epididymis is craggy and beaded, with a sinus or cold abscess on the posterior aspect of scrotum, associated with seminal vesiculitis. The latter may be diagnosed by the typical suprapubic pain, experienced during ejaculation and supraprostatic tenderness, during digital examination of the rectum.

d) Salpingitis, oophoritis, synovitis, arthritis, mastitis etc have been rarely described.

The secondary infection with pyogenic bacteria rapidly supervenes, producing cellulitis, abscess formation, bacteremia and rarely septicemia.

2. *Lymphatic obstruction with varicosity*

Secondary to fibrosis of lymph nodes draining an area, due to endolymphangitis obliterans, the proximal lymph vessels or nodes may become varicose and enlarged. The examples are:

i) Lymph varix (syn: diffuse hydrocele of the cord): The lymphatics (usually of the spermatic cord) become diffusely enlarged and dilated.

ii) Lymphadenovarix: Enlarged and softened

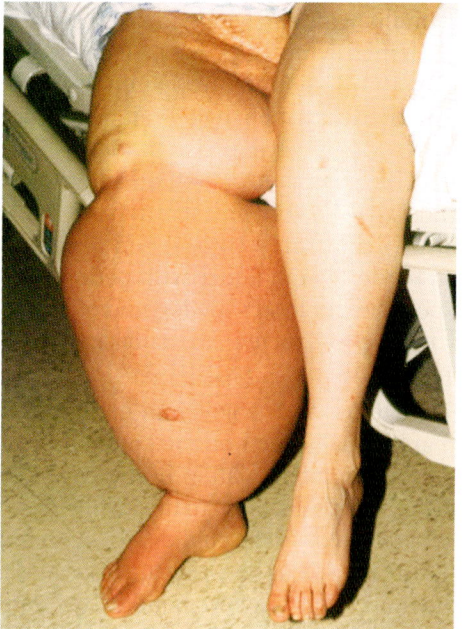

Fig. 41.1. Massive elephantiasis of lower limb
(courtesy: Dr K R Reddy, Kakinada)

lymph nodes, usually of the inguinal group, often a painless sequel to recurrent inflammations and outflow obstruction.

iii) Hydrocele: Collection of fluid in the tunica vaginalis secondary to lymphatic obstruction. Although usually clear, the fluid may be milky and turbid and may even contain microfilaria.

iv) Lymph scrotum: The varicosity of the lymphatics affects the skin of the scrotum and results in multiple vesicles containing clear or slightly turbid fluid. Rupture of these causes a lymph ooze (lymphorrhea or lymphorrhagia) from the skin and predisposes to infection.

ELEPHANTIASIS

Stagnation of lymph in the tissue causes a pitting edema initially, which waxes and wanes with each attack of inflammation. With the passage of time, the interstitial fluid with rich protein content, excites an intense tissue response and fibroblastic activity. The edema is at first partially reversible, but eventually becomes irreversible and hard. Finally the skin becomes irregular, thickened and warty areas of lymphorrhagia and ulceration may supervene.

ELEPHANTIASIS OF SCROTUM AND PENIS

Scrotum is a common site, as the draining nodes (inguinal) are those most frequently involved in the process; the swelling is maximal in the dependent portion. Between the hypertrophied skin and the testis (often with a hydrocele), is a rubbery mass of tissue (blubber). In case of the penis, distortion and thickening of the skin and subcutaneous tissue causes a *ram horn penis*. Sometimes the penis is totally buried intrascrotally.

ELEPHANTIASIS OF LIMBS

The lower limb is most commonly affected, with occurrence of the same process as described for scrotum. Superadded cutaneous fungal infection (often with Epidermo-phyton floccosum) and bacterial infection compound the edematous process in the limbs.

ELEPHANTIASIS OF VULVA AND BREAST

Besides filariasis in endemic areas, lymphogranuloma venereum (esthiomene) and irradia-

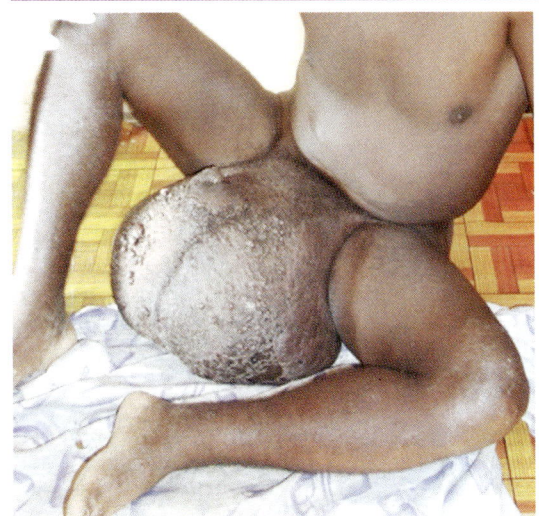

Fig. 41.2. Massive filarial scrotum with lymph vesicles and burried penis
(courtesy: Dr. C J Reddy, Gudur)

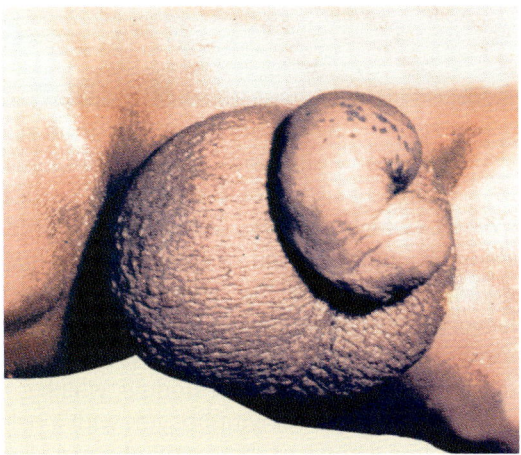

Fig. 41.3. Ram-horn penis
(courtesy: Prof T Gunasagaran, Chennai)

tion of groin/axilla for cancers are the common causes of elephantiasis in these sites.

3. *Lymph rupture*

When intra-lymphatic tension is too high, rupture may occur, resulting in escape of chyle or lymph (depending on the obstruction being above or below the cisterna chyli).

TYPES OF CHYLORRHAGIA

a) Chyluria: After some straining, the patient passes 'milky urine', sometimes admixed with blood (hematochyluria). The cause is retroperitoneal lymphatic rupture into the renal pelves and ureters. The condition is usually self resolving. This phenomenon may also be seen in genitourinary tuberculosis.

b) Chylocele: Milky fluid in the tunica vaginalis, rarely with microfilaria, which has to be differentiated from a spermatocele.

c) Chylous diarrhea: Rupture into the mucosa of the alimentary tract causes this rare condition.

d) Chylothorax (pleural cavity) and chylous ascites (peritoneal cavity) also may occur.

Investigations: see chapter 43

Treatment

Medical: see chapter 43

Surgical treatment is indicated only for gross deformities.

Elephantiasis of scrotum

It involves either partial excision and reconstruction or total excision of scrotum, the latter being followed by implantation of testes in the thighs.

The principles are: removal of all the blubbery tissue through large anterior elliptical incisions, and debulking of elephantiasis, as the posterior scrotal skin is rarely involved. Eversion or excision of the tunica is performed to prevent/treat hydrocele, as well as to help the 'accomodation' problem to an extent. The remaining skin is sutured either in 'X' or 'inverted Y' (Mercedes) manner. If the entire scrotal skin requires excision due to extensive involvement, the testicles may have to be implanted in the thighs.

Ram-horn penis

This is the lymphedema of penis, usually associated with that of scrotum, its peculiar shape earning that name. It may also be treated by either

(a) partial excision and reconstruction or

(b) total excision of penile skin and skin grafting; the former is more popular, since it preserves the all-important cutaneous sensations of the organ.

42 Lymph Nodes

A normal lymph node is about 3mm size (size of a pin head), clinically impalpable, consisting of a peripheral portion (*cortex*), which receives lymph via afferent channels, and a central or hilar portion, (*medulla*), from where the efferent lymphatics leave. Other lymphoid organs include spleen, tonsils and thymus; their characteristic structural feature is the *follicle* or nodule, which is a spherical collection of lymphocytes with a pale central area, known as the *germinal center*. The thymus and spleen have no afferent lymphatics. Isolated lymphoid follicles are also seen in the walls of gastrointestinal and respiratory tract, more aggregated in the ileum, known as *Peyer's patches*. The *gut associated lymphoid tissue* (GALT) is probably the largest lymphoid mass in the body. Of the 800 or so lymph nodes in the body, more than 300 are placed in the neck and it is often the presenting feature of generalized adenopathy.

There are two types of lymphocytes in the lymphoid tissue, B-type, derived probably from bone marrow and the T-type, from thymus. Apart from these, the lymphoid organs contain phagocytic cells (macrophages and histiocytes), as part of the larger reticuloendothelial (monocyte-macrophage) system. The defense mechanisms of the body include phagocytosis, a nonspecific engulfing process, and the immune response, a specific reaction to various antigens, such as microorganisms, foreign proteins etc. The immune response is of two types,

(a) humoral antibody response, mediated by B-cells, producing protein molecules known as antibodies, which combine with antigens, to form complexes, to be destroyed by phagocytes and

(b) cell-mediated response, carried out by T-cells, producing specific cells that circulate in blood to destroy the antigens and activate

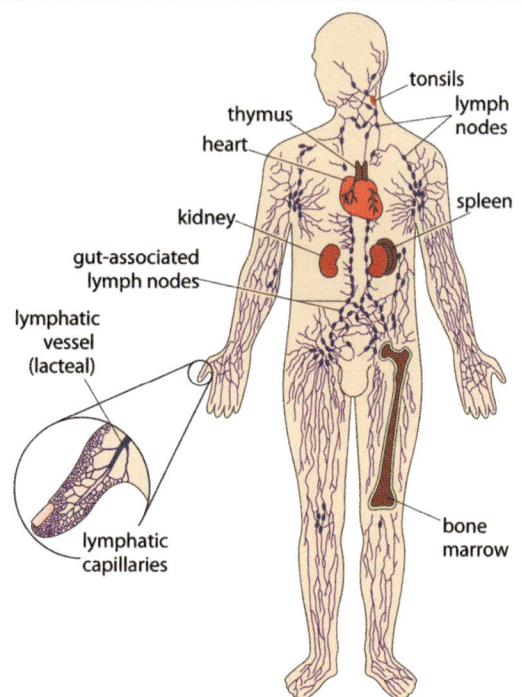

Fig. 42.1. The distribution of lymphatic tissue

phagocytes. The B-cells also become transformed into plasma cells, to produce various *immunoglobulins*, like IgG, IgM etc. This ability to produce one particular antibody in large quantities has paved the way for the development of the *monoclonal antibody* concept, to identify specific antigens. The discovery of some types of B-cells known as, plasma cells and B-memory cells and in the T-cells, T-helper, T-suppressor, T-killer and T-memory types, have opened new avenues for the rapid growth of the fascinating subject of immunology.

The causes of lymph nodal enlargement may be classified as:

Inflammatory

Acute nonspecific

nonsuppurating or pyogenic infections, septicemia*

(* associated with enlargement of several groups of lymph nodes)

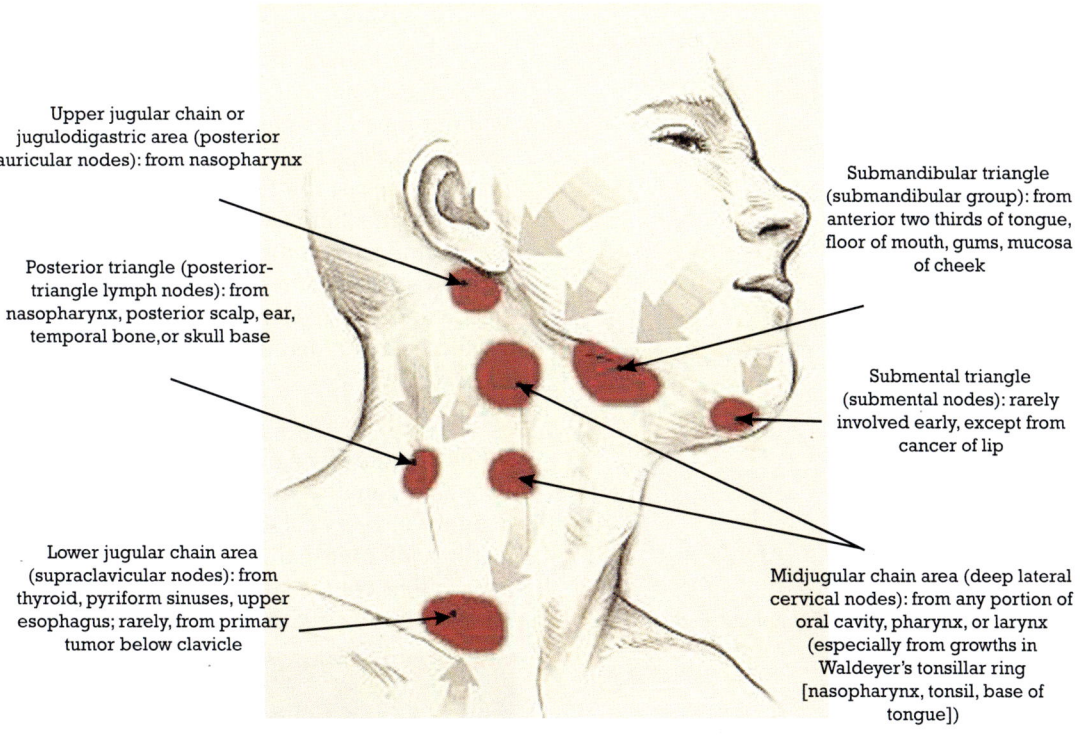

Upper jugular chain or jugulodigastric area (posterior auricular nodes): from nasopharynx

Submandibular triangle (submandibular group): from anterior two thirds of tongue, floor of mouth, gums, mucosa of cheek

Posterior triangle (posterior-triangle lymph nodes): from nasopharynx, posterior scalp, ear, temporal bone, or skull base

Submental triangle (submental nodes): rarely involved early, except from cancer of lip

Lower jugular chain area (supraclavicular nodes): from thyroid, pyriform sinuses, upper esophagus; rarely, from primary tumor below clavicle

Midjugular chain area (deep lateral cervical nodes): from any portion of oral cavity, pharynx, or larynx (especially from growths in Waldeyer's tonsillar ring [nasopharynx, tonsil, base of tongue])

Fig. 42.2. Common primary cancers metastasizing into various groups of cervical nodes

Group of nodes	Level	Drainage area
Prelaryngeal (Delphian)	L-6	Larynx, thyroid (true vocal cords have no lymphatics)
Pretracheal & Paratracheal	L-6	Thytoid, trachea
Submental & submandibular	L-1	Ant 2/3 of tongue, floor of mouth, lips, cheek
Upper anterior (jugulo-digastric)	L-2	Tonsil, post 1/3 of tongue, oropharynx, pyriform sinus parotid, external ear
Upper posterior	L-2	Adenoids, posterior pharynx, retropharyngeal area
Middle deep cervical	L-3	Thyroid, supraglottis, cricopharyngeal region
Lower anterior (jugulo-omohyoid)	L-4	Tongue, thyroid, subglottis
Supraclavicular (Virchow)	L-4	Abdominal & thoracic viscera, breast
Lower posterior	L-5	Thyroid, postcricoid, esophagus, lungs, breast

Table - 42.1 Drainage areas for neck nodes

Specific
tuberculosis*, infectious mononucleosis*, bubonic plague*, LGV

Chronic nonspecific
pyogenic, sarcoidosis*, autoimmune disorders*

Specific
Bacterial

tuberculosis*, syphilis*, brucellosis*

Viral
LGV, cat-scratch disease

Parasitological
filarial*, toxoplasmosis*

Fungal
blastomycosis, histoplasmosis, cocci-

(* associated with enlargement of several groups of lymph nodes)
Note: tuberculous lymphadenitis may have either acute (less common) or insidious presentation

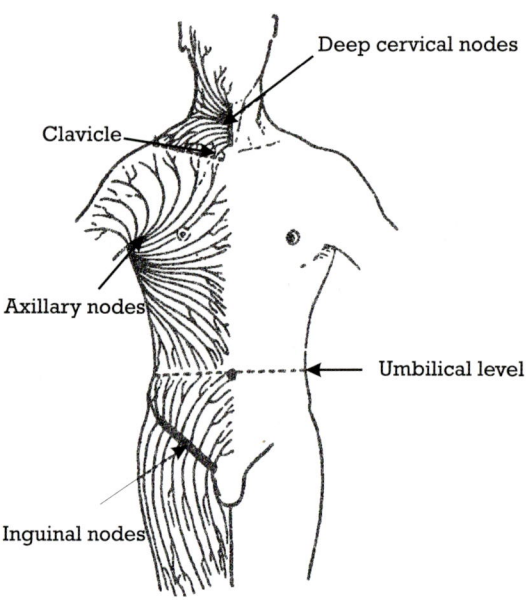

Fig. 42.3. Pattern of lymphatic drainage.

diodomycosis

Neoplastic

Secondary carcinoma*
Lymphomas*: Hodgkin's disease, NHL
Lymphatic leukemia*

Miscellaneous

Lymphadenopathy as a part of generalized disease and HIV etc.

Are they lymph nodes?

The lymph nodes are clinically identified by their *location* in the normal anatomical sites of lymph nodes and their *multiplicity* causing nodularity. Except in areas such as liver or thyroid, a nodular swelling generally implies enlarged lymph nodes, unless proved otherwise.

Jewels of Gyan - 42.1

Are they lymph nodes?
Multiple nodular swellings situated in the anatomical areas where lymph nodal groups normally exist, have to be considered as lymph nodes, unless proved otherwise.

Is the nodal enlargement significant?

It is well known that soft, flat, nontender cervical/inguinal lymphadenopathy can exist, without much clinical significance. A progressively enlarging, tender and/or hard node, even in these areas, particularly with a primary disease in the drainage fields, should be considered significant. Comparison with the opposite side provides another important clue to their significance, hence lymph nodes on both sides should be examined even in unilateral disease of extremity.

Lymph node biopsy

While planning for a node biopsy in generalized lymphadenopathy, such as lymphoma, the inguinal and cervical sites are better avoided, as features of preexisting chronic inflammation may often confuse the histopathology. The node to be excised for biopsy should not be

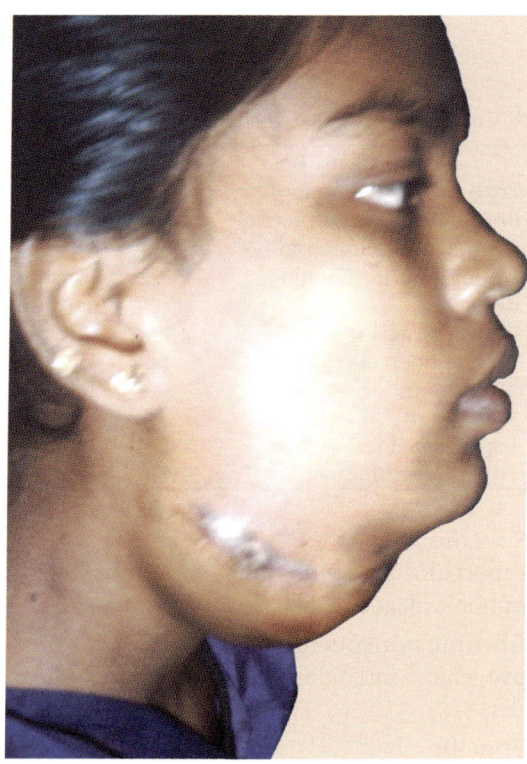

Fig. 42.4. Scrofuloderma over tuberculous submandibular lymphadenitis (courtesy: Lifeline Hospitals, Chennai)

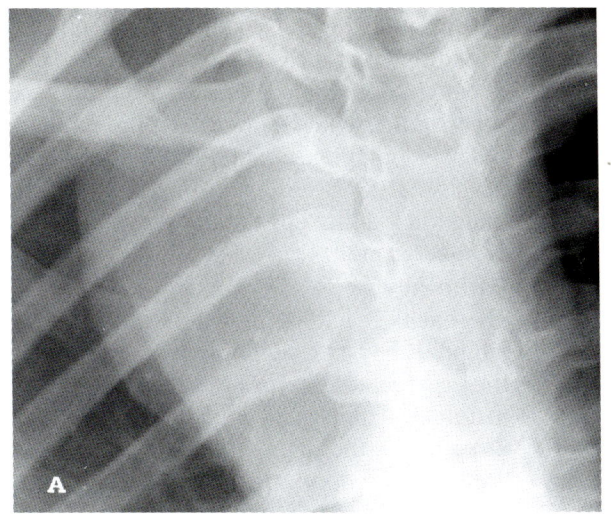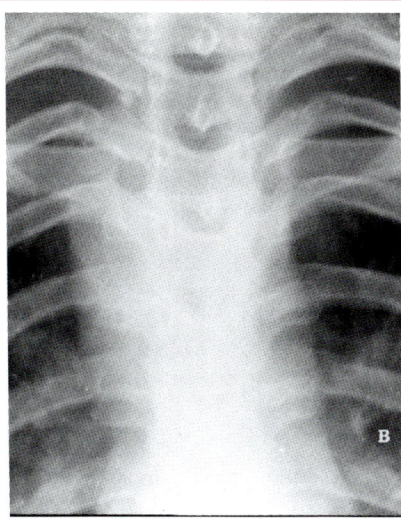

Fig. 42.5. (a) Massive superior mediastinal tuberculous lymphadenopathy, confirmed by core needle biopsy, in a 16 yr. old woman, causing SVC compression; (b) near total resolution with six months of chemotherapy (courtesy: Halsted Surgical Clinic. Chennai)

crushed with instruments, but handled gently by picking it with periglandular areolar tissue. If some traction is needed to facilitate dissection, it may be done by a fine suture placed through the node. It should be kept in a saline soaked gauze swab for microbiology (if indicated) and *formalin* (37% solution of formaldehyde gas in water) fixative for histopathology. As a matter of routine, the nodes are stripped of all the fatty tissue around them and only 'skeletonized' nodes are sent to the pathology department, putting different groups in separate containers

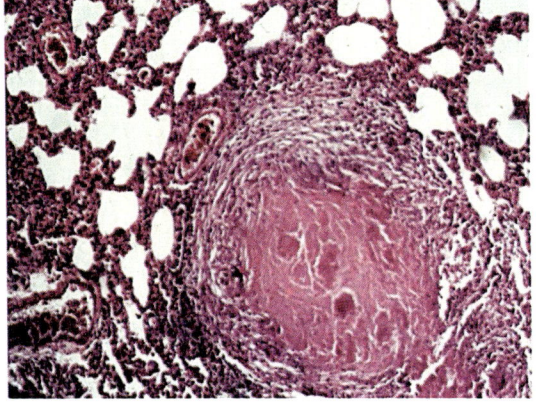

Fig. 42.6. Histology of tubercle
(courtesy: Prof Sandhya Sundaram, Chennai)

and labelled accordingly. It is easy to identify the nodes embedded in soft fat in a fresh surgical specimen, but it may not be so, if it is hardened in formalin.

ACUTE NONSPECIFIC LYMPHADENITIS

This is the result of a septic focus in the drainage area and presents as painful, warm, tender enlargement of one or more lymph nodes, associated with constitutional features. The diagnosis is obvious, if the primary site of infection is evident, which responds promptly to appropriate antibiotics and NSAIDs, but it may evade detection in areas such as the mediastinum and retroperitoneum. The natural course of this disease may be one of the following:

a) resolution

b) suppuration and abscess formation which may form a sinus on breaking down (or surgical incision)

c) drift into chronicity.

ACUTE SPECIFIC LYMPHADENITIS is seen in

conditions such as filariasis, infectious mononucleosis, tuberculosis, lymphogranuloma venereum (LGV), syphilis, bubonic plague etc. they are described under appropriate sections.

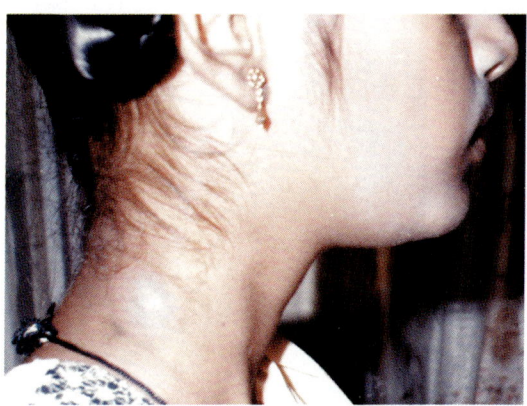

Fig. 42.7. Cold abscess neck
(courtesy: Lifeline Hospitals, Chennai)

CHRONIC NONSPECIFIC (SIMPLE) LYMPH-ADENITIS

Neck nodes are usually involved from smouldering sepsis in the teeth, tonsils, or pediculosis capitis. The inguinal nodes in bare-foot walkers may also be a seat of this disease. Generally a single anatomical group is involved, with a tendency to resolve with or without antibiotic therapy. Suppuration leading to an abscess formation is a common complication, besides causing diagnostic difficulty with other types of chronic lymphadenopathy, such as lymphoma or tuberculosis.

Careful search for a focus of sepsis should be done and for neck nodes, the scalp, ENT/ dental examinations should be routinely done, before a 2-week course of wide spectrum antibiotics is started, covering mixed infections. NSAIDs are generally avoided, unless severe local pain exists, since they mask signs of inflammation and delay detection of an abscess. If an abscess is suspected, it may be confirmed by needling or USG and adequately drained, by Hilton's method, collecting the pus for microbiology (Gm stain and culture), to guide further chemotherapy. With adequate local treatment and eliminating the focus of sepsis, total resolution can be expected in this disease.

CHRONIC SPECIFIC LYMPHADENITIS TUBERCULOSIS

This is the commonest etiology among this group, affecting the young (though no age is exempt), with tonsils and pharynx as the portal of entry for the organism, *Mycobacterium tuberculosis*, which then reaches the submandibular, submental, upper/middle deep cervical *(levels 1,2 & 3)* groups. The usual source of infection is either open pulmonary tuberculosis or infected milk.

Pathology

The bacilli reaching the lymph nodes through lymphatics, excite a granulomatous reaction in the cortex, with the formation of typical histological units, called *tubercles* (by which the disease gets the name), consisting of a central area of *caseation* necrosis, surrounded by lymphocytes, epitheloid and giant cells and finally by fibrosis. The giant cells (*Langhan*), with bits of nuclei eccentrically placed in both poles, are typical but not pathognomonic of the tuberculous process, since they are basically of foreign body type and may be seen in other granulomatous diseases.

The inflammation spreads to adjacent nodes, causing *periadenitis*, responsible for the classical matting of nodes. It differs from infiltrative diseases, such as NHL or metastatic carcinoma, when adjacent nodes may get fixed to each other, by the nodes being flat and distinct grooves being palpated between them. Caseation softens the nodes, 'pus' coming out of them, to form a *cold abscess*, giving the typical variable consistency. Initially developing under the investing cervical fascia, the pus tracks out through the points of entry of vessels and nerves, to lie in the subcutaneous plane, forming the *dumb-bell* or *collar-stud abscess*. If left untreated, the overlying skin gets indurated and ultimately breaks down to form a sinus discharging serous fluid. Hypertrophy of skin with scarring around the sinuses, leads to a condition known as *scrofuloderma*.

Clinical features

Classically seen in patients under 20, as enlarged painful nodes, usually in the upper neck, associated with systemic features like evening fever, night sweats, malaise and loss of apetite/weight. On examination, enlarged, matted lymph nodes are seen, often with signs of local inflammation, such as redness, warmth and tenderness. Presence of associated pulmonary tuberculosis is only an exception and not the rule.

Differential diagnosis other causes of chronic lymphadenopathy

Investigations and treatment: see under especially after an acute lepra reaction to result in a cold abscess.

Investigations

Aspiration of cold abscess, bacteriology of the aspirate (Gm stain and culture) and x-ray of the involved bone are the additional studies, rest as described under abdominal tuberculosis.

Treatment

Basic treatment is 4-drug anti-tuberculous chemotherapy, following diagnostic aspiration.

Therapeutic aspiration at a nondependent site, advocated earlier, has been very unsatisfactory, because the caseous pus is too thick to be retrieved even through the widest bore needle employed. The current practice is to incise, drain and curette (under cover of anti-tuberculous therapy), which has the following advantages:

(a) removing the thick caseous materal helps faster resolution of the swelling

(b) occasionally there may be associated secondary pyogenic infection, which is better treated by liberal drainage, than by aspiration.

(c) often, cold abscess is diagnosed clinically, hence examining the curettings provides clinching histological evidence.

If the patient is adequately covered by anti-tuberculous therapy, the risk of developing a persistent sinus is minimal. Orthopedic treatment for spine disease should be provided on the merits of the situation.

Neoplastic diseases of lymph nodes

There are virtually no benign tumors in relation to lymph nodes; the malignant disease may be primary (lymphoma/ leukemia) or secondary, the latter being more common.

LYMPHOMAS

'Nowhere in pathology has a chaos of names so clouded clear concepts as in the lymphoid tumors' (Willis). The earlier classification of lymphoproliferative disorders into Hodgkin's disease, lymphosarcoma, reticulum cell sarcoma and giant follicle lymphoma (Brill-Symmers disease), has been replaced by the Rappaport classification, based on therapeutic and prognostic considerations, which may be simplified as follows:

1. *Hodgkin's lymphoma* (HL): after Butler & Rye (in general, has better prognosis than NHL)

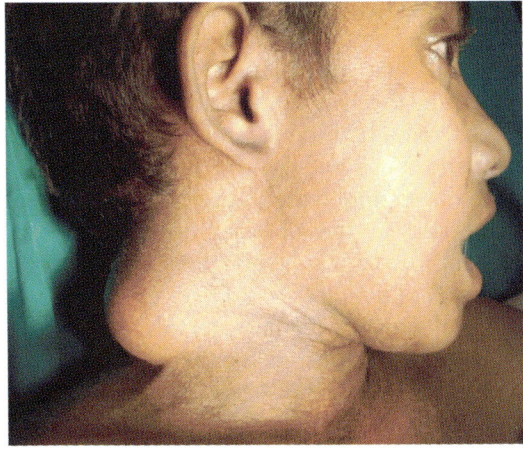

Fig. 42.8. Cold abscess neck
(courtesy: Laxmi Hospital, Kakinada)

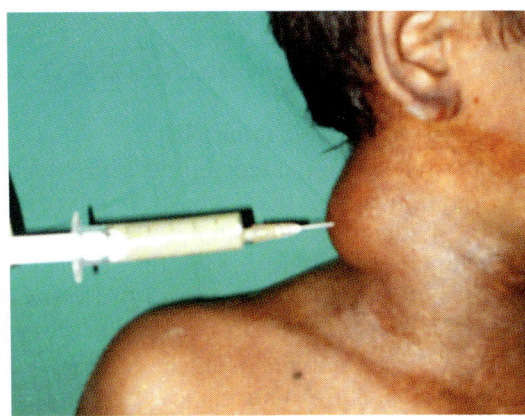

Fig. 42.9. Diagnostic aspiration of a cold abscess

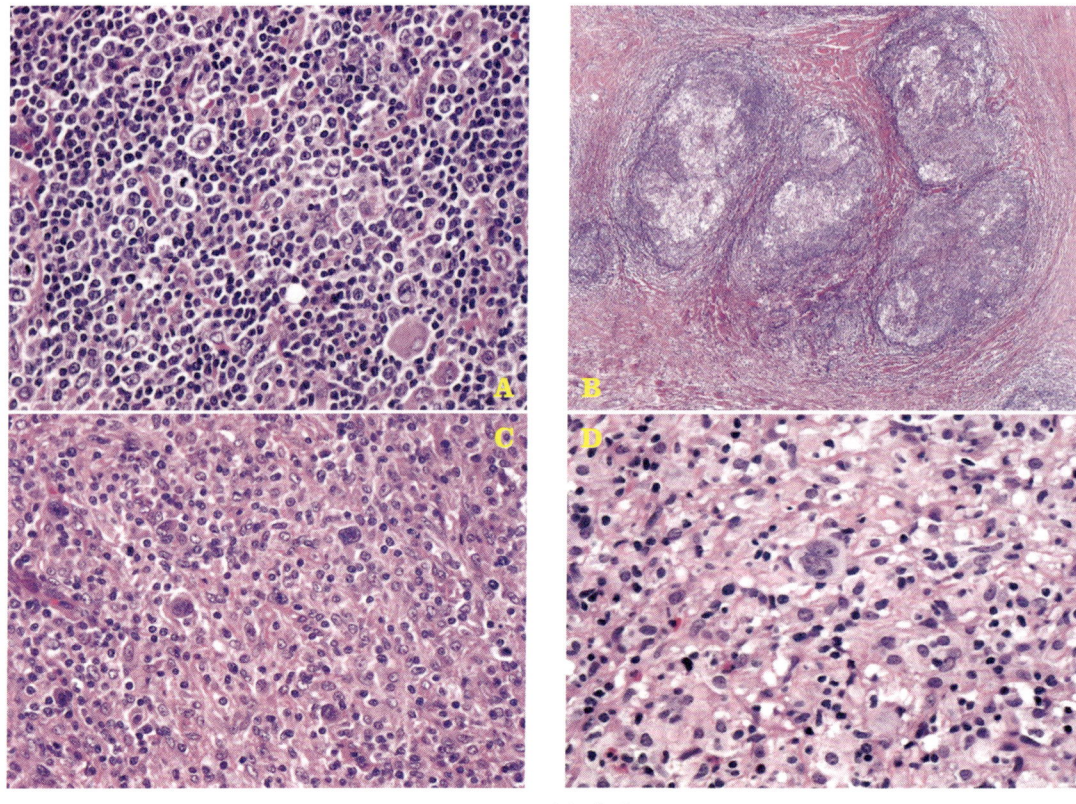

Fig. 42.10. Hodgkin's disease
A. Lymphocyte predominant **B.** Nodular sclerosis
C. Mixed cellularity **D.** Lymphocyte depletion
(courtesy: Prof Sandhya Sundaram, Chennai)

a) lymphocyte predominant (earlier known as paragranuloma, carries best prognosis)
b) nodular sclerosis
c) mixed cellularity
d) lymphocyte depletion (worst prognosis, among HL)

2. *Non-Hodgkin's lymphoma* (NHL)
   a) well differentiated (Broder's I), which may be lymphocytic, histiocytic or mixed
   b) moderately differentiated (Broder's II)
   c) poorly differentiated (Broder's III)
   d) undifferentiated (Broder's IV), a variant of this type is the Burkitt's lymphoma.

3. *Hodgkin's sarcoma*, which has mixed histological features and clinical behavior, a term not much preferred by contemporary pathologists.

HODGKIN'S DISEASE (syn: Hodgkin's lymphoma HL)

Pathology

This is the commonest type of lymphoma, with bimodal age distribution. Macroscopically, except in the lymphocyte depletion type, the nodes remain discrete and rounded, with a rubbery consistency and a fish flesh appearance on section, fixity to each other occurring quite late in the disease. Pruritus may be present due to skin involvement. The periodic fever (*Pel-Ebstein*), considered to be due to tumor necrosis at regular intervals, observed in high grade lesions, is neither constant nor typical of Hodgkin's disease. Previous infection with infectious mononucleosis (Epstein-Barr virus) and HIV may be associated with higher incidences of the disease.

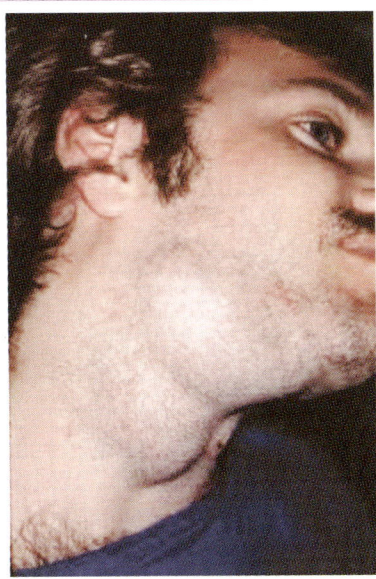

Fig. 42.11. Cervical lymphadenopathy in Hodgkin's disease
(courtesy: Dr C M Kishore, Chennai)

Histologically, four types are described (see above), with progressively worsening prognosis. Cellular pleomorphism and typical mirror-image nucleated Reed-Sternberg (R-S) giant cells are the important features in the diagnosis, besides eosinophilic infiltration. The R-S cells are not the actual cancer cells, represent local tissue response to malignant cells, but have diagnostic and prognostic significance (more the cells, worse the prognosis).

Lymphocyte predominant: nodal architecture is replaced by normal appearing small lymphocytes, with infrequent R-S giant cells.

Nodular sclerosis: frequent bands and collagenous septa, with a population of eosinophils, plasma cells and lymphocytes, in between. Occasional R-S cells seen.

Mixed cellularity: same as the preceding, but without bands and septa and more R-S cells.

Lymphocyte depletion: nodal architecture is totally effaced, with abundant R-S cells. Minimal lymphocytes and disorderly fibrosis are seen.

Clinical staging (Ann Arbour)

Stage 0:   The only lymph node clinically present has been excised for biopsy, leaving no gross residual disease.

Stage I: Involvement of a single group of lymph nodes (90% - 10yr. survival)

Stage II: Involvement of more than one group on one side of diaphragm (90% -10yr. survival)

Stage III: Involvement of groups on either side of diaphragm (75% - 10yr. survival)

Stage IV: Disseminated foci or multiple extra-lymphatic involvement (65% - 10yr. survival). Involvement of one extra-lymphatic site, liver or spleen may not alter the clinical stage.

Involvement of extra-lymphatic sites (E), hepatic (H), spleen (S), bone marrow (M), bone (O), or pleura (P) are indicated with appropriate suffixes to them, like I-E, II-ES etc. Each stage is further subdivided depending upon the absence (A) or presence (B) of constitutional features, such as fever, anorexia, weight loss(>10%), anemia, pruritus, night sweats and bone pains. Suffix of 'X' indicates bulky nodal mass more than 10cm size.

Clinical features

It occurs in the young (2nd and 3rd decades), with a slight male preponderance. Typically painless progressive enlargement of lymph nodes,

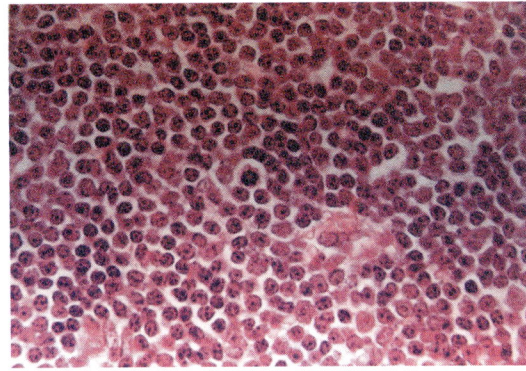

Fig. 42.12. Histology of diffuse large cell lymphoma
(courtesy: Lifeline Hospitals, Chennai)

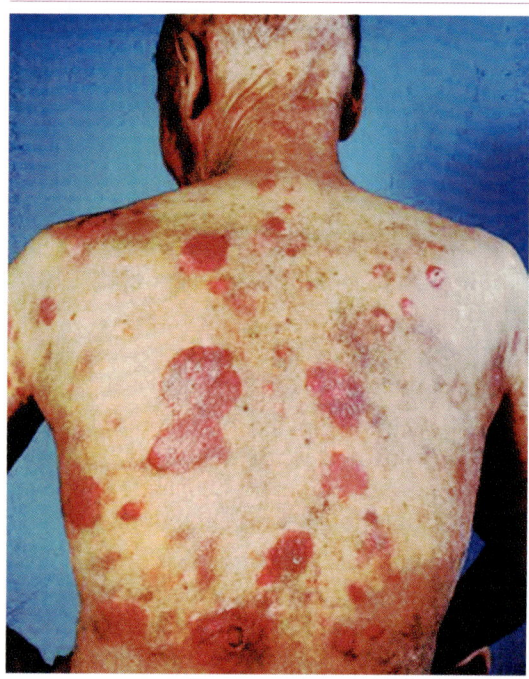

Fig. 42.13. Mycosis fungoides

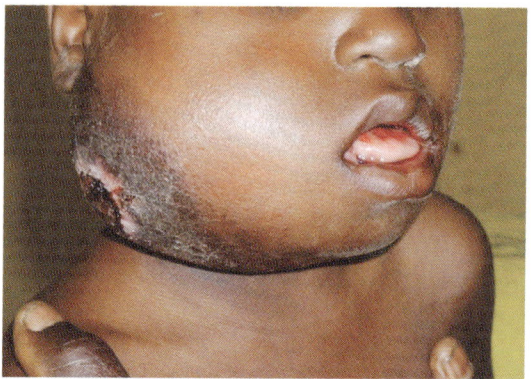

Fig. 42.14. Burkitt's lymphoma

usually the cervical group, followed by axillary and mediastinal groups (the so called centrifugal distribution) is seen, in a contiguous manner with or without the constitutional symptoms mentioned above. Local pain, induced by consumption of alcohol, is a peculiar, but unexplained phenomenon in this disease. Pressure symptoms, such as superior venacaval obstruction (mediastinal disease) or paraplegia (vertebral disease) are not uncommon. Skin involvement may lead to intractable pruritus. Minimal enlargement of liver/spleen is commonly seen. Hyperabduction of both arms causes venous engorgement in the neck, in any SOL compressing the superior vena cava (SVC), such as mediastinal nodes or goitre (Pemberton's sign).

History of reduction in the size of nodes, following some nonspecific treatment by the

	Feature	Hodgkin's	N H L	Tuberculosis	Sarcoidosis
1	Age incidence	Bimodal	>40	<20	20-50
2	Nature of lesion	Malignant	Malignant	Granuloma (caseating)	Granuloma (non-caseating)
3	Fever	Rare	Rare	Common	Rare
4	Weight loss	Common	Common	Common	Rare
5	Nodal distribution	Centrifugal	Centripetal	Often cervical	Hilar
6	Character of nodes	Discrete	Adherent	Matted	Discrete
7	Consistency of nodes	Rubbery	Firm/hard	Variable	Firm
8	Discharging sinuses	Never	Never	Common	Never
9	Hepatosplenomegaly	Common	Rare	Rare	Rare
10	Pulmonary infiltration	Rare	Rare	Common	Common
11	Visceral involvement	Occasional	Common	Occasional	Rare
12	Corticosteroids	Effective	Effective	Not useful	Specific
13	Immunosuppressives	Useful	Useful	Harmful	Not useful
14	Prognosis	Good	Fair	Excellent	Excellent

Table – 42.2. Differentiating features of common types of chronic lymphadenopathy

family physician, does not automatically exclude malignancy, since dramatic resolution may be seen in lymphomas, following *steroid therapy*.

Differential diagnosis

1) tuberculosis: constitutional symptoms, matting, caseation (producing variable consistency) and sinus formation are present. The age, typical distribution and characteristics of the enlarged nodes, make the diagnosis easy in most of the cases.

2) non-Hodgkin's lymphoma: older age, firm/hard, fixed nodes with centripetal distribution

3) Boeck's sarcoidosis: besides hilar nodes, it affects lungs, skin, eyes and intestines and Kveim-Siltzbach skin test is positive.

4) nonspecific lymphadenitis: due to a focus of sepsis

Investigations

Blood examination for anemia and eosinophilia, specific studies include, node biopsy and immunohistochemistry (IHC), chest x-ray, USG of abdomen, CT scan of chest. Currently PET-CT and Gallium scan are being increasingly employed for a comprehensive staging of the disease.

Gordon's biological test: production of encephalitis in rabbits, by intracerebral injection of the extract of the lymph node of Hodgkin's disease, is not routinely done.

Markers of worse prognosis

a) tumor bulk
b) stage
c) histopatholgy (grade)
d) presence of constitutional symptoms (B-stage)
e) low hematocrit at presentation (bone marrow involvement)
f) high LDH (liver involvement)

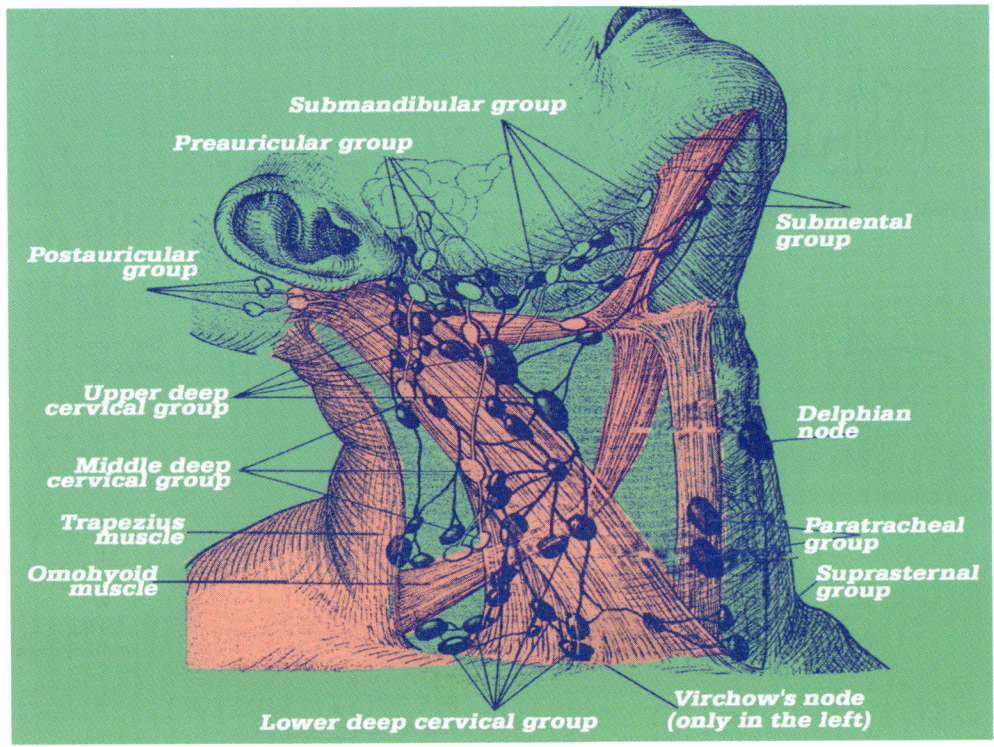

Fig. 42.15. Various groups of cervical lymph nodes

Staging laparotomy: Once very popular, but now sparingly performed, owing to the advent of noninvasive imaging methods. Realization that systemic chemotherapy should be given in all stages of the disease, has also made detection of some tiny intra-abdominal focus, therapeutically insignificant, obviating such an operative diagnostic exercise.

Even by its proponents, it is recommended only for those patients with histologically aggressive disease and without obvious infra-diaphragmatic disease, when positive findings may alter staging/therapy/prognosis. It consists of thorough exploration of all the abdominal viscera and lymph nodes (removed for biopsy, if necessary), liver biopsy, splenectomy, iliac bone biopsy and in women, median fixation of ovaries (to keep them away from the radiation field). Nowadays, in those few situations where it is felt necessary, it has been replaced by minimally invasive (diagnostic) laparoscopy.

Mediastinal lymphadenopathy

For mediastinal lymphadenopathy, earlier practiced mediastionoscopy is given up since its yield in establishing the diagnosis is only 50%. Instead, a contrast-enhanced CT (CECT) and transbronchial needle aspiration (TBNA), with or without the aid of endobronchial ultrasound (EBUS) are currently employed to establish the diagnosis.

Treatment protocol in a nut-shell:

a) Role of surgery:

   (i) to establish diagnosis

   (ii) strictly localized and easily removable nodes may be excised for 'debulking' advantage, upto stages I and II.

b) Role of radiotherapy: as curative upto stage III-A, including cervical, axillary, mediastinal, abdominal and ilioinguinal groups (mantle or inverted 'Y' field), protecting the vital organs

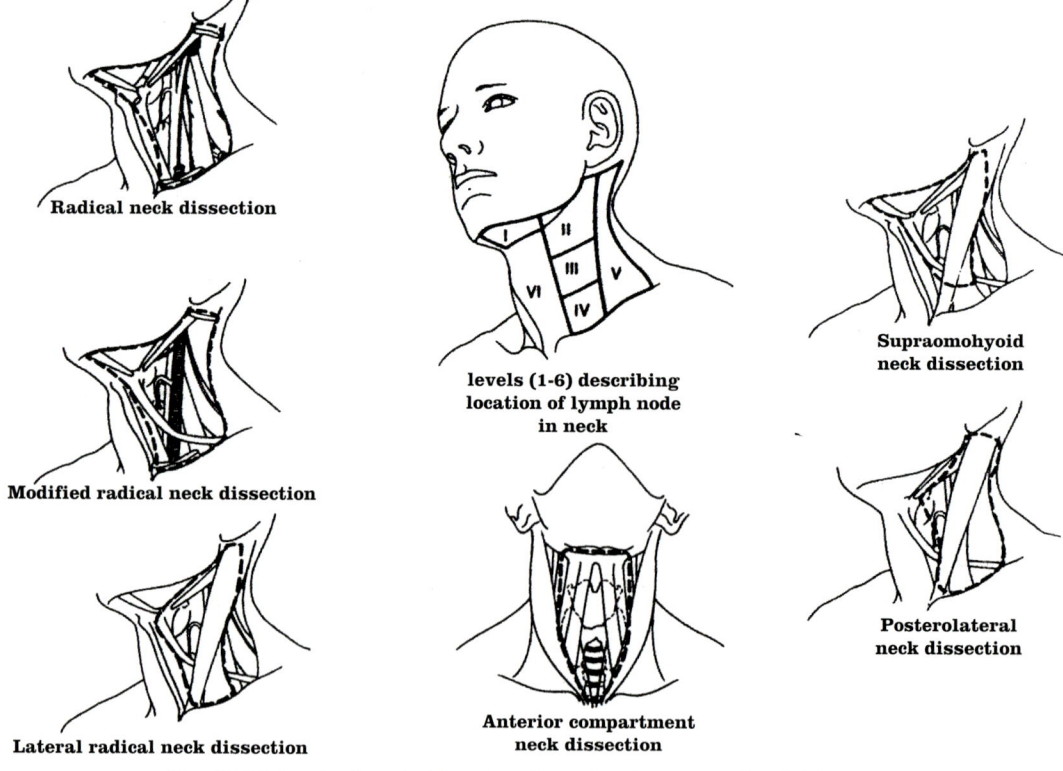

Radical neck dissection

Modified radical neck dissection

Lateral radical neck dissection

levels (1-6) describing location of lymph node in neck

Anterior compartment neck dissection

Supraomohyoid neck dissection

Posterolateral neck dissection

Fig. 42.16. Levels of cervical lymph nodes and various types of nodal dissection

with lead shields. Only palliative form of RT is given for III-B and IV disease. The two common modalities of RT are involved field radiotherapy (IFRT) and extended field radiotherapy (EFRT)

c) Role of chemotherapy: *This is given in all stages*, realizing the systemic nature of the disease. Cyclical combination chemotherapy for 6-9months, either with Mechlorethamine (nitrogen musturd), Oncovin (vincristine), Prednisolone and Procarbazine (MOPP) as first line and Adriamycin, Bleomycin, Vincristine and Prednisolone (ABVP) as second line regime.

It is a highly radiosensitive and chemo-sensitive disease, with >80% cure rate, if treated early.

The causes of death in lymphomas are:

(1) immunosuppresion leading to opportunistic infections

(2) conversion into acute leukemia, under the influence of cytotoxic therapy. Other complications include: anemia/thrombocytopenia, pulmonary fibrosis, infertility etc. The second line (ABVP) regime is preferred to MOPP by many, because of the high risk of developing myelodysplasia or acute myeloid leukemia (AML) with the latter.

(3) other complications of radio/chemotherpy.

Management of advanced/recurrent disease: Aggressive chemo-radiation, made possible by autologous bone marrow transplantation (BMT), may be attempted to achieve cure

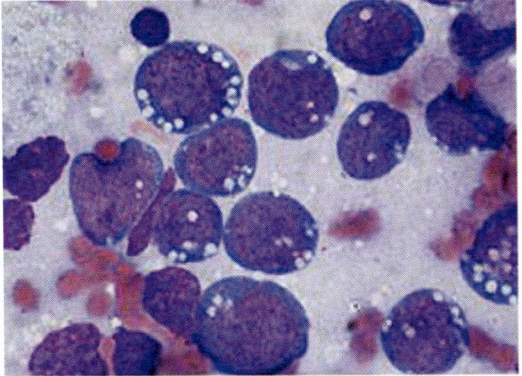

Fig. 42.17. Histology of Burkitt's lymphoma
Note "starry sky" appearance

(rarely) or remission (often). Complications of such aggressive therapy include hypothyroidism, infertility, avascular necrosis of femoral head, secondary neoplasms and neurological complications (due to radiation &/or vincristine).

NON-HODGKIN'S LYMPHOMA (NHL)

The clinical presentation, differential diagnosis, investigations and management of early or advanced disease, is similar to Hodgkin's disease; only salient differences are mentioned here. The working classification of NHL is largely based on pattern (follicular or diffuse), cell type (small or large, lymphocytic, immunoblastic or lymphoblastic) and nuclear cleaving (small or large cleaved). Tumors with follicular pattern, small lymphocytic type, with small cleaved nuclei carry favorable prognosis. With the advent of immunohistochemistry (IHC) and molecular biology, Revised European American Lymphoma (REAL) classification, based on clinical, morphological, genetic features and surface markers, has been proposed. More sophisticated WHO classification is also currently available. Primary cutaneous lymphoma, known as *mycosis fungoides*, is a rare phenomenon, involving T-lymphocytes; lymph nodes and viscera may be involved later. This may also be encountered in Hodgkin's disease; sometimes circulating malignant cells with convoluted nuclei are seen, known as Sizary cells. Certain infections have been incriminated in the etiology of NHL, such as H pylori for bowel and Borrelia for skin involvement.

Occuring in older age group, centripetally distributed, high prevalence to soft tissue and visceral involvement, firm/hard nodes, with early fixity by perinodal infiltration and carries a poor prognosis compared to HL.

It has been observed that those with NHL of testes, paranasal sinuses and bone marrow have special predilection for CNS involvement, hence CSF analysis/cytology should be done in such cases, to consider intrathecal chemotherapy, if necessary.

Treatment

A combination of Cyclophosphamide, Oncovin, Prednisolone and Procarbazine (COPP) is the first line and ABVP (as for Hodgkin's) is the second line chemotherapeutic regime. Administration of targeted therapy using monoclonal antibodies, in the recent times has improved overall results (see chapter 34 on chemotherapy)

Follow up protocol: the patients in remission, after initial treatment should be reviewed once in 3 months for 2 years and 6 monthly thereafter. Thorough physical examination, routine blood counts, liver function tests (LFT) and chest skiagram, are performed during each visit, with USG/CT/ PET scan, if warranted.

Differences between common diseases presenting with generalized lymphadenopathy are given in Table 42.2

BURKITT'S LYMPHOMA (syn: malignant lymphoma of Africa, Burkitt's tumor)

Initially this disease of children was reported as endemic in Africa and Guinea, but it is now known to occasionally occur in other parts of the world. Its incidence appears to overlap that of malaria, but their relation is unclear, and is possibly a heightened immunological response. Reciprocal translocation of chromosomes 8-14 has been linked with this disease.

Pathology

A vectored *Ebstein-Barr* virus, similar to one that causes infectious mononucleosis, is responsible for this predominantly extranodal 'infective lymphoma'. It is a rapidly growing highly undifferentiated B cell tumor of multicentric origin, primarily affecting the jaws and kidneys. Other organs often involved are CNS, gonads, vertebrae, breasts and thyroid, but peripheral lymph nodes are rarely affected. Untreated, it may prove rapidly fatal, but spontaneous regression has occasionally been reported.

Microscopically dense masses of darkly stained primitive lymphoid cells, interspersed with large clear histiocytes, giving an appearance of a *starry night*.

Clinical features

Mostly seen in children between 4 and 8 and rare after 20, with male preponderance (2:1), presenting as facial, abdominal tumors and CNS manifestations, such as headache, cranial nerve palsies, altered sensorium etc. Painless skeletal involvement occurs in vertebra, femur, humerus, tibia and ilium.

Differential diagnosis

1. osteogenic sarcoma: occurs at slightly older age, unifocal, painful and rapidly metastasizing.

2. other types of lymphomas

Investigations

Soft tissue and skeletal survey by nuclear imaging, x-rays and biopsy to establish tissue diagnosis.

Treatment

It is highly radio/chemosensitive and combination therapy is recommended, as RT alone may induce development of tumors in other parts. Role of surgery is limited to establishing diagnosis (biopsy) or removal of large ovarian tumors.

Jewels of Gyan - 42.2

Rules of 80% for neck nodes

80% of neck mases are malignant

80% of neoplasms occur in men

80% of neoplasms are metastatic

80% of patients with metastatic nodes are elderly

80% of metastatic nodes in neck are from primaries located above clavicle

Tumors	Suggested Immunohistochemistry
Large round cell	Keratin
	Leukocyte common antigen (LCA)
	S100
Small round cell	LCA
	Keratin
	Desmin
	Vimentin
	Chromogranin
Spindle cell	S100
	HMB 45 (Melanoma-specific antigen)
	Keratin
? Mesothelioma	Keratin
	Carcinoembryonic antigen (CEA)
	Leu M_1
Adenocarcinoma? site	Cystic disease fluid protein
	Thyroglobulin
	Prostatic acid phosphatase
	Prostate-specific antigen (PSA)

Table 42.3. Immunohistochemical stains to aid in identifying unknown primary tumors

SECONDARY CARCINOMA

As oral and pharyngeal cancers are among the commonest cancers in India, secondary malignant lymphadenopathy of the neck is extremely common. In the first four decades of life, thyroid and nasopharyngeal malignancies are responsible, but beyond 50, oral, pharyngeal and laryngeal cancers form the common primary sites for metastatic neck nodes.

The predilection for a tumor to spread to lymphatics appears to be decided by the presence of a specific complementary molecule in it.

Distribution of cervical lymph nodes

The main lymph nodes in the neck, called the deep cervical lymph nodes, are all arranged vertically along the carotid sheath and internal jugular vein, and they drain the afferent lymphatics from various lymphatic zones. These are broadly divided into superior, middle and inferior deep cervical groups. *Waldeyer* had earlier classified the nodes graphically into one vertical chain of nodes on either side (deep cervical) and two horizontal circles namely the outer and the inner rings (of Waldeyer). The

inner ring comprises the tonsils (lingual and faucial), lymphoid tissue around the Eustachian tube and the adenoids. The *outer ring* comprises of the sublingual, submental, submandibular, jugulodigastric (upper deep cervical), retropharyngeal, preauricular, retroauricular and the occipital group.

It is now customary to describe the cervical nodes by levels:

Level-I: *Submental* group: Nodes between two anterior bellies of digastric and the hyoid bone and the submandibular group of nodes bounded by posterior belly of digastric and body of the mandible.

Level-II: *Upper deep jugular* group: Lymph nodes around the upper third of the jugular vein and adjacent spinal accessory nerve extending from the level of carotid bifurcation to the skull base. Tonsillar node is included in this group.

Level-III: *Middle deep jugular* group: Nodes around middle third of the internal jugular vein extending from level, carotid bifurcation superiorly to the cricothyroid notch inferiorly.

Level-IV: *Lower deep jugular* group: Lymph nodes located around the lower third of the internal jugular vein extending from the cricothyroid notch to the clavicle.

Level-V: *Posterior triangle* group: Nodes located along the lower half of the spinal accessory nerve and the transverse cervical artery. The supraclavicular (*Virchow's*) nodes are also included in this group, located between the anterior border of trapezius and the posterior border of SCM muscle.

Level-VI: *Anterior compartment* group: Lymph nodes in relation to the midline structures of the neck extending from the hyoid to suprasternal notch, between the two SCMs, consisting of the perithyroid, paratracheal, prelaryngeal (*Delphian*), precricoid lymph nodes and those in suprasternal space (of *Burns*).

It should be realized that level of nodes is only for *anatomical identification* and has no relevance to the stage of the disease.

Virchow's node

These are left supraclavicular nodes, located in relation to the termination of the thoracic duct, at the confluence of the internal jugular and subclavian veins, in front of scalene muscles, best palpated between the sternal and clavicular heads of the SCM, against the background of scalene muscles, either by standing behind (preferable) or in front of the patient. Involvement of these lymph nodes indicates advanced malignancy of abdominal/thoracic viscera (*Troisier's sign*), stomach being the

commonest organ. This is considered to be due to the retrograde embolization of tumor cells into these nodes, from the obstructed termination of the thoracic duct.

Clinical staging of cervical metastatic nodes:

Nx	lymph nodes cannot be assessed
N0	no metastasis
N1	metastasis in a single node, homo-lateral <3 cm size
N2a	metastasis in a single node, 3 - 6 cm size
N2b	multiple nodes on the same side
N2c	bilateral nodes <6cm size
N3	any node >6 cm and fixed.

Clinical features

Besides the painless lump in the neck, the patient may present symptoms suggestive of primary disease, such as nasal block/ epistaxis (nasopharynx), dysphagia (posterior tongue/ hypopharynx), hoarseness of voice (larynx/ thyroid), hemoptysis (larynx) etc. In late stages, the nodes may ulcerate, bleed or fungate, with offensive odor, adding to the malady. Each group of nodes is inspected/ palpated systematically and findings noted. A very useful maneuver to palpate minimally enlarged nodes under SCM is to pinch the muscles with fingers and move the hand up and down, to feel for the nodes slipping under the fingers.

They are usually multiple, hard and mobile in early stages, but get fixed later on. It should be realized that in most situations, when we say

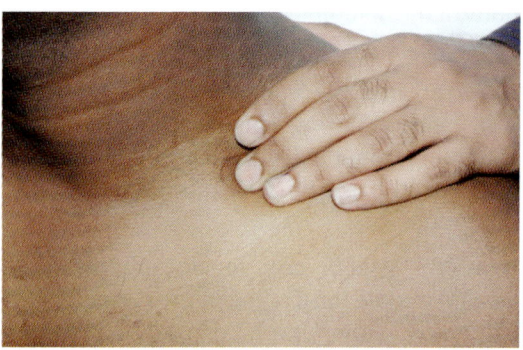

Fig. 42.18. Palpation of Virchow's node

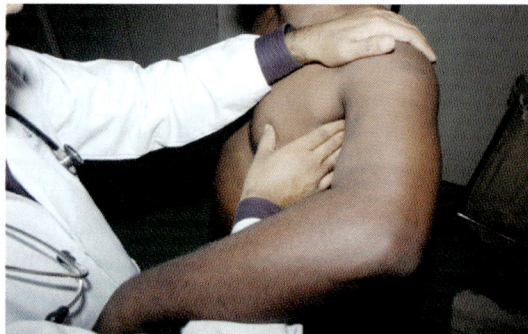

Fig. 42.19. Palpation of axillary nodes

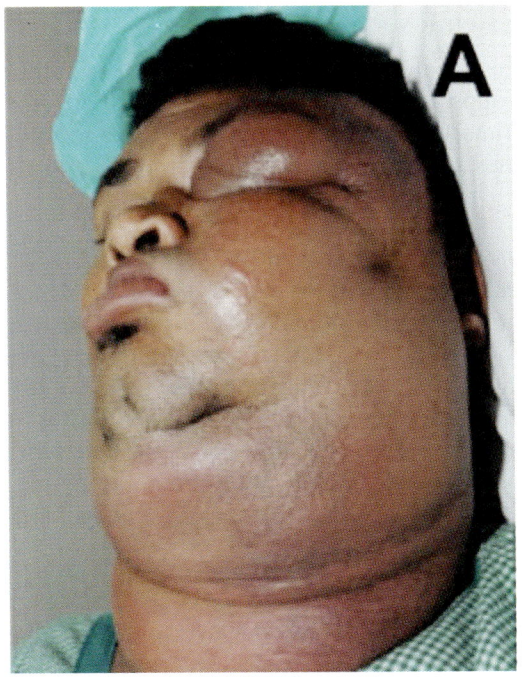
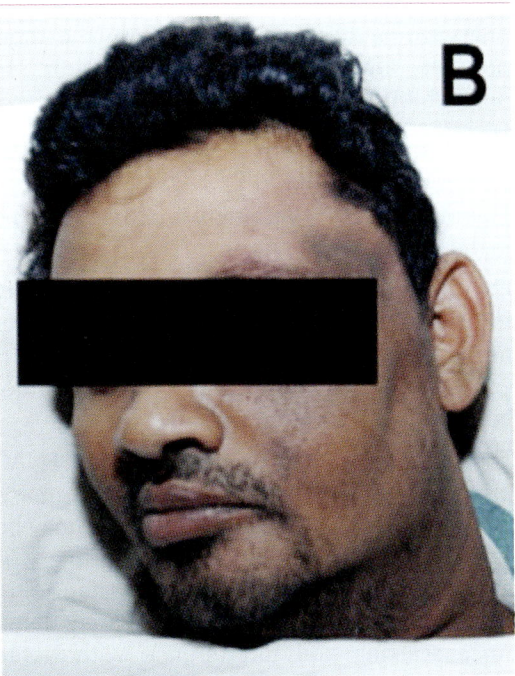

Fig. 42.20. A. Acute left submandibular lymphadenitis due to dental sepsis, causing extensive cellulitis of the neck and face; **B.** Near total resolution with high antibiotics for two weeks
(courtesy: Lifelife Hospitals, Chennai)

the nodes are 'fixed', it implies fixity to the adjacent bone, since some movement can always be appreciated even if there is infiltration into fascia, muscle, vessels etc. In the neck however, owing to proximity of vital structures, restricted movement of a large mass, may be taken as 'fixity', to denote non-resectability. Infiltration into the prevertebral fascia/muscles, may also grossly limit the movement, to the point of 'fixity'. A laryngeal crepitus, elicited by side-to-side movement of the larynx by two fingers, in normal individuals, may be lost in hypopharyngeal growth or any SOL, which separates the larynx from the vertebral column (*Bocca's sign*).

Differential diagnosis

a) inflammatory nodes are soft, bilateral and usually <3 cm size, with an identifiable focus of sepsis.

b) lymphoma: they are firm/hard in NHL and rubbery in HL, other groups such as axillary or inguinal may be involved.

c) tumors of lower pole of parotid, tend to have the upper border merge with the main gland, over the mandible.

d) tumors of the submandibular gland exhibit bidigital palpability, but when only the external part is involved, it may be clinically indistinguishable from an enlarged lymph node. Multiplicity may be the only feature in favor of nodes.

e) carotid body tumors are rubbery, with a typical location and transmitted pulsations owing to the relation to the carotid fork. These lesions also have a very indistinct upper border.

f) Branchial cyst has a typical location, cystic consistency and occurs in the younger age.

Investigations

Laryngoscopy: Standard indirect or direct laryngoscopy, for the valleculae, epiglottis, vocal cords, has to be done, but they have several 'blind spots', such as pyriform sinuses, subglottic larynx etc. Flexible, video-guided pharyngo-laryngoscopy is currently the most popular and foolproof investigation, to detect/biopsy occult malignancies.

CT/MRI: these are valuable in deep-seated primaries, such as nasopharynx.

Thyroid scintiscan, if primary is suspected to be in the gland.

FNAC: This has 90% sensitivity and specificity for a neck mass. The largest node, without necrosis should be chosen and if the report is equivocal, it may be repeated by using a wide-bore needle (Tru-cut).

The ideal approach is to complement the FNAC of the secondary with a biopsy of primary, though when one is positive, the other may be superfluous, but tissue from the primary is always preferable, to that of a metastatic site. Open biopsy of the lymph node is rarely done, since scarring and interference with tissue planes may compromise the subsequent lymph node dissection, if needed. By breaking the fascial barriers that hold the cancer invasion, open biopsy increases the chances of local recurrence, following subsequent excision. It is to be realized that squamous head and neck cancers rarely spread beyond the neck and the usual cause of death in these patients, is hemorrhage from carotid invasion due to local recurrence, hence the general resentment against open biopsy, for neck nodes.

If a complete head and neck physical examination is nonrevealing, a more detailed visual and digital examination of the neck, mouth, pharynx and larynx under anesthesia, as well as aerodigestive endoscopy should be done. If this also draws a blank, blind biopsies from nasopharynx, tonsils, tonsillar beds, base of tongue and pyriform fossa are performed, with >10% yield of detecting primary, in such situations. However, in recent times, such 'wild-goose chasing' is largely obviated by the use of CT/MRI/PET imaging, which not only locate, but delineate the relation of the lesion to vital structures, to enable appropriate therapeutic strategy to be worked out.

Systemic survey

This should include examination of other groups of lymph nodes and search for the primary as mentioned above and other secondaries, visceral or skeletal.

Cervical nodes with occult primary

The occult primary (30%) indicates that the secondary metastatic nodes arise from a primary that is too small to be clinically made out. About 50% of them are SCC, 25% are adenocarcinoma and the rest (25 %) are anaplastic tumors. The occult primary sites in the order of frequency are: nasopharynx, tonsil, base of tongue, floor of mouth, thyroid, larynx, pyriform fossa, broncho-esophagus and stomach.

Branchiogenic carcinoma?

A node without an obvious primary (after thorough investigations) was often labeled empirically as a branchiogenic carcinoma (carcinoma arising from a branchial remnant), but such a diagnosis is acceptable only if:

a)   there is survival without recurrence for 5 years after surgical extirpation (ex: out; stirps: root) of the nodes.

b)   a biopsy from the sites mentioned above were negative for malignancy

c)   histological proof of origin from tissues in branchial vestiages can be obtained.

d)   the tumor is anterior to the upper third of SCM muscle.

However, *no documented case of 'branchiogenic carcinoma', satisfying these criteria is available to date*; it is possible that heterotopic squamous epithelium in the lymph node is the site of origin of such a pathological curiosity.

Treatment of neck secondaries

Without clinically palpable metastasis (N0)

There is considerable debate regarding *prophylactic* neck dissection (before clinically palpable nodes appear); earlier consensus against it, is being questioned in light of current experience.

Factors in favor of prophylactic nodal surgery are:

a) incidence of microscopic spread in N0 is around 10-15%.

b) morbidity and recurrence rate is higher when dissection is done for clinically palpable nodes

c) block dissection carries negligible mortality

d) neck disease is the common cause of death, in head and neck cancers

Factors against such aggressive approach are:

a) vast majority (85-90%) of them never require neck surgery later

b) filtering advantage of nodes is lost, in case of local recurrence or development of a second primary

c) prophylactic surgery does not totally eliminate the possibility of later nodal secondaries

d) there is no hard proof that it improves overall survivals

Unilateral lymph nodes (N1)

The earlier practise of functional neck dissection, sparing the SCM, spinal accessory nerve and internal jugular vein, has been given up in preference to standard block dissection, except for papillary thyroid carcinoma (PTC).

Metastasis in multiple nodes (N2a/b)

The treatment is radical neck dissection followed by postoperative radiotherapy.

Bilateral neck nodes, under 6cm size (N2c)

These occur in 5% of cancers and are of unfavourable prognostic significance, with only 5% survivals after 5years. If mobile, bilateral neck dissection at the same sitting is an acceptable approach. The most important complication is raised intracranial tension (ICT). It is shown that following ligation of one internal jugular vein, there is a three fold increase in the ICT, lasting for 12 hours, which reaches to five fold, lasting much longer, when the second one is also interrupted at the same time. Some methods to avoid this complication include infusion of

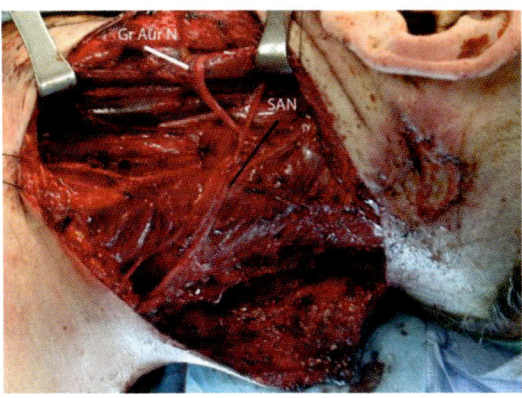

Fig. 42.21. Appearance at the completion of right sided neck dissection, preserving IJV.

mannitol (acceptable), avoiding tight compressed postoperative dressing (acceptable), keep the patient in erect/sitting position (impractical), removal of CSF (dangerous, may precipitate coning)

Nodes above 6cm and fixed (N3)

If the metastatic nodes are fixed to the deeper structures &/or there is distant metastasis, palliative radio/chemotherapy therapy is the only option available. In locally advanced disease, without distant spread, this may downstage the disease, allowing subsequent salvage surgery.

Types of block dissection in the neck

a) Standard unilateral or bilateral block dissection (Crile), from mandible to clavicle

b) Functional modification of standard dissection (Bocca), limited at the present time, to papillary carcinoma of thyroid or prophylactic nodal dissection in clinically N0 status.

c) Selective neck dissection, depending upon the primary site

i) supraomohyoid dissection - removing submental, submandibular, upper/mid-jugular groups (levels I, II & III), for tumors of lip, anterior tongue, floor of mouth and cheek

ii) posterolateral dissection - removing suboccipital, retroauricular, upper/mid-jugular and posterior triangle groups (levels II, III, IV & V), for tumors of naso-pharynx or posterior scalp

iii) lateral dissection - upper, middle and lower jugular groups (levels II, III & IV), for tumors of pharynx and larynx

iv) anterior compartment - dissection removing perithyroidal, paratracheal, prelaryngeal and precricoid nodes (level VI), for thyoid cancers

v) node (berry) picking operation - done for papillary carcinoma of thyroid, earlier practiced, has been given up in preference to functional neck dissection.

Functional neck dissection (Bocca)

This has been introduced during the evolution of cancer surgery in the last 4 decades, where more radical and mutilative procedures (such as commando operation) have been abandoned in preference to limited but adequate clearance and adjuvant chemo/radiotherapy. The additional morbidity of sacrificing the SCM, internal jugular vein and spinal accessory nerve has not translated into improved cure rates, similar to the experience of radical mastectomy for breast carcinoma. *However, at the present time, it is limited to papillary carcinoma of thyroid, prophylactic nodal dissection for N0 status in head and neck cancers and on the lesser involved side, during bilateral radical dissection, to retain at least one of the internal jugular veins.*

There are three types of modified (functional) neck dissection

Type 1: sparing spinal acces. nerve (SAN)
Type 2: sparing SAN + int. jugular vein (IJV)
Type 3: sparing SAN + IJV + SCM muscle

Technique of standard block dissection: All the strap muscles, groups of nodes and node-bearing fat, omohyoid, SCM, scalenus anticus, internal jugular vein, spinal accessory nerve and submandibular salivary glands are removed. The acronym for the order of dissection is IPADS: inferior, posterior, anterior, deep and superior. Several incisions have been used for the standard dissection, 'T' shaped (Crile), 'Y' shaped (Ward), double 'Y' (Martin) and ladder (MacFee) incisions.

The principle of all these incisions is to give maximum exposure to the underlying structures, while preserving the vascularity of the flaps. The flaps are raised from the inferior incision and entire fibroareolar tissue from the anterior border of trapezius to the posterior border of the SCM is elevated. The lower end of the SCM is cut, then the omohyoid is severed and the phrenic nerve, coursing in front of scalenus anticus is identified and preserved, while dividing the scalene muscle. The internal jugular vein is dissected from the common carotid and vagus, ligated at the lowest point and reflected upwards dissecting all the nodes along with it. Then the attention is directed towards the posterior border and all the fibroareolar tissue from the base of the floor of the posterior triangle is cleared up to the mastoid process.

This is followed by dissection of the anterior compartment. The main aspect of this is the submandibular salivary gland dissection along with dissection of submental/submandibular nodes, dissection is done until the anterior midline, from symphysis menti to suprasternal space (of Burns). In the fourth step the deep dissection is done and scalenus anticus is removed. The internal jugular vein and the nodes are dissected upwards upto the hypoglossal nerve. Then the spinal accessory nerve is sacrificed, only if it is involved in the tumor process. The operation is finally com-

Jewels of Gyan - 42.3

The advantages of functional modification are:

a) lesser procedure

b) better neck and shoulder functions

c) protection of carotids by the muscle, reducing the risk of secondary hemorrhage

d) since internal jugular vein is not disturbed, bilateral dissection is possible at the same time

pleted by clearing the superior border, with its submental and submandibular connections and this is carried posteriorly over the lower pole of the parotid to the mastoid process and is completed by transecting the jugular vein at the upper border. The following nerves are preserved vagus, hypoglossal, lingual and the mandibular branch of the facial nerve.

Complications of radical neck dissection

The major complications, their prevention and treatment are much the same as inguinal nodal dissection, namely flap necrosis, lymph collection, lymphorrhea, lymphedema of the limb and secondary hemorrhage, their prevention and treatment are described in chapter 33. Muscle flap of intact SCM or divided/rotated levator scapulae, is fixed over the carotid sheath, to protect the vessels and to prevent secondary hemorrhage. Free tissue grafts have also been tried to cover skeletonized vessels, but they are less effective and not popular.

Other causes of lymphadenopathy

BOECK'S SARCOIDOSIS (Schaumann's disease)

It is a non-caseating, non-infectious granulomatous disease seen in young adults, with widespread involvement of mainly lymphoreticular system and also lungs, eyes, skin and intestines, of uncertain etiology.

Clinically several groups of lymph nodes are enlarged, firm, discrerte and nontender. Hilar adenopathy and pulmonary infiltration are characteristic. Other organs involved include, liver, spleen, heart, parotid glands and central nervous system.

Differential diagnosis

Hodgkin's disease, tuberculosis, bronchogenic carcinoma, Sjogren's syndrome, Crohn's disease etc.

Investigations

Chest x-ray, intradermal test (Kveim-Siltzbach) and node biopsy. Serum angiotensin converting enzyme (ACE) is elevated in 60% of patients. Gallium-69 scintiscan will reveal activity in lymph nodes, lung and salivary glands. In patients with active disease, bronchoalveolar

lavage (BAL) fluid will show increased lymphocytes, particularly CD-4 positive, T-helper/inducer cells.

Treatment

Corticosteroids are specific and often curative. Topical steroids are useful in skin/eye disease. Agents, such as methotrexate, hydroxychloroquine, azathioprine or chlorambucil also have been tried in refractory cases.

Syphilitic lymphadenitis

It is primarily an STD, though congenital and non-sexual/extragenital types are present, caused by a delicate spirochete, *Treponema pallidum*, in which lymph nodes are involved in all the three stages. The classical lymph nodes of *primary* syphilis are firm, shotty, painless and discrete, without signs of local inflammation or suppuration, associated with a Hunterian genital chancre. In the adenopathy in extragenital chancres, however, secondary pyogenic infection may sometimes supervene. *Secondary* syphilis, generalized painless shotty lymphadenopathy occurs, with predilection for epitrochilear, suboccipital and postauricular nodes. Pink, macular, non-itching, symmetrical, cutaneous erruptions usually accompany lymphadenopathy and mucocutaneous lesions like condylomas (perianal) or snail-track or serpiginous ulcers (oral/anal) are also seen. Very rarely lymph nodes are seen in the *tertiary* stage, although it predominantly affects the CVS or CNS.

Investigations

They are described in chapter 54 on tongue. Treponema pallidum may also be demonstrated in the scrapings of the chancre or mucocutaneous lesions.

Treatment

Penicillin is the treatment of choice; macrolides (erythromycin), tetracyclines and ceftriaxone, may be used as an alternative in patients, hypersensitive to penicillin.

Filarial lymphadenitis (see under filariasis, chapter 41)

It is due to a combined pathology, infection

257

occurring because of the filarial parasite, complicated by secondary bacterial infection.

The treatment of choice is a combination of anti-filarial and broad spectrum antibiotics.

Lymphogranuloma venereum (LGV)

It is a systemic STD, seen in tropics, caused by *Chlamydia trachomatis* (Chlamydia A), same organism responsible for chlamydial urethritis. Occasional transmission by non-sexual contact, formites or laboratory accidents have been reported.

Clinical features

Three stages are recognized: primary (local), secondary (inguinal) and tertiary (anogenital) stages.

The primary genital lesion develops from 3-20 days after exposure, as a small painless vesicle or non-indurated ulcer or papule over the penis. It heals in a few days without a scar. In women and in homosexuals, primary anal or rectal infection develops after receptive anal intercourse. From the primary site. the organism spreads via lymphatics, commonly presenting in heterosexual men as the inguinal syndrome, characterised by painful inguinal lymphadenopathy, associated with constitutional symptoms, beginning 2 to 6 weeks after exposure.

The inguinal adenopathy, known as *bubo* (boubon: groin), may be unilateral or bilateral and may involve iliac nodes also. The nodes are initially discrete but progressive periadenitis converts them into a matted mass of nodes, which get liquefied and become fluctuant. The overlying skin becomes fixed, inflamed, thin and finally breaks down, to form nonhealing sinuses. Extensive enlargement of the chain of inguinal nodes both above and below the inguinal ligament results in the *grooving sign*, which although not specific, is most commonly seen in LGV.

In late stages, there is lymphatic obstruction and anorectal inflammation. Perineal lymphedema may produce masses or genital elephantiasis (esthiomene), with susceptibility to perianal suppuration and recto-vaginal fistula, ultimately leading to scarring and *anal strictures*.

Histology

Infected nodes are found to have characterisic, small, stellate abscesses surrounded by histiocytes, which often contain inclusion bodies (Levinthal-Cole-Lilly), diagnostic of chlamydial infection. These abscesses coalesce to form large, necrotic foci.

Investigations

1) Isolation of the causative organism, by culturing the aspirate from the bubo, on McCoy cells.

2) Complement fixation test (CFT) is specific when progressively rising titres are demonstrated during the disease process.

3) Immunoglobulin-M microimmunofluorescence (MIF) test is more sensitive than CFT.

4) Frei's test is less frequently done nowadays, but may be of some value in ruling out LGV. This is a skin test using antigen made from the exudate of a suppurated lymph node. Erythema and induration after 48 hours indicate a positive reaction.

Complications

1. Rectal stricture due to the fibrotic response.

2. Genital elephantiasis and ulceration, due to lymphatic obstruction of the draining nodes, known as esthiomene (esthiomenos: eroded).

3. Multiple sinuses and fistulae, involving the penis, urethra or the rectum.

4. Perianal suppuration

Treatment

Antibiotic combinations including sulphonamides, tetracyclines, macrolides or quinolones, are effective. Aspiration of the bubo may be done to reduce tension and pain, as incision invariably results in a troublesome sinus.

Infectious mononucleosis (syn: glandular fever, 'kissing' disease)

An acute febrile illness due to Ebstein-Barr virus (EBV) with generalized lymph node enlargement, associated with fever, sore throat, splenomegaly, abdominal pain (mesenteric lymphadenopathy), headache and neck stiffness. The 'mono' syndrome consists of fever, fatigue, adenopathy, splenomegaly and pharyngitis. It is transmitted by droplet infection (and also by kissing amongst youngsters, hence the name 'kissing' disease). Cervical adenopathy especially involving the upper deep cervical and the suboccipital nodes is the most prominent feature. Hypertrophy of lymph nodes without loss of architecture is the classical histopathology with lymphoid cells and macrophages filling the sinuses of the lymph nodes. Suppuration does not occur unless superadded infection occurs.

Investigations

Lymphocytosis and atypical monocytosis are very characteristic

Positive *EBV titres* (IgG or IgM) are highly specific.

Paul Bunnel test for heterophile antibodies: identification of agglutinins for sheep's RBC, during the active phase of the disease, is diagnostic upto 70%. Thrombocytopenia, disturbed liver functions, hypergammaglobulinemia may be the other features of the disease. *Monospot* test is used for rapid screening of the disease. A fibrin ring granuloma is seen on histology of a lymph node.

Treatment

There is no specific antiviral drug; secondary infection is best treated by tetracyclines or fluoroquinolones. Steroids are sometimes used to treat complications such as, tracheal compression, hemolytic anemia and thrombocytopenic purpura. A newer antiviral agent, valacyclovir is found to be effective against EBV.

Cat-scratch disease (syn: benign inoculation lymphoreticulosis, cat scratch fever)

Common in the west, neither a cat nor a scratch is always found in this disease, which is due to a chlamydial organism akin to LGV, known as *Bartonella henselae*, occurring in children. A primary lesion, a small pustule is often missed and a prominent secondary lymphadenitis, usually cervical, which may suppurate and form crust, is a common finding. CNS features like aseptic meningitis/encephalitis, cranial nerve palsies may be seen, as also purpura, conjunctivitis or parotitis.

Diagnosis is made either from the history of the cat scratch, a specific skin test or a biopsy of the lymph nodes which will show in early stages follicular and histiocyctic proliferation and in the late stages, formation of microabscesses.

Treatment

It is a self-limiting disease, does not warrant any treatment, but associated secondary infection, may be treated with a short course of tetracyclines or fluoroquinolones.

Brucellosis (syn: undulant fever)

Also known as a 'disease of mistakes', it is chracterised by waxing/waning fever, caused by *Brucella melitensis*, a Gm negative, nonmotile coccobacillus. In the prodromal period, malaise, gastrointestinal symptoms, and headache are seen and after a few weeks irregular fever and progressive paresthesia dominate the clinical picture. Hepato-splenomegaly and lymphadenopathy, mostly cervical and mediastinal, are almost always present. Other associated features are, weight loss, cystitis, epididymo-orchitis, skin rash/purpuric spots, visual, pulmonary and neuropsychiatric disturbances,

Investigations

Anemia, thrombocytopenia and leukopenia are commonly seen. Node biopsy may show large cells which resemble the Reed-Sternberg cells of Hodgkin's disease (vide supra). Blood culture is positive in 70% in acute cases. The specific serologic tests such as, brucella antibody complement fixation test and brucella standard tube agglutination (STA) test and ELISA are diagnostic, while elevated IgM and IgG titres may be useful after several weeks.

Treatment

Broad spectrum cephalosporins or fluoro-quinolones may be given. Alternate drugs are, doxycycline, co-trimoxazole (sulfamethoxazole+trimethoprim) and rifampicin.

Toxoplasmosis

This is caused by an intracellular parasite, *Toxoplasma gondii*, which multiplies within the endothelial and other cells of the host. It may be congenital (mother to child) or acquired and is of four clinical types:

1. *CNS* type: presents with meningoence-phalitis, fever, marked headache, delirium, convulsions, loss of hearing and vomiting. It also develops as an opportunistic infection in patients with HIV, producing an SOL in the brain.

2. *Exanthematous* type: presents with fever, widespread maculopapular skin rash and sometimes pneumonitis and myocarditis.

3. *Lymphatic* type: presents as enlargement of single/multiple groups of lymph nodes, associated with constitutional features

4. *Latent* type: presents with bizarre manifetations, to be diagnosed only by a biopsy.

TORCH syndrome: toxoplasmosis, rubella, cytomegalovirus and herpes simplex.

Investigations

Demonstration of the organism in blood, body fluids or tissues is confirmatory

Increased T-suppressor lymphocyte count in adults is seen. In the acute stage, ELISA technique may identify the toxoplasma antigen. IgM and IgG levels may be supportive; Sabin-Feldman dye test is both specific and sensitive to IgG antibodies, but not done in many laboratories, as it requires live toxoplasma organism. Double-sandwich IgM ELISA is more popular, as it is equally sensitive and specific in making the diagnosis.

Treatment

An infected mother should be counseled about the risk to the fetus. Sulfadiazine-pyrimethamine combination is useful as the primary form of therapy. Alternate drugs are spiromycin, clindamycin, azithromycin, clarithromycin and atovaquone. Steroids may be given for ocular or CNS involvement.

43 Lymphedema

(lympha: spring water)

Anatomy: The lymphatic system is composed of:

1. Lymphatic capillaries which absorb lymph from the interstitial compartment in various tissues in the body (except CNS, which has no lymphatics)

2. Collecting lymph vessels for transport

3. The lymph nodes which act as mechanical filters and also play an immunological role.

About 2-4 litres of lymph is drained into the venous system per day.

Forces propelling lymph forwards in their channels:

1. Gravity

2. Pulsatile flow in the arterial tree

3. Tissue interstitial fluid pressure (normal -5-10mmHg)

4. Transient increase in tissue pressure due to muscular contractions or external compression

5. Presence of valves in the system, preventing reflux.

Definition: Lymphedema is interstitial edema of lymphatic origin, results from the obstruction of lymphatic flow. It may be due to various causes, broadly classified into primary and secondary types.

Primary lymphedema is due to developmental anomalies of lymphatics, they are:

1. Milroy's disease
2. Lymphedema praecox
3. Lymphedema tarda

Secondary lymphedema is acquired, due to an identifiable cause and is more common. Loss of venoarteriolar reflux (VAR), which is believed to protect capillaries in dependent parts of the body (legs) from excessive hydrostatic forces, may be a contributory factor.

1. Inflammatory

a) Filariasis (commonest cause in tropical countries).
b) Recurrent nonspecfic infection.
c) Streptococcal cellulitis.
d) Tuberculosis.
e) Lymphogranuloma venereum

2. Neoplastic (commonest cause in developed countries)

a) Due to infiltration of lymph nodes and their afferent/efferent channels.
b) Following radical lymph node dissection.
c) Post irradiation fibrosis.

Malignancies associated with lymphedema

Carcinoma

Squamous cell Ca
Basal cell Ca
Malignant melanoma

Sarcoma

Lymphangioma sarcoma (Stewart-Treves syndrome).
Kaposi's sarcoma
Malignant fibrous histiocytoma (MFH)
Liposarcoma
lymphoma

3. Arterial insufficiency, particularly of acute nature in the limbs, produces lymphedema due to cessation of pulsatile flow in arterioles. This, in association with swelling of infarcted tissue,

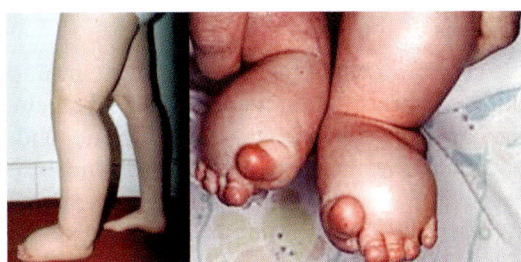

Fig. 43.1 & 2. Milroy's disease

creates a vicious cycle, by increasing the tissue pressure and compressing the venous channels, making edema worse. Ultimately it may reach a stage of arterial compression, within a closed (osteofascial) compartment, threatening the viability of the limb, unless immediate surgical decompression by a liberal fasciotomy is carried out. This is known as compartment syndrome commonly encountered in the leg, following injury or acute ischemia.

4.   Acute deep vein thrombosis (DVT) also produces lymph stasis; though the precise mechanism is not clear, associated lymphangitis is an accepted cause. Very often simple ligation of a major vein does not result in significant edema, whereas in acute deep thrombophlebitis, it can be massive, which is considered to be due to lymphatic obstruction acting in synergism with venous obstruction.

5.   Post-traumatic sympathetic dystrophy may also produce lymphedema.

6.   Turner syndrome (44-X or monosomy X)

The causes of lymphedema may be remembered as APLASIA

Aplasia or hypoplasia
Parasitic (filariasis)
Lymphatic obstruction (malignancy)
Altered lymph motility
Surgicial excision of lymphatics
Inflammatory or infectious
After radiotherapy

PRiMARY LYMPHEDEMA

a)   Milroy's disease or lymphedema congenita presents at birth, without sex predilection, transmitted by autosomal dominant trait (chromosome-5).

b)   Lymphedema praecox presents around puberty, starts as spontaneous swelling over the foot or ankle worsened by activity or dependency, may be unilateral or bilateral and progresses to involve the entire limb over period of several years. There is an arbitrary limit of the age of 35 years for this disease, after which it is termed lymphedema tarda.

c)   Lymphedema tarda presents in adult life, after 35. (The latter two are sometimes referred to as Meige's disease)

All these probably represent different parts of the spectrum of developmental anomalies of the lymphatics, such as aplasia, hypoplasia or varicose dilatation. The commonest is hypoplasia, affecting females more than males.

There are many other syndromes associated with lymphedema, such as Turner's, Klippel-Trenaunay, Weber's, Noonan's syndromes etc.

FILARIAL LYMPHEDEMA

This is the commest cause of lymphedema of the lower limb in tropical countries caused by Wuchereria bancrofti or Brugia malayi, transmitted by a mosquito vector, Culex fatigans. This disease is endemic in certain parts of India.

Pathology

Primary problem is obstruction to lymphatics and subsequent fibrosis. The sequence of events are, recurrent filarial fever, lymphangitis, lymph stagnation and lymphedema. With each attack of lymphangititis, obstruction of more and more lymph channels develops, which may resolve to some extent in the interim periods, though return to normal size of limb may not occur. The edema is initially pitting and reversible, but the extravasated tissue fluid excites inflammation, leading to fibrosis making it hard, nonpitting and fixed. The skin and subcutaneous tissue get enormously thickened, mostly confined to leg, foot and toes, often forming a jackfruit sized dead weight, developing uneven contours and papillary excrescences. Eventual necrosis and ulceration due to strangulation of their blood supply may occur, providing favorite sites for maggots to breed and thrive.

Clinical features

History of repeated attacks of fever with chills and rigors associated with regional (usually inguinal) lymphadenopathy.

According to the progress of the disease the lymphedema can be divided into four clinical stages:

Stage-1: The limb or the affected part feels heavy after an attack and with succeeding attacks becomes uniformly swollen, the edema is pitting, totally reversible and completely relieved by rest and elevation. No skin changes are present.

Stage-2: The lymphedema does not fully subside with the rest or elevation. The edema is partly pitting and reduced by elastic compression. Regional lymphadeonopathy is present but no skin changes.

Stage-3: Severe nonpitting edema is present, with little reduction by rest or elevation. There is considerable thickening of the skin and subcutaneous tissue.

Stage-4: Edema is gross with dense subcutaneous fibrosis, thick and hyperkeratotic skin, warty projections with ulceration, The edema is nonpitting and unaltered by rest, elevation or elastic compression.

The structures usually affected are lower limbs (mostly below knee), scrotum, penile skin and upper limb, but breast, vulva are also rarely involved.

Differential diagnosis

It should be remembered that unilateral limb edema is due to local causes, like venous or lymphatic obstruction, whereas bilateral involvement is often due to a systemic cause, such as cardiac, renal, hepatic, nutritional, endocrinal etc. rarely, a unilateral factor present on both sides, may produce bilateral edema.

1. Chronic venous edema of the lower limb - this resolves within a day or two of bed rest and elevation, while lymphedema takes several days or it may never.

2. Lymphangioma - this does not resolve with rest; small lymphatic vesicles may be observed by a magnifying lens.

3. Diffuse neurofibromatosis - associated with von Recklinghausen's disease; other areas may be involved and features like pigmented café au lait spots may be seen.

4. Lipedema - a rare condition characterised by diffuse nonpitting enlargement of the subcutaneous tissue of both the extremities, seen in patients with obesity, hypothyroidism etc.

Specific investigations

1) Eosinophilia may be seen in filarial infestation.

2) Night blood smear for microfilaria see chapter 41.

3) Complement fixation or immunoflorescence tests for filariasis

4) Lymphangiography (Kinmonth) to diagnose lymphedema, malignant disease in the iliac/paraaortic lymphnodes and to demonstrate the nature of lymphatic abnormality. By preliminary subcutaneous injection of a dye into the dorsum of foot, the tiny lymphatics are identified and cannulated by an incision, using a magnifying loupe. Slow injection of a water soluble contrast (Lipoidol ultrafluid) about 30ml, is done, using a gravity injector, taking around six hours. X-rays of calf, thigh, ilioinguinal and paraaortic regions are taken, to identify the pathology. Direct injection of the contrast into the superficial inguinal nodes may also be given (lymphadenogram), to study the retroperitoneal region, up to the diaphragm.

Small metastatic deposits in the nodes cause filling defects due to obliteration of lymph nodal sinuses. Large deposits cause larger filling defects and generalized enlargement of nodes, while lymphoma causes foamy or reticular pattern with enlargement.

5) High resolution ultrasound.

6) CT scan, these two will detect any SOL or venous thrombosis.

7) Doppler/Duplex imaging to study the deep venous system.

8) Isotope lymphangiography (lymphoscintigram), using ^{99m}Tc labeled sulfur colloid or human serum nanoalbumin (HSA), being totally noninvasive and equally informative, has largely replaced lymphangiography for a functional assessment of the lymphatic system of the limbs. In this study, the isotope can be

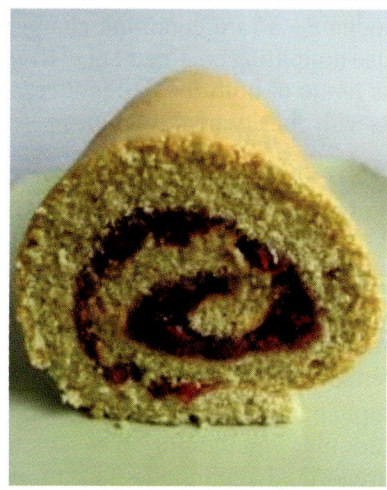

Fig. 43.3. Swiss roll

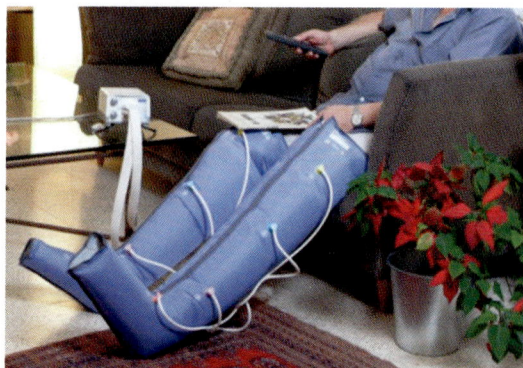

Fig. 43.4. Pneumatic compression pump for lymphedema for an ambulatory patient

directly injected into the subcutaneous tissue of a web space, without the need for cannulating the lymphatics.

9) Analysis of tissue fluid: It can be aspirated or collected by placing a polythene tube with multiple perforations in subcutaneous plane. Typically lymphedema fluid has a higher protein content (>1.5gm%) and A/G ratio. It is not routinely done due to technical difficulties and lack of reproducibility.

10) Simple injection of a highly diffusible dye, such as patent blue or sky blue into the web space, has been attempted, with an aim of delineating the dermal lymphatics. Dermal backflow, following massage of skin and active joint movements, producing a 'marbled' appearance, is indicative of obstruction to deep lymphatics.

Treatment

Medical

I)   bed rest
ii) elevation, above the heart level or by 10°
iii) elastic support, may be given by 'old-fashioned' crepe bandage (less effective) or custom-made pressure-gradient elastic stockings, while on their feet. During night they may be removed and legs kept elevated. The ideal pressure required by the stockinet in the foot is 50mmHg; at ankle 40; in the midcalf 30 and at knee 20, with a gradient of 30mm.

iv) centripetal massages, either by manual or by sequential pneumatic compression pump and multilayered lymphedema bandaging (MLLB) with non-elastic compression are employed for faster resolution.

v) antifilarial therapy , with DEC or ivermectin, latter is given as a single dose in combination with albendazole, orally once in six months

vi) antibiotics, usually against Gram positive cocci

vii) antiedema drugs

viii) specific vaccine against strepto/staphylococci of filarial origin, to prevent the so called 'filarial attacks' due to secondary bacterial infection

ix) fluorides have been given as long term parenteral therapy, to discourage parasitic activity, with some success. Its rationale is not clear, but the observation that filariasis is rare in areas endemic for flurosis (due to increased fluoride content in drinking water), is the basis for this empirical therapy.

x) an antifibroblastic agent, stanozolol (the 'Olympic steroid') is also helpful in reducing the fibrosis of subcutaneous tissue, which is considered to be the reason for converting reversible (pitting) edema into irreversible and hard (nonpitting) swelling, in the long run.

xi) a benzopyrone compound, coumarin (Lympedim) is found to be very effective in increasing the number and activity of tissue macrophages, disintegrating the macro-molecules and reducing the viscosity of intersti-tial fluid, for better absorption. It has no antico-agulant property like dicoumarol.

Surgical: indications are:

1. Clinical stages 2, 3 & 4.
2. Skin changes.
3. Functional impairment.
4. Physical and cosmetic considerations.

The surgical treatment consists of:

1. Lymphangioplasty (operations to promote lymph drainage)

a. Subcutaneous implantation of silk threads, multifilament Teflon or polythene tubes, which act as capillary wicks and facilitate lymph flow .

b. Removal of strips of deep fascia to divert the lymph flow through it, by establishing commu-nications with deep lymphatics (Kondoleon's operation)

c. Omental transposition, from the abdomen into the thigh.

d. Nodo-venous shunting (Niebowicz) by anastomosing the cut surface of a lymph-node proximal to obstruction, with intact afferents, with a lateral opening made in the long saphenous vein. Alternately a lympho-venous shunt, wherein a dilated lymph channel is dis-sected in the groin and pulled through into a tributary of saphenous vein and anchored (Cockett).

e. Enteromesenteric bridge (of Kinmonth) uses the submucous lymphatic plexus of the small bowel and the mesenteric lymphatics as a pedicle.

These procedures are attempted only if the edema is reversible to some extent but have not

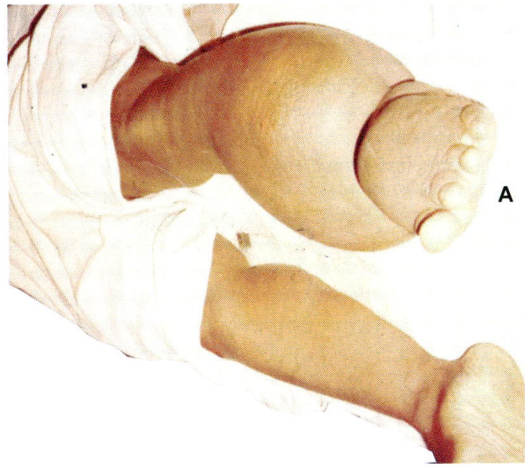

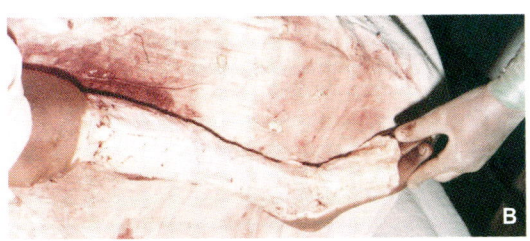

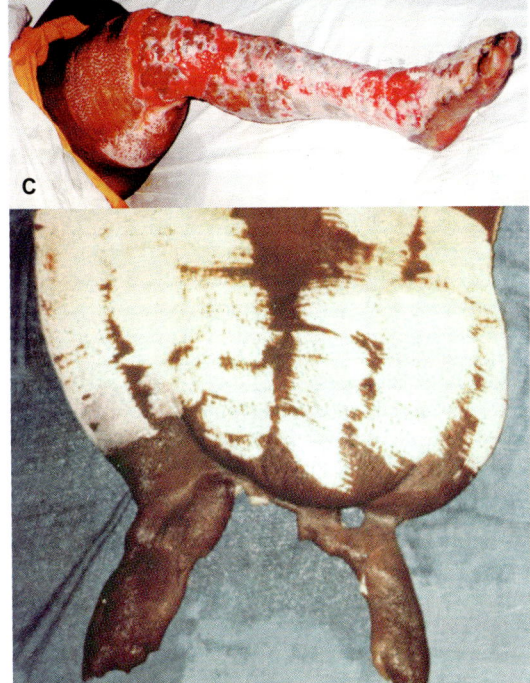

Fig. 43.5. Steps of Charles' operation

A. 4th degree lymphedema left leg   B. Excision of skin & subcutaneous tissue
C. Final result after skin grafting   D. Excised specimen
(courtesy: Halsted Surgical Clinic, Chennai)

been very successful in the hands of majority of surgeons.

2. Excision operations

These operations remove the elephantiatic tissues and the patient is dramaticaly relieved of the 'dead weight' in the limb. As the underlying lympho-obstructive pathology exists, recurrence to an acceptable magnitude may occur; hence the importance of continuing medical treatment cannot be overemphasized.

a) Excision and primary closure (reduction plasty of Homan): is the simplest, by tailoring redundant skin and subcutaneous tissue, to optimal size. Since it involes considerable undermining of skin flaps, only one hemicircumference of the leg is reduced at a time, to avoid avascular necrosis of skin.

b) Charles' operation (total excision and skin grafting): Both these operations are done under a tourniquet, to minimize blood loss. Initially split skin grafts are collected from the affected leg and thigh, the hypertrophied dermal and subdermal tissues are excised upto the deep fascia and the skin graft is wrapped around the

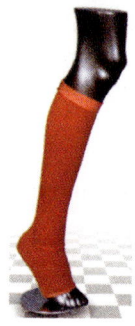
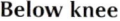
Below knee

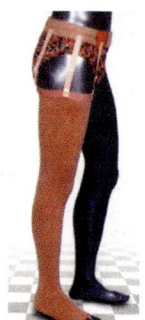
Full leg

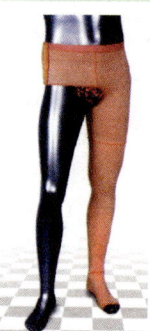
Unilateral pantihose

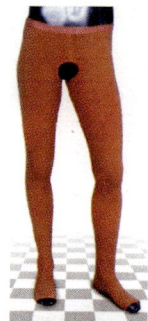
Bilateral pantihose

Fig. 43.6. Custom-made pressure-gradient elastic stockings
(courtesy: Norma D.N.D. Products, New Delhi)

	Feature	Venous edema	Lymphedema
1	Geographical	More in the west	Tropical countries
2	Distribution	Commonly whole limb	Mostly below knee
3	Recurrent fever/chills	Rare	Common
4	Lymphadenopathy	Rare	Common
5	Nature	Pitting and reversible	Becomes nonpitting soon
6	Pigmentation/dermatitis	Common	Never
7	Ulcers	Around ankle	Anywhere due to secondary infection
8	Skin excrescences	Not seen	Common
9	Massive swelling of leg	In acute stage	In chronic stage
10	Doppler evidence	Deep vein dysfunction	No DVD
11	Tests for filariasis	Negative	May be positive
12	Analysis of tissue fluid	Low protein/normal A-G ratio	High protein/raised A-G ratio
13	Lymphangiogram (conventional or isotopic)	Normal	May show lymphatic obstruction
14	Response to therapy	For venous disease	For lymphatic disease

Table-43.1 : Differences between venous and lymphedema

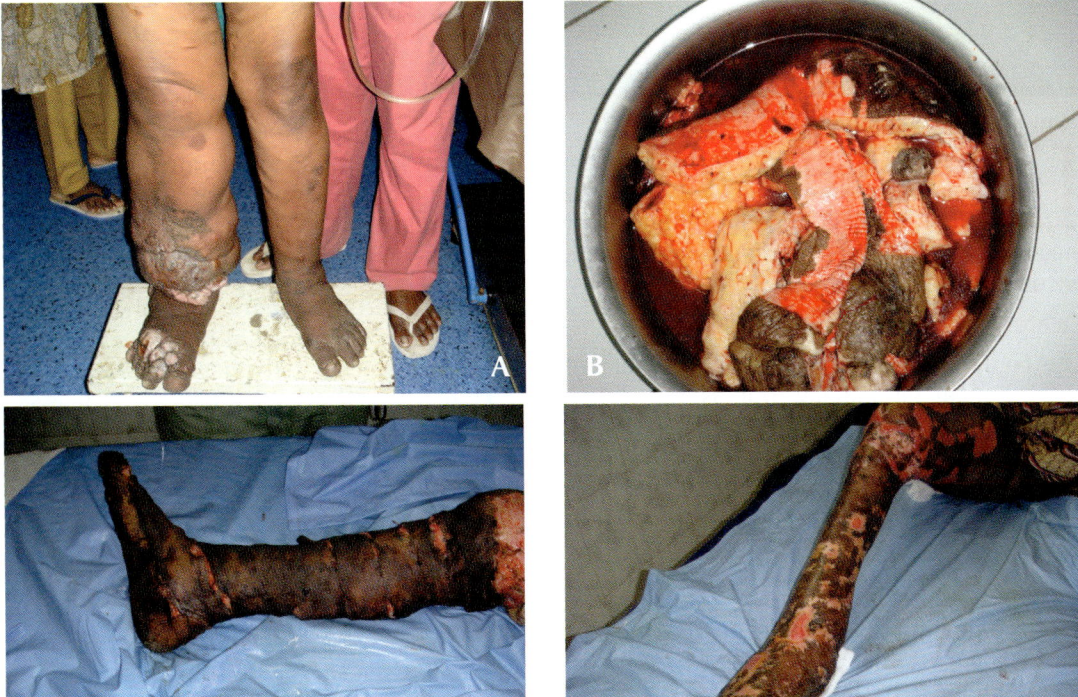

Fig. 43.7.
A. Filarial lymphedema 4th degree **B.** Excision of skin and subcutaneous tissue, after harvesting the skin for grafting
C. Wrapping the skin graft around the foot and leg   **D.** Final result after three weeks
(courtesy: Halsted Surgical Clinic, Chennai)

denuded leg, in a spiral manner. Before the release of tourniquet, adequate elastic compression is given over the foot and leg, to prevent undue bleeding, which is maintained for 72-96 hours, when the wound is inspected. External compression also helps neovascularization of the grafted skin.

Complications include sensory loss, failure of graft, ulceration, aggravation of edema distal to excision, hypertrophic scar etc. Since there is not much of subcutaneous tissue in the foot and toes, results of this operation are unsatisfactory in these areas, compared to leg and thigh. Thromboembolic complications of deep veins may occur, but rare.

c) Thompson's operation (buried dermal flap): After excision of subcutaneous tissue and parts of deep fascia, retaining the redundant skin flaps, the shaved edges of which are buried deep into muscles, allowing communication between superficial and deep lymphatics as well as muscular venules to develop. This is also known as 'swiss roll' operation, by its ultimate shape.

d) Amputation is rarely required, if the patient had 'earned' it, after all conservative procedures are to no avail, to provide necessary comfort, usually for a disabling disease of foot.

(syn: fatty hernia of linea alba)

Definition: This is a hernia occurring through the linea alba between the xiphoid process and the umbilicus. It may be congenital, seen in infants or acquired, occurring in middle age.

Contents

The contents are usually a small globule of preperitoneal fat initially, but as the defect enlarges, a complete peritoneal sac may develop, to house omentum or bowel. Generally the falciform ligament of liver prevents visceral herniation in epigastric defects.

Clinical features

It may be symptomless, discovered during routine examination by a doctor or may present with a palpable parietal nodule above the umbilicus, tethered to the linea alba.

A dull aching pain is often present because of traction on the omentum (when it is a content); this is exaggerated after food, and causes pain akin to acid-peptic disease (APD).

Although usually solitary, more than one defect may be seen. Reducibility may be observed but there is no impulse on coughing in the initial stages.

Differential diagnosis

Lipoma, neurofibroma or other parietal soft tissue benign tumors.

Midline incisional (ventral) hernia: history and scar of previous surgery will be present

Acid peptic disease (APD): as mentioned earlier, lack of associated symptoms, such as epigastric burning, eructations etc. should help, but both may often coexist.

Strangulation is a rare complication of epigastric hernia.

Investigations: No specific studies are necessary for diagnosis, but only to exclude other abdominal diseases causing dyspepsia and for anesthesia fitness.

Treatment

It is always advisable to operate on this condition as it is often symptomatic and if left alone, it may progressively enlarge.

Procedure (epigastric herniorrhaphy)

Through a vertical midline incision, the sac is reduced, the edges of the defect in the linea alba are dissected out and closed with a '8' stitch of a nonabsorbable material, such as silk or polypropylene (prolene). If a definite sac is present, the contents are reduced and herniotomy is done, before carrying out repair. Employing mesh repair was rare till the recent evidence favored it. Laparoscopic mesh plasty is now catching up fast and the elegance of an intraperitoneal onlay mesh (IPOM) is only offset by its cost. Special, adhision-resistant meshes (Proceed or Physiomesh by Ethicon and Parietex by Covidien) are currently available for use.

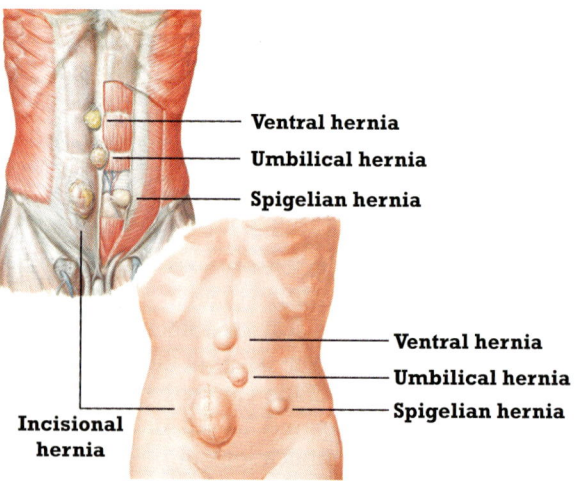

Ventral hernia
Umbilical hernia
Spigelian hernia

Ventral hernia
Umbilical hernia
Spigelian hernia

Incisional hernia

Fig. 44.1 Common herniae of anterior abdominal wall

45 Umbilical Hernia

CONGENITAL UMBILICAL HERNIA (syn: omphalocele, exomphalos) is the failure of the primitive midgut to return into the celom (abdominal cavity) in early fetal life and due to failure of the formation of the anterior abdominal wall to a variable extent (see rotation gut), by the nonfusion of the lateral folds forming the celomic cavity. There is a higher incidence of this disease in infants with mucopolysaccharidoses, such as Hurler's and Hunter's syndromes.

Hunter's syndrome is an x-linked genetic disorder affecting male children, due to the deficiency of enzyme, iduronate-2-sulfatase (I-2-S), leading to build up of glycoaminoglycans (GAG), earlier called mucopolysaccharides, in various tissues such as CNS, CVS, blood cells, fibroblasts etc. interfering with their functions.

Hurler's syndrome is also a genetic disorder, transmitted by an autosomal recessive trait, occurring in both genders, due to deficiency of α-L-iduronidase, with similar manifestations. These are progressive, life-limiting diseases, with no specific treatment.

1. *Exomphalos minor*: Here a small sac is seen, with the cord attached to the summit and is reduced easily by strapping after returning the contents into the abdominal cavity, the strapping being maintained for at least 2 weeks.

2. *Exomphalos major*: In this condition the defect is large and the thin sac over it is liable to

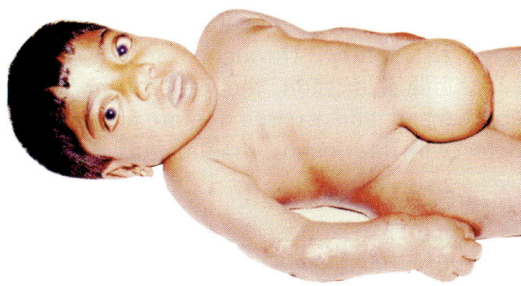

Fig. 45.2. Large umbilical hernia in an infant (with Hunter's syndrome)
(courtesy: Lifeline Hospitals, Chennai)

burst; the umbilical cord is attached to a large swelling which contains small and large gut or sometimes even the liver. In contrast to exomphalos minor, the cord is attached at the periphery of the sac.

Treatment

After adequate nutritional support, hydration, antibiotic cover and blood transfusion if necessary, urgent surgical intervention is carried out, creating large skin flaps on either side, to cover the sac. Tension releasing lateral incisions of the rectus sheath may be performed to permit good closure. Sometimes, only skin can be closed initially, creating a hernia, requiring fascial reconstruction later.

UMBILICAL HERNIA IN INFANTS

Sometimes following umbilical sepsis after birth, the umbilical cicatrix becomes weak and thin resulting in herniation, but spontaneous cure may occur in a few months. A smooth hemispherical swelling over the umbilicus, becoming apparent only on coughing or crying, with intact skin and typical reducibility is unmistakable.

Conservative management

The earlier method was strapping a large coin or a round piece of plastic on the umbilicus, for a few weeks, after reducing the hernia. Many surgeons feel no treatment is necessary for this

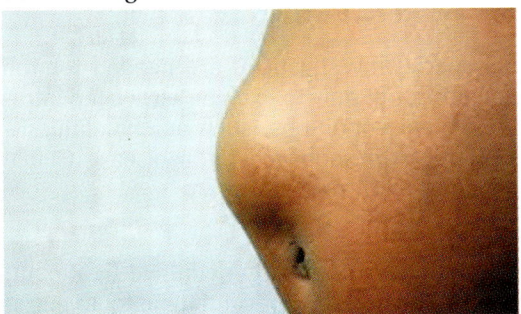

Fig. 45.1 Supra-umbilical hernia

condition, as it often disappears once the infant starts crawling on the tummy.

Surgery

This should be done only if the hernia persists after 12 months. Through a small, curved subumbilical incision, the neck of the sac is approached and excised, before closing the defect with fine nonabsorbable sutures.

UMBILICAL (PARAUMBILICAL) HERNIA IN ADULTS

In adults, the so-called umbilical hernia, is a herniation occurring not through the umbilical cicatrix but either just above (supraumbilical) or below (infraumbilical); hence a better term is paraumbilical hernia. Although omentum is the usual content of the sac, small or large gut may also be present. They quickly become irreducible because the neck is usually narrow and the omental contents develop adhesions to the sac.

Predisposing factors: same as for a ventral hernia - such as obesity, attenuation of the abdominal wall muscles, repeated pregnancies, gross ascites etc.

Symptoms

Painful swelling is the commonest presentation, rarely intestinal obstruction, if bowel is housed

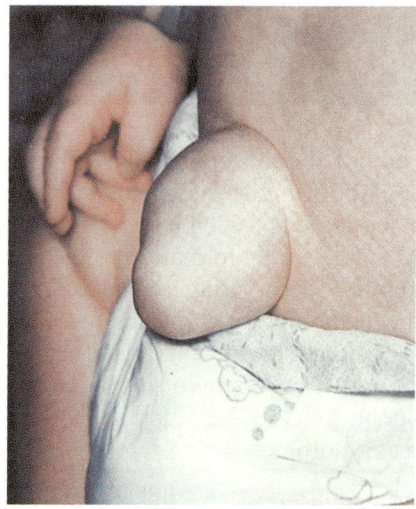

Fig. 45.4. Large umbilical hernia in a child
(courtesy: Lifeline Hospitals, Chennai)

in the sac. It should be remembered that even after strangulation, the patient may not develop typical features of intestinal obstruction, if only omentum is involved, though reflex vomiting may be seen. If omentum is adherent to the sac, traction may cause postprandial discomfort, mimicking acid-peptic disease (APD).

Signs

A globular hernial buldge is seen in relation to the umbilicus and on palpation the granular feel of omentum may be appreciated. If bowel is present, the mass may be resonant to percussion and peristaltic sounds may be heard by auscultation. They may be partially reducible with some impulse felt on coughing in uncomplicated hernia. If reducible, a circular defect in the linea alba may be appreciated by finger invagination.

Investigations

No special investigations are needed for the diagnosis, but only to exclude associated intra-abdominal conditions, such as cholelithiasis, APD or gastroesophageal reflux disease (GERD) and to assess fitness for surgery.

Treatment

Early surgery is the only definitive treatment, after observing same precautions as for a ventral hernia.

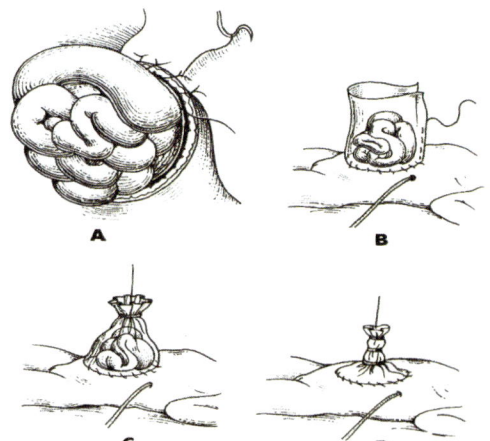

Fig. 45.3. Staged repair of omphalocele
A. Silastic mesh secured all around the defect
B. The mesh closed creating a cylinder.
C. End of the mesh tied with tape
D. Tapes tied down by inching, reducing the viscera

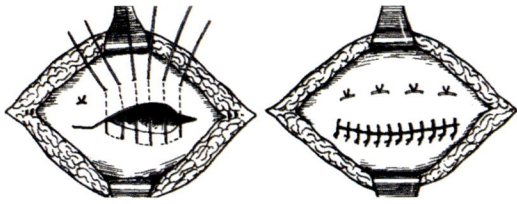

Fig. 45.5. Mayo's double-breasting operation for umbilical hernia

Surgery Mayo's operation

This repair consisting of double-breasting the fascia, through a transverse elliptical incision around the bulge, the neck of the sac and the rectus sheath are exposed. The sac is opened and contents reduced (or excised), after releasing the adhesions, if present. The redundant sac is excised and edge approximated with a running catgut stitch. The oval or circular defect in the linea alba is converted into a transverse ellipse by cutting away triangular bits in the corners and a series of horizontal overlapping mattress sutures, using prolene or any nonabsorbable material, are inserted, so that the upper margin of the linea alba overlaps the lower flap, by about 1-2cm. A few interrupted sutures are used to secure the overlap and the fat and skin are closed in layers. If the umbilicus needs to be excised, a neo-umbilicus may be fashioned as described under ventral hernia, for esthetic reasons.

Drawbacks of Mayo's repair

1. Double-breasting increases the tension on suture line
2. Best healing of fascia takes place, when it is

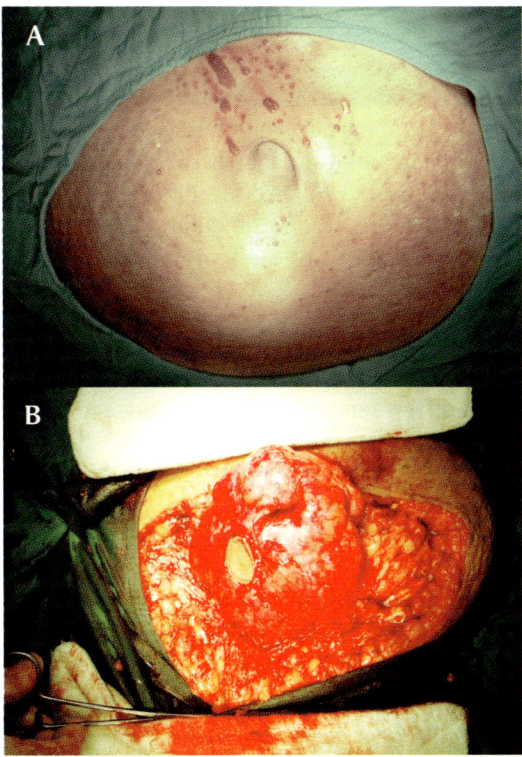

Fig. 45.6 Large infraumbilical hernia
A. Draped for surgery B. Large sac contaning omentum dissected for excession

apposed edge to edge; here it is apposed surface to surface, which is not physiological.

Repair by simple approximation of edges, using continuous nonabsorbable suturing, is equally popular with modern surgeons, obviating these drawbacks of the Mayo's method.

An onlay mesh repair or laparoscopic intraperitoneal mesh plasty (as described in the previous chapter) is now gaining momentum for defects larger than 2cm, though the current evidence is clearly in favor of using a mesh for all umbilical defects.

Jewels of Gyan - 45.1

True Umbilical Herniae are seen only in infants

Mesh repair favored for all but the smallest (2 x 2 cm) hernia.

In children, repair umbilical hernia after 12 months (but inguinal hernia as early as possible).

46 Femoral Hernia

Femoral hernia is much less common than the inguinal (1:10), with a female preponderance (5:1) and rare before puberty. It carries a high risk of strangulation because of the sharp margins of the femoral opening and its narrow neck.

Anatomy

The femoral canal is the most medial compartment of the femoral sheath, about 2cm long, extending from the femoral ring above to the saphenous opening (fossa ovalis) below, the base directed upwards. It contains the lymphatics leaving the thigh to enter the pelvis, a lymph node of Cloquet, some fat and areolar tissue. It is closed above by the septum tranversalis and below by the cribriform (sieve-like) fascia.

The femoral ring is bounded anteriorly by inguinal (Poupart's) ligament, laterally by a thin areolar septum separating it from the common femoral vein, posteriorly by pectineus muscle, fascia and ligament of Cooper and medially by the lacunar (Gimbernat's) ligament.

The saphenous opening is situated 4cms below and lateral to the pubic tubercle with a thick upper outer falciform (sickle-shaped) margin, known as Hey's ligament, which explains the upward inclination of the femoral hernia once it enters this plane, conferring the classical retort shape to it. Repeated flexion of the hip joint, pressing the groin fold, may also be responsible for the upward tilt of the fundus.

Occasionally the obturator artery takes an abnormal origin from external iliac or inferior epigastric artery (instead of anterior division of hypogastric) and descends down behind the lacunar ligament to enter the obturator foramen. At this point it is vulnerable for injury if the lacunar ligament is cut to reduce a femoral hernia, as the other sides of the ring cannot be divided. More is said about this artery than actually experienced, hence the saying 'more ink is spilt than blood about this artery'.

The reasons for female preponderance (5:1) are:

1. relative: since inguinal hernia is rare in women (no testicular descent), the femoral appears more common

2. absolute: poor development of iliopsoas muscle (which fills the lateral part of the gap between the inguinal ligament and the ilio-pubic arch), allowing lateral displacement of the neurovascular structures, creating

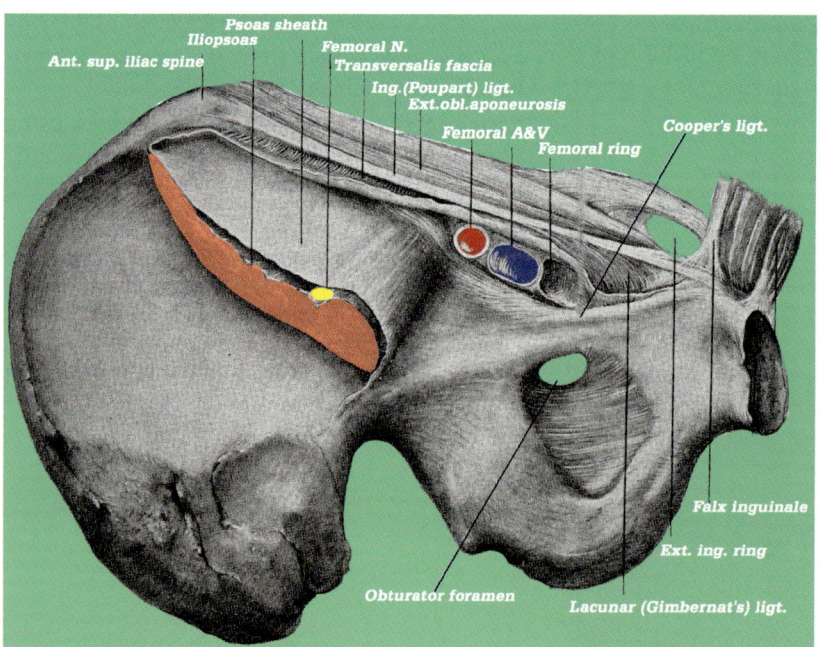

Fig. 46.1. Contents of the left femoral arch viewed from the pelvis

Labels in figure: Psoas sheath; Iliopsoas; Ant. sup. iliac spine; Femoral N.; Transversalis fascia; Ing.(Poupart) ligt.; Ext.obl.aponeurosis; Femoral A&V; Cooper's ligt.; Femoral ring; Falx inguinale; Ext. ing. ring; Obturator foramen; Lacunar (Gimbernat's) ligt.

laxity of the femoral ring.

Secondly, the less acute angle of attachment of the inguinal ligament to the pubic bone, results in a wider femoral ring, in females.

Special (rare) types of femoral hernia

1. Cloquet's hernia: when it passes between the pectineus muscle and Cooper's ligament

2. Laugier's hernia: when it passes through a defect in the Gimbernat's ligament

3. Hesselbach's hernia: when it passes lateral to the femoral artery

4. Narath (prevascular) hernia: when it descends in front of the femoral artery, behind the inguinal ligament, sometimes found in association with congenital dislocation of hip - CDH (syn: developmental dysplasia of hip - DDH).

5. Serafini (postvascular) hernia: when it passes behind the femoral vessels (rarest)

Clinical features

A tender lump in the groin fold, in a middle-aged woman, is the commonest presenting symptom. It is often irreducible but the presence of severe pain should be considered as an indication of strangulation. In view of the nar-

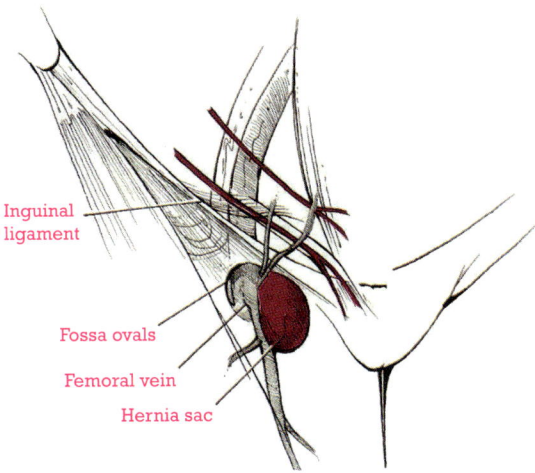

Inguinal ligament

Fossa ovals

Femoral vein

Hernia sac

Fig. 46.3. Relations of right femoral hernia

row opening, only a part of the circumference of the bowel gets into the canal, hence strangulated Richter's hernia is very common in this situation. Since the lumen of the bowel is not totally obstructed, the patient continues to pass flatus (a deceptive feature) even after the bowel wall is necrosed, but typically with bleeding into the lumen.

Patient may experience vague postprandial discomfort because of the traction on the adherent omentum following a meal. It is not rare for the hernia to be detected by an alert clinician only after strangulation, driving home the importance of examining the groins in cases of intestinal obstruction.

Local examination

A globular swelling, sometimes difficult to detect as it is buried in the fat, may be seen or felt below and lateral to the pubic tubercle. The classical reducibility and expansile impulse on coughing are rarely observed, because of the tight ring, omental adhesions and tortuous course of the hernia.

Gaur's sign: dilatation of superficial epigastic and circumflex iliac veins due to compression by the herniation.

Differential diagnosis

1. Inguinal hernia: Located above and medial

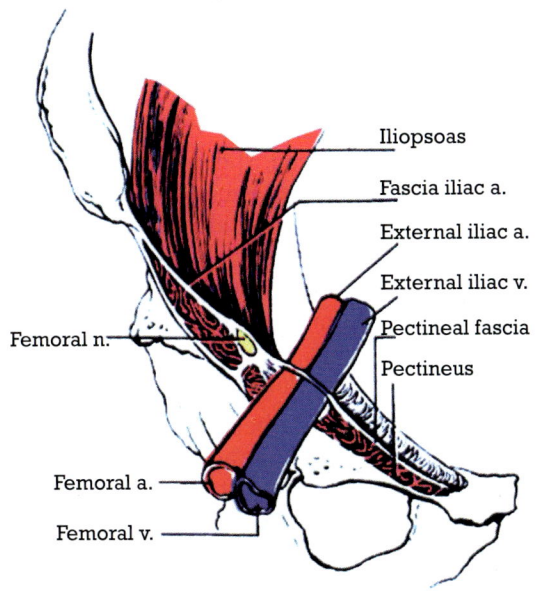

Iliopsoas

Fascia iliac a.

External iliac a.

External iliac v.

Pectineal fascia

Pectineus

Femoral n.

Femoral a.

Femoral v.

Fig. 46.2. Structures under the inguinal ligament

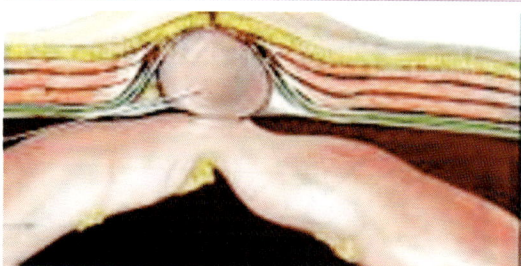

Fig. 46.4. Richter's hernia

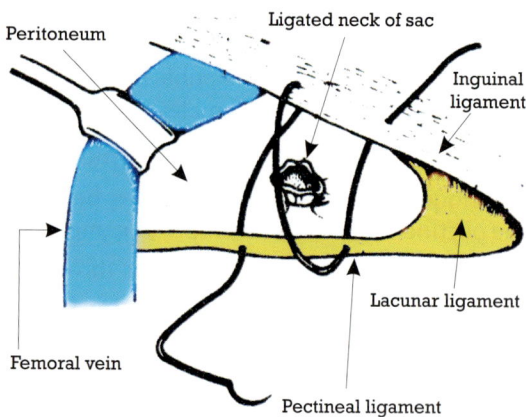

Fig. 46.5. Lockwood (low) repair of femoral hernia

to the pubic tubercle, often descends into the scrotum, reducible and exhibits cough impulse. Three finger (Zieman's) test will identify the impulse over the fossa ovalis. Normal size of external inguinal ring detected during attempted digital invagination, is against the diagnosis of inguinal hernia. It should not be forgotten that the patient may be having both inguinal and femoral hernia, confusing the picture.

2. Inguinal lymphadenopathy: Often multiple, the diagnosis may be clinched if a primary disease in the drainage area of inguinal nodes, is evident.

3. Saphena varix: Huge dilated venous island presenting as a compressible swelling at the saphenous opening with a thrill appreciated on coughing (Morrisey's sign), associated with long saphenous varicocities in the leg. This swelling will disappear if the patient is examined in Trendelenburg position.

4. Lipoma or neurofibroma.

5. Psoas abscess: Presents as a tender, cystic swelling in the groin and in the right iliac fossa, with cross fluctuation, associated with flexor spasm of the hip and constitutional symptoms.

6. Femoral artery aneurysm: Either the patient is elderly atherosclerotic or gives history of injury to the groin, presents as a pulsatile compressible swelling, sometimes with absent distal pulses, due to embolization.

Investigations

There are no specific investigations to diagnose femoral hernia, but only those aimed at evaluating the patient for anesthesia and surgery. A

radiological study by injecting a contrast into the peritoneal cavity, to demonstrate the sac (peritoneography or herniography), is rarely needed. High resolution USG or a CT scan may be helpful in obese patients, with equivocal physical findings.

Treatment

In view of the inconvenient location there is no possibility of using a truss for femoral hernia. The only definitive treatment for it is surgery, for which five approaches are possible.

1. Low or femoral (Lockwood) approach: This is the easiest and most popular for treating uncomplicated femoral hernia. An incision is made about an inch below the inguinal ligament, over the swelling. The sac is dissected up to the femoral ring and excised after reducing the contents. After proper identification of the anatomical structures, the femoral ring is obliterated by 2 or 3 interrupted nonabsorbable sutures approximating the inguinal and Cooper's ligaments, carefully protecting the femoral vein, while taking the lateral bites.

2. Mid or inguinal (Lotheissen) approach: This is preferred if the patient also has an inguinal hernia. Through an inguinal incision, posterior wall of the canal (fascia transversalis) is exposed, which is incised to identify the neck of the sac. The sac may be excised either from inside or outside before similar repair of the

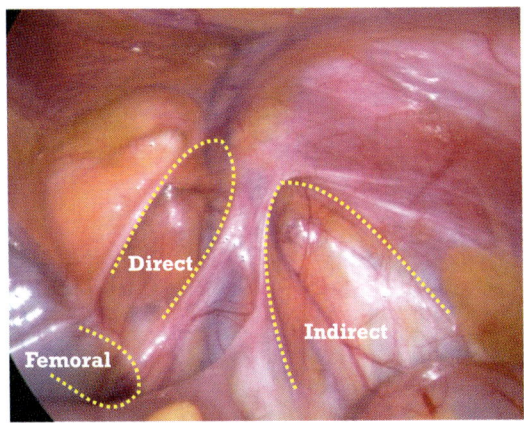

Fig. 46.6. Laparoscopic view in a patient with triple herniae
(courtesy: Dr M Muralidharan, Chennai)

Summary of the types of repair

1. Common, uncomplicated: low repair
2. Associated with inguinal hernia: inguinal approach
3. Strangulated: high or abdominal approach
4. Bilateral: Henry or extraperitoneal repair
5. Expertise availble: laparoscopic method

ring is carried out from within. The inguinal hernia if present, may also be dealt with appropriately.

3. High or abdominal (Mc Evedy) approach: This is the ideal approach for strangulated femoral hernia, allowing resection of bowel if necessary, by laparotomy through a lower paramedian incision. If no bowel resection is required the hernia may be repaired by a properitoneal approach, as in Henry technique for inguinal hernia.

4. Properitoneal (Henry) approach: By a low midline incision, the peritoneum is pushed away, to reach the sac, from inside, which is excised and the canal repaired from above. It requires some anatomic orientation, but the advantage is that bilateral hernia can be repaired through the same incision.

5. Laparoscopic repair is a recent addition, fixing a mesh against femoral ring from inside, in the properitoneal plane, after reducing the contents. Its advantage over the standard open femoral approach, requiring 5cm incision and 24 hours hospitalization, is questionable. The learning curve of laparoscopic mesh plasty (total extraperitoneal prosthetic mesh - TEP) for femoral hernia is quite steep, but once crossed, it is a very physiological repair.

Complications

a) Femoral hernia has a very high incidence of strangulation (Richter's type), the treatment for which has already been outlined.

b) Injury to the common femoral vein, during surgery requiring repair by fine vascular sutures, should be meticulously avoided by keeping a finger over it while taking the most lateral bite on the Cooper's ligament.

c) Postoperatively there may be collection of lymph or frank lymphorrhea from the wound.

d) Lymphedema of the limb is a possibility if lymphatics entering the pelvis, through the femoral canal are damaged during the repair.

e) Periosteitis pubis, producing adductor spasm, may be a troublesome complication.

f) Injury to abnormal obturator artery, coursing behind the lacunar ligament, has been described.

47 Inguinal Hernia

Anatomy: The inguinal canal extends in an oblique manner from the deep to the superficial inguinal ring, parallel to the inguinal (Poupart's) ligament. The superficial (external) inguinal ring is a triangular aperture in the external oblique, lying 2cm above and medial to the pubic tubercle. It normally does not admit the tip of a finger; if forcibly attempted, the patient resists due to discomfort. The deep (internal) ring is a 'U' shaped defect in the transversalis fascia, 2cm above the mid point of the inguinal ligament (between anterior superior iliac spine and pubic tubercle).The inferior epigastric arteries, from the external iliacs, pass up medial to the deep ring, to enter the rectus sheath, behind the rectus abdominis, raising a peritoneal fold on either side, in the anterior abdominal wall, termed lateral umbilical ligaments.

Boundaries: The floor is formed by the inguinal ligament, the posterior wall by the transversalis fascia and more medially by the conjoint tendon. The roof of the canal is formed by arching fibres of the conjoint tendon, the anterior wall,

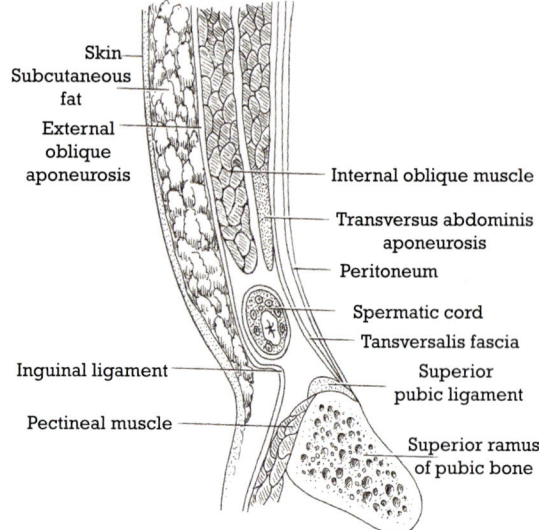

Fig. 47.3.Vertical section of inguinal region of abdominal wall

by the external oblique aponeurosis, assisted laterally by a portion of internal oblique muscle.

Hesselbach's triangle: It is a weak area of the anterior abdominal wall through which a direct inguinal hernia presents itself, bounded later-

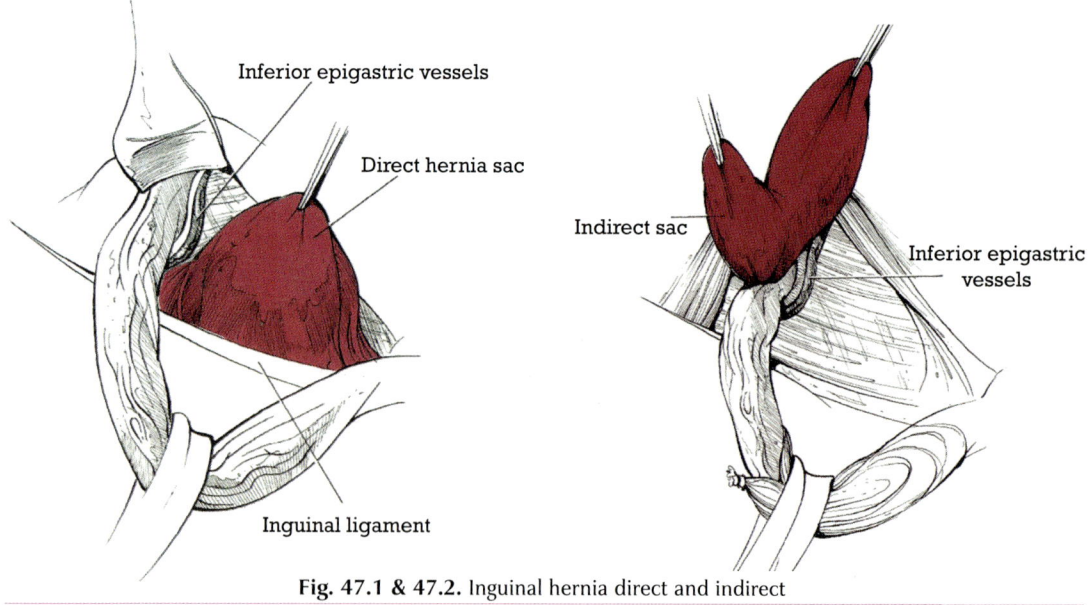

Fig. 47.1 & 47.2. Inguinal hernia direct and indirect

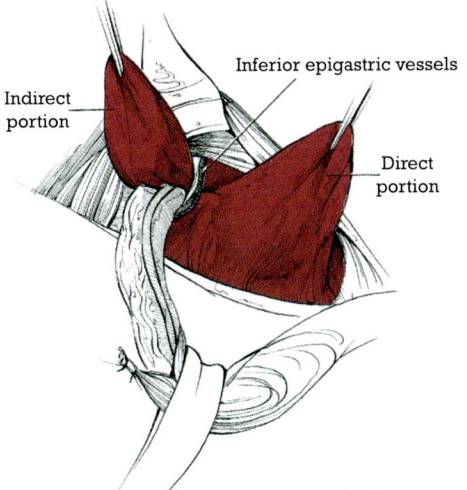

Fig. 47.4. Inguinal hernia with direct and indirect sacs double hernia of saddle type (pantaloon hernia)

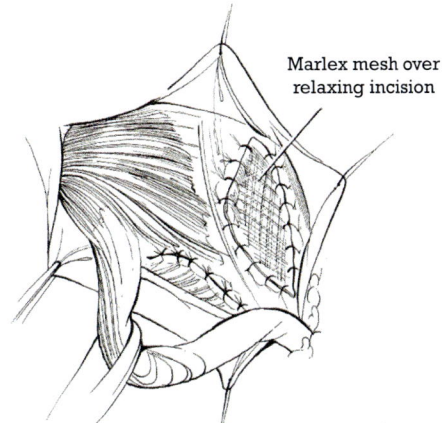

Fig. 47.5. Bassini repair of inguinal hernia Mesh is sutured to close the fascial defect following Tanner's muscle slide

ally by inferior epigastric vessels, medially by the lower part of the lateral border of the rectus abdominis and inferiorly by the medial third of the inguinal ligament. The floor is formed by transversalis fascia and is bisected by the medial umbilical ligament, formed by the obliterated umbilical artery.

Externally from the skin, the two layers of super-

Jewels of Gyan - 47.1

Peritoneal Folds

There are five peritoneal folds in the lower anterior abdominal wall converging towards the umbilicus.

The median umbilical ligament, formed by the obliterated urachus, extends from fundus of the bladder to the umbilicus.

Two medial umbilical ligaments, representing obliterated umbilical arteries, raising peritoneal folds, bisecting the Hesselbach's triangles

Two lateral umbilical ligaments are the peritoneal folds raised by inferior epigastric vessels on either side forming the lateral boundary of the triangles and lying medial to the internal inguinal rings.

---

ficial fascia, superficial fatty (*Camper's*) and deep membranous (*Scarpa's*) fasciae and a thin areolar layer immediately over the external oblique aponeurosis, known as *fascia innominatum of Gallaudet*, covering the inguinal canal.

Contents

The canal contains the spermatic cord and the ilioinguinal nerve (L-1). The cord contains:

1. cremasteric muscle (from the internal oblique muscle)
2. internal spermatic fascia (from transversalis fascia)
3. vas deferens
4. accompanying arteries to the vas (artery to vas from vesical arteries and cremasteric artery from the inferior epigastric)
5. testicular artery (from aorta)
6. pampiniform plexus of veins (to form the spermatic or testicular veins)
7. fat
8. lymphatics (draining testis and epididymis)
9. genital branch of the genitofemoral nerve (L-1, 2)
10. obliterated processus vaginalis
11. autonomic nerve fibers, along the vessels

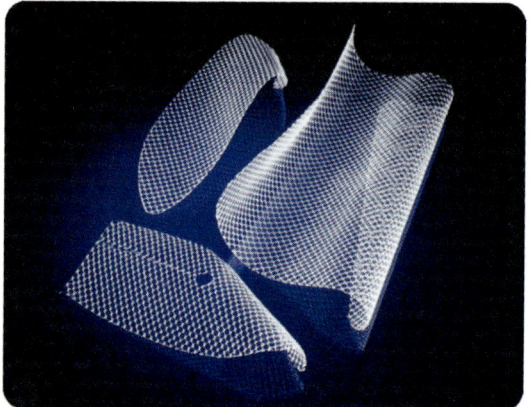

Fig. 47.6. Polypropylene hernia mesh

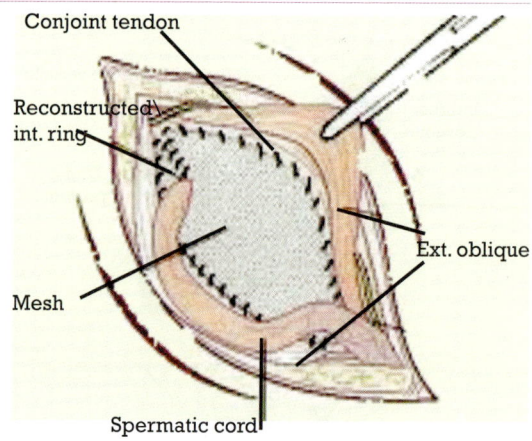

Fig. 47.7. Lichtenstein's tension-free mesh repair

Actually, the spermatic cord is complete, only after it acquires the outer cover, external spermatic fascia, from external oblique aponeurosis, as it leaves the inguinal canal. In females, it is replaced by the round ligament (ligamentum teres) of the uterus, derived from the gubernaculum ovarii.

The inguinal hernia may be *indirect* (oblique) or *direct*. An indirect hernia comes through the deep ring, anterolateral to the cord structures while a direct one comes through the posterior wall, medial to the deep ring and inferior epigastric vessels; the *Hesselbach's triangle* (vide supra). It must be stressed that both types of inguinal herniae occur due to a weakness of the transversalis fascia, whereas the indirect one has an additional factor, the imperfectly obliterated processus vaginalis, providing a 'ready-made' sac.

Normal mechanisms preventing the development of hernia: In spite of the definite weakness of the inguinal canal created by the testicular sojourn, only few men develop hernia; thanks to some defense mechanisms in that region, coming into action whenever there is abnormal increase of intra-abdominal pressure.

i) *Shutter-valve* mechanism, by the obliquity of the canal, anterior and posterior walls of the canal get jammed against each other.

ii) *Pinch-cock* mechanism, by the arching fibers of the conjoint tendon, encircling the internal ring, shutting off any gap in the transversalis fascia.

iii) Condensation of tranversalis fascia at the internal ring, closes the ring effectively

iv) The bulk of cremaster muscle firms up, by contraction, filling the extra space in the canal

v) Both crura of external ring come together during muscular contraction

The first two are considered important and explain why sometimes, the hernial contents do not emerge in the supine position, as these mechanisms come to play before the contents reach the internal ring, to enter the canal.

Complications: are the same as for any hernia, such as:

1. irreducibility, often they become partially irreducible due to adhesions, but expansile cough impulse can still be appreciated on careful examination

2. incarceration, no different from the former, a term generally not preferred

3. obstruction, to the bowel lumen, requires urgent surgical intervention

4. strangulation, obstruction associated with impairment of blood supply to the contents. This is a serious complication, with a time-bound bowel necrosis, unless relieved within 6 hours.

It is not always easy to differentiate obstruction

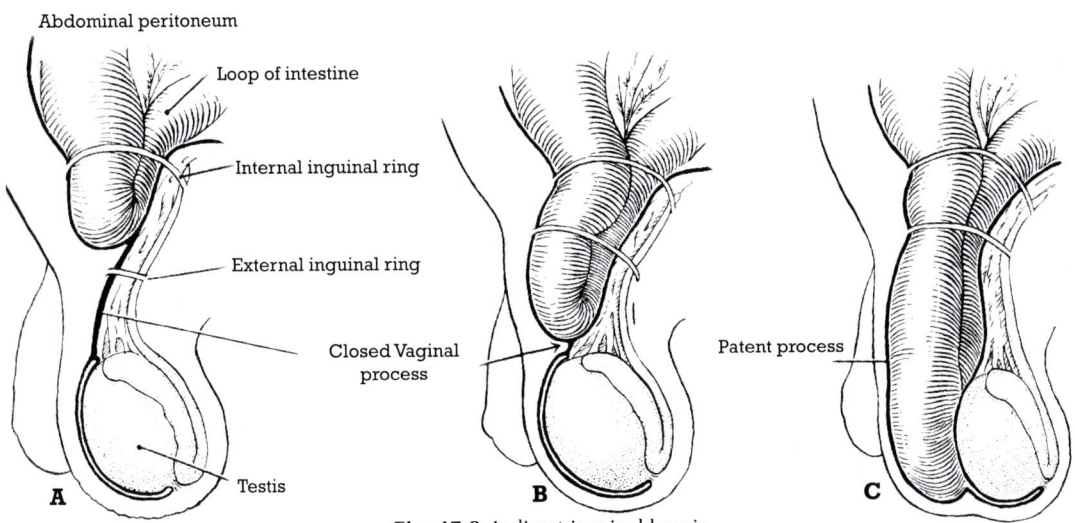

Fig. 47.8. Indirect inguinal hernia
A. Bubanocele B. Funicular type C. Complete (congential)

from strangulation, particularly in early stages. Local pain and tenderness may be more in strangulation, whereas on careful examination, some cough impulse may be detected in simple obstruction. However in a clinical context, it is always safe to presuppose strangulation and proceed expediently, as nothing is lost if it turns out at surgery to be only an obstructed hernia.

	Feature	Indirect	Direct
1.	Age	Children and young adults	Elderly
2.	Sex predilection	Male predominance (20:1)	Rare in females
3.	Side	Commoner on right	No such preference
4.	Bilaterality	Occasionally	Usually (upto 50%) bilateral
5.	Shape	Inguinoscrota l and pear or retort shapped due to preformed sac	Incomplete and globular, has no preformed sac
6.	Direction	Downwards and medial	Forwards
7.	Spontaneous reduction	Uncommon	Common
8.	Zieman's three finger Test	Impulse felt over the int ernal. ring	Felt over the ext ernal ring
9.	External ring invagination Test	Impulse felt by the tip of finger	Felt by the pulp of finger
10.	Topography	Descends readily into scrotum	Does not
11.	Internal ring occlusion Test	Hernia does not come out	Comes out thro ugh Hess elbach's triangle
12.	Risk of irreducibility or strangulation	Considerable	Minimal

Table-47.1: Differences between indirect and direct inguinal hernia
Most surgeons feel that this academic exercise is unnecessary and has no practical significance, since it can be determined at the time of surgery. In USA, this difference is rarely discussed.

INDIRECT INGUINAL HERNIA: These are basically considered to be congenital, in the sense, the defective or nonobliterated peritoneal processus, is blamed for its predisposition. They occur in younger individuals with a high male preponderance, attributable to testicular descent. They are commoner on the right side, because of the later descent of the right testis. Topographic types are:

i) *bubonocele*: (boubon: groin) here the processus vaginalis is obliterated up to the level of the external ring. Therefore, this presents as a swelling confined to the inguinal canal only or jetting out of the external ring.

ii) *funicular* hernia , in which the processus is closed at the level of the epididymis, the testis lies immediately below the hernial contents.

iii) *complete* hernia is one in which the hernial sac comes up to the tunica vaginalis, the testis itself becomes a content and is felt behind the other contents of the hernia. Since the entire processus vaginalis is patent, it is also known as 'congenital' hernia.

DIRECT INGUINAL HERNIA

A direct hernia protrudes through the posterior wall of the canal, medial to the inferior epigastric vessels i.e., through the Hesselbach's triangle. The contents of the sac lie separate from and usually behind and medial to the cord

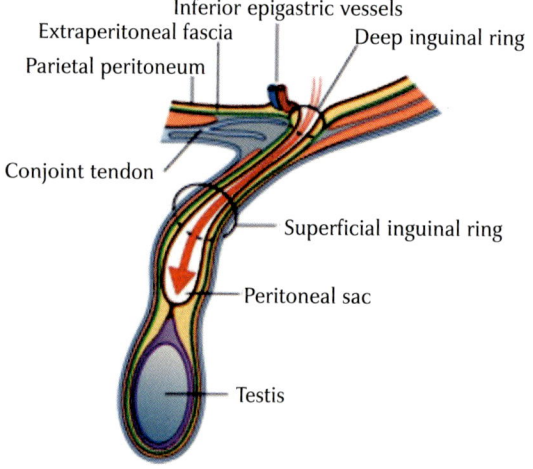

Inferior epigastric vessels
Extraperitoneal fascia
Parietal peritoneum
Deep inguinal ring
Conjoint tendon
Superficial inguinal ring
Peritoneal sac
Testis

Fig. 47.9. Indirect inguinal hernia

structures. The neck of the direct hernia is medial to the inferior epigastric artery, in contrast to the indirect, which is lateral. Strangulation is rare here as the neck of the sac is often wide. As it does not descend into the scrotum, it usually does not attain a large size.

A direct hernia is acquired and tends to be bilateral. A rare variety of congenital direct hernia occurs in a defect in the conjoint tendon, just before its insertion (Ogilvie hernia).

History of previous surgery

In the past history, operations in relation to the ilioinguinal and iliohypogastric nerves (L-1), such as appendectomy through Mc Burney/Lanz incision, lumbar sympathectomy, sigmoid colostomy, surgery on kidneys/ureters, including transplantation and perinephric/psoas abscess, extended low transverse (Pfannenstiel) incision for pelvic operations, are important, as injury to those nerves may weaken conjoint tendon, predisposing to the development of inguinal hernia years later.

Symptoms

1. Asymptomatic swelling discovered during routine medical examination

2. Dragging pain in the groin is often the commonest symptom. This discomfort may antedate the appearance of the hernia and may be referred to the testis. Pull on the omentum or mesentery may cause epigastric pain. If a hernia is very painful and tender it should be assumed that either irreducibility, obstruction or strangulation is imminent.

3. A painless lump, appearing and disappearing, is a pathognomonic feature of an uncomplicated hernia.

4. Other symptoms: Any cause of incre-ased intra-abdominal pressure like chronic constipation, chronic obstructive pulmonary/rinary disease should be enquired into.

5. Obstructive symptoms: As obstruction supervenes within the hernia, colicky abdominal pain, vomiting, constipation and distension will appear.

6. In delayed, neglected cases of strangulation, signs of septicemia may be associated with intestinal obstruction.

Signs

Patient is examined in the standing as well as in supine positions, because sometimes an early hernia may not come out, if examined in supine position. *The two classical signs of an uncomplicated hernia are expansile cough impulse and reducibility.*

1. Position - if it is inguino-scrotal, obviously it is an inguinal hernia, but if it is below and lateral to the pubic tubercle, going into the thigh, it is a femoral hernia.

2. Scrotal or inguinoscrotal - the root of the scrotum is held between thumb and fingers and if the examiner is able to *get above the swelling*, it is a scrotal swelling, usually a vaginal hydrocele. If the upper pole of the swelling cannot be appreciated (cannot get above the swelling), it is an inguinoscrotal swelling. For hydroceles, for which upper pole can not be reached, see chapter on hydrocele.

3. Cough impulse - while inspecting or palpating, either at the root of the scrotum (felt between the fingers) or at the superficial ring (with the thumb), the patient is asked to cough, for an expansile impulse which is indicative of an uncomplicated hernia.

4. Consistency - it may be elastic or doughy in an enterocele, with bowel sounds heard on auscultation. Soft or granular feel is in favor of an omentocele. If it feels tensely cystic and tender, strangulation has to be suspected.

5. Reducibility - methodical reduction of a hernia is also known as taxis; *the best person to reduce a large hernia is the patient himself*, having improvised his own 'technique' usually by thigh flexion and medial rotation. The clinician

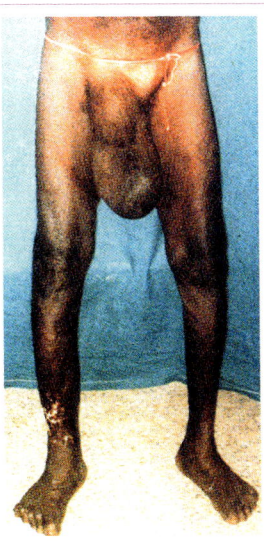

Fig. 47.10. Large right scrotal hernia and left bubonocele (courtesy: Halsted Surgical Clinic, Chennai)

may carry it out, by a similar method, in difficult cases. An enterocele produces a gurgling sound while being reduced. Forcible or rough attempts to reduce should not be done, for fear of the following complications:

(a) friable bowel in the sac may be traumatized or perforated

(b) nonviable or gangrenous loops of bowel may be reduced inadvertently and

(c) the whole hernia is simply pushed into the abdominal cavity, with the strangulation of loops persisting, within the tight-necked sac, termed *reduction en masse*. The latter two complications may create 'euphoria' in both patient and doctor alike, but can be disastrous in outcome, if left unrecognized.

6. *Internal ring occlusion test*: after reduction of the hernia, thumb is pressed over the deep ring and the patient is asked to cough. An indirect hernia will not pop out of the abdominal cavity, whereas a direct hernia will bulge medial to the occluding thumb. In a rare contingency, if the internal ring is larger than the thumb, even an indirect hernia may appear on coughing, a fallacy to reckon with.

7. *External ring invagination test*: after reduction of the hernia, the little/index finger is invaginated, borrowing skin from the bottom of the scrotum, into the superficial ring. The size of the ring is initially assessed, weak posterior wall may be noted in a direct hernia and finally the patient is asked to cough, to identify where the impulse is felt (by the pulp of the finger in direct and by the tip in indirect hernia). This is neither reliable nor comfortable and is generally not used (except, of course, in the examinations!) in practice (refer Jewels of Gyan 47.2).

8) *Zieman's three finger test:* The patient is asked to cough, with ring, middle and index

fingers placed over the surface markings for internal, external rings and saphenous opening respectively. Depending upon where the impulse is felt, it may be indirect, direct inguinal hernia or femoral hernia, in that order

9) Testis can be felt separate from the contents, a point of differentiation from a vaginal hydrocele.

10) How to identify the type in an irreducible inguinal hernia: Since it warrants immediate surgery, this academic distinction is not crucial; however, the following points may be noted: the very fact that it is irreducible, its retort shape and the inguinoscrotal disposition, all go in favor of an indirect variety.

11) Garnall's maneuver is done to bring out a hernia in children, when other methods have failed. The child is held on the abdomen from behind by both hands of the clinician and the child is lifted up, to increase the intra-abdominal pressure (as well as to make the child cry!).

Enterocele Vs omentocele or (epiplocele)

In an enterocele, visible peristalsis may be present, and it has an elastic feel, with a resonant note on percussion due to bowel gas. Peristaltic sounds may be heard on auscultation. It reduces with a gurgle, being more difficult initially, it is

easily accomplished in the later stage. In an omentocele, often due to omental adhesions, the later part of the reduction is more difficult, if not impossible.

Abdominal examination: it is important to look for any mass, causing constipation. In an elderly patient presenting with an inguinal hernia, incipient bowel obstruction, particularly colonic malignancy, should be excluded, since it may be a heralding manifestation and some surgeons insist on a colonoscopic evaluation, before operating on a hernia, in the elderly.

Secondly, assessment of the tone of the lower abdominal musculature must be done, either by simple inspection of the area, with the patient standing up or by putting the abdominal muscles to contraction by head/leg rising test (*Carnett's test*) or straining against a closed glottis (Valsalva maneuver). Oval-shaped diffuse bulges seen between the anterior superior iliac spine and the rectus muscle, just above the inguinal ligament, corresponding to the area of the conjoint tendon, known as *Malgaigne bulges*, indicate attenuation of the muscles required for repair, with a high likelihood of requiring a hernioplasty. It should be realized that they are neither diagnostic of a hernia nor does their presence automatically imply that a good herniorraphy cannot be performed.

Perineal and rectal examination: is essential to identify urethral/anal stricture (in young) and prostatic enlargement (in elderly), requiring primary attention before treating the hernia.

If an enlarged prostate is detected by digital examination, a detailed history regarding micturition should be elicited and residual urine in the bladder has to be measured, either by USG or by catheterization. Normally there should be no residual urine, but in the elderly, with a weak detrusor, <50ml is allowed as 'normal' and when it is more, further

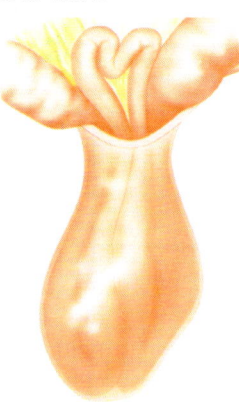

Fig. 47.11. Maydl's hernia with strangulated internal loop

studies, such as uroflowmetry (urodynamic study), IVU, cystoscopy etc. are warranted, to clinch the existence of obstructive pathology, due to prostatic enlargement. Tumor markers, like serum acid phosphatase and prostate specifc antigen (PSA), for malignancy, have to be done to plan appropriate treatment.

Chest examination to exclude conditions producing chronic cough, bronchospastic &/or obstructive pulmonary diseases (COPD), is mandatory. Not only should they be treated as precipitating factors, but they increase the risk of postoperative respiratory complications, such as atelectasis, pneumonitis or retained secretions.

Special types of inguinal hernia (based on the contents and the topography)

1. Richter's hernia - where only a portion of the circumference of the gut is involved, is very rare in inguinal hernia. It is dangerous as it can be easily overlooked, since the patient passes flatus and feces, despite ongoing bowel necrosis and features of intestinal obstruction may not appear till late.

2. Littre's hernia - when Meckel's diverticulum is found in the sac.

3. Maydl's hernia (syn: hernia-en-W, retrograde strangulation) - where there are two loops of bowel within the sac, the intervening loop remaining in the abdomen and vulnerable for strangulation. This is very dangerous because two 'healthy' looking loops of bowel are found in the sac and are inadvertently reduced. It is imperative to inspect the entire stretch of bowel loop, for vascularity and viability.

4. Amyand's hernia - when the appendix, along with the cecum descends into the (right) hernial sac.

5. Sliding hernia or hernia-en-glissade - is defined as a hernia, where a viscus forms part of the sac. Usually the cecum (on the right), sigmoid colon (on the left) or bladder (on any side), slide down along the sac; this phenomenon is seen in a long standing hernia of any type. By its

medial location, urinary bladder slides very often into a direct hernia. Other examples of sliding hernia are: esophageal hiatal hernia, cystocele or rectocele in women, often seen with uterine descent.

6. Interstitial hernia - The hernial sac lies between the muscle layers of the abdominal wall. It can lie between the peritoneum and transversalis fascia (*preperitoneal*) or between the oblique muscles (*interparietal*) or in the subcutaneous tissue, outside the external oblique (*extraparietal*).

7. Saddle or *pantaloon (Romberg) hernia* - both direct and indirect types are present, 'saddled' by the inferior epigastric vessels.

Differential diagnosis

a) vaginal hydrocele: oval, cystic, transilluminant, confined to the scrotum, without cough impulse or reducibility, testis cannot be felt separate

b) encysted hydrocele of the cord

c) varicocele: classical feel of 'bag of worms' and it fills from below when the patient stands up after occluding the superficial ring.

d) funiculitis: secondary to filariasis or sexually transmitted disease, with local and systemic signs of inflammation apparent

e) inguinal (canalicular) or retractile testis

f) diffuse lipoma of the cord

g) femoral hernia: location and Zieman's three finger test

h) lymph varix of the scrotum:, due to lymphatic obstruction, usually filarial. Features are very similar to a varicocele, but without side preponderance nor a thrill felt on coughing. It is transilluminant, though not easy to elicit.

i) psoas abscess: cystic swelling above and below inguinal ligament, with cross fluctuation and systemic/local signs of inflammation

Investigations

There are no specific investigations for an inguinal hernia, except those needed to certify fitness for anesthesia. USG abdomen to exclude obstructive uropathy and a large bowel study (barium enema or colonoscopy), in cases of progressive constipation to exclude an obstructing lesion, may be necessary in appropriate cases. In children, when the presence of hernia is in doubt, a contrast study (celiography, peritoneography or herniography), may reveal the scrotal sac. This is performed by injecting contrast into the peritoneal cavity through a polythene tube and taking an x-ray of the groin, after allowing the child to play around for a few minutes. A *CT/MRI may also be helpful, in adults with persistent groin pain, to exclude occult hernia.*

Treatment

Operation is the only definitive treatment. *The truss has harmed more patients than it helped*, hence its use should be strongly discouraged. The problems encountered in the use of a truss are: cumbersome nature, pressure complications of skin, higher incidence of strangulation and difficult subsequent surgery due to local tissue attenuation. If the hernia pops out, with the truss in place, as it prevents it from going in, there is a high probability of bowel injury or strangulation. Since operation for hernia can be done under local/field-block anesthesia, no patient should be considered unfit for surgery. Furthermore, if someone is deemed unfit for elective surgery, it would be even more hazardous to do an emergency operation on the patient, in the event of strangulation.

Operative management: three types of standard operations are available.

1. herniotomy
2. herniorrhaphy
3. hernioplasty

1. Herniotomy: In this operation, the neck of the sac is transfixed and ligated at its highest point; it is done as the sole procedure in infants and children with normal abdominal musculature and where the only pathology is a patent processus vaginalis. In all other herniae, it is done as a preliminary step, before repairing the defect. Some surgeons perform a digital exploration through the opened peritoneal sac, to

feel for any other defects and the integrity of the inguinal musculature. Very often, in direct hernia, the sac is not excised, for fear of injuring the urinary bladder, if it is sliding into it. It is simply inverted into the abdominal cavity by a 'purse-string' suture of prolene, over which a standard repair is carried out.

2. Herniorrhaphy: This is repair of the posterior wall of the inguinal canal by various methods of apposition, by using the structures of the vicinity, usually following herniotomy. It is very commonly performed in adults, with good muscular tone.

3. Hernioplasty: This is repairing the musculofascial defect, using extraneous structures, (either autologous or synthetic), which are not the components of the vicinity.

Indications for hernioplasty are: poor muscle tone, in recurrent hernias with wide defect, or in other words, it should be done whenever a satisfactory herniorraphy cannot be done, due to anatomical reasons. It also implies that an attempt to repair the defect with local tissue is always made, before deciding in favor of plasty and under normal circumstances, decision for hernioplasty is made only during surgery and not preoperatively. *However primary hernioplasty is being increasingly preferred world over, as it is tension free, with less postoperative pain and lowest long term recurrence rates.* The additional operating time, cost and fear of infection, were the main objections to such a 'blanket' indication earlier; however meta-analyses of large studies are now in favor of mesh plasty.

Operations
Herniotomy

A 5cm incision is made just 2cm above and parallel to the medial half of the inguinal ligament, the Camper (superficial fatty) and Scarpa (deep membranous) fasciae are divided and the external oblique is exposed. Anatomical landmarks, external ring, inguinal ligament etc. are identified before the inguinal canal is laid open, by cutting the external oblique aponeurosis, in the direction of its fibres, in a manner by which a cloth is cut by a pair of scissors, without moving its jaws. An incision is made on the fascial envelope of the cord and the sac will then be seen on the antero-lateral aspect of the cord structures. This is separated from the cord structures and then the sac is dissected upto the neck where it emerges from the deep ring. Here the structures to be noticed are the small pad of extra peritoneal fat and inferior epigastric artery. The sac is opened and the contents are reduced. It is then transfixed and ligated as high as possible so that the transfixed stump will disappear under the conjoint tendon.

Herniorrhaphy

In addition to the steps performed above, the posterior wall is strengthened using a variety of techniques, following the two cardinal principles for any hernia repair, namely use of nonabsorbable sutures and approximating the edges of the defect without tension.

a) In the standard Bassini repair the posterior wall is reinforced by suturing the conjoint tendon, (the lower margin of the internal oblique and transversus) along with the lower felted margin of transversalis fascia to the shelving edge of the inguinal ligament by a series of nonabsorbable sutures, the most medial one passing from the conjoint tendon to the periosteum of the pubic tubercle. The main drawback of this procedure is that, suturing a muscle (conjoint tendon) with fascia (inguinal ligament), is *not* considered physiological, but it has stood the test of time and some of the poor results reported are believed to be more related to the operating surgeon rather than the technique. There are several modifications of the Bassini repair, mostly unauthorized and self-styled and such an expression is better avoided. Suturing only the conjoint tendon to the inguinal ligament, is commonly referred to as the 'modified Bassini repair, leaving the transversalis fascia untouched, probably explaining the inferior results

	Indications for TEP	Contraindications for TEP
1.	Recurrent hernia	Obstructed /strangulated inguinal hernia
2.	Bilateral hernia	Ascites
3.	Multiple herniae	Bleeding disorders
	Technique of TEP	
	Landmarks to be identified for TEP	Principles in TEP
4.	Pubic bone midline	Head down supine position
5.	Inferior epigastric artery	Surgeons standing opposite side of hernia
6.	Cooper`s ligament	Camera person placed on opposite side of hernia
7.	Iliopubic tract	Monitor at foot end
8.	Cord and vas deferens Muscle and nerves in relation	Catheterise/empty the bladder properly prior to TEP
		Adequate wide space creations
		Careful dissection of cord and sac
		Ligate indirect sac
		Mesh should not be fixed laterally
		Size of mesh is 15x15cm
		Two point of fixation -one at pubic bone other at Cooper`s ligament by tacks/staplers

Table-47.2 Totally extraperitoneal mesh placement (TEP)

reported with this procedure. One very effective modification is to employ *continuous* monofilament suture, such as prolene, for the repair, allowing distribution of tension equally through the entire length of repair.

b) Another low recurrence herniorrhaphy is the *Shouldice* repair, where the transversalis fascia is slit open mediolaterally. The upper leaf is double-breasted onto the lower leaf and this is followed by double-breasting the conjoint tendon and internal oblique on to the inguinal ligament; thus 4 double-breasting layers are used to approximate the roof to the floor of the inguinal canal.

c) In *Devlin* repair the external oblique is also double breasted in front of the four layered Shouldice repair.

d) *Halsted* repair is useful in dealing with a large direct hernia, where additional support of the posterior wall is desirable, by suturing the external oblique behind the cord, positioning the cord subcutaneously. Loss of obliquity of the inguinal canal is considered its main disadvantage, making the normal 'shutter-valve' mechanism ineffective.

e) *Willi Meyer* repair is to double-breast the external oblique aponeurosis, when it is unusually lax and redundant. A modification of this is to create a 'neo-inguinal canal' between the two layers of the overlapping fascia, in which cord is placed.

f) *Ferguson* repair is placing the spermatic cord deep to the posterior wall repair, shifting the internal ring medially; this is not a popular operation.

g) *Henry* repair is an extraproperitoneal approach, by a low midline incision, accessing both inguinal regions from within, effecting bilateral operation at the same time.

h) *Lotheissen* repair is used, if there is associated femoral hernia, where the conjoint tendon is sutured down to pectineal (Cooper's) ligament, closing both inguinal and femoral defects.

i) *Lytle* stitch: to narrow the internal ring, is sometimes used alone in children, for whom standard repair is not necessary. A figure of '8' stitch of nonabsorbable material is placed, just medial to internal ring. In adults this step is used when the internal ring is abnormally patulous and has the advantage of displacing the spermatic cord laterally.

j) *La Roque's* technique: used for sliding hernia, where a good herniotomy cannot be done, owing to bowel adherence. A mini-laparotomy is performed just above the internal ring, by a grid-iron incision, the redundant sac of hernia is pulled into it and amputated, without bowel coming in the way and the wound closed. The hernia without the sac, is repaired by any standard method.

Hernioplasty: Three drawbacks of hernioplasty, which may not be significant under the present context, are:

(a) time consuming,
(b) cost of the prosthetic mesh
(c) being a foreign body, infection can be disastrous. The popular types of hernioplasty are:

1. *Lichtenstein's* (tension-free) hernioplasty in which the gap in the posterior wall of the inguinal canal is filled up with a polypropylene or PTFE (Gore-tex) mesh, which is sutured above to the conjoint tendon and below to the inguinal ligament, with a window placed laterally, permitting the spermatic cord to traverse. This is

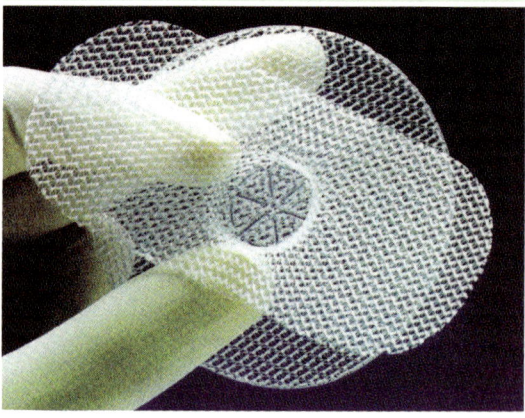

Fig. 47.12. Trilaminar prolene hernia system

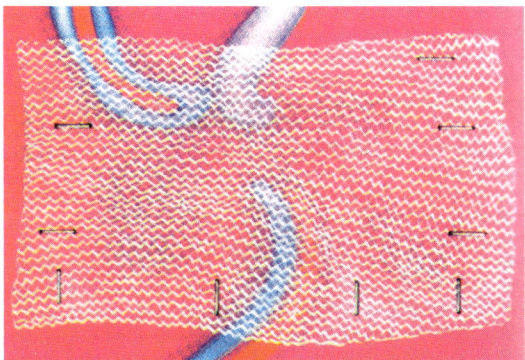

Fig. 47.13. Transparent prolene mesh for laparoscopic hernioplasty

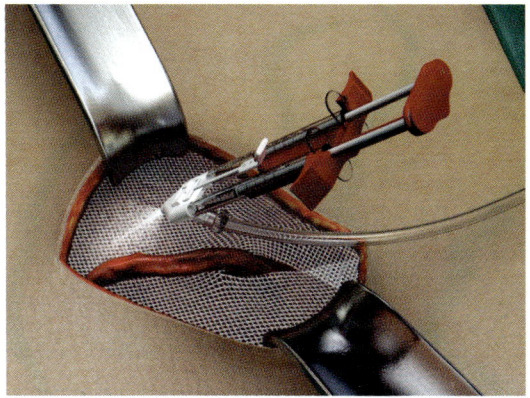

Fig. 47.14. Inguinal hernia mesh fixation by fibrin glue

the most popular in the current set up, easily done and credited with the lowest reported recurrence rate and minimal postoperative discomfort. Recently 'plug and patch' type of prosthesis (Perfix), which has an obturator part dipping into the internal ring, thus obliterating it, while the remaining part is used as a regular patch, is being used.

2. *Trilaminar prolene* hernia system (PHS) or ultrapro hernia system (UHS) involves one circular layer of mesh behind the transversalis fascia, a connector that acts as a plug and an external layer, superficial to transversalis fascia, thus combining laparoscopic mesh plasty with Lichtenstein's repair. This is credited with no recurrence and useful for recurrent complex hernias.

3. *Preperitoneal (Nyhus)* hernioplasty in which an incision is made well above the inguinal canal and the preperitoneal space is entered. The internal ring is identified, hernial sac pulled into the abdomen and inverted with a purse-string suture. A large prosthetic mesh is inserted against the internal ring, between the transversalis fascia and transversus abdominis muscle. It is fixed in place by a few anchoring stitches, before closing the wound.

4. *Laparoscopic* hernioplasty has now increasingly become popular and can be done transperitoneally or extraperitoneally. In the former, the posterior wall of the inguinal canal is approached through the peritoneal cavity, the

peritoneum around the internal ring is incised and a mesh is stapled anterior to the peritoneum, onto the inguinal ligament and conjoint tendon. The peritoneal flaps are then approximated. Care should be taken to avoid stapling or dissecting in the *triangle of doom* (bounded by the vas medially and gonadal vessels laterally and containing the external iliac vessels) and the *triangle of pain* (bounded by the inguinal ligament and gonadal vessels, transmitting the femoral nerve, anterior and lateral cutaneous nerves of thigh). This can also be done entirely through the extraperitoneal route, an easier procedure with lesser morbidity. The comparability of long term results with standard surgery continues to be under debate, to justify the additional cost and expertise involved in these 'high-tech' procedures.

Transabdominal Pre Peritoneal Mesh Repair (TAPP) using Laparoscope

This is used in large indirect hernia or reducible inguinal hernia. 10mm umbilical port is used for laparoscope. 5mm ports are placed one on each side on pararectal point at or above the level of umbilicus so as to achieve adequate triangulation. Contents of the hernia are reduced. Hernial sac is dissected in preperitoneal plane after making horizontal incision at the upper part of the sac. The vas, gonadal vessels, pubic bone, inferior epigastic vessels are identified. Once sac is dissected and excised, a prolone/vipro/ultrapro mesh of

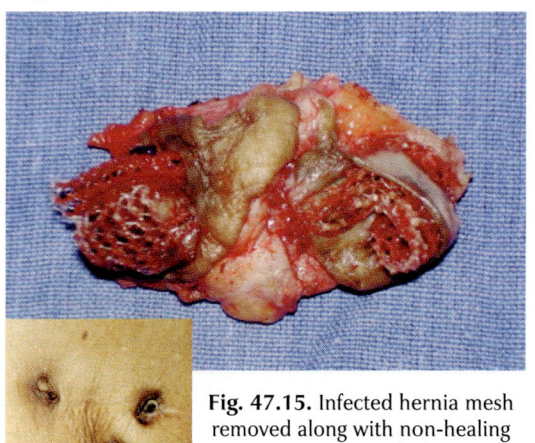

Fig. 47.15. Infected hernia mesh removed along with non-healing sinuses (shown below) (courtesy: Lifeline Hospitals, Chennai)

15x12cm size is placed in the peritoneal space and fixed to pubic bone using tacks. Peritoneum is closed over the mesh with continuous absorbable suture.

Totally extra peritoneal repair (TEP) repair

This technique is gaining more popularity then TAPP. After introducing the standard 3 ports (10, 5 & 5mm), dissection is carried out carefully, first downwards, then medially up to the public tubercle, iliopectineal ligament and laterally to iliac and inferior epigastric vessels. Once adequate space is created, a 15x15cm mesh is placed and spread behind the inguinofemoral area, without any folds. Mesh may be sutured to iliopectineal ligament. Migration of a mesh is not common and bilateral hernia may be treated effectively, using a larger mesh.

Difficulties and complications in TEP repair

Difficulty in dissecting indirect sac
Cord/vas injury

Inadvertent opening of the sac/peritoneum and interference with pneumoperitoneum.

Injuries to major structures like iliac vessels - 0.5-1.0%

Displacement of mesh or erosion into structures like urinary bladder (rare)
Nerve injury

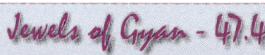

Characteristics of ideal mesh

1. Should be chemically inert and infection free
2. Should be easily sterilized
3. Should produce minimal foreign body reaction
4. Should not be carcinogenic
5. Should not mechanical strains
6. Should not react with body tissue
7. Should not react with fluids
8. Should develop adhesions with tissue soon after its implantation

Formation of seroma/hematoma
Infection

Recurrence

Advantages of TEP repair

Approach is totally extra peritoneal
Small incision
Proper placement of mesh in right space, i.e., preperitoneal space
peritoneal cavity is intact and not opened

Kugel patch repair

An oval shaped piece of mesh is inserted behind the hernia defect through a small incision .The mesh is held open by a memory recoil ring. A single absorbable suture holds the mesh in place.

Benefits

1. Less pain
2. Lower recurrence rate
3. Does not require general anesthesia

Complications of mesh

1. Infection
2. Mechanical failure
3. Pain
4. Foreign body Reaction
5. Adhesions and Intestinal complications
6. Nerve damage
7. Cost

Disadvantages

1. Risk of nerve injury
2. Not appropriate for contaminated case.

5) *Laparoscopic slip mesh*, by total extra-peritoneal placement of prosthesis (TEPP), to obliterate the defects of entire lower anterior abdominal wall (*myopectineal orifice of Fruchaud*) is a recent addition for multiple groin herniae.

Meshes used in hernioplasty: Although fascia lata, external oblique aponeurosis, anterior rectus sheath or even skin were earlier used in hernioplasty, they are almost never used in the current surgical scenario, readily available prosthetic meshes having taken their place. Some popular ones are the Marlex and Prolene, which are made up of knitted, monofilament polypropylene. They are inert, semielastic and semirigid. The Merselene mesh is made up of braided polyester, Dacron. It is less popular than prolene meshes. Expanded polytetrafluoroethylene PTFE (Gore-tex), is expensive and not considered ideal because it is smooth and has no microscopic pores to allow fibroblastic growth. All these meshes should not be placed intraperitoneally in contact with bowel, as they could cause adhesive obstruction. Infection is a major dissuader of mesh repair, in low volume peripheral centres.

Anatomical considerations for laparoscopic repair of groin hernia

1. Preperitoneal space is the potential space infront of the peritoneum, behind the transversalis fascia and rectus muscle. Below infront of the urinary bladder it is called space of Retzius medially and Space of Bogros, laterally. Three fossae lying in relation to the peritoneal folds - supravesical and medial fossae are located medial to lateral umbilical ligaments, the sites of direct hernia. The lateral fossa are lateral to lateral umbilical folds and are the sites for the indirect hernia.

2. The myopectineal orifice of Fruchaud is bounded medially by the lateral border of rectus abdominis, laterally by iliopsoas, superiorly by conjoint tendon and inferiorly by pectin pubis. This area is the site for groin hernias, which should be covered by mesh of adequate size to strengthen the defect and to prevent recurrence. Iliopubic tract is analogue of the inguinal ligament, extends from Cooper's ligament to anterior superior iliac spine which divides endoscopic view of preperitoneal space into superior compartment (containing inferior epigastic vessels, Hesselbach's triangle, cord structures and is this site for indirect hernia) and inferior compartment (containing femoral canal, iliac vessels, iliopsoas muscle, genitofemoral nerve, lateral femoral cutaneous nerve). External iliac vessels lie in a triangle formed by gonadal vessels laterally, vas deferens medially and peritoneal reflection inferiorly (triangle of doom).

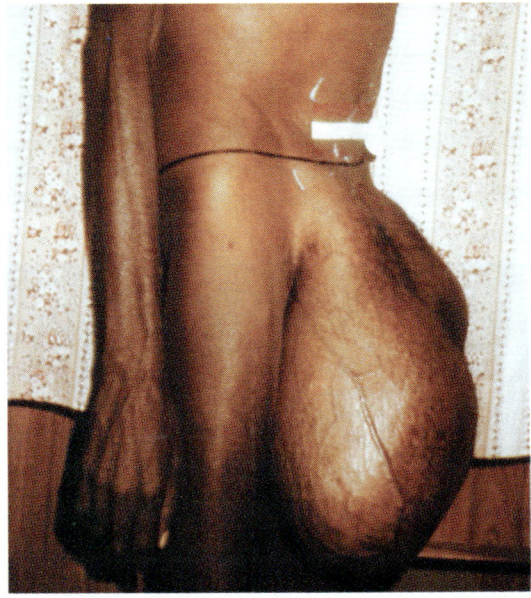

Fig. 47.16. Huge inguinal hernia, reaching the knees (preliminary pneumoperitoneum was used to expand abdominal volume, to facilitate reposition during surgery)
(courtesy: Halsted Surgical Clinic, Chennai)

3. Aberrant obturator artery is an occasional branch of inferior epigastric artery replacing its pubic branch, travels across Cooper's ligament, which during fixation of the mesh, can cause

troublesome hemorrhage (corona mortis). Triangle of pain is formed by gonadal vessels medially, illio pubic tract laterally and peritoneal reflection below. Genitofemoral nerve and lateral cutaneous nerve of thigh traverse this triangle. Injury to these nerves either by dissection or by tacks, may cause postoperative neuralgia, hence, tacks or staplers should not be placed in this triangle.

In conclusion, it may be stated that mesh repair for all types of hernias is currently the gold standard with least rates of recurrence. With experience, the operating time is no longer than tissue repair, nor the infection rate any higher. The debate between open versus laparoscopic approach, however continues, the latter preferred in high volume centres.

Why herniorrhaphy or plasty for indirect hernia? There is no doubt that in an indirect hernia the basic problem is the sac, but there is always some laxity of both internal and external rings and weakness of tranversalis fascia, the latter seems to be a common factor in all groin hernias. If a single stitch is used to tighten the muscular internal ring, it may simply cut through, hence a row of sutures are placed starting from the medial end; the most lateral of them makes the internal ring 'snug' around the cord. In other words, the rest of the sutures in the 'repair' are only to support the lateralmost one. Similarly while approximating the leaves of external oblique from its lateral corner, the most medial stitch decides the size of the external ring. Admittedly the size of the external ring is of no great consequence in terms of the strength of the inguinal canal, but during a medical examination for a job, sometimes the size of external ring is checked, to certify 'fitness'.

Adjuvant procedures to facilitate hernia repair:

i) *Tanner's relaxing incision* or slide: this is used if there is a wider defect with the anticipated tension being more than ideal for the repair. In this, the external oblique is retracted medially, to expose its line of fusion with other two mus-

cles of abdominal wall, to form the rectus sheath. The latter two are incised vertically in a paramedian line, exposing the rectus muscle. This aponeurotic 'slide' permits a relatively tension-free approximation of conjoint tendon to the inguinal ligament, though in a modern context, such a case calls for a mesh plasty.

ii) *Debulking* the spermatic cord: may be done, when it is very thick, preventing snug closure of the rings. Sometimes, an associated diffuse lipoma or rarely a lymph varix of the cord may also be excised, for the same purpose.

iii) *Koontz's excision of spermatic cord:* The inguinal part of spermatic cord can safely be excised, without affecting the blood supply to the testis. Hence in difficult repairs, this step comes handy, so that both rings can be totally obliterated, but it is important not to disturb the testis in its place nor deliver it into the inguinal wound, since it is nourished by scrotal/septal blood supply, through the tunica. For the same reason, bilateral Koontz's resection is not advisable at the same time. The advantage of surgery in women is that the round ligament may be totally excised in all cases, closing the rings permanently.

iv) *Orchidectomy* is the best option in the very elderly, in large sliding hernias or indeed in any difficult situation, allowing total obliteration of rings.

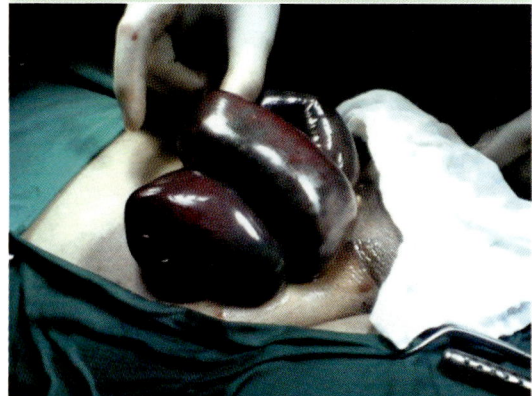

Fig. 47.17. Gangrenous loops of bowel in a strangulated inguinal hernia courtesy: Dr K R Reddy, Kakinada

v) *Fusion* of inguinal canal can be performed, following the above two procedures, by approximating the anterior and posterior walls of the canal, converting the area into a solid bar of tissue, virtually eliminating any chance of recurrence.

vi) *Omentectomy* may sometimes be necessary, before herniotomy, if chronically adherent and knotted omentum cannot be reduced.

vii) Transfixation of the stump to the conjoint tendon, using a nonabsorbable stitch, is sometimes done for large, bulky sacs, to prevent 'stump recurrence'.

viii) Artificial tension *pneumoperitoneum* to expand the volume of the abdominal cavity preoperatively may become necessary in large scrotal hernia, the so-called 'scrotal abdomen', to obviate an accommodation problem, during surgery. A polythene tube is introduced under strict aseptic conditions, into the peritoneal cavity, a few days prior to surgery and air is injected under pressure, to the point of tolerance, which may be about 1-2 litres, depending upon the size of the patient. This is carried out daily till the day of surgery, to facilitate reduction of the herniated omentum/bowel in the abdomen, during the operation. This method may be used for large ventral hernias also, for the same purpose.

Bilateral hernia: There is no consensus about simultaneous single sitting repair. Avoiding additional cost and the need for a second surgery are the main attractions of synchronous repair, whereas increased operating time, a higher incidence of infection, a higher recurrence rate and the remote possibility of creating a femoral weakness (due to tension on the transversalis fascia), are the main objections. If the surgeon opts for a synchronous repair, Tanner's relaxing incisions on both sides, or a mesh hernioplasty would eliminate undue tension (in the surgeon's mind also!) and consequent higher incidence of recurrence.

Associated hydrocele: is not uncommon and both may be safely operated upon at the same time. As a principle, whenever two procedures have to be done for a patient at one sitting, the cleaner of them should be done first, before the potentially contaminated one. Hence hydrocele surgery should follow hernia repair, either delivering it into the inguinal wound or by a separate scrotal incision. However, if the hydrocele is obviously complicated by infection (pyocele), it is wise to treat it first to eradicate sepsis, deferring hernia repair to a later date.

Strangulation: Patients present with irreducibility and severe pain with or without features of intestinal obstruction, but reflex vomiting may be seen due to omental involvement. A tender, tensely cystic inguinoscrotal swelling, which cannot be reduced and exhibits no cough impulse, makes the clinical diagnosis straightforward. If bowel is involved, signs of intestinal obstruction (vomiting, colicky abdominal pain, distension and obstipation) may be present. In late or neglected cases with bowel gangrene, signs of peritonitis and/or septicemia may be evident, with considerable morbidity and mortality.

Investigations

As it is a surgical emergency, only essential investigations such as routine blood and urine, chest skiagram, an ECG, serum biochemistry (including electrolytes if necessary), should be done for anesthetic evaluation, expediently correcting any abnormalities detected.

Treatment

Preoperative care: nasogastric decompression and intravenous fluids with antibiotics may be needed, if intestinal obstruction is suspected.

Anesthesia: For a fit and stable patient, any conventional anesthesia, like general or spinal may be employed. Otherwise, surgery can be comfortably performed under ilioinguinal field-block with lignocaine; hence *no patient should be considered unsuitable for urgent intervention*.

Surgery

Essential differences in the steps of operation from the standard operation are: inguino-scrotal incision, opening the sac first, to let out the sequestrated toxic fluid and to get hold of the involved loop, before the constricting ring are divided. This step is important because, if the constricting band is released before opening the sac, not only does the toxic fluid in the sac drain into the peritoneal cavity, but the loop of bowel involved may also slip inside, making it virtually impossible to retrieve the same segment of bowel for inspection, often necessitating an avoidable laparotomy. The usual constricting bands are external ring and the neck of sac at the internal ring; use of Childe's hernia director, may sometimes be necessary while dividing the constriction, to avoid injury to subjacent bowel. After dividing these, some more loops of bowel are drawn into the field, to inspect the afferent and efferent segments for viability. (see Maydl's strangulation)

The signs of bowel viability are:

(a) color

(b) peristalsis

(c) pulsations at the mesenteric border.

If doubt exists, 100% oxygen may be given by mask to the patient, to see if the color improves. If it is still equivocal, sticking the bowel wall with a fine needle, to see the bleeding or injecting 0.5ml of prostigmine into the mesentery, to stimulate the segment of bowel go into spasm, have been suggested, but most of the surgeons prefer to play safe, by resecting the devitalized bowel, at this point.

Rest of the operation is the same as the elective procedure. Of course, if bowel is resected, nasogastric aspiration and intravenous fluids should be continued till the intestinal functions return, which may be for 48 hours. A rare cause of intestinal stricture and obstruction, months or years after delayed reduction of a strangulated hernia, is segmental ischemia of the bowel at its entry and exit points at the neck of the hernial sac, usually 6-12" apart, due to prolonged pressure of constriction, going to cicatrization (intestinal stenosis of Garre).

Causes of recurrence of a hernia: They may be very much the same as those of any hernia elsewhere, which may be divided into three groups:

a) preoperative causes: these are more related to the patient, such as persistence of cough, urinary obstruction and constipation, obesity, diabetes mellitus, anemia, hypoprotenemia, avitaminosis, immunosuppression, untreated septic focus, improper local hygiene etc.

b) operative causes: these are mostly technical, such as selection of wrong procedure, not doing high ligation of sac, using absorbable material for repair, not considering plasty when required, improper hemostasis or leaving dead space, resulting in wound hematoma, bilateral synchronous repair, not employing prophylaxis against infection etc.

c) postoperative causes: wound infection, pulmonary complications leading to persistent cough (relentless smoking), unrelieved obstructive uropathy or constipation, too early return to work involving physical strain etc.

Complications specific to surgery for inguinal hernia

1. Nerve injury: Ilioinguinal and genital branch of genitofemoral nerve traverse the inguinal canal. They may be inadvertently severed leading to anesthesia or paresthesia of the groin or scrotum. More troublesome complications is their entrapment in a stitch or tacker, causing intractable neuralgia, occasion-

ally requiring re-exploration to divide (neurotomy) or release (neurolysis) the nerve. This is more commonly encountered in mesh repair of hernia, hence the caution, 'no fixation of the inferolateral part of the mesh'.

2. Secondary hydrocele: Injury to the lymphatics or veins of the spermatic cord, may lead to secondary hydrocele. If the rings are made too tight during herniorrhaphy, compression of these structures may be another reason.

3. Bowel injury: In sliding hernia, there is a danger of causing bowel injury or ischemia, if an over-zealous attempt is made to separate the bowel from the peritoneal sac. Bowel loop may also be cought in the herniotomy stitch, while doing 'high' ligation of sac. In strangulation, an error of judgement in missing a non-viable loop and reducing it, may be disastrous

4. Mesh infection, foreign body reaction or migration may occur. If not properly 'peritonealized' the mesh may get adherent to a bowel loop, leading to obstruction or fistula.

5. Periosteitis pubis: This is a rare, but troublesome complication, due to the most medial stitch of repair, including the pubic periosteum. Patient develops persistent local pain, tenderness and spasm of adductor muscles of the thigh, attached to the pubic bone, which may persist for several weeks.

6. Injury to external iliac vessels. While taking a bite in the inguinal ligament, it should be remembered that the vessels lie very close to it and vulnerable for injury; vein more than the artery. It is advisable, as the midinguinal point is reached, to depress the floor of the canal with a finger (or more safely using an instrument) to push the vessels away from the ligament and needle bite.

7. Fournier's gangrene of scrotum (rarely)

The concept of triple neurectomy

In cases of intractable post hernioplasty neuralgia, due to suspected nerve entrapment, re-exploration and division of three nerves (iliohypogastric, ilioinguinal and genital branch of genitofemoral) may offer relief. A preliminary injection of bupivacaine (Sensorcaine) into the inguinal canal is given, to confirm the diagnosis. Prophylactic triple neurectomy during all inguinal mesh repairs, advocated by some centres, has not gained universal acceptance.

A concluding word of caution: It may be surprising to know that a candidate who gets a case of inguinal hernia in the examination, statistically has only 50% chances of satisfying the examiners! Being a very common condition/operation seen or done in practice, no mistakes are accepted, in contrast to difficult cases like an abdominal mass or a soft tissue malignancy. Keeping this experience in mind, every attempt has been made in this chapter to exhaustively cover all of the points likely to come up for discussion in a case of a hernia, acknowledging that some areas still might be left uncovered, considering the horizons of the subject!

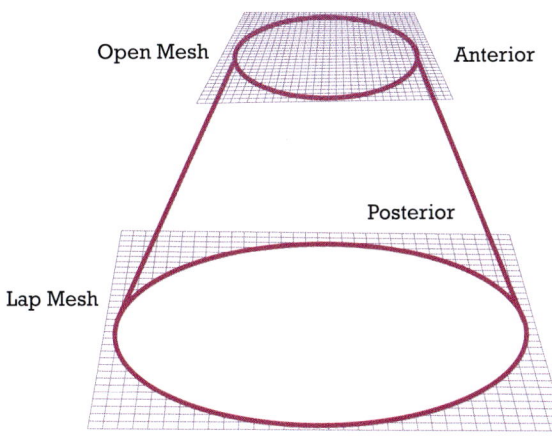

Fig. 47.18. The inguinal canal is a truncated cone. Therefore, lap mesh has to be large (15 x 12 cm), whereas open mesh can be small (6 x 8 cm)

48 Incisional Hernia

(syn: ventral hernia, postoperative hernia)

Definition: A hernia occurring through a separation of the edges of a musculo-apneurotic surgical suture line. The sac may contain bowel, omentum or both.

Etiology

Several general and local etiological factors predispose to the development of an incisional hernia.

It may be realized that the vast majority of these are preventable, if standard principles of surgery are meticulously observed. Even laparoscopy and enterostomy (colostomy, ileostomy etc) wounds are not immune to this complication.

a) General factors: mostly factors related to patient

Obesity, chronic cough, malnutrition, hypoproteinemia, avitaminosis, jaundice, ascites, excessive abdominal distension, steroid use, connective tissue disorders, immune deficiency etc.

b) Local factors: mostly related to technique of surgery

1. Inadequate amount of musculo-apneurotic layer of the anterior abdomical wall.

2. Poor technique of wound closure including usage of absorbable sutures.

3. Inadequate suture/wound length ratio (4:1 or 6:1 is ideal)

4. Wound dead-space and hematoma.

5. Wound infection.

6. Injury to the nerves of that area, e.g. Battle`s pararectal vertical incision for appendectomy may injure the ilioinguinal nerve predisposing to a hernia.

7. Tube drainage brought out through the main laparotomy wound itself.

8. Highest incidence of ventral hernia is seen in lower abdominal incisions in women, due to attenuation of muscles and fascia by repeated pregnancies. Hence gynecological and obstetric operations are notorious for this complication, unjustifiably earning them a bad reputation.

9. Muscle-splitting incisions, such as McBurney (grid iron) incision for appendix or flank incision for ureter or lumbar sympathetic chain, have the least incidence of incisional hernia.

Symptoms

The early signs of a disrupted wound is a serosanguinous discharge through the lapartomy wound around 3rd postoperative day. Whatever be the reason, when the wound scar formation is very weak, it makes the wound vulnerable for developing a hernia.

The usual presentation is a painless swelling, located in the vicinity of a scar of a previous laparotomy/laparoscopy/enterostomy, appearing during coughing or in the erect position. Irreducibility, pain and vomiting may signify adhesions of omentum and loops of bowel within the sac, with or without obstruction. Strangulation is rare, but possible in hernias with a narrow neck and sharp edges of the fascial defect.

Signs

A globular swelling is seen arising from the scar, soft or doughy and reducible with a cough

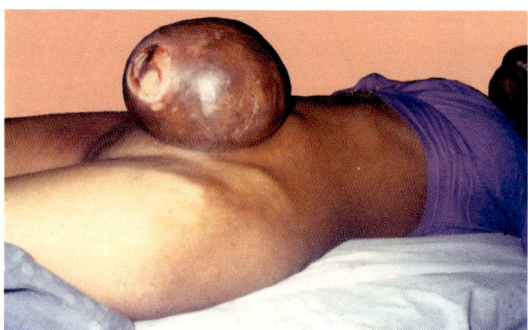

Fig. 48.1. Huge ventral hernia, with gravid uterus as its contents (Cesarean section and herniorrhaphy were done at the time of delivery)
(courtesy: Halsted Surgical Clinic, Chennai)

impulse. If loops of bowel are present in the sac, it may be resonant and reduces with a gurgle. A weak and flabby abdominal musculature may be made out. The margins of the fascial defect are usually felt, by dipping the fingers into the hernia, after reducing it.

A very useful maneuver for the surgeon is to perform head/leg rising test, after reducing the hernia and his fingers invaginated deep into the defect. If the lateral edges of the strong fascia come together, jamming against the dipping fingers, a comfortable herniorrhaphy can be accomplished, but if a wide gap persists even after putting the abdominal muscles to contraction, the need for hernioplasty is imminent.

Often, in the standing position, a large fold of skin and fat, called panniculus (membranous sheet of tissue) abdominis, hangs like an apron, particularly in obese patients with long standing hernia. This may require excision at the time of surgery (panniculectomy).

Differential diagnosis

i) Irreducible hernia may look like a benign/ malignant soft tissue tumor, a hematoma or a chronic abscess. The history, its location, visible peristalsis and resonant note over the swelling and the gurgling will help to identify it.

ii) Hematoma of rectus sheath, classically seen in hypertensives or those on anticoagulant therapy, presenting as a paramedian, tensely cystic mass of acute onset, in the intermuscular plane, fixed to rectus muscle/sheath, associated with echymosis of the overlying skin. It is due to rupture of inferior epigastric vessels, as a result of trivial injury or violent muscular contraction. It may also be rarely seen during the 3rd trimester of pregnancy. The quantity of blood collected may sometimes be so great as to cause hypovolemic features.

Iii) Phantom hernia: this is due to paralysis of anterior abdominal muscles, usually due to anterior poliomyelitis (in children) or injury to intercostal, subcostal, ilioinguinal or iliohypogastric nerves. One classical example is a subcostal (Kocher's) incision, which cuts across the intercostal nerves, denervating the upper quadrant of the abdominal wall on that side, leading to a diffuse bulge in that region.

Iv) Divarication of recti: this is also a phantom hernia, more common in lower abdomen of mutliparous women, producing a linear midline swelling, without definite fascial edges (as in a hernia). It becomes more prominent by head/leg rising (Carnett's) test or Valsalva maneuver. The gap is so large that normal abdominal/pelvic viscera can be palpated by invagination and it never strangulates.

Investigations

There are no specific investigation to diagnose a ventral hernia, but only those needed to exclude other conditions, such as desmoid, hematoma or an abscess as well as those needed for anesthetic evaluation.

An USG of abdomen is very useful, to detect any incidental diseases like cholelithiasis, uterine fibroids, ovarian cysts, so that if the situation allows, they may also be tackled at the same time, obviating the need for another surgery, soon after.

Treatment

Non-operative: There is hardly any role for conservative management of ventral hernia, except in very elderly fragile individuals, with a low risk of strangulation due to a large neck. Unless some serious contraindication exists, as a rule, all hernias should be repaired, since morbidity and mortality in those patients may be unacceptably high if they require urgent surgery for obstruction/ strangulation

Preoperative precautions

1) weight reduction.
2) correction of anemia, hypoprotenemia and other metabolic abnormalities.
3) if chronic bronchitis, urinary obstruction or constipation are present, they should be attended to.
4) colonic lavage is given to prepare the bowel in the event of inadvertant injury, if extensive adhesions are anticipated.

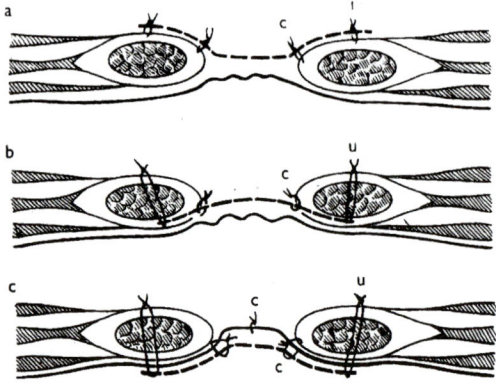

Fig. 48.2. Placement of the mesh in ventral hernia repair
a. Onlay **b.** Extraperitoneal **c.** Intraperitoneal

5) artificial pneumoperitoneum may be necessary in obese patients with large herniae (see chapter 47).

Operative treatment (ventral or incisional herniorrhaphy)

The hernia is approached through a long, elliptical incision including the previous scar and redundant, atrophic and unhealthy skin. The skin flap is dissected off from the sac and the sac is opened around the neck. The contents are reduced after releasing omental/bowel adhesions, sometimes excising the omen-tum, if needed. A herniotomy is then performed by excising the sac and closing it with a continuous catgut stitch, as any perito-neal closure. In obese patients with fatty abdominal wall, it may be difficult to identify small defects in other areas, which when overlooked, may result in 'recurrence'. The fool-proof method is to feel the entire anterior abdominal wall from inside, before peritoneal closure, for 'dimples', often with omental adhesions guarding them.

The musculoaponeurotic defect is dissected out and the edge

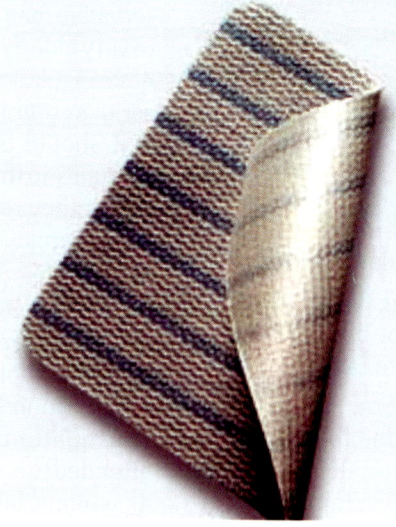

Fig. 48.3. Proceed mesh used for repairing large vental hernia

freshened, till good strong fascia is reached. These steps are common to all hernias, various types of repair differ only from here onwards:

Types of repair

1. *Anatomical*: It is possible, if the defect is small enough, to bring the edges together without undue tension. In this, the individual layers of the anterior abdominal wall are sutured to restore original anatomy, using nonabsorbable material for muscle and fascia.

2. *Cattell's* repair: is not much different from the preceding, applying the basic principle of layered approximation.

3. *Mass closure*: The margins of the defect are approximated (in full thickness), in one layer, with through and through interrupted, nonabsorbable sutures, taking liberal bites from the edges.

4. *Keel* operation: (keel is the midline longitudinal metal support at the bottom of the entire ship, projecting down as a ridge) In this operation the unopened hernial sac is reduced en masse into the abdomen, inverting it in several layers, ultimately reaching a good strong fascia. The margins of the fascia are then sutured with nonabsorbable suture, turning in more of parietes, so that at the end, it looks like the keel of a ship, when viewed from within.

5. *Peter Jones repair*: In this repair, interrupted sutures are used, but the suturing is done in such a way as to invert the edge of the defect, with a gap of about 1cm between adjacent sutures.

6. *Nuttall's* operation: This is meant for lower midline defects; the principle of this repair is to detach the lower insertions of both recti abdo-

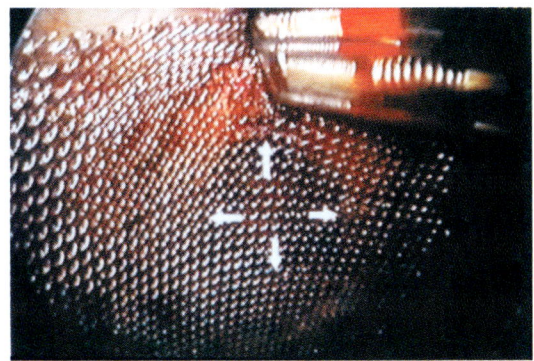

Fig. 48.4. Laparoscopic hernioplasty mesh being stapled to the fascial defect
(courtesy: Lifeline Hospitals, Chennai)

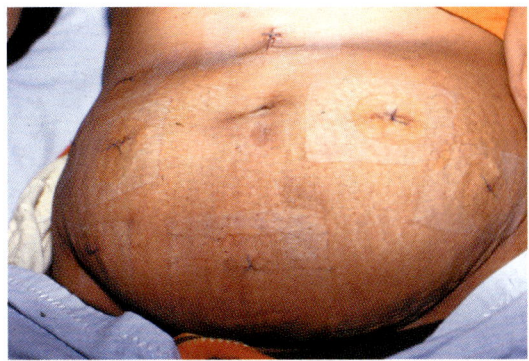

Fig. 48.5. Healed port wounds following Laparoscopic ventral hernioplasty
(courtesy: Lifeline Hospitals, Chennai)

minis from the symphysis pubis and to reattach them to the pubic tubercles of the opposite side, overlapping each other providing strength. The rectus sheath is sutured in front, with nonabsorbable sutures.

7. *Mesh repair* (hernioplasty): This is becoming increasingly popular, for its lowest recurrence rate, bridging fascial gap with a synthetic mesh, such as polypropylene (Prolene), Dacron, Marlex, or PTFE (Goretex). The mesh may be placed extraperitoneally, deep to fascial sheath (inlay) or superficial to it (on lay). Progressive ingrowth of fibroblasts within the lattice work of the mesh occurs, strengthening the abdominal wall. Infection, extrusion of the mesh and bowel adhesions (if not concealed by peritoneal layer) are the main complications of this procedure.

8. The *Stoppa's* repair (GPRPVS - giant prosthetic replacement of previsceral space) consists of implantation of a large sheet of mesh to completely cover the abdominal wall. This is placed in the preperitoneal space of Nyhus in order to prevent adhesions with the bowel loops and fistulation.

9. The *bipedicled mesh plasty* (Ramirez's procedure) is used if there is

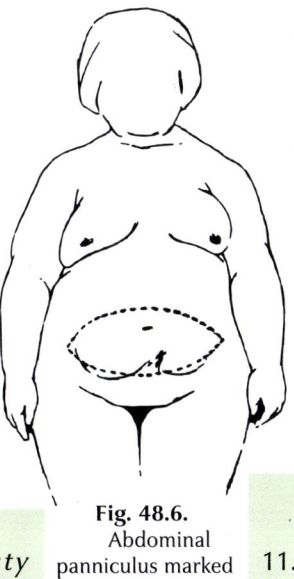

Fig. 48.6.
Abdominal panniculus marked for excision

need to cover the mesh or if there is a fear of infective sequelae. A large curvilinear incision on either flank is used to release the tension of the anterior abdominal wall. Even a large central midline defect can be covered by bringing both the edges together. The resultant lateral defects are covered by a mesh by continuing to raise the skin flap from the midline. This covers the lateral areas with a mesh but does not open up the mesh to the exterior.

10. **Abdominoplasty (or 'tummy tuck'):** If an excessive panniculus abdominis is present, it is better to excise it, by a transverse elliptical incision, at the time of hernia repair, for physicial and cosmetic advantage. Sometimes, this can be carried upto the upper abdomen, leaving a disc of skin around the umbilicus, which ultimately fits into a circular window made in the mobilized upper skin flap, to restore the normal appearance of the 'belly button'. In view of the extensive mobilization and undermining of flaps, an ambulant suction drain (Redivac or Hemovac) is employed, to prevent collection of blood/lymph in the dead space created.

11. Creation of **neo-umbilicus** is done, if the umbilicus has to be

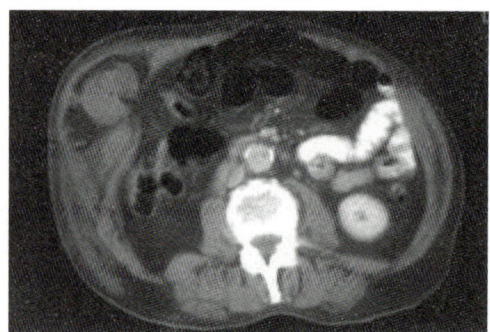

Fig. 48.7. CT scan - Spigelian hernia left side

excised, during repair. Using a fine nonabsorbable stitch, dermis from the upper flap, devoid of subcutaneous fat, is snugly anchored to linea alba or line of fascial repair in the midline, creating a depression or dimple, mimicking the umbilicus, for esthetic purposes.

Recent trials of placing an absorbable polyglactin mesh, to strengthen normal abdominal wound closure, with an aim of preventing herniation, in the 'high risk' group, were not shown to be beneficial in providing necessary wound support, during the crucial period of fascial healing.

Since faulty collagen cross linkng is being blamed for the development of postoperative hernia, mesh repair has become mandatory. In open surgery, a regular polyproplene mesh is deployed, where as in laparoscopic repairs, specially designed meshes, such as Proceed, Parietex etc. are used for intraperitoneal onlay mesh placement (IPOM).

Postoperative care

a) Prophylactic intravenous bactericidal antibiotics should be started, before the incision is made, to be given for about 6hrs after surgery (*Burke*), but if the bowel is inadvertently opened while releasing adhesions, they have to be continued for at least 72hrs.

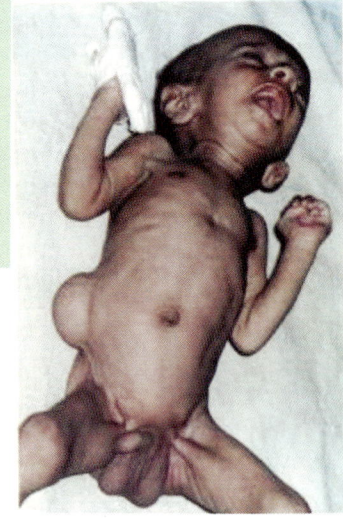

Fig. 48.8. Lumbar hernia in a neonate
(courtesy: Dr S Ramesh, Chennai)

b) If large sized hernia is repaired, naso-gastric decompression and IV fluids should be given, till the intestinal peristalsis is established.

c) Drains may be removed after 48hrs, if not much soaking seen.

d) DVT prophylaxis, early movements of the legs and ambulation (to prevent thromboembolism).

e) Chest physiotherapy in obese elderly is extremely important in the early postoperative period.

f) Fluid (lymph) collection under the flaps may require aspiration under strict aseptic conditions.

RARE TYPES OF HERNIAS

1. SPIGELIAN HERNIA

This is a rare paramedian hernia of the anterior abdominal wall developing through a weakness in the Spigel's fascia, which is formed by the fusion of internal oblique and transversus aponeuroses, before the formation of the rectus sheath, at the semilunar line. It commonly occurs in obese patients above 50, at the level of the arcuate line (of Douglas), where the fascial fibers are more or less parallel and split. The hernia is usually intraparietal, as the sac is under the external oblique aponeuro-sis, seen as a diffuse bulge at a point of intersection of semi-lunar line with the spino-umbilical line and often goes unrecognized in the early stage.

USG/CT may be necessary to detect a small Spigelian hernia. After exposing the sac under the external oblique and performing a herniotomy, smaller defects can be repaired by simple closure, but the larger ones may need a mesh repair.

2. INTERSTITIAL or INTRA-PERIETAL HERNIA

The hernia sac dissects its way into the layers of abdominal parietes, as an extension of groin (inguinal or femoral) hernia. It is more common in males and except vague discomfort over the site of hernia, neither the patient nor the physician appreciates a distinct swelling, leading to delayed diagnosis, till it strangulates. Recently, with liberal use of CT/MRI for abdominal diagnosis, more and more of these conditions are detected before they complicate. Depending upon its relation to the musclular layers of the abdominal wall, they are classified as:

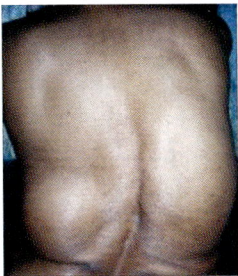

Fig. 48.9. Left Petit's hernia

I. Properitoneal type (20%): it is generally a diverticular extension from a groin hernia and sometimes diagnosed during surgery for them. The suprainguinal bulge becomes less prominent on putting the abdominal muscles to contraction.

ii. Intermusclular type (60%): this is a bilocular extension of an inguinal hernia, usually passing between external and internal oblique muscles and presents as a supra-inguinal bulge, besides the parent (inguinal) hernia. The size of the swelling may remain unaltered on leg rising test.

iii. Subcutaneous or inguinosuperficial type (20%): The sac dissects its way into sub-cutaneous plane. The swelling becomes more prominent on putting the abdominal muscles to contraction.

Treatment: Since most of them present with acute intestinal obstruction, minimum essential investigations and immediate surgery is mandatory.

3. LUMBAR HERNIA

Most of them come out through the inferior lumbar triangle (of Petit), bounded below by the iliac crest, medially by latissimus dorsi and laterally by external oblique. Rarely it may be seen in relation to superior lumbar triangle (of Grynfeltt), bounded above by the 12th rib, laterally by internal oblique, medially by sacrospinalis and covered by latissimus dorsi. The floor of these triangles is formed by

lumbodorsal fascia. A hernia may also develop in the loin in relation to incisions made for operations, such as lumbar sympathectomy, drainage of psoas abscess, nephro or uretero-lithotomy etc.

Differential diagnosis

Benign/malignant soft tissue tumors, cold abscess and phantom hernia due to muscular paralysis.

Treatment: As for other hernias, surgical repair is the only curative treatment. In view of the fact that bony structures form boundaries for lumbar triangles, simple repair is not possible and implanting a mesh may be imperative. For the postoperative hernias in that region, local tissue repair may be sufficient for smaller defects, but larger ones require mesh plasty.

4. OBTURATOR HERNIA

More common in females above 60, the hernia passes through the obturator canal meant for obturator vessels and nerve, to present in the femoral region, under the pectineus and adductor brevis muscles, hence not clinically detected. The sac exerts pressure on the obturator nerve, resulting in pain experienced over the medial aspect of thigh and knee. The pain precipitated by coughing or straining, but not during hip movements is typical of this hernia, more so when it is obstructed or

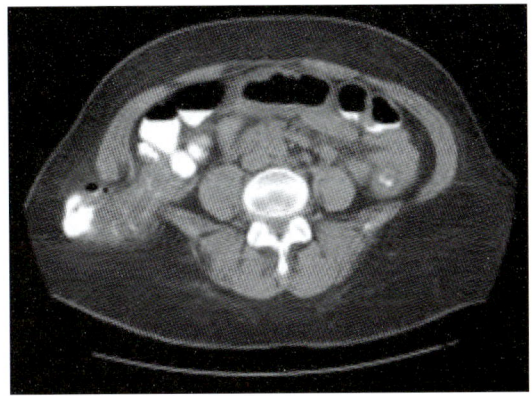

Fig. 48.10. CT scan showing lumbar hernia

strangulated (Howship-Romberg sign).

Uncomplicated obturator hernia probably goes undiagnosed. Usually patient presents with intestinal obstruction and before the days of CT scan, preoperative diagnosis was seldom made.

Treatment: Surgery is the only definitive treatment for this condition. Pelvic laparotomy

is performed, hernial contents reduced, if necessary by widening the constricting fascial ring and the defect closed, carefully protecting the nerve. Larger defects may be closed either by using a mesh or the broad ligament (if it is present) pulled anteriorly and sutured to cover the gap. Alternately a strip of fascia lata may be used for the repair.

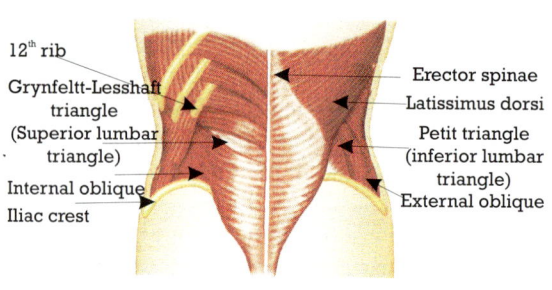

Fig. 48.11. Grynfeltt-Lesshaft triangle (superior lumbar triangle)

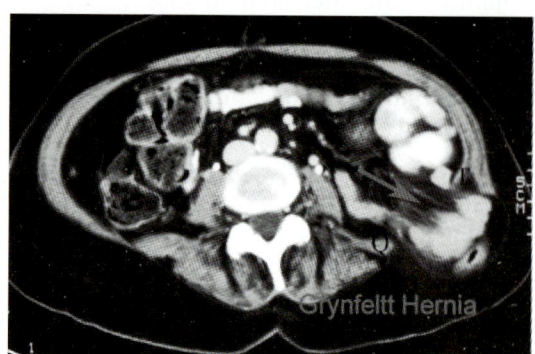

Fig. 48.12. CT scan showing Grynfeltt hernia

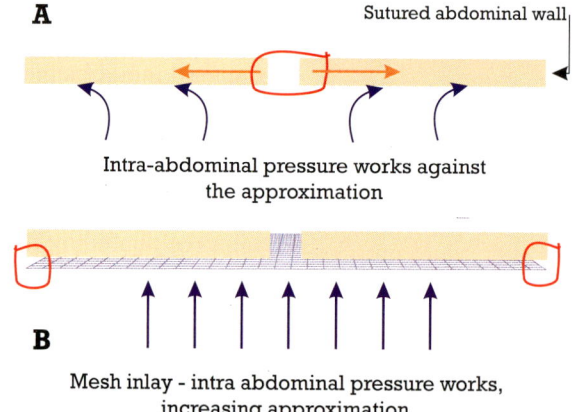

Fig. 48.13. Laplace's law in hernia surgery (using physics to advantage)

49 Burst Abdomen

(syn: abdominal wound dehiscence)

Incidence: About 1% of all laparotomy wounds develop this potentially fatal complication, between the 5th and 8th postoperative days, with the abdominal wound bursting open and extrusion of the viscera. The actual disruption, due to failure of the deep sutures apposing the abdominal wall layers, precedes the dramatic clinical event.

Etiopathogenesis

The major factors are:

a) General condition of the patient: Obesity, jaundice, malignant disease, hypoproteinemia, anemia, immune suppression, pregnancy etc.

b) Postoperative high intra-abdominal pressure: violent spells of cough and vomiting, due to any reason, as also protracted paralytic ileus and vigorous postoperative ventilation.

c) Choice of incisions: Transverse incisions have a lower rate of dehiscence, compared to vertical ones. Incisions in the upper abdomen are more prone for dehiscence than those in the lower abdomen.

d). Technique of wound closure:

i. Suture material: Non-absorbable sutures like polyamide (Nylon) and polypropylene (Prole-ne) have a much lower rate of dehiscence than absorbable sutures like catgut or polyglycolic acid (vicryl).

ii. Method of closure: Interrupted fascial suturing has a lower rate of wound dehi-scence than continuous. Interrupted 'far and near'(Peter Jones)

closure method is recommended for the patient who is prone to develop this complication. When continuous suturing is done, the length of the suture material should be at least four times the length of the wound (vide ventral hernia).

iii. Drainage tubes: Drainage tubes brought out through the main wound cause a higher incidence of burst abdomen.

iv) Too tight or too loose suturing

e) Nature of underlying disease:

Peritonitis: Heavy infection in the deeper layers of the wound causes cutting through and dehiscence.

Pancreaticoduodenal operations: Leaks after such operations cause digestion of tissue and absorbable suture materials by the powerful proteolytic enzymes.

Clinical features

A serosanguineous discharge (pink) from the wound, considered pathognomonic of dehiscence, is a forerunner of disruption in the majority of cases, signifying extraperitoneal displacement of viscera through the separated dee-per layers. Often patients volunteer the

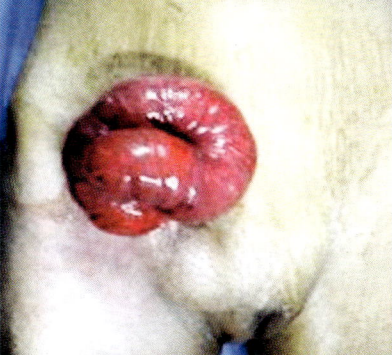

information that they felt something 'give way', usually following a violent coughing/vomiting spell. Pain and shock are conspicuously absent; symptoms and signs of intestinal obstruction may be present. Bowel or omentum prolapsing out of the wound is the end result, a frightening sight indeed.

Fig. 49.1. Burst abdomen of right lower paramedian incision for a perfotated appendix

Investigations

Before undertaking an urgent reoperation, some

Six 'S': Causes for burst abdomen

Surgery: peritonitis, leak of intestinal juices, pancreatitis

Sepsis: florid wound infection

Sutures: use of absorbable material for fascia

Straining: coughing or vomiting

Sickness: malignancy, diabetes, immune deficiency, uremia

Surgeon: expertise and expediency

investigations have to be done, to see the fitness for anesthesia and surgery.

Abdominal USG is a simple, expedient study, that gives a lot of information such as, abscesses in the peritoneal cavity or within the solid viscera or defect in the deeper layers of the suture line and collection of fluid in Morrison's hepatorenal pouch (most dependent of all peritoneal spaces, in recumbent position) or pelvis. The identification of these problems influences the treatment strategies. Hematology, serum proteins, renal/liver function tests and serum electrolytes may be necessary, more so if the patient has features of intestinal obstruction.

Treatment

Immediately after noticing the condition, no attempt to reposition the bowel loops into the abdomen should be made. The area is rinsed with warm saline and covered with a sterile sheet, while waiting to be shifted to the operation room. A good IV line started, analgesic, anxiolytic and antibiotic agents should be administered. Nasogastric aspirations and urinary output monitoring by an indwelling catheter are essential.

After stabilizing the patient's condition, an emergency operation is required to replace the bowel, relieve any obstruction and resuture the disrupted abdominal wound.

Preoperative (summary)

i. Reassurance of patient

ii. Wash and cover area with sterile towels

iii. Nasogastric aspiration

iv. Indwelling urinary catheter

v. Intravenous fluids

vi. Medication to relieve pain and anxiety

vii. Antibiotics

viii. Blood transfusion, if necessary

Operative procedure

Under general anesthesia with adequate relaxation every protruding loop of intestine is washed gently with warm saline solution and returned to the abdominal cavity. Any collections of pus are carefully looked for, in all possible spaces, drained and irrigated. Protruding greater omentum is treated similarly and spread over the intestines. The abdominal wall is irrigated, cleansed and all layers approximated in a single layer, supported by traditional 'deep tension sutures' of interrupted through and through nonabsorbable material (prolene or nylon) and with a soft plastic collar to protect the skin from pressure necrosis.

The abdominal wall may be supported by adhesive plaster encircling the anterior two thirds of the circumference of the trunk. Wide spectrum antibiotics, nasogastric decompression, IV fluids, indwelling urinary catheter for monitoring the output etc. have to be continued. Contrary to expectation, peritonitis rarely supervenes, so also skin infection and healing is usually satisfactory. Thanks to collagen stimulation following repair of dehiscence, the final wound strength is actually better than normal; a second dehiscence or incisional hernia rarely occurs, if proper closure is performed.

Recent advances: Antibiotic impregnated meshes to replace the central portion of the wound are now being used in some centres.

Zipper mesh laparostomy: In the presence of gross peritonitis, the abdominal wound may be closed with a 'zipper' in place, to enable inspection and irrigation of the viscera frequently, till the infection is totally eliminated, when regular closure may be done.

50 Tumor Markers in Surgery

This *term is used in clinical parlance, to denote a chemical measurable in serum or urine, which helps to diagnose and monitor the progression of the neoplasm, which secretes it.* These are products of the metobolic activity of tumors and are either tumor-derived or tumor-associated, although not necessarily tumor-specific. They may be secreted (into blood, urine or other body fluids) or expressed (at the cell surface) in quantities larger than those in normal tissue. Their concentrations in body fluids are measured by radio-immunoassay or detected on the cell surface (in paraffin sections, smears or fresh biopsy tissue), by histochemistry. Recently, more and more genetic markers (oncogenes) for several malignancies are being identified, making this a complex, but useful subject.

Classification

1. Clinical
2. Biochemical
3. Radioisotopic
4. Immunological
5. Histochemical

An ideal tumor marker should have the following features:

1. high specificity and sensitivity
2. levels should correlate with the tumor mass
3. useful for screening, diagnosis, prognostication and detecting residual/recurrent disease
4. possible to estimate in most of the laboratories at reasonable cost.

Note that these hormones may be *ectopic* (i.e. their production is inappropriate to the tissue of origin of the tumor) or *eutopic* (i.e. appropriate to the tissue of origin).

However certain common markers in routine clinical use are discussed here:

Ectopic hormones

ACTH and MSH (melanocyte stimulating hormone) - bronchogenic carcinoma

ADH (antidiuretic hormone) - bronchogenic carcinoma

Hypothalamic releasing factors - bronchogenic carcinoma

PTH (parathormone) - bronchogenic carcinoma

Calcitonin - bronchogenic and breast carcinoma

Prostaglandins - colon and breast carcinoma

Entopic hormones

Thyroglobulin in differentiated (papillary and follicular) thyroid cancers

β-hCG (human chorionic gonadotrophin) choriocarcinoma and teratoma

5-HIAA (5-hydroxy indole acetic acid) for carcinoid tumor

PSA (prostate specific antigen) - prostatic carcinoma

SAP (serum acid phosphatase) - prostatic carcinoma

Calcitonin in medullary thyroid carcinoma (MTC)

Catecholamines and vanillyl mandelic acid (VMA) in pheochromocytoma

Urinary homovanillic acid in neuroblastoma.

Oncofetal products and antigens

CEA (carcino-embryonic antigen) - GI tract, breast, gonads and pancreas

AFP (α-fetoprotein) - hepatoma and teratoma
Ferritin - many
Cancer basic protein - all
Pregnancy associated proteins - breast and teratoma
Placental type enzymes - many

Clinical applications

Those suitable for routine management and

general screening are very limited. They include the following:

Human chorionic gonadotropins (hCG)

Produced by placenta (reaching maximum concentration in the eighth gestational week) and abnormal trophoblastic tissue. It is composed of non-specific and specific subunits. It increases in chorionic carcinoma and can detect a tumor mass of 1mg; it is therefore used as a screening test in all cases of hydatidiform mole after uterine evacuation to judge the progress, to monitor chemotherapy and to detect early metastases. β-hCG (above 10 i.u/l) is found in 50% of testicular teratomas and in few pure seminomas. False high levels may occur after orchidectomy and hypogonadism owing to high LH (luteinising hormone), identical to β-hCG subunit, and retesting after testosterone administration is therefore needed. hCG may be increased also in carcinoma of the pancreas, stomach and bronchus.

α-Fetoprotein (AFP)

This is a protein synthesized by yolk sac, liver and GI tract and is the major serum protein of the fetus. Normal range 1-16 ug/l in adults; levels above 40ug/l are found in 60% of teratomas

Cancer type	Marker(s)	Main uses
Colorectal	CEA	Prognosis, postoperative surveillance, monitoring therapy
Germ cell	AFP, HCG, LSH (prognosis only)	Prognosis, postoperative surveillance, monitoring therapy
Trophoblastic	HCG	Prognosis, postoperative surveillance, monitoring therapy
Ovarian	CA-125	Monitoring therapy, differential diagnosis of benign and malignant massesin postmenopausal women
Prostate	PSA	Screening, prognosis, postoperative surveillance, monitoring therapy
Breast	ER, PR	Predicting response to hormone therapy, prognosis
	HER-2	Predicting response to trastuzumab and lapatinib, prognosis
	uPA, PAI-I	Prognosis in nose-negative patients
	CA I5-3, CEA	Postoperative surveillance, monitoring therapy
Hepatocellular	AFP	Diagnostic aid, prognosis, postoperative surveillance, monitoringtherapy
Thyroid (differentiated)	Thyroglobulin	Postoperative surveillance, monitoring therapy

Abbreviations: CEA – Caricinoembryonic antigen, AFP – α-fetoprotein, HGC – Human Choriogonadotrophin, LDH – Lactate dehydrogenase, PSA – Prostate-specific antigen, ER – Estrogen receptor, PR – Progesterone receptor, uPA – urokinase plasminogen activator, PAI – Plasminogen activator inhibitor

Table-50.1 - Some of the most useful markers currently available, and their clinical utility.

and although the elevation of AFP is nonspecific, its assay in conjunction with β-hCG gives positive results in 75-95% of testicular teratomas and both levels are crucial in the subsequent management.

Staging: Preorchidectomy high marker levels that fall to normal postoperatively, suggest stage-I while persistently high levels after orchidectomy suggest undetected stage-II (retroperitoneal lymph nodes) or Stage-III (supradiaphragmatic nodes) and slow fall in AFP levels may indicate a residual AFP-producing tumor.

Assessing prognosis: Levels of hCG $<5 \times 10^4$ iu/l and AFP <500ug/l are associated with low mortality whereas levels $>1 \times 10^5$ i.u/l and 1mg/l respectively carry high mortality in metastatic teratoma (the marker level is proportional to the bulk of the tumor).

Monitoring therapy: 80% of metastatic teratomas undergo remission on combined chemotherapy, the duration of which is judged by assay of markers (if they become normal, there is no need for maintenance therapy). If marker levels fall to normal, but there is static or residual disease evident on chest X-ray or CT scan and if biopsy of the residual lesion shows differentiated teratoma or necrotic tissue, no further therapy is indicated. On the other hand, advancing disease with static marker levels indicates loss of marker-producing property of the tumor and change of therapy is indicated.

AFP, β-hCG, and lactate dehydrogenase: these are mandatory in determining prognosis in patients with germ cell cancer and the former two are useful in surveillance and monitoring treatment. Following curative treatment for non-seminomatous germ cell tumors of the testis, consistently rising AFP or β-HCG levels with or without radiological or clinical findings, suggest active disease and should lead to the initiation of treatment, provided causes of false positive marker levels are excluded.

Carcino-embryonic antigen (CEA)

A glycoprotein synthesized by tumor cells and by normal colonic epithelium, is carried on the cell surface membrane and normally shed with feces but in cancers it escapes into the interstitial fluid. Although raised levels are nonspecific, it is present in 65% of all colorectal cancers, which depends on:

1. tumor stage: CEA is raised in 30% of patients with Duke's stage-A tumor and in 90% of those with hepatic metastases

2. tumor site: CEA levels are low or absent in right colonic and rectal tumors and higher in left colonic, particularly sigmoid cancer

3. degree of differentiation

4. Functional hepatic status

CEA therefore has no role in screening of general population; however, it is used as a prognostic indicator (very high preoperative levels suggest a poor prognosis) and as an indicator for second-look surgery for cure in early recurrence of colonic carcinomas. In monitoring therapy, falling CEA levels suggest a response to chemo/radiotherapy.

Its role in colorectal cancer (CRC)

1. determining prognosis

2. surveillance following curative resection

3. monitoring therapy in patients with advanced disease

Preoperative levels of CEA should be determined because they may provide independent prognostic information, influence surgical management, and provide a baseline level for subsequent follow-up. Preoperative levels, if elevated, may also help identify high risk node-negative patients that could benefit from adjuvant chemotherapy. Following curative surgery for CRC, several meta-analyses have shown that the use of an intensive follow-up regime that included regular determinations of CEA resulted in a modest but statistically significant better survival rate than with no or minimal follow-up.

CA-125 in ovarian cancer

The main uses of CA-125 are in the differential diagnosis of benign and malignant pelvic masses in postmenopausal women and in monitoring chemotherapy in patients with ovarian cancer. If a postmenopausal woman presents with a pelvic mass and elevated CA-125, she should be promptly referred to a specialized gynecological oncology unit. It should also be used in monitoring chemotherapy in patients with ovarian cancer. However, its role in the follow-up of asymptomatic (apparently disease-free) patients who have completed treatment for ovarian cancer is under evaluation.

While evaluating a female patient with ascites, CA-125 has to be used with caution, since it may also be elevated in peritoneal tuberculosis

Biomarkers in breast cancer

Estrogen and progesterone receptors as prognostic and predictive markers

Measurement of both estrogen (ER) and progesterone receptors (PR) is used for predicting the response of invasive breast cancers to hormonal therapy. However its role to assess endocrine therapy in patients with ductal carcinoma-in-situ is less clear. Although primarily used to identify endocrine sensitivity, ER may also be used for determining prognosis in newly diagnosed breast cancer patients, with the following limitations:

(1) the beneficial effect of its presence only lasts only for 6-7 years and

(2) its value in patients with node-negative disease is questionable. Despite these limitations, it is recommended that ER and PR be included in the risk classification scheme for newly diagnosed breast cancer patients.

HER-2 as a predictive and prognostic marker

(**H**uman **e**pidermal growth factor **r**eceptor) The primary use of HER-2 in breast cancer is to employ anti-HER-2 therapy, such as trastuzumab and lapatinib. Like ER, HER-2 can be both predictive and prognostic in patients with breast cancer. HER-2 positive patients with lymph nodal disease have a worse outcome compared with HER-2 negative patients, unless adjuvant anti-HER-2 treatment is given.

Urokinase plasminogen activator (uPA) and plasminogen activator inhibitor (PAI)-1 as

prognostic markers: The prognostic impact for these two proteins in lymph node negative breast cancer patients has been validated in both a multicenter prospective randomized trial and a pooled analysis of individual data from over 8,000 patients. The results from both these (level I evidence) studies showed that lymph node negative breast cancer patients with low levels of uPA and PAI-1 have a minimal risk of disease recurrence and we may be able to avoid potentially toxic adjuvant chemotherapy for them. The requirement of fresh or freshly frozen tumor tissue, however, limits their routine use.

CA 15-3 in postoperative surveillance and monitoring therapy: The role of serial measurements of CA 15-3 and CEA in the postoperative monitoring of asymptomatic and clinically disease-free patients, treated for breast cancer is controversial.

However, CA 15-3 and CEA may be used in combination with radiology for monitoring therapy in patients with advanced breast cancer. These markers are particularly useful in monitoring therapy in patients that are difficult to evaluate using imaging modalities.

"Omics": The "omics" technologies involve genomics (the study of an organism's entire genome), transcriptomics (the study of an organism's entire mRNA), and proteomics (the study of an organism's entire protein). Of these three technologies, transcriptomics, or gene expression profiling, has emerged as being the most clinically useful. Gene expression profiling involves simultaneous measurement of multiple mRNA species. This may be accomplished by using either microarray (gene chips) or multiplex reverse transcriptase polymerase chain reaction (RT-PCR). The main clinical application of gene expression profiling to date is in determining the prognosis in patients with newly diagnosed cancer. Although prognostic signatures have been reported for several types of cancer, it is in breast cancer where the most extensive investigations have been carried out.

Two profiles, in particular, have undergone detailed studies in this malignancy:

1. MammaPrint: it is a 70-gene profile that was originally shown to predict outcome in lymph node negative breast cancer patients under the age of 55. Subsequently, the prognostic signature was both internally and externally validated and shown to predict outcome independent of the classical prognostic factors for breast cancer. In 2007, MammaPrint was cleared by the US FDA for predicting outcome in lymph node negative breast cancer patients younger than 61 years of age. Currently, it is undergoing prospective validation as part of the ongoing research.

2. Oncotype DX test: it measures the expression of 21 genes (16 cancer-related and 5 control genes) using multiplex RT-PCR in paraffin-embedded and formalin-fixed tumor tissue. Based on the relative expression of the 16 cancer-related genes, a recurrence score is calculated. Currently, the main use of the test is for predicting the risk of recurrence in newly diagnosed breast cancer patients without nodal disease and ER positive, under treatment with adjuvant tamoxifen. In contrast to gene expression profiling, the use of proteomics to provide clinically useful information has to date been disappointing. Although multiple preliminary reports have claimed that one form of proteomics known as surface-enhanced laser desorption and ionization can detect several cancer types with considerably enhanced sensitivity and specificity compared with existing markers, few

of these findings have been confirmed using external validation studies. As such, at present, there is no role for the proteomics either in the detection or in the routine management of patients with cancer.

Prostate-specific antigen in prostate cancer

Although widely used, the effect of prostate-specific antigen (PSA) screening on reducing mortality from prostate cancer remains to be established. Thus, guidelines from expert panels on PSA screening vary; most expert panels agree, however, that prior to screening, the patient must be adequately counseled regarding the potential benefits, limitations, and pitfalls associated with this biomarker. PSA can provide prognostic information in patients with prostate cancer in several ways. These include the use of absolute pretreatment levels (the higher the PSA level, the worse the outcome), a combination of pretreatment levels and established prognostic factors to generate nomograms, and the use of serial levels to calculate either PSA velocity or PSA doubling time. The wide variability in PSA levels, however, may limit its ability to determine velocity and doubling time. Finally, serial PSA estimations may be more useful than a single value in the post-therapy surveillance.

The specificity of PSA is around 75% and it may be elevated in about 25% of patients with benign hyperplasia. Recently, estimation of the fraction of PSA that is unbound to plasma proteins (free PSA) and its ratio to total PSA has improved its specificity in malignancy (<15% is considered significant). It is not influenced by rectal examination and is more specific and sensitive than serum acid phosphatase, which is elevated only after the tumor has breached the capsule of the prostate.

Conclusions

1. Lack of specificity and sensitivity of the most of the tumor markers preclude their routine use in detection of early malignancies

2. They may be of some value in certain situations in aid differential diagnosis (e.g. CA

125 in pelvic mass of a postmenopausal woman) or in identifying unknown primary (e.g. AFP, hCG for germ cell tumors and PSA for prostate cancer)

3. ER, PR status for identifying endocrine sensitivity and Her-2 for predicting response to trastuzumab (Herceptin) in breast carcinoma, have great practical significance.

4. Markers useful in post-therapy surveillance are: AFP, hCG in NSGCT and trophoblastic tumors; CEA in colorectal carcinoma; thyroglobulin in differentiated thyroid cancers; calcitonin in MTC; PSA in prostatic Ca; CA 125 in ovarian Ca.

5. Gene expression microarray and proteomics may be the markers of the future.

Currently, the most frequent application of tumor biomarkers is in postoperative surveillance and monitoring therapy in patients with advanced disease.

There are, however, a number of points that should be borne in mind when using markers in these settings.

1. With the possible exception of hCG in patients with trophoblastic disease, none of the available biomarkers is elevated in serum from *all patients* with a specific cancer, even in the presence of advanced disease. In certain situations, therefore, a second-line biomarker may be required.

2. Therapy should not be altered following a single increase or decrease in a biomarker level. All increases and decreases in marker levels should be confirmed with a second sample.

3. Transient increases in biomarker concentrations can occur following the start of specific therapy. The spurious increases or spikes are probably due to therapy-mediated apoptosis or necrosis of tumor cells and not due to tumor progression.

4. Benign diseases may give rise to elevated biomarker concentrations. These increases may be transient or persistent, depending on the specific abnormality. Increases found in benign diseases, however, are rarely of the same magnitude as that seen in advanced cancers.

5. The impact of measuring serial levels of tumor biomarkers on patient outcome is unclear in many malignancies. The use of CEA as part of a surveillance strategy in patients who have had curative surgery for CRC does, however, have a modest but significant impact on patient survival.

6. Finally, it is important to state that many of the other tumor markers currently available do not satisfy evidence-based criteria for their clinical utility.

These include:

CA 19-9 in pancreatic cancer

Cytokeratin in SCC

NSE, chromogranin and calcitonin in neuroendocrine tumors

Specific cytokeratins in several different types of carcinomas.

Some of the commonly used immuno-histochemical tumor markers are:

Epithelial and colorectal: cytokeratin
Lymphoma: CD-3 & 20
Ovary: CA-125, CK-20
Melanoma: S-100
GIST: CD-117

51 Salivary Glands

Embryology: Solid proliferation of cells from the oral cavity, which later canalize, forming the ducts and gland tissue.

Parotid gland is ectodermal in origin, hence dermoid cyst can occur in it (from first branchial cleft). Submandibular and sublingual glands are endodermal.

The direction of the ducts and the location of their orifices are nondependent, predisposing to calculus formation, more so in the submandibular duct. This is due to the erect posture acquired by man as against quadrupeds, who have their face looking down, facilitating free flow of saliva into the mouth.

Anatomy
Parotid gland

(par: near; otis: ear)

This lobulated inverted pyramidal shape gland lies in front of the mastoid, behind the mandible and below the external acoustic meatus. It has a true capsule which is a condensed peripheral fibrous tissue of the gland, and a false capsule which is given off from the investing layer of deep cervical fascia, known as the parotidomasseteric fascia, which covers the gland and is attached above to the lower border of the zygomatic arch. Deep to the parotid gland this fascia thickens, becomes cord-like, and runs up to the styloid process, as stylomandibular ligament. The parotid fascia is particularly thick, and it is imprudent to wait for fluctuation in cases of parotid abscess, as it occurs very late in the disease process.

Structures within the gland

The facial nerve is the most important structure, with prefound clinical and legal implications. After emerging from the stylomastoid foramen, it enters the gland in the posteriomedial surface and passes forwards and downwards through the gland, to divide into two primary divisions, zygomaticotemporal and

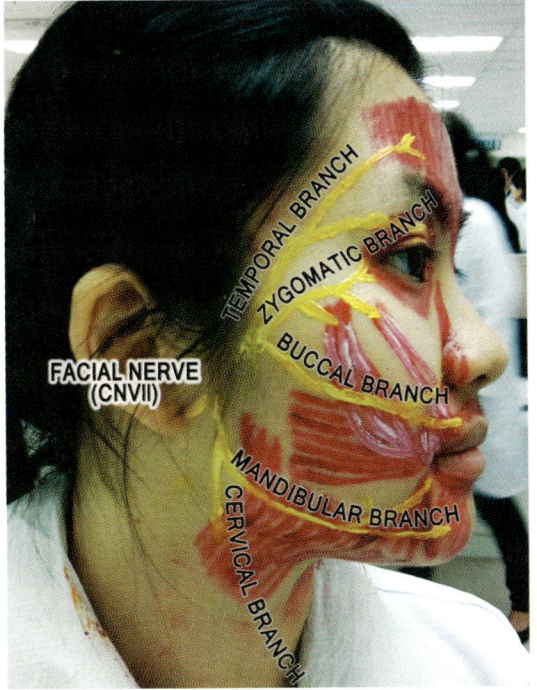

Fig. 51.1. Branches of facial nerve

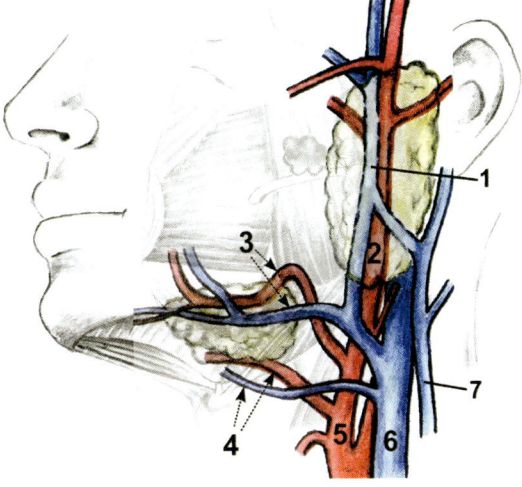

Fig. 51.2. Arteries and veins in relation to parotid gland

1. retromandibular vein   2. external carotid artery,
3. facial artery and vein,   4. lingual artery and vein,
5. external carotid artery,   6. internal jugular vein,
7. external jugular vein.

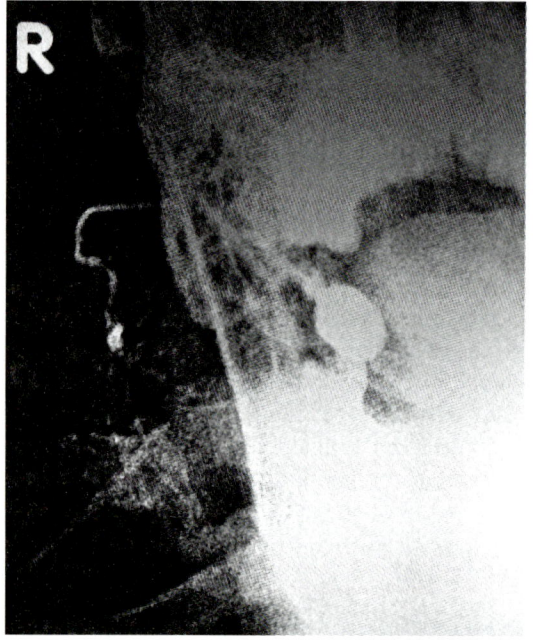

Fig. 51.3. Normal parotid sialogram

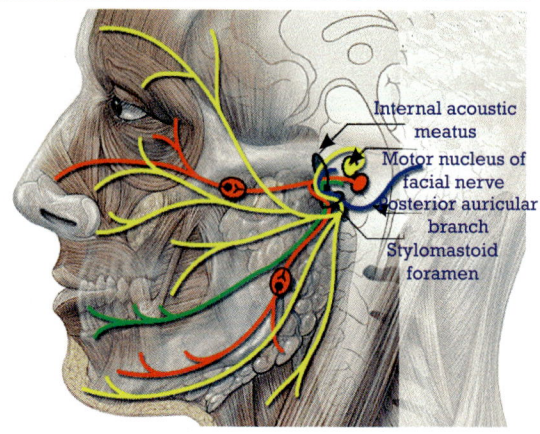

Fig. 51.5. Branches of the facial nerve

cervicofacial. The former further divides into zygomatic and temporal branches while the latter into the buccal, marginal mandibular and cervical branches. All these branches create an arbitrary division of the parotid into a larger superficial and a smaller deep portion as they exit from the anteriomedial surface of the parotid, to innervate the muscles of face. Sometimes, the primary division of the nerve may take place before it enters the gland.

Immediately deep to the facial nerve runs the retromandibular vein, formed by the union of maxillary and superficial temporal veins in the upper part of the gland, traversing through the gland in the same plane as the facial nerve, known as the *facio-venous plane of Patey*. From the lower border of parotid, this vein divides into anterior and posterior branches. The posterior one joins the posterior auricular vein to form the external jugular while the

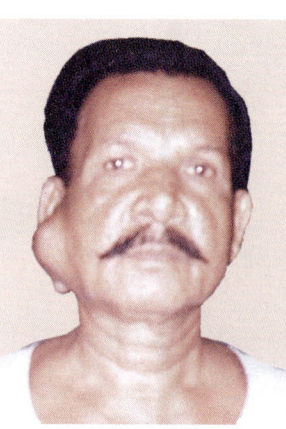

Fig. 51.4. Mixed parotid tumor (courtesy: Halsted Surgical Clinic, Chennai)

anterior one joins the facial vein. *If venous bleeding occurs during superficial parotidectomy, it is likely that the dissection has gone deeper to the branches of facial nerve.*

The deep portion of the parotid lies in a quadrangular space, called retromandibular canal, bounded above by the base of skull, below by the stylomandibular ligament, behind by the mastoid and styloid processes and in front by the vertical ramus of mandible. Its deep relations are the three muscles, stylohyoid, styloglossus and stylopharyngeus and the lateral wall of pharynx. It is important to realize that the external carotid artery divides into its terminal branches, namely, superficial temporal and internal maxillary, *within the substance* of the deep part of the parotid. Torrential bleeding occurs during any surgery on the deep lobe, such as a dumb-bell tumor, which can only be prevented by preliminary control of the external carotid artery, at its origin (C M K Reddy & K K Ramalingam).

The parotid duct, described by Stensen (who subsequently became the father of modern geology), runs from the upper medial part of the gland, first anteriorly upto the anterior border of masseter and then curves sharply inwards through the buccinator muscle to open into the mouth, its orifice situated opposite to the upper second molar tooth. Palpation of the duct against a contracted masseter, is an essential step in the examination of the parotid gland.

The most common developmental anomaly of the parotid gland is the accessory parotid lobe. This arises from the horizontal part of the parotid duct as it goes past the anterior border of the masseter. It is important to note this, as any disease of the main gland can also involve the accessory lobe.

Submandibular gland

This gland situated in the submandibular region, is divided into deep and superficial parts by the mylohyoid, but are continuous with each other along its posterior border. The superficial part of the gland is covered by skin, platysma, investing layer of deep cervical fascia, which is attached to the lower border of mandible. The facial artery courses through the gland substance.

The deep part of the gland lies between the mylohyoid muscle inferolaterally and stylo-glossus and hyoglossus medially. The lingual nerve and submandibular ganglion are superior to it and the hypoglossal nerve and the deep lingual vein are below.

Submandibular (Wharton's) duct comes out from the deep part of the gland running between the mylohyoid and hyoglossus and it lies between the lingual and hypoglossal nerves. It is crossed by the lingual nerve near the anterior border of the gland (second molar region) and then runs upwards and forwards along the floor of the mouth, to open on the side of the frenulum linguae, where the papilla of the orifice is readily visible.

Sublingual gland

This is the smallest of the three, flattened and almond-sized, situated in the anterior floor of the mouth, in the submucous plane over the mylohyoid muscle. Lying in relation to the inner surface (sublingual fossa) of the mandible, it

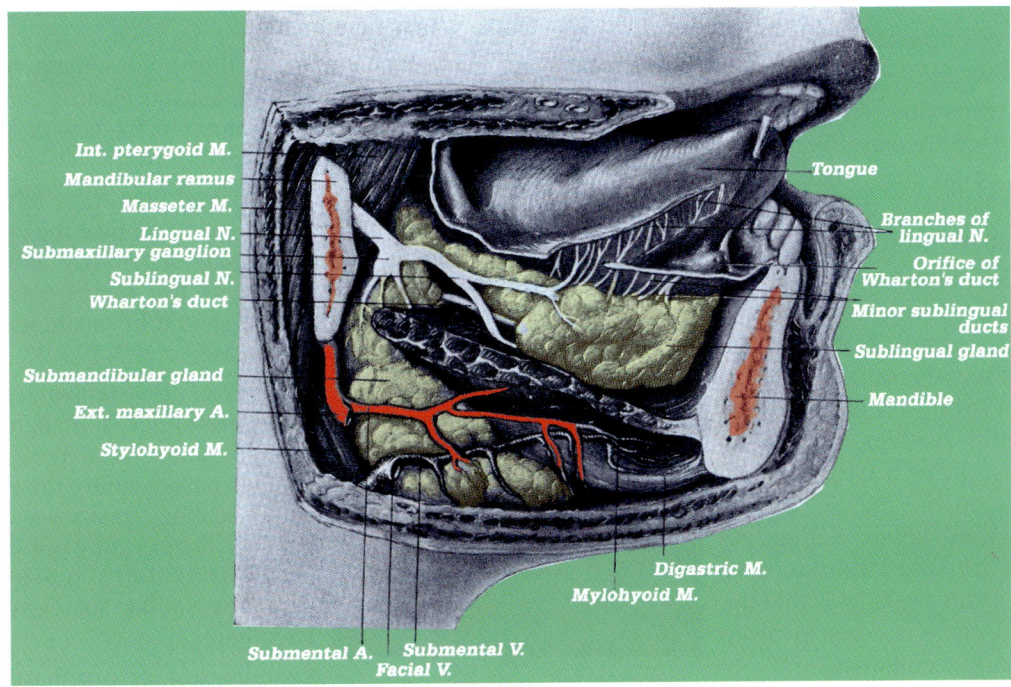

Fig. 51.6. Lateral view of the sublingual region (body of the mandible removed)

raises sublingual folds on each side of the symphysis. Posteriorly it is related to the deep portion of the submandibular salivary gland, laterally to the mandible and medially to the genioglossus muscle, which separates it from the Wharton's duct and lingual nerve. It has multiple short ducts, some opening into the Wharton's duct and the rest directly into the floor of the mouth, through which the mucoid secretions are discharged.

Examination of salivary glands

Standard pattern is to examine the gland, its duct, the draining lymph nodes, the other glands, and facial nerve in case of parotid gland, followed by systemic examination.

Hobsley's dictum: *In inflammations the entire gland is uniformly enlarged, whereas neoplasms cause localized, asymmetrical enlargements.* Thus, in parotitis, for example, all the poles of the parotid are evenly enlarged, whereas, a tumor arises only from one of the poles. This dictum is mostly true in respect to all other organs in the body.

Some important points in clinical examination

On inspection, swelling of the parotid gland often obliterates the hollow just below the lobule of the ear, between the mandible and mastoid process.

As the parotid is encased in a tough parotidomasseteric fascia, contraction of masseter muscle restricts the freedom of movement for a parotid swelling within the fascia, giving a false sense of 'fixity' to the muscle, but an important differentiating feature between benign and malignant swellings is that the facial nerve is never involved in benign conditions.

Bidigital palpation between

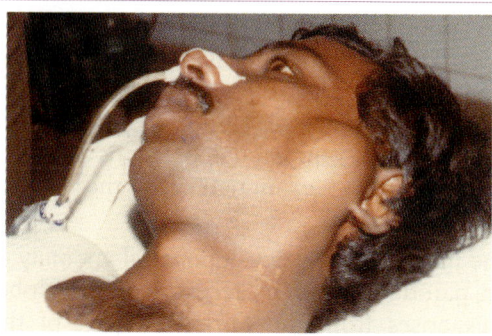

Fig. 51.8. Mixed parotid tumor
(courtesy: Dr C J Reddy, Gudur, AP)

the index finger inside and fingers of the other hand placed outside the floor of the mouth, is an excellent way of palpating the submandibular/sublingual glands. While doing so, four possibilities have to be kept in mind.

1) it is appreciated better with the inner finger: enlarged sublingual or deep part of submandibular salivary gland and calculus in the Wharton's duct.

2) it is appreciated better by external fingers: enlarged submandibular/submental lymph nodes or superficial part of submandibular salivary gland.

3) it is felt equally well by both: enlargement of entire submandibular salivary gland.

4) it is found to be immobile: fixed to or arising from the jaw.

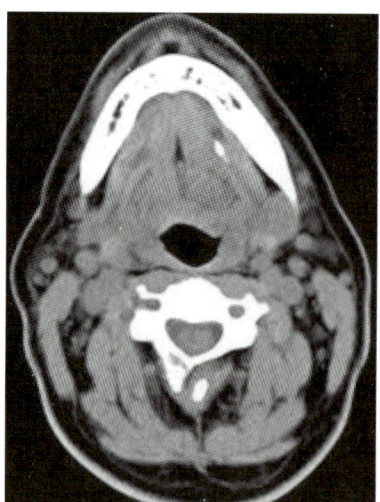

Fig. 51.7. CT scan - calculus in Wharton's duct

The parotid duct, best felt by rolling the finger over the tightened masseter muscle and its orifice at the upper second molar, should be examined in every case.

If the facial nerve is involved, it indicates either a malignant parotid tumor or a previous surgical misadventure (beware of preexisting facial palsy due to childhood meningoencephalitis, Bell's palsy or cerebrovascular accident in later life).

Examination of oropharynx, for enlargement of deep lobe

of parotid (dumb-bell tumor), which displaces the soft palate to the opposite side, is very important.

Lymph nodes - preauricular, parotid, retro-mandibular, submandibular and submental nodes have to be routinely examined. In advanced malignancy, the deep cervical chain may also be involved.

Sialography - The Stensen's duct orifice is cannulated by a fine plastic cannula and dilute lipiodol is injected, to demonstrate the ductal and acinar pattern. Dilatation or obstruction of the ducts, calculi, dilatation of acini, filling defects due to SOL in the gland etc. may all be made out on sialography. In recurrent parotitis of childhood (*sialectasis*), snowstorm appearance of the dilated acini is made out and in a parotid fistula it helps to localise if it is communicating with a major duct (ductal fistula) or the gland tissue (glandular or acinar fistula).

ACUTE SUPPURATIVE PAROTITIS

Although acute parotitis is commonly a viral disease (mumps), acute suppurative parotitis is often seen in the hospital environment. Staphylococcal aureus and streptococcus viridans are the usual infecting organisms, and background factors predisposing to such an infection are:

Poor oral hygiene
Suboptimal nutrition
Reduced blood flow owing to dehydration
Radiotherapy
Partial obstruction to the duct, leading to impaired drainage of secretion, predisposing to calculus formation.

Fortunately with improved postoperative oral hygiene and effective antibiotics this is rarely seen nowadays. However another type of acute ascending bacterial parotitis, *idiopathic parotitis*, occurs in otherwise healthy young adults, without any obvious cause.

Clinical features

A painful diffuse swelling of acute onset is seen, with systemic features, such as fever, malaise and regional lymph nodal enlargement. There is local warmth and tenderness, the gland feeling edematous and brawny, with overlying cellulitis. The orifice of Stensen's duct may be edematous and hyperemic and on pressure over the parotid region, turbid or purulent saliva is seen issuing out, clinching the diagnosis of suppuration, but as indicated, typical fluctuation may be absent.

Investigations

Sialography should not be done in the acute stage and undertaken only after the inflammation has settled. Ultrasound scan will demonstrate acinar/ductal dilatation, abscess or calculus, if present.

Treatment

Adequate hydration, wide spectrum antibiotics and NSAIDs must be started if an abscess has not formed. Meticulous oral hygiene is observed and soft diet allowed. If fluctuation has appeared or if there is brawny induration and suspicion of parotid abscess, it should be drained following a diagnostic aspiration, employing a cosmetically acceptable incision in front of the tragus and coming down to the lobe of the ear. Although the skin and subcutaneous tissue are cut vertically along with the incision the deep fascia is opened horizontally in line with the facial nerve (Hilton's method). After the pus is drained a soft penrose or glove drain is inserted to permit total resolution.

MUMPS

(syn: epidemic parotitis).

Caused by a virus known as paramyxovirus (PMV), is a self limiting acute infection of parotid glands.

It has an incubation period of 2-3 weeks and the disease lasts for about 1-2 weeks. It may be bilateral (90%), associated with orchitis (30%), pancreatitis and rarely meningitis.

It is common in children with poor oral hygiene or following some debilitating illness, typically with enlarged painful salivary glands, high fever and headache, rarely requiring confirmatory tests, such as elevated serum amylase and polyvalent chain reaction (PCR).

No specific therapy is available, NSAIDs give symptomatic relief. Sialogogues, including acid foods or beverages increase salivary secretions and cause local discomfort, hence not advisable. Mumps can be prevented by vaccination in childhood, generally combined with measles and rubella (MMR vaccine). Aspirin has to be avoided in mumps due to the possible link with Reye's syndrome, which is highly lethal involvement of CNS and liver, following any viral infection, of unclear etiology. Predilection for this serious complication following aspirin therapy in viral infections has been established in 1963.

CHRONIC SIALADENITIS

This occurs much more frequently in the submandibular gland than in the parotid gland, because:

1) secretions are mucoid, with higher protein content, whereas saliva from the parotid is more serous and less viscous.

2) nondependent drainage of the submandibular duct

3) rich lymphatics in and around the submandibular gland predispose to infection especially in the presence of oral sepsis.

4) a common etiological factor causing submandibular sialadenitis is the presence of a stone in the Wharton's duct, which is rare in parotid.

Clinical features

Recurrent bouts of pain swelling and tenderness in the submandibular region, exaggerated on taking food or sialogogues (like citric acid, juices, etc) is the hallmark of this disease. The waxing/waning course is typical, with a bidigitally palpable, diffuse swelling of the gland. The lymph nodes may be enlarged either discrete or adherent to the gland. Wharton's duct should be examined, for the inflamed papilla and pressure on the submandibular gland may expel turbid material. Palpation of the gland and along the duct may reveal a calculus.

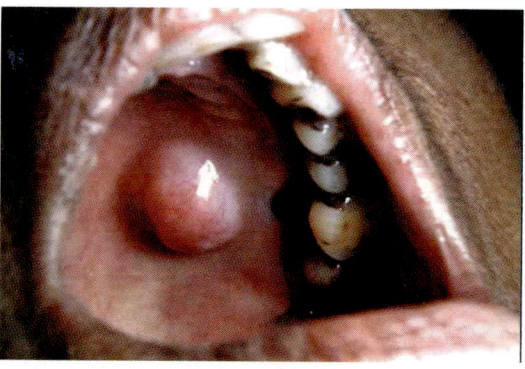

Fig. 51.9. Pleomorphic adenoma from a minor salivary gland of palate

Investigations

Apart from baseline investigations, a plain x-ray of the floor of the mouth often reveals a radio-opaque stone. Sialography is also useful to localise the obstructing element, but may not be needed in the presence of calculus.

Treatment

If the chronic inflammation is only due to a ductal stone, especially if it can be palpated along its length, one can make an attempt to remove the calculus from the intraoral segment of the duct. The duct is fixed by stay sutures on either side of the stone and an incision is made over it, which is removed. There is no need to close the ductal incision.

If there is recurrent sialadenitis without an obvious calculus or persists after removal of a ductal calculus, defying medical therapy, sialadenectomy may be necessary.

RECURRENT PAROTITIS OF CHILDHOOD
(syn: sialectasis)

Occurring between the ages of 3 and 6 years, this condition is marked by recurrent episodes of pain and swelling of the gland usually on one side, along with fever. Each attack of inflammation lasts for about a week and responds to antibiotics and NSAID therapy. Recurrent episodes occur at regular intervals, may be once in 3 months and this process goes on till puberty when spontaneous resolution is the rule.

Clinically, a diffuse swelling of the parotid is made out which is tender to touch. The duct orifice appears normal. The draining lymph nodes are often enlarged. No other features of systemic illness are present.

Investigations

Besides the baseline studies, the investigation of choice is sialography, after acute inflammation resolves. This shows a classic punctate sialectasis (snow storm) appearance. Multiple acinar dilatation is the underlying pathology with stagnant salivary secretions, favoring infection.

Treatment

Attention to oral hygiene
Prevention of dryness of the mouth by adequate hydration
Mucolytic agents
Sailagogues, such as lime, peppermint, chewing gum or drugs like cisapride
Broad spectrum antibiotics
NSAIDs
Reassurance to the patient

Sialography may be not only diagnostic, but often has a therapeutic benefit of causing resolution of disease

Surgery is not required except in the rare occurrence of a parotid abscess

RECURRENT PAROTITIS OF ADULTS

(syn: chronic interstitial parotitis)

This occurs in the setting of intermittent obstruction by a calculus in the Stensen's duct (unilateral) or due to an autoimmune cause (often bilateral).

Clinical features

History of recurrent attacks of pain, swelling and purulent saliva is present. Examination reveals diffuse swelling of the parotid glands, and palpation of the Stensen's duct sometimes reveals the obstructing stone.

Management

An x-ray should be taken to confirm the presence of a stone in the duct. Sialography may be performed after the subsidence of acute inflammation.

Treatment

As in submandibular salivary gland, if there is recurrent infection of the gland with no obvious obstructing stone, it is best excised (parotidectomy). If a stone is found in Stensen's duct, it is best approached by the oral route. Sometimes idiopathic stricture of the parotid duct causes recurrent infection. This is dealt with by ductoplasty and dilatation by the buccal approach. If a gland is to be excised for an inflammatory reason, then it is better to remove both the lobes, conserving the facial nerve (total conservative parotidectomy) as the superficial parotidectomy may leave an area of inflammation in the deep lobe which may be very difficult to access subsequently.

Other conditions causing chronic acalculus sialadenitis:

Granulomatous sialadenitis

Tuberculous disease of the parotid and submandibular salivary gland is not uncommon in India and often the diagnosis is made needle biopsy or after surgical excision.

Radiation sialadenitis: If the parotid glands are within the radiation field of head and neck cancers, acute radiation parotitis, usually self-limiting, develops within 24 hours of commencement of RT.

Syphilitic parotitis: Rarely, in tertiary syphilis, the parotid gland may be involved with gummatous changes and dense fibrosis of the glands.

Sarcoidosis

This is a systemic granulomatous disease of unknown etiology, probably of autoimmune nature (involving T-helper lymphocytes and mononuclear phagocytes infiltration) with a predilection for salivary tissue. It manifests as bilateral parotid and submandibular swelling (one of the causes of Mickuliz's syndrome). Here the parotid or submandibular glands are involved as part of a generalized process. Rarely isolated enlargement of a single gland, the so-called *'sarcoid pseudotumor'*, is seen and the diagnosis can be made by excision biopsy of the affected gland. *The Heerfordt's syndrome* comprises of parotid enlargement, iridocyclitis, fever and sometimes facial nerve involvement, seen in sarcoidosis. (see chapter 42)

Wegener's granulomatosis: This midline granulomatous disease involves destruction of the oropharynx, nasopharynx and can rarely involve the salivary glands.

Etiology: granulomatous vasculitis of unknown etiology, probably autoimmune. Other systems affected: CVS, pulmonary, renal, gastrointestinal, neurological, skin etc.

In this condition, HLA-B8 may be elevated and presence of antibodies to neutrophil cytoplasmic antigens (cANCA) may be diagnostic.

The enlargement of the salivary gland is a minor feature of the disease and not a presenting one. The treatment is cytotoxic chemotherapy and prognosis is dismal.

Fungal infection

Salivary mycosis usually occurs in immuno-compro-mised patients and is seen in the setting of HIV disease. Rapid swelling of the salivary gland followed by cystic changes and necrosis occurs. Treatment is by appropriate systemic anti-fungal therapy.

Toxoplasmosis

Due to the protozoan toxo-plasma gondii, this condition occurs as an acute febrile illness, headache, sore throat, lymphadenopathy and malaise. Sometimes unilateral parotid swelling may occur necessitating even a parotidectomy. If diagnosed along with the systemic features of the illness it resolves spontaneously in a few weeks or months. A serum test (Sabin-Seldman) is pathognomonic for this disease (see also under lymph nodes, chapter 42).

Acute necrotizing sialometaplasia

This benign lesion is important because it closely resembles carcinoma. Found usually in heavy smokers, it occurs in the hard palate in the posterior paramedian region and is thought to be an irritative response of the minor salivary glands of the palate to the toxic constituents of cigarette smoke. The lesion resembles a large molluscum contagiosum with a central necrotic ulcerative area and indurated and elevated margins. The differential diagnosis is that of carcinoma palate, also common in smokers, which can be clinched only by biopsy. With cessation of smoking and local astringent applications, resolution may be expected in 4-8 weeks.

Mucocele

Mucous retention cyst may occur in any salivary gland but is more common in the minor salivary glands as a result of an obstruction to the duct draining the small glands. It is very common in the lower lip but may occur anywhere in the mouth. A ranula is one such lesion arising from the subling-ual gland (vide supra, under ranula, chapter 53)

Sialosis is diffuse enlargement of salivary glands for metabolic reasons, such as diabetes mellitus, acromegaly etc. and in obesity attributed to fatty infiltration. No specific treatment is necessary, except to identify the underlying cause and to differentiate it from other causes of enlargement of salivary glands.

SIALOLITHIASIS

Denotes various types of calcific masses that form in the ducts or parenchyma of the salivary glands. They are more common in males (2:1), and usually stem from the calcification of an intraluminal organic nidus, i.e., dried secretions, cellular debris or intraductal

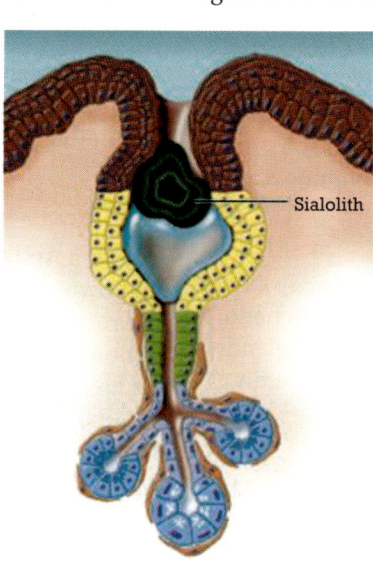

Sialolith

Fig. 51.10. Sialolithiasis

bacterial clumps. The calculi are most commonly seen in relation to the subman-dibular gland (80%), because of the following reasons:

1) The salivary flow from the submandibular gland is non-dependent

2) Secretions are more alkaline with a tendency to precipitate calcium

3) The mucin and protein content of sub-mandibular secretions are high compared to parotid

4) The Wharton's duct is wider in diameter and longer than the Stensen's duct, leading to stasis of secretions. Thus a combination of high viscosity and nondependent drainage gives a propensity to stone formation.

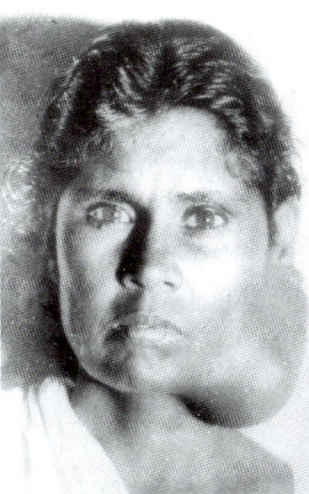

Fig. 51.11. Large parotid pleomorphic adenoma (courtesy: Prof T Gunasagaran, Chennai)

Most submandibular stones (80%) are radio-opaque whereas most parotid gland stones are radiolucent. The latter also tend to acquire a *stag-horn* shape, as they commonly form at the confluence of main ductal system. Unlike renal calculi, the formation of salivary stones is not related to metabolic disorders of calcium or phosphate, but may be related to uric acid (gout). In ductal calculi, a vicious cycle is produced; calculus ⇒ stasis ⇒ infection ⇒ calculus, worsening the pathology. They have a high recurrence rate following surgery, eventually requiring removal of the gland, for permanent cure. Other contributory diseases are: poor oral hygiene, chronic sialadenitis, cystic fibrosis and Sjogren's syndrome.

Clinical features

The main symptoms are pain and swelling beneath the jaw, aggravated during meals and lasting for an hour or so later. This picture is typical of total obstruction but some swelling and discomfort is seen in the much commoner incomplete obstruction, where symptoms are precipitated by secondary infection. Often the swelling is the principal complaint because it precedes and persists long after the pain subsides. The disease may rarely be bilateral. The patient may be relieved of his symptoms by pressure or massaging the gland, with discharge of purulent saliva into the mouth. The stone sometimes passes via naturalis, resulting in spontaneous remission.

An almond shaped submandibular mass in relation to the mylohyoid muscle, with or without local warmth and tenderness, is seen. The surface is smooth or uneven due to lobulation and fibrosis, with distinct edges, except the upper, which is wedged between the mandible and mylohyoid. The skin is freely mobile over the gland and although the gland itself can be moved a little from side to side, most movements are restricted due to tethering to the underlying muscles. It is best felt by bidigital palpation, both fingers appreciating it equally well. Regional lymphadenopathy is indicative of secondary infection. The submandibular duct should always be inspected/palpated and the stone in the duct may be sprouting through the orifice or may be palpated as the duct runs along the floor of the mouth. Gentle pressure on the gland will often expel the 'tell-tale' turbid discharge from the orifice.

Differential diagnosis

1. Sjogren's syndrome (chapter 52)
2. Mikulicz's syndrome (chapter 52)
3. Submandibular neoplasm
4. Acute viral and bacterial sialadenitis

Investigations

Plain x-ray may show a large calculus in the duct. Intraoral occlusive films may show calcification in the area of Wharton's duct. If calculi are not identified on a plain film, a sialogram or CT/MRI scan may be useful.

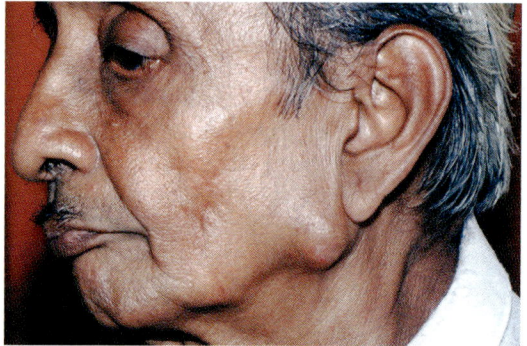

Fig. 51.12. Carcinoma parotid with impending skin break down
(courtesy: Lifeline Hospitals Chennai)

Treatment

It consists of the treatment of the stone and the gland.

Treatment of the calculus depends upon its location. In the floor of the mouth, it can be easily approached intraorally under local anesthesia. Between stay sutures, the duct is opened and the calculus removed, bearing in mind, the lingual nerve which crosses the duct opposite to the second molar tooth. If a stone is impacted at the orifice, a meatotomy/extraction can be performed, followed by meatoplasty. In case of multiple stones, especially if located within the substance of the gland, a formal sialadenectomy offers cure.

SALIVARY NEOPLASMS

Most salivary gland neoplasms are benign and even the malignant tumors are relatively slow growing. The commonest tumor of the parotid is the pleomorphic adenoma. The features of malignancy in a parotid tumor are:

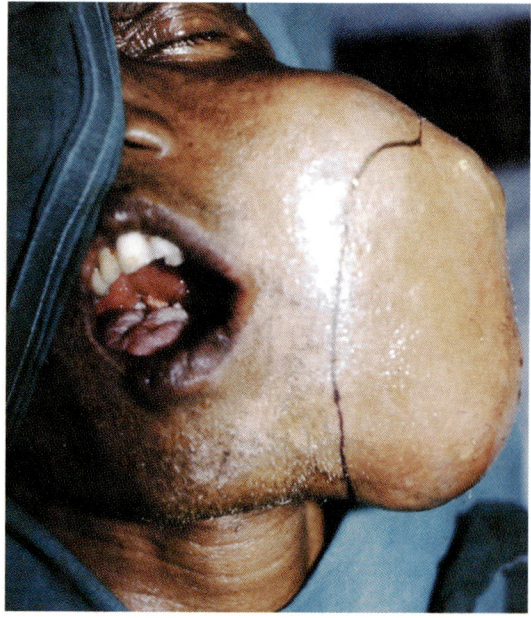

Fig. 51.13. Recurrent carcinoma parotid
(courtesy: Dr K Sreekanth, Chennai)

1. fast rate of growth
2. local pain
3. fixity
4. facial nerve involvement
5. secondary skin changes
6. spread to regional/distant sites

Classification (WHO-1991)

Epithelial tumors: benign:
    Pleomorphic adenoma (mixed tumor)
    Monomorphic adenoma
        Oxyphil adenoma
        Basal cell adenoma
        Adenolymphoma (Warthin's tumor)

Feature	Pleomorphic adenoma	Warthin's tumor
Incidence	Very common (90%)	Rare (10%)
Gender	More in females	More in males
Number	Single	Often bilateral
Consistency	Firm	Soft cystic (pseudo)
Histology	Pleomorphism	Epithelial and lymphoid structures
^{99m}Tc scan	Cold spot	Hot spot
Treatment	Superficial parotidectomy	Excision or enucleation
Recurrence	Can occur	Never
Malignant change	Can occur	Never

Table-51.1 Difference between pleomorphic adenoma and Warthin's tumor

Malignant:

    Acinic cell carcinoma

    Mucoepidermoid carcinoma

    Adenoid cystic carcinoma

    Papillary adenocarcinoma

    Squamous cell carcinoma

    Undifferentiated carcinoma

    Carcinoma ex pleomorphic adenoma

Nonepithelial tumors: benign:

    Hemangioma

    Lymphangioma

    Neurofibroma

    Neurilemmoma (Schwannoma)

Malignant: Lymphoma

Unclassified

Pathology

Pleomorphic adenoma (syn: mixed salivary tumor)

This is the most common salivary tumor, the histogenesis of which is still disputed, occurring usually in the 5th decade, with a slight female preponderance. Gross examination shows a firm lobulated or elastic mass with some cystic areas. It possesses a thin and flimsy capsule with several breaches through which the tumor tissue protrudes, forming 'pseudopodia'. These two factors account for the high incidence of recurrence following enucleation or simple excision of the tumor and the multicentric nature of their recurrence. Microscopy reveals proliferation of epithelial cells in strands or ducts, separated by myoepithelial-like cells and mucoid secretions. The secretions are often compressed to give a semblance of cartilage (pseudo) and the typical pleomorphism. Some pathologists believe that they are actual islands of cartilaginous tissue, but this is still a focus of dispute. In long standing pleomorphic adenoma, an adenocarcinoma may develop which is known as carcinoma ex pleomorphic adenoma.

Warthin's tumor (syn: adenolymphoma, papillary cystadenoma lymphomatosum)

Incidence of Warthin's tumor is 10% of all salivary tumors with male preponderance. This classically presents as a slowly growing, soft, fluctuant (pseudo) swelling occupying the lower pole of the parotid (rarely other salivary glands) in men over 40, with a high degree of bilaterality. Multifocal tumors on one side have also been reported. Histogenesis of this tumor is not clear; the most accepted theory is that it is developed from lymphoid inclusions in the form of hamartomas in the parotid, since such inclusions are never found in the other salivary glands. If this developmental explanation is accepted, it remains to be understood why they are rare in children.

Gross examination reveals a well capsulated, smooth asymmetrical enlargement of the gland. Histologically a double-layered epithelium is seen lining cystic spaces, but it is more solid than cystic and the fluctuation elicited is often false. The epithelium has columnar cells as the inner lining and cuboidal cells as the outer layer. It is inverted into the cystic cavities, appearing as multiple papillary projections, with stroma containing lymphoid tissue. *The combination of squamous metaplasia and microinfarcts*, seen in *needle biopsy is considered diagnostic of this lesion*. [99m]Tc scan clinches the diagnosis as this tumor produces a 'hot' spot, whereas all others produce a 'cold' defect.

Acinic cell carcinoma

They occur almost exclusively in the parotid gland and present as soft cystic tumors in middle aged women. Macroscopically they are well encapsulated and have a relatively benign appearance, but may occasionally metastasize and locally invade, causing facial palsy. Histopathology shows a clump of cells in a glandular pattern very similar to a serous cyst adenoma. Treated by a formal superficial parotidectomy.

Mucoepidermoid carcinoma

This exhibits the hardest consistency amongst parotid tumors. It is usually slow growing and invades local tissues to a limited degree. However it is known to metastasize to bones, lungs, skin and lymph nodes. It is difficult to make out the aggression of an individual tumor histologically and it is only done by clinical correlation. Each tumor has its individual degree of differentiation, rate of growth and spread. Histopathologically as the name implies, there are areas of mucus secreting cells and sheets of cells resembling the epidermoid and epithelial cells. The background stroma, myxomatous tissue and cartilage-like appearance of mucin, so characteristic of a pleomorphic adenoma, are absent in this tumor.

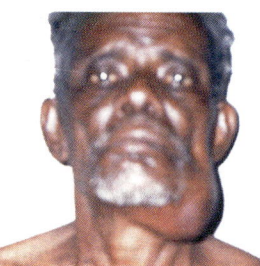

Fig. 51.14. Submandibular mixed tumor (courtesy: Lifeline Hospitals, Chennai)

Adenoid cystic carcinoma

It differs from mucoepidermoid and acinic cell tumor, in that, following initial slow growth, sooner or later *node involvement occurs characteristically*. This is manifested as pain or areas of anesthesia of the skin or motor paralysis of muscles in relation to the involved nodes. This is uncommon in the parotid, but is seen often in relation to the minor salivary glands. The cancer cells of this tumor have a propensity to spread along the perineural spaces, making total eradication quite difficult in the later stages. The cells are also known to travel along adjacent tissues and periosteum of the bone causing significant bone resorption. Classical histopathology shows both ductal epithelial cells as well as myoepithelial cells, accumulating within the basophilic background matrix and are scattered in such a way as to give them a cribriform or lace like appearance. The ductal component of the cells forms strands and cords and like cysts filled with eosinophilic material. This also enhances the cribriform appearance, which is the hallmark of adenoid cystic carcinoma. The treatment is wide excision or total radical parotidectomy.

Incidence of malignancy

It is inversely related to their size, highest in the minor salivary glands, less in the submandibular and least in the parotid. Thus any possible nodule arising from the minor salivary

gland in the palate should be looked at with a high index of suspicion. Although over 80% of all salivary epithelial tumors arise in the paro-tid, only 15% of them are malignant, whereas 30% of submandibular and 60% of minor salivary gland tumors are malignant.

Symptoms

Neoplasms of the salivary glands are described together because the pathology, investigations and management are identical. Only the local anatomical and surgical details differ and they are discussed separately.

Parotid

The patient usually presents with a painless, slowly growing swelling in the region of the parotid. Local pain may be a feature secondary to infiltration of sensory nerves (commoner with adenoid cystic carcinoma and acinic cell tumor), which may also be referred to the ear, through the auriculotemporal nerve. *Facial nerve involvement*, early in the course, is a typical sign of malignancy. Another symptom occasionally seen, is a type of paresthesia, known as *formication*, a feeling of ants crawling over the skin. Ulceration and fungation occurring from rapidly growing malignancies, may also be seen in salivary cancers.

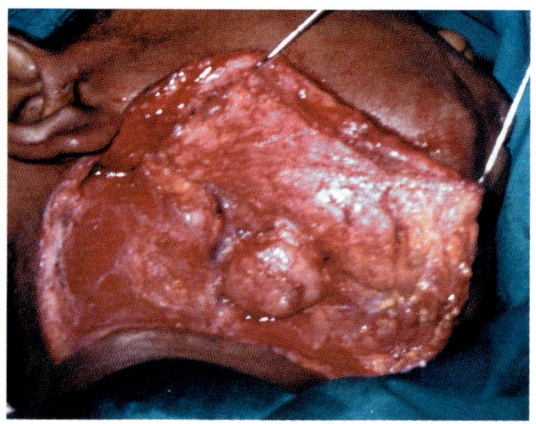

Fig. 51.15. Exposed mixed parotid tumor (courtesy: Lifeline Hospitals, Chennai)

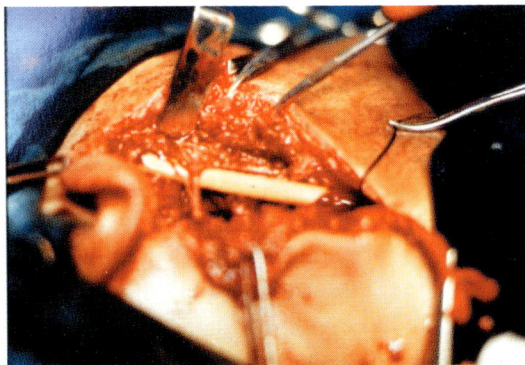

Fig. 51.16. Exposed facial nerve and branches during superficial parotidectomy
(courtesy: Halsted Surgical Clinic, Chennai)

Signs

The classical sign of a parotid neoplasm is elevation of the ear lobule and obliteration of the retromandibular hollow. The commonest tumor is the pleomorphic adenoma and the commonest site is from the superficial lobe of the gland. Invoking the Hobsley's dictum, an asymmetrical lump arising from any salivary gland is always a neoplasm, and a diffuse enlargement of the gland is most probably nonneoplastic. Regional lymph nodes (upper deep cervical or level-2) are enlarged only in malignancy. Other salivary glands and lachrymal glands should be examined, since generalized involvement occurs in Sjogren's, Mikulicz's syndrome, etc.

Submandibular/sublingual tumors

The classic presentation of a submandibular salivary tumor is a swelling under the lower border of the horizontal part of the mandible and a sublingual tumor, a paramedian swelling in the floor of the mouth. Diseases of minor salivary glands usually present as a submucous or ulcerated nodule, usually over the palate and lips and rarely over the cheek and floor of the mouth.

Investigations

Apart from routine baseline investigations, high frequency USG and CT/MRI are useful imaging techniques for both parotid and submandibular gland tumors, helping to define the mass, identify relation to adjacent structures, involvement of deep lobe and to plan definite surgical therapy. Sialogram has no role in the management of salivary gland tumors.

Open biopsy is contraindicated in parotid and submandibular gland, the reason being that they are most often pleomorphic adenomas, which have a thin capsule and high incidence of tumor implantation into the operative wound, whereas it is an excellent tool for minor salivary gland tumors, to plan subsequent definitive surgery. While performing preoperative biopsy of these tumors, it is important to plan in such a manner as to include the area in subsequent definitive excision.

Needle biopsy, especially an FNAC is now

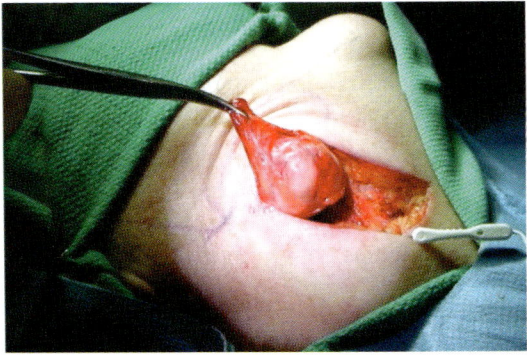

Fig. 51.17. Right submandibular sialadenectomy

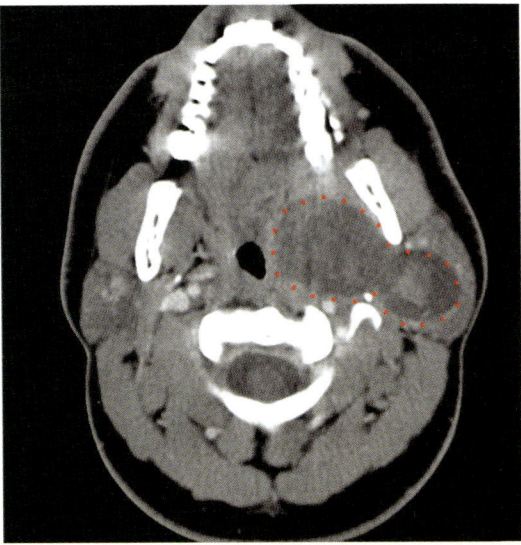

Fig. 51.18. CT scan showing dumb-bell tumor of deep lobe of left parotid (marked in red dotted line)

accepted as a viable alternative to open/ wedge biopsy, especially in suspected malignancy or Warthin's tumor. Large studies have shown that there is no significant risk of spreading tumor cells along the track of the needle, provided a thin (22-24) gauge needle is employed. Notwithstanding the opponents for preoperative biopsy, the advantage of having a tissue diagnosis in hand before surgery outweighs possible disadvantages, such as tumor implantation, facial nerve injury etc. The decision regarding the extent of resection or sacrificing the facial nerve, during surgery is more comfortably taken, if the nature of the disease is known earlier. However the sensitivity and specificity of an FNAC, largely depend upon the expertise available.

Treatment

Adequate surgical clearance is the sheet anchor in their management.

Parotid gland

1) Extracapsular enucleation of FNAC-proved Warthin's tumor.

2) Superficial conservative parotidectomy is excising the superficial lobe, sparing the facial nerve, commonly done for mixed tumors of superficial lobe.

3) Total conservative parotidectomy is removing the entire parotid, preserving the facial nerve, done for dumb-bell mixed tumor of the deep lobe.

4) Radical parotidectomy is done for malignancy and includes removal of the entire gland, the facial nerve and the regional lymph nodes.

Pleomorphic adenoma: If it is located in the superficial part of the gland, superficial conservative parotidectomy is the procedure of choice. Management of a dumb-bell tumor is discussed later.

For malignant tumors, total parotidectomy with (radical) or without (conservative) sacrificing the facial nerve, has to be performed, following histological confirmation. It should be realized that adequate cancer clearance is more important than preserving the facial nerve, but removing the facial nerve 'for the sake of removing', is unwarranted, if it does not interfere with tumor clearance.

If lymph nodes are enlarged, a 10-day course of antibiotics, to cover mixed infection, is given, to see if they regress. If they persist, metastatic disease is presumed and a radical neck dissection has to be performed. A preoperative FNAC of the nodes will be helpful in that situation.

MINOR SALIVARY GLAND TUMORS

The minor salivary glands are situated in and around the oral cavity, about 4-500 in number. They are mostly mucus-secreting, hence small (subcentimeter) mucus retention cysts can occur in relation to these glands, commonly over the gums and lips.

90% of tumors araising from these glands are malignant. Typically a minor salivary tumor starts as submucous nodule, to ulcerate later; an important differentiating feature from carcinoma of buccal mucosa, which starts as an ulcer. The ulcerated lesion bleeds to touch and the regional lymph nodes may be involved either by metastasis or secondary infection.

After confirming the diagnosis by a punch biopsy of the edge, wide excision, using either diathermy of laser is the treatment. If the lymph nodes donot regress with a course of antibiotics, they have to be excised enbloc, preferably after FNAC confirmation.

Minor salivary gland tumors of the cheek or palate are excised with 0.5-1.0cm margin in all three dimensions, and subjected to histopathology. Adjuvant RT may be needed, if the margins of clearance are not adequate or if the tumor is poorly differentiated.

Nonepithelial tumors

Hemangiomas and lymphangiomas are the commonest nonepithelial salivary gland tumors in childhood, whereas neurofibromas and neurilemmomas are common in adults. In children, progressive growth of a spongy compressible swelling, with some local warmth, makes the diagnosis easy, but the adult tumors are solid and usually diagnosed after parotidectomy.

Spontaneous regression may occur in a hemangioma developing under the age of three, but such involution may not be seen in lymphangiomas. Sclerotherapy may be tried in these lesions for a few sittings, failing which, complete surgical excision is the treatment of choice.

Lymphomas

Salivary gland lymphomas may either arise from lymphoid tissue entrapped within the capsule or more rarely denovo from the glands themselves. These are also known to occur as a complication of HIV infection or Sjogren's syndrome. They are usually non-Hodgkin's lymphomas (NHL), with a predilection for the females and the parotids. Diagnosis is by USG/CT/MRI, confirmed by needle biopsy and followed by investigations for staging. The treatment is as for NHL elsewhere, with radio/ chemotherapy (COPP or CHOP regime), for 6-9 cycles. The prognosis is excellent, with a potential for cure.

Parotid and HIV

An unusual feature seen in HIV positive patients is multiple parotid cysts. A classical MRI/CT appearance is that of Swiss cheese with multiple large cystic lesions. Apart from the cosmetic reasons, relevant only in long term survivors on chemotherapy, there is no indication for surgery. These glands do not become painful nor does xerostomia supervene. Rarely infection of these cysts may require surgical drainage.

DUMB-BELL TUMOR OF PAROTID

Parotid neoplasms arising from the deep lobe show minimal external swelling, instead progressively enlarging between the styloid process and the mandible, to present as a swelling in the lateral wall of the pharynx at the posterior pillar of the fauces, displacing the soft palate to the opposite side. Patients are often seen in ENT department for dysphagia or dysphonia initially. If there is a preauricular swelling, bimanual palpation of the tumor may be done, to establish its continuity with the parapharyngeal mass, which may be confirmed by a CT/MRI scan and transoral needle biopsy. Examination under anesthesia may show a lobulated lump palpable in the lateral pharyngeal wall, with free movement of mucosa over the tumor. A growing tumor of the deep lobe in the retromandibular canal (vide supra) assumes an hour-glass constriction, producing the typical dumb-bell shape.

Superficial conservative parotidectomy (also known as super-facial parotidectomy)

The standard incision used earlier was 'Y' shaped, the fork enclosing the ear, but now many prefer an 'S' (Sistrunk's) or 'C' shaped incision running infront of the tragus and turning vertical below the ear. In large tumors, a postauricular extension, converting into a 'Y' may be necessary.

The skin flaps are raised on either side, exposing the entire superficial surface of parotid. The dissection is carefully carried to the depth, avoiding injury to the great auricular nerve. The insertion of SCM into the mastoid process is identified, exposing the cartilaginous external auditory meatus and posterior belly of digastric, both serving as landmarks for the facial trunk, as it emerges from the stylomastoid foramen. Another method of locating the facial nerve is by pulling the lobule of the ear backwards, creating a sharp angle at the tip of the tragus. The nerve trunk is situated about 1 cm deep to the tip of the tragus when the pull is maintained. The nerve may also be located by deep dissection between the styloid process (identified by the posterior belly of digastric) and the bony part of external meatus.

After ascertaining the nerve branches lying deep to the tumor , the gland is gently seprated by opening a curved hemostat (Crile's), inserted

---

Jewels of Gyan - 51.1

Hobsley's Dictum in Parotid

Inflammation: Whole parotid swollen

Neoplasm: A part of the gland is swollen

into the gland substance, inching along the twigs. A proper plane of dissection (facio-venous plane of Patey) is developed and the entire gland above to this plane is removed in superficial parotidectomy. In tumors of deep lobe, the branches may be splayed superficial to the mass. The diagnosis is established by CT scan and trans-oral needle biopsy. With soft slings, the branches of facial nerve have to be gently lifted, to approach the tumor underneath.

Surgery for dumb–bell tumor

A preliminary ligation of external carotid artery at its origin is carried out, before the gland exposed by standard incision, the exposed facial nerve branches are lifted by slings, to expose the deep part of the gland. The styloid process digitally fractured and the stylomandibular ligament is divided, to open up the constricting part of retromandibular canal (vide supra), when the capsulated tumor in the deep lobe may be easily delivered into the field by digital enucleation. After removal of the tumor-bearing deep lobe, the external carotid arterial control is released and meticulous hemostasis is established before closure of wound, leaving a suction drain.

Complications of parotid surgery: 5-Fs, facial nerve injury, Frey's syndrome, fistula, fluid collection and flap necrosis.

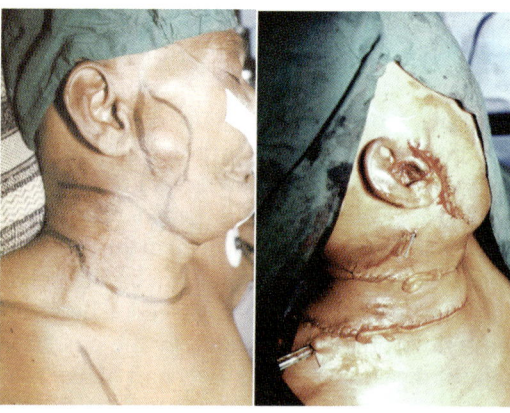

Fig. 51.19. Carcinoma parotid
Total parotidectomy and radical nodal dissection by step-ladder (MacFee) incision
(courtesy: Lifeline Hospitals, Chennai)

Jewels of Gyan -51.3

**Parotidectomy Complications
The Five Fs!**

Facial nerve injury
Frey's syndrome
Fistula salivary
Fluid collection
Flap necrosis

1) Injury to the facial nerve is the most feared and commonest complication, the probabilities of which warrant adequate preoperative counseling, to avoid litigations. In view of the relation of the nerve to the deep part of the gland, this complication is more seen following total parotidectomy. The injury may be deliberate or inadvertent, former is justified in biopsy-proved malignancies and the latter is either neurapraxia/axonotmesis (70%), due to handling/retraction of the nerves or neurotmesis (30%). Routine identification of the facial trunk and its primary divisions, early in the course of dissection, using the posterior belly of digastric and cartilaginous external auditory meatus as the important landmarks, has largely reduced nerve accidents. Blunt dissection of the gland substance in a proper plane, in postero-anterior direction is essential. Intra-operative use of the galvanic nerve stimulator is a useful, but not essential addition.

Management: If the nerve has been severed or partly removed, either direct perineural suturing or nerve grafting, using a segment of great auricular nerve, may be done. The practice followed in some centers, to harvest a segment of great auricular nerve, as a routine in all cases, before the dissection is deepened, has limited subscribers. If the facial weakness is identified in the postoperative period, wait and watch policy is the best, to see if recovery takes place within a few weeks (neurapraxia or axonotmesis), before planning further management. Facial strapping, electrical stimulation and steps to prevent exposure keratitis, such as lateral tarsorrhaphy, may be useful in the meantime. In late cases, either static sling operations, with fascia lata strips or dynamic slings, with temporalis muscle/fascia, to restore closure of lids and reform nasolabial fold, may be considered.

2) Frey's syndrome (syn: auriculotemporal syndrome or gustatory sweating): This is due to partial injury to auriculotemporal nerve, with malregeneration of its autonomic fibers. Secretomotor postganglionic parasympathetic fibers (from the otic ganglion) join sudomotor sympathetic and common sensory fibers of the nerve. There is flushing, hyperhidrosis and hyperesthesia in the area of distribution of the auriculotemporal nerve, (in front of and above the external ear) during meals. This is not a serious problem; patients improve with reassurance and symptomatic treatment. Topical antiperspirants, such as aluminium chloride hexahydrate, may also provide symptomatic relief. Rarely, for chronic disabling symptoms, the extreme step of auriculotemporal neurectomy will be required. After all, why venture a second operation for symptoms that can be handled with a kerchief at the dining table! Injection of botulin toxin (botox) into the affected skin has shown some benefit in interactable cases.

3) Salivary fistula may be from the remaing gland or a major duct. There is discharge of saliva from the suture line, usually from the 4th postoperative day onwards, pouring out more during mastication. They may be seen following partial excision of the parotid, penetrating wounds or drainage of a parotid abscess. Given time, the majority of them heal by conservative treatment with anticholinergic drugs, such as propanthe-line bromide, oxyphenonium bromide or dicyclomine hydrochloride, to reduce secretions.

In refractory cases persisting for 3-6 months, a lipiodol sialogram is done to identify if it is glandular or ductal, as it is the latter type that often fails to resolve. The following therapeutic options are available in such cases, but the first two are more popular:

a) converting an external fistula into an internal one
b) auriculotemporal neurotomy, to reduce secretions
c) low dose radiation (2000 r) to the parotid region
d) ductal reconstruction (Newman-Seabrook's operation), with tantalum wire or polythene stent
e) completion (total) parotidectomy, least preferred and should be avoided, for fear of creating another complication in the processs

4) collection of saliva/lymph under the flaps is very common, with an intact suture line. All that is needed, is to aspirate under strict aseptic conditions and administer anti-secretory agents.

5) necrosis of skin flaps is rare and occurs only when a lot of skin undermining is done or if the external carotid artery is ligated to control

Jewels of Gyan - 51.2

The rule of '2' in submandibular sialadenectomy

Two common indications for surgery: calculus and tumor
Two inches long incision is made, two finger breadths below the jaw
Two superficial nerves to protect: cervical and mandibular branches of facial
Two deep nerves to preserve: lingual and hypoglossal
Two-point ligation of facial artery
Two muscles to divide: platysma and mylohyoid
Two lobes of the gland to be excised

bleeding during surgery for large tumors. Incisions with acute angles, such as 'Y of 'T' are more prone to necrosis at the tips, hence those with gentle curves ('C' or 'S') are preferred.

Submandibular sialadenectomy

The incision is made about two finger breadths (3 cms) below the inferior border of mandible in order to avoid damaging the looping mandibular branch of the facial nerve. It is deepened up to the investing layer of deep cervical fascia and flaps raised at that depth. The upper flap will contain the mandibular branch of the facial nerve. The anterior facial vein is clamped overlying the submandibular gland and the superficial lobe is then mobilised all around. The facial artery which enters the submandibular gland is identified, ligated and divided at two points, both below and above the gland. Multiple small vessels which may be running from the facial artery or deep facial vein to the gland are also dealt with progressively. After freeing the entire superficial lobe of the gland it is retracted posteriorly to reveal the groove between the superficial and deep lobes, occupied by the posterior

border of the mylohyoid muscle. This is retracted forwards and the deep lobe is then accessed and mobilised. Small veins draining the deep part of the gland, joining the deep lingual veins are controlled by pressure or cautery. After the gland is freed from the vessels, it is retracted and can be seen to be in close relation to the lingual nerve, which runs on the hyoglossus muscle with the submandibular ganglion suspended from it. The fibres between the nerve and the gland are carefully transected, freeing the entire gland except the duct, which is then tied and divided as far anteriorly as possible.

1) Mandibular branch of facial nerve (superficially, and is preserved by the flap containing three cms of skin and platysma below the inferior border of mandible).
2) The lingual nerve (tackled last by dividing only a few fibres between the nerve and the gland)
3) Hypoglossal nerve (lying inferior to the lingual nerve on hyoglossus and preserved by keeping the dissection away from the muscle)
Tumors of sublingual salivary gland are treated by transoral sialadenectomy.

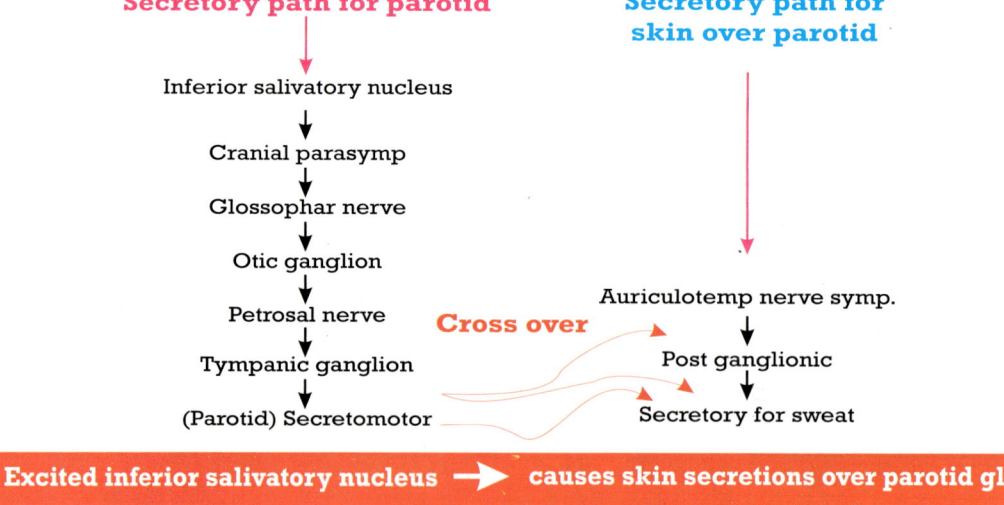

Fig.51.20. Anatomical basis of Frey's syndrome

52 Mikulicz Disease and Sjögren's Syndrome

Mikulicz disease, a rare autoimmune disease is considered a benign lymphoepithelial lesion, characterised by the triad of

1. symmetrical enlargement of all the salivary glands

2. symmetrical enlargement of both the lacrimal glands, causing narrowing of the palpebral fissures

3. xerostomia and xerophthalmia

This disease is characterized by infiltration of the salivary and lacrimal glands with T and B cell lymphoid population and the presence of epimyoepithelial islands. This is usually considered a variant of *Sjogren's syndrome*, without its arthropathy (rheumatoid).

MIKULICZ SYNDROME is a combination of bilateral salivary and lacrimal gland enlargement seen in many systemic diseases, like sarcoidosis, leukemia, lymphoma etc and Sjögren's syndrome. It is due to infiltration of these glands by round cells and loss of acinar epithelium.

Investigations

Routine studies and those to exclude underlying autoimmune process, to be confirmed by needle biopsy.

Treatment

Any identifiable underlying disease should be treated on its merits, otherwise it is only symptomatic. Sialagogues NSAIDs, steroids and immunosupressants have been tried for palliation, but the routine indication of the latter two is debatable.

Treatment of xerophthalmia (dry eyes): The lacrimal puncta may be obliterated by diathermy or laser, resulting in retention of a thin film of secretions over the eye ball. Eye drops of methyl cellulose solution (0.5%) may also be useful (artificial tears).

Treatment of xerostomia (dry mouth): Meticulous oral hygiene with chlorhexidine mouthwashes and dental flossing is necessary, as also methyl cellulose mouthwashes. A prokinetic parasympathomimetic drug,

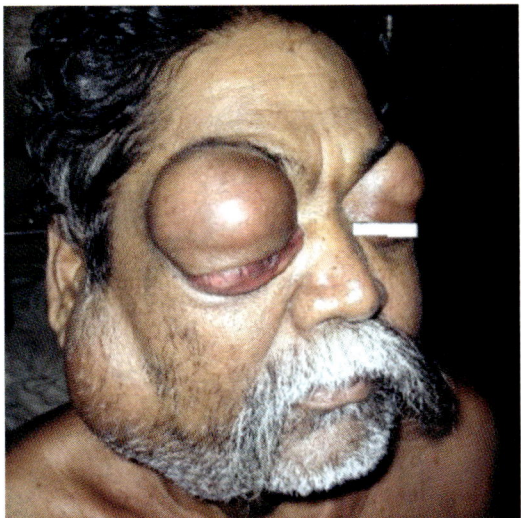

Fig. 52.1. Mantle-cell NHL presenting as Mikulicz syndrome

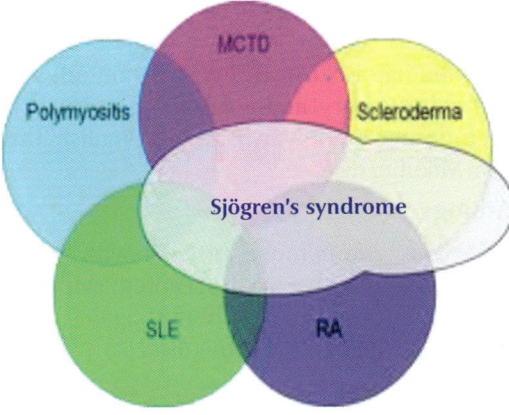

MCTD: Multimodal connective tissue disorder
SLE: Systemic lupus erythematosus
RA: Rheumatoid arthritis

Fig. 52.2. A disease model of Sjögren's syndrome in a minor salivary gland

cisapride is found to be a useful sialagogue (agogos: leading), in such conditions.

SJÖGREN'S SYNDROME

It is a disease with both inflammatory and neoplastic characteristics with female preponderance (9:1), commonly seen in postmenopausal women. It is a chronic progressive autoimmune disease, characterized by exocrine gland (salivary and lacrimal) involvement by lymphocytic infiltrate, associated with hypergammaglobulinemia. Systemic manifestations are seen in a third of patients and a small number develop keratoconjunctivitis sicca (sicca: dry) and NHL, as observed in relation to Hashimoto's thyroiditis. It may be seen in isolation (primary) or in association with connective tissue disorders (see below).

Clinical features

The triad of xerostomia (dry mouth), xerophthalmia (dry eyes) and arthritis is classical. The dryness of eyes and mouth, due to insufficient secretions by lacrimal/salivary glands is also termed sicca syndrome. It may be associated with dysphagia due to lower esophageal dysmotility.

The disease may be unilateral, with or without significant enlargement of lacrimal and salivary glands. Associated connective tissue disorders like rheumatoid arthritis (most common), systemic lupus erythematosus, polyarteritis, scleroderma or polymyositis, distinguish this from Mikulicz disease.

Etiology

Not clear, autoimmune process with B-cell hyperactivity, is the most accepted, with the demonstration of autoantibodies against salivary tissue in patients with this disease.

Pathology

Atrophy of acinar tissue, with lymphoplasmocytic infiltration of all the glands affected. Adding to the confusion in terminology, Mikulicz syndrome also has similar histological findings. Finding myoepithelial islands, due to metaplasia of ducts, clinches the diagnosis and distinguishes this from lymphoma. This disease may predispose to the development of NHL of salivary glands.

Investigations

Identification of autoantibodies (antiSS-A & B) and tissue diagnosis by needle biopsy, may be needed in atypical cases. Investigations for collagen disorders are supportive.

Treatment

Same as Mikulicz syndrome; steroid therapy has been tried in intractable cases, with uncertain response.

IV immunoglobulins may be useful in primary Sjögren's to relieve neuropathy.

Also interferon alfa is found to improve neuropathy.

Rituximab, a monoclonal antibody is found to be promising in treating associated vasculitis.

Artifical tear substitutes, such as autologous serum tears are lately being used.

An immunosuppressant, cyclosporine eye drops (Restants) reduces lacrimal gland inflammation and causes improvement in ocular symptoms.

Surgery, total or subtotal excision of salivary glands has been attempted in some patients for cosmetic reasons as well as a preventive step against development of a lymphoma.

To clear the confusion in nomenclature, it may be broadly stated that in a clinical context, if only lacrimal/salivary glands are enlarged, it is called *Mikulicz disease*.

If the enlargement is seen in other systemic diseases, such as sarcoidosis, lymphoma, leukemia, tuberculosis etc. it is known as *Mikulicz syndrome*.

If it is associated with connective tissue disorders, it is known as *Sjögren's syndrome*.

There is reluctance by some pathologists to discriminate between these conditions and they believe that these are manifestations of one and

53 Mouth

The oral cavity is lined by stratified squamous epithelium, most of it is non-keratinized, except over the alveolar process and the retromolar trigone of hard palate, where it is keratinized (masticatory mucosa).

BUCCAL or MUCOUS RETENTION CYSTS

Definition: Cysts in the cheek or lips due to blockage of the ducts of the minor mucous glands lining oral cavity, are known as mucous retention cysts. They are, in fact, mucoceles of the minor mucous glands.

Clinical symptoms

These cysts can occur at any age with equal sex distribution. Commonest presentation is a painless small, smooth, rounded, pinkish, freely mobile lump on the inner aspect of the cheek or lip. They may get bitten during mastication, and become secondarily infected, giving rise to a submucous abscess. As the cyst is so tiny, usually under 5mm. transillumination and fluctuation are not easy to demonstrate.

Differential diagnosis

Tumor of a minor salivary gland and mucosal polyp

Treatment

Depending on the size, either excision of the cyst or marsupialization may be done under local anesthesia, but endotracheal general anes-

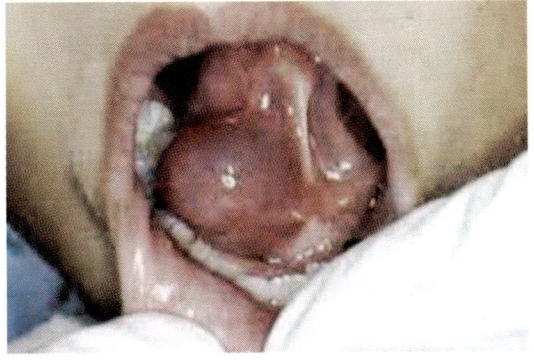

Fig. 53.1. Ranula

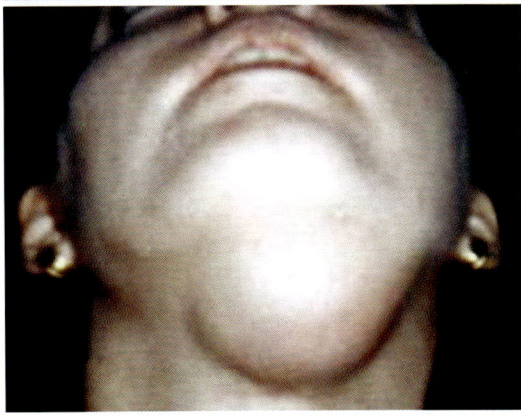

Fig. 53.2. Plunging ranula

thesia may be necessary for large posteriorly placed cysts, to prevent aspiration of saliva/blood during surgery.

RANULA

Definition: (rana: frog) The most accepted is a large retention cyst from a mucous gland of the floor of the mouth, communicating with a minor salivary glands (glands of Blandin and Nuhn). The disease derives its name by the appearance to that of a frog's belly (Hippocrates). A persistent cervical sinus or posterior minor salivary gland communication are postulated to be the causes of a plunging type of ranula.

Pathology

A delicate fibrous capsule, lined by a layer of macrophages and externally by the buccal mucous membrane, containing thin mucoid fluid.

Clinical features

It presents as a painless, progressively enlarging, rounded mass in the floor of the mouth, usually on one side of midline. Pain denotes either a fast rate of growth or infection. 'Waxing and waning' are well known, as spontaneous rupture and refilling occur often.

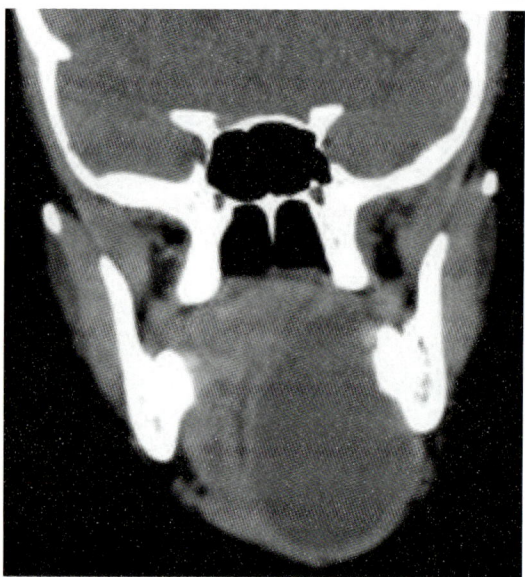

Fig. 53.3. CT scan of a plunging ranula

Signs

A brilliantly transilluminant, smooth cyst in the floor of the mouth, over which the Wharton's duct may be seen coursing, is unmistakable. It is not warm or tender, soft cystic in consistency; the mucosa is movable over the swelling, but by its size and location, it appears to be relatively fixed to the soft tissue underneath. Movements of the tongue are usually affected and there is no regional lymphadenopathy.

Plunging ranula: Some ranulae have a communication into the neck, along the posterior border of the mylohyoid. If a swelling is visible in the submandibular region as well, bidigital palpation should be done and if pressure from below is directly transmitted to the intraoral finger (*cross fluctuation*), the diagnosis is confirmed.

Differential diagnosis

1) Lymph cyst: it may be virtually impossible to distinguish between the two, except that the fluid contained is slightly thinner than in a ranula. However, this is largely academic, since the treatment is the same.

2) Sublingual dermoid cyst:

(a) often situated in the midline and
(b) tensely cystic without translucency, are the helpful features to identify this condition.

Complications: Infection, rupture, interference with mastication, movements of tongue and speech.

Treatment

The ranula may be dissected out through the oral route, under local or general anesthesia and completely excised, along with the affected salivary gland, if possible. An alternative procedure which is equally effective and is popular is marsupialization or saucerization, by liberally deroofing the cyst, since it is relatively simpler and avoids possible injury to Wharton's duct or lingual nerve.

Deep or plunging ranula may also be treated by one of the methods above, ensuring good drainage of the cervical extension and avoiding a cosmetically undesirable cervical incision.

Inflammations

These may be:
1. stomatitis
2. gingivitis
3. gingivo-stomatitis

The oral cavity contains many organisms, but they are prevented from becoming pathogenic by:

a. regular desquamation
b. constant washing of the oral cavity by saliva so that the organisms are swallowed and destroyed in the stomach
c. mild antimicrobial activity of saliva

Predisposing factors

a. vitamin and nutritional deficiencies
b. Candidial infection
c. epidermolysis bullosa
d. cytotoxic drugs
e. reduced ability to deal with secondary infection, as in cyclical leukopenia, agranulocytosis (granulocytopenia), aplastic anemia, hypogammaglobulinemia, chronic adreno-

cortical therapy or HIV infection

f.   autoimmune mechanism

g.   lichen planus

h.   metallic toxins such as mercury, sulphur, bismuth and lead poisoning.

Treatment

O.2% aqueous solution of chlorhexidine as mouth wash, along with treatment of the specific etiology.

Specific types of stomatitis

APHTHOUS STOMATITIS (syn: dyspeptic ulcers)

Recurrent minor aphthous ulceration

Recurrent major aphthous ulceration

Herpetiform aphthous ulceration

Minor aphthous ulcers

Either single or multiple recurrent painful ulcers, occurring more in women, usually 5-10mm size, oval in shape with a yellow base and red margin. They are found over the nonkeratinized areas and usually heal within 1-2 weeks.

MAJOR APHTHOUS ULCERS

These are similar to minor aphthae except larger in size, and taking a longer time to heal, with resultant scarring.

Treatment

Mouthwashes with 0.2% aqueous chlorhexidine solution or gel for local application, in combination with metronidazole and lignocaine are popularly used. Major aphthae are treated with triamcinolone acetonide, and choline salicylate as oral gel is applied for minor ulcers. Immunostimulants, such as levamisole, arabinoxylan etc are useful in reducing relapses. Anabolic steroids, blood component therapy are found effective in intractable cases. Diclofenac topical applications are used for relief of local discomfort.

Behcet's syndrome

Seen in young males, with genital, conjunctival and oral ulcerations, skin rashes, arthritis, thrombophlebitis, colitis and neurological

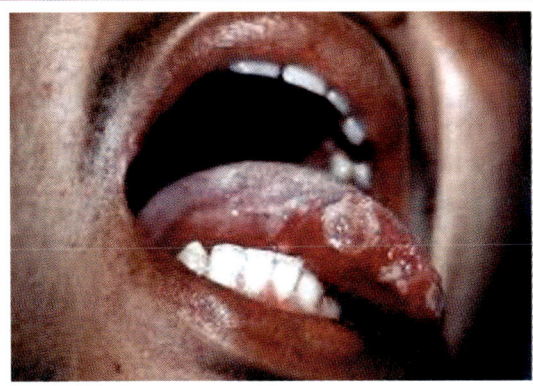

Fig. 53.4. Behcet's syndrome

symptoms, considered to be due to autoimmune vasculopathy.

Reiter's syndrome

Nongonorrheal urethritis, arthritis, conjunctivitis and oral ulcers.

Herpes simplex

Usually subclinical; many small vesicles appear which rapidly break down to form small yellow ulcers with bright red margins. These may also occur over the cheeks. The patients are usually toxic, with fever and submandibular lymphadenitis.

Treatment

Soft diet, analgesics and 0.2% aqueous chlorhexidine mouth washes. Given early in the course, specific antiviral therapy (acyclovir) may be useful.

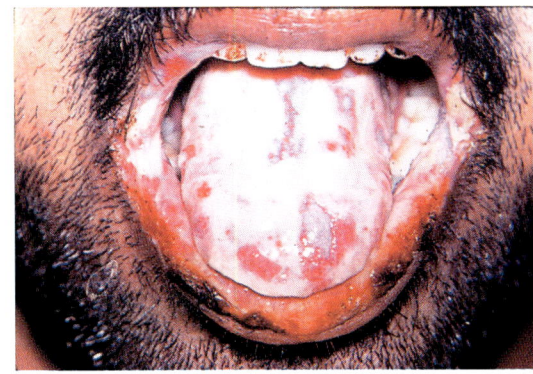

Fig. 53.5. Oral candidiasis
(courtesy: Prof T Gunasagaran, Chennai)

Herpes labialis

This is due to periodic reactivation of herpes virus in response to cold wind, bright sunlight or a febrile illness. Kissing may transmit the virus; hence such gestures should be avoided (by the patient and the doctor!).

Transfer of infection to the eyes results in herpetic keratitis and possible permanent opaque corneal scarring.

Monilial stomatitis

The following are the clinical forms of candida infection:

a) Acute pseudomembranous candidiasis (syn: thrush)

This usually occurs in debilitated infants and also in chronically ill, elderly and patients on steroids and cytotoxic drugs.

Treatment

Miconazole gel 1% topical application and amphotericin-B lozenges.

b) Acute hypertrophic or hyperplastic candidiasis

Presentation is as above; in addition, tongue is also involved.

c) Acute atrophic candidiasis

This occurs as a complication of the use of broad spectrum antibiotics.

d) Chronic atrophic candidiasis: (denture sore mouth)

This is characterized by a painless patch of red edematous mucosa over the area covered by an upper denture, seen in patients with poor dental hygiene.

Treatment

1. Dentures should not be worn at night.
2. Amphotericin-B lozenges.
3. Nystatin cream may be applied to the inside of the denture.

e) Chronic hypertrophic or hyperplastic candidiasis and speckled leucoplakia.

Angular cheilosis: (syn: angular stomatitis)
Moist infected and crusting cracks are seen at the angle of mouth. This may be due to

a. leak of saliva at the angles of the mouth and the moist skin becoming infected by candidiasis.
b. in children who suck the finger
c. when dentures cause occlusion deformity during mouth closure
d. loss of canine eminence
e. avitaminosis

Treatment

Nystatin, miconazole, fusidate or mupirocin ointment

VINCENT'S ACUTE ULCERATIVE GINGIVITIS: (syn: acute ulcero-membranous stomatitis, vincent's angina)

This is due to *Borrelia vincenti* and *Bacteroides fusiformis* (called Vincent's organisms) and starts at the interdental papillae, progressing to form a deep crater covered with a greenish gray necrotic tissue. It may start around the wisdom tooth or tonsil, spreading to adjacent areas in severe cases, but does not affect the edentulous mouth (see phagedenic ulcer- chapter 15).

Clinical features

Fever and persistent severe ache in the affected part.

Treatment

Strict oral hygiene and frequent antimicrobial mouth washes, supported by therapy for the underlying disease with metronidazole and penicillin for two weeks.

Rhagades

This occur in the corners of the mouth in congenital syphilis, leaving scars when healed.

Burns

Thermal burns produced by hot food, electrical burns if the socket is kept in the mouth and chemical burns due to suicidal/accidental ingestion of acid/alkali can occur.

Treatment

Topical hydrocortisone application

Analgesics and antibiotics in severe cases.

Microstomia, if it occurs, may require surgical correction.

Single oral ulcer

This is usually caused by sharp tooth/denture. It may also be tuberculous, fungal, malignant, or due to Wegener's granuloma, eosinophilic granulona and lymphoproliferative disorders.

Treatment

Sharp tooth or ill fitting denture has to be attended to.

Biopsy and microbiological examination may be required for refractory ulcers.

An overview of oral cancers (covers the chapters of Tongue, Lips and Cheek)

Head and neck cancers in India account for 30% of all cancers in males in various cancer registries. Nearly 80,000 oral cancers are diagnosed every year in our country. Nearly two thirds of these are located in the tongue and gingivo-buccal complex where the betel 'quid' is kept.

Squamous cell carcinoma (SCC) is the most common histologic type seen in more than 90% of these tumors. Alcohol and tobacco abuse are common etiologic factors. Because the entire aerodigestive tract is exposed to these carcinogens, patients are at increased risk for developing second primary neoplasms of the head and neck, lung, esophagus, hence a comprehensive clinical, endoscopic and radiological evaluation of the entire head and neck and chest is warranted.

Human papillomavirus (HPV) infection is now well accepted as a risk factor for the development of SCC of the head and neck, particularly cancers of the lingual and palatine tonsils, and base of tongue. A strong causal relationship has been established between HPV-16 and the development of these cancers and finding of HPV genome in the cancer cells is associated with favorable prognosis.

The management of patients with head and neck cancer is complex, the evaluation requires a multidisciplinary approach by the health care providers with expertise in caring for these patients The initial evaluation includes a detailed history and physical examination of the head and neck region; mirror and fiberoptic examination as clinically indicated, biopsy to clinch the diagnosis, CT/MRI of primary and neck as indicated and chest imaging. Moreover, managing and preventing sequelae of radical surgery, radiotherapy, and chemotherapy (e.g. pain, xerostomia, speech, swallowing and nutrition problems) require professional management. Patients should also be strongly encouraged to stop smoking and alcohol consumption, because these may impair the immune response, efficacy of treatment and adversely affect the prognosis.

Treatment modalities

Single modality treatment with either surgery (for well differentiated) or radiotherapy (for moderately differentiated) is generally recommended for the patients who present with early stage oral cavity cancers. In contrast, combined modality therapy (neoadjuvant or adjuvant radiotherapy and chemotherapy) is generally recommended for the patients with poorly differentiated cancers or resectable loco-regionally advanced disease. Definitive chemoradiation is considered for inoperable loco-regionally advanced cancers or as neoadjuvant therapy to down-stage the disease.

Principles of surgery
Primary t

Surgical resection should be planned based on the extent of the oral tumor as ascertained by clinical examination and careful interpretation of appropriate radiographic images. Perineural invasion should be suspected when tumors are adjacent to motor or sensory nerves. When invasion is suspected, the nerve should be dissected both proximally and distally and resected to obtain clearance of disease.

Marginal or segmental resection of the mandible may be necessary to encompass the cancer with adequate tumor free margins. Segmental resection should be considered in tumors that grossly involve mandibular periosteum (as determined by tumor fixation to the mandible) or show evidence of direct tumor involvement of the bone at the time of operation or through preoperative imaging.

The extent of mandibular resection will depend on the degree of involvement accessed clinically and in the operating room. An adequate excision is defined as clear resection margins with at least 1.5cm from the gross tumor. A pathological clear margin is defined as the distance from the invasive tumor front that is 5mm or more from the resected margin. In view of high risk of developing osteoradio-necrosis following RT, if the jaw is invoved, RT as the only modality of curative treatment is not recommended, but it may be given as neoadjuvant therapy, followed by surgery to resect jaw or to palliate nonresectable tumors.

Primary closure is recommended when appropriate but should not be pursued at the expense of obtaining wide, tumor free margins, by established principles of cancer surgery. Reconstructive closure with split-thickness skin grafts, local/regional flaps, free tissue transfers with or without mandibular reconstruction is performed at the discretion of the surgeon. Primary reconstruction is preferable to improve the quality of life for these patients, if the surgeon is satisfied with the adequacy of tumor resection.

Management of the neck

Historically neck dissections have been classified as "radical" or "modified radical" procedures. The modified radical procedures preserved the SCM muscle, jugular vein, spinal accessory nerve. It is preferable to classify cervical lymphadenectomy using current nomenclature as either "comprehensive" or "selective."

A comprehensive neck dissection is one that removes all the five lymph nodal groups that would be included in a classic radical neck dissection. Whether the SCM muscle, IJV or spinal accessory nerve are preserved does not affect whether the dissection is classified as comprehensive. A selective neck dissection is one that removes a selective lymph node groups.

The surgical management of regional lymph nodes is dictated by the extent of tumor at initial tumor staging. The type of neck dissection is defined according to preoperative clinical staging and is determined at the discretion of the surgeon, based on the initial preoperative staging. In general a selective neck dissection of at least levels I to III is indicated in clinically negative necks (N0) and a comprehensive neck dissection is done for clinically node positive disease. Patients with advanced lesions involving the anterior tongue or floor of mouth which approximate or cross the midline, should undergo contralateral submandibular dissection (level-1) as necessary to achieve adequate tumor resection.

Adjuvant postoperative radiation or chemo-radiation is prescribed in all locally advanced tumors and in early tumors with microscopic residual tumor or any other adverse tumor factor. All patients should have regular follow-up visits to assess for symptoms and possible tumor recurrence, nutrition, dental health, speech and swallowing function and ultimate quality of life (QOL).

54 Tongue

Embryology Anterior 2/3: Lingual swelling (buds) from the floor of the first branchial arch and a midline structure just posterior to them called *tuberculum impar.*

Posterior 1/3: Cranial part of the *hypobranchial eminence* from 2nd, 3rd and 4th branchial arches called the cupola, just behind the foramen cecum (cecum: blind). The caudal part of the eminence becomes the epiglottis, just in front of the tracheal groove. The two parts of the tongue are separated by the sulcus terminalis. The musculature is derived from the *occipital myotomes*, and hence draws its nerve supply from the hypoglossal nerve. The sensory (general and special) supply for the anterior 2/3, is derived from the first arch nerves, lingual branch of mandibular and chorda tympani, whereas glossopharyngeal (nerve of 3rd arch) supplies both sensations to the posterior third.

Pain from the tongue is generally referred to the ear, since both lingual and auriculotemporal nerves are branches of the posterior division of the mandibular nerve.

Anomalies of tongue

Anterior end may be unfused (*bifid tongue)* seen commonly in South American races.

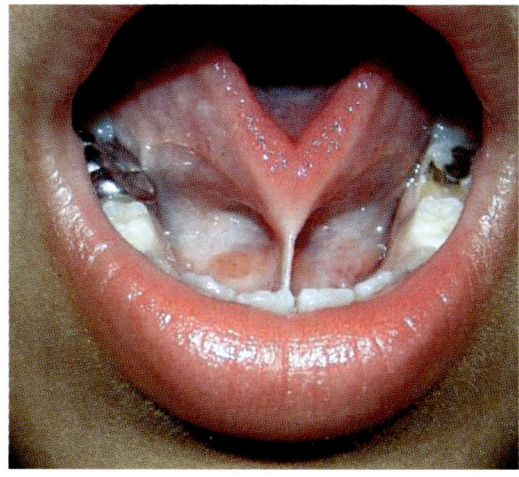

Fig. 54.1. Tongue-tie

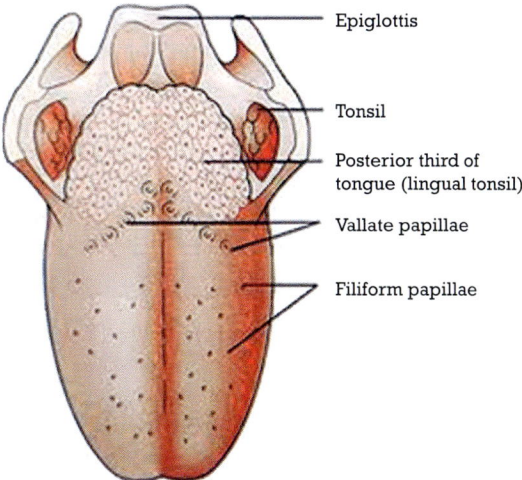

Fig. 54.2. Anatomy of tongue

Ankyloglossia: the congenital type (syn: tongue-tie) is due to a long frenulum adhering to the ventral aspect of the tongue almost to its tip, preventing full protrusion, causing problems of phonation. The acquired type is due to cancer infiltration, associated with other 'tell-tale' features.

Treatment

Frenuloplasty for the congenital type: Lysis of the ventral synechiae and release of tongue-tie, by dividing the frenulum transversly and suturing it vertically. This is done as early as possible (around 12 months age) to allow the development of normal phonation.

Superior ankyloglossia is a rare condition seen in association with cleft palate.

Lingual thyroid: (see chapter 87 on thyroid)

Macroglossia: It is a painless diffuse enlargement of the tongue; the causes are:

i) hamartomas, such as hemangioma, lymphangioma or neurofibroma
ii) cretinism (hypothyroidism in children)
iii) arteriovenous malformation (AVM)
iv) amyloidosis (rare)
v) diffuse infiltrating carcinoma (rare)

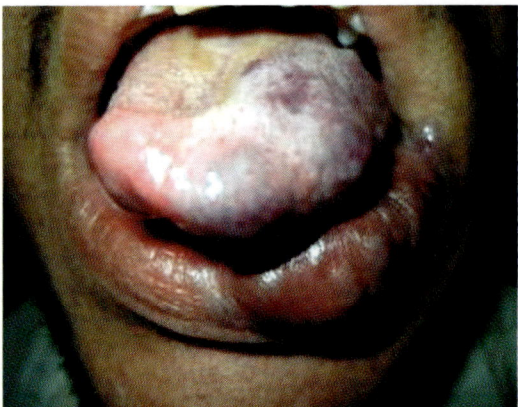

Fig. 54.3. Lymphangioma of tongue and lower lip

Hemangioma: see chapter 80

LYMPHANGIOMA: This is a hamartoma with multiple dilated lymphatic spaces, causing total or segmental macroglossia and protrusion, seen in children or rarely at birth. The tongue may be ulcerated because of repeated dental trauma, leading to infection or bleeding.

Features: soft compressible swelling of tongue, without bluish hue. Ulceration may be seen over the dorsum and margins.

Differential diagnosis

Other causes of macroglossia

Treatment is difficult; sclerotherapy, excisional surgery using cryo/laser with reconstruction if necessary, are the available options.

In *cretinism*, diffuse infiltration of the tongue muscle with myxoid and mucopolysaccharide material is responsible for its enlargement; a protruding tongue from a partially open mouth is typically seen in hypothyroid facies. Besides hormonal therapy, resection and reconstruction may also be occasionally necessary to restore the size/habitus of the tongue.

ULCERS OF TONGUE

This is a very common clinical condition; precise diagnosis sometimes taxes even an experienced clinician. Some important types are discussed here:

i)   APHTHOUS ULCER (syn: dyspeptic ulcer)

This is the commonest, presenting as a small, shallow circular ulcer with a layer of whitish slough in the floor, surrounded by a hyperemic border. Often multiple, extremely painful, located near the tip, lateral margins and under surface of tongue, *without induration of the base*. Usually with a positive family history, it starts around adolescence and typically runs an intractable waxing/waning course, healing and reappearing in different places, defying treatment. Commonly seen in smokers, alcoholics and those with immune deficiency states, these ulcers never become malignant. Diseases often associated with these ulcers are acid-peptic disease (APD), amebiasis, helminthic infestations, avitaminosis, inflammatory bowel diseases (IBD) and *Behcet`s syndrome* (a vasculitis of unknown etiology - see chapter 53)

Differential diagnosis

Other benign ulcers of tongue

Investigations: only to exclude predisposing/associated conditions mentioned

Treatment

There is no permanent solution to this nagging problem. Primary attention to any underlying disease is logical and generally effective. In idiopathic ulcers local treatment with emollient intraoral creams or carbonoxolone lozenges may offer symptomatic relief. Anabolic steroids, blood component transfusions and immunomodulators, such as levamisole (Vermisol), and arabinoxylan are found to be very useful in intractable cases, but may have to be given for several weeks.

ii)   DENTAL ULCER

As the name implies, faulty dentition, sharp tooth or ill fitting denture may be responsible for traumatic ulceration. It closely resembles an aphthous ulcer but is more elongated, occurs at the margins exposed to teeth, and never in the central area of the dorsum of the tongue, without induration of base. By their origin due to chronic irritation, they carry some malignant potential.

Differential diagnosis

Other ulcers of tongue, benign and malignant.

Investigations

i)   Dental evaluation is necessary in all cases

ii)   Edge biopsy, if not responding to conventional therapy and has borderline features of SCC.

Treatment

Proper dental care should help to prevent such ulcerations. Primary attention to the culprit tooth or denture is essential for cure. Local emollient therapy may be useful.

iii) CARCINOMATOUS ULCER

This is the commonest nonhealing ulcer in the anterior two thirds of the tongue in elderly individuals, due to SCC. The margins of the tongue are often involved. Painless initially, there is hypersalivation and local and referred pain later, with or without lymphadenopathy. Involvement of the lingual nerve may refer pain to the external ear, through the auriculo-temporal nerve, as both are branches of the posterior division of the mandibular. Being most often an SCC, it typifies such a lesion elsewhere, with raised, everted edges, slough covering the floor, indurated base fixed to the muscles of tongue and cervical lymph nodal enlargement, either due to secondary infection or to tumor spread.

Differential diagnosis, investigations and treatment: vide infra

iv) TUBERCULOUS ULCER

Young patients, with open tuberculosis (in the lungs or larynx) may develop these ulcers, which are multiple, painful, situated anteriorly with undermined edges and angry-red granulation tissue in the floor, occasionally with enlarged, matted cervical lymphnodes.

Differential diagnosis

Other benign and malignant ulcers

Investigations

Besides routine studies, ESR, chest x-ray, Mantoux, IgA, IgG, IgM and an edge biopsy if necessary.

Treatment

6-9 months of antituberculosis chemotherapy.

v)   SYPHILITIC ULCER (syn: Great pox)

Syphilis is named after a sheaperd, who suffered from the disease

Caused by a spirochete, *treponema pallidum;* ulcers can occur over the tongue in all three stages of syphilis: extragenital chancre (*primary*), snail-track ulcers (*secondary*) and gummatous ulcer (*tertiary*). Of these, the latter is most common, associated with superficial glossitis and other syphilitic stigmata.

Differential diagnosis

Other ulcers of the tongue

Serological diagnosis of syphilis

Nontreponemal tests

VDRL (Venereal Disease Research Laboratory) slide test is a nonspecific test using sheep cardiac muscle extract, cardiolipin, which is antigenically identical with Treponema pallidum.

RPR (rapid plasma regain) test

TRUST (toluidine red unheated serum test)
These are very sensitive and useful for routine screening, but may give false positive results in many other granulomatous disease, such as leprosy, sarcoidosis, collagen disorders and some viral infections due to cross reactivity.

False negatives can also occur due to prozone reaction. When there is high concentration of target antibodies, due to disproportionate AB/AG ratio, the interpretation may be 'non-reactive'. If the test is repeated after diluting the serum (1:16), it may turn positive.

Treponemal tests

TPHA: Treponema pallidum hemagglutination

FTA-ABS: (Fluorescent treponema antibody absorption) test

EIA: Enzyme immunoassay

> ### *Jewels of Gyan - 54.1*
>
> ### Common ulcers of the tongue
>
> | Painful | Painless |
> |---|---|
> | Aphthous ulcer | Carcinomatous |
> | Dental ulcer | Syphilitic ulcer |
> | Tuberculous ulcer | Systemic diseases |
> | Smoker's ulcer | Monilial ulcer |
> | Herpetic ulcer | |
> | Ictal ulcer | |

TPPA: Treponema pallidum particle agglutination

TPI: Treponema pallidum immobilization

DFM: Dark field microscopy

Western blot

These are more specific and sensitive, but may not detect endemic syphilis (yaws and pinta)

If CNS involvement is suspected, CSF study may provide better yield.

Hutchinson's triad in congenital syphilis are Moon's teeth, interstitial keratitis and perceptive progressive bilateral deafness.

Treatment

Penicillin is the sheet anchor in the treatment of syphilis, macrolides being used in resistant cases as an alternative as well as for those who are hypersensitive to penicillin.

vi) ictal and post pertussis ulcer (ictus: stroke or seizure)

These are present in epileptics and in children with whooping cough respectively and occur due to repeated jerky movements between the teeth and the tongue. The ulcers are typically located on the under surface of the tongue close to the frenum. They require only symptomatic treatment, besides attention to the underlying disorder.

vii) HERPETIC ULCER

Herpetic neuritis of the lingual nerve causes very painful, multiple, small, shallow and circular ulcers. These develop from an initial vesicular lesion and confluence of adjacent ulcers may produce an advancing and circinate edge.

Treatment

Systemic and topical acyclovir therapy along with neurotrophic vitamins and NSAIDs are very helpful in reducing the morbidity, particularly if given at an early stage.

viii) *Smoker's ulcer* (syn: nonspecific ulcer)

A nonspecific ulcer could develop on a background of chronic superficial glossitis usually on the dorsum of the anterior $2/3^{rds}$ of the tongue. A high predilection to smokers has earned its name. Abstinence from smoking and local emollient creams are all that are required for cure.

Fissures of tongue

Congenital fissures are rare, mostly disposed transversely as against those due to chronic superficial glossitis or syphilis, wherein they are longitudinal.

Median rhomboid glossitis is probably due

to candidiasis. A rhomboid or oval mass develops in the dorsal midline, just in front of the foramen cecum, with a smooth surface, bereft of papillae. It is innocuous and needs no treatment except nystatin or clotrimazole mouth washes. Its importance lies in its similarity to malignancy.

Hairy tongue is due to a fungal infection by Aspergillus niger, resulting in hypertrophy of papillae and bacterial proliferation giving rise to a black furry appearance. It is also treated by mouthwashes with fungicides and 40% urea in water.

Neoplasms of tongue

Benign tumors

a) PAPILLOMA

This is the commonest benign tumor of the tongue and may be sessile or pedunculated. It presents as a small (about 5mm) painless, warty growth in the anterior $2/3^{rd}$ of the tongue especially the tip. Ulceration due to repeated trauma may occur giving rise to bleeding and regional lymphadenopathy. Occasionally, the 'head' of the lesion may be avulsed by accidental dental injury, leaving a bleeding base, which may or may not regrow.

Clinical features
1. presence of a warty lesion on the tongue
2. ulceration (due to dental trauma)
3. bleeding
4. regional lymphadenopathy(rare)

Differential diagnosis
Other benign lesions of the tongue and SCC

Treatment
No specific investigations are necessary; if submental/submandibular lymph nodes are enlarged, a course of antibiotics to cover mixed infections, may be given for 10 days, to ascertain their benignancy, before embarking on surgery for the tongue lesion.

Surgery
Under local anesthesia the tumor is excised by an elliptical incision, including a few mm of normal tissue at the base and sent for routine histopathology, to exclude a preinvasive malignancy. Recurrence is rare following adequate excision.

b) HEMANGIOMA
This is mostly a hamartomatous malformation, usually of cavernous type arising from the venous chanels, with all the features of hemangioma elsewhere, such as bluish color, indistinct borders, irregular surface, compressibility (sign of emptying) etc. Recurrent ulceration and bleeding are frequent and troublesome problems in this location due to trauma by occluding teeth and hard ingredients of food. Some contemporary workers consider this lesion as a benign tumor, with a rare potential to turn sarcomatous.

Differential diagnosis
Other benign lesions of tongue

Treatment
I) *Sclerotherapy*, with the usual sclerosants, given into and around the lesion, at multiple sittings under short general anesthesia, at 4-6weekly intervals, is curative in the majority of cases (see under lip) or at least makes subsequent surgery easier.

ii) *Surgery*: Preferably under nasotracheal general anesthesia, the lesion is excised, realizing its 'ice-berg' nature. A posterior oral pack with a roller gauze is very useful, to prevent blood choking the airway. Use of cryo or NdYAG laser knife, to obtain a bloodless field of excision of these vascular malformations is a recent introduction, providing comfort to patient and surgeon, besides improving the results. Preliminary bilateral control of external carotid arteries is extremely useful in extensive lesions, before excision.

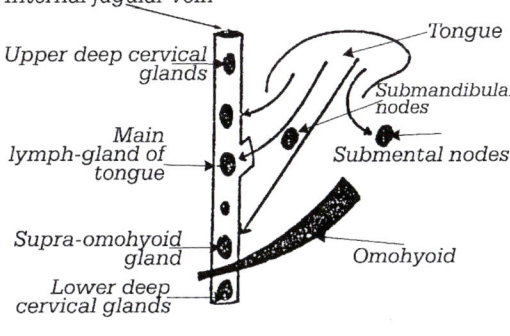

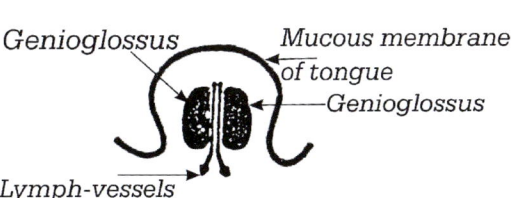

Fig. 54.4. Lymphatic drainage of tongue

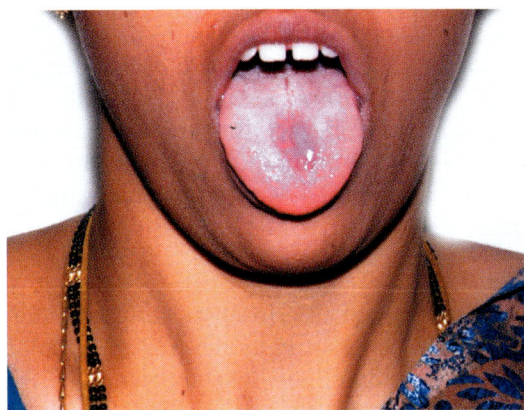

Fig. 54.5. Erythroplakia of tongue
(courtesy: Lifeline Hospitals, Chennai)

Other rare benign lesions include lymph-angioma, lipoma, neurofibroma, lingual thyroid, hematoma, ectopic salivary tumor, amyloidosis etc. An osteoma is a rare tumor, probably due to calcification of a branchial cartilage, developed around foramen cecum. These are treated essentially by surgery, on their individual merits.

CARCINOMA TONGUE

This is a disease of special importance because of its higher incidence in developing countries, essentially SCC, which accounts for nearly $1/5^{th}$ of all head and neck cancers.

Etiology

Men over 50 are usually affected, predisposing factors being the seven 'S's.
1. Smoking
2. Sharp tooth
3. Sepsis
4. Spirits (alcohol)
5. Spices
6. Syphilis (now uncommon)
7. Susceptibility, with or without any of the above.

Precancerous conditions

Erythroplacia, leukoplakia, hyperkeratosis, chronic superficial glossitis and benign tumors (papilloma). The causes of leukoplakia and dyskeratosis are the above mentioned seven 'S's.

The use of tobacco and betelnut (holding the quid for sometime in the mouth) in India, is a major factor in predisposing to oral malignancies, so also chronic superficial glossitis and leukoplakia of tongue. Other etiological factors are *Plummer-Vinson* (Kelly-Patterson) syndrome, avitaminosis-A and infections by human papillomavirus (HPV) and herpes simplex.

Pathology

Most of them are SCC from the surface epithelium; rarely adenocarcinoma from the minor salivary glands or the mucous glands of the tongue, the latter being more common in the posterior third. Other clinical curiosities include rhabdomyosarcoma and metastatic melanoma etc. Macroscopically ulcerative, fissured, exophytic (or warty) and plaque types of carcinomas are present. The prognosis of SCC tongue is worse than that of SCC of cheek or lip, putatively due to the following reasons:

1) biologically more aggressive tumor
2) crossed bilateral lymphatic drainage
3) constant movements of the tongue facilitating earlier lymphatic/hematogenous spread

Ulcer type is the commonest (vide supra), located at the margins, with all the features of SCC. The induration that is palpable beyond the visible lesion, gives the clinician the true size of the tumor.

Fissure type occurs typically in the chronic superficial glossitis of syphilis where progressive dysplasia and fissuring occur. The tumor cells invade deep into the muscular substance of the tongue, producing induration, which is never seen in benign fissures. The diagnosis is often delayed, till much of the tongue is involved or nodal spread occurs.

Exophytic or warty type: Like the SCC of penis, an exophytic, cauliflower like protrusion can sometimes occur especially when malignancy supervenes in a papilloma or in a patch of leukoplakia.

Plaque type: Rarely a submucous plaque with diffuse infiltration may be seen, progressively enlarging the tongue (vide macroglossia).

Microscopy of this lesion shows an SCC, i.e., cell nest formation depending upon the degree of differentiation. In general, they are less well differentiated than in the lip, accounting for the worse prognosis. In the posterior third, as the superficial layer stratification and cornification is much less, there is more of a glandular and lymphocytic infiltration of the tumor, earning names such as transitional cell epithelioma, lymphoepithelioma etc.

Spread of tumor

i) *Contiguous* spread

Invasion of the mandible could occur from

tumors of the margin and invasion of the floor of the mouth from under surface cancers. The median septum of the tongue is usually respected for quite some time and invasion across the midline rarely occurs. Malignant involvement of the floor of the mouth or the mandible usually results in immobility of the tongue (malignant ankyloglossia). Posterior tumor spreads to the oropharynx, tonsils and epiglottis.

ii) *Lymphatic* spread

As these tumors are usually poorly differentiated and aggressive, early lymphatic spread is the rule, more by embolization than by permeation. This is also facilitated by constant movement of the tongue. Though some anatomical preferences in terms of lymphatic drainage, are known, variations and exceptions are too many to be dogmatic. Generally, the tip drains into the submental and upper deep cervical or jugulodigastric group, anterior 2/3 into the submandibular and mid deep cervical group and posterior 1/3rd into the retromandibular and lower deep cervical (juguloomohyoid) group of nodes on the same side. Paramedian tissue however has bilateral drainage, due to crossover of channels.

iii) *Hematogenous* spread is rare and occurs more often in poorly differentiated tumors from the posterior third.

Symptoms
(see also under ulcers of tongue)
i) A painless nonhealing ulcer or a lump over the tongue is the commonest symptom.
ii) Excessive salivation due to local irritation and discomfort while swallowing
iii) Halitosis due to ulceration and secondary infection
iv) Pain in the later stages, locally and referred to the ear, through lingual-auriculotemporal pathway.
v) Dysphagia (or odynophagia) may be present in posterior tumors.
vi) Ankyloglossia or restricted mobility of the tongue, due to tumor infiltration into floor of mouth or mandible.
vii) Hoarseness of the voice if laryngo-pharynx is involved.
viii) Lump in the neck, due to enlarged cervical lymphnodes.

Signs
Majority occur in the anterior 2/3 of the dorsum, about 20% occur in the posterior third and 10% on the margins, tip and ventral aspect. Depending upon the type of carcinoma

(1) an irregular ulcer with an everted edge,

(2) a warty papilloma-like lesion, with an indurated base,

(3) a hard lump within the tongue with an indistinct edge and an irregular surface

(4) a deep linear fissure with basal induration, may be seen. Adjacent structures like the floor of the mouth, gums and tonsils may be involved. Lymphnodes, i.e., submental, submandibular and deep cervical (upper, middle and lower) groups may be involved.

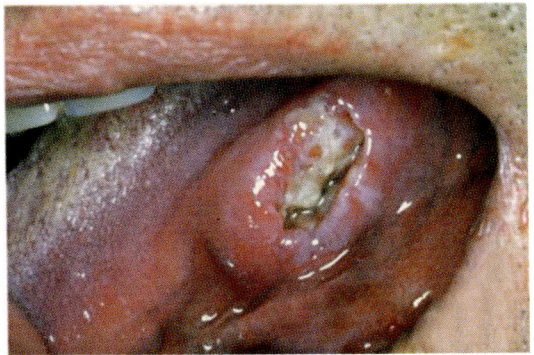

Fig. 54.6. Early carcinoma tongue

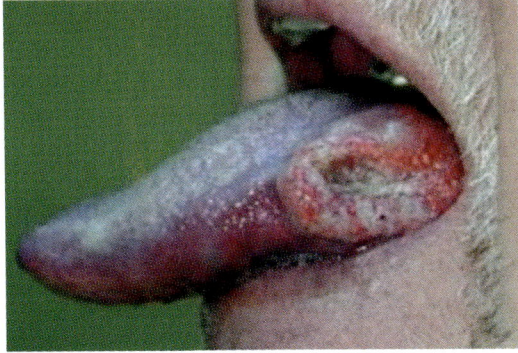

Fig. 54.7. Carcinoma tongue

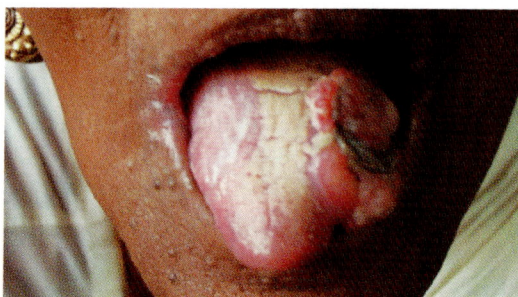

Fig. 54.7. Advanced carcinoma tongue

Investigations

There is room for error in clinical diagnosis, hence it should be established by an edge/punch biopsy of the lesion. For doubtful lesions of the tongue, *toluidine blue* (a supravital dye that stains carcinoma-in-situ lesions) staining is an adjunct to early detection. In the presence of enlarged lymphnodes, a trial course of antibiotics is given while awaiting the histopathology report and any further doubts about their status must be settled by an FNAC. Besides the routine investigations, an x-ray of chest and the jaw should be done, to identify the extent of tumor. A fibreoptic endoscopy of oro/laryngopharynx may be needed for posterior tumors.

Staging: TNMG (tumor, nodes, metastases and histological grade) staging is popularly used by oncologists (see under SCC). MRI is currently the most popular study for proper locoregional staging.

Treatment

The two modalities of curative treatment either radical surgery or radiotherapy (for early lesions) or in combination (for advanced tumors). Chemoradiotherapy is used before (neoadjuvant) or after excisional surgery (adjuvant) and for nonresectable or recurrent tumors (palliative).

Surgery

Indications: Considerations such as operative risk, postoperative disfigurement, loss of function, grade of tumor differentiation, availability of infrastructure and expertise will influence the choice. For T-1 lesions (<2cm), a wide surgical excision with a three-dimensional clearance of 1 cm is adequate. T-2 lesions (<5cm) can be managed equally well by partial glossectomy or irradiation. In larger tumors, when surgery is required, a composite resection involving

(1) the primary tumor, amounting to hemi or subtotal glossectomy,

(2) the affected nodes by standard block dissection and

(3) resection of the mandible (Commando operation) was once very popular. However now the mandibular resection is currently advocated only when the growth infiltrates the floor of the mouth and reaches close to the jaw (hemimandibulectomy or segmental resection). Current awareness that the mandible is involved directly and not through the lymphatics, except in elderly edentulous people, makes mandibular resection unnecessary, even if there is a 5mm gap from the gross tumor to the bone.

Following jaw resections, some form of internal stabilization, with a rib graft or Kirschner wire may be necessary, to avoid collapse and disfigurement. It should be realized that removal of the anterior (central) segment of the mandible is associated with loss of support of the tongue with the risk of its falling back and obstructing the air passage in the immediate postoperative period. In patients with cancer of the anterior part of the tongue with involvement of the floor of the mouth, a pull through procedure (by delivering the tongue between the mylohyoids) can be done if the mandible is free. For posterior third cancers, an excellent access is obtained by dividing the mandible in the midline and 'bivalving' the tongue.

Reconstruction

Small lesions can be treated adequately by wide surgical excision and repair. For larger lesions the defect is reconstituted by using a forehead flap based on the superficial temporal artery and brought into the mouth under the zygomatic arch. Such procedures are rarely required in view of the remarkable power of regeneration of the tongue, which leaves no trace of resection, if examined a few months after subtotal glossectomy!

Radiotherapy

SCC is a radiosensitive tumor and T1 or T2 lesions can be cured by brachytherapy, by implanting radium needles, iridium or tantulum wires into the tumor. For lesions with >1cm depth, teletherapy is the treatment of choice. A high incidence of osteoradionecrosis is observed whenever a diseased jaw (either by tumor invasion or secondary to dental sepsis) is irradiated; hence radiotherapy as the only form of curative treatment is not given if tumor involves the jaw, but it may be given before a planned resection of the jaw or to palliate advanced cancers. Extraction of all the teeth is routinely done before radiotherapy, for two reasons: to eliminate septic foci in their roots, and secondly they are going to fall off anyway following RT, by its effect on mesodermal elements such as odontoblasts and cementum.

Although cobalt-60 (^{60}Co) could also be used for radiotherapy, the linear accelerator has many advantages including a shorter treatment time, deep and homogenous tissue penetration, creation of a sharper field margin and sparing of the surrounding normal tissue from radiation injury. For large tumors with nodal involvement, combination therapy is used with preoperative irradiation of the tumor and node bearing area, followed by radical excision. Intensity modulated RT (IMRT) is another recent addition to the field of RT.

Treatment of secondary lymph nodes (see also under lymph nodes)

i) if not clinically enlarged (N-0), regular follow up is all that is required.

ii) if enlarged nodes are obviously involved by tumor (confirmed by FNAC), the treatment of choice is block dissection at the time of excision of primary tumor, with or without resection of the mandible (see Commando operation)

iii) if the nodes are fixed and nonresectable, palliative chemo/radiotherapy is the only option. As part of the mandible can be resected without much of functional or cosmetic defects, a curative procedure may still be possible even if the tumor is fixed to the jaw.

Controversies in the management of nodal secondaries

I) Clinically negative neck nodes (N-0). Some workers strongly advocate the performance of an elective neck dissection in all cases based on the observation that upto 30% of patients without palpable nodes in the neck have positive nodes on histopathological examination. The current consensus, however recommends an elective neck dissection when the primary tumor is large (T-3 and above) and of high grade. In all other situations a careful wait and watch is recommended, reserving block dissection for clinically enlarged nodes.

ii) Radical (Crile) vs functional (Bocca) neck dissection: Postoperative morbidity after radical neck dissection is due to the removal of structures like the spinal accessory nerve, internal jugular vein and SCM. In fact, all tumor-bearing nodes can be radically cleared without sacrificing these structures and the presence of SCM muscle is a safeguard against secondary hemorrhage from the carotids. However most workers feel that except for papillary carcinoma of thyroid or prophylactic nodal dissection in clinically N-0 disease, standard radical dissection is preferable to the functional modification.

iii) Supra-omohyoid neck dissection: In this operation, the submental, submandibular and upper deep cervical lymph nodes are cleared only upto the level where the central tendon of the omohyoid intersects the internal jugular vein. This operation is justified only in cases with well differentiated and small (<T-2) tumors with minimal lymph node enlargement. However, the observation that middle and lower deep cervical nodes are sometimes involved skipping the upper groups is a strong argument against this limited node excision, and it is best given up.

Technique of radical neck dissection: see under

lymph nodes (chapter 42)

Bilateral nodal secondaries

These have a poor prognosis. Bilateral neck dissection sparing one internal jugular vein (on the less involved side) may be done either simultaneously or in two sittings.

Chemotherapy

Generally the rate of response and duration of effectiveness are depressingly low. Methotrexate, Cis-platin, Bleomycin, 5-FU have all been tried with varying success. High dose methotrexate with leucovorin (citrovorum factor) rescue has shown a marginal benefit, as has Cis-platin (response rate 25%). Bleomycin is an effective drug against the SCC but carries a high incidence of pulmonary fibrosis. Chemotherapy is also given prior to surgery (induction or neo-adjuvant therapy) with the aim of reducing the tumor load, rendering it resectable and possibly preventing growth of viable tumor cells spilt during surgery.

Recurrent carcinoma

Post-RT recurrence: The ideal option for cancer recurring after radiotherapy is wide field resection, monobloc lymph node excision and reconstruction, often using a myocutaneous flap swung from an unirradiated area onto the resultant defect.

Post-surgical recurrence: For the majority of these patients, radiation therapy is the treatment of choice, if not given earlier. More aggressive local resections have been attempted with a hope of eradicating the disease, but additional morbidity outweighs possible advantages in the long run.

Prognostic factors in oral/lingual carcinoma

As in any cancer, the following factors influence the ultimate outcome:

A) Tumor size

For T-1 tumors, the cure rate is 90%, falling to 10% in T-3.

B) Nodes

The single most important factor is lymphatic metastasis. Even one histologically positive lymph node reduces the prognosis by 45% and multiple nodes, size >3cms, mid, lower deep cervical or contralateral nodal disease and capsular invasion are all indicate grave prognosis. Histologically 'stimulated' nodes (showing sinus histiocytosis) carry a better prognosis than the lymphocyte depleted type.

C) Histological criteria

Jacobson's combination is one of *structural factors* i.e. nuclear pleomorphism, nucleolar number etc., and *tumor-host relationship factors* i.e. mode of invasion, stage of invasion, cellular response and vascular invasion.

D) Immunological factors

Positive DNCB (dinitro-chlorobenzene) test or a high serum glycoprotein indicate good immunity. Low absolute lymphocyte count, low T-lymphocyte count, increased IgA and decreased IgE, have been shown to confer a poor prognosis.

Neoplasms of the lip may be benign or malignant.

Benign neoplasms

The common benign tumors of the lip are:

i) papilloma
ii) hemangioma
iii) nevus
iv) ectopic salivary tumor

Other soft tissue tumors like a lipoma or neurofibroma also may occur.

a) Papilloma

It is described in greater detail in chapter 11. A warty lesion, 0.5-1 cm size, seen on the outer aspect of the lip (early presentation). Mostly pedunculated, the common symptoms are bleeding and ulceration, due to dental trauma. Occasionally the head of the wart is caught between the occluding teeth and may be avulsed and fall off, but if the base is intact, it may regrow.

Differential diagnosis

mucous retention cyst, ectopic salivary tumor, hamartoma or carcinoma.

Treatment

Excision or coagulation (diathermy or laser), may be performed.

b) Hemangioma is a very common lesion of the lips; presentation and management is as for such lesions elsewhere (see chapter 80)

c) Nevi: Nevi of the lip are parallel in appearance and treatment to nevi elsewhere. Thus junctional, compound and intradermal nevi are present, with similar biological behavior as observed elsewhere (vide supra), including premalignant nature of the junctional type, capable of turning into a melanoma in response to chronic irritation. Bleeding, itching, ulceration, regional lymphadenopathy or rapid growth in a lip nevus, especially one without hair, are the ominous signs.

d) Ectopic salivary tumor is a common solid swelling occurring around oral cavity and the vestibule. Tiny salivary glands line the border of the lips and may be the seat of a pleomorphic tumor. Recognition of these is vital since they show a higher potential for malignancy here than in the major salivary glands. Excision biopsy should be done as a preliminary step, but if a carcinomatous change is detected, wider excision, with at least 5mm. margin, should be done followed by appropriate lip reconstruction as per the principles of cosmetic surgery.

MALIGNANT NEOPLASMS

They are SCC, BCC and melanoma in order of frequency.

Etiology

The predisposing factors are smoking, tobacco quid kept in the vestibule, syphilis, spices and irradiation. Exposure to sunlight, especially in light-skinned people may be contributory, as seen by the higher incidence of lip cancers in farmers and outdoor labourers exposed to actinic radiation. Lower lip is most often affected.

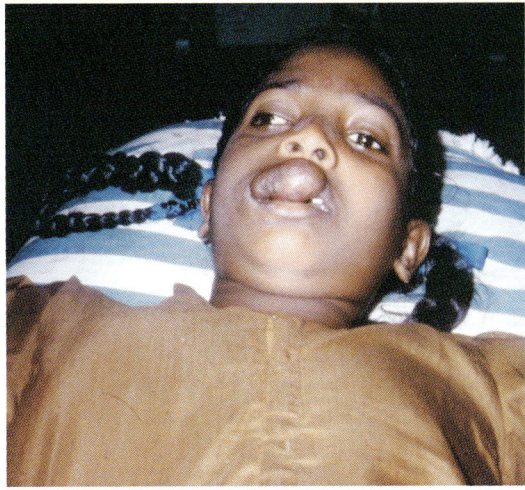

Fig. 55.1. Cavernous hemangioma upper lip (courtesy: Halsted Surgical Clinic, Chennai)

Pathology

A nonhealing ulcer, a fissure or an ulcerated nodule are the types of presentation of SCC, which is the commonest tumor of the lip, usually beginning at the mucocutaneous junction, and exhibiting all the features of SCC elsewhere.

Spread: Contiguous spread to the neighbouring areas of the cheek and face can occur. The mandible may also be involved both by direct or by retrograde lymphatic spread. Lymphatic spread to submental and sub-man-dibular nodes, followed by the upper deep cervical nodes is seen early in the course. From the upper lip the spread may occur to the preauricular and submandi-bular nodes, whereas from the angle of the mouth, it may reach any group of nodes described above. Lower lip lesions spread to submental/submandibular lymph nodes on either side, due to crossed drainage. Enlarged lymph nodes not responding to a course of antibiotics, may not be 'inflammatory' and warrant further investigations. Contact spread from one

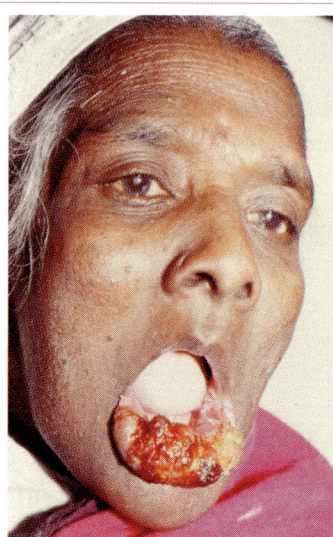

Fig. 55.3. Advanced carcinoma lower lip
(courtesy: Prof T Gunasagaran, Chennai)

lip to the other may occur, the so called 'kiss cancer'.

Mandible involvement: Contiguous spread and via the lymphatics along the mental nerve.

Hematogenous spread occurs to the lungs, liver and bone, but rare and late, seen in poorly differentiated tumors.

Clinical features

1. Non healing ulcer.
2. Ulcerated nodule.
3. Foul smelling discharge and bleeding.
4. Swellings under the chin and upper neck (lymph nodes).

Physical findings

Location: mostly lower lip, a contact lesion may be seen in the upper

Size: depends upon the duration of lesion, usually 2-4cm.

Edge: everted, raised and friable.

Floor: large amount of slough and necrotic tissue present, bleeds to touch.

Base: indurated, may involve all layers of lip, skin, muscle and mucosa

Discharge: watery, foul smelling.

Mobility: mobile in early cases; may be fixed to the gum (mucoperiosteum) or bone later.

If the tumor is infiltrating the jaw, bony erosion/thickening may be noticed

All the lymph nodes mentioned should be carefully examined for enlargement, but they may be due to either metastasis or secondary infection. Size (>2cm), consistency (firm/hard), fixity to surrounding tissue or adjacent node, absence of features of inflammation (pain, warmth, tenderness etc) would help to identify nodal secondaries.

In carcinoma of lower lip or jaw, loss of central part of mandible results in pouting of lower lip

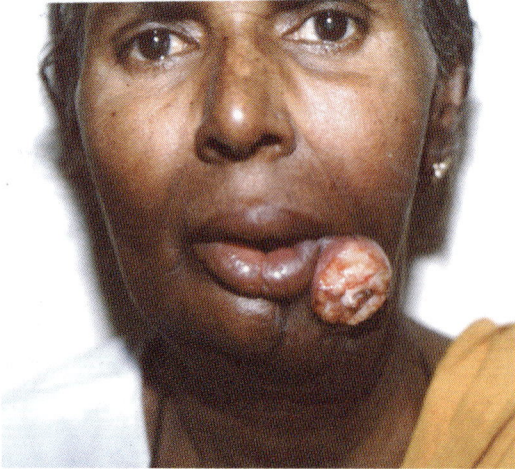

Fig. 55.2. Carcinoma lower lip
(courtesy: Dr K Sreekanth, Chennai)

and drooling of saliva, known as Andy Gump deformity.

Differential diagnosis

1. Hunterian chancre.
2. Pyogenic granuloma.
3. Kerato-acanthoma.

Treatment

1. *Surgery*: Local resection with a margin of 5mm followed by reconstruction is all that is required for lesions less than 2cms. For larger lesions, wider excision with appropriate reconstruction, involving free or rotation flap, may be needed.

If palpable regional nodes persist after a course of antibiotics, they should be biopsied or excised; many prefer the latter, at the time of surgery for primary lesion. Supra-omohyoid dissection may be sufficient for early well differentiated lesions with <4 nodes, whereas standard radical neck dissection will be necessary for larger tumor or with >4 nodes, especially if deep cervical nodes are involved. It should be noted that the supra-omohyoid dissection is unacceptable for the carcinoma of the tongue, which is more malignant; this procedure has some place in early tumors of lip and cheek.

2. Radiotherapy (RT): As in other locations, for epithelioma (SCC), radiotherapy is equally effective and less mutilating, without the morbidity of anesthesia. This is favoured by many as the first line therapy, 4-5000 rads given over 4-5 weeks. For small lesions, cure rate is similar to surgery, however for lymph nodal disease, surgery is preferred if they are mobile, as they are less radiosensitive than the primary tumor. As in SCC elsewhere, RT is also employed for palliation or to down-stage the disease preoperatively (neoadjuvant therapy).

3. Chemotherapy: Bleomycin, cis-platinum, methotrexate, 5-FU have been used in various combinations, as adjuvant or neo-adjuvant therapy and for palliation in disseminated cases(rare).

Other lesions of the lip

a. *Pyogenic granuloma*: This is a sessile polypoid growth of granulation tissue secondary to trauma and pyogenic infection *(see chapter 14)*

b. *Leucoplakia*: Elevated white papular lesion on the lip(also seen on tongue, palate, cheek etc). The diagnostic point is that these patches cannot be removed by direct pressure, in contrast to oral moniliasis(thrush). If predisposing factors like tobacco/betel abuse, sharp/septic tooth are present they should be addressed, including good oral/ dental hygiene. A reassuring edge biopsy may be done, to exclude preinvasive malignancy. Immune stimulants, such as levamisole (Vermisol), tinocordin (Immu Mod) have been found to be useful in the long run. Excisional surgery is rarely needed for this condition, but close follow up is mandatory, because of its premalignant potential.

c. *Kerato-acanthoma*: Although this resembles a carcinoma it is a benign superficial cutaneous tumor arising from the follicle-bearing area of the lip. It is much commoner in elderly Caucasians, probably as a sequel to chronic actinic exposure.

It presents as a small hemispherical lesion with a well marked edge; the central portion of the dome eventually breaks down, extruding the core of keratinic tissue, leading to healing of the ulcer gradually. This is important because

1) it mimics a tumor and

2) the resultant scarring may produce deformity of the lip.

Treatment

Limited excision by a 'V' cut and primary closure, submitting the tissue for histopathological examination to confirm the diagnosis.

d. *Mucous cysts* are retention cysts of the minor salivary glands (described under Cheek)

e. *Primary (Hunterian) chancre and mucocutaneous snail-track ulcers* of secondary syphylis (described under Tongue)

f. *Herpes simplex* infection (herpes labialis) may ioccur,usually in children following some febrile illness, leaving tiny shallow ulcers after the visicles over the lips rupture, with tendency for spontaneous healing. Oral and topical acyclovir help faster resolution.

g. *Macrochelia* is swelling of the entire lip seen in a hemangioma, lymphangioma, neuro-fibroma and rarely a recurrent type may be due to Melkersson-Rosenthal syndrome, sometimes preceded by Bell's palsy. A granulomatous involvement of the lips may be occasionally seen in association with Crohn's disease.

h. *Pigmentation of lips* and buccal mucosa is seen in smokers, Addison's disease and Peutz-Jeghers syndrome. The latter syndrome, inherited as autosomal dominant trait, is associated with adenomatous polyposis of small bowel, with a predilection for intussusception and rarely malignant transformation.

Buccal mucosa spreads between the two alveolar ridges, the angle of the mouth anteriorly and the retromolar region posteriorly, upto the anterior pillar of fauces. Subjacent structures include the buccal pad of fat, buccinator muscle and the Stenson's duct opening into the cavity. Although discussed separately, carcinoma of the cheek, tongue and the rest of the oral cavity have several features in common, such as the same type of premalignant lesions, geographical incidence (very high in Indians), and similar histological features, with surgery and radiotherapy being the two main options.

Benign lesions of the cheek

1) Hamartomas, such as hemangioma, lymphangioma or neurofibroma

2) Ectopic salivary tumors: present as firm/hard nodules, usually under 10mm size, mobile and discrete. They may be located anywhere in the vicinity of oral mucosa (from mandible to zygoma), including the palate. Mostly they are pleomorphic adenomas, with a high tendency to turn malignant.

3) Mucous retention cysts or lymph cysts

4) Precancerous lesions, such as leukoplakia, erythroplakia, submucous fibrosis (vide infra)

5) Aphthous ulcers (earlier called dyspeptic ulcer)

6) Sebaceous cyst, lipoma, papilloma etc

CARCINOMA CHEEK

About 5% of all oral cancers arise from the buccal mucosa and despite several advances made in the understanding of oncogenesis, early diagnosis and treatment modalities, the overall cure rates of oral and oro-pharyngeal malignancies *have not improved considerably*, over the last decades, probably because of two reasons:

1. The phenomenon of 'multiple primary tumors'. The entire aerodigestive tract becomes vulnerable to malignancies and a patient who survives his intitial malignancy may still develop another SCC in the ENT regions, esophagus and bronchi.

2. It was once believed that blood borne metastasis rarely occurs in SCC, but it is now realized that a good number of these patients develop hematogenous secondaries.

Etiology

1) Male predominance (3:1), except in the verrucous type, which is seen more in women

2) Tobacco/betel/pan chewing especially the quid being retained in the cheek. Nicotine and nornicotine are precursors of carcinogenic nitrosamines. Tobacco also contains nitrates which are converted to nitrites by the enzyme, nitrate reductase, present in the normal bacterial flora of the mouth. When tobacco is held in the mouth for a long time, there is sufficient time for these chemical steps, to form nitrosamines.

3) Alcohol consumption potentiates the effect of tobacco, in inducing malignancy.

4) Repeated dental trauma, during occlusion.

5) 'Chutta' cancer (see chapter 19).

6) Human papilloma-virus (HPV) is associated with verrucous carcinoma.

7) Precancerous lesions, such as

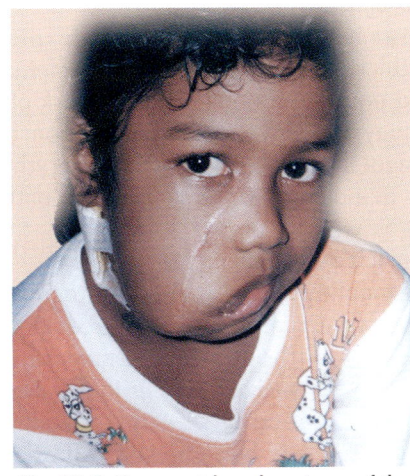

Fig. 56.1. Recurrent lymphangioma of the cheek
note the scar of previous surgery
(courtesy: Lifeline Hospitals, Chennai)

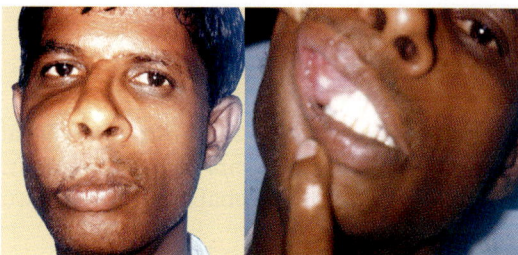

Fig. 56.2 & 56.3. Carcinoma right cheek
(courtesy: Halsted Surgical Clinic, Chennai)

a) leukoplakia
b) erythroplakia
c) oral submucous fibrosis
d) hyperplastic candidiasis

Other conditions, associated with higher incidence of oral cancer but the causal relationship has not yet been fully established, are:

1) Oral lichen planus.

2) Plummer-Vinson (Kelly-Patterson) syndrome or sideropenic dysphagia.

3) Discoid lupus erythematosis

4) Syphilitic glossitis.

5) Dyskeratosis congenita.

a) Leukoplakia

This is defined by the WHO, as *any white patch or plaque that cannot be characterised clinically or pathologically as any other specific disease*. It has manifestations ranging from a small circumscribed white plaque to diffuse thickened white patches. From its name, it need not be understood that it is always white; it may also be yellowish or grey. It ranges from the totally innocuous type of homogenous lesion to a dangerous speckled leukoplakia presenting as a thick irregular infiltrating/ulcerating lesion. It is differentiated from oral candidiasis by the inability to rub off the lesion. Histologically, varying degrees of hyperkeratosis are seen with or without dysplasia, which may progress to a preinvasive (carcinoma-in-situ) or invasive cancer. Leukoplakia of a homogenous pattern may be observed by regular follow-up; suspicious areas could be subjected to *toluidine blue* staining and subsequently biopsied. If the leukoplakia is of the speckled or ulcerating type, it is best treated by local excision by a CO_2 laser or by cyrotherapy. *Although the overall incidence of malignancy in leukoplakia was once thought to be as high as 30%, it is now realized that the average risk is much less (<10%).*

Management

1. Detailed clinical examination of the rest of the aero-digestive tract.

2. Tobacco/betel or alcohol consumption should be stopped immediately, which by itself may make the mucosal abnormality resolve in up to 50% of the cases, but it might take several months.

3. Excision of the lesions manifesting with dysplasia or carcinoma-in-situ is the treatment of choice. For larger areas, if the mucosa can not be closed, following excision, it may be allowed to heal by secondary intention.

b) Erythroplakia

In recent years it has been demonstrated that erythroplakia has a much higher incidence of malignant potential than leukoplakia. By definition it is *any bright red velvety plaque in the oral cavity which cannot be characterised clinically or pathologically as any other recognizable condition.*

Histological presentation: Red shiny velvety plaques sometimes manifesting a nodular surface. The risk of malignancy is much higher in this condition than in leukoplakia; hence all patches of erythroplakia should be excised and sent for histopathology.

c) Oral submucous fibrosis (SMF)

This is a progressive disease, endemic in Asia, in which areas of fibrosis occur just beneath the buccal mucosa. Contraction of the fibrous bands occur in the next stage limiting opening of the mouth and tongue movements. This seems to be present in the patients who chew betel and areca nut. Hypersensitivity to spices and tobacco has also been hypothesised as a cause of SMF. One of the most accepted theories postulates

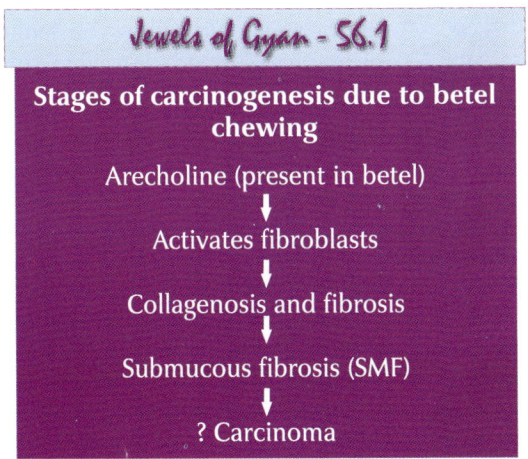

Jewels of Gyan - 56.1

Stages of carcinogenesis due to betel chewing

Arecholine (present in betel)
↓
Activates fibroblasts
↓
Collagenosis and fibrosis
↓
Submucous fibrosis (SMF)
↓
? Carcinoma

hypersynthesis of fibroblasts and collagenosis due to an alkaloid present in the betel nut , arecoline.

Histology

Severe fibrosis under the epithelial layer with progressive atrophy of the epithelium is seen, which seems to predispose to malignant change. The multiple fibrotic bands that prevent movement of mouth can be treated by intra lesional steroids or by excision and grafting. Although this helps in the trismus and ankyloglossia, treating the fibrotic bands does not seem to decrease the incidence of squamous cell carcinoma.

d) Hyperplastic candidiasis

This is often found at the angle of the mouth and the parts of the cheek just beneath the labial corner. Multiple dense white plaques which are larger and thicker than the leukoplakic patches are seen in this condition. They can be partially rubbed off, differentiating this condition from leukoplakia. It is now believed that an invasive candidal infection might cause leukoplakia and some decrease in the local mucosal immunity, predisposing to local malignancy, favoring long term treatment with antifungal therapy. Of course doubtful lesions should be biopsied, so as not to miss a preinvasive cancer.

e) Other potentially premalignant lesions are syphilis and oral/cutaneous lichen planus.

Plummer-Vinson syndrome predisposes to postcricoid carcinoma; however there seems to be a slightly higher incidence of oral carcinoma as well.

f) Discoid lupus erythematosis causes papular white well demarcated patches in the mouth and cheek. There is a small but definite incidence of carcinoma in this lesion. The syndrome of *dyskeratosis congenita* is one of oral and cutaneous atrophy, sometimes associated with oral malignancy.

Clinical features

Leukoplakia precedes carcinoma in the cheek more frequently than in any other part of the oral cavity. Depending on the macroscopic type, an ulcer, a fissure or a proliferating growth may be seen. A foul smelling discharge is sometimes present. Many patients present late either because of the lack of pain (pain occurs if the lesion invades afferent nerve fibres or secondary infection supervenes) or the lesion is mistaken for denture-related ulceration. Nodal spread occurs much later compared to tongue and lip carcinoma, submental, submandibular and retro-mandibular groups being the primary drainage areas.

Pathology

It is usually a well differentiated SCC, falling into three types, in order of worsening prognosis, namely; *papilliferous* (or proliferating or verrucous type), *fissure* type and the *ulcerative* type. Buccal mucosa is the commonest site for the verrucous type of low grade SCC, virtually without metastatic potential. Secondary infection is common in carcinoma of the cheek because the lesion is vulnerable to trauma by the occluding teeth. Posterior extension involves the palatoglossal arch and the soft palate. Spread through the layers of the cheek involves the overlying skin and may lead to formation of an orocutaneous fistula or involvement of the adjacent gum, though actual infiltration into the jaw is a rare and late event.

Investigations

The diagnosis of this disease is primarily clinical but it should be confirmed by an edge biopsy under local anesthesia, including the most suspicious area as well as the adjacent normal mucosa. FNAC may be applicable to a suspicious lymph node rema-ining after a trial course of antibiotics. Plain skiagraphy is of limited value and may detect involvement of the alveolus, but an orthopanto-mogram (OPG) is more informative. CT and MRI are useful in cancers of the cheek with retromolar extension to identify possible extension to the base of the skull or tonsillar fossa.

Treatment

As these are radiosensitive tumors, the choice between surgery and RT is quite debatable. Small lesions confined to the buccal mucosa are best treated with a wide excision including the underlying bucci-nator muscle. Reconstruction is performed with a quilted split skin graft or the raw area is just allowed to epithelialize.

If the lesion extends posteriorly to the retro-molar area or the palatoglossal area, wide excision is done followed by reconstruction with a free radial forearm flap, which permits adequate mandibular reconstruction, if needed. Another viable alternative is to use the forehead flap of McGregor which is based on the superficial temporal artery. It is a reliable flap but the main problem is the cosmesis. The principle is to free the forehead skin, tunneling under the zygomatic arch to line the inner aspect of the cheek. Split skin graft is used to cover the donor site of the forehead. Alternately, Narayanan's folded skin flap from the temple may be employed.

If the lower alveolus has been involved, mandibular resection and restoration of continuity of

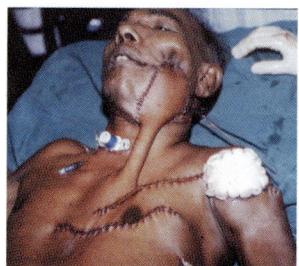

Fig. 56.4. Deltopectoral flap to close the cheek defect

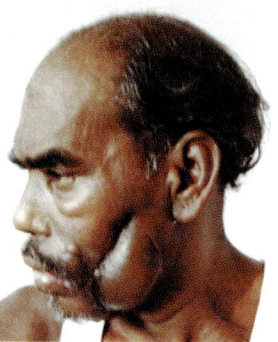

Fig. 56.5. Final result after disconnection (courtesy: Dr K Sreekanth, Hyderabad)

the bone should follow the same principles outlined for tongue carcinoma, using either rib or radius or iliac crest grafts.

Primary versus delayed reconstruction

In patients with less than ideal nutritional status, the resection of tumor is initially done, allowing the general health to improve and subsequently plan for reconstruction of the orocutaneous fistula. However the physical and esthetic considerations of such ghastly facial defects have prompted primary reconstruction, provided adequate 'cancer clearance' is achieved. The fact that many patients with a large orocutaneous fistula never improve enough to permit second stage surgery, is another strong factor in favor of primary repair. If cure cannot be achieved, it offers the best palliation, by improving the quality of life.

Nodal secondaries

The management of the neck secondaries of carcinoma of the cheek is identical to that of carcinoma of the tongue, with one exception i.e. neck dissection need not always be undertaken in T2:N0:M0 tumors. The lymphatic metastasis is much slower in these tumors as compared to the tongue or lips. The rest of the management is identical to SCC elsewhere.

Salient points in the management of oral cancers are:

1. Involvement of the retromolar areas and skull base was once thought to indicate inoperability; however skull base surgery using facial osteotomy techniques have now rendered them resectable.

2. Reconstruction of the defects with either muscle flaps like latissimus dorsi, pectoralis major, radial forearm flap or transfer of free

tissue based on microvascular technique, produce excellent cosmetic and functional results.

3. The morbidity of radiotherapy has been considerably reduced by improved techniques of delivery.

4. Osteo-radionecrosis is quite uncommon; however routine dental extraction before RT is still practiced.

5. Implantations of Iridium for T1/2 tumors help by delivering high dose radiation with excellent local control.

6. Hyperfractionation radiotherapy is another recent advance, wherein smaller fractions of radiation are given over a longer period, with a higher dose delivered to the tumor but minimal damage to adjacent normal tissue.

7. Chemotherapy has not been shown to improve survival; platinum-based regimes seem to be helpful in fungating or painful tumors, but more often it is used as neo-adjuvant therapy, to down-stage the disease.

	Feature	Surgery	Radiation
1.	Preferred in	Well dif. tumors	Poorly dif. tumors
2.	Aim	Curative	Curative or palliative neoadjuvant or adjuvant
3.	For lymph nodal disease	Preferred	Not as radiosensitive as primary lesion
4.	Mutilation	Present	Absent
5.	If jaw is involved	Preferred	RT as the only form of curative therapy should not be given, but may be given for palliation or as neoadjuvant treatment
6.	Risk of anesthesia	Present	Absent

Table-56.1. Comparison between surgery and RT for cancer cheek

57 Cleft lip

Embryology: The face, lips and palate develop between the 6th and 7th weeks of intrauterine life. The failure of mesodermal penetration into the epithelially bilayered face of the embryo is the currently accepted theory, for the development of cleft lip and palate. Five processes fuse around the stomodeum (primitive mouth):

a. one frontonasal process - central

b. two maxillary processes - lateral

c. Two mandibular processes - lateral

The central part of the upper lip is formed from the medial nasal process (derived from the frontonasal process) and the lateral aspect (rest of the upper lip) is formed from the maxillary process. Thus, cleft lip is almost always paramedian, due to defective fusion of the medial nasal process with the maxillary process. True central 'hare lip', normally seen in rabbits, is extremely rare in humans.

Etiology

1. Trimethoprim or other teratogenic drugs used in the first trimester of pregnancy

2. Increased maternal age

3. Smoking

4. Viral infections (e.g. rubella), during pregnancy

5. Parents with cleft lip

6. Hypervitaminosis-A in pregnancy

7. Steroids intake

8. Diabetic mothers

9. Consanguineous marriages

10. Hypoxic insult to the fetus like threatened abortion

11. Maternal radiation during first trimester

12. Exposure to solar eclipse in first trimester (it is also called 'grahana soola'; grahana: eclipse; soola: stroke)

13. More common on the left (see under cleft palate)

Anatomic classification

Central (very rare): due to failure of fusion of the bulbous extremities of the median nasal process and globular processes.

Lateral: Defective fusion of the median nasal process with the maxillary process, which may be unilateral or bilateral.

It may be *incomplete*, the posterior bridge is known as Simon Art's band

The term *complete* cleft lip is used if the cleft extends to the floor of the nose, often with increased width of the ipsilateral nostril.

Compound cleft lip is one associated with a cleft in the alveolus.

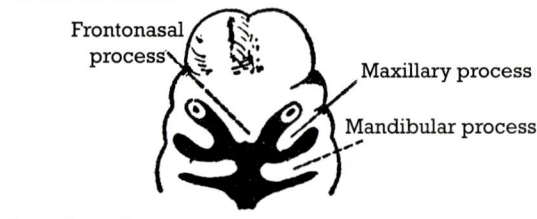

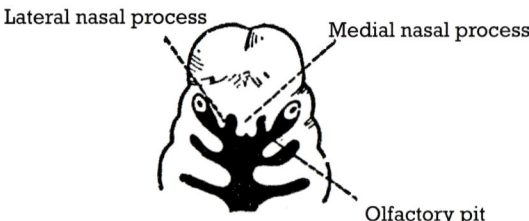

The development of face

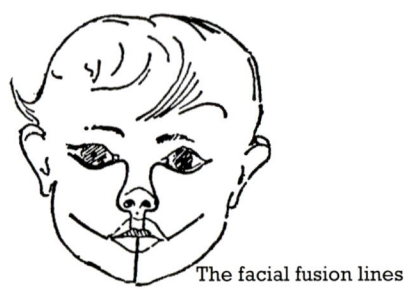

The facial fusion lines

Fig. 57.1. Stages of development of face

Complicated cleft lip is one associated with a cleft palate.

Inferior labial sinuses are two small blind tubes in the lower lip associated with cleft lip

Cleft lower lip is an extremely rare anomaly due to failure of fusion of the two mandibular processes.

Incidence: One in 750 live births, out of them:

    Cleft lip alone 25%
    Cleft palate alone 25%
    Combined 50%
    Unilateral cleft 65%
    Left sided more common.(see under cleft palate)

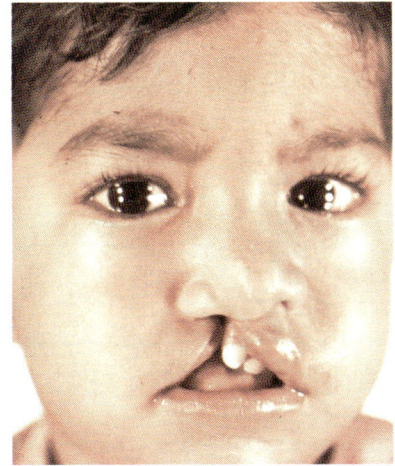

Fig. 57.2. Cleft lip
(courtesy: Prof T Dorairajan, Chennai)

Problems

1. *Cosmetic* disfigurement
2. *Suction* problems: Orbicularis oris muscle ring around the mouth is not complete; a vacuum is therefore not created for effective suction. This eventually affects the nutritional status. For improved milk delivery, the hole of the rubber teat (in the bottle feed) should be enlarged.

3. *Dentition*: The upper lateral incisors may be absent, small, or duplicated. The maxilla is smaller, causing a relative mandibular prognathism.

4. *Speech*: The *labial* syllables, namely B,F,M,P,V which need proper apposition of the lips, are imperfect.

Treatment

Timing of repair: The repair should be undertaken before the age of 3 months, i.e. well before primary dentition, for optimal results.

Reasons

a) The baby's general condition will permit safe anesthesia and surgery

b) The lip elements are larger, and lend themselves to easier and more precise approxima-

tion.

c) Post operative feeding is easier with the dropper.

d) Defective speech is avoided.

e) The alveolar gap lessens (thereby favoring normal development of the alveolus) after the repair of a compound cleft lip.

f) When associated with cleft palate, early lip reconstruction will lessen the palatal gap to some extent.

Interim treatment, while waiting for surgery

a) other congenital malformations (e.g. cardiac) should be looked for.

b) presurgical orthodontic treatment with acrylic splints if necessary to align the alveolus.

Operative technique: Only broad principles of surgery are outlined here:

a) Surgery for cleft lip is done under endotracheal general anesthesia, using an 'L' shaped Oxford tube.

b) Repair of the cleft lip to maintain normal shape and symmetry.

c) Adequate mobilization of flaps from either side to avoid suture line tension.

d) Paring of the edges for perfect union.

e) Layered apposition of the tissues (mucous membrane, muscle and skin)

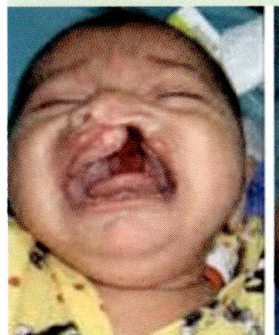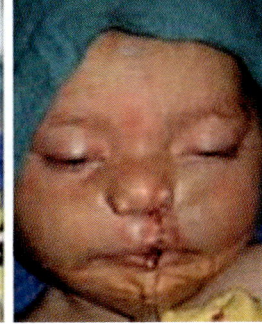

Fig. 57.3. cleft lip-before and after surgery

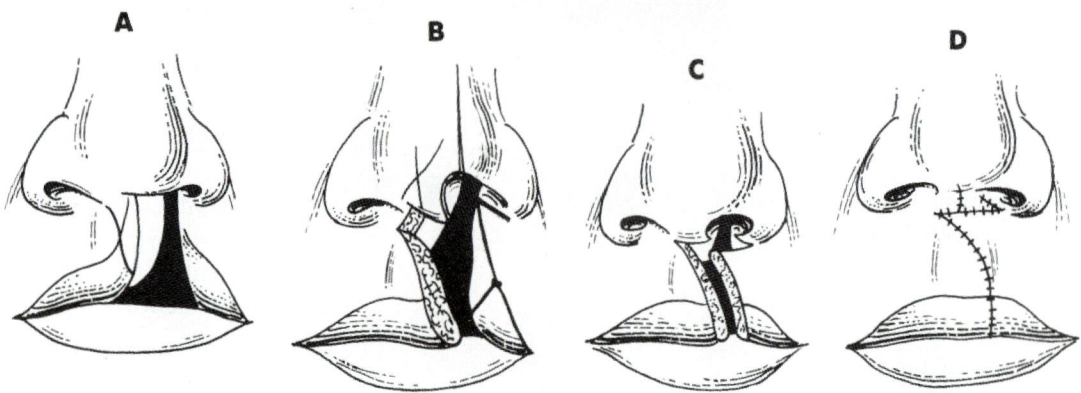

Fig. 57.4. Rotation-advancement technic of repair of unilateral cleft lip

f) Increased vertical length of the upper lip from the floor of the nostril to the vermilion border of the lip, to exactly match the opposite side. All the described methods differ only in this step.

Millard's technique is the 'rotation down and advancement closure' of the lip elements.

Mirault-Blair's operation:

I Stage: Mobilization of the lip (lateral to the cleft) and a part of the cheek. The medial part is dissected off the maxilla.

II Stage: The margins are cut in full thickness and triangulated.

III Stage: Resuturing of the flaps to get a continuous red margin of the lip (Cupid's bow).

Bilateral cases and those associated with cleft palate, require more complicated procedures.

Post operative measures

a) *Logan's bow* to be applied on the operated site, to prevent trauma and relieve tension.

b) Elbows should be splinted, to prevent interfering with the dressings by the child

c) Nutrition by dropper feeding.

d) Antibiotics.

e) Sutures to be removed on 5th day, preferably under short general anesthesia.

Normal breast/bottle feeding is allowed after three weeks.

Jewels of Gyan - 01.1

Millard's rule of 10

According to this, the operation is ideally carried out when

1. the baby is 10 weeks old
2. the weight is at least 10 pounds
3. the hemoglobin is above 10gm%

58 Cleft Palate

Embryology: The hard palate develops from two sources.

a) The two palatine processes, arising from the maxillary process on either side, fuse to form the primary palate.

b) The secondary palate, i.e. the premaxilla, which is a part of the median nasal process.

Cleft palate is due to a failure of fusion of these three process. Both cleft lip and palate are more common on the left, probably because the left palatal process is the last to assume the horizontal position.

As the fusion takes place from before backwards, the uvula is always involved.

The cleft palate is associated with:

Apert's syndrome

Treacher Collins syndrome

Down's syndrome

It may also be commonly associated with disorders, such as nerve deafness, otitis media and problems of speech and dentition.

Anatomic classification

1. Incomplete
   a) Bifid uvula: cleft of the uvula only

   b) Cleft of the soft palate along its entire length

   c) Cleft of the entire soft palate and the posterior part of the hard palate.

2. Complete cleft palate: cleft of whole of soft and hard palate, so that the nasal and oral cavities become one.

In front, the gap may extend on one side of the premaxilla (bipartite cleft palate). If the

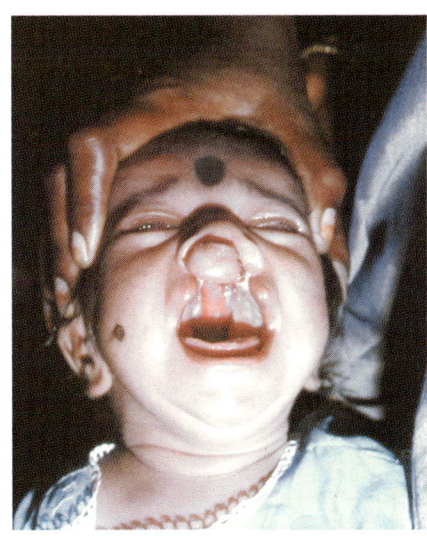

Fig.58.1. Bilateral cleft lip and palate (courtesy: Prof T Dorairajan, Chennai)

gap extends on both sides of the premaxilla, it is a tripartite cleft palate.

Occult submucosal cleft palate is caused by defective fusion of the muscle masses although the mucous membrane is intact. This causes the child to have a typical 'cleft palate speech'.

Problems

a) Speech: Palatal consonants, B,D,K,P,T will be pronounced with a nasal intonation. During normal speech the palate moves to the posterior pharyngeal wall to shut off the nasal cavity from the mouth; this is called velopharyngeal closure. In cleft palate, air escapes into the nose and causes the 'hyper-nasal' speech.

b) Sucking: Negative pressure in the mouth cannot be generated

c) Regurgitation: Reflux of liquid food into the nose

d) Deafness: Inflammatory changes of the pharyngeal mucosa will impede drainage of the Eustachian tube. Accumulation of this exudate predisposes to acute and chronic suppurative otitis media and defective hearing.

e) Dentition: Irregular development of the alveolus causes various problems of dentition like irregular incisors and mandibular prognathism.

f) Olfaction: Contamination of nasal mucosa by oral bacteria causes a chronic rhinitis.

g) Respiratory infections: aspiration pneumonitis and lung abscess may occur.

Treatment

Timing of repair: it is ideally done before the child devel-

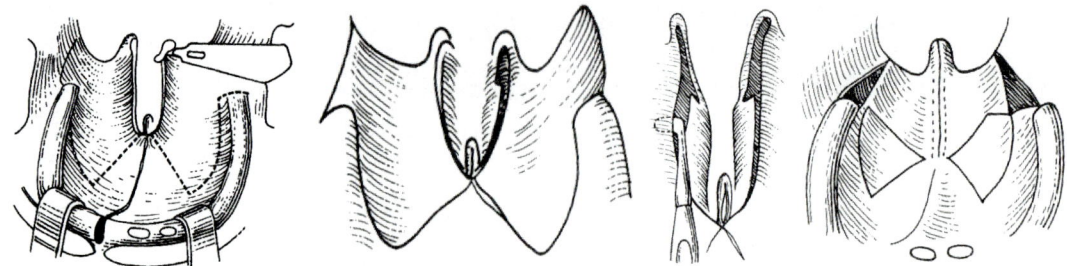

Fig. 58.2. Wardill-Kilner (V-Y) palatoplasty for cleft soft palate

ops nasal speech (before 12 months) and after secondary dentition has taken place, since too early repair may cause maldevelopment of the maxillae. Until then, a plate should be constructed to cover the palatal gap and to facilitate feeding. At intervals, fresh plates are made to help mould the palate until the alveolar processes are in apposition ready for repair.

Operative technique

These operations are also done under endotracheal general anesthesia, using an 'L' shaped Oxford tube. Only broad principles of surgery are outlined here:

1) *von Langenbeck's* operation: The margins of the defect are freshened, bipedicled mucoperiosteal flaps based on greater palatine vessels are raised on either side and the flaps sutured in layers. Fracturing both the pterygoid hamuli will facilitate relaxation of the flaps.

2) *Wardill's* operation: In this operation, the problems of tension and avascularity of the flaps, common in von Langenbeck's operation are overcome by dividing the two flaps on either side, to create four flaps, in a 'W' manner. These are brought to the midline and sutured in a 'V-Y' fashion, to increase the length of the palate. The posterior flaps are also pulled back-wards, to increase the length further and to diminish the space between the oropharynx and the nasopharynx. The mucosa, muscles and mucoperiosteum are sutured with interrupted sutures.

3) *Furlow's* operation: This is a double-apposing 'Z-plasty' technique, preferred by many surgeons.

Bilateral defects require more sophisticated surgical and dental procedures.

Postoperative care

1. The child's elbows are splinted

2. Oral cleanliness is maintained.

3. Airway is kept clear.

4. Oral feeding is started as soon as possible.

5. Dedicated speech therapy is mandatory to normalize speech postoperatively.

6. Secondary dental problems occur in later childhood and these will require orthodontic correction.

Breakdown of closure will result in a palatal fistula, allowing ingested fluid to escape into the nose and cause speech disturbances. Smaller ones may be closed by raising adjacent flaps but larger fistulas may require flaps of gingiva or tongue.

(epulis: gumboil, upon the gum)

Definition: A localized swelling arising from the gum. They may be inflammatory or neoplastic, related to the epithelium or underlying connective tissue, since gum is a mucoperiosteal cover.

Classification

1. Congenital (vide infra)

2. Acquired

   i) fibrous (commonest) (firm)
   ii) granulomatous (soft)
   iii) myeloid (firm)
   iv) carcinomatous (hard)
   v) sarcomatous (hard)

The first two are inflammatory, the myeloid epulis is of borderline malignancy, whereas the last two are frankly malignant. The terms, carcinomatous and sarcomatous epulis are not preferred by contemporary pathologists, instead they are called carcinoma and sarcoma of the gum respectively.

Clinical features

Naturally vary according to the type; in general they present as pink, soft, vascular, partially compressible swellings over the anterior part of the gum of the lower jaw (more than the upper).

FIBROUS EPULIS: This is the most common type, arising from the periosteum near the premolar or incisor teeth. It is not a true neoplasm but tissue hyperplasia in response to chronic irritation from the sharp margin of carious cavity and as it grows, it dislodges the tooth itself.

Pathology

it is composed of mainly fibroblasts with neovascularisation.

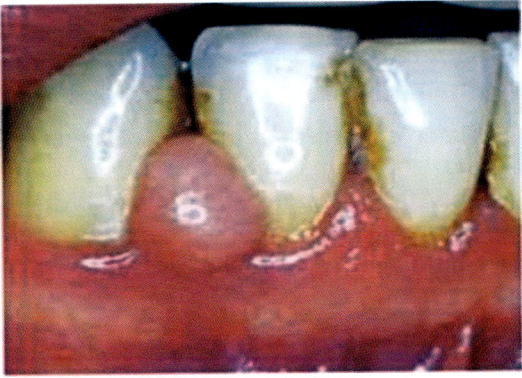

Fig. 59.1. Fibrous epulis

Rarely it may become sarcomatous. (vide infra)

Clinical features

It is a slow growing, non-tender, soft to firm nodule, covered by pink mucous membrane, usually located at the rim of a dental socket and may be pedunculated, without ulceration or regional lymphadenopathy. Rapid growth indicates malignant transformation.

Differential diagnosis

The other types of epulis, odontomes, metabolic or dysplastic bone cysts, osteomyelitis, actinomycosis, brown tumor of hyperparathyroidism etc.

Treatment

Excision, along with the socket of the culprit tooth, is curative. The tissue should be examined by the pathologist.

GRANULOMATOUS EPULIS

This is an exuberant granulation tissue in relation to a septic tooth, in effect a pyogenic granuloma of the gum.

Clinical features

Often associated with a carious tooth, ill-fitting denture or poor

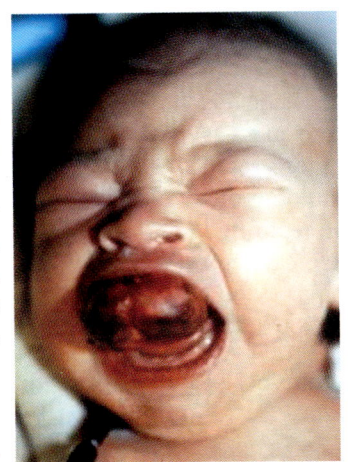

Fig. 59.2. Congenital epulis

oral hygiene; the swelling looks light red and vascular, bleeding to touch and associated with enlarged, tender submandibular/submental lymph nodes.

Differential diagnosis: same as fibrous type

Treatment

Extraction of the carious tooth associated with the swelling, proper oral/dental hygiene and attention to the denture fitting, may all be helpful. The granulation tissue is scraped and is examined histologically or it may be cauterized by diathermy or laser.

MYELOID EPULIS

(syn: giant cell epulis, peripheral giant cell reparative granuloma) is a benign giant cell tumor arising from the gingiva, displacing the teeth, less common than the fibrous and granulomatous types. It develops due to constant irritation from an adjacent infected socket or at the site of a shed primary tooth, but with morphological features of a benign osteoclastoma and behaves like a locally aggressive lesion.

Pathology

Microscopically the stroma consists of fibrovascular tissue and multinucleated giant cells, similar to a giant cell tumor (osteoclastoma), but true giant cell tumors almost never occur in the jaws.

Clinical features

Though the underlying mass is hard due to expansion of the marginal bone under cover of the mucoperiosteum, yet the gum covering it is hyperemic, edematous and soft. The mass is sessile, plum-colored and exhibits more rapid growth than the fibrous and the granulomatous epulides. The adjacent tooth may be separated or loosened. X-ray may show the typical soap bubble appearance of an osteoclastoma.

Complications: Ulceration and hemorrhage.

Differential diagnosis: same as other types of epulis.

Treatment

A small swelling can be treated by simple curettage and filling the cavity with cancellous bone chips from the iliac crest. In case of large tumor, wide excision of the bone should be performed, the gap being filled by bone graft, from the rib or iliac crest.

CARCINOMATOUS EPULIS (carcinoma of gum)

It is an epithelioma of the gum seen in the elderly, usually arising from the alveolar margin, but it may be located in relation to the socket of a tooth. As in epithelioma elsewhere, it may infiltrate the jaw, fungate, secondarily infected or spread to regional nodes. A wedge biopsy would clinch the matter and x-ray jaw may reveal bony involvement, to plan proper treatment.

Clinical features and management is the same as SCC in other areas.

Sarcomatous epulis (sarcoma of gum) is the rarest and most malignant of all and its features and management are dealt under STS.

Epulis of the newborn

It is a rare congenital gingival 'tumor' that most commonly occurs along the alveolar ridge of the maxilla in newborn girls, usually without any abnormalities of the teeth or additional congenital malformations. The actual etiology is unknown and may require excision and the gum recontoured.

Pregnancy epulis occurs either due to poor dental hygiene or hormonal changes during pregnancy (sometimes in adolescence in both genders) and managed in line with granulomatous variety.

Drug-induced epulides: Prolonged use drugs such as phenytoin (an anticonvulsant), nifedipine (calcium channel blocker and coronary vasodilator) etc, have been associated with diffuse or localized enlargement of gums. If they do not regress with the withdrawal of the drug, excision is needed.

60 Jaw Swellings

Cyst of the jaws are quite common; the majority are radicular cysts of inflammatory origin. They are classified as follows:

1. Odontogenic developmental cysts (syn: follicular cyst) arising from the dental follicle, namely dental, dentigerous and keratocysts.

2. Fissural cysts, in relation to bony suture lines, such as nasopalatine, nasolabial, median mandibular, globulomaxillary cysts.

3. Odontogenic tumors, such as odontoma and adamantinoma (syn: ameloblastoma)

DENTAL CYST (syn: radicular or apical periodontal cyst)

This is a sequel of dental inflammatory disease and the commonest cyst of the jaw. It usually develops from chronic apical infection of a tooth, stimulating the epithelial rests of Malassez to proliferate, undergoing cystic degeneration. It is lined by stratified squamous epithelium derived from the epithelial debris. The contents may be fluid or semifluid consisting cellular debris, cholesterol crystals and foreign body giant cells. The cyst continues to grow at the expense of surrounding tissues and causes expansion of the alveolus. If there is persistent infection, the epithelium is destroyed and replaced by a fibrous wall. It has the following features:

1) It tends to occur most frequently in the upper jaw, where it attains a large size and may encroach upon the antrum or even open into it, mimicking carcinoma.

2) This cyst may appear at any age, but commonly seen in 3rd decade of life.

3) Once formed, the cyst enlarges slowly with resorption of the adjacent bone, expanding the jaw. In the lower jaw, the greater part of the mandible, including the ramus, may be involved.

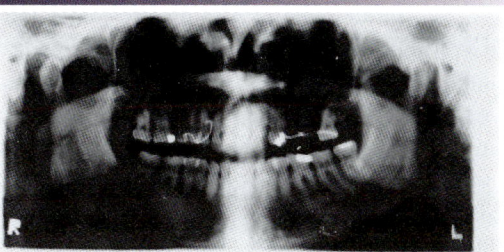

Fig. 60.1. Orthopantomogram (OPG)
(courtesy: Halsted Surgical Clinic , Chennai)

4) It is usually painless, unless infected.

5) When the bone is thinned out, there may be`egg shell' crackling and if the bone is completely destroyed exposing the cyst wall, it may become fluctuant.

6) Radiography is helpful in diagnosis. A circular radiolucent area is seen in relation to the apex of the affected tooth, sometimes with a sclerosed margin.

Differential diagnosis

Odontogenic tumors and other odontogenic cysts

Treatment

1) Oral and dental hygiene must be maintained and any carious tooth attended to.

2) Through an intraoral route, the entire epithelial lining is removed, the cyst wall is curetted and the cavity obliterated by pushing the soft tissue in, before the gum is closed.

DENTIGEROUS CYST: (syn: follicular odontome or cyst)

This is associated with an unerupted permanent tooth; hence it often contains the tooth, commonly the mandibular 3rd molar and maxillary canine, lying obliquely in the viscid fluid of the cyst.

Pathology

It arises from the separation of the enamel epithelium from the surface of the crown of an erupting tooth, after the development of enamel, with accumulation of fluid. The tooth is displaced deep into the jaw and prevented from erupting normally. The cyst has an internal epithelial lining of stratified squamous or columnar and an outer dense fibrous connective tissue covering. The contents are similar to that of the dental cyst (fluid or semifluid with cholesterol crystals and foreign body giant cells), in addition to the culprit tooth. It may attain a large size or occasionally the epithelium gets destroyed due to infection, so that the cyst remains small. Changes such as hyperplasia, degeneration, inflammation, calcification, dysplasia and neoplasia (ameloblastoma) have been identified in the epithelium of dentigerous cysts.

Clinical features

1) it usually occurs in young adults, often detected by routine dental skiagraphy.
2) the common locations are mandibular (last molar) and maxillary (canine).
3) the cyst may grow larger and expand the outer table of the jaw causing 'eggshell' crackling.
4) it is a painless swelling unless infected.
5) cyst of the jaw with a missing tooth is highly diagnostic.
6) x-ray of jaw shows a well defined radiolucenct cyst with part or whole of the unerupted tooth lying within. The larger cysts may be multilocular, sometimes giving a pseudotrabecular or soap-bubble appearance.

Differential diagnosis: same as for dental cyst

Treatment

Total excision of the cyst wall, as in a dental cyst, is imperative, including the tooth lying inside. If it is very large, total excision may not be possible, when it can be marsupialised after deroofing and curetting the lining epithelium, partly filling it with oral mocosa.

Keratocyst: This is a rarer condition, sometimes multiple, arising from residual strands of epithelium derived from the dental lamina, in the retromolar region. Occasionally it may envelop a tooth, mimicking dentigerous cyst in the x-ray, but however remains separated from the crown of the tooth or tooth follicle, hence also known as extrafollicular dentigerous cyst. It is seen commonly in the 4th decade and around the 3rd molar region of the mandible. Multiple keratocysts form part of the nevoid basal cell carcinoma (Gorlin's syndrome).

Pathology

The lining of the cyst has an outer fibrous coat and an inner stratified squamous epithelium of keratinising variety (which develop keratin). The epithelial lining is so thin and delicate that it may be easily torn during excision, portions of which left behind, explaining the high rate of recurrence in this type.

Treatment

Complete removal of the cyst with its lining epithelium has to be done, if necessary with the resection of involved bone, to prevent recurrence.

FISSURAL CYST: These occur near the lines of bony fusion and include nasopalatine, nasolabial, median mandibular cyst etc. which are quite rare compared to the odontogenic developmental cysts. They are also lined by an outer fibrous and an inner stratified squamous epithelial lining, with mucoid content and capable of attaining a large size, if untreated.

Treatment

Excision of the cyst, along with the lining membrane, obliterating the space with mucosal flaps.

ODONTOGENIC TUMORS

Odontogenic tumors are of three types: epithelial, mesenchymal and mixed.

Epithelial: ameloblastoma (adamantinoma or Eve's disease) and odontogenic adenomatoid tumor

Mesenchymal: fibroma and cementoma
Mixed: odontomas

AMELOBLASTOMA (syn: adamantinoma, Eve's disease)

It is a true epithelial neoplasm of the enamel-forming cells (ameloblasts), akin to basal cell carcinoma of the skin, occurring most often in the molar mandible.

Pathology

Gross: Ameloblastoma starts as a solid soft tissue tumor but goes on to form a multilocular cyst. Lower jaw and molar region are the commonest sites; the maxilla may also be rarely involved. By destruction of the root, the overlying tooth gets loose and may fall of. It is a locally invasive tumor, with a great potential for recurrence but does not metastasize.

Microscopic: The picture may vary but the main feature is the nests of vacuolated ameloblastic epithelium lying in dense connective tissue stroma, with cystic degeneration, which occasionally may enclose the crown of an unerupted tooth to mimic a dentigerous cyst.

Other sites for adamantinoma: stalk of pituitary and tibia may rarely be the seat of this tumor, but the nomenclature in these locations is disputed, consensus being towards BCC.

Clinical features

Is a rare tumor, seen in all ages, with the peak incidence being in middle age, and a slight female preponderance. It is a slow growing, painless swelling located in the molar mandible, initially hard, becomes cystic, with eggshell crackling on palpation, expands the outer table of the jaw more than the inner. Uncontrolled bleeding following extraction of a 'loose tooth' overlying the tumor, may be a presenting feature.

X-ray shows large loculations with small multiple translucent areas separated by fine bony trabeculae, giving rise to a honey-comb appearance. Disintegration of the overlying tooth is typical.

Differential diagnosis

1. Osteoclastoma or giant cell tumor affecting the mandible.
2. Giant-celled reparative granuloma.

Treatment

Since it is a locally invasive tumor, simple local excision or curetting is insufficient, leading to invariable recurrences. Such an adamant behavior of the tumor (due to inadequate surgery), recurrences showing up even decades after excision, had earned the tumor the name adamantinoma.

It is not radiosensitive, hence the definitive treatment is wide excision, with the portion of the jaw bearing the tumor, with appropriate reconstruction. If the tumor is very large, affecting the major part of the mandible, hemimandibulectomy may be necessary; the resultant defect is made good by a prosthesis or bone graft.

ODONTOMAS

These are actually hamartomatous lesions rather than true neoplasms and their classification seems more an exercise for the surgical pathologist than clinically significant. Majority are calcified, hard odontomas, containing all dental tissues, seen as circumscribed lesions in the x-ray. The dental tissues may form a compound composite odontoma or may be arranged haphazardly to form complex composite odontoma. Soft odontomas are composed of fibrous or fibromyxomatous elements. The simplest classification of them is:

I. Connective tissue odontomas (arising from connective tissue elements)
- a. Fibrous odontoma
- b. Cementoma
- c. Fibromyxomatous odontoma
- d. Sarcomatous odontoma

II. Composite odontomas (arising from both epithelial and connective tissue elements)
- a. Radicular odontoma.
- b. Compound composite odontoma
- c. Complex composite odontoma

Osseous tumors of the jaws

Benign tumors
- a. Fibroosseous group
- b. Paget's disease of bone

c. Fibromyxoma
d. Giant-celled reparative granuloma

Malignant tumors

a. Osteosarcoma
b. Adeno/squamous cell carcinoma of the maxillary antrum.
c. Burkitt's lymphoma (see under lymph nodes, chapter 42)
d. Secondary carcinoma by direct invasion from tongue, cheek, lips, floor of mouth or lymph nodes.

GIANT-CELLED REPARATIVE GRANULOMA

This is not a neoplasm and occurs due to hemorrhage within the marrow of the jaw.

Pathology

Macroscopically, it consists of opaque semi-solid dark-red material. It occurs entirely in the jaw either in the mandible or in the maxilla. Presents as a lobulated tumor and gradually erodes the cortex, whch is covered with a thin layer of subperiosteal new bone.

Microscopically, the tumor has a stroma of plump connective tissue cells and scanty collagen, with many thin walled blood vessels and quite a number of osteoclast-like multinucleate giant cells. These giant cells are distributed unevenly in the stroma.

Histiocytes may be found scattered throughout the lesion. It is often difficult to distinguish this lesion from giant cell epulis and the so called brown tumor of hyperparathyroidism.

Clinical features

1. It occurs more often between the ages of 10 and 25 years.
2. Females are frequently involved than males.
3. The swelling is painless.
4. It often involves the mandible rather than the maxilla.
5. X-ray shows round or oval lobulated area of radiotranslucency. It expands and thins out the cortex but does not perforate it, as there is always a thin layer of subperiosteal new bone.

Differential diagnosis

1. Osteoclastoma
2. Adamantinoma.
3. 'Brown tumor' of hyper parathyroidism; serum calcium level must always be determined to exclude this condition. X-ray of other parts of the skeleton is also necessary.

Treatment

1. Thorough curettage through an external incision is the treatment of choice. The bone cavity should not be opened into the mouth (chronic osteomyelitis may result from intra-oral microbes).
2. The condition usually does not recur; if it does, the diagnosis may have to be reviewed.
3. Recent reports of success with calcitonin therapy, achieving near total regression, have appeared.

Carcinoma maxillary antrum is an SCC and presents as a mass projecting upwards (into the orbital fossa), downwards (into the hard palate), inwards (into the nasal cavity) or outwards (onto the face). Those exposed to industrial hardwood dust are vulnerable to develop an adenocarcinoma in the antrum. The features depend upon the direction of tumor growth:

1) upwards into the floor of the orbit: diplopia or numbness due to maxillary nerve involvement
2) inwards into the nose: nasal block/discharge or epistaxis
3) outwards: facial swelling and deformity, rarely ulceration/fungation
4) downwards: dental pain or intraoral ulcerated mass
5) backwards: involvement of multiple cranial nerves and base of skull

Diagnostic and therapeutic methods are like SCC elsewhere. Excision of maxillary tumor involves much mutilation of the face, which may be made good by a prosthetic implant.

Osteomyelitis of the jaw

It may be acute suppurative, chronic suppurative and chronic sclerosing types.

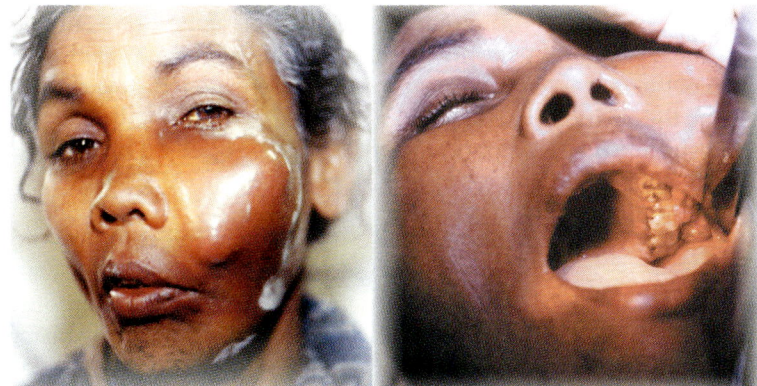

Fig. 60.2. Carcinoma of maxillary antrum, external swelling and intraoral projection
(courtesy: Dr K Sreekanth, Hyderabad)

X-ray may initially show periosteal reaction, but a lytic lesion may be a late feature.

Treatment

Antibiotics aiming at mixed infection, must be started immediately, pending the microbiology report and be continued or modified depending upon the antibiogram and clinical response by then. If a subperiosteal abscess is formed, it should be liberally deroofed, while extracting the affending tooth.

a) Acute suppurative osteomyelitis

It is rare considering the incidence of apical abscess. It actually starts as an infection of a dental root, commonly in the mandible, leading to an apical or alveolar abscess. Primary bone infection is virtually never seen. Some of the predisposing conditions for this are:

1. Malnutrition
2. Exanthematous fevers, such as measles, scarlet fever etc
3. Dental caries
4. Injuries of the mandible with mucosal breach (treated as compound fracture).
5. Immunosuppresion
6. Diabetes mellitus

Clinical features

As acute osteomyelitis elsewhere, throbbing pain, swelling of the overlying gum, with loosening of the culprit tooth, associated with constitutional symptoms, such as fever, malaise etc., are characteristically seen. The abscess formed may surface externally over the face or internally into the oral cavity and rupture, forming a sinus, with prompt relief of pain. Subperiosteal new bone formation (involucrum) may form, around the necrosed bone (sequestrum), supporting the jaw, hence external disfugurement is rare. Maxillary involvement with much periorbital cellulitis is common in infants.

b) Chronic suppurative osteomyelitis

This is the result of inadequately treated acute infection. As in osteomyelitis elsewhere, there may be involucrum (new bone formation), surrounding the sequestrum (dead bone) and discharging sinuses will be seen in the exterior in the face or chin. At this stage it is difficult to treat the condition with antibiotics only due to reduction in blood supply to the affected area.

Clinical features

There is pain, swelling and tenderness at the affected site. Increased pressure in the dental canal compresses the inferior dental nerve and this will cause numbness of the chin. On palpation one can easily feel the irregular, thickened and tender affected portion of the jaw. Once the sinus has developed, it is fixed to the diseased bone with sprouting granulation tissue in its opening suggesting the presence of sequestrum inside.

X-ray will show irregular involucrum and necrosed bone (sequestrum) inside. Such a findng is a late feature.

Treatment

Once chronic osteomyelitis has developed, it requires saucerisation of the involucrum and removal of the entire sequestrum (sequestrectomy). A suitable incision is made at the dependent part of the affected area of the mandible, the involucrum is chiselled and the cavity is laid open, removing any sequestrum. The cavity is packed lightly with petroleum jelly gauze and appropriate antibiotics should be given (see chapter 111).

c) Chronic sclerosing (non-suppurative) osteomyelitis

It is a condition in which neither pus nor sequestrum is formed, but the involved jaw becomes sclerosed with small cavities containing granulation tissue.

Clinical features

The disease starts insidiously with recurrent, subacute episodes of soft tissue swelling over the involved jaw, with increased pain and warmth over the affected segment. The affected jaw becomes thickened, irregular and tender. The cause of this condition is not definitely known, though radiation and chemical necrosis in the form of phosphorus, arsenic or mercury poisoning may cause such an osteomyelitis. Even tuberculosis, syphilis and actinomycosis have been incriminated, but some pathologists claim that it occurs due to infection by anaerobic organisms. The condition is almost like Brodie's abscess with sclerosis surrounding an osteolytic lesion in the skiagram.

X-ray may also reveal periosteal reaction and local osteitis.

Treatment

Antibiotics, such as clindamycin and anaerobicidals like metronidazole have been used with some success in this condition, but the majority of these cases do not respond either to antibiotics nor even repeated decortication; jaw resection appears to be the only definite solution.

ACTINOMYCOSIS

Actinomycosis, a common infection in the West, but not so in the East, is caused by an anaerobic or microaerophilic, filamentous, Gram positive and weakly acid-fast organism, Actinomyces israelii. This organism is a normal commensal in tonsillar crypts and dental cavities in healthy individuals, but becomes pathogenic, producing a subacute pyogenic inflammation, whenever intraoral bacterial infection or trauma (dental surgery) devitalises the tissues and reduces their oxidation potential to a level compatible with the growth of these anaerobes.

Predisposing factors

1. Trauma
2. Presence of carious tooth
3. Secondary bacterial invasion
4. Hypersensitivity

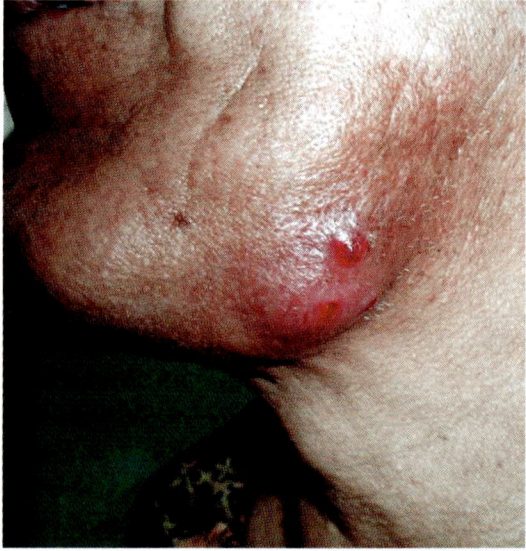

Fig. 60.3. Actinomycosis of the lower jaw with multiple sinuses
(courtesy: Lifeline Hospitals, Chennai)

Jewels of Gyan - 60.1

The 5 'S's of Actinomycosis

Swelling of
Skin and
Subcutaneous tissue with
Sinuses discharging
Sulphur granules

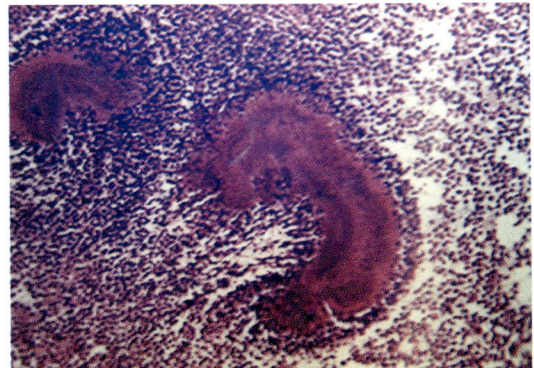

Fig. 60.4. Histology of 'ray fungus'
(courtesy: Lifeline Hospitals, Chennai)

Pathology

In tissues the actinomyces grow in the form of yellow colonies. There is a dense central mass of tangled threads surrounded by radiating, sometimes terminally clubbed filaments that create a fuzzy border to the colony formation. This colony is grossly visible thus giving rise to the characteristic yellow and sometimes grey, sulphur granules, also known as fish-roe bodies. If one of these granules is crushed under a cover glass and examined unstained, two elements can be distinguished; branching mycelial filaments and club forms. The filaments constitute the greater part of the body and radiate from the central part of the granule, whereas the clubs are pear-shaped bodies which form fringes round the periphery of the colony. These clubs probably represent a means of defense against the protective forces of the tissues and are produced as deposition of lipid material derived from the host tissues. Hence, the filaments are Gram positive, whereas the clubs are Gram negative. The characteristic radial arrangement is responsible for the familiar term, ray fungus.

Microscopy: The picture is that of a suppurating granuloma, consists of a pus-filled core in which there may be a number of mycelial colonies. More peripherally there is cellular infiltration which consists of mononuclear histiocytes, lymphocytes and occasional giant cells. Dense scar gradually replaces all other elements and imparts the characteristic woody, indurated nature to the lesion. It must be remembered that mycelia may not be found in sections of the tissue and should not be accepted as the only point of diagnostic value. Mycelia are more often seen in soft areas and in the pus rather than in a piece of hard tissue.

Spread

1. Spread by lymph stream is practically unknown; so if the draining lymph nodes are enlarged, secondary infection must be considered.

2. Spread by blood stream is uncommon but very rarely a lesion may 'invade' into a vessel and give rise to mestatasis in distant organs. Commonly liver, brain and heart, but rarely kidney, spleen and the ovaries may be the organs of such involvement.

Four main clinical forms of actinomycosis are seen:

(1) cervicofacial; discussed here in detail

(2) thoracic

(3) ileocecal and

(4) foot; one of the causes of mycetoma foot, the other and more common being madura mycosis (see chapter 70).

CERVICOFACIAL ACTINOMYCOSIS

Tissues of the face and neck including the tongue and mandible are mainly affected. The mandible is more frequently affected adjacent to a carious tooth.

Clinical features

1. The swelling is mostly seen over the angle of the mandible, often adjacent to a carious tooth.

2. The onset is insidious

3. The condition is painless.

4. The gum and the adjacent soft tissue becomes swollen and indurated. In course of time a large woody swelling develops over the angle of the jaw, known as 'lumpy jaw'.

5. The hard induration eventually becomes soft and fluctuant, due to central suppuration.

6. Periostitis and osteomyelitis with extensive destruction of bone are common accompaniments.

7. The overlying skin of the affected face and neck becomes bluish in color.

8. Abscesses develop and eventually burst to cause multiple sinuses. Chronicity, dense induration and sinuses surrounded by bluish skin are the most characteristic features of cervico-facial actinomycosis.

9. The pus discharging through the sinuses is usually thin and may contain tiny sulphur granules. These granules are most readily found in the pus of a newly opened lesion, but not in older lesions. In such cases it is best to allow a considerable amount of secretion to collect before examining it. The grains may be recognised at the bottom of such a collection.

10. X-ray appearance is characteristically negative in early stages but this distinguishes it from osteomyelitis of other reasons. Some amount of sclerosis may be seen in long standing cases, at multiple sites.

Treatment

Treatment of this condition is mainly medical. Actinomyces are sensitive to penicillin, tetracycline and lincomycin. An intensive course of penicillin (6-10 mega units IV/day) is given for a month, followed by IM or oral administration for 6 months. Supplementation with iodide in the form of tincture iodine and an antifibroblastic agent, stanozolol, are helpful in resolving fibrosis. Antimycotic drugs, such as nystatin, myconazole, clotrimazole, ketaconazole, flucytocine, fluconazole, amphotericin-B etc. have all been used in various combinations to eradicate actinomycosis.

Role of surgery: it is restricted to chronic and resistant cases not responding to antibiotics properly. Drainage of the abscesses should be performed by widening the openings of the sinuses and loosely packing the cavities with roller gauze soaked in tincture iodine (2%).

In some resistant cases, radiotherapy has been tried, but neither has it proved beneficial nor does it stand to logic; besides it may be oncogenic (delayed development of differentiated tumors of thyroid, mainly papillary carcinoma).

61 Cancer Screening

The aim is to detect and treat the disease in the population at an early curable stage in order to reduce cancer morbidity and mortality.

Advantages

1. Improved prognosis.
2. Less radical curative treatment.
3. Reassurance for those with negative test results.
4. Resource savings from less radical treatment.

Disadvantages

1. Longer morbidity for those with unaltered prognosis.

2. Overtreatment of borderline abnormalities.

3. False reassurance for those with false negative results.

4. Anxiety and morbidity for those with false positive results.

5. Cooperation from population to accept screening and carry out repeated tests cannot be relied on.

6. Hazards of screening tests.

7. Resource costs from screening, diagnosis, investigations and over treatment.

In the absence of effective methods of primary prevention or effective treatment of symptomatic tumors, screening offers the best hope of controlling the mortality from some cancers. Health education promoting self examination is also a form of screening, e.g. breast cancer, skin melanoma and testicular cancer. Medical follow-up, e.g. hydatidiform mole by β-hCG assay for chorion epithelioma is another form of screening.

The *sensitivity* of a test is the number of positive tests per 100 patients with the disease. The *specificity of a* test is the number of negative tests per 100 patients who do not have the disease.

Mass screening

1) Uterine cervix

Exfoliative cytology with 80% sensitivity and very high specificity, is a very popular screening test (Papanicolaou). It has the disadvantage of over-treatment of borderline abnormalities. Colposcopic biopsy and laser excision of affected epithelium may reduce this disadvantage. The age and frequency of screening is controversial. Yearly 'pap smear' for women >40 is generally recommended up to the age of 70.

Women who have had a total hysterectomy (removal of the uterus and cervix) may also choose to stop having Pap tests, unless the surgery was done for invasive or pre-invasive cervical cancer. Women who have had a subtotal hysterectomy (without removal of the cervix) should continue to have Pap tests.

Some women, with postive history or those harbor chronic cervical sepsis or erosion, may

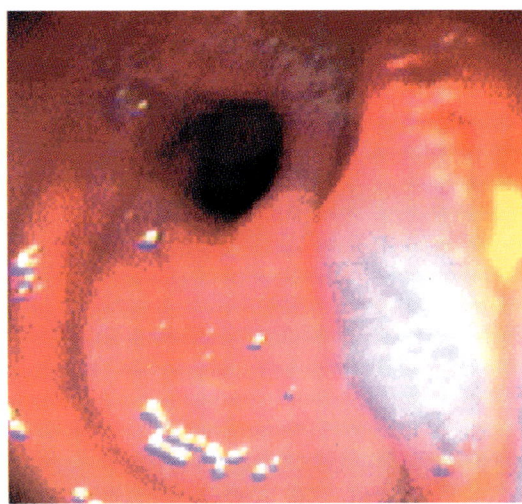

Fig. 61.1. Endoscopic detection of early gastric carcinoma in a patient who had gastrojejunostomy done for chronic duodenal ulcer
(courtesy: Lifeline Hospitals, Chennai)

need a closer screening schedule for cervical cancer.

2) Stomach

Double-contrast barium meal detects early gastric carcinoma. It carries a radiation hazard and is very non-specific with almost 25% of screened individuals requiring further investigations involving fluoroscopy, cytology, and endoscopy. Mortality has been reduced by 20% since the test was introduced, but the natural history of this disease is illunderstood and it is argued that both incidence of and mortality from gastric cancer are showing a decline. In high risk patients (1st degree relative with gastric cancer, endemic population, A+ve blood group etc.) endoscopic screening with supravital dyes helps in the pick up of early neoplastic foci. However, its cost-effectiveness in mass screening, in developing countries, is debatable.

3) Breast

This is the only cancer in which screening reduces the mortality rate (proven in randomized controlled trials), in women above 40. Annual mammography (by a single oblique view) is highly sensitive and specific with low radiation hazard and cost: 20% of detected cancers are preinvasive. Breast self examination (BSE), which should commence form 3rd decade of life, needs greater publicity in the general population. Although widely advocated, its sensitivity, specificity and effectiveness in reducing overall mortality, lack statistical support at the present time. MRI may be more sensitive but its availability and cost precludes its routine application, except in distinctly high risk group.

4) Lung

The multifocal, often bilateral, distribution of lung cancers along with their rapid growth rate make attempts to control mortality by screening, disappointing. Chest x-ray and sputum cytology combined and repeated at 4-monthly intervals detect nearly 90% of cases especially in high risk groups. Neither of them is sufficiently sensitive on its own; x-rays lack specificity whereas with cytology localization of lesion is difficult. Health education aimed at primary prevention and measures to curtail cigarette smoking seem much more profitable means of control.

5) Large intestine

a. Identification and treatment of premalignant conditions, e.g. polyposis coli.

Jewels of Gyan - 61.1

General guidelines to reduce cancer risk

- Consumption of tobacco in any form to be avoided
- Optimal weight (BMI) has to be maintained
- Regular physical activity to be maintained
- Plenty of fruits, vegetables and fibre to be consumed
- The quantity of alcohol (if habituated) has to be watched
- Skin has to be protected against direct exposure to sun
- The level of radiation received in profession has to be watched
- Hormones, such as contraceptives, HRT etc have to be used with extreme caution
- Any benign lesion noticed, must be reviewed by a physician
- Knowledge about yourself, your family, predecessors
- Regular check-ups as recommended for cancer screening have to be carried out

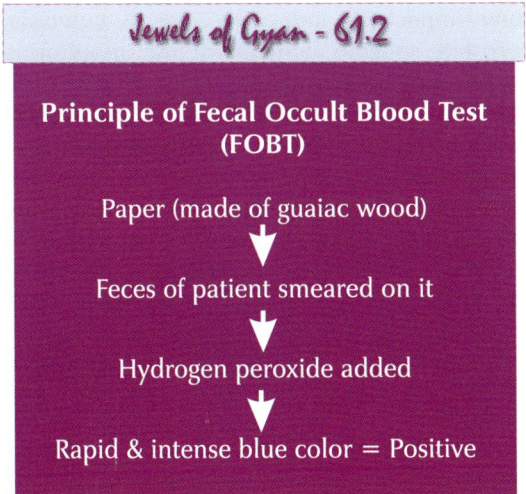

Jewels of Gyan - 61.2

Principle of Fecal Occult Blood Test (FOBT)

Paper (made of guaiac wood)

↓

Feces of patient smeared on it

↓

Hydrogen peroxide added

↓

Rapid & intense blue color = Positive

b. Routine sigmoidoscopic/colonoscopic screening (practised in USA) is not very cost effective and not acceptable to the general population. However, annual screening is essential for those who had colonic cancer resected or polyp excised.

c. Guaiac-impregnated filter paper test for occult blood (do-it-yourself test) is a promising new screening tool. The specimen can be mailed to a laboratory for analysis. The test lacks specificity (bleeding gums after brushing the teeth may give false positive results, often leading to upper/lower GI endoscopy, which are neither pleasant to get done nor cost-effective. Low compliance because of disinclination for taking a fecal sample is another problem.

d. Immunology-based hemoccult tests are most sensitive and specific in detecting occult GI hemorrhage.

General recommendations for Colorectal cancer (CRC) and polyps

Beginning at age 50, both men and women should follow one of these protocols:

Tests that find polyps and cancer, carried every 5 years:

Flexible sigmoidoscopy or colonoscopy
Double-contrast barium enema, and

CT colonography or virtual colonoscopy

A CT scan of the abdomen and colonoscopy should be included while investigating for unexplained weight loss or anemia, above the age 40.

Tests that primarily find cancer carried every year:

Fecal occult blood test (FOBT)

Fecal immunochemical test (FIT)

Stool DNA test (sDNA), interval uncertain, may be less frequent

Of course, if any of the above tests is positive, a colonoscopy should be done.

6) Urinary bladder

Workers exposed to carcinogenic chemicals in their occupation (e.g. rubber and dye industry) may be screened by urinary cytology at 6-monthly intervals. Its sensivity, specificity and effectiveness need to be evaluated. Detecting frank or microscopic hematuria warrents cystopic evaluation. So also those who were treated for bladder carcinoma need annual examination.

7) Thyroid

First-degree relatives of patients with medullary thyroid carcinoma (MTC) may be screened by measuring calcitonin levels (20% of these carcinomas have a familial history with an autosomal dominant inheritance). The role of thyroglobulin estimation in detecting early differentiated cancers is not well established, probably it is more useful in postoperative surviellance.

8) Endometrial (uterine) cancer

The American Cancer Society recommends that at the time of menopause, all women should be informed about the risks and symptoms of endometrial cancer. Women on longterm tamoxifen therapy may increase the risk of developing endometrial cancer. Postmenopausal spotting has to be viewed with high suspicion. Routine annual hysteroscopic endometrial biopsy recommended by some

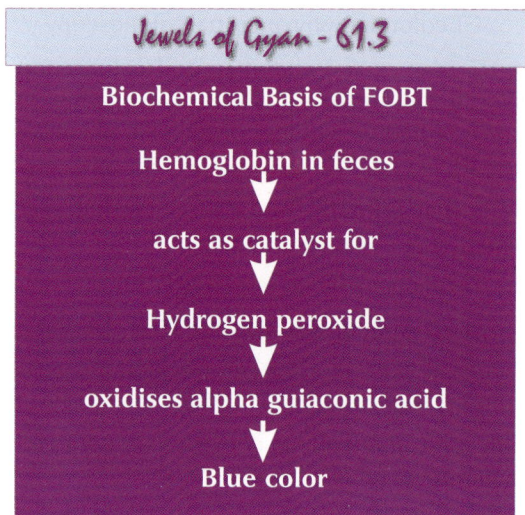

Jewels of Gyan - 61.3

Biochemical Basis of FOBT

Hemoglobin in feces

↓

acts as catalyst for

↓

Hydrogen peroxide

↓

oxidises alpha guiaconic acid

↓

Blue color

any impact in improving overall survivals, prostate-specific antigen (PSA) monitoring appears to be sensitive and cost-effective test for early detection. The trend of elevation in serial estimation may be more significant than a single measurement. More aggressive screening may be needed for the subgroup having benign enlargement and if father or brother had prostate cancer, before the age of 65. It is important that blood sample for PSA and acid phosphatase estimation should be drawn, before carrying out digital rectal examination, if the index of suspicion of cancer is high, since prostatic massage may release these markers into blood stream, giving false high values.

oncologists, may be ideal, but not considered practical for general population and limited to high risk (and affordable) group.

9) Prostate

Notwithstanding the ongoing debate, if screening tests for prostate cancer had made

Ultimately it has to be realized that 'paranoid' health consciousness of general public and exercising high index of suspicion by the physician are the key factors in early detection of malignancies, thereby improving the prospects of potential cure.

62 Volkmann's Ischemic Contracture

Definition: This is an ischemic fibrosis and contracture of the muscles and tendons in the flexor compartment of the forearm usually following a supracondylar fracture of the elbow, also known as *anterior compartment syndrome* of the forearm.

Clinical background

This is a sequel to a tightly applied plaster of paris (PoP), after reduction of a fracture around the elbow, more readily seen in patients who are hypotensive due to other reasons, with decreased effective perfusion pressure. The increase in pressure causes first venous and then arterial obstruction at the elbow, causing acute ischemia of the entire muscles of flexor compartment of forearm. The ischemic necrosis (infarction) is followed by fibrosis and contracture of the affected muscles.

Normal tissue pressure is less than 10mm Hg and if it exceeds 30, perfusion to soft tissue in including muscle, is impaired.

3 stages of pathology (Tsuge and Green).

Acute stage of vascular crisis (about 24 hrs).

Subacute evolutionary or parietic stage (up to 6 months).

Chronic stage of established contracture,

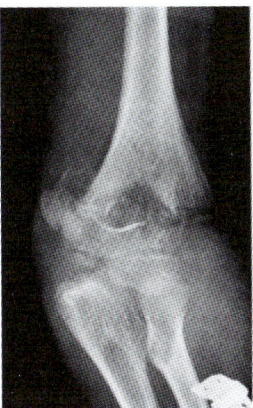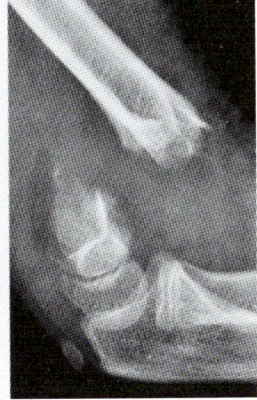

Fig. 62.1. Grossly displaced supracondylar fracture of humerus, vulnerable for VIC

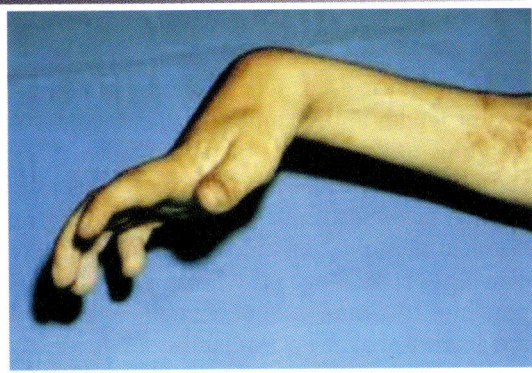

Fig. 62.2. Volkmann's deformity

classified as mild, moderate and severe types.

If the muscle damage is minimal, patient may develop features of effort-induced compartment syndrome in due course, experiencing pain and paresthesia on exercise.

Clinical features

Following the closed reduction and application of an above-elbow cylindrical cast, for a fracture (commonly supracondylar humerus), the patient complains of pain and coldness of the forearm and hand, with impaired capillary filling of nail beds and digital pulps. The movements of wrist and fingers are painful and restricted, particularly passive extension of the latter. These manifestations, along with paresthesia, appearing a few hours after immobilization in PoP, should ring the warning bells, calling for immediate decompression.

Absence of radial pulse may be a late sign, because of its superficial course in forearm and anterior interosseous artery is the first to be affected. However, if the radial pulse is clinically absent, angiographic evaluation may be helpful to identify injury to brachial artery, related to original trauma. Altered sensation due to ischemia of nerves is noticed within 30 min. Ischemia more than 4 hours is critical and irreversible damage occurs after 12 hours.

Liberal fasciotomy on either side of forearm

(sometimes dorsum of hand), may be necessary, if decompression by PoP release is not yielding desirable revascularization.

If the situation is allowed to persist, irreparable ischemic damage occurs in the volar forearm and hand muscles, as seen by motor weakness, loss of length and volume, the flexor tendons standing out in the distal forearm. The sensations are usually unaffected unless the median nerve also suffers ischemic injury. The classical sign of Volkmann's contracture is the clawing of all fingers, whose extension is possible to some extent, when wrist and metacarpo-phalangeal (MP) joints are passively flexed, in contrast to ulnar/median clawing; where such a maneuver makes extension of fingers ineffective, by relaxing the interrossei and lumbricals.

Volkmann's effect: when wrist is extended, fingers go into flexion and when the wrist is flexed, fingers can be extended

Bunnell deformity: wrist flexed, forerarm pronated, thumb is adducted.

Tsuge's classification:

I) mild form: only deep flexors of forearm are involved.

ii) moderate form: deep and superficial groups are affected.

iii) severe form: flexors and extensors are affected.

Differential diagnosis

Ulnar claw with or without median component (vide supra), absence of quick movements and sensory loss pertaining to the area of the nerve affected are the clinching features in the diagnosis of peripheral nerve lesions.

Dupuytren's contracture: The movements of the wrist is not affected, nor do they influence the attitude of the fingers. Medial fingers are affected more often and extensors are never involved.

Prevention

This condition is best prevented by careful observation during the first 12 hours after elbow immobilization, when the edema is expected to occur. Many prefer to use a PoP slab, to a cylindrical cast, initially, to avoid circumferential compression, till the traumatic swelling subsides, to be replaced by a full cast, a week or so later. If early ischemic changes indicated above are seen, the POP should be slit open for decompression of the compartment, immediately. The flexion of elbow should be reduced till good vascularity is restored, before further immobilization, with liberal cotton padding. Elevation and antiedema therapy are useful adjuncts for optimal results.

Treatment

In patients seen late, because of initial delay in identification of such a complication, subcutaneous fasciotomy has to be carried out without procrastination, to break the chain of events; more ischemia ⇒ more edema ⇒ more compression ⇒ more ischemia and further vascular compromise.

In established cases of Volkmann's contracture, a *muscle sliding procedure* (of Max-Page), by releasing and shifting distally the common flexor origin from the medial epicondyle of humerus, to gain length for the major tendons along with long term physiotherapy, can reduce disability. Other procedures employed are excision of the fibrous parts of the flexor muscles and rarely arthrodesis of wrist, in the functional position.

Recent additions: Tendon transfer to motorize the flexor pollicis longus (FPL) and digitorum longus (FDL) or functional free transfer of gracilis muscle, to restore wrist and finger movements, are currently employed in some centres.

63 Hand

Surgical principles: The hand is an organ of grasp, sensation and expression and requires a combination of movements at the shoulder, elbow and wrist to place the hand in an optimal position for function, hence the hand should never be treated in isolation from the upper limb.

The problems of the hand demand careful assessment based on a thorough understanding of anatomy and functions. Surgery, for other than ischemia and infections, is preferably done under a pneumatic tourniquet, to achieve a dry field allowing precise dissections. For fingers, a soft silastic band is the best tourniquet. Regional block, such as brachial, axillary, Bier's (intravenous), wrist or digital block, is ideal for cooperative patients, but a general anesthetic is preferred for children as well as in acute infections. *Adrenaline* should never be mixed with lignocaine used for digital block, for fear of inducing lasting vasoconstriction and digital ischemia.

Deep palmar spaces

These are potential spaces wherein infection may occur and pus collects, situated between the interosseous aponeurosis (covering the interossei and metacarpals) posteriorly and long flexor tendons and their lumbricals anteriorly. The middle palmar space lies between the 3rd metacarpal bone to the hypothenar eminence and separated from thenar space by a strong fibrous septum. The thenar space lies between the 3rd metacarpal bone and tendon of flexor pollicis longus. Best access for these spaces, to avoid synovial bursae and neurovascular structures, is through the corresponding webspace.

Surgery on the hand is delicate, the importance of necessary techniques of accurate suturing and atraumatic handling of tissues, with specially designed fine instruments, can never be overemphasized. Carefully applied dressings, with adequate padding with fluffed gauze or cotton wool held with gentle elastic

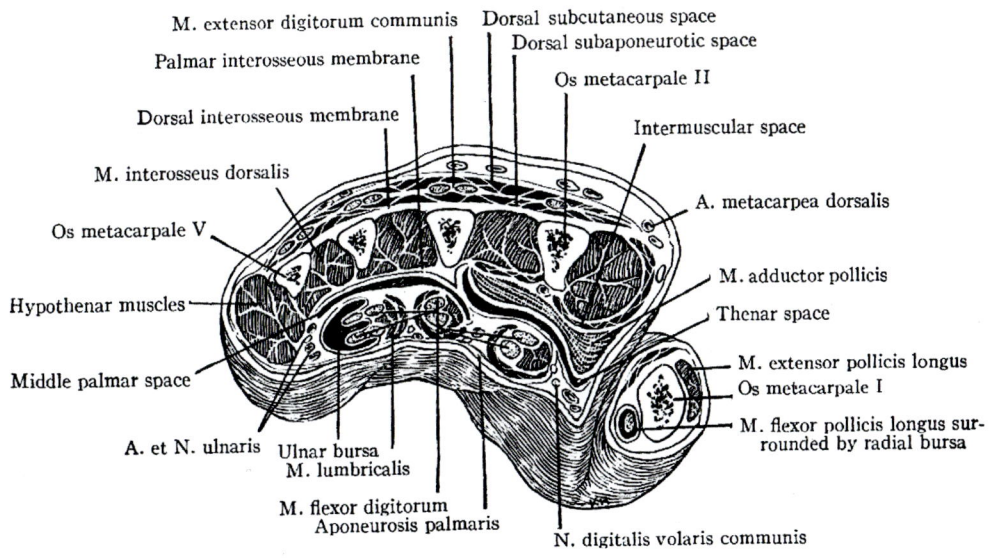

Fig. 63.1. Cross section of the hand showing palmar spaces

bandage in a comfortable and physiological position and postoperative elevation, by hanging the hand to a saline stand, are essential routines in hand surgery. The optimal position of immobilization is the James position which is 90° flexion of metacarpophalangeal (MP) joints, slight flexion of interphalangeal (IP) and dorsiflexion of wrist joints with the thumb in the neutral position. This is best achieved by a well padded volar plaster slab extending up to the tips of the fingers. A forearm sling is essential for an ambulatory patient.

Incisions should not cross flexor creases, as the resultant scar may restrict movements. They should be placed obliquely across the lines or in neutral areas, such as lateral aspects of fingers. Precise orientation of neurovascular anatomy is important during sharp dissections, while under a tourniquet eliminating arterial pulsations, which normally help to identify the vascular pedicles.

Infections

Acute suppurative infection of hand and fingers is known as a *whitlow*.

Etiology

i)   manual laborers, house wives and tailors
ii) diabetes mellitus
iii) ischemia, as in thoracic outlet syndrome
iv) neurological diseases such as syringo-myelia, tabes dorsalis etc.

They are mostly due to staphylococcus aureus, streptococcus pyogenes and Gm negative bacilli. Suppuration can be prevented by aggressive treatment with wide spectrum antibiotics, in the stage of cellulitis, but having once occurred, early detection, localization and adequate drainage, under continued antibiotic cover, guided by microbiological study, is of utmost importance.

Clinical types

1. Acute and chronic paronychia

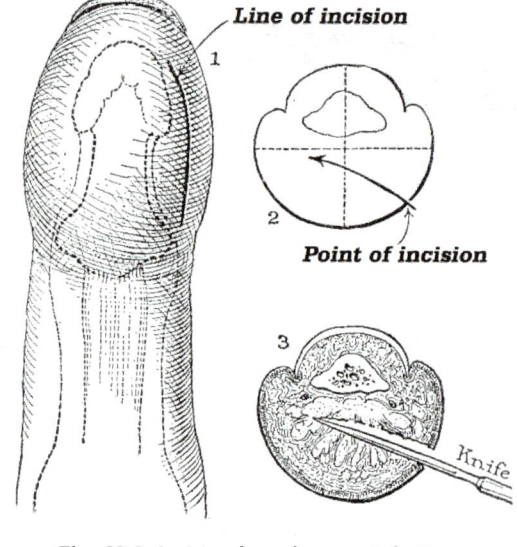

Fig. 63.3. Incision for pulp space infection of the finger

2. Pulp space and subungual infections
3. Infection of the web space
4. Acute suppurative tenosynovitis and infection of the space of Parona
5. Subcutaneous infection and abscesses
6. Osteomyelitis and septic arthritis

Morvan's disease is the recurrent whitlow seen in syringomylia.

ACUTE PARONYCHIA

It is the commonest hand infection, which is subcuticular and under the eponychium; it arises from the nail bed. Suppuration usually follows with adherence of the eponychium to the base of the nail. The pus tends to track around the cutaneous margin and in 40% of cases under the nail.

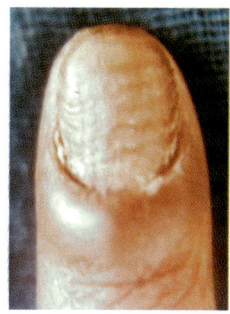

Fig. 63.2. Acute paronychia (courtesy: Prof T Gunasagaran, Chennai)

It is treated by draining the pus under a digital block with 2% lignocaine, but a general anesthetic is preferred by many, in view of possible cellulitis or lymphangitis at the base of the digit. The eponychium is gently and completely stripped from the nail. Often parts of the eponychium and nail fold need excision and the wound is allowed to granulate. Floating nail is probably nonviable, and should be eased out, allowing a new one to grow.

CHRONIC PARONYCHIA

Mostly seen in housemaids due to various etiologies (e.g. yeast, fungus) The chronic process has an occasional flare up and it does not respond to antibiotics or local antifungal ointment, but systemic antimycotic agents may be effective. Rarely ablation of the nail bed is necessary to eradicate infection.

PULP SPACE INFECTION (syn: felon)

It is the second most common infection of the hand and usually develops from a pin/thorn prick or infected pulp hematoma, due to repeated trauma, as seen in those using percussion musical instruments.

Surgical anatomy of the space

This space is separated from the middle pulp space by the attachment of deep fascia, to the base of the distal phalanx and is traversed by multiple fibrous septa. The arterial branches to the epiphysis of distal phalanx do not transverse this space. So the epiphysis is unaffected when the infective process leads to osteomyelitis of distal phalanx, due to thromboarteritis of the arterial twigs in this space.

Clinical features

Dull pain, worse at night and exaggerated in dependent position of the limb, is seen with indurated/fluctuant pulp. An untreated abscess may take the shape of a collar-stud, with subcuticular extension. Regional lymph nodes become enlarged and tender. It has to be differentiated from herpetic whitlow, sometimes seen in dental workers.

Treatment

Given early enough, wide spectrum antibiotics may prevent suppuration or cause localization of pus. Drainage is done by incising the abscess at the point of maximum tenderness, but an incision over the volar aspect should be avoided, as it leaves a tender scar. Some essential points during drainage are:

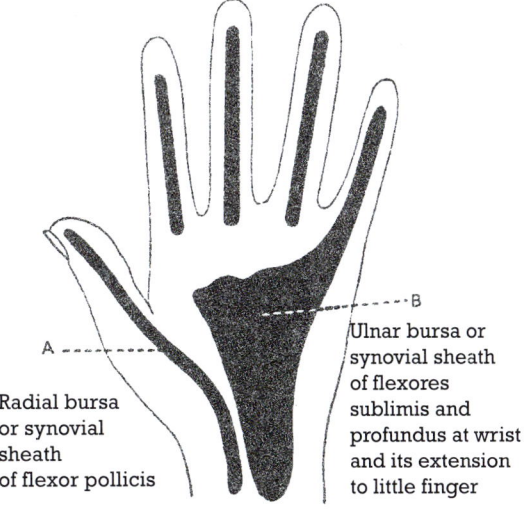

Fig. 63.4. Fascial spaces and synovial bursae of the hand

i) lateral incision of the pulp space
ii) all fibrous septa should be divided as the pus is multiloculated, by making a through and through cut across the pulp
iii) not to damage the periosteum of terminal phalanx
iv) all slough should be removed
v) closure of the wound to be avoided

Serial radiographs are necessary if osteomyelitis of the terminal phalanx is suspected.

Acute subungual infection

This usually results from an infected subungual hematoma from a pin prick or broken splinter and the condition is often termed an apical abscess. The margins of the nail become exquisitely tender. Treatment is by broad spectrum antibiotics along with V shaped excision of the nail edges. This can be prevented by draining the hematoma in a novel manner; the tip of an open safety pin is made red hot in a candle flame and the nail (which has no sensations) over the blood clot is punctured, creating exit for the tense hematoma, with prompt relief of pain.

Web space infection

The web spaces are the three triangular regions between the dorsal and volar aspects of skin, filled with loose fat, which bulges between the

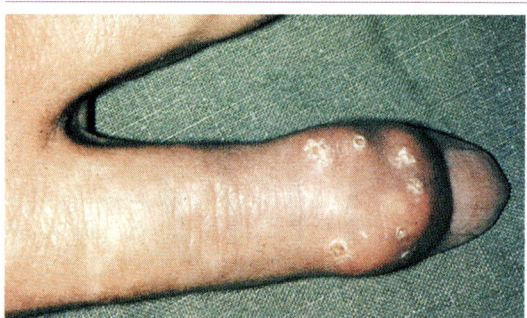

Fig. 63.5. Fungal granuloma of digit
(courtesy: Lifeline Hospitals, Chennai)

divisions of the palmar fascia. Infection in these spaces usually originate from punctured wounds, when pus accumulates here, saddling the deep transverse ligament, it finds the dorsal skin least resistant for pointing.

Clinical features

The base of the fingers is swollen and the adjacent fingers are separated in severe cases. The maximum tenderness is found in the web. If untreated the pus can track to the adjacent web space. Drainage of pus is done by a transverse incision on the palmar aspect of the space. When it communicates with a dorsal pocket, a counter incision may be necessary. If two web spaces are affected, they should be drained by separate incisions.

Acute suppurative tenosynovitis

Features

Acute suppurative tenosynovitis involves the whole sheath rapidly and is the most feared of all infections of the hand. There is uniform swelling of the entire finger and tenderness along the sheath, with slight flexion of all joints due to pain, which is aggravated by extension of the digit (hook sign). Pus within the tendon sheath destroys the gliding mechanism, creates adhesions and consequently restricts movements.

Treatment

Always surgical, under general anesthesia, approach is normally made by a mid-axial incision (along the axis of joint motion). However, the recent technique for exposing these flexor sheath infections is by double incisions, one in the distal palm over the proximal sheath at the level of the distal palmar crease and a second mid-axial incision, at the distal end of the sheath at the DIP joint and to irrigate the sheath with normal saline by introducing a small intravenous catheter, which is left in-situ for postoperative antibiotic irrigation.

Complications

Involvement of the forearm (Parona's space) from the hand, is due to bursting of abscess either into the radial or ulnar bursa proximally and the pus is bounded ventrally by the long flexor tendons and dorsally by the pronator quadratus muscle. Extension of the abscess into the forearm can be identified while draining an abscess in the palm, by applying pressure above the wrist, to see if pus comes out, when another incision should also be made in the forearm to drain the space of Parona, leaving a soft (Penrose) drain.

Perpetuation of the suppurative process is probably due to extension of sepsis to the fascial spaces. Suppurative arthritis of a rela-ted joint with stiff digit, may even need an arthrodesis or amputation of the digit occasionally. Median nerve palsy may occur, which can be prevented by early decompression of the carpel tunnel.

Deep palmar abscess

Modes of infection include penetrating wound, infection of a hematoma by blood borne organisms and extension of infection from suppurative tenosynovitis.

Surgical anatomy

The deep spaces of the hand are located between the deep flexor tendons and the interossei and metacarpals dorsally. This subtendinous palmar area is divided into a thenar space and the mid palmar space.

Clinical features

Localized swellings, redness and tenderness present. The patient is invariably a manual worker. The edematous swelling of the dorsum of the hand is so great, that it is often referred to as the 'frog hand'. Extension of MP joints is very painful, but extension of IP joints are both painless and free and this differentiates it from suppurative tenosynovitis As tension mounts the normal concavity of the palm becomes flattened and gradually the palm become convex.

Treatment

Under general anesthesia, a central transverse incision is made in the line of the flexion crease passing across the middle of the palm. Should pus be encountered beneath the aponeurosis, then location of pus at a deeper plane should be made, by probing of the palmar fascia by a sinus forceps and drained.

Subcutaneous infection

These can occur on the dorsal and volar surfaces at various level and the varieties are intraepidermal abscess, intradermal abscess, subcutaneous abscess, collar-stud abscess.

Other infections
Madura mycosis

This is due to infection with Norcardia madurae and is similar to madura foot (chapter 70).

Orf (syn: contagious pustular dermatitis)

It is a viral infection of the hands, transmitted in the saliva of sheep, running a self-limiting course (3-6 weeks), the red papules becoming nodules of reddish blue turning grey. Treatment is conservative.

Pilonidal sinus described in chapter 26.

Barber's pilonidal sinus is due to the customer's clippings penetrating the skin, most frequently the web between ring and middle fingers of the left hand. In the non-inflamed state the lesion is marked by a small black dot with a collarette of epithelial scales around it. A cyst like nodule can be palpated beneath the visible lesion. Recurrent attacks of subacute or acute inflammation in the sinus prompt the patient to seek relief by excision.

Common tumors of digits

SCC and Melanoma: described in chapters 20 and 22.

Glomus tumor (syn: chemodectoma, glomangioma, angioneuromyoma)

They arise from specialized tissue called glomus apparatus consists of tortuous arterioles directly communicating with venules, surrounded by network of small nerves and large clear cells (glomus cells). These chemosensitive organs are purple in color, found in limbs, especially the nail beds, regulate the temperature of skin. It is a small compressible nodule, with pain out of proportion to the size, sometimes triggered by the exposure of limb to sudden changes in external temperature. They grow very slowly with low potential to turn malignant.

Inflation of a BP cuff over the limb proximal to the tumor elicits severe pain at the site of the lesion, since it is highly vascular. If the cuff is inflated above the systolic pressure, the pain gets relieved, to reappear while it is being deflated (Hildreth's sign).

Treatment: Excision is curative. It is not a radiosensitive tumor.

syn; chronic tenovaginitis or enthesopathy

This is due to thickening of the fibrous sheath leading to difficulty/limitation of movements of the tendons within it and may be considered a type of 'tunnel syndrome'. Common sites for this disease are at the wrist (de Quervain's disease) and in the palm (trigger finger).

Certain conditions like hypothyroidism, diabetes mellitus, focus of sepsis etc may be associated, though their causal relation is unclear. Autoimmune connective tissue disorders may be complicated by these conditions.

De QUERVAIN'S DISEASE

Definition: This is an idiopathic inflammation of subacute nature, affecting the tendons of the abductor pollicis longus (APL) and extensor pollicis brevis (EPB), in their common sheath, running in a groove on the lateral aspect of the distal radius, under the extensor retinaculum of the wrist (first extensor compartment).

Etiology: It is considered to be due to an autoimmune disorder and recurrent trauma may determine the site of affection. A fibrous sheath loosely holds these two tendons as they travel along the lateral border of the lower third of the

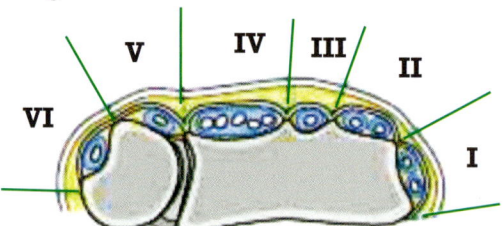

Fig. 64.1. Extensor compartments over the back of the wrist

I   Abductor pollicis longus and extensor pollicis brevis.
II Extensor carpi radialis longus and brevis.
III Extensor pollicis longus.
IV Extensor digitorum longus and extensor indicis.
V   Extensor digiti minimi.
VI Extensor carpi ulnari

radius and the inflammatory process narrows the osteofascial tunnel, causing stenosis or entrapment. Progressive degenerative diseases of fascia and tendons, such as senile enthesopathy (enthesis: insertion of muscles and tendons), may also be a contributory factor.

Clinical features

Just above the radial styloid process, a tender lump is palpable, resembling an exostosis, occasionally with a crepitus, produced by movements of the tendons (wet leather sign). Careful proximal and distal palpation often reveals the two tendons, involved in a nonspecific inflammation. As can be expected, abduction and extension of thumb will be restricted and forcible ulnar deviation (adduction) of the wrist causes severe pain, due to the stretching of these tendons (*Finkelstein's sign*).

Differential diagnosis

i)   Exostosis: bony swelling, not tender
ii) Ganglion: circumscribed, cystic, non-tender, swelling, tethered to the underlying joint capsule, typically located in the middle of the wrist posteriorly.
iii) Aschoff bodies (rheumatic arthropathy) and tophi (gout).
iv) Heberden's nodes (bony thickening of DIP joints) and Bouchard's nodes (thickening of PIP joints) seen in osteoarthrosis.
v)   Benign tumors arising from the sheath of the tendons such as synovioma, fibroma etc.
vi) Tuberculous tenosynovitis
Vii) Arthritis of first carpo-metacarpal joint

Specific investigations

X-Ray wrist: to rule out bony lesion. No other specific investigations are required to diagnose this condition. As there is a slightly higher incidence in autoimmune diseases, like rheumatoid arthritis, the necessary investigations may be done, if other features exist. Diabetes mellitus, myxedema, hyperuricemia etc. have to be routinely excluded.

Treatment

1. Rest, splinting wrist in abduction
2. Local injection of depot steroids like triamcinolone acetate and vigorous physiotherapy to the limbs may be helpful. Systemic administration of NSAIDs to relieve pain and stanazolol (the Olympic steroid) to discourage unwanted fibroblastic activity, have been found to be beneficial in these patients.
3. If these measures fail to resolve the process, surgery may be required, but rarely. Under regional block and a tourniquet, the constricting sheath is exposed through a vertical incision on the lateral border of distal radius, which is slit open or partially excised and the two tendons are released. At the conclusion of the surgery a long acting steroid is infiltrated into the sheath, to prevent postoperative fibrosis and recurrence. After releasing the tourniquet and proper hemostasis, the wound is closed in layers and compression dressing applied.

TRIGGER FINGER
(syn: snapping finger)

This is due to stenosing tenosynovitis of the fibrous sheaths or pulleys of the long flexors of fingers or nodular thickening of these tendons (typically the sublimus tendon), forming a trigger-like resistance to their free movement during flexion and extension; sometimes the latter movement is possible only by the help of the other hand.

It occurs in middle age with female preponderance. The etiology is not clear, repeated trauma, diabetes, rheumatoid arthritis have been incriminated.

Trigger thumb

This is a rare condition due to congenital construction of tendon sheath of flexor pollicis longus at the level of first MP joint. It may be bilateral. The child keeps the IP joint of the thumb in flexion and attempt at forcible extension suddenly releases the thumb into full extension with a 'click'. A small nodule may be palpable over the tendon at that level.

Clinical features

It may be seen in children, when the thumb is often involved, whereas in adults, the long flexors of ring, middle index and little fingers are affected in that order of frequency. The patient experiences a painless snap during the movements of the finger, once past the constricting point, the rest of the movement is normal. A tender thickening or nodule may be felt, at about the level of the MP joint (distal palmar crease) of the affected digit.

The flexed finger can be unlocked by passively flexing the MP joint and extending the IP joints (Lapidus test)

Investigations

Same as de Quervain's disease

Treatment

Medical therapy with NSAIDs, ultrasound massage, local infiltration of steroids may relieve any discomfort, but have no curative role, in this disease.

Surgery, by open or closed division of flexor pulley, gives excellent results; under regional block, using a tourniquet, the fibrous sheath of the flexor tendon is exposed, by a transverse skin incision (over distal palmar crease) and a longitudinal incision of the palmar aponeurosis (to avoid injury to neurovascular structures). The thickened constriction around the tendon is identified and is 'deroofed', by partial excision. The movements of the finger are tested, to satisfy the free slide of the tendon in that area, before the tourniquet is released. Only skin is sutured, a boxing glove compression dressing is applied and hand kept elevated for 24hours, following which active and passive movements of the finger are begun.

65 Carpal Tunnel Syndrome

Definition: Symptom-complex of median nerve compression, seen when there is increased pressure in the carpal tunnel of the wrist, under the flexor retinaculum.

Etiology

Occurs more in middle-aged women, obesity, hypothyroidism, acromegaly, osteoarthrosis, fracture/dislocations around the wrist, tenosynovitis of flexor tendons, fibrositis related to a focus of sepsis and autoimmune connective disorders, such as rheumatoid arthritis, have all been incriminated in causing this condition. Rarely it is also seen in pregnancy, congestive cardiac failure (due to fluid retention) and as an occupational disease in those performing forceful and repetitive movements of the hand. It may be feature in Hunter's or Hurler's syndromes.

Pathology

The median nerve coursing under the flexor retinaculum (transverse carpal ligament), along with long flexors is vulnerable for compression, with the slightest encroachment of the narrow space, due to any of the reasons mentioned above, resulting in specific sensory and motor disturbances.

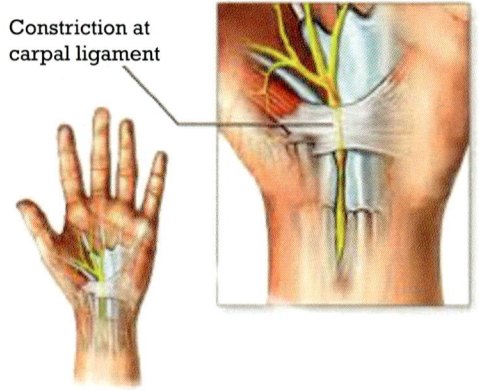

Constriction at carpal ligament

Fig. 65.1. Anatomy of the carpal tunnel

Clinical features

i) Pain and *paresthesia* occurring more at night, along the distribution of the median nerve, over the lateral 3½ fingers, are seen. The thenar emimence is not involved, since this area is supplied by its palmar branch, arising from median nerve at a higher point, travelling superficial to the retinaculum. The pain may radiate to the whole arm.

ii) weakness and wasting of thenar group of muscles, typically with loss of opposition of thumb and clumsiness of the fine movement of the hand. LOAF: lumbricals (radial two), opponens pollicis, abductor pollicis brevis and flexor pollicis brevis are affected.

iii) Tinel's sign: digital pressure over the flexor retinaculum aggravates symptoms within 30 seconds.

iv) *Phalen's maneuver* is gravity-induced wrist flexion which reproduces symptoms within a minute.

Differential diagnosis

Cervical spondylosis, cervical cord compression, nerve injuries, brachial neuralgia, thoracic outlet compression, Hansen's disease etc.

The ulnar nerve, which passes superficial to the retinaculum, is encased in a canal (of Guyon), in relation to pisiform bone, by a slender slip of fascia, known as the superficial part of the retinaculum, which may occasionally cause compression of the nerve.

Investigations

They are done more to exclude other conditions. Nerve conduction studies and CT/MRI scan are diagnostic. A routine x-ray, including the 'carpal tunnel view' is equally informative and cost-effective.

Treatment

Conservative: Treatment of any predisposing condition (vide supra) is important, along with symptomatic therapy with NSAIDs and antiedema agents. Local infiltration of deposteroids may be tried, which rarely cures but makes the patient request for surgery, since the injection into the nerve may sometimes worsen symptoms !

Splints to maintain neutral or slightly extended position of wrist, worn more at night may offer symptomatic relief, if they are associated with other predisposing diseases.

Surgery

This requires complete division of the transverse carpal ligament, by a longitudinal incision, distal to the wrist crease, upto the cardinal line of Kaplan (a line drawn across the palm, at the level of distal border of the hyperextended thumb, to indicate the level at which the median nerve gives off its muscular branches in the hand), under regional anesthesia, using a tourniquet. Careful identification of the palmar branch and twigs to thenar muscles and protection is important. The median nerve often shows an hourglass contriction at the compression point, which should be left untouched, to avoid neurapraxia and adhesions.

A single port endoscopic division of the ligament is becoming increasingly popular, but has a slightly higher incidence of injury to the nerve branches mentioned and incomplete division of the retinaculum, hence requires further evaluation.

Unrelieved symptoms after surgery are due to:

i)   incomplete division of the retinaculum

ii) inaccurate preoperative diagnosis

iii) overlooked functional component in the symptoms

This may be avoided by careful preoperative electrophysiological and if necessary psychiatric evaluation, complemented by meticulous surgery.

66 Dupuytren's Contracture

Definition: This is a diffuse proliferative disorder involving the palmar aponeurosis, resulting in nodularity and shortening of its longitudinal fibers and flexion deformity of metacarpophalangeal (MP) and proximal interphalangeal (PIP) joints, mostly involving the ring and little fingers. The thumb, index and middle (lateral three) fingers are rarely involved.

Etiology

Mostly seen in Caucasians with familial transmission as an autosomal dominant trait with variable penetrance. It is seen in the fourth decade, often bilateral, with a male preponderance. Repeated micro trauma leading to myofibroblastic contracture may be a factor. The disease may start in the fascia and extends to the overlying skin or vice versa, hence considered as fascio-dermal disease (Hueston). Conditions seen in association with this disease are:

i)   alcoholic cirrhosis

ii) diabetes mellitus

iii) Peyronie's disease of penis

iv) keloids and scar hypertrophy

v)   plantar fasciitis and fibromatosis

vi) epilepsy on phenytoin therapy

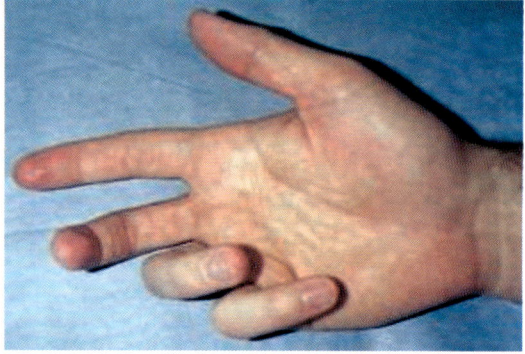

Fig. 66.1. Dupuytren's contracture

Pathology

The disease has three stages, namely proliferative, involutional and residual (Luck). It is essentially an inflammatory fibrosis of the aponeurosis and tissue overlying it, leading to contraction of newly formed collagen. Similar nodules may also appear in other locations, such as dorsal aspect of PIP joints, fascia over anteromedial forearm (covering the flexor carpi ulnaris), tendocalcaneus (Achilles tendon). An autoimmune process has been incriminated in its pathogenesis, without concrete evidence.

Clinical features

In established disease, there is no difficulty in diagnosis, but it may not be so in early stages. Typically seen in a male, between 30-50, with bilateral involvement, though not symmetrical, presenting with progressive flexion deformity of MP and PIP joints of medial two fingers, the so-called *coachman's hand*. Nodularity and obvious shortening of the palmar aponeurosis, making it stand out, when a passive attempt is made to straighten the fingers, are pathognomonic. Typically the joint deformities are unaffected by wrist movements, in contrast to ulnar/median clawing or Volkmann's contracture. Knuckle (Garrod's) pads over the affected PIP joints, related to constant pressure and friction, may be seen.

Associated conditions and nodules in other areas indicated(vide supra) are of corroborative value to the diagnosis.

Differential diagnosis

i)   Volkmann's ischemic contracture

ii) ulnar/median nerve palsy with clawing

iii) severe degree of trigger finger

iv) deformity due to trauma or infection

Investigations

As in trigger finger, studies are only to identify associated disorders

Treatment

Conservative therapy should be tried in the early stages, with NSAIDs, active and passive extension movements of the involved digits, in an attempt to avoid or defer surgery as far as possible.

Poor prognostic features:

Early age of onset

Presence of Garrod's knuckle pads

Number of rays involved

Coexistent epileptic condition

Alcoholism

Indications for surgery:

Painful nodules

Involvement of skin

Contracture of MP or IP joint more than 30°

Surgical procedures

i)   Subcutaneous (closed) fasciotomy of Luck

ii) Partial excision of palmar aponeurosis

iii) Meticulous total excision of the aponeurosis and decompression, is the definitive treatment

iv) Dermofasciectomy with full thickness skin graft.

Common surgical dilemma: too little or too much surgery ?

Postop splinting of the fingers in extension and active movements from 3rd PO day
Passive stetching from 7th day onwards.

v)   Arthrodesis or Amputation of fingers, rarely resorted to, for an insoluble problem to the finger.

67 Ganglion

Definition: A ganglion is mucoid degeneration of a tendon sheath or a joint capsule, which may or may not communicate with the underlying joint, containing clear, gelatinous fluid.

Etiology

Synovial herniation and the bursacular (ganglion arising from a bursa) theory were earlier popular, but now it is believed to be a degeneration of capsular and perisynovial tissue in relation to a joint, causing progressive accumulation of myxoid tissue within a fibrous capsule. Thus every ganglion arises in the vicinity of a joint. Several extensions of the ganglion (like 'pseudopodia') may occur, giving rise to its notoriously high recurrence rate, following excision. Common sites are, around the wrist, ankle and foot (dorsum commoner than ventral, as the dorsal retinacula are thinner than the ventral).

Symptoms

The commonest presentation is a rounded lump adjacent to the joint, pain felt only in later stages with increasing tension, more so with acute movements of the related joint or due to pressure on an underlying nerve (e.g. ulnar nerve).

Signs

It is usually a circumscribed, small (10-15mm), slightly mobile, tensely cystic, smooth, nontender swelling, without local warmth. Its relationship to the underlying tendon can be demonstrated by further restriction of mobility when the related muscle is contracted. The skin is free over the swelling, which exhibits limitation of intrinsic mobility in the axis of the tendon.

Differential diagnosis

1. exostosis
2. sebaceous cyst
3. tumor arising from synovial sheath
4. neurofibroma
5. implantation dermoid cyst
6. arterial aneurysm (clotted)

Investigations

Generally no specific investigations are needed to diagnose a ganglion, in its typical locations. If a situation warrants, the investigation of choice is an MRI, which will delineate the cyst, differentiate it from other swellings and demarcate its attachment to a particular tendon or joint space. Other investigations like an x-ray of the affected joint, etc are directed at ruling out other diagnoses.

Treatment

i) The biblical treatment of direct heavy pressure on the ganglion rupturing it (hitting with a bible!), is still followed by some, but is not very pleasant and has an unacceptably high rate of recurrence.

ii) Sclerotherapy with a sclerosant-steroid combination, after aspiration, is another treatment which also has a high recurrence rate, besides the possibility of introducing infection.

iii) Surgical: Complete excision of the ganglion with all its 'pseudopodia', is definitive and is usually done under regional anesthesia (brachial/axillary or Bier's block), as 'day-care' surgery. Using a tourniquet, the entire swelling is dissected out from the underlying tendon and traced down to the communication to joint space and amputated. Sometimes, deliberate

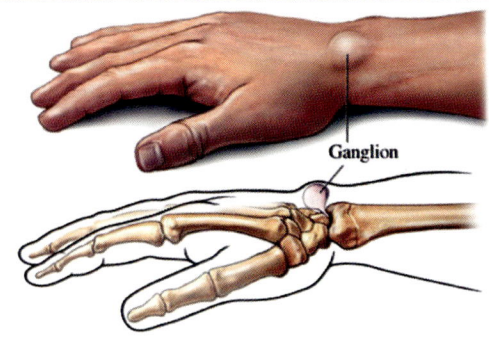

Fig. 67.1. Ganglion, dorsum of wrist

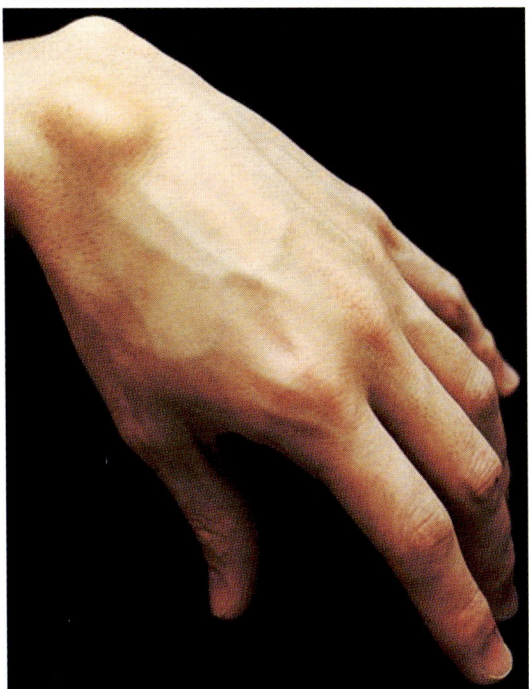

Fig. 67.2. Ganglion dorsum of the left wrist

rupture of the cyst during the initial stage facilitates easy dissection. The resultant gap in the capsule may either be left open or closed with a 'figure of 8' stitch of absorbable material. The excised tissue is subjected to routine histopathological examination, so as not to miss a masquerading tumor of the synovium.

COMPOUND PALMAR GANGLION

Definition: This is a dumb-bell shaped swelling of the common flexor synovial sheath of the wrist, due to chronic inflammation, with a swelling appearing on either side of the flexor retinaculum (transverse carpal ligament). This sheath located in the space of Parona in the lower forearm, extending into the palm, is known as *the ulnar bursa*.

Pathology

The commonest cause is *tuberculosis*, others being connective tissue diseases such as rheumatoid arthritis. Inflammation of the ulnar bursa causes synovial effusion with formation of loose granulomatous bodies, known as *melon*

seed bodies. Initially the process is confined to the forearm, but extends gradually into the palm, under the retinaculum, as the synovial inflammation (pannus) proceeds distally, causing corresponding swelling in the palm. In course of time, the bursa will be lined by granulation tissue and weaken the affected tendons causing their rupture, due even to trivial trauma.

Symptoms

A painful swelling over the forearm and palm in a patient with a background of tuberculosis (young age) or rheumatoid arthritis (middle age) is unmistakable. Constitutional symptoms related to the etiology may be present.

Signs

A tender, cystic swelling over the forearm and palm, with typical transillumination and cross-fluctuation, leads to the clinical diagnosis. Due to inflammatory compression within the carpal tunnel, there may be a sensory/motor deficit, related to median nerve distribution. Spontaneous or traumatic rupture of the affected tendon and wasting of the hand muscles due to disuse and nerve damage may occur.

Differential diagnosis

i) pyogenic infection of the ulnar bursa (pain, fever, warmth, tenderness and history of penetrating injury).

ii) synovial sarcoma of the flexor sheath, usu-

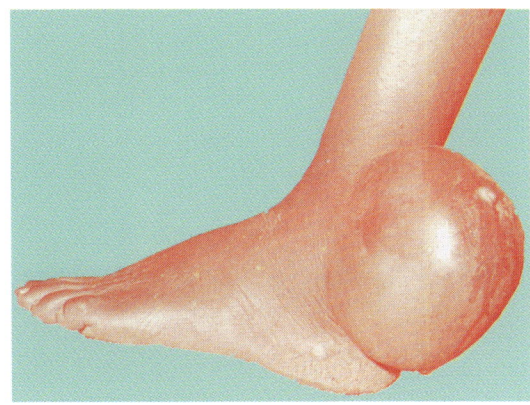

Fig. 67.3. Large ganglion, ankle
(courtesy: Prof. T Gunasagaran, Chennai)

ally dumb-bell shaped, solid without fluctuation, showing appreciable growth.

Investigations

Chest x-ray, ESR, Mantoux, IgA, IgG, IgM and PCR to rule out tuberculosis. Rose Waller test, x-rays of other joints, may be done to detect rheumatoid arthritis.

Treatment

The treatment depends upon the etiology. Repeated aspirations under cover of anti-tuberculous therapy for 6-9months is generally curative. Total excision of the affected synovium, which may turn out to be a tedious exercise, is reserved for failure of adequate medical therapy, producing severe functional disability.

If rheumatoid arthritis is the underlying disease, a total synovectomy may be needed because the pathology originates from the affected synovium (pannus). Unlike in tuberculous compound palmar ganglion, the recurrence rate is much higher in rheumatoid disease.

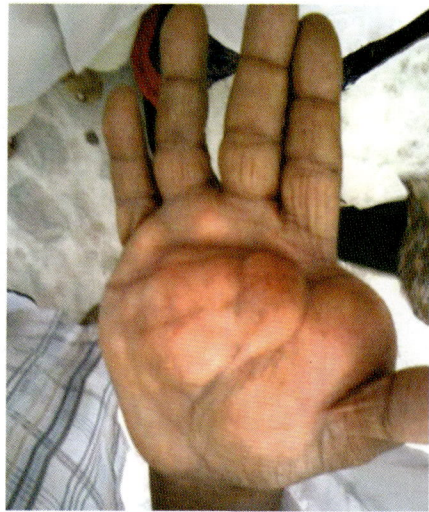

Fig. 67.4. Compound palmar ganglion in tuberculous tenosynovitis
(courtesy: Lifeline Hospitals, Chennai)

Active physiotherapy is essential in all cases, to retain hand/finger movements, which may be affected due to adhesions (synechia) developing within the sheaths, binding the tendons.

68 Bursa

(Bursa: wine-skin, a bag made from animal skin, for holding or dispensing wine)

A *true* bursa is a physiological cystic collection of synovial fluid in relation to a joint or in the interface between a bone and a muscle sliding over it. An *adventitious* (also known as supernumerary) bursa is a pathological collection, without a true synovial lining, acquired in relation to a point of friction, usually against a bony prominence, by the repeated shearing effect on overlying tissues. Unless they are inflamed or infected, bursae are helpful to reduce friction during joint/muscle movements.

Bursae around the knee: These are divided into the anterior, medial, posteromedial and lateral groups.

i) Anterior group

1. Suprapatellar bursa - in front of the lower end of the femur.
2. Prepatellar bursa in front of lower end of the patella.
3. Superficial infrapatellar bursa - in front of the ligamentum patellae and tibial tuberosity.
4. Deep infrapatellar bursa between the ligamentum patellae and tibia.

Of these, the suprapatellar bursa communicates with the knee and swells up in progressive osteoarthrosis of the joint.

Housemaid's knee: Due to frequent kneeling at work, the prepatellar bursa gets enlarged, producing a soft cystic swelling between the skin

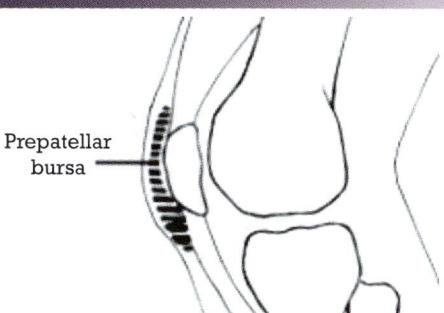
Fig. 68.2. Prepatellar bursa

and the patella. Sebaceous cyst, lipoma, neurofibroma and synovial tumor are the differential diagnosis. Except aspiration of the synovial fluid, which is both diagnostic and therapeutic, no specific investigations are necessary. Following aspiration, to exclude frank infection, local rest and NSAIDs would suffice in most of cases, surgical excision is required only in refractory bursitis.

Preliminary course of appropriate antibiotics should be given, if examination of aspirate reveals infection.

Clergyman's knee: In those who habituate the

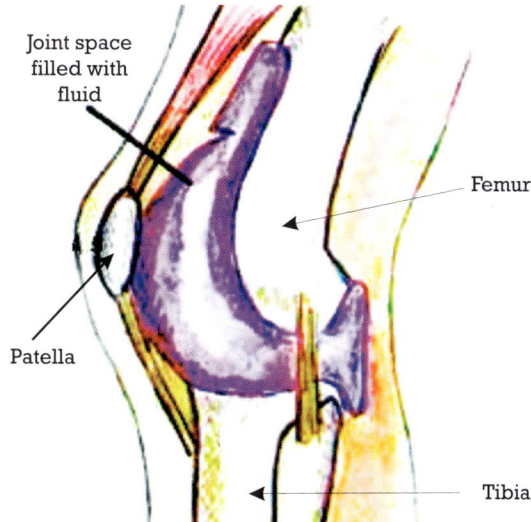

Joint space filled with fluid

Femur

Patella

Tibia

Fig. 68.3. Suprapetaller bursa, as extension of synovial cavity of the knee joint

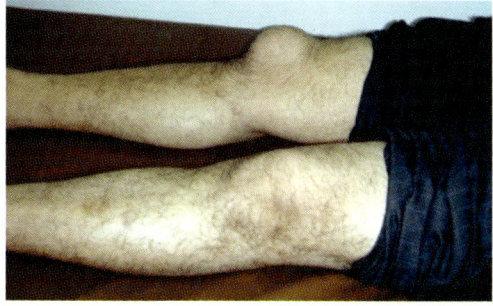
Fig. 68.1. Prepatellar bursa

upright kneeling posture, the infra-patellar area is subjected to repeated pressure, causing deep infrapatellar bursitis. The management is similar to the above condition.

Suprapatellar bursitis occurs, secondary to osteoarthrosis and is actually an extension of synovial effusion of knee joint. This is important since careless needling or similar intervention may introduce infection into the knee joint. Management is as for osteoarthrosis; aspiration under strict aseptic conditions may be done for diagnosis and for symptomatic relief.

ii) Posteromedial group

1. *Medial collateral bursa:* This bursa is immediately deep to the medial collateral ligament of the knee joint and is related to the insertion of the semimembranosus tendon and medial meniscus. It typically occurs as a result of a torn tibial collateral ligament/medial meniscus complex and rarely as an isolated disease. The treatment is repair of the ligament and meniscus, on their merits.

2. The *semimembranosus bursa* lies between the insertion of the semimembranosus tendon and the medial condyle of tibia, which is sometimes involved in connective tissue diseases like rheumatoid arthritis. Because of its clinical importance when enlarged, it has been described in detail, later in this chapter.

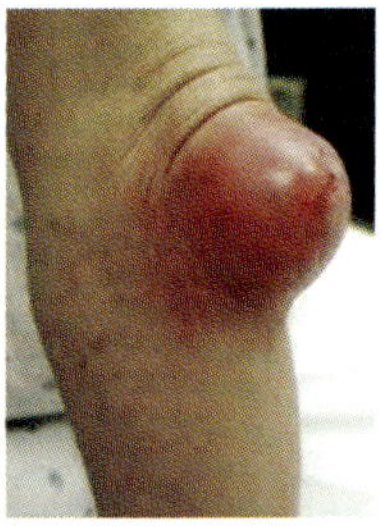

3. The medial gastrocnemius bursa lies between the gastrocnemius tendon and the capsules of the knee joint and like supra-pateller bursa, this may communicate with the knee joint and could be a route of infection.

4. The *bursa anserina* (resembles goose's foot) lies superficial to the tibial collateral ligament and in between the three tendons of insertion into the anteromedial

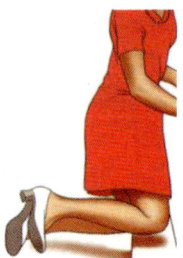

Fig. 68.4. Picture showing the cause of 'housemaid' knee

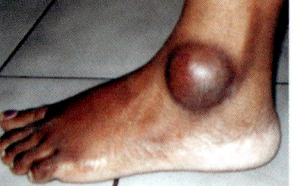

Fig. 68.5. Inflamed prepatellar bursa

Fig. 68.6. Inflamed adventitious bursa over the lateral malleolus

surface of the tibia, namely sarto rius, gracilis and semitendinosus.

iii) Lateral group

1. The superficial fibular collateral bursa lies between the biceps femoris tendon and fibular collateral ligament.
2. The deep fibular bursa lies between the fibular collateral ligament and popliteus tendon.
3. The lateral gastrocnemius bursa lies between the lateral head of gastrocnemius and capsule of knee joint.

Most of these bursae may be of interest to the anatomist, but only two are important to surgeon, viz: the semimembranosus bursitis and Morrant Baker's cyst: these will be described here:

Semimembranosus bursitis (syn: gamekeeper's knee): This deep bursa lies between the medial condyle of the tibia and the medial head of the gastrocnemius on the deeper aspect and the semimembranosus tendon superficially; it may communicate with the knee joint. This presents as a swelling in the posteromedial aspect of the knee joint.

With a higher incidence in professionals who walk with their knee in a semiflexed position, the lump is usually painless but may become painful in acute bursitis or if infected. It becomes conspicuous when the knee is made straight or the semimembranosus tendon gets tightened, flexion of the knee decreases the tension in the bursa. It is soft cystic, fluctuant, not warm or tender and may be associated with effusion of the knee, in the communicating type, though the cyst can not be totally emptied into it.

Differential diagnosis

1. Morrant Baker's cyst (vide infra)
2. Popliteal aneurysm: elderly atheros-clerotic, expansile pulsations, midposterior position and distal ischemia are diagnostic.
3. Lipoma: lobulated, mobile, not

cystic nor fluctuant, no change with movements of the knee.

Treatment

A smaller asymptomatic swelling is probably best left alone. Aspiration of the bursa followed by a compression bandage and use of NSAIDs may suffice for moderate sized cysts. If it is large, painful and restricting knee mobility, it should be excised by a transverse incision, under regional anesthesia, carefully identifying and ligating a communication with the knee joint if present.

MORRANT BAKER'S CYST

This is a synovial cyst which develops due to a herniation of popliteal synovium through a deficiency in the capsule of the knee joint posteriorly, due to any exudative disease of the knee, such as osteoarthrosis or rheumatoid arthritis.

Clinical features

Unlike the semimembranosus bursa, this is almost always due to inflammatory pathology of the knee, increasing the tension within and forcing a herniation. It clinically presents as a soft cystic, nontender swelling behind the knee joint, in a much deeper plane than the previous type, as a rule associated with effusion of the knee, movements of the knee alter its size, flexion makes it almost disappear, because of the communication with the joint space.

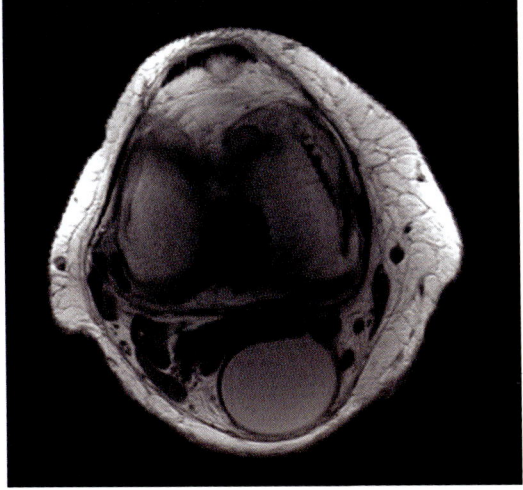

Fig. 68.7. Morrant Baker's cyst

Movements of the knee joint are usually painfully restricted due to the underlying disease.

The cyst tends to leak or rupture due to trivial injury, producing local cellulitis, not unlike that seen in an abscess, deep vein thrombosis (DVT) or a leaking popliteal aneurysm.

Investigations

The only specific investigation is x-ray of the knee joint which will show the changes of osteoarthrosis or rheumatoid arthritis.

Treatment

The primary pathology must be addressed. Aspiration of the cyst with injection of long acting steroids may help. If conservative treatment does not help, excision of the cyst with or without synovectomy, has to be done, along with repair of the defect in the posterior capsule of the knee joint. Recurrence following excision warrants search for some underlying joint pathology.

Adventitious bursae: A few examples of these bursa are:

1. Weaver's Bursa: A bursa develops superficial to the ischial tuberosity in patients who are professional weavers and who spend long periods sitting on their bottom.

2. Student's elbow: A bursa develops in the subcutaneous plane over the olecranon process, called olecranon bursa, in those who sit with elbows resting on desks, such as students and computer operators.

3. Bunion: A bursa develops over the medial aspect of the head of the first metatarsal, in patients with halux valgus. A bunionette or tailor's bunion is a similar cyst over the lateral aspect of fifth metatarsal bone, both of these are seen more in patients with broad foot, wearing tight, pointed shoes.

4. Porter's shoulder (syn: Billingsgate hump, after the fish market in London): a bursa develops in laborers who carry large weights on their shoulders.

69 Bleeding in Surgery

Bleeding during or after an operation is due either to local causes or to a hemostatic failure.

It may be primary, secondary or reactionary.

Primary hemorrhage is the one occurring during surgery.

Reactionary hemorrhage, occurs within 24 hours (usually 4-6 hours), which may be due to a slipped ligature or clot dislodgement after cessation of the reflex vasospasm.

Secondary hemorrhage occurs 7-14 days after surgery and is usually due to infection.

The causes of bleeding may be local or general.

Local causes

1. Slipped ligature: controlled with artery forceps and religation (or diathermy coagulation applied to small bleeding vessel.

2. Profuse bleeding of scalp: direct pressure (applying and everting a series of forceps to the epicranial aponeurosis)

3. Bleeding from cerebral or lumbar vessels may be controlled by silver (Cushing) clips.

4. Uncontrollable bleeding: may be underrun or transfixed with a figure of '8' stitch. If the continuity of a main vessel is to be restored, fine atraumatic (e.g. 5 or 4/0 prolene) suture is used for the anastomosis.

5. Bleeding after embolectomy or vascular grafting: pack pressure using rolls of gauze or peanut gauze held by forceps for a few minutes. Sometimes a piece of muscle is cut; mashed and used to seal bleeding from the arteriotomy.

6. For continuous oozing: knitted absorbable fabric with oxidized cellulose (Oxycel or Surgicel), absorbable gelatin sponze (Gelfoam) or gauze soaked in 1:1000 solution of adrenaline.

7. Oozing bone: dealt with by bone wax

8. Bleeding spleen is controlled by splenectomy or splenorrhaphy, while a bleeding from

kidney is treated conservatively.

9. Bleeding from tonsillar fossa: simple pressure, bipolar diathermy, sliding a ligature or topical astringents, such as tannic acid.

10. Bleeding from prostatectomy: pressure with hot packs, diathermy or hemostatic suturing.

11. Bleeding during hepatobiliary surgery: digital compression of the portal triad in the free border of gastrohepatic (lesser) omentum at the foramen of Winslow (Pringle maneuver) and try to locate and control the bleeding point.

12. Bleeding from extremities: elevation (if possible) is sufficient for venous and tourniquet application for arterial bleeding.

General causes

a) Purpura due to vascular defects

   1. Henoch-Schonlein purpura

   2. Scurvy

   3. Severe infections complicating meningococcal and rarely staphylococcal, Escherichia coli and Hemophilus influenzae septicemia

   4. Abdominal rose spots in typhoid fever

   5. Splinter hemorrhages of the nail beds in subacute bacterial endocarditis

   6. Purpura in many viral diseases such as small pox, measles and chicken pox.

   7. Drug reaction

   8. Macroglobulinemia and hereditary hemorrhagic telangiectasia

b) Purpura due to platelet abnormalities

   1. Primary idiopathic thrombocytopenia

   2. Secondary thrombocytopenia- seen in blood dyscrasias as side effect of drugs in thrombotic thrombocytopenic purpura (triad of thrombocytopenia, purpura and acute hemolytic anemia along with transient neurological signs), in systemic lupus erythematosus, in acute infections, in extensive hemangiomas in infants (Kasabach-Merritt syndrome) and following massive blood transfusions.

3. Thrombocytopathic purpura due to defective platelet function as seen in renal and hepatic failures and in macroglobulinemia.

4. Thrombocythemic purpura (hemorrhagic thrombocythemia) is a rare disease due to excessive but dysfunctional platelets, causing severe GI tract and postoperative bleeding.

c) Defects in the clotting mechanisms

1. Hemophilia (VIII deficiency), Christmas disease (IX deficiency), Von Willebrand's disease (VIII and platelet abnormalities)

2. Hypoprothrombinemia (V, VII and X deficiencies) occurs either as an inherited autosomal recessive disease or as an acquired disease, with the primary problem of vitamin K deficiency; seen in liver failure, malabsorption syndrome, obstructive jaundice, hemorrhagic disease of the newborn and in those on anticoagulant therapy

3. Hypofibrinogenemia- congenital or acquired. The acquired cases are seen in the defibrination diseases, such as fibrinolytic syndrome and disseminated intravascular coagulation (DIC).

4. Perioperative administration of anticoagulant or antiplatzlet agents.

5. Due to augmented plasminogen activity, there is slight increased bleeding tendency in women during the menstrual cycle, more so on the first day, hence elective major surgery, including dental procedures, may be avoided around that period.

Fibrinolytic syndrome: Activation of the plasmin system when large amounts of tissue activator are released into the blood, e.g. in cardiopulmonary operations, abruptio placentae, prostatic carcinoma, acute leukemia, liver disease and congenital heart disease. In these conditions, the plasmin disintegrates fibrinogen, making the blood unable to coagulate and the resulting degradation products can be detected in blood.

Treatment: Eliminating the cause, replacing clotting factors, use of epsilon aminocaproic acid (EACA) and other styptics.

Disseminated intravascular coagulation (DIC)

(syn: consumption coagulopathy)

Occurs as a result of the release of clotting factors into the blood stream and/or extensive endothelial damage leading to fibrin formation which produces vascular obstruction and micro-infarction and activates the fibrinolytic system. The extensive intravascular coagulation consumes the clotting factors, leading to afibrinoginemia, thrombocytopenia and microangiopathic hemolytic anemia seen in the blood film. The final two paradoxical effects are infarction and bleeding respectively.

DIC may be seen in several situations: abruptio placentae, intrauterine retention of a dead fetus, asphyxia neonatorum, erythroblastosis, incompatible blood transfusion, after severe trauma, fat embolism, open heart surgery with extracorporeal circulation and extensive lung operations in the newborn, severe infections (as in Waterhouse-Fredreichsen syndrome and generalised Schwartzman reaction after endotoxin blockage of reticuloendothelial cells), purpura fulminans, metastatic cancer especially prostate, thrombotic thrombocytopenic purpura, malignant hypertension etc.

Clinically there is postoperative bleeding, ecchymosis and bleeding from several orifices, Treatment is with platelet and fresh blood and/or fibrinogen, Heparin should be given as a continuous infusion of 10 unit/kg. EACA is contraindicated since clots are unlysable and it may cause acute renal necrosis in DIC.

Circulating anticoagulants (antithromboplastins): encountered in patients with hemophilia and Christmas disease who have developed antibodies after repeated transfusions of factors VII and IX respectively and also found in pregnancy, systemic lupus erythematosus and following ionising radiation.

Practical points

Clinical assessment is important. Past history of Local vascular diseases: The commonest cause of regional bleeding is local vascular disease, e.g.

bleeding from the umbilicus after childbirth, following circumcision, tooth extraction or tonsillectomy suggests a bleeding disorder. Other factors are family history (of clotting defects and hereditary hemorrhagic telangiectasia) and drug history. Examination may reveal petechial hemorrhages or purpura (suggests platelet/generalised vascular disorder) or ecchymoses &/or hemarthrosis (suggests factors VII or IX clotting defects).

Laboratory investigations include platelet count, prothrombin time (PT-which tests extrinsic system, i.e. factor VII and common pathway, i.e factors X, V and prothrombin) and partial thromboplastin time (PTT- which tests intrinsic system, i.e factors XII, XI, IX, VII and common pathway). To summarize:

PT	PTT	Defect
Normal	Normal	platelets or capillaries
High	High	common pathway
Normal	High	intrinsic system
High	Normal	factor VII def. (rare)

as a result of badly ligated blood vessels or secondary infection, rather than a generalised bleeding disorder, Epistaxis is usually due to a vascular abnormality in the nose and hematuria is due to a urinary tract lesion, e.g. lithiasis, tumor or prostatic enlargement, Severe postoperative regional bleeding may be due to platelet deficiency (either quantitative or qualitative)or to an impairment of the clotting mechanism but is rarely caused by generalised vascular damage acting on its own.

Principles of therapy

1. Blood volume maintenance.
2. Treatment of the underlying disorder (as in DIC)
3. Replacement therapy. Platelet transfusions should be given if the count is less then 50,000/cmm in a bleeding patient (given in the form of platelet concentrates or fresh blood. ABO compatibility is essential since platelets carry ABO antigens). Clotting factors are replaced, e.g. factor VIII in hemophilia given in

the form of cryoprecipitate bags or fresh frozen plasma (FFP) is also given (20ml/kg) in:

a. liver disease (with vitamin K)

b. DIC (with platelets with or without fibrinogen; the latter carries a significant risk of hepatitis).

c. massive transfusion.

d. oral anticoagulant therapy (with im/iv. vitamin K,10mg). Bleeding with heparin, neutralisation by protamine (1mg per 100u of unfractionated heparin) is necessary. For streptokinase, EACA is the specific antidote- 100mg/kg iv. over 30 min.

Local/Topical hemostatic agents

Thrombin: obtained from bovine plasma, it is applied as dry powder or fresh solution on the bleeding surface, very useful in GI bleeding, hemophilia, neurosurgery etc

Fibrin: prepared from human plasma, it is available as sheets or foam, for packing the bleeding surface. It gets absorbed in a few days. It is also available as a spray to be applied on the cut edge of liver etc.

Gelatin foam: Gelatin made into sponge, moistened with saline of thrombin solution and packed over the oozing surface. It gets absorbed in about a month.

Cellulose: oxidised regenerated cellulose (Surgicel), which is rich in collagen, is a powerful local hemostatic.

Russels viper venom: Rich in thromboplastin, applied over the bleeding surface

Vasoconstrictors: 1% solution of adrenaline soaked gause used to pack the bleeding wound Astringents: Tannic acid in glycerol is used to stop bleeding gums, hemorrhoids and tonsillar fossa after tonsillectomy

Feracrylum is a cyanoacrylate product, very useful in controlling diffuse oozing during surgery, by its property in sealing off the bleeding minute vessels. Due to its high

molecular weight (over 100,000 daltons) it is not systemically absorbed, hence exerts very little effect on the functions of internal organs. It is only for topical application and should not be used parenterally.

Injectables

Vitamin K (phytonadione, menadione) Fat soluble vitamin, promotes synthesis of factors VII, IX and X. After parenteral administration, it may take about 24 hours to restrore coagulation factors.

Fibrinogen fraction of human plasma (Fibrinal) is employed to control bleeding in hemophiliacs and in acute afibrinogenemic states. When combined with antihemophilic factor from pooled plasma (Fibrinal-H) it is found to be more effective.

Adrenochrome monosemicarbazone reduces capillary fragility, control oozing from microvessels, may be given orally or parenterally.

Aminocaproid acid is an analogue of amino acid lysine is effective inhibitor certain enzymatic process in fibrinolysis and useful to reverse the action of tissue plasminogen activator (tPA)

Tissue extract: extract of lung parenchyma (Clauden), rich in thromboplastin and platelet aggregation activator.

Ethamsylate is water soluble non-steroidal agent, is known to maintain capillary integrity, probably by promoting polymerization of mucopolysaccharide in vessel wall. It also inhibits action of prostacycline on platelets. Prostacycline, through thromboxane-2 pathway, prevents platelet aggregation.

Tranexamic acid is a potent anti-fibrinolytic agent, prevents converstion of plasminogen to plasmin and is considered several times more effective than alfa-aminocaproic acid. It may be given by oral or parenteral route.

African cobra venom (Botrops jararaca) extract has powerful styptic property and has been available commercially for parenteral use (Botropase).

Principles of perioperative anticoagulant therapy

The guidelines proposed by the American College of Chest Physicians:

In performing non-cardiac surgery on patients on anticoagulation, major concern is to balance between excessive bleeding during and after surgery and thromboembolic phenomenon, for which the anticoagulation was prescribed in the first place. The risks have to be weighed against the benefits of continuation or otherwise of anticoagulation during the procedure.

The other option is to switch from oral medication to heparinization (socalled heparin bridge) during the perioperative period, so as to have better control on the therapeutic level of the agent and facility for reversal, if such contingency arises. It naturally depends on the annual risk of thromboembolism and the nature of surgery, in terms of additional morbidity arising out of hemorrhagic tendency. For example, patient who had undergone prosthtetic heart valve implant carries high risk of thromboembolism (60%), if there is no adequate anticoagulation, as also a thrombophilic patient. Whereas in a patient undergoing intraocular or intracranial surgery, even a trivial bleeding may be disastrous. Similarly there is a difference in handling anti-platelet therapy in patients who have bare metal stents in their coronary arteries and those with drug-eluting stents.

N-acetylcysteine, an agent used to reduce reperfusion injury and perioperative inflammation, is also known to impair coagulation. Its use has increased the risk of bleeding and required replacement of blood products more than in the control group.

Three options available to surgeon, based on the risk of thromboembolism, are:

1. Minimal risk: withdraw anticoagulant &/or antiplatelet therapy 4-5 days before elective surgery and restart 2-3 days after surgery
2. Moderate risk: switch to perioperative use of heparin bridge with LMWH

3. High risk: continue the same level of anticoagulant &/or antiplatelet therapy through the procedure

For vast majority of general surgical procedures, there is no statistically significant additional bleeding or required blood replacement, when the oral anticoagulation is continued. However, under such circumstances, expediency of the operating surgeon and meticulous hemostasis during the procedure may be of great significance.

Recent advances

Recombinant factor VIIa is found to be useful in patients with hemophilia (A & B) who developed inhibitory antibodies to factors VII and IX:

1. to stop bleeding after warfarin/heparin therapy.

2. to control expansion of the hematoma in raised intracranial pressure.

Hypotensive anesthesia may be used to reduce bleeding during surgery.

Blood salvage procedures: the spilled blood in thoracic cavity or abdominal cavity is salvaged, processed and reinfused into the patient.

Surgical tourniquet

It is a compressing or constricting device used to control limb circulation for a short period; pressure applied circumferentially over the skin, is transmitted to occlude veins (first) and arteries (later). Since Joseph Lister (1864) introduced it for clinical use and later improved by exsanguination by limb elevation, prior to the application of tourniquet, it was extensively used in war injuries to control hemorrhage.. Friederich von Esmarch developed a rubber bandage, which can exsanguinate and control bleeding at the same time and Harvey Cushing introduced (1904) pneumatic cuff for the same purpose, which can be inflated and deflated as necessary. Richard von Volkmann demonstrated that its prolonged use can lead to limb ischemia and paralysis. August Bier (1908) used it to induce IV regional anesthesia (IVRA). Simple rubber bands are also used to achieve bloodless field during surgery on digits.

Special points regarding tourniquet use

1. Limb occlusion pressure (LOP) must be higher than arterial systolic pressure, but minimum effective pressure has to be employed

2. Cushioning by cotton roll is essential to prevent injury to nerves and muscles

3. Though irreversible ischemic changes may occur after 6 hours, it is safe to limit its use to 60-90min or release and reapply, if longer periods are required

4. It is ineffective when applied in the forearm or leg, where there are two bones, preventing vascular occlusion by external pressure

5. Ischemia reperfusion injury (IRI - see chapter 77) or thromboembolism may occur

6. If surgical hemostasis is inadequate, rebound bleeding can occur

7. It may be retained inadvertently, leading to disastrous loss of limb. Some surgeons tie the device to the operating table, so as not to overlook removing it after the procedure

8. Post-tourniquet syndrome (PTS) consists of pain, numbness, paresis, edema, stiffness etc. which may last for few hours to days, sometimes leading to compartment syndrome

Jewels of Gyan - 69.1

Increased bleeding during surgery is often the first sign of a mismatched blood transfusion

70 Madura Mycosis

(syn: Nocardiasis, Madura foot, mycetoma foot)

This is a chronic infective granulomatous disease caused by a filamentous, aerobic, inconstantly acid-fast organism, a transition form between bacteria and fungi, called *Nocardia madurae* and a fungus, *Madurella mycetomi*. This is common in tropical countries and was first described from Madurai, South India in 1842, hence the name.

Etiopathogenesis

The organism enters the body through a crack or puncture in the sole of the foot. At the site of its entry, a granulomatous response occurs, resulting in the formation of a subcutaneous nodule. Very slow radial growth of the organism in the subcutaneous and subfascial planes results in the formation of multiple nodules and vesicles all around the primary lesion. These vesicles then break open to discharge granules that are either yellow, black or red. It should be noted that it is a mixed population of organisms that causes Madura foot. The black color producing organisms limit the infection to the subcutaneous space but those of yellow and the red tend to progressively involve tendons, fascia and adjacent bone. Later on, secondary infection with pyogenic organisms occurs and this tends to spread along the tendon sheaths and bones. The infection excites a dense fibrous reaction and is extremely resistant to medical treatment.

Clinical features

Common in bare-footed farmers, presenting with swelling and flattening of the concavity of the foot and a bulge on the dorsal aspect (due to secondary infection). The entire sole is soon indurated and riddled with multiple nodules, vesicles and sinuses, to attain a huge size.

The sole of the foot is predominantly affected with the infection extending to the dorsum and multiple nodules and sinuses spread all over. These can often be felt fixed to the bones and adjacent tendon sheaths, which is difficult to appreciate because of the induration. The pedal pulses are normal and arterial/venous circulation is unaffected. Secondary infection, which is invariably present, is responsible for the involvement of regional lymph nodes and sometimes lymphangitic streaks.

Differential diagnosis

Tuberculous granuloma, STS and SCC

Investigations

Apart from general investigations, x-ray of the foot may show destruction of bones and joints. Gm stain and culture of the purulent discharge from the sinus will usually show mixed infec-

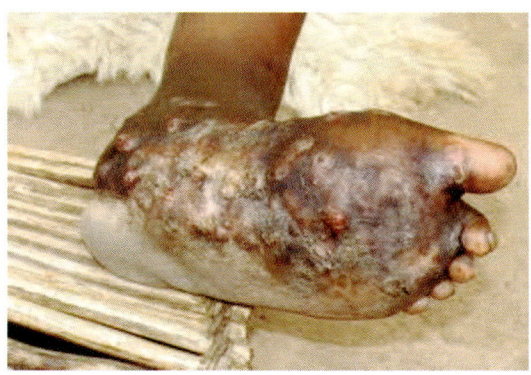

Fig. 70.1. Madura foot with multiple sinuses

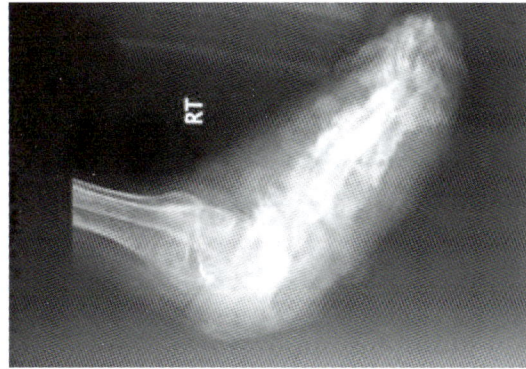

Fig. 70.2. Bone involvement in Madura mycosis

tion. Acid-fast bacilli (Nocardia) are sometimes made out by Ziehl-Neelsen stain.

Wedge biopsy is done to establish the diagnosis, but not always needed; it may be useful to exclude underlying malignancy. Alternately a sinus track may be curetted and the retrived material subjected to HPE. Special fungal studies also may be done from tissue preserved in normal saline.

Treatment: Medical

i) In the early cases, 6 months of therapy with diamino diphenyl sulphone (DDS, Dapsone) may help.

ii) Long term rifampicin has also been used successfully in some cases.

iii) Third generation cephalosporins and broad spectrum antibiotics are given to treat the secondary infection.

Surgical: Basically two types of operations are described, excision of soft tissue disease and amputation for skeletal (bone and joint) involvement. Unfortunately at the time of presentation, most cases of Madura foot have extensive skeletal (tarsal/metatarsal) involvement of the foot, forming the main indication for amputation, under cover of chemotherapy. The level may depend upon the area of skeletal disease, e.g. midtarsal for forefoot disease, Syme's for tarsal involvement and higher amputation for more extensive involvement of entire foot.

Complications

1. spreading cellulitis

2. pyemic complications

3. metastatic abscesses

4. reactive arthritis

5. amyloidosis.

6. rarely STS in longstanding disease

71 Fissure-in-Ano

Definition: This is a linear fissured ulcer in the anoderm, which may be acute or chronic. Conventionally any fissure existing for more than 6 weeks, is termed chronic.

Etiology

Several factors have been implicated in the pathogenesis of an anal fissure.

1) A *hard bolus* of fecal matter propelled downwards from the anorectal angle causes a traumatic tear of the anoderm. A history of constipation and straining of stools frequently precedes the development of this acute, painful condition.

2) *Acute infective* conditions like amebic/bacillary dysentery can sometimes be followed by the development of an anal fissure. Acute/recurrent anal fissure may be seen in HIV infected patients.

3) *Chronic inflammatory* bowel diseases (IBD), such as Crohn`s disease and ulcerative colitis have a high incidence of anal fissure.

4) *Ischemia*: The most accepted theory is that the median (both posterior and anterior) zones are the least vascularized portions of the anal circumference. The distribution of the two primary divisions of superior hemorrhoidal artery, is at 3 and 9-o' clock positions and the watershed zones are at 6 and 12-o' clock positions.

Angiographic studies have also confirmed the ischemic nature of most chronic fissures. High anal tone due to spasm of the internal anal sphincter seems to be a contributory factor, by compression of the arteries that penetrate the anal sphincter, which explains why a division of internal sphincter (sphincterotomy) or a stretch allows fissure healing (vide infra).

This also accounts for severe pain associated with anal fissure, relieved promptly by sphincterotomy.

Clinical features

In *acute* fissure, the patient complains of painful defecation, constipation and passing blood-streaked motion, due to direct contact between the fecal bolus and the fissure. Profuse bleeding is not the rule and should alert the possibility of co-existent hemorrhoids or tumor. In *chronic* fissure, apart from all these symptoms, features of chronic constipation, abdominal distension and left iliac fossa fullness/discomfort due to the unevacuated sigmoid colon, may also be present. In early childhood, this may result in faulty bowel habits and occasionally lead to a megacolon (acquired).

In >95% of cases they are in the posterior midline position; the remaining are anteriorly located. Fissures present off the midline may suggest some specific underlying pathology such as Crohn's disease, HIV, syphilis or malignancy, requiring detailed evaluation.

Careful anal inspection reveals a canoe-shaped (canoe: light boat with pointed ends) ulcer in the 6-o' clock (or 12-o' clock) position, with a skin tag seen at the inferior end of the ulcer, known as sentinel pile (sentinel: guard). This is pathognomonic of a chronic anal fissure, generally signifying the need for surgical intervention.

Digital examination may be extremely painful and often resisted; hence it should be done with the gentle introduction of a well lubricated

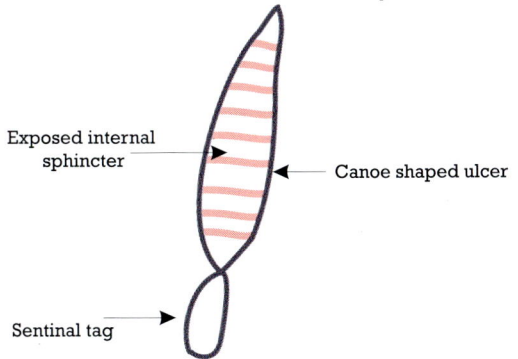

Exposed internal sphincter

Canoe shaped ulcer

Sentinal tag

Fig. 71.1. The triad of chronic fissure-in-ano

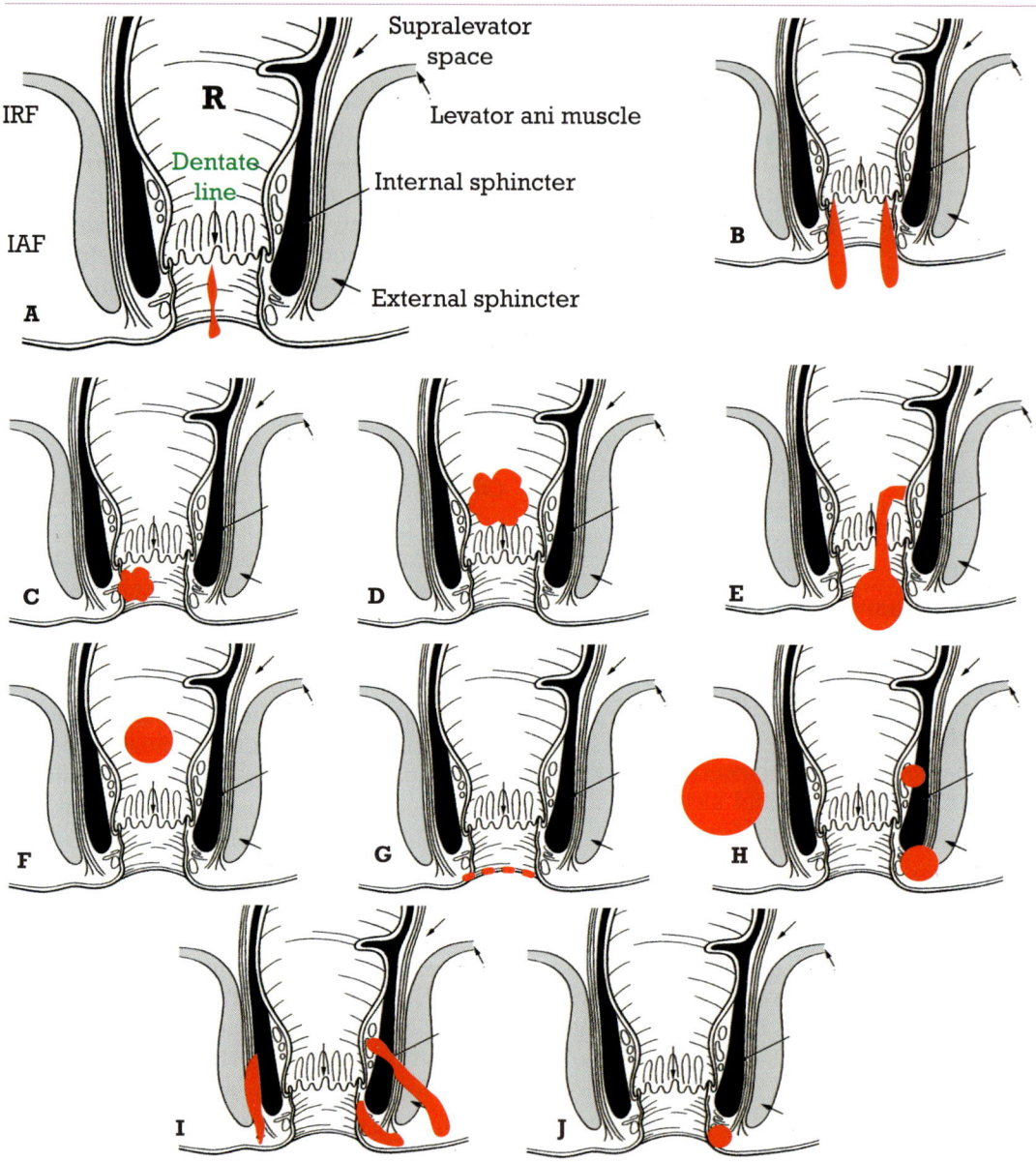

Fig. 71.2 .Diagramatic topography of various anorectal conditions
A. Fissure-in-ano with a sentinel pile B. Hemorrhoids C. Carcinoma anal canal
D. Carcinoma rectum E. Pedunculated rectal polyp F. Solitary rectal ulcer G. Anal warts H. Perianal abscesses (submucous, ischiorectal and subcutaneous) I. Fistulae-in-ano (low, intersphincteric and high) J. Thrombotic pile or perianal hematoma

(with lignocaine jelly) finger. Besides assessing the extent of sphincteric spasm and induration along the ulcer, it excludes lesions higher up in the rectum. Proctoscopic examination is virtually impossible in an office setting and done only in the operating room under anesthesia.

Differential diagnosis

Perianal abscess, inflamed/thrombosed piles, acute proctitis etc.

Treatment

Proctocolitis due to amebiasis, giardiasis, ulcerative colitis or Crohn's disease, should be identified and treated appropriately. Most acute fissures settle with conservative management, i.e., high fibre diet, bulk laxatives and anesthetic/lubricant topical applications (lignocaine jelly). Local heat by sitz baths and NSAIDs also provide symptomatic relief.

The agents for chemical sphincterotomy aim to create a reversible reduction in the abnormally high resting sphincter pressure, until the fissure has healed, but have much higher recurrence rates than surgery.

Surgical treatment

The main principle of surgery is temporary disruption of the internal sphincter apparatus to reduce its resting tone and permit the fissure to heal. They are:

i) Manual anal dilatation (MAD or Lord's procedure)

In this done under short anesthesia, the internal sphincter is manually stretched upto 4-finger breadths, rupturing the muscle fibers, permitting the fissure to heal. In diabetics, in the elderly and in those with some neurological diseases, it may take several weeks for the restoration of normal sphincter mechanism, with interim troublesome fecal incontinence. The recent review on this procedure seems to caution against excessive dilatation, particularly in

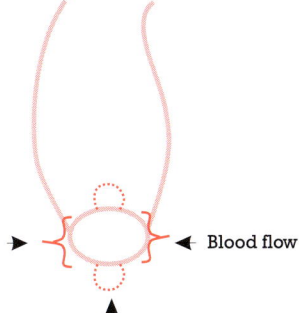

Fig. 71.3. Vascular cause of 6-o'clock and 12-o'clock fissures

---

Jewels of Gyan – 71.1

Surgical error to be avoided

Carrying internal sphincteromy above the dentate line (anorectal ring)

▼

Permanently weakens involuntary sphincter mechanism

▼

The external sphincter is switched off during sleep when the anal continence is maintained by the internal sphincter

▼

Anal incontinence develops allowing escape of rectal mucus outside

▼

Causes nocturnal soiling and pruritus ani

the above group, as they are vulnerable for intractable anal incontinence, inviting litigations.

ii) Internal sphincterotomy (Eisenhammer)

Division of the internal sphincter is a more controlled operation than the preceding one and is done by two methods, open and closed, based on the principle that division of the internal sphincter at any one point is totally safe, in terms of continence. However for optimal results, the precautions to be observed are:

a) it should not be divided at two points

b) a part of the sphincter should not be removed.

c) The anorectal ring (highest part of internal sphincter) should not be divided

d) The vertical extent of the sphincterotomy should stop at the dentate line

e) Lateral sphincterotomy is preferable to the posterior one, since the latter favors guttering of the 6-o'clock part of the anal canal, leading to entrapment of fecal material and pruritus ani.

In open lateral sphincterotomy (Notaras), an ellipse of skin is excised at the anal verge, preferably at the 3 or 9-o'clock positions, exposing the lower border of the internal sphincter, which stands out as white glistening fibers.

Separating it from the external sphincter outside and the mucosa inside, the internal sphincter is divided in its lower 4/5th, leaving the top fifth, which forms the anorectal ring, intact. After hemostasis, loose vaseline dressings into the wound and cylindrical gauze pack into the anal canal are kept for a few hours, till the first sitz bath is given. The sphincterotomy may also be done at the 6-o'clock position, with equal comfort.

In closed sphincterotomy, the blade of a knife is inserted by a stab wound, between the internal and external sphincter and by swivelling it for 90° (Notaras technique), the lower 4/5^{ths} of the sphincter is divided as in the open method. It is important to preserve the anorectal ring, which is necessary for continence.

Contraindications for IS: Patients with preoperative incontinence, irritable bowl syndrome, women with prior obstetric injury. Patient with high risk of continence disturbance should be evaluated by anorectal manometry and ultrasound before surgery is offered. As an alternate to dividing sphincter, anal advancement flap is employed in women and those with low resting anal pressures.

Prevention

Recurrence of a fissure may be prevented by high bulk diet and avoiding constipation, by using agents like isaphagul husk, methyl cellulose, psyllium, bran etc., as necessary. Prompt treatment of the predisposing conditions mentioned, particularly amebiasis, should also prevent development of fissures in the long run.

Recent advances

1. Nitrate creams: the knowledge that they decrease the resting anal sphincteric tone has led to the deployment of nitrate creams as local applications to relax the sphincteric muscles, to break the vicious cycle of pain $\Rightarrow$ spasm $\Rightarrow$ ischemia $\Rightarrow$ pain. This is also the treatment of choice in HIV-induced anal fissures, since surgery may worsen the disease.

2. Clostridium botulinum toxin (Botox) injection into the internal sphincter, which causes relaxation due to paralysis for 6-12 weeks, enabling fissure healing.

3. Oral nifedipine is also shown to produce sphincteric relaxation and heal fissures.

72 Hemorrhoids

syn: piles (pilus: pillar or a ball)

HEMORRHOIDS (Haima: blood; rhoias: flowing) are varicosities of the middle and inferior hemorrhoidal (rectal) venous plexuses. The most frequently observed anal disease is hemorrhoids or piles, atleast 50% of all individuals complain of hemorrhoids atleast once in their life time. This disease has been recognised and treated since antiquity and it is on record that Hippocrates himself suffered from piles!

Anatomy

When the anus of the patient is viewed in the lithotomy position, the pile masses commonly present at 3, 7 and 11-o'clock positions, corresponding to the divisions of the superior hemorrhoidal (rectal) artery, one on the left and two on the right.

They may be external or internal, referring to their relation to the pectinate (Hilton's or dentate) line. Hence the former are lined by anoderm and seen readily outside, whereas the latter covered by anal mucosa, prolapse out only in late stages. This division may be arbitrary, since most of them are lined by both mucosa (above) and skin (below), to a variable extent.

Accessory hemorrhoids: Apart from the main

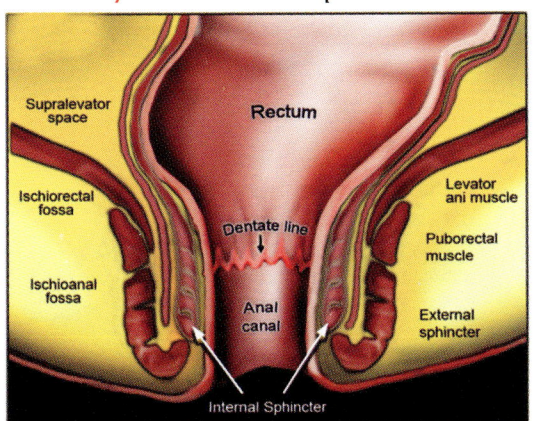

Fig. 72.1. Anatomy of anorectum

pile masses indicated, in chronic neglected cases, due to increased pressure in the wall of the rectum, muco-venous bulges develop in between, known as accessory piles, making them appear circumferential.

Etiology

They may be primary or idiopathic and secondary due to an identifiable cause.

It is well known that they have a hereditary predisposition, occur probably due to inherent weakness of venous wall, similar to varicose veins of the le.g. The superior rectal vein, which continues as the inferior mesenteric, draining into the portal system, has no valves and this has also been blamed for the development of hemorrhoids. The pathogenesis involves a number of factors, resulting in venous engorgement and downward displacement of the anal cushions, progressively affecting the entire circumference of the anal canal.

The current concept of genesis of primary hemorrhoids, is that the mucosa and submucosa at these three sites (3,7 and 11-o' clock) are occupied by longitudinal anal cushions, from early infancy and are present in normal individuals. Increased pressure within these cushions seems to cause downward displacement, with the development of hemorrhoids at the corresponding locations. As these cushions prolapse out, the internal sphincter grips them and further increases the venous engorgement, an important point to be realized, in the management of this condition. It is now understood that a glomerular apparatus exists in the hemorrhoids with afferent and efferent arterioles (hence the distinct *arterial* type of bleeding from piles).

Causes for secondary hemorrhoids are:

i)   chronic constipation/diarrhea
ii) chronic urethral obstruction
iii) carcinoma rectum or rectosigmoid, by compressing the venous plexuses

iv) any pelvic 'SOL', such as a large ovarian or adnexal tumor, for the same reason

v) pregnancy, due to increased pelvic venous circulation, sphincteric relaxation under influence of hormones and compression of superior rectal (or inferior mesenteric) vein by the enlarging uterus

vi) portal hypertension, since communications between superior (portal) and middle/inferior rectal (systemic) veins occur in the submucosa of anorectum.

vii) congestive cardiac failure, due to increased systemic venous pressure

viii) chronic proctitis, leading to hyperemia and congestion of anorectum

Clinical features

Uncomplicated hemorrhoids are painless. Mass projecting and recurrent frank bleeding per rectum, at the end of defecation, are the classical symptoms. A mucoid discharge may frequently accompany, due to mucosal congestion, causing pruritus ani. Prolapse occurs as a progression of the hemorrhoidal process, initially they get reduced spontaneously (first degree), later requiring manual reduction (second degree), and ultimately reaching a stage where they cannot be reduced or they pop out soon after (third degree). Prolapsed, complicated (inflamed, thrombosed, ulcerated, gangrenous etc.) piles may be considered as fourth degree disease.

Thrombosed/inflamed piles and associated fissure are the two common reasons for 'painful' hemorrhoids. Anemia resulting from recurrent, silent bleeding from the piles is a very common presentation in developing countries.

In secondary hemorrhoids, the features of primary disease have to be identified and treated appropriately. Overlooking a high rectal malignancy before carrying out 'hemorrhoidectomy' can be disastrous to the patient as well as to the doctor's credibility.

Internal hemorrhoids commence just below the anorectal ring, appear as bright red globular swellings, when viewed through a proctoscope. External hemorrhoids are the continuation of the above, seen below the pectinate line upto the anal margin and beyond, covered by anoderm. The pedicle is the most vascular part of the pile and can sometimes show compressibility and expansile pulsations (visible/palpable), due to its communication with a branch of the superior rectal artery (arterial pile). In such cases, bleeding can be profuse, the patient often describing it as a 'jet from a syringe', due to the arterial nature of bleeding.

Investigations

Besides the routine investigations, a rectal examination and a proctosigmoidoscopy are essential. An abdominal USG and a colonoscopy may be needed in certain cases.

Rectal examination: Second and third degree piles may be visible outside, but first degree is difficult to identify by digital examination unless thrombosed/inflamed. It helps to exclude associated conditions, such as fissure, fistula or malignancy.

Proctosigmoidoscopy: Besides visualizing first degree internal piles, this will exclude associated diseases of rectosigmoid, requiring primary attention.

Colonoscopy: This is indicated if doubt exists about the presence of the proximal bowel pathology, but its routine use is neither necessary nor cost effective. It is however, an essential investigation to evaluate a patient with persistent post-hemorrhoidectomy bleeding.

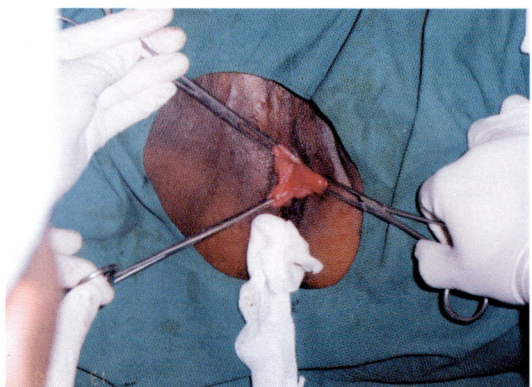

Fig. 72.2. Hemorrhoids in classical positions
(courtesy: Lifeline Hospitals, Chennai)

Differential diagnosis

i) *genital/perineal warts*, identified by multiple papilliferous excrescences, history of anal receptive intercourse etc. (see chapter 34, on penis)

ii) *perianal hematoma*, also termed 'thrombotic pile', is an acute thrombosis of the perianal venous plexus usually after straining or trauma. It appears as a small, pink, painful, cystic swelling just outside the verge. In the majority of cases it settles down with symptomatic therapy, but definitive treatment is evacuation of the hematoma by lancing it, which can be often done in the office, followed by dramatic relief from discomfort.

iii) rectal *polyp* may be seen in any age, but common in children, presents as a rounded, often pedunculated and ulcerated mass, around 1-3cm in size, poping in and out of the anal verge. This is the commonest cause of persistent rectal bleeding in children.

iv) *carcinoma* of the anal canal is identified by an indurated, ulcerated mass, with typical raised everted edges, bleeding easily to touch and associated with inguinal lymphadenopathy.

v) *prolapse* of rectum, which may be partial (mucosal) or total (procedentia). It appears as a tubular projection, covered by mucosa, circumferential, appearing while straining or squatting and getting reduced spontaneously or by manual effort. This may mimic a much rarer condition, a colocolic *intussusception*, but mucocutaneous continuity all around is the clue to identify prolapse.

Indications for addition of colorectal investigations:

Iron deficiency anemia
Positive fecal occult blood test
Age >50

Family history of adenoma or colorectal cancer

Suspicion of cancer or inflammatory bowel disease (IBD).

Complications

I) *bleeding:* Severe anemia may be seen in chronic occult bleeding from hemorrhoids, but acute severe bleeding may also occur, which may not correlate with the size of the pile masses. This is often precipitated by straining at stools or trauma produced by hard stools and is typically arterial in nature.

ii) *thrombosis:* Acute clotting of the pile mass may occur, producing a tender painful swelling with perianal edema, which is often a complication of strangulation.

iii) *strangulation:* Sometimes prolapsing internal hemorrhoids are gripped above by the internal sphincter resulting in venous congestion, severe pain and edema, ultimately leading to ulceration or gangrene.

iv) *ulceration*: This occurs as a consequence of prolapse or strangulation, often confusing with the diagnosis of carcinoma.

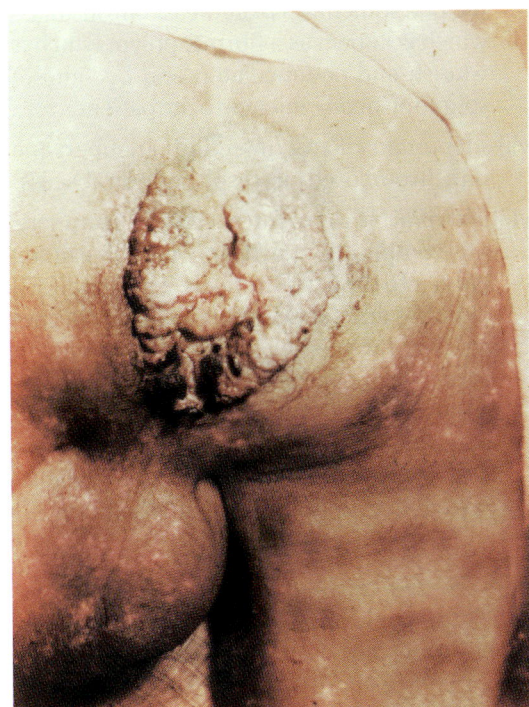

Fig. 72.3. Genital warts around the anus (condylomata acuminata)
(courtesy: Dr C J Reddy, Gudur, AP)

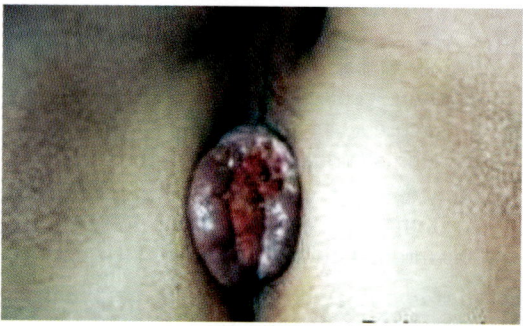

Fig. 72.4. Prolapsed piles

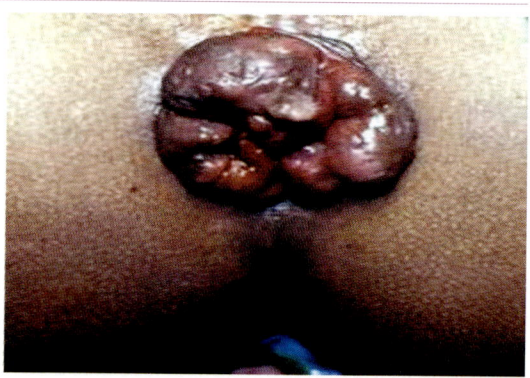

Fig. 72.5. Prolapsed thrombosed piles

v) *gangrene:* If strangulation is progressive, the venous edema causes obstruction of arterial blood supply, leading to gangrene. The pile mass may slough, producing ulceration, bleeding or portal pyemia. A pleasant but rare event, the patient may be cured of his piles, following sloughing and auto-amputation.

vi) *fibrosis:* After strangulation and thrombosis the pile sometimes becomes a fibrous mass which is known as a fibrous polyp, which is whitish and pedunculated and becomes a source of inconvenience to the patient.

vii) *suppuration:* Rarely infection can supervene on a thrombosed pile resulting in an abscess.

viii) *pyelephlebitis* or *portal pyemia:* This is a serious complication, pyogenic emboli gaining entry into the portal radicals. Abnormal LFT, jaundice and septicemia may follow in succession, threatening life. This is a sequel to suppuration/gangrene of piles or ill-timed surgery for grossly infected piles. Use of high antibiotics following blood culture and liberal local drainage may tilt the balance favorably, in a potentially fatal situation.

Treatment of hemorrhoids

Conservative treatment: consists of laxatives and local application of proprietary creams, suppositories are useful in early hemorrhoids where constipation is the major precipitating factor. However except a local emollient effect, these creams have no permanent curative effect on the pile masses.

Non-operative treatment of hemorrhoids

This may be tried for 1st and 2nd degree hemorrhoids or for those waiting for surgery for some reason, aiming for symptomatic relief:

1. Bowel regulation and avoiding constipation, if necessary with appropriate medication, are very essential

2. Topical creams with emollient and local anesthetic agents for symptomatic relief

3. Diosmins (natural or synthetic): there are micronized flavonoid agents administered orally, which increase venous tone and decrease capillary permeability

4. Calcium dobesilate: it also has similar action. Further, it inhibits platelet/erythrocyte aggregation and releases tissue plasmino gen activator (tPA), thus augmenting fibrinolytic activity. However it does not interfere with

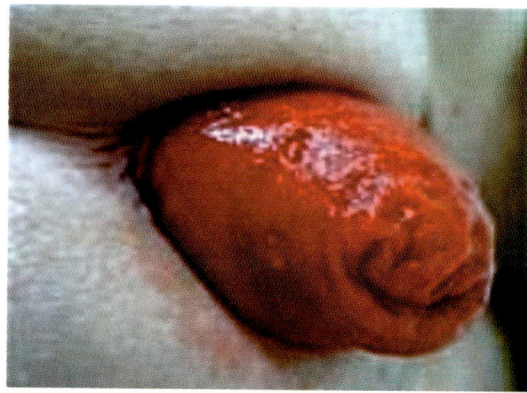

Fig. 72.6. Total prolapse (procedentia) of rectum

normal clotting functions of blood. Oral and topical preparations of dobesilate are in clinical use

5. Troxerutin (hydroxyrutosides) is a mixture of semisynthetic flavonoids

6. If bleeding present, styptic agents and topical astringent preparations may be useful

7. Associated fissure and consequent sphincteric spasm has to be treated on the merits (see chapter 71)

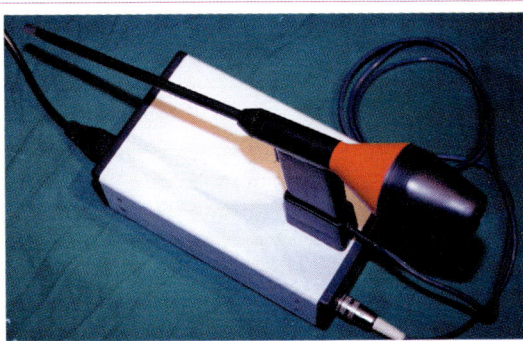

Fig. 72.8. Infra-red coagulator
(courtesy: Lifeline Hospitals, Chennai)

Surgical treatment

i) *Anal stretch* (Lord's procedure)
The principle that congestion of piles occurs secondary to a tight anal sphincter is utilized in this procedure of manual anal dilatation (MAD). This is said to relieve the pressure on the anal cushions and decongest the pile. In order to maintain the hypotonia of the sphincter the patient is taught self dilatation with an anal dilator of the St. Mark's type, for a few weeks (see chapter 71).

First degree hemorrhoids, especially when accompanied by a fissure, may be elegantly treated by this technique or its modification, which is most often a lateral internal sphincterotomy (vide supra).

ii) *Injection sclerotherapy* (Mitchell)
For first and second degree hemorrhoids, injection sclerotherapy offers a vital alternative outpatient therapy. A side-open proctoscope is introduced past the hemorrhoids up to the pedicle and the obturator is removed permitting the pedicle portion to bulge into the lumen. A Gabriel's syringe is used for injection of the sclerosant (5% phenol with gingely oil or almond oil) into the submucosal plane, about 2ml at each site, with an objective of obliterating the hemorrhoidal pedicle. Deep anterior injection of sclerosant may induce chemical prostatitis.

iii) *Banding* (Baron)
For larger 2° piles avascular necrosis can be induced by applying a rubber band to the base of the pedicle of each pile, with the help of a special apparatus called Baron's banding gun. The largest two piles are banded at each sitting and repeated after 3 weeks if necessary to deal with the smaller ones. Pain, bleeding and persistent anal discharge are the drawbacks of this procedure.

The above two types of treatment, namely sclerotherapy and banding, although known for their simplicity and ease of performance as office procedures, have a very high recurrence rate compared to standard surgery.

iv) *Cryotherapy*
A cryo probe with a temperature of -196°C at its tip, is applied directly to the base of the internal hemorrhoids. The low temperature is attained by compression of nitrous oxide to create liquid nitrogen. This causes coagulation necrosis of the hemorrhoidal tissue. The main draw back of cryotherapy is that it causes an offensive

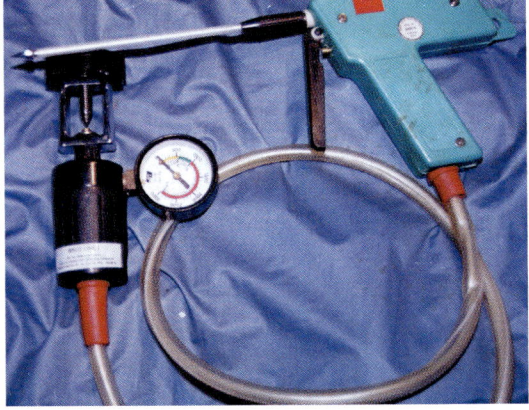

Fig. 72.7. Cryotherapy apparatus
(courtesy: Lifeline Hospitals, Chennai)

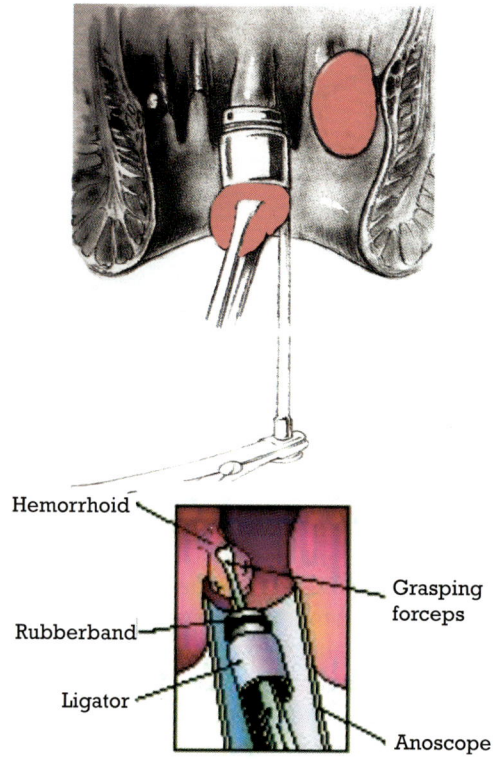

Fig. 72.9. Baron's band applicator

Hemorrhoid

Grasping forceps

Rubberband

Ligator

Anoscope

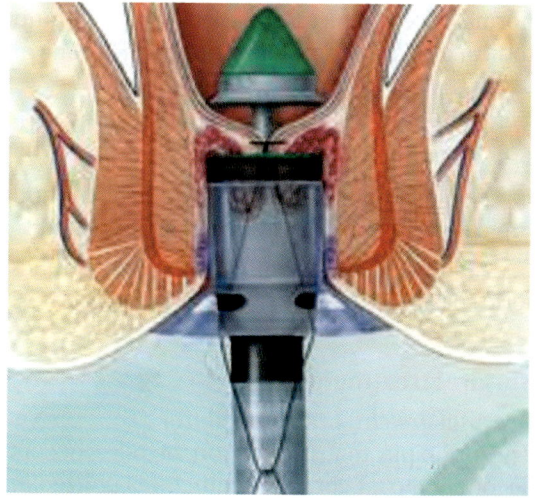

Fig. 72.10. Longo's stapling of hemorrhoids

mucous discharge for a few weeks.

v)   *Infrared* coagulation (IRC)
The same principle of thermal coagulative necrosis is applied but here it is heat therapy. The infrared probe, at about 200°C temperature is kept in direct contact with the base of the piles, causing rapid coagulation of the pedicle. The main advantages of IRC over cryotherapy is the short (30-60sec. as against cryo which requires 4-6min.) duration of contact and much less mucous discharge, because of the limited area of necrosis.

vi)   *Laser* photocoagulation
This is the most effective and painless way of photocoagulating the pile masses, using either a contact or a non-contact Laser (Nd: YAG). The selective absorption of the laser energy by the blood in the anal cushions results in a controlled thermal exposure of the target tissue. The disadvantages are high cost and risk of injury to the eyes of the operator. Inexperienced handling of

the energy delivering probe may result in perforation of the rectal wall, which is very rare with IRC.

vii)   *Stapling* the pedicles (Longo) is yet another recent introduction, using a circular stapling gun. A purse-string suture is placed just above the anorectal ring, excluding the muscular layer of the rectum, with the help of a side-open speculum. This is tied around the central rod of the stapler, with the anvil pushed beyond it. This also pulls the mucocutaneous junction upwards, eliminating the bulging masses to some extent. The 'gun' with two rows of staples, is then 'fired', excising a *single* doughnut. Placement of the purse-string at the right place and depth is the key to this operation; total lack of pain and day-care procedure are the main attractions, whereas indications limited to 1st and 2nd degrees, cost, expertise and high incidence of secondary hemorrhage are its drawbacks.

viii)   *Excisional* surgery
For prolapsed or complicated piles and those not cured by other methods, standard open hemorrhoidectomy, under local/spinal/general anesthesia, is the treatment of choice. Three positions are in use, in order of preference, lithotomy, left lateral (Sim's) or jack-knife (prone).

ix) Doppler-guided hemorrhoidal artery ligation (HAL) (Morinaga): The earlier belief was that there are 3 hemorrhoidal branches, but using Doppler, usually 5 or 6 arterial branches are identified and transfix-ligated, above the dentate line. Perioperative withdrawal of anti-coagulant or antiplatelet agents may be necessary to avoid postoperative bleeding.

Types of surgery

a. Milligan-Morgan (open) hemorrhoidectomy
b. Park's submucosal (closed) hemorrhoidectomy
c. Whiteheads operation
d. Laser/Diathermy hemorrhoidectomy

1. Open (standard) technique: An open-ended self-retaining bivalve speculum is very useful for this procedure. By grasping the base of the pile mass, a 'V' cut is made over the skin and mucous membrane, the mass is dissected upto its root and the pedicle is then transfixed and amputated. The stump and the mucosal edges are fixed to the underlying sphincter, for some distance, leaving some raw area at the muco-cutaneous border. When all the three masses are so excised, a clover leaf appearance is seen at the end, with mucosal bridges interposed. If there are secondary masses making them circumferential, their excision should be followed by primary muco-cutaneous suturing, to pre-

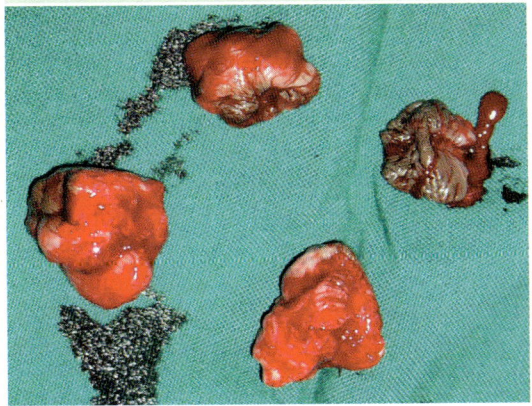

Fig. 72.11. Four large pile masses excised (courtesy: Halsted Surgical Clinic Chennai)

vent a continuous raw area all around and a consequent stricture. A cylindrical pack rolled in paraffin gauze is kept inside for a few hours (till the first sitz bath), as a tamponade against reactionary bleeding. Earlier practice of using silk ligature for the pedicle is not popular, only plain catgut is used instead (for reasons not clear, use of chromic catgut for piles operation is associated with high incidence of stricture).

Complications

i) Reactionary hemorrhage is the commonest postoperative complication and usually stops with pressure packing. Rarely reexploration to transfix the pedicle is warranted.

ii) Retention of urine occurs in the early postoperative phase usually secondary to reflex inhibition or spinal anesthesia. Removal of the anal pack, giving sitz bath and reassurance are generally successful, rarely urethral catheterization may be required. Possibility of overlooked prostatic disease, causing retention has to be remembered.

iii) Anal stenosis may occur if the muco-cutaneous bridges are insufficient, causing progressive fibrosis of the wound, which can usually be treated by repeated anal dilatations. In a small proportion of cases a plastic procedure (skin advancement anoplasty) may be needed to restore an adequate anal orifice. Prevention of stricture is the primary objective in modern surgery for piles.

2. Closed technique

In this operation two radial incisions are made in the mucosa of the anorectum, and the hemorrhoids are dissected out from the underlying sphincter, after raising mucosal flaps. This is facilitated by submucosal injection of saline and adrenaline. After the pedicle has been tied and the pile mass excised, the flaps are approximated with a running absorbable suture. The main virtue of this technique is that the muco-cutaneous approximation avoids raw area and prevents stricture. The main drawback is infection under the flaps leading to submucosal abscess formation. However, experience has failed to show any major difference between the two methods, in terms of postoperative pain or healing time. Furthermore this method may not be suitable for very large hemorrhoids.

3. *Laser/diathermy hemorrhoidectomy*

The contact variety of the Nd:YAG laser 'knife' may be used to directly dissect out the hemorrhoids, just as in an open operation, but instead of ligation/transfixion, the pedicle is laserized and cut. As sealing of the sensory nerve endings occurs with the laser knife there is much less postoperative pain, though total healing time may be the same. The same may be performed with a diathermy probe or harmonic knife as well.

The main disadvantages are
- a. high incidence of reactionary hemorrhage from the laserized pedicle.
- b. cost and expertise

4. *Whitehead's operation*

In this type the entire prolapsing skin and mucosa are excised in toto along with the pile mass, the mucosa and skin are sutured together circumferentially around the anus. This *open* operation is mentioned only to be condemned, as it causes an *unacceptably high rate of anal stricture*. However, combining with standard excision of major piles, the secondary pile masses may be treated by primary mucocutaneous suturing following excision, to avoid circumferential raw area, thus minimizing the risk of developing a stricture.

Treatment of complications (strangulation, thrombosis, gangrene or acute prolapse)

The conventional therapy has been rest, icepacks and antibiotics to reduce the edema, to prepare for semi-elective surgery and to minimize the risk of pyelephlebitis or portal vein thrombosis. But in this era of powerful antibiotics, such a fear is probably unnecessary, the consensus favoring early surgery.

Hemorrhoids in special situations
Pregnancy

This is an all too common complaint, reassurance and stool softeners are enough to keep them decongested till delivery, when they usually regress. If they persist and become symptomatic, they may be treated by any of the methods described above.

Inflammatory bowel disease (IBD)

Crohn's disease and ulcerative colitis are often associated with hemorrhoids, fissures and fistulae. They heal as usual following surgery, unless receiving large doses of steroids as a treatment for IBD.

Portal hypertension (PH)

Described nearly a century ago, the spectrum of dilated porto-systemic anastomoses seen in PH, includes the hemorrhoidal plexuses, occurring in <5% of the patients. The superior hemorrhoidal vein draining into the inferior mesenteric vein (portal system) and the middle and inferior veins draining into the tributaries of the hypogastric (internal iliac) vein, form a submucous plexus in the anorectum. The treatment for this fortunately infrequent complication of PH is no different from the standard nor does it significantly add to the morbidity of PH, unless associated with severe coagulopathy or hypoproteinemia.

Pruritus ani

Intractable perianal itching experienced, may be due to several causes.

1. Poor local hygiene, hyperhidrosis, wearing nonabsorbant clothes etc
2. Perianal discharge and persistent moisture, due to fissure, piles, prolapse, polyp, proctitis, warts etc. Sometimes, vaginal discharge due to Trichomoniasis, may cause problems in the 'neighborhood'
3. Local skin allergic conditions and dermatosis, such as urticaria, hay fever, lichen plannus, reaction to drugs, soaps, ointments etc
4. Fungal skin infections (epidermophytosis)
5. Worm infestation (thread worm), scabies, pediculosis
6. Psychoneurosis, may be considered

after reasonably excluding the above mentioned organic causes, but the possibility of secondary phychosis due to the unrelenting troublesome itching also has to be remembered.

Treatment: Any identifiable cause has to be appropriately treated. Nonspecific measures, like improving local hygiene, hair clipping, antiperspirant spray, topical steroids, eliminating moisture by strapping the buttocks apart, may all be beneficial. Ultimately psychotherapy and counseling may be resorted to, after addressing the treatable organic conditions.

73 Perianal Abscess

It is now recognized that perianal abscess and fistula are two phases of the same disease, namely perianal suppuration and they should be regarded as the parts of same pathology. However for therapeutic reasons they are considered separately.

PERIANAL ABSCESS

Etiology

The commonest cause of a perianal abscess is crypto-glandular sepsis. The anal glands, situated in the inter-sphincteric space, empty their mucous secretions through ducts piercing the internal sphincter and open into the base of anal crypts, situated at the level of the pectinate line, more densely distributed in the posterior half of the anus. Obstruction to their ducts causes retention of secretions and cyst formation in the intersphincteric plane (akin to a sebaceous cyst), which gets infected by gut specific organisms, forming an abscess. Secondary infection of a deep-seated hematoma, due to some injury (two-wheeler riders) to the perineum, is yet another causative factor for abscess formation. There is a distinct male preponderance.

However, perianal sepsis may also occur in a wide variety other situations, such as local skin lesions like hidradenitis suppurativa, localized pyoderma or an infected sebaceous cyst. It may also follow surgical or penetrating wounds in that region or injection sclerotherapy of piles. Diabetes mellitus, obesity and inflammatory bowel diseases (IBD) are associated with high incidence of perianal suppuration.

Spread

From the inter-sphincteric plane, it may track downwards to open out just close to the anal verge (subcutaneous abscess) or it may go upwards leading to an intramural or intramuscular abscess or outside the gut wall above the levator ani (pararectal) or below the muscle, leading to an ischiorectal abscess. Circum-ferential spread in this plane all round the rectum and anal canal may result in a horse-shoe abscess, connecting both ischiorectal fossae. Although a pelvirectal abscess may also rarely be produced by a similar process, more often it is a sequel of peritoneal sepsis. These various locations of abscesses form the main basis of their classification (Parks).

Complications

i) fistula formation by their natural tendency to burst through the skin(externally) or anorectal wall (internally)

ii) septicemia, especially in large ischio-rectal or horse-shoe abscess

iii) necrotizing skin and fascial infection

iv) clostridial infections (tetanus and gas gangrene) rarely.

Clinical features

History of purulent perianal/anal discharge or previous surgeries may provide a vital clue to the diagnosis. The main symptoms are throbbing

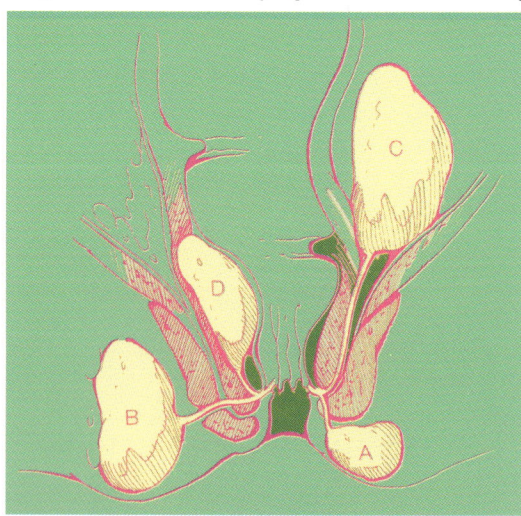

Fig. 73.1. Types of anorectal abscess
A. Subcutaneous (perianal)
B. Ischiorectal
C. Supralevator (pelvic)
D. Intersphincteric or submucous

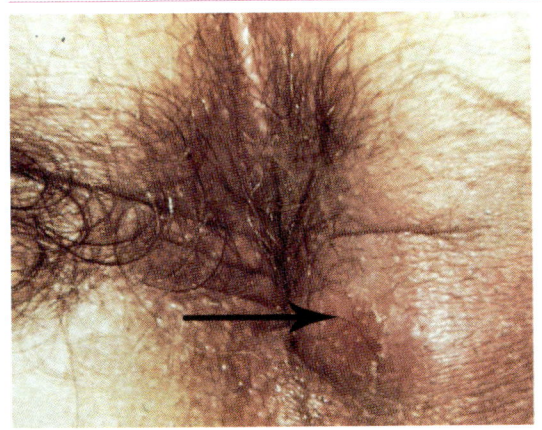

Fig. 73.2. Perianal abscess

perianal pain and swelling aggravated by sitting, walking and defecation. Systemic features like fever, chills and tachycardia are seen frequently with deep-seated large abscesses.

Most often an obvious swelling, tenderness, induration, redness or signs of cellulitis in the perianal area are seen by external/digital examination. Inguinal lymph nodes may be enlarged. Sometimes a small intersphincteric abscess may be very painful, similar to an acute anal fissure, requiring examination under anesthesia, to clinch the diagnosis. An anterior abscess should be distinguished from periurethral abscess in men and Bartholin's abscess in women. Careful examination, if necessary with a blunt malleable probe, will often reveal an internal fistulous opening in many patients, during surgical drainage of an abscess.

Investigations

Besides routine investigations, proctoscopy if permitted by the patient, not only may show purulent discharge from the internal opening, on pressing over the abscess, but it excludes other incidental conditions, such as hemorrhoids, polyp or stricture. Predisposing conditions like diabetes, IBD, including amebic proctitis have to be screened for, in all cases. A source of sepsis elsewhere, e.g. urogenital tract, pyogenic skin/bone infections, tonsillitis, suppurative otitis/sinusitis etc. should be looked for.

Treatment

Except to treat the overt infection and to relieve pain, medical therapy is of no avail; furthermore, administration of wide spectrum antibiotics without drainage of the sepsis often creates more complex fistulous lesions. Spontaneous healing and complete resolution is very rare; hence surgery is the treatment of choice.

For optimal results, employing general/spinal anesthesia, early surgery to drain pus, laying open all the loculations and adequate saucerization of the wound are essential. A fistulous tract opening into anorectum, must be always looked for and laid open, whenever possible (in high fistula, above the anorectal ring, this is not possible).

A cruciate skin incision is initially made over the induration to drain pus, usually under tension and with an offensive odor, the edges of which are liberally excised, to make the wound wider than deeper. By digital exploration, all loculations are broken and drained, before packing the wound with paraffin gauze. Patient is started on sitz baths and allowed normal diet and activity, from the day of surgery.

INTER-SPHINCTERIC ABSCESS

To drain such an abscess a disc of the mucosa is excised up to the level of the dentate line. The internal sphincter fibres, below the cavity are divided upto the top of the cavity and the intersphincteric space is curetted, to remove unhealthy granulation tissue and the infected culprit anal gland.

ISCHIORECTAL AND PARARECTAL ABSCESS

Through a radial incision made in the perianal tissue and continued into the ischiorectal fossa the drainage is performed. If a bidigital examination confirms the extension into the pararectal space, the levator muscle fibres are separated to allow free drainage of the roof of the abscess cavity.

PELVI-RECTAL ABSCESS

A pelvirectal abscess caused by pelvic disease

such as pelvic appendicitis, salpingitis or perforated diverticulitis, is felt as a cystic bulge in the anterior wall of rectum, by digital examination. it may also follow general peritonitis due to any reason, such as enteric or peptic ulcer perforation, leaked bowel anastomosis or bowel injury (see pelvic abscess in chapter 7). If a loop of small bowel is caught in the cavity, features of intestinal obstruction may be evident. The aims of treatment are to drain the abscess and to attend to the primary pathology. In males it is best drained through the anterior wall of rectum, after confirming its presence by needling under vision using a bivalve rectal speculum. In females the rectovaginal pouch (of Douglas) may be effectively drained through posterior fornix of vagina.

HORSE-SHOE ABSCESS

For a horse-shoe abscess or a deep posterior anal abscess a single or multiple radial incisons radiating from the anal verge are used to enter the abscess cavity. If a fistulous tract is found then a seton is placed using a polyamide (nylon) suture, to allow easy identification of the tract at a later stage. The consensus no longer recommends

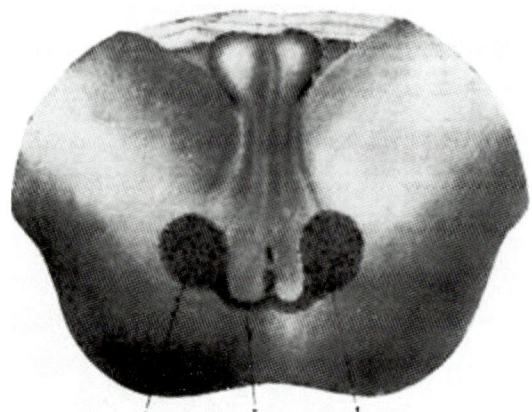

Fig. 73.4. Horse-shoe shapped perianal abscess

primary suture of perianal sepsis, as recurrence is unacceptably high.

Role of colostomy

Occasionally ischiorectal abscess may lead to serious, life-threatening complications, such as septicemia, pyemia, renal failure or Fournier's gangrene. It has been observed that the morbidity (and mortality) may be high in those with anemia, hypoproteinemia, azotemia (or uremia) or scrotal involvement; a defunctioning colostomy may be life-saving in these circumstances.

> **Jewels of Gyan – 73.1**
>
> **35% of perianal abscesses**
> ↓
> are actually fistulas.
> When in doubt, get an
> MRI scan of perineum!

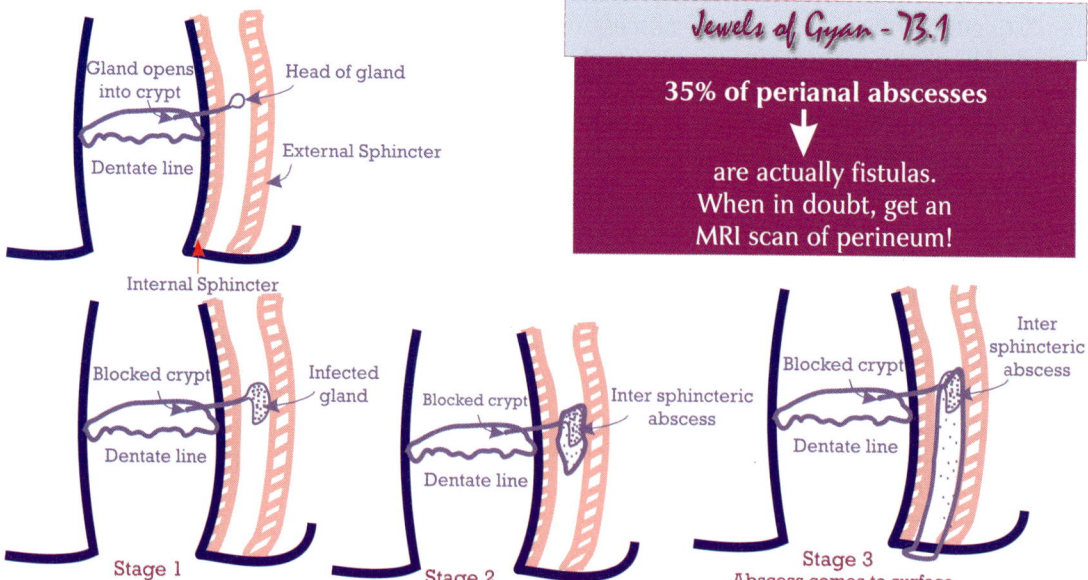

Fig. 73.3. Pathogenesis of perianal suppuration

74 Fistula-in-Ano

Etiology: Ninety percent of the ano-rectal fistulae have a crypto-glandular origin exactly similar to that of an abscess, the remaining may have specific etiology, such as IBD, tuberculosis, amebiasis etc. Conditions which may predispose to fistula in ano:

a) post-surgical

    1) fissurectomy
    2) hemorrhoidectomy
    3) episiotomy
    4) prostatectomy
    5) low anterior resection of rectum
    6) injection sclerotherapy for piles

b) specific infections

    1) tuberculosis
    2) actinomycosis
    3) lymphogranuloma venereum (LGV)
    4) amebiasis

c) inflammatory bowel diseases (IBD)

d) malignancy of anus and low rectum

e) post irradiation

f) trauma

    1) penetrating injuries
    2) impalement
    3) enema injury

As mentioned earlier, untreated progression of anorectal abscesses almost always leads to anorectal fistulae.

In a fistula with multiple external openings, the following conditions have to be considered;

1. IBD, especially Crohn's disease
2. Lymphogranuloma venereum (LGV)
3. Tuberculosis
4 Colloid carcinoma of rectum
5. Actinomycosis (rare)

Clinical features

Recurrent purulent/serosanguinous/fecal/ gaseous discharge with perianal skin irritation is the commonest presenting symptom. Intermittent

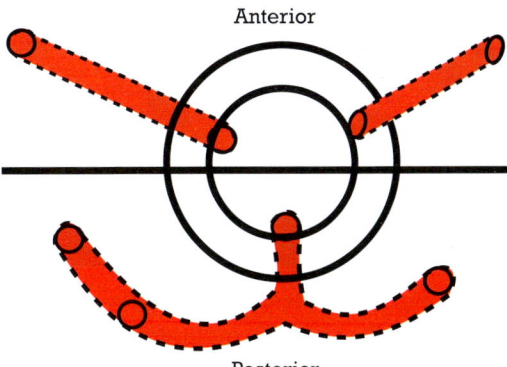

Fig. 74.1. Goodsall's rule for internal opening

swelling, pain and fever sometimes occur due to blocked orifice and retention of secretions in the fistulous tract, spontaneously open under pressure, with relief of local/systemic features. Multiple branching secondary openings in the perineum, may give rise to a 'watering can' appearance.

If there is no abscess or cellulitis, palpation is

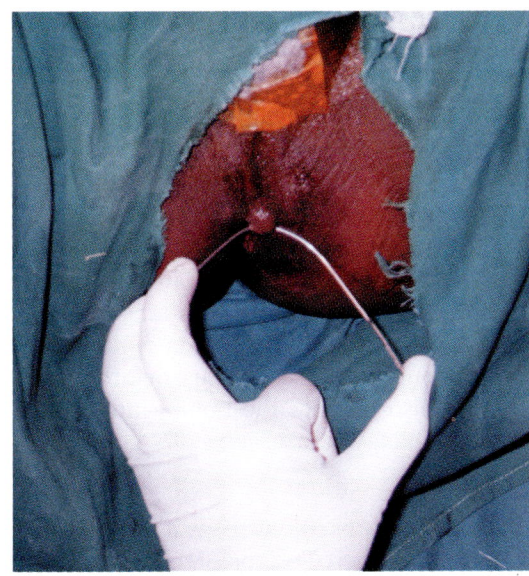

Fig. 74.2. Superficial fistula with a probe
(courtesy: Lifeline Hospitals, Chennai)

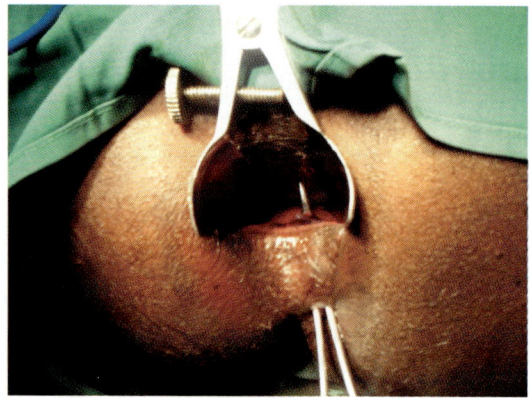

Fig. 74.3. Midsphincteric fistula-in-ano

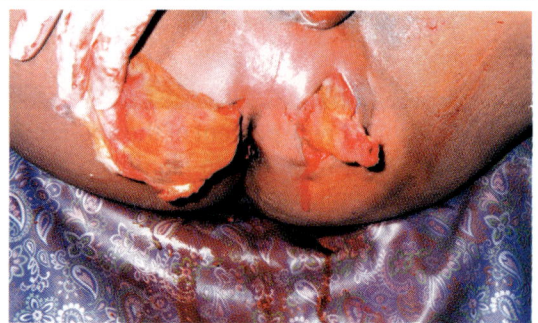

Fig. 74.4. Bilateral fistulectomy
(courtesy: Lifeline Hospitals, Chennai)

painless and a cord like indurated track can be palpated more or less radially between the external opening and the anal canal, unless the fistula is of the high variety. Bidigital examination is useful to appreciate the tract crossing the external sphincter. However, in vast majority of cases, the internal opening is located around the level of anal crypts.

Goodsall's rule: Fistulous openings in front of an imaginary line dividing the anus transversely have a direct radial course to the anus, while those with an external opening behind this line have a curved course and usually reach the anal canal in the midline (6-o'clock position). However, if the anterior opening is located more than an inch away from the anal verge, its tract also may be curved.

Gentle exploration with a blunt probe or injection of methylene blue, helps to identify the fistulous track and the internal opening, if it is done under direct vision through an open-ended bivalved rectal speculum. The latter is preferred by many, for fear of creating a false passage by overzealous probing. If done just before surgery, the dye also outlines the ramifications of the track, enabling total excision.

Other investigations

Sigmoidoscopy or colonoscopy if a suspicion of malignancy, tuberculosis or IBD exists.

Fistulography with lipiodol in recurrent/complicated/high fistulous tracts to identify the anatomy of the tract and internal opening.

Endoanal ultrasonography, CT or MRI, combined with fistulography would provide precise 3-dimensional orientation of complex fistulous tracts and help to exclude a rare possibility of osteomyelitis of coccyx.

MRI fistulogram, of late, has become the most preferred investigation to delineate complex fistulae, horse-shoe tracks, etc. to ensure total elimination of the disease at surgery.

Park's classification

Low type (extrasphincteric, below the internal sphincter)

Mid type (inter and trans-sphincteric)

High type (suprasphincteric, above the anorectal ring)

Treatment

Surgery is the only option. As 90% of them are due to crypto-glandular infection, excision of the complete tract along with the infection source, i.e. the gland and the duct is desirable. Surgery must achieve the following goals:

Deroofing or excision of the intersphincteric abscess

Laying open of the primary tract

Drainage of any secondary tracts

Minimal or no division of the internal sphincter to prevent incontinence

Healthy healing from the depth with minimal scarring

Although laying open a fistula (fistulotomy) is

still widely practiced, excision of the tract with its ramifications (fistulectomy) and the dense fibrous tissue is the ideal procedure, following the same geometrical principle for abscess deroofing, the ultimate wound should be wider than deeper, to avoid premature skin healing. Fistulectomy and fistulotomy are easy to perform in cases of low and mid fistula; however if the fistulous opening is above the anorectal ring, the latter(with less sphincter damage) is preferred.

Another method using a seton (seta: bristle) is also popular for high fistula, in which a thick monofilament nylon is threaded into the fistulous tract, brought out through the anal canal and then tied on to the perineum. It is gradually tightened every day, to cut the rectal wall below it, while the part above heals, so that finally the track is eliminated or converted into mid/low fistula, amenable for conventional surgical excision. This cumbersome process may take 4-8 weeks, but has the greatest advantage of avoiding division of entire sphincter at once, thus eliminating the possibility of developing incontinence or nocturnal soiling.

In intractable high fistula, certain cure is possible only with preliminary defunctioning sigmoid colostomy, before excision of tract and repair of rectal wall in two layers. The colostomy may be eliminated within weeks following total healing of the wound. This extreme step is rarely required nowadays.

Other procedures

1) Primary suture: This is recommended only for low fistula, following complete excision of the tract and fibrous tissue, if the patient is extremely 'time-conscious', but fully aware of the high risk of recurrence. This is

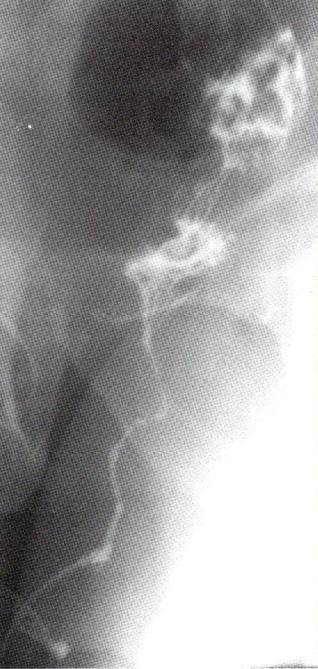

Fig. 74.5. Fistulogram showing contrast entering the rectum (courtesy: Halsted Surgical Clinic, Chennai)

unsound in principle, because of the risk of hematoma formation due to dead space in the depth, which may get infected, leading to recurrence.

2) Sometimes a spilt skin graft is advocated for the fistulectomy wound, in order to shorten healing time, but has the disadvantage of leaving a concave deformity, besides the uncertainty of its survival under such unhygienic conditions and lack of adequate immobilization, even if it is quilted.

3) Re-routing of a high fistulous tract (Mann & Keton) is not a very popular staged procedure in which the extra sphincteric part of the tract is moved inward to a site where it can be layed open without sacrificing the sphincter.

4) Sliding flap advancement: In this technique all the fistulous tracts are cored out completely from the external to the internal opening. The intersphincteric space is curetted and the gap through the sphincter is closed by separate stitches of absorbable material. Then a flap of mucosa is undermined and sutured around the opening.

5) Horse-shoe fistula is one of the difficult types to treat; its primary fistulous opening is usually in the posterior midline crypt. By preliminary injection of a dye, the entire tract is excised by a semilunar incision and the cavity is deroofed through a sagittal incision to the tip of the coccyx. The postanal space is opened and that portion of the tract below the ano-coccygeal raphe is excised. The remaining tract is drained through the seton on both sides. After the lateral wounds have healed the seton tract may be excised or cored out.

Recent advances

After coring out the unhealthy granulation tissue, *cyanoacrylate glue* is injected into a sinus/fistulous tract, totally obliterating it, obviating the need for troublesome surgery. If it is proved equally effective by experience, it may replace all other forms of therapy in the future, in the treatment of fistula-in-ano, which is notorious for recurrences following surgery and often responsible for earning ill reputation (and giving ulcers!) to the surgeons.

Fibrin glue for complex fistula-in-ano: Described by Hedelin in 1982, its mode of action is by stimulating the growth of fibroblasts and pluripotent endothelial cells into the tract and seal it off. The glue, a mixture of fibronectin and collagen, is deployed after curetting the fistulous tract, preferably without an internal opening in the high pressure zone of anorectum. This method may be suitable in fistula due to Crohn's disease, which have high failure rate following conventional surgery and has a cure rate of about 40%.

Anal fistula plug: It is made from biomaterial derived from submucosa of swine small bowel. This is made into a conical plug, which is rail-roaded into the tract by a probe in the internal opening and the excess material projecting out of the external opening is trimmed. This is done as a day-care procedure, provides a scaffolding for the native fibroblasts to proliferate and fill up the tract and has a reported cure rate over 80%.

Recent advances

Video-assisted anal fistula therapy (VAAFT): a fine caliber endoscope is inserted into the external opening of the fistula and all the ramifications of the disease are visualized. The entire lining is cauterized and the internal opening is either sutured or stapled. The long term cure rate is under evaluation.

Another intrusion by minimal access surgery!

Feature	Fistulotomy	Fistulectomy
Tissue excision	Minimal	Liberal
Healing time	Minimal	Considerable
Sphincter injury	Minimal	Significant
Incontinence	Rare	Considerable
Tissue for HPE	Not possible	Possible
Recurrence rate	High	Low ?
Preference for	High type	Low & mid type

Table- 74.1. Differences between fistulotomy and fistulectomy

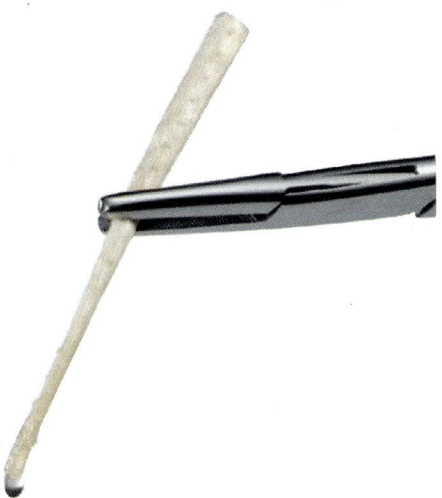

Fig. 74.6. Biomaterial plug to treat fistula-in-ano

75 Solitary Rectal Ulcer Syndrome

Definition: An inflammatory lesion occurring in the mid-rectum, typically around 5-10cm from the anal verge, which is often a large solitary ulcer. It may, however appear like a granular patch of proctitis, a carpet of pseudopolypi, or sometimes multiple confluent ulcers; it is commonly seen in women between 30 and 60.

The name SRUS itself is a misnomer, as these are often multiple, can occur even in the proximal colon and are often polypoid without ulceration.

Etiopathogenesis

Although it was earlier grouped under inflammatory bowel diseases (IBD), it is now known that the *solitary rectal ulcer syndrome* (SRUS) is a definite and separate entity. Many patients with this lesion seem to have a recto-rectal/recto-anal intussusception/prolapse and the primary pathology appears to be a motility disorder of the anorectum, causing increased pressure on the anterior rectal mucosa. This has emerged as the single important factor influencing the treatment of this condition. An earlier suggestion that it was due to trauma of repeated digital evacuation of hard feces, necessitated by severe constipation, may also be relevant in some instances. Microscopy shows a microvillous mucosal configuration with fibrosis of lamina propria.

Clinical features

The commonest symptom is tenesmus and passage of blood and mucus per rectum, with perianal soiling and pruritus ani. History of chronic constipation is almost always present. Digital examination may detect prolapse or intussusception of the rectum. Usual location of the ulcer by digital examination: anterior wall of rectum, centered on a rectal fold, at a distance of 5-10cm from the anal verge.

Investigations

Examination of stools for ova and cysts is helpful, but not clinching, since amebiasis may coexist and be unrelated to the ulcer or serve as a perpetuating factor.

Proctosigmoidoscopy may reveal either a large ulcer, confluent small ulcers or multiple

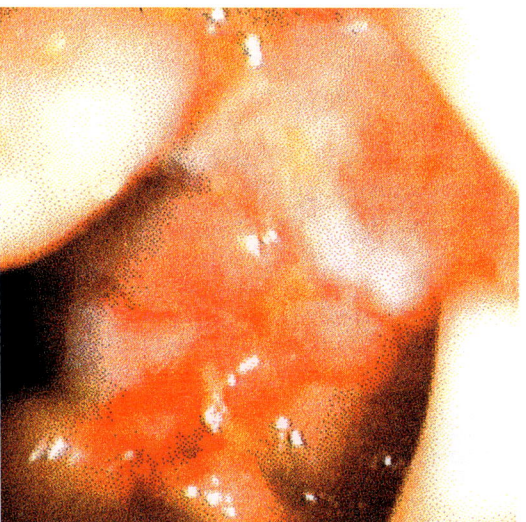 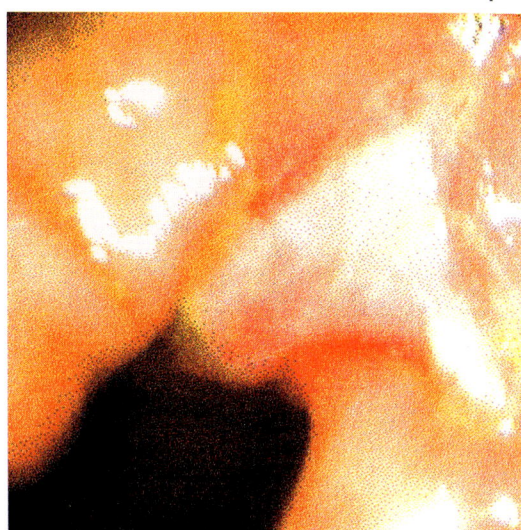

Fig. 75.1. Proctoscopic view of solitary rectal ulcer (courtesy: Lifeline Hospitals, Chennai)

pseudopolypoidal mucosal elevations and rarely a picture of granulomatous proctitis. After excluding other proximal lesions by colonoscopy, multiple edge or punch biopsies of the ulcer should be done to rule out malignancy. The ulcers may be multiple in about 30% of patients.

The other useful, but infrequently done investigations in this condition are:

1. defecatory proctogram with thin barium for intussusception.

2. rectal manometry: very high luminal pressures are recorded in some segments of the rectum in patients with this syndrome. An incoordinate sphincter complex, with a loose external sphincter and a tight internal sphincter has been implicated as a causative mechanism of SRUS.

3. endoanal ultrasonogram.

4. barium enema.

Differential diagnosis

1. Other ulcers of the rectum, e.g. amebic ulcers (multiple, flask shaped, short history, attacks of dysentery and lower abdominal cramps, relieved by bowel movement).

2. Carcinoma of rectum (everted edge, large and indurated, evidence of secondaries). This dreaded possibility has to be meticulously excluded by adequate multiple biopsies, on more than one occasion, if warranted.

3. Crohn's disease (evidence of small bowel disease, waxing/waning course, ulceration is rare).

Treatment

Depending upon the etiology, in patients with rectal prolapse or recto-anal intussusception, an anti-descent procedure (rectopexy) will suffice to prevent recurrent trauma causing SRUS. Combining sigmoid resection (either open or laparoscopic) may add to the cure rate of this disease. Thus a subset of patients with abnormalities seen on a defecatory proctogram will benefit with this approach.

For those without obvious correctable disorders, the treatment is expectant and conservative, consisting of a high fibre intake, biofeedback training and salicylate or steroid enemas. Laserization (with an Nd:YAG laser) has recently emerged as a viable therapeutic modality, as also thermocoagulation with an Argon plasma coagulator.

Severe unrelenting symptoms or foci of dysplasia are indications for resectional surgery which is usually a low anterior resection of the rectum. Recent reports indicate a small incidence of malignancy (adenocarcinoma) in these ulcers, if left untreated.

(syn: shock lung, traumatic wet lung, pump lung)

Definition: Acute condition characterized by bilateral pulmonary infiltrates and severe hypoxemia in the absence of evidence of cardiogenic pulmonary edema.

Acute lung injury (ALI): Partial arterial O_2 pressure (PaO_2)/Functional inspiratory O_2 pressure (FiO_2) ratio 200-300 (milder form of ARDS)

ARDS: PaO_2/FiO_2 ratio < 200
Pulmonary capillary wedge pressure (PCWP) is < 18mmHg in ARDS patients.

Pathophysiology

1. ARDS is characterised by increase in permeability of alveolar capillary barrier, leading to influx of fluid into the alveolar space. A variety of insults results in damage either to vascular endothelium or to the Alveolar epithelium leading to ARDS.

The main site of injury may be focused on either vascular endothelium (e.g. sepsis) or Alveolar epithelium (e.g. aspiration of gastric contents).

Damage to type I epithelial cells results in decreased production of surfactant with resultant decreased compliance and Alveolar collapse.

2. Neutrophils appear play a key role in pathogenesis of ARDS, as suggested by studies of broncho alveolar lavage (BAL) and lung biopsy specimens in early ARDS, but it may be reactive rather than causative.

3. Cytokines (TNF, Leukotrienes, Microphage inhibitory factor) along with platelet sequestration and activation are important in development of ARDS. An imbalance of pro- and anti-inflammatory cytokines is thought to occur after an inciting event such as sepsis. Prostaglandins, 5-hydroxytryptamine (serotonin), histamine and lysosomal enzymes also are found to play a part in the patho-genesis of ARDS.

4. ARDS causes marked increased intrapulmonary shunting leading to severe hypoxemia: High FiO_2 is required to maintain adequate tissue oxygenation and life. High FiO_2 levels cause diffuse alveolar damage (DAD) by the O_2 free radicals and related oxidative stress, called oxygen toxicity.

Generally, O_2 concentration >65% for prolonged periods can result in DAD, membrane formation and eventually fibrosis.

5. ARDS is associated with pulmonary hyper tension. Pulmonary artery vasoconstriction contributes to ventilation-perfusion mismatch leading to hypoxemia in ARDS.

Normalization of pulmonary artery pressure occurs as the syndrome resolves.

The development of progressive pulmonary hypertension (PHT) is associated with poor prognosis.

Many causes have been identified for setting a cascade of events in motion:

Direct lung injury

Pneumonia
Aspiration
Near drowning
Air/ Fat embolism
Inhalation of fumes or hot air
Indirect lung injury
Bacteremia
Sepsis, shock
Poly trauma
Extensive burns
Massive transfusion
Drug over dose
Acute pancreatitis
Post-perfusion injury after cardiopulmonary bypass.
Head injury and Increased intracranial tension (ICT).

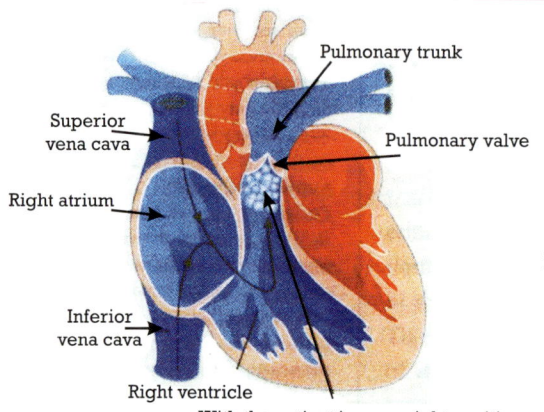

Pulmonary trunk

Superior vena cava

Pulmonary valve

Right atrium

Inferior vena cava

Right ventricle

With the patient in an upright position, air bubbles travel through the right atrium and to the top of the right ventricle, lodging near the pulmonary valve obstructing the blood flow to the lungs

Fig. 76.1. Air embolism locking the pulmonary artery in supine position

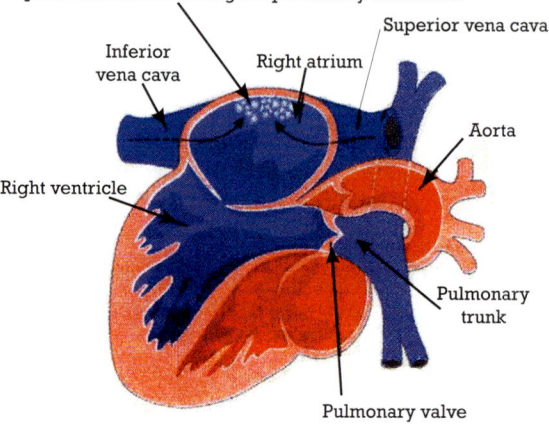

With the patient in the left Trendelenburg position air bubbles rise in the right atrium and are, therefore, prevented from entering the pulmonary circulation

Superior vena cava

Inferior vena cava

Right atrium

Right ventricle

Aorta

Pulmonary trunk

Pulmonary valve

Fig. 76.2. Air trapped in right side of the heart in left Trendelenburg position

Clinical features

Patients developing ARDS are critically ill, often with multisystem organ failure, illness develops 12-48hrs after the inciting event, although rarely it may take up to a few days. With the onset of lung injury; patients initially develop dyspnea, tachycardia, tachypnea, anxiety and agitation.

Physical examination

Febrile or hypothermia

Hypotension
Peripheral vasoconstriction with cold extremities
Cyanosis of lips, nail beds
Lung signs: bilateral diffuse rales

To rule out cardiogenic pulmonary edema, the signs of CCF or intravascular volume overload have to be looked for, such as:

raised JVP
cardiac murmur or gallop
hepatomegaly
edema

Investigations

ABG: Initially shows respiratory alkalosis, if sepsis present metabolic acidosis with or without respiratory compensation.

PaO$_2$/FiO$_2$ ratio, as indicated above.
Hematologic: Septic patients: leucopenia or leukocytosis, thrombocytopenia, features of DIC.

Renal: RFT to rule out ATN probably from renal ischemia

Liver: LFT abnormalities noted in hepatocelullar injury or cholestasis.

Cytokines 1L-1, 1L-6 and 1L-8 are raised in patients at risk for ARDS.

Chest x-ray: Initially, the infiltration may have a patchy peripheral distribution, but soon progresses to diffuse bilateral involvement with ground glass appearance or frank alveolar infiltration, with normal costophrenic angles.

CT Chest: It is more sensitive in detecting pulmonary interstitial emphysema, pneumothorax, pneumomediastinum, pleural effusion, cavitation and mediastinal lymphadenopathy.

Echocardiography: Transesophageal echography in supine position, to exclude cardiac causes.

Invasive hemodynamic monitoring: To rule out cardiogenic pulmonary edema, hemodynamic monitoring with pulmonary artery (Swan-Ganz) catheter introduced into a

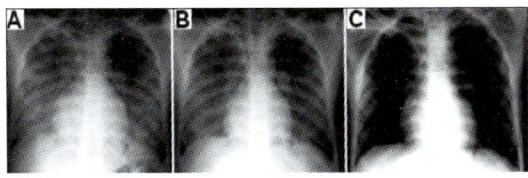

Fig. 76.3. X-ray chest in ARDS
A.   At the time of admission
B.   Partial resolution with treatment
C.   Complete resolution

central vein usually right internal jugular or subclavian vein may be required for continuous pressure monitoring. Pulmonary artery occlusion pressure (PAOP)<18, indicates non-cardiogenic pulmonary edema.

Bronchoscopy is done to:
evaluate possibility of infection
perform broncho-alveolar lavage (BAL)

Histologic findings:

Initially exudative phase
Interstitial edema
Alveolar hemorrhage and edema
Alveolar collapse
Pulmonary capillary congestion
Hyaline membrane formation

Normal pressure ranges (mmHg)

Vessel	Systolic	Diastolic
Central venous pressure (CVP)	3-8	
Rt Ventricle	15-30	3-8
Pulmonary artery	15-30	4-12
Pulmonary vein or capillary wedge pressure (PCWP)	2-15	
Lt Ventricle	100-140	3-12

TREATMENT OF ARDS

1. Any identifiable causes has to be treated first, on their merits.

2. Fluid management: Fluid conservative strategy improved oxygenation index and lung injury score and an increase in ventilator free days without an increase in Non-pulmonary organ failure. It is important to distinguish between initial resuscitation for early goal directed therapy and maintenance fluid therapy. CVP guided fluid therapy will be preferred. An ARDS clinical trials network study of fluid conservative strategy versus fluid liberal strategy found no statistically significant difference in 60 day mortality between 2 groups. However patients treated with fluid conservative strategy had an improved oxygenation, index, lung injury score and increase in ventilator free days. Intake output to be closely monitored, and in oliguric patients hemodialysis (HD) with ultrafiltration or continuous veno-venous hemodialysis (CVVHD) may be required.

3. O_2 inhalation

4. Non-invasive Ventilation: In ALI or mild ARDS, continuous positive airway pressure (CPAP) or noninvasive positive pressure ventilation (NIPPV) may be advantageous.

5. Mechanical Ventilation: The aim in mechanical ventilation in the ARDS patient is to maintain adequate oxygenation and preventing complication of oxygen toxicity and mechanical ventilation. Patient treated with low tidal volume (6ml/kg) had significantly lower mortality rate. Higher levels of PEEP may be required to open up collapsed alveoli and to drive fluid out of them, with careful monitoring of haemodynamic status. Muscular paralytic agents should be used judiciously. If high inspiratory pressures are required to deliver even low tidal volumes, pressure controlled ventilation may be initiated. Increasing the normal inspiration/expiration (I:E) ratio of ventilation (1: 2) may be tried if oxygenation problem persists. High frequency ventilation (jet or oscillatory) is a mode which uses low tidal volume and high respiratory rate. Partial liquid ventilation has also been tried in ARDS. Some 60-75% of patient with ARDS have significant improvement in oxygenation when turned from supine to prone (prone ventilation). Improvement is possibly related to recruitment of dependent lung zone, increased functional residual capacity (FRC), improved diaphramatic excursion, increased cardiac output and improved VQ matching. In patients

requiring prolonged ventilation tracheostomy may be required. Other strategies, such as extracorporeal membrane oxygenation (ECMO) remain a potential heroic measure in select cases.

6. Drugs found to be useful

Antibiotics, large dose steroids, artificial surfactants, mucolytic (bromhexine) and ciliokinetic agents (ambroxol)

FAT EMBOLISM

This phenomenon usually follows major fractures, but may be rarely seen during over zealous administration of intravenous fat (in TPN) and following lymphangiogram with a fat soluble contrast. Conditions such as acute pancreatitis, extensive burns diabetes mellitus and steroid therapy may be associated with fat embolism syndrome.

Clinical features

Fever out of proportion to injury is a common feature. Urine examination may reveal fat globules, but it is not pathognomonic, since such a finding is not uncommon following major trauma, without fat embolism syndrome. Corroborative findings in this disease are, drop in hematocrit, thrombocytopenia, hypocalcemia, hypoalbuminemia and elevated serum lipase. Chest x-ray may reveal diffuse parenchymal infiltrates ('snow-storm' appearance) and arterial blood gases analysis shows hypoxia and respiratory acidosis. Isotope pulmonary scan is very useful in this condition; it may show multiple areas of hypoperfusion.

Treatment

Besides general and ventilatory support, use of heparin, low molecular dextran, antiplatelet agents and fat solvents (IV), such as ethyl alcohol (which also reduces lipase activity and production of free fatty acids) are recommended.

AIR EMBOLISM

Air may be accidentally injected into the veins (artificial pneumoperitoneum or pneumothorax or IV infusion under pressure), tubal insufflation and attempted abortion or through a large vein opened in the neck during surgery or cut throat injuries. An estimated 4-5ml/Kg of air (approximately 200-300ml) is required to cause death, though smaller volumes may cause morbidity.

When air enters the right atrium, it is churned up and enters the right ventricle choking the pulmonary arteries (air lock). Dyspnea, cyanosis and acute right ventricular failure may be seen. If it enters the left ventricle either due to punctured pulmonary arteries, arteriovenous shunts or paradoxical embolism, it may embolize into coronary or cerebral vessels, with serious consequences.

Treatment

It is largely prevented by the use of plastic infusion bags and acute awareness of this possibility during air insufflation and venotomy.

Tilting the patient immediately into Trendelenburg position with a left lateral tilt; facilitates the trapped air to pass into lower limb veins and into the apex of the ventricle. Oxygen administration and ventilatory/circulatory support as necessary may be instituted. In severe cases either needle aspiration or direct evacuation of air from the ventricle by a thoracotomy may be needed.

Caisson's disease

Also known as acute decompression disease, it may affect divers, those who work in compressed air chambers or deep mines and those who ascend in open aeroplanes to high altitudes. When the decompression is too rapid, nitrogen in the blood and tissues gets converted into minute bubbles and occlude microvasculature. Patient may develop symptoms of acute ischemia in multiple areas, such as muscles, CNS, lungs etc. producing bizarre manifestations. Tightness of chest or dry cough (the 'chokes') may indicate pulmonary involvement.

It requires urgent supportive therapy, inhalations of 100% oxygen, recompression and gradual decompression. High altitude victims are relieved by gradual descent. If appropriate remedial measures are employed in time, outcome is excellent, but in cases of CNS involvement or delayed institution of treatment, residual symptoms may be long lasting.

Recent advances

Extracorporeal lung assistance (ECLA) is used in some centres and has shown an edge over conventional treatment protocols, similar to extracorporeal membrane oxygenation (ECMO), which has made a small but significant difference in the outcome of acute pulmonary insufficiency in infants.

77 Lower Limb Ischemia

ISCHEMIA of the lower limb is far more common than that of the upper limb; it may be acute, acute-on-chronic or chronic. The causes may be classified as follows:

1) Acute:

i) thromboembolism
ii) trauma
iii) frostbite
iv) toxic (e.g. insect bite)

2) Acute-on-chronic: thromboembolism developing in an artery with preexisting occlusive intimal disease. This is probably the commonest presentation of occlusive arterial disease.

3) Chronic:

i) atherosclerosis
ii) vasculitis

   a) thromboangiitis obliterans (TAO)
   b) collagen vascular diseases
   c) nonspecific aorto-arteritis (NAA)
   d) allergic/toxic

iii) diabetic angiopathy
iv) popliteal artery diseases (e.g. entrapment, adventitial cystic disease)
v) arteriovenous fistula/malformation (AVF or AVM)
vi) vasospastic diseases (e.g. ergotism, acrocyanosis, livido reticularis, causalgia etc)
vii) Thrombophilia, such as homocysteinemia, antiphospholipid syndrome (e.g. antibodies against lupus anticoagulant and cardiolipin) etc.

Clinical features

These depend upon the type of presentation, either acute, chronic or more commonly acute-on-chronic.

The classical features of *acute* occlusion are unmistakable (7 Ps): all are self explanatory

i) pistol-shot onset
ii) pain
iii) pallor
iv) pulselessness
v) paresthesia
vi) paralysis
vii) poikilothermia (cold extremity)

In *chronic* ischemia, on the other hand, various clinical stages (Fontaine classification) may be seen, such as

(i) claudication (claudicare: to limp),
(ii) rest pain,
(iii) pregangrene
(iv) gangrene.

The term 'limb failure', referring to the latter three stages, was used during the period when the subject of vascular surgery was evolving, to identify those requiring surgery, but such a distinction is no longer relevant, since disabling claudication interfering with normal activities also constitutes limb failure, requiring intervention. Such a degree of limb-threatening ischemia is currently referred to as critical limb ischemia (CLI). The claudication ('cry of starving nerves'), may be graded (Boyd) according to its severity;

(1) pain comes on walking, but is partially relieved on further walking, due to vasodilatation induced by ischemia, washing away the 'pain-producing' metabolites and the patient continues to walk

(2) on walking the pain appears and persists, but the patient manages to walk

(3) pain is so severe and unrelenting, that the patient has to stop for a few minutes, before he can walk further.

In any arterial occlusive disorder, it is essential to look for evidence of ischemia in other parts of the body, such as cerebral (transient ischemic attacks-TIAs), coronary (angina pectoris), mesenteric (abdominal angina), renal (secondary hypertension) etc. This is necessary not only for assessing the extent of systemic involvement, but also in terms of planning out treatment strategies.

The signs of chronic ischemia of a limb are:

i) dependent rubor or Buerger's sign (blanching of the foot on elevation of the limb and blushing on lowering to dependency), as a result of vasomotor instability

ii) thin shiny skin

iii) loss of hair

iv) reduced volume, due to wasting of muscles and fat

v) brittle, grooved nails

vi) trophic ulceration

Vii) ischemic tissue necrosis and gangrene

Acute-on-chronic occlusion: This is the most common variety of 'acute' occlusion, where some thromboembolic process shuts off the vessel, with preexisting intimal disease and compromised lumen. In view of the therapeutic implications, the identification of the type of occlusion is of considerable significance.

Peripheral pulses: Except in cases of microangiopathy, absent peripheral pulses is vital to the diagnosis of limb ischemia and clinical assessment of the level of arterial occlusion; hence the importance of palpating at standard anatomical points is obvious. They are conventionally recorded in 4 grades:

grade 0:   no pulse (0)
grade 1:   very low volume pulse (1+)
grade 2:   subnormal volume (2+)
grade 3:   normal volume (3+)

Parvus et tardus pulse: Low volume, low tension with slow upstroke, seen in the post-stenotic arterial segments, e.g. aortic stenosis or incomplete occlusion of a major artery.

The *abdominal aorta* may be palpated by deep digital pressure, in not-so-obese patients, more easily in the umbilical than the epigastric region, due to the normal lumbar lordosis. Absent pulsation of the abdominal aorta indicates high (suprarenal) occlusive disease. When both femorals are absent, in the presence of aortic pulse, it may indicate aorto-iliac disease. The *common femoral* pulse is readily felt in the groin fold, in the midinguinal point and for a distance of 5cm. below, before it disappears into the subsartorial (Hunter's or adductor) canal.

The *popliteal* pulse is the most difficult to feel in the lower limb, as it runs between the two femoral condyles and the heads of the gastrocnemius and is best palpated against the popliteal surface of tibia, with knee semiflexed (patient either in supine or prone position), both hands of the clinician encircling the leg, thumbs just below the tibial tubercle, other eight fingers spread flat, applying firm pressure over an area, covering about 5x5cm in the lower popliteal fossa.

Dorsalis pedis, the continuation of the anterior tibial artery, enters the foot midway between the two malleoli, runs lateral to the extensor hallucis longus tendon, to the base of the first intermetatarsal space, where it dips into the sole, to join the lateral plantar artery forming the plantar arch. It may be palpated lateral to the tendon, in the proximal half of the foot. The *posterior tibial* artery, the larger of the two terminal branches of the popliteal, lying in line with it, passes under the flexor retinaculum of the foot, where it divides into medial and lateral plantar arteries. It is felt immediately behind and below the medial malleolus, about 3cm in front of the tendo calcaneus (Achilles' tendon).

Crossed leg sign (of Fuchsig)

This is to identify the presence of pulsatile popliteal artery, which is ofen diffcult to detect by direct palpation. The patient is made to sit on a chair with legs crossed, keeping the leg to be

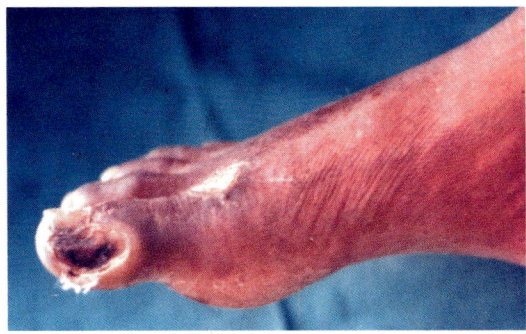

Fig. 77.1. Ischemic ulcer great toe due to
sup.fem.artery occlusion
(courtesy: Dr C J Reddy, Gudur, AP)

Feature	Arterial	Venous	Neurogenic
Location	Foot & calf	Foot	Entire leg
Low backache	Absent	Absent	May be present
Incidence	Common	Rare	Rare
Relieving factors	Rest	Elevation	Rest with knee flexed
Peripheral pulses	Absent	Present	Present
Edema	Absent	Present	Absent
Pigmentation	Absent	Present	Absent
SLR Test	Negative	Negative	Positive
Sensory/motor deficit	Absent	Absent	May be present
Trophic changes	Present	Absent	May be present
Diagnosis	Duplex/angio	Duplex	MRI of lumbar spine

Table-77.1 Differences between various types of claudication

examined above the other. Fine oscillatory moments of the leg/foot, synchronizing with peripheral pulse, are noticed, due to transmission of popliteal pulse (if it is of sufficient amplitude) through the calf muscles, against the opposite patella.

Pathology of chronic ischemia

Intermittent claudication occurs when blood flow to the muscles is unable to meet the increased metabolic demands during exercise, while it may be sufficient at rest. The pain is due to abnormal accumulation of metabolites within the muscle, not cleared because of inadequate perfusion. During exercise the muscular arterioles dilate enormously, reducing the peripheral resistance, but the arterial pressure is maintained due to autonomic redistribution of flow in normal conditions, whereas this is not possible in arterial occlusion; hence the effective *perfusion pressure* drops in the distribution channels beyond the point of stenosis.

Depending upon the level of occlusion, the claudication may be gluteal (aorto-iliac), femoral (ilio-femoral), crural (femoro-popliteal) or pedal (tibial). The claudication distance not only indicates the severity, but the progression of the disease as well. Initially the patient may continue to walk with pain, but as the disease progresses, only resting for a few minutes relieves the pain, before further walking is possible. Rest pain, pregangrene (dusky hue, with Raynaud's phenomenon) and frank gangrene are features of worsening ischemia of the limb, in that order.

Hemorrheology (rheos: current) is the study of flow properties of blood. The size of the capillaries is much smaller than the diameter of the RBC, hence the latter take all sorts of shapes, such as tear drops, dumb-bell, cone etc. which is largely influenced by the ATP content of the RBC. Drugs like pentoxiphylline, are known to increase the intracellular ATP of RBC, thus improving their 'flexibility'. Unfortunately all rheological factors in an occlusive arterial disease, will adversely influence the outcome. They are:

i) hypercoagulability
ii) increased viscosity
iii) increased platelet activity
iv) reduction in flow velocity

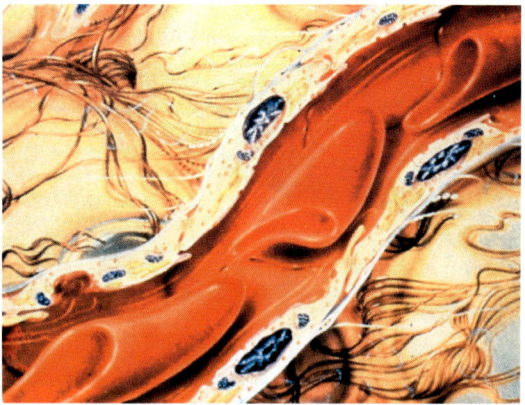

Fig. 77.2. Cone shaped RBC passing through narrow capillaries demonstrating their extreme deformability

Differential diagnosis

i)   Venous ulcer and claudication (described in chapter 82)

ii)   Neurogenic claudication, due to lumbo-sacral root compression, can very closely mimic that of ischemia. Absence of features of chronic ischemia of limb, pain appearing at rest, with normal peripheral pulses, evidence of sensory and motor deficit in the limb, paraspinal pain and muscle spasm and positive *straight leg rising* (SLR) sign, all should support the diagnosis of sciatica. If suspected, full neurological evaluation is warranted, the diagnosis may be clinched by CT/MRI of lumbar spine. The possibility of both of them coexisting should not be over-looked.

Investigations

Routine: Urine, blood examination, including lipid profile, chest/abdomen x-ray, electrocardiogram and echocardiogram. Plain x-ray of the affected region may show calcific vessels

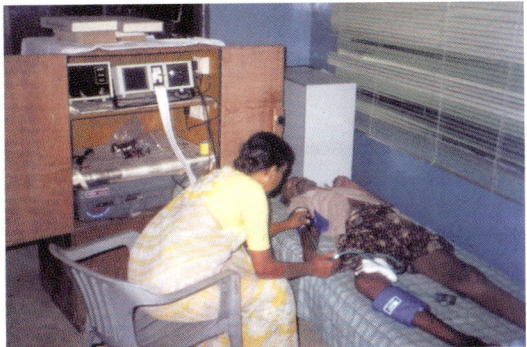

Fig. 77.5. Segmental pressure recording using a Doppler probe
(courtesy: Halsted Surgical Clinic, Chennai)

(Monckeberg degeneration or atherosclerosis).

Specific

1)   Venous filling time gives a rough index of severity of ischemia, which is the time taken for the appearance of veins, when an elevated limb is restored to dependent position. Normal is <15sec; above 30sec. the limb is clearly ischemic and if it is more than 45sec. there is a threat to the viability of limb.

2)   Claudication distance gives a fair indication of the severity of ischemia and its progressive reduction indicates worsening ischemia. This may be accurately measured by the use of a computerized treadmill or digitalized pedometer.

3)   Buerger's test: With the patient in the supine position, the leg is elevated slowly to 45°, the angle at which the limb turns pale (blanching due to vasoconstriction) is noted. This angle is called Buerger's vasomotor angle. Then the limb is dropped down, with patient sitting on the edge of stool and look for a cyanotic hue (desaturated blood passing through the limb) and finally dependent rubor (blushing due to reactive hyperemia). This denotes vasomotor instability in chronic ischemic states, particularly if there is significant vasospastic component, as seen in Buerger's disease.

4)   **Doppler** examination is a noninvasive ultrasonic study, to detect the proximal point of occlusion, collaterals and distal run-off. The physical principle that the frequency of sound emitted by a moving source is increased if the

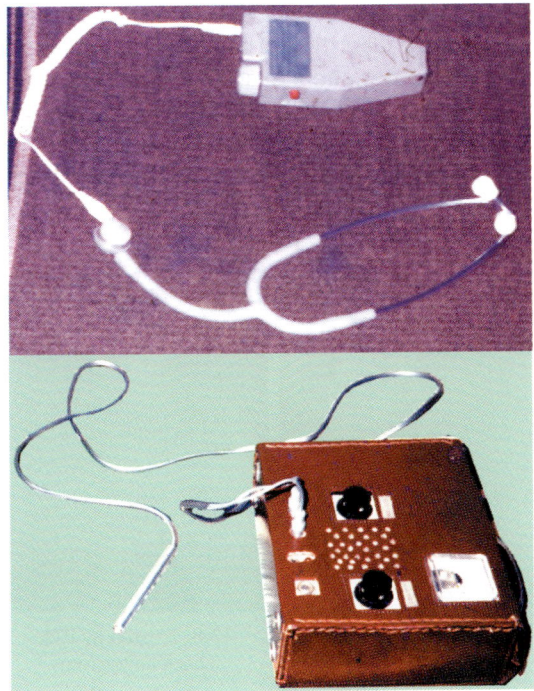

Fig. 77.3 & 77.4. Portable Doppler machines
(courtesy: Halsted Surgical Clinic, Chennai)

429

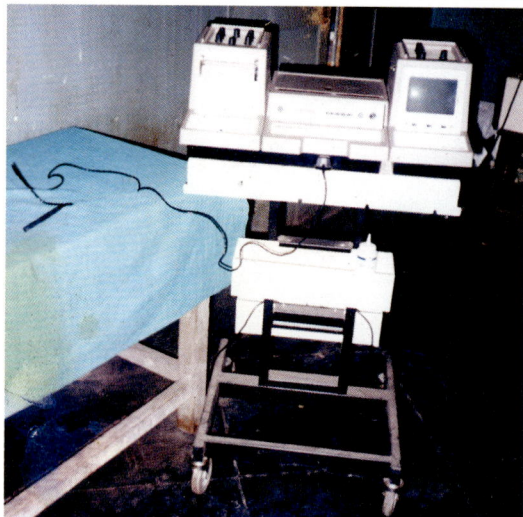

Fig. 77.6. Bidirectional waveform Doppler recorder (courtesy: Prof M Raghuram, Chennai)

source is moving towards the receiver and reduced if the source is moving away, is known as the *Doppler effect*. Sound waves beyond audible range (ultrasound beam), with a frequency usually between 2-10MHz, are sent inside, and the reflection is received by a pair of piezoelectric crystals and converted into audible signals, by a computer (human audible range of sound: 20Hz to 20KiloHz or 20,000Hz).

The character of the sound waves received depends upon the medium through which they pass; if it is static, they return unaltered and if it is moving (flowing blood), they produce different signals (*Doppler shift*) by which various clinical conditions may be identified. A waveform Doppler is to print the amplitude of a pulse wave on a graph, for analysis.

5) Duplex imaging: (it is so-called since it records both anatomical details and flow characteristics in a vessel) is a real time B-mode (brightness mode) ultrasonography, by which the image of the object being scanned is seen or can be recorded and may be considered as an improvised noninvasive angiogram. The information on the thickness of the vessel wall, extent of occlusion, lumen available for flow etc. is sufficient in most of the cases to carry out recon-

structive procedures, thus avoiding a conventional angiography.

6) Color coding is yet another improvement; by processing larger volumes of tissue at a time, the velocity and direction of flow (towards or away from the probe) in a vessel may be arrived at.

7) Segmental pressure recording using a Doppler probe is a very important investigation, in the day to day evaluation of arterial occlusion. Normally brachial and ankle blood pressures are equal, with an *ankle/brachial index* (ABI) of 0.9-1.1; less than 0.6 is considered critical and under 0.3 is grave. False high pressure reading may be seen in atherosclerotic/calcified peripheral vessels, requiring greater compression for occlusion. Normal systolic pressures recorded in the thigh: 130-140, below-knee: 120-130, at ankle: 110-120 and toe pressure: 80-90mmHg. Toe pressure <50 or an *ankle/toe gradient* >50 in the young and >60 in the elderly indicates critical ischemia. While calculating ABI, the highest pressure of the 3 vessels at the ankle has to be considered.

8) Post-exercise pressure recording may detect subclinical but critical proximal stenosis, as the drop in the peripheral resistance after exercise, produces reduction in blood pressure (common) or disappearance of pulse (rare), beyond occlusion, only to reappear after 10 minutes (sign of disappearing pulse).

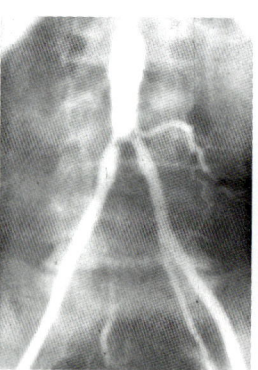
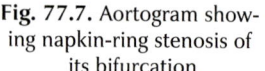
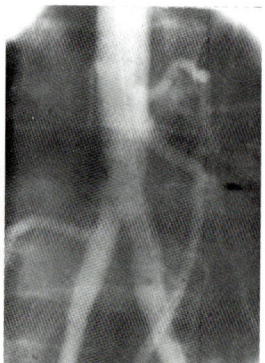

Fig. 77.7. Aortogram showing napkin-ring stenosis of its bifurcation

77.8. Treated by PTA check angiogram

(courtesy: Dr K N Reddy, Chennai)

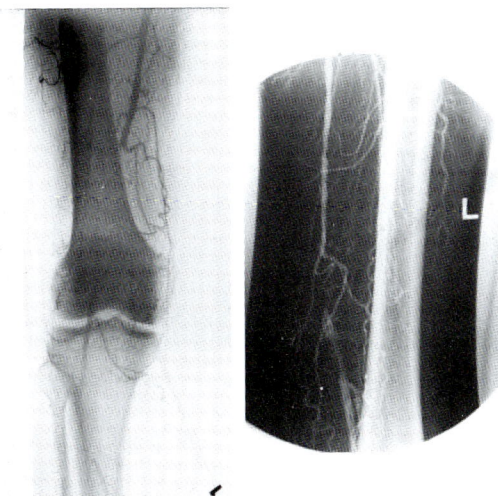

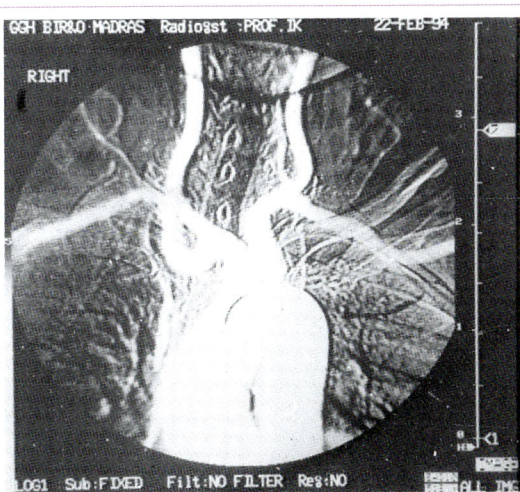

Fig. 77.9. Femoral angiograms showing distal femoral block with popliteal reformation (good distal run-off) (courtesy: Halsted Surgical Clinic, Chennai)

Fig. 77.11. Digital subtraction angiogram (DSA) of aortic arch and its branches (courtesy: Prof M Raghuram, Chennai)

9) *Transcutaneous oximetry* is the intracutaneous oxygen tension ($TcPO_2$) measured by placing a polarographic electrode (Clark) over the skin, which appears to correlate with arterial values and the degree of ischemia. The main drawback of this measurement is the interference by the body temperature, skin thickness, and local edema/cellulitis; hence it is not routinely done, but used only to predict the healing potential of an ulcer/ wound, on an ischemic background. The normal foot has a $TcPO_2$ of 50-60mmHg; under 30 indicates significant ischemia.

10) *Plethysmography* and *Xenon*[133] muscle clearance studies have limited clinical applications and are not routinely done.

11) *Angiography* is the 'gold standard' investigation in arterial occlusions, but is needed only if direct arterial surgery is indicated/contemplated, for which several techniques are available. They are:

i) Conventional, known as retrograde femoral/axillary aortography

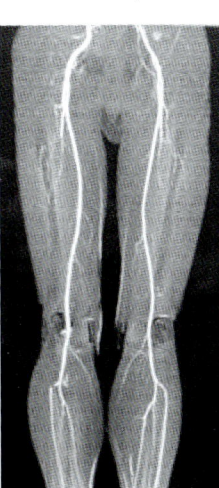

Fig.77.10. CT angiogram of both lower limbs. Note the occlusion at the origin of right anterior tibilal artery, with good distal run-off

ii) Digital subtraction angiography (DSA), which may be intravenous or intra-arterial

iii) CT (standard or multislice) angiography

iv) Magnetic resonance angiography (MRA)

v) Isotopic angiography, with ^{99m}Tc

i) Conventional angiogram (*Seldinger technique*) is done by puncturing the femoral/axillary/radial artery percutaneously and a guide wire is introduced through the needle (*Cournand's*), over which a catheter is threaded into the vessel and the wire withdrawn. Under monitoring with a C-arm image intensifier, the catheter tip can be negotiated to the desired level, before injection of a contrast, such as iothalamate meglu-mine (Conray) or gadolinium; the latter is preferred in the presence of renal dysfunction. Manual injection may be sufficient for peripheral vessels, but a programmed pressure injector, with serial filming or video recording is necessary for aortic study. Initial injection of a small test dose will not only identify iodine sensitivity, but also ascertain proper placement of the catheter. With experience, a pig-tail catheter can be negotiated into any

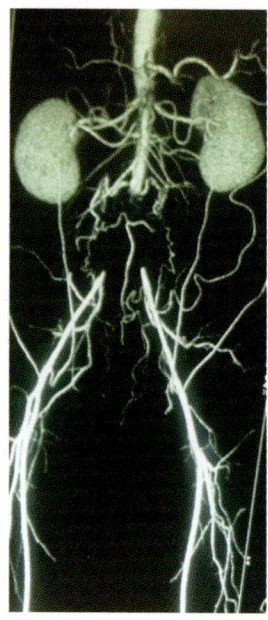

Fig. 77.12. CT aortogram showing aorto-iliac occlusion (Leriche) with good distal run-off.

branch of aorta, such as coronaries, carotid, subclavian, hepatic, mesenteric, renal etc, called selective angiography, so that minimum contrast can be used to derive maximum information. Higher incidence of lactic acidosis is associated with the use of iodized contrast while the patient is on metformin therapy for diabetes. The following points have to be noted in an angiogram:

a) proximal level of occlusion

b) length of stenosed/occluded segment

c) state of proximal vessel

d) distal run-off

e) collateral vessels

f) direction of flow in a vessel (e.g. reversal of flow in vertebral artery in subclavian steal syndrome)

g) patency of a bypass graft

h) post-stenotic or anastomotic aneurysm

ii) multislice helical CT (MSCT) angiogram is emerging as a highly sensitive method of diagnosing of vascular injuries.

iii) Digital subtraction angiogram (DSA) is a novel imaging technique using a computer. An x-ray image of the part to be studied is initially taken, which goes into the memory. The contrast is then injected and pictures are taken. The computer subtracts the first image from the second, eliminating bone and other soft tissue opacities from the picture, retaining only the vessels filled with contrast. The resolution is so good that the contrast may be given intravenously, obviating the need for an arterial puncture.

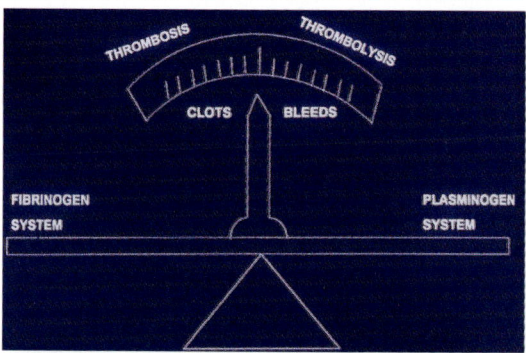

Fig. 77.13. Delicate balance between fibrinogen and plasminogen systems

iv) magnetic resonance angiography (MRA) can be done without giving any contrast, a totally noninvasive and safe procedure.

v) Isotope angiography using ^{99m}Tc labeled RBC, is useful in children to study AVM, to avoid invasive investigations, but the resolution is inferior to the other types of angiography.

If both femorals are absent, the aorta may be accessed either through axillary arteries (trans-axillary aortogram) or by direct percutaneous puncture of the aorta (trans-lumbar aortogram); the latter, being a blind procedure, is least preferred nowadays.

Differences between arterial and venous ulcer (see chapter 82 on varicose veins).

Treatment

Management of acute occlusion

As already indicated, it is crucial to identify a simple acute occlusion from the acute-

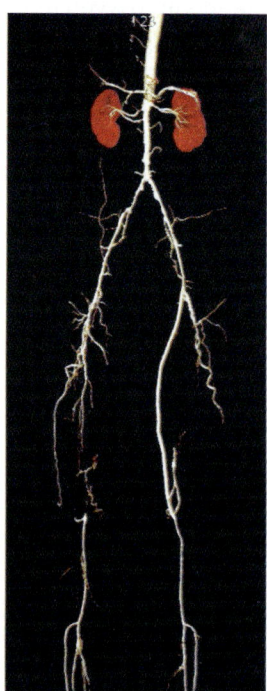

Fig. 77.14. CT angiogram showing bilateral multisegmental occlusions. Fem-pop bypass grafting was done for left SFA

on-chronic type. Prior history of claudication, features of chronic ischemia of the limb, and evidence of arterial insufficiency in the other limb, would help identify the latter, in which no urgent surgical intervention is indicated. An expedient search for source of embolus should be done, such as cardiac chambers/ valves, atheromatous plaques (athero-embolization) from major vessels and aneurysms, with special reference to *silent cardiac infarction* with mural thrombosis. However a definite source can be identified only in <50% of them. In the rest, it is believed to be a *pathological accident*. *Paradoxical embolization* arising from the venous system, passing through an ASD/VSD, and getting lodged in the peripheral arteries is a rare clinical event.

The general principles of treatment are:

a) anticoagulation with heparin, either unfractionated or fractionated. In acute occlusions, heparin is preferred because of its immediate (within 5min) action (vide infra).

b) antiplatelet agents

c) rheological therapy with low molecular dextran, to improve microcirculation

d) if thromboembolectomy is planned, assessment of cardiac status, to withstand reperfusion effects, is mandatory

e) *Fibrinolytic agents*, such as urokinase, streptokinase or tissue plasminogen activator (tPA), ideally given within 72 hours of thromboembolism, for optimal results.

f) If occurring on a previously healthy vessel, urgent thromboembolectomy is carried out, while continuing the medical regime.

Procedure: Though an angiogram may be very useful, it is not essential and may consume time, delaying surgery. Doppler/duplex recording is generally sufficient for purposes of planning surgery. It can be done comfortably under local or spinal anesthesia; the latter gives an additional benefit of 'sympathectomy effect' to the limb. The vessel is surgically exposed and arteriotomy is made distal to the pulsating segment, after proximal and distal control of the vessel by silastic loops or vascular clamps. Using a Fogarty balloon catheter, both proximal and distal clots are systematically retrieved, introducing a suitable sized catheter, distal clearance upto the ankle is possible, to restore good proximal pulsations and brisk retrograde bleeding.

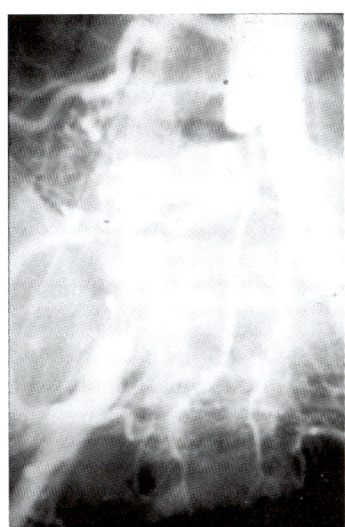

Fig. 77.15. Extensive acute iliac occlusion (right)

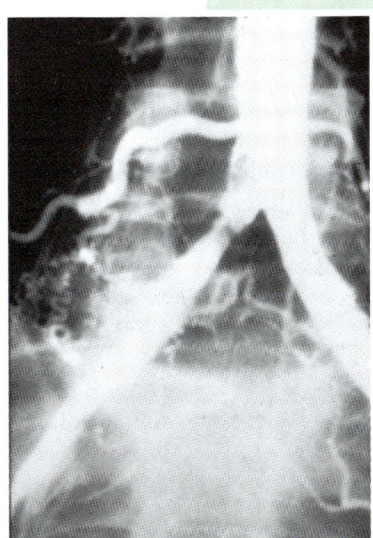

77.16. After infusion of thrombolytic agents, showing the culprit stenosis
(Courtesy: Dr P J Reddy, Texas, USA)

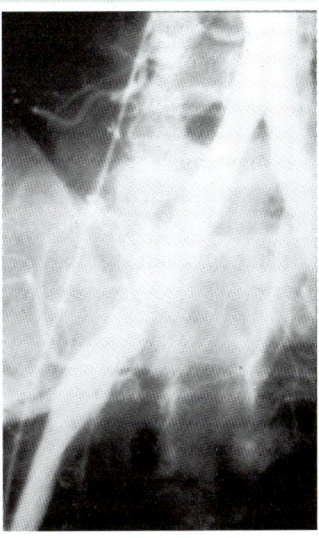

77.17. Angiogram after the stenosis treated by transluminal angioplasty (PTA)

Compartment	Sensory deficit	Motor deficit	Movement painful
Anterior	First web space	Toe extension	Toe flexion
Lateral	Dorsum of foot	Foot eversion	Foot inversion
Superficial posterior		Plantar flexion	Dorsiflexion
Deep posterior	Sole of foot	Toe flexion	Toe extension

Table-77.2. Compartment syndrome of leg

Transverse arteriotomy is preferable for medium-sized vessels, to avoid hour-glass constriction following closure.

The arteriotomy is then closed with fine nonabsorbable material (aorta: 4-0; iliac/femoral: 5-0; popliteal: 6-0 and for tibials:7/8-0). In delayed cases, where propagation of clots into the small distribution channels is expected, intra-arterial thrombolysis may be employed to clear them and a 'check angiogram' is taken on the table, at conclusion. Some centres use intraoperative angioscopy for this purpose. A subcutaneous fasciotomy (Mubarak) of the calf, covering all the 3 compartments (medial, anterior and posterior), should be done at the end, if compartment swelling is anticipated, due to reperfusion effect.

Reperfusion injury refers to the local and systemic effects of embolectomy, seen more in delayed cases. Ideally restoration of flow should be done within 6 hours, to prevent irreversible tissue changes, but that appears to be a luxury in a clinical set up. Earlier, a 72-hour 'dead-line' was given for doing successful embolectomy, but experience has disproved it, especially in patients on anticoagulation earlier, as is the case most often. Successful embolectomy has been carried out even after 6 weeks of occlusion, in a patient who was convalescing from a cardiac infarction.

Normal tissue pressure is under 10mm Hg and if it exceeds 30, a cascade of pathological events is set in motion, ultimately culminating in an osteo-fascial compartment syndrome.

Ischemia-reperfusion injury (IRI)

When there is acute limb ischemia, the tissue energy sources are exhausted and if it is prolonged over 6 hours, a series of biochemical events is set in motion. The process is actually initiated within 3 hours and becomes irreversible after 6 hours. The cell membrane becomes more permeable, calcium enters the cell and potassium comes out. The cell edema and transudation of fluid increases tissue pressure, compressing lymphatic and venous channels, producing compartment syndrome, which is worsened by sudden revascularization, increasing the input into the limb.

The systemic manifestations may be more serious and life-theatening. Because of anerobic glycolysis, there is metabolic acidosis and rhabdomyolysis leads to the release of myoglobulin, precipitating renal tubular dysfunction and life-threatening hyperkalemia. With reperfusion all the stagnant toxic metabolites, including inflammatory mediators such as platelet activating factor (PAF), tumor necrosis factor (TNF-alfa) are released into general circulation, causing widespread tissue damage. It also brings in new supply of oxygen, which reacts with hypoxanthine to form xanthine and provide oxygen free radicals, activating the platelets and leukocytes, producing microthrombi, further jeopardizing the microcirculation. All these events ultimetely lead to systemic inflammatory

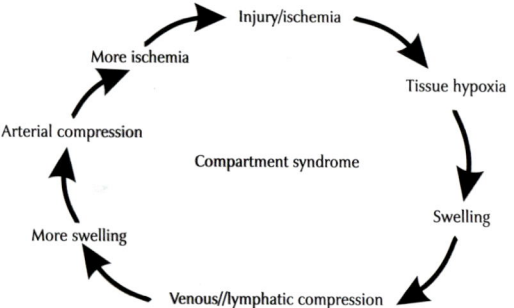

Fig. 77.18. The vicious cycle of compartment syndrome

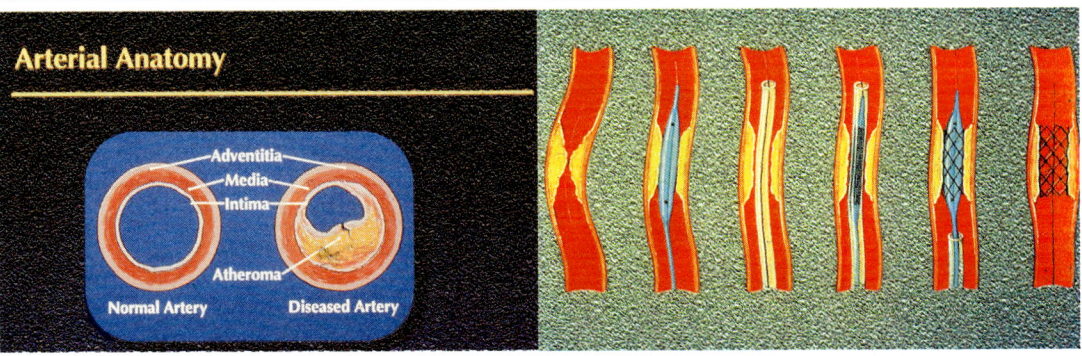

Arterial Anatomy

Adventitia
Media
Intima
Atheroma
Normal Artery   Diseased Artery

Fig. 77.19. Atheromatous occlusion of arterial lumen & **77.20.** Dilatation and stenting by PTA
(courtesy: Dr. P.J. Reddy, Texas, USA)

response syndrome (SIRS) and later to multiorgan dysfunction syndrome (MODS), with high mortality, depending upon the number of malfunctioning systems.

Several agents have been in use to blunt the local and systemic effects of IRI, such as antioxidants, N-acetylcysteine, ACE inhibitors, calcium channel blockers, allopurinol, iron/potassium chelating agents, nitric oxide (NO) donors, mannitol, adenosine and catalase. Preconditioning for ischemia appears to reduce the severity of the pathology, as seen in cases of acute-on-chronic ischemia, where the limb is exposed to gradually worsening attacks of transient ischemia. Naturally, the earlier the vascularity is re-established, lesser the local and systemic

complications and better the ultimate outlook.

Effect of stagnated blood returning to the circulation may be disastrous to the heart, so that many workers feel that if a patient has compromised cardiac status, it may not be safe to carry out embolectomy, especially if delayed, and instead advise amputation as expedient and life saving, under such circumstances. It should be stated at this juncture that the overall in-hospital mortality in patients with major arterial emboli is over 25%, the majority attributable to their underlying cardiac status.

Fat and air embolism: see chapter 76 (ARDS)

Vascular trauma

Blunt and penetrating injuries or high velocity missiles, may cause injury to blood vessels, threatening life or the viability of limb. Iatrogenic injuries also are on the increase in the recent times due to the liberal application

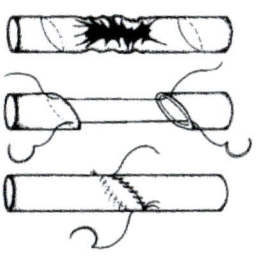

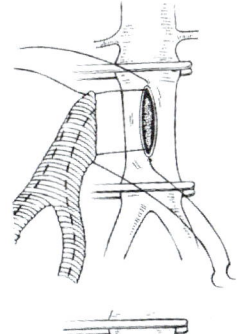

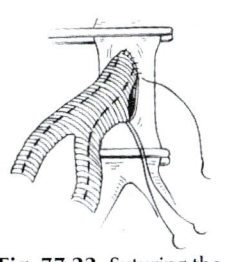

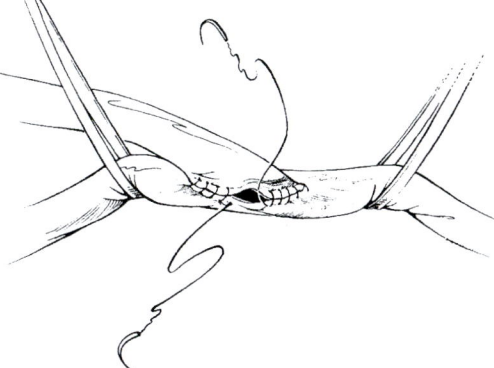

Fig. 77.21. Bevelling the ends to prevent stenosis of the vascular end-to-end anastomosis

Fig. 77.22. Suturing the stem of the bifurcated graft to infrarenal aorta

Fig. 77.23. End-to-side vascular anastomosis

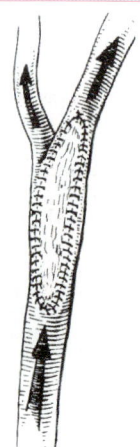

Fig. 77.24. Patch angioplasty, to prevent hour-glass constriction following arteriotomy

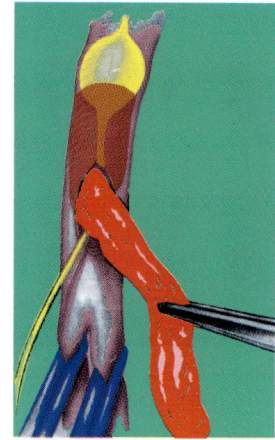

Fig. 77.25. Thrombo-embolectomy using a Fogarty balloon catheter (courtesy: Halsted Surgical Clinic, Chennai)

as to the anticipated outcome in terms of limb and life, considering the availability of infrastructure and expertise in the institution, to avoid 'after thoughts' and litigations. As most of those cases tend to be medico-legal in nature, proper documentation is essential and the appropriate authority has to be notified immediately on admission.

3. Institute supportive therapy, including blood volume replacement and higher antibiotics. Vital functions, including oxygen

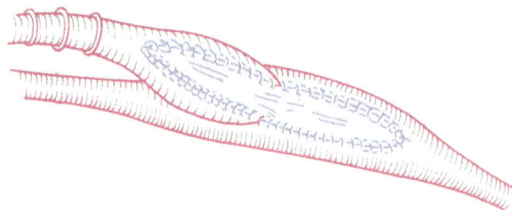

Fig. 77.26. Patch angioplasty, to prevent anastomotic stenosis

of endovascular procedures, for various vascular diseases.

Major vascular injury has to be suspected if there is:

1. Rapidly expanding hematoma
2. impaired peripheral pulse
3. features of acute ischemia of limb
4. hemodynamic instability

The vascular injury may be in the lumen (thrombus), in the vessel wall (intimal injury with subintimal hematoma) or vessel disruption, either partial or total. External compression, due to a displaced fracture or compartment syndrome, may also occlude blood vessels.

The following principles may be observed in the management of vascular trauma:

1. General evaluation for other major visceral injuries, preexisting vascular disease and for purposes of anesthesia, if required. Any life-theatening injury should receive priority attention, remembering 'life is more important than limb'. Relevant investigations, which may influence the management and ultimate outcome, have to be immediately carried out.

2. Adequate patient counseling is important,

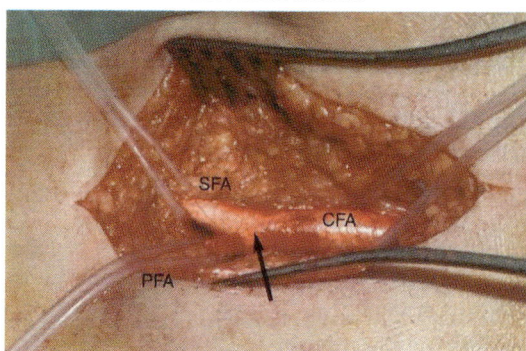

Fig. 77.27. Bifurcation of common femoral artery controlled with soft loops before arteriotomy for embolectomy

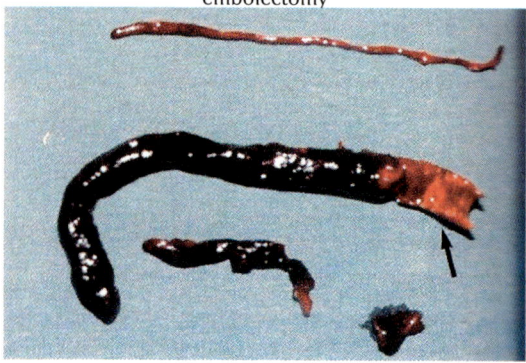

Fig. 77.28. Clots retrieved by Fogarty embolectomy

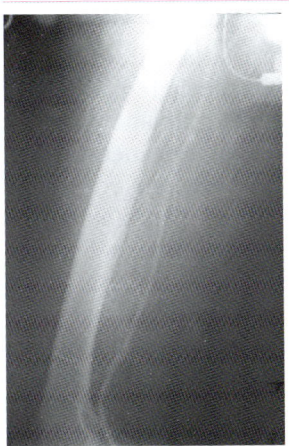

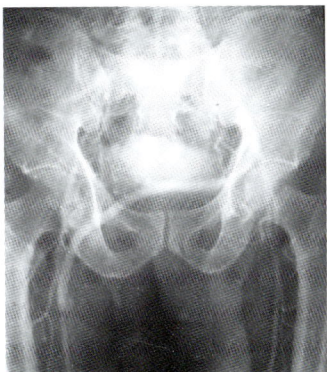

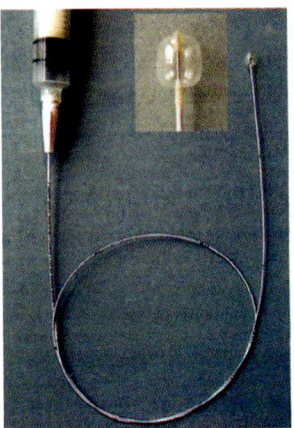

Fig. 77.29. Postoperative angiogram of long fem-pop bypass using reversed saphenous vein (courtesy: Halsted Surgical Clinic, Chennai)

Fig. 77.30. Postoperative angiogram of crossover ilio-femoral bypass (courtesy: Halsted Surgical Clinic, Chennai)

Fig. 77.31. Fogarty balloon embolectomy catheter

saturation (pulsoximentry) and urine output (indwelling catheter) have to be monitored.

4. Urgent angiography either conventional, Duplex or Multislice Helical CT (MSCT)

5. If a fracture is present in that region, it should be appropriately immobilized, before attempting vascular repair

6. Anticoagulation (heparinization), if there is no contraindication due to other injuries and hemorrheological agents, such as low molecular dextran or cilostazol

7. Urgent exploration and appropriate vascular repair. It may be expedient to ligate the not-so-critical artery, such as a terminal branch of popliteal or brachial artery, which may be well compensated by collaterals. If any graft is required to replace the injured vessel, synthetic conduits should be avoided as far as possible, in view of high potential for infection and subsequent occlusion.

8. Post-procedure angiogram to check the repair as well as outflow vascular tree

9. Appropriate measures to prevent thrombosis of the repaired artery and also deep vein thrombosis (DVT), vulnerable as a result of injury or immobilization.

Medical therapy of chronic ischemia, common to all types:

i)   Abstinence from tobacco in any form is essential; the patient can have either his cigarette or his leg, but not both.

Tobacco and vascular disease

Relationship of smoking and vascular disease was established almost century ago by placing omentum of anesthetized monkey under a microscope and giving inhalations of tobacco smoke. Spasm of the fine omental vessels were observed, reversible on cessation of tobacco inhalation.

Actions

1. Increased permeability of arterial wall due to carboxy-hemoglobin-induced hypoxia and spasm of vasavasorum

2. Nicotine sensitizes sympathetic end organs to circulating catacholamines, inducing vasospasm

3. Increased platelet count and activity through prostaglandin-thromboxane-A2 pathway

4. Tobacco glycoprotein (TGP) causes hypersensitivity reaction, endothelial injury and thrombotic tendency

5. Lowers HDL apoproteins

6. Interferes with macrophage activity and local immunity

Note: *Tobacco in any form is harmful and tremendous moral boost to a smoker, is a smoking doctor!* Passive inhalation of cigarette smoke is as bad as regular smoking.

i) Healthy alternative: E-smoking has been developed recently, incorporating a lithium battery and automizer which produces fumes of propyl glycol with variable proportion of nicotine, as well as a glow at the end, mimicking actual smoking in many respects, but without its harmful effects.

ii) Attention to obesity, diabetes mellitus etc.

iii) Dyslipidemia (increased cholesterol or tri-glycerides) may be controlled by any of the 'statins', such as lovastatin, simvostatin, atorvastatin or rosuvastatin.

iv) Graded (Buerger's) exercises, to open up new collateral channels

v) Anticoagulants oral or parenteral, the latter is by unfractionated (regular) or fractionated (low molecular weight-LMW) heparin. Oral anti-coagulants produce therapeutic level of anticoagulation (prothrombin time should be 2-3 times the control) by about 48hrs. and their effect may be countered by administration of

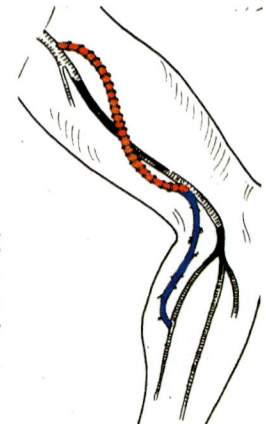

Fig. 77.32. Femoro-tibial bypass using a composite graft (ringed PTFE and reversed saphenous vein)

vitamin K1. The regular (unfraction-ated) heparin has a half-life of 2hrs and the dose (IV or deep intramuscular) is titrated by serial estimations of clot-ting time, to maintain it atleast around twice its normal. Overdose of heparin may be countered by protamine sul-fate (1mg for every 100u. of heparin). Fractionated (LMW) heparin is long acting, given IM, once a day, needs no titration and has minimal risk of hem-orrhagic complications, hence most preferred in current practice.

The principle of LMWH is selective retention of factor I and II blocking (anticoagulant) effect, without the anti Xa (pro-hemorrhagic) property of unfractionated heparin.

vi) Antiplatelet agents (e.g. aspirin, dipyri-damol, ticlopidine, clopidogrel, prasugrel etc)

vii) Hemorrheological agents: Rheology is study of flow properties of a fluid. When it is applied to blood, it is called hemorrheology and agents altering the flow properties of blood are in clini-cal use. (e.g. pentoxiphylline, cilastazol, cinarazine, low molecular weight dextran etc). The RBC with larger diameter (7-8μ) require to alter their shape, as they pass through capillaries with smaller diameter. The energy for this flexi-bility is dervied from ATP and these agents increase the intracelluar ATP of RBC. Pentoxi-

Feature	Oral	Heparin	
		Regular	LMW
Onset	2-3 days	5 min	30 min
Half-life	48 hrs	2-4 hrs	12-24 hrs
Mode	Antiprothrombin	Antithrombin	Antithrombin
Monitor	INR	APTT	Not needed
Administration	OD	Q4-6H	Q12-24H
Reversal	Vit K	Protamine	Protamine
Mol wt		15,000	<8,000
Bleeding	Possible	Possible	Rare
Action	Fact II, VII, IX & X (Vit K depedent)	Fact I,II,IX & Xa	Fact I & II
Platelet function	No effect	Inhibits	Minimal

Table-77.3. Comparison between oral and heparin anticoagulation

phylline (Trental) also lowers plasma fibrinogen level, viscosity and platelet aggregation.

Low molecular weight dextran (LMWD-Lomodex): It is a high polymer of dextrose with a molecular weight of 40,000. By expanding blood volume, it reduces viscosity. It coats the RBC and platelets with electronegative charge, thus preventing rouleaux formation and aggregation, an anti-sludging property. It also normalizes elevated factor VIII and fibrinogen, induced by surgical stress and has mild antilipemic property.

viii)   Vasodilators (e.g. papaverine, nicotinic acid, isoxsuprine, nilidrine, cyclandilate etc): Their systemic use is controversial, as there is already vasodilatation as a result of ischemia. Systemic administration of vasodilators may only dilate the vessels in other areas, stealing blood away from the affected limb, which may worsen the condition. Hence regional (intra-arterial) administration of drugs like papaverine (short acting), reserpine or guanethidine (long acting) is preferred, if a significant vasospastic component is suspected in the causation of ischemia.

ix) prostaglandin analogues are being used to improve the microcirculation by vasodilatation, to treat nonhealing ischemic ulcers. Alpostin 60mcgm/kg is infused as slow IV drip to run for about 6hrs, everyday for 6days.

Surgical treatment may be direct or indirect arterial surgery

1)   Direct arterial surgery - three types:

i)   Thrombo-endarterectomy, eminently suitable for major vessels with short stenotic segments; the plane of dissection to remove the obstructing pathology is within the layers of tunica media (the entire intima and part of the media are removed).

ii)   Angioplasty means widening a stenotic segment, by one of the two methods:

a)   an open method, making a longitudinal arteriotomy over the stenosis and fixing an elliptical patch of vein or PTFE over it, effec-tively increasing the lumen. The origin of profunda femoris is a favourite site for this procedure (profundaplasty).

b)   Percutaneous transluminal angioplasty (PTA) of Gruntzig, is best suited for short segment stenosis of inaccessible vessels, such as coronary, renal, common iliac etc. Though the original method is by a controlled compression of the atheromatous tissue projecting into the lumen using a balloon catheter, several endovascular innovations have come in, such as stenting, laser vaporization, laser-assisted balloon angioplasty (LABA), angioscopic atherectomy, rotablator atherectomy, and many more. With accumulating experience, more and more areas are being included within the purview of these minimally invasive, day-care procedures, preferred by both patient and vascular interventionist. (see chapter 84)

Drug-eluting stents (DES)

(elute: wash out or release)

One important reason for the failure of bare metal stents (BMS), following transluminal angioplasty in a low flow system like coronary arteries, is the accumulation of macrophages around the stent, as a foreign body reaction leading to proliferation of endothelium and fibroblasts, triggering thrombosis &/or restenosis of the vessel. It has been shown that if the stents are coated with antimitotic or cytostatic drugs, which prevent tissue proliferation, the incidence of restenosis and need for re-intervention is less.

The metals used in the stents: either stainless-steel or nitinol (an alloy of nickel and titanium).

The common drugs currently used with slow release technology are:

paclitaxel (antimitotic), everolimus, biolimus and zotarolimus (cytostatic), the latter (limus) group being currently favored.

However, the main drawback of DES is inhibition of formation of neo-intima over the stent, leaving the surface thrombogenic for

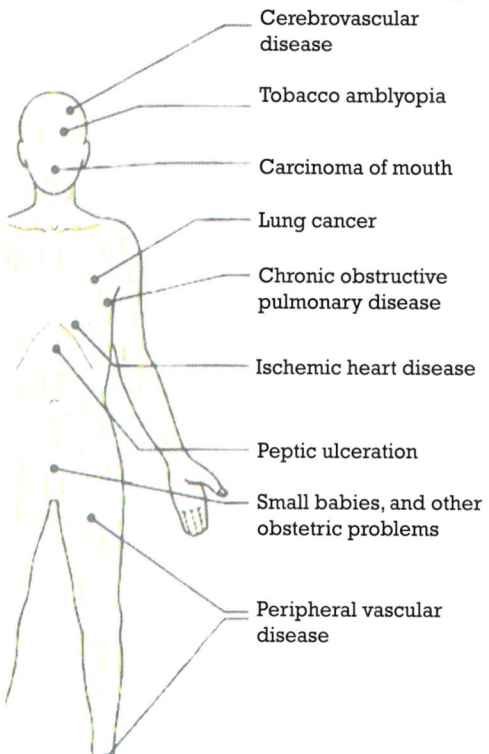

- Cerebrovascular disease
- Tobacco amblyopia
- Carcinoma of mouth
- Lung cancer
- Chronic obstructive pulmonary disease
- Ischemic heart disease
- Peptic ulceration
- Small babies, and other obstetric problems
- Peripheral vascular disease

Fig. 77.33. Tobacco-related diseases

several months. The theoretical advantages claimed and the additional cost of these devices have not translated into significant overall survival benefit, compared to BMS.

Currently biodegradable, heparin-coated or antibiotic-coated stents are also available.

iii) Bypass grafting, using autologous vein, synthetic material (e.g. Teflon, Dacron, PTFE etc) or from biological source (bovine artery or human umbilical vein), made immunologically inert by appropriate chemical treatment. Most preferred conduits among them are the long saphenous vein for low flow systems, such as coronaries, renal or infragenicular vessels and PTFE (polytetra-fluoroethylene) or Dacron for high flow segments, like

aortic, iliac or femoral segments. The basic techniques of vascular control and surgery have been described by Carrell in 1903, which are followed even by contemporary vascular surgeons.

The drawbacks of synthetic grafts are:

a) They are stiff and non-compliant, not ideal conduits for low flow system.

b) more thrombogenic; since it takes a few days for pseudointima formation, both early and late graft failures are more than a vein graft

c) infection can be disastrous, often leading to inevitable removal of the graft.

d) whenever it crosses a joint, constant bending may cause injury by 'graft fatigue'

e) foreign body reaction

f) high cost

Reversed vs in-situ vein grafts: Conventionally, when a vein is used as a conduit, it is *reversed* so as not to allow valves interfere with the flow of blood through them. Alternately the vein is being used *in-situ*, without harvesting, after destroying the valves with a *valvulotome*. The proponents for in-situ grafting say that it avoids damage to vasavasorum and endothelium, with better long-term patency rates. The size-match is also better with the arteries, since when it is reversed, the wider side of the vein is anastomosed to the narrower (distal) artery. However, the main drawback of this method is that it cannot be done, if the ipsilateral vein is unsuitable for use (or earlier removed) and secondly, the claims of better patency have not been substantiated universally.

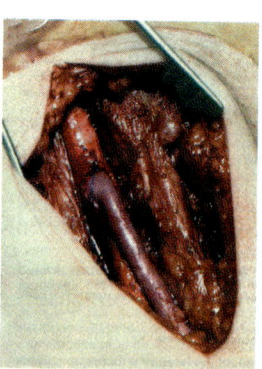

Fig. 77.34. Reversed long saphenous vein anastomosed end-to-side to common femoral artery

Depending upon the level of the distal anastomosis in the lower limb, these procedures are known as infrainguinal, infragenicular or inframalleolar bypasses.

1) Extra-anatomical bypass is directing the blood flow through a conduit, which is routed different from that of normal course of blood vessels; examples are:

a) axillo-femoral bypass
b) carotid-subclavian
c) crossover ilio-femoral or ilio-popliteal
d) spleno-renal

This method is useful whenever there is extensive occlusive disease of the proximal vessel unsuitable for implanting the graft.

2) Indirect arterial surgery is done to improve the collateral flow, when direct surgery is not feasible. They are:

i) Lumbar sympathectomy: Sympathetic stimulation in a limb causes cutaneous vasoconstriction and muscular vasodilation; the reverse occurs following sympathectomy. Thus, sympathectomy may not improve claudication, but is very effective for skin ulcers and digital gangrene. However, plethysmographic studies showed overall increased blood flow into the limb following sympathectomy, indirectly improving muscle perfusion, which explains the relief from claudication pain often observed. As ischemia causes local vasodilatation, a strong argument against sympathectomy exists, that it can not produce any further dilatation in such a limb. All factors considered, the consensus however is in its favor, when there is a definite vasospastic component or when no direct arterial surgery is possible.

Prediction of effect of sympathectomy: The earlier method of estimating the Brown's vasomotor index is too cumbersome and not very reliable. Ankle-brachial index (ABI) of >0.3 has been consistently shown to correlate with favorable results after sympathectomy.

Contraindications for sympathectomy

1. Gross tissue necrosis
2. Patients above 50
3. Severe peripheral neuropathy (e.g. diabetes mellitus).

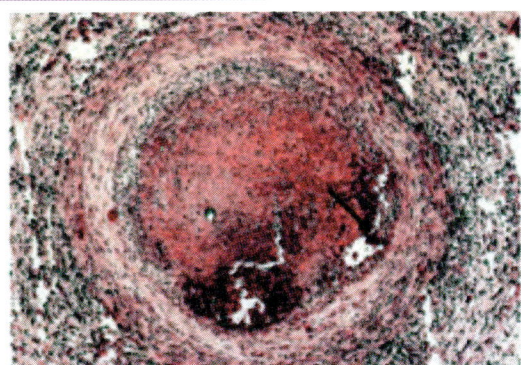

Fig. 77.36. Section of an artery in Buerger's disease showing recanalization of organized thrombus and prominent cellular infiltrates

It should be realized that sympa-thectomy can never be a substitute for direct arterial surgery, when feasible, though it may be used as an adjuvant.

Technique: consists of excision of L2-4 (preganglionic) para-aortic sympathetic ganglia through which entire lower limb is supplied (cells of origin are in the sacral gangia), by extraperitoneal approach. The effect is immediate, seen within a few hours and lasts for a variable period of time, ranging from weeks to years. The reasons for such a temporary effect are: alternate channels of sympathetic flow get established in due course and denervated sympathetic end organs become hypersensitive to circulating catecholamines, as in upper motor neuron lesions.

Complications of lumbar sympathectomy

a) Injury to lumbar veins and IVC is common on the right side, due to shortness of the former and proximity of the latter. Digital or pad compression generally controls the bleed; rarely a lateral tear of the IVC may need repair using fine vascular suture, with the help of a partially occluding curved Satinsky vascular clamp.

b) Injury to ilioinguinal/iliohypogastric (L1) nerves while splitting the internal oblique, may produce weak-

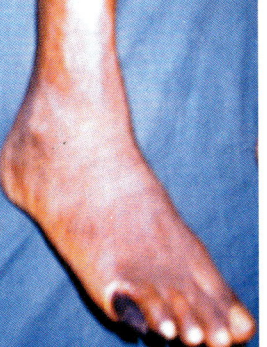

Fig. 77.35. TAO with gangrene little toe
(courtesy: Halsted Surgical Clinic, Chennai)

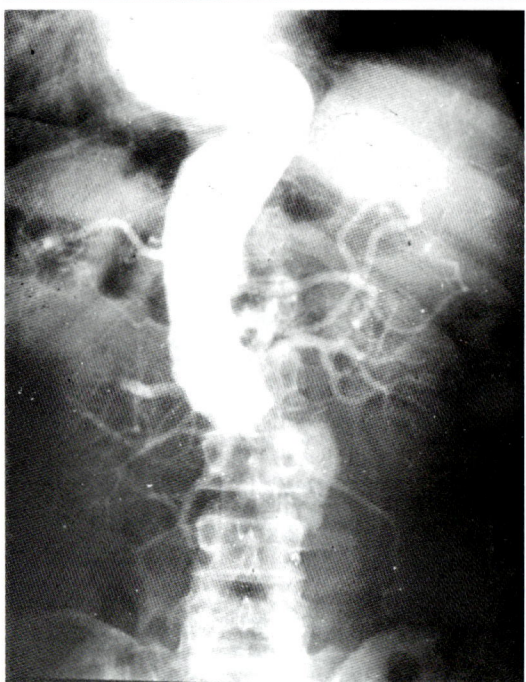

Fig. 77.37. Aortogram showing total occlusion of proximal abdominal aorta in NAA (courtesy: Halsted Surgical Clinic, Chennai)

ness of the conjoint tendon, predisposing to inguinal hernia.

c) Removal of L1 ganglion, which supplies ejaculatory nerve and internal vesical sphincter, may lead to either dry or retrograde ejaculation, leading to infertility (blissfully transient). Hence, bilateral excision of L1, which has no additional benefit in terms of limb blood flow, should be avoided in the young.

d) Injury to genitofemoral nerve (coursing in front of the psoas muscle) and ureter, while pushing the posterior peritoneum medially, to reach the antero-lateral surface of vertebral bodies.

e) Inadvertent opening of the peritoneum is very common, but not harmful; it can simply be closed with catgut, as soon as it is noticed.

f) Wound hematoma is also a common problem, since many of these patients are on anticoagulant/antiplatelet drugs, for the limb ischemia

Chemical sympathectomy

This is done by injecting absolute alcohol or phenol into the lumbar sympathetic chain, under imaging guide. Special care has to be taken not to enter into inferior venacava (on right) or aorta (on left), before delivering the chemical. Immediate warming of the limb may be expected, if the injection is effective, which may last for several days or weeks. Same objections for standard sympathectomy hold good for this procedure. Besides the drawbacks of any such injection, if it has not produced desired result, the dilemma exists whether the injection was given in the proper place.

(i) Omentopexy is done by lengthening the greater omentum and bringing it into the thigh, almost upto the knee and fixing in the subfascial plane, to create neovasculature supplying the muscles, similar to the Vineberg's procedure for myocardial revascularization. This operation is subjected to more debate than sympathectomy, with very few proponents claiming long term benefits in terms of claudication and limb salvage.

iii) other less popular operations include laying the tibial marrow open to develop neovasculature, feeding the muscular vessels (Ilizirov's procedure) and implantation of human placenta in the thigh, the rationale for which is unclear, may be related to release of prostaglandins.

Specific conditions

Atherosclerosis: (athere: gruel; sklerosis: hard) This is a progressive systemic disease of the aged, characterized by intramural deposition of lipids, blood cells, fibrin, calcium and foam cells loaded with lipids. The etiological factors are: male preponderance, genetic predilection, dyslipidemia by increased low density and very low density lipoproteins(LDL & VLDL), hypertension, smoking or other forms of tobacco abuse, diabetes mellitus, increased platelet activity, sedentary life style and strenuous mental activity.

Thrombophilia is a state of hypercoagulability of the blood, leading to thromboembolic disorders, described in detail under venous diseases (chapter 85).

Homocystinemia, an inborn error of sulfur aminoacid metabolism, due to deficiency of a liver enzyme, cystathionine, is recognized to be another factor, responsible for hypercoagulable state and premature development of atherosclerosis. It is characterized by elevated plasma methionine and homocystine and large amounts of urinary homocystine (*homocystinuria*). Homocystine is an aminoacid, that can oxidize LDL cholesterol, by which endothelial dysfunction and proliferation of vascular smooth muscle cells occur, leading to early atherosclerosis. The clinical manifestations (mental retardation, cardiovascular and skeletal disorders, hepatomegaly, ectopia lentis etc) resemble Marfan's syndrome. Besides genetic factors, it is interesting that elevated homocystine levels may be seen in deficiency states of vitamin B-6, B-12 and folic acid and its metabolic harm can be blunted to some extent by giving these agents.

Atherosclerosis is known to occur virtually in every artery in the body, though more commonly seen in the aorta and its main branches, including coronaries, superficial femoral in the adductor canal, bifurcations of carotid, iliac, femoral and popliteal arteries. The clinical picture and the management naturally depend upon the site and tempo of occluding pathology.

Leriche syndrome is a triad of claudication of one or both legs, sexual impotence and absent or weak femoral pulses, seen in aorto-iliac occlusion. The claudication may be gluteal, if the hypogastric occlusive process is extensive.

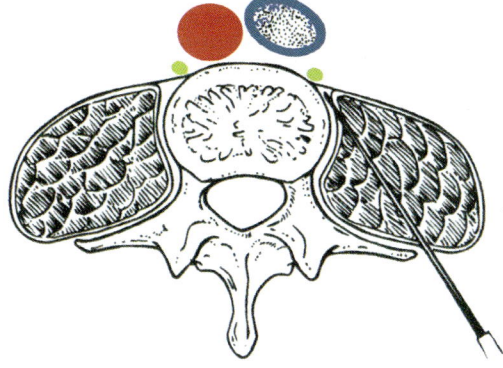

Fig. 77.38. Percutaneous lumbar sympathetic block

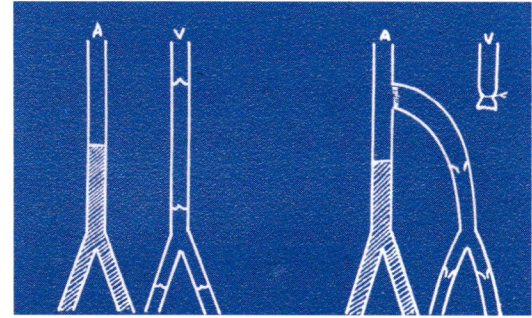

Fig. 77.39. Schematic diagram of arterialisation of popliteal vein

History of impotence is often elicited during interrogation and not complained of by the patient, because the inability to walk even a few yards attracts their primary attention (after all if one cannot walk to the girl, the question of potency does not arise!). The aorto-iliac disease is classified (Leriche) into type-I: confined to distal aorta and common iliac arteries, type-II: disease extending to external iliacs and type-III: multisegmental aorto-ilio-femoral occlusions.

Acute Leriche syndrome refers to a saddle embolus lodged at the aortic bifurcation, occluding both common iliacs, usually from mural thrombus of a recent cardiac infarction and it requires urgent embolectomy through both femorals, generally under local anesthesia, with good results.

THROMBOANGIITIS OBLITERANS (syn: Buerger's disease, TAO)

Definition: It is an inflammatory obliteration of terminal arteries, with involvement of accompanying veins and nerves, occurring in young smok-

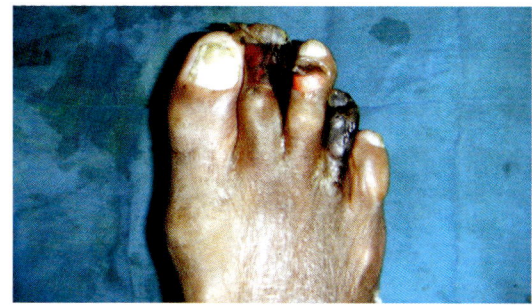

Fig. 77.40. Buerger's disease with gangrene of toes

ers, commonly affecting the infragenicular vessels of the leg (small and medium sized arteries).

Etiology

Occurring mainly in the lower socio-economic population, with a male predominance (9:1), in the 2nd and 3rd decades of life. Beedi smokers are more affected than those who smoke cigarettes with refined tobacco. They have a hypercoagulable state, due to an increase in serum fibrinogen level, platelet activity and tendency for aggregation. Interestingly, smoking filter cigarettes or pipe is less injurious and hookha is virtually harmless with reference to arterial disease.

Exogenous factors: smoking, usually more than 20 cigarettes/day for several years may predispose to some immune-mediated vascular injury, through nicotine, carbon monoxide, tobacco glycoprotein (TGP) etc.

Endogenous factors: sympathetic overactivity: Nicotine from smoking seems to sensitize the sympathetic nerve endings to the circulating catecholamines, causing vasospasm. An auto-immune process has also been suggested in view of the increased complement factors and anticollagen antibodies detected in patients with TAO. A hypercoagulable state of the blood contributes to thrombosis of the involved vascular tree.

Pathology

It is a *panarteritis*, involving all layers, disease starting mostly from the toes and foot and working proximally, without much distal run-off; hence this occlusive process is generally considered non-reconstructable. Firm thrombus is seen occluding the affected vessels, which may contain blood cells, giant cells and microabscesses, ultimately leading to dense fibro-

	Feature	TAO	ASO
1.	Age	<40	>50
2.	Smoking	Invariably present	May be present
3.	Socioeconomic	Low & middle	Middle & high
4.	Hypercoagulable state	+++	No
5.	Sympathetic hyperactivity	+++	No
6.	Autoimmune factors	May be present	Absent
7.	Diabetes & hypertension	Absent	Usually present
8.	Caliber of vessels	Small & medium	Large & medium
9.	Layers involved	Diffuse panarteritis	Atheromatous intimal disease
10.	Microabscesses	Present	Absent
11.	Migrating thrombophlebitis	May be seen	Absent
12	Raynaud's phenomenon	May be present	Usually absent
13.	Onset of gangrene	Very early	Late
14.	Angiogram	Cock-screw collaterals seen	Usually not seen
15.	Reconstructability	Rare	Common
16.	Involvement of other vessels (carotid, coronary, renal etc)	Rare	Common
17.	Progress	Arrests with cessation of tobacco use and sympathectomy	Relentlessly progressive disease involving other areas

Table-77.4. Differences between thromboangiitis obliterans and atherosclerosis obliterans (ASO)

sis. It may also affect upper limb as well as other arteries in the body, such as mesenteric, coronary and cerebral. There may be migrating superficial thrombophlebitis, attributable to hypercoagulable state. The vascular pathology is reversible to a considerable extent, if the patient totally abstains from *tobacco* in any form, in the early stage of the disease.

Using electrophysiological technique, utilizing the level of sudomotor activity, the sympathetic tone in any segment of skin can be measured (CMKReddy & Vijay Jayakar), which clearly demonstrates the following:

i) increased basal sympathetic tone in normal lower limbs in erect posture, especially in the feet and toes.

ii) there is still higher sympathetic activity in the limbs affected by TAO

iii) considerable drop in the tone to subnormal levels following adequate sympathectomy

iv) there is return of normal tone usually within a few weeks or sometimes longer

Since TAO is primarily a disease of sympathetic system, it manifests first in the toes and foot, where maximum sympathetic activity is normally seen; only rarely other regions are affected.

Clinical features

The primary symptom is *intermittent claudication*, which is initially pedal, later becomes crural and rarely femoral or gluteal. This may progress to rest pain, pregangrene or frank gangrene, usually of the dry type, *early tissue necrosis* being typical of TAO. If arteries of other areas are involved, symptoms referable to those organs, such as abdominal angina (mesenteric), angina pectoris (coronary), TIAs (cerebral) etc. may be seen. When there is rest pain, the patient prefers to hang the foot to dependency, for some relief and often they sleep sitting. Features of chronic ischemia of the limb may be present.

There is bilateral absence of pedal pulses, though symptoms may be on one side, as the disease need not be symmetrical. Very often

digital ulceration/gangrene are seen, long before the obliteration of the popliteal pulse and are invariably seen, when the popliteal pulse is absent. In fact, it may be stated that absence of tissue necrosis, with absent popliteal or femoral pulse, is against the diagnosis of TAO. Involvement of upper limb vessels (positive Allen's test), attacks of superficial thrombophlebitis with edema of extremity and features of Raynaud's phenomenon, are corroborative to the diagnosis.

Differential diagnosis

i) Atherosclerosis occurring in young (juvenile atherosclerosis), as in progeria (pro: advance; geras: senility). This is very difficult to distinguish, to the extent that some western workers feel that there is no such entity as TAO and they are actually variants of atherosclerosis. In a clinical context, whenever the presentation of 'TAO' is atypical, this condition has to be considered.

ii) Thromboembolism has an acute presentation and is usually localized to one limb. The source of emboli can be identified only in <50% of cases of acute arterial occlusions.

iii) *Popliteal artery entrapment* disease is to be suspected in young males (male to female ratio is 15:1), which may be bilateral in 25% of cases. In this condition, the popliteal artery, instead of coursing between the two heads of the gastrocnemius, passes medial to the medial head or popliteus muscle, causing compression during muscle contraction, leading to secondary thrombosis and permanent occlusion. In those with unobliterated distal pulse, popliteal angiogram with and without plantar flexion of foot (medial deviation of the artery, occlusion and poststenotic aneurysm), clinches the diagnosis. A CT scan is helpful in occluded cases, to identify the abnormal placement of the artery.

iv) *Adventitial cystic disease* of the popliteal artery is a rare condition of unclear etiology, most accepted being cystic degeneration of the vessel wall, due to the collection from mucin-secreting developmental rests (derived from the adjacent synovium) in the adventitia, resembling a ganglion, causing luminal occlusion. Seen in middle age, arteriogram (smooth lateral filling defect), USG and CT are helpful in establishing the diagnosis.

v) Nonspecific aorto-arteritis (NAA) is a disease causing occlusion of aorta or its branches in young nonsmokers, due to uncertain etiology, similar to the *pulseless disease* of Takayasu. Hypersensitivity to agents such as tuberculous protein and autoimmunity are putative etiological factors. Isolated involvement of the femoro-popliteal segment is rare and identification of occlusion of aorta and/or its main branches is diagnostic.

Screening for underlying thrombophilic state has to be done and treated appropriately. High incidence of associated myocarditis may influence overall treatment.

Immunosuppressant agents, such as cyclophosphamide, methotrexate or mycophenolate have been used with some success in arresting the progression.

vi) Diabetic angiopathy and gangrene (see chapter 17 on Gangrene)

vii) Systemic collagen vascular disorders, such as polyarteritis nodosa, scleroderma, giant cell arteritis etc. may cause progressive arterial occlusion, due to autoimmine process, associated with digital ischemia and loss of toes in succession over the years. Involvement of other visceral arteries, elevated ESR and detection of antibodies against nuclei or mitochondria provide the clue to the diagnosis, clinched by arterial biopsy.

Investigations for TAO

There are no specific laboratory tests for TAO, except to rule out other types of vasulitis which mimic the disease. ESR, C-reactive protein (CRP), rheumatoid factor, antinuclear or mitochondrial antibodies (ANA/AMA) for collagen vascular disorders, antineutrophilic cytoplasmic antibodies (ANCA), more specific for autoimmune vasculitis, may be routinely done. Also the screening for thrombophilia,

such as serum homocysteine, antiphospholipid antibodies, to help overall management of the disease, may be done. In cases of atypical presentation, tests for rarer conditions, such as anticentromere antibody (ACA) for scleroderma, serologic markers for CREST syndrome (calcinosis, Raynaud's disease, esophageal disease, sclerodactyly and telangiectasia) may be considered. Circulating immune complexes against type I and III collagen have also been detected in some cases of TAO, but most of these tests appear to be of academic significance than helpful to the diagnosis.

Doppler/Duplex recordings will provide sufficient information to arrive at the diagnosis, but if direct arterial surgery is contemplated, angiography (as a road map) is necessary. Cardiac source of emboli should be excluded by an echocardiogram.

Angiography (conventional, multislice CT or DSA): Involvement of small and medium sized vessels, diffuse or segmental in nature, more in the lower limbs, is typical. Relatively normal proximal vessels and spiraling (cock-screw) collaterals with poor distal run-off are supportive of the diagnosis. However, it should be realized that there are no pathognomonic arteriographic findings in TAO.

Treatment

Medical treatment, as described earlier, with strict abstinence from tobacco in any form is helpful in claudicators, with or without pedal pulses.

Jewels of Gyan - 77.1

Angiographic features in TAO

Involvement of small and medium arteries
Healthy proximal vessels
Segmental distribution of disease
Abrupt termination of main vessels with tree-root appprearance
Cock-screw collaterals due to dilated vasa-vasora
Poor outflow channels and distal run-off
Bilateral disease, often unequal degree

Prostaglandin analogues (vide supra) and calcium channel blockers may be effective

Surgical

i) *Lumbar sympathectomy* on the affected side provides good symptomatic relief, often 'tiding over the crisis'. It is eminently suitable for digital ischemia and skin ulcers, but its role in claudication is questionable. Notwithstanding the nonbelievers of this operation, experience has shown that the patients are 'cured' of their disease following this procedure, provided it is done early enough, before the development of frank gangrene and the patients quit consuming tobacco in any form. The only patients who develop recurrent symptoms are those who restart smoking ! (technical considerations of sympathectomy are detailed earlier)

ii) If angiogram reveales some run-off and hope of revascularization by direct arterial surgery, it may be attempted, as per the options available.

iii) *Arterialisation of vein* (Vira Reddy) is an interesting concept, utilizing the veins as arterial conduits, beyond the occluded arterial tree. The popliteal vein is divided just above the level of the arterial occlusion, the proximal end ligated and the distal end is anastomosed to the side of the pulsating popliteal artery, ligating as many venous tributaries as possible, through the popliteal incision, favouring blood flowing to distal regions. The important considerations are:

a) lower the level this is done, the better it functions, with less systemic/local AVF effects.

b) it should be done before gross tissue necrosis sets in

c) patient should be a nondiabetic and quit smoking totally

d) not associated with obvious venous insufficiency of the limb

e) being unconventional and a controversial procedure, it is done for only those, in whom all other methods of treatment have failed and the limb committed to amputation, as such failure of limb salvage after this operation need not be regretted.

f) the success of this operation is observed within first 24 hours, as a healthy equilibrium is established between input/output of blood to the limb.

The main objections expressed for this procedure are:

a) how can the veins be used, since in TAO, both arteries and veins are diseased?

b) will valves not interfere with distal flow of blood?

c) what happens to the venous return of the limb?

d) how do the venules function as arterioles at the cell level?

It has been observed at surgery, that the popliteal vein is never involved in the disease. When the vein is exposed to arterial pressure, it balloons out, making the valves incompetent. There are many veins, other than the main popliteal, to carry out the venous functions in the leg. It is however, not clear at the cellular level, how the capillary circulation is rearranged, but the fact remains that the operation saves about 25% of limbs from being amputated, if properly selected and carried out.

iv) Other less popular procedures are omentopexy in the thigh and leg, implantation of human placenta and Ilizirov's operation.

v) Below-knee amputation is the last resort.

Amputations in the lower limb: This indicates ultimate failure of the art and science of vascular surgery, the reasons for which can be multiple, related to educational, socio-economic and inherent problems of patients as well as available infrastructure and expertise of institutions.

Amputation of a toe for a gangrene due to major arterial occlusion, should not be done, as it invariably leads to loss of foot or leg, unless preceded by some form of revascularization (see chapter on Amputation).

Recent advances

1) Intraoperative check, hitherto done by postprocedure angiogram, is being largely replaced by angioscopy and intravascular ultrasound (IVUS).

2) To prevent restenosis following a PTA, agents such as PGI$_2$ inhibitor (Ciprostene), **p**henylanyl **p**ropyl **a**rgininic **c**hloromethyl **k**etone (PPACK), colchicine, anti-angiogenic drug (AGM-1470), a platelet integrin receptor antagonist, adciximab (ReoPro) and gene therapy are being tried, in different centres.

3) Drugs to improve efficiency of muscle metabolism, such as carnitine, naftidofuryl (an anti-serotonin agent) etc and a potent antiplatelet, vasodilator and prostacycline analogue, homedin, are found to improve claudication distance.

4) Endoscopic vascular surgery is being attempted, but no large successful series have been reported so far.

Tissue–engineered vascular conduits (TEVC)

Small diameter artificial vascular conduits with patency rates of native vessels has been a dream, ever since bypass surgery was popularized in 1960. The concept of biological 'living' grafts implies the ability to respond to immediate environment, to be remodeled by the host, with a potential for viscoelastic property and self-repair, if injured and should be least thrombogenic, while interfacing with circulating blood. The creation of TEVC involves the harvest of desired cells, cell expansion in culture, seedling onto a scaffold and implantation of the construct back into a living environment (such as peritoneal cavity), that induces tissue regeneration. Of course providing a vasoactive anti-thrombotic endothelium, that can withstand arterial sheer stress, is the key step in the process and development of stem cell technology should come handy in this connection.

Angiogenic factors

Angiogenesis is the physiological process involving the growth of new blood vessels from pre-existing vessels and is a normal and vital process in growth and development, as well as in wound healing and in granulation tissue. However, it is also a fundamental step in the transition of tumors from a dormant to an active state, leading to the application of angiogenesis inhibitors.

Regarding the mechanism of action, pro-angiogenic methods can be differentiated into three main categories: gene therapy, targeting genes of interest for amplification or inhibition; protein therapy, which primarily manipulates angiogenic growth factors like fibroblastic growth factor (FGF) or vascular endothelial growth factor (VEGF); and cell-based therapies, which involve the implantation of specific cell types.

The modern clinical application of the principle of angiogenesis can be divided into two main areas: anti-angiogenic therapies, which angiogenic research began with, and pro-angiogenic therapies, to promote wound healing and for neovascularization of ischemic parts. Whereas anti-angiogenic therapies are being employed to fight cancer and malignancies, which require an abundance of oxygen and nutrients to proliferate, pro-angiogenic therapies are being explored as options to treat cardiovascular diseases, a leading cause of death in the world.

The role of stem cell therapy from autologous bone marrow for limb salvage, in otherwise hopeless situation, is under evaluation.

MICROVASCULAR SURGERY

This relatively recent addition to vascular restorative surgery, involves repairing or anastomosing small vessels using an operating microscope, commonly employed in reimplantation of dismembered parts of the body and for free tissue transfer. They are highly specialized procedures done only in dedicated teams in specialized centres, often taking several hours to perform, using special instruments and very fine suture materials.

Areas suitable for reimplantation procedure

1. Parts of limbs, either by macro (proximal to wrist or ankle) or microimplantation (distal)
2. scalp

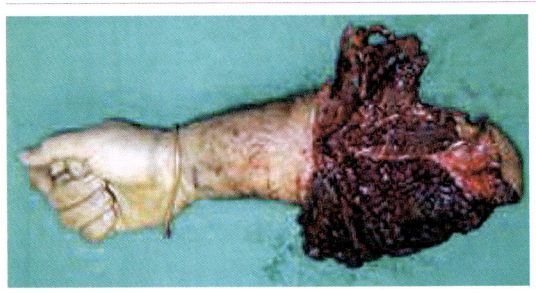 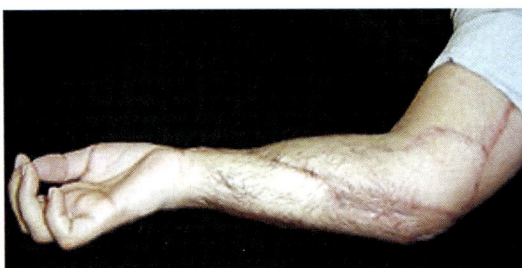

Fig. 77.41 & 42. Microvascular reimplantation of severed forearm

3. external ear
4. penis
5. facial tissue.

Guidelines to the primary physicians on the spot, when reimplantation is considered

Ensure that no other life-threatening injury to the patient is present, requiring primary attention.

Control wound bleeding by pressure, avoid clamping and further damage to vessels.

Wash the wound with warm saline and cover with sterile dressings.

Give tetanus prophylaxis and start an appropriate antibiotic.

Contact the nearest centre for microvascular surgery and transfer the patient without delay.

The dismembered part is kept in a polythene bag, which is transported in a container with ice cubes placed around it. The tissue should not

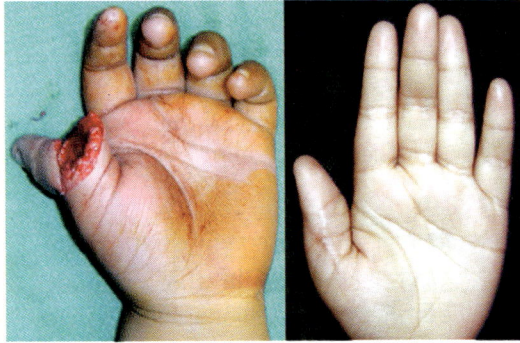

Fig. 77.44 & 45. Microvascular reimplantation of severed thumb

be frozen by bringing in direct contact with the ice cubes.

The patient should reach the specialized unit as early as possible, after attending to the medicolegal formalities, preferably within 6 hours (from the time of the incident), for injuries proximal to the wrist and before 12 hours for distal injuries.

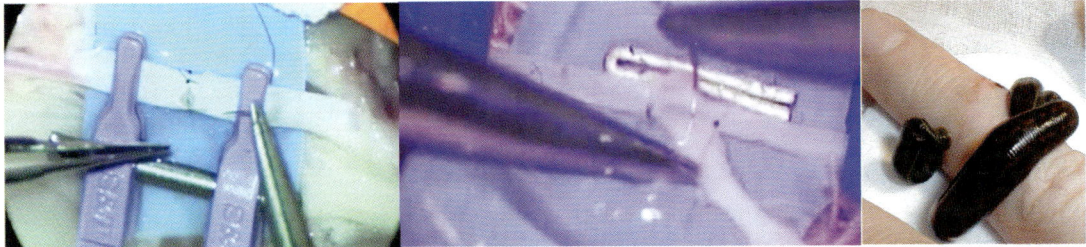

Fig. 77.43. A: Microvascular anastomosis, end-to-end; B: End-to-side anastomosis; C: Leech therapy (see footnote)

Today leeches (Hirudo medicinalis) are bred in captivity in many institutions including Bristol Zoo Gardens. Leeches have found new fame in microsurgery, where doctors require the precision of the leech to drain congested blood from wounded sites, complemented by the anticoagulant, hirudin, in their saliva. Plastic surgeons are particularly grateful for the contribution made by the leech, due to their use in the treatment of difficult grafts and reconstructive microsurgery.

78 Thoracic Outlet Syndrome (TOS)

Definition: Also called thoracic inlet syndrome, it is due to compression of the brachial plexus, subclavian artery and/or subclavian vein, due to a variety of causes, namely:

- (a) cervical rib syndrome
- (b) scalenus anticus syndrome
- (c) first rib syndrome
- (d) costoclavicular syndrome
- (e) hyperabduction syndrome
- (f) pectoralis minor syndrome
- (g) Pancoast's syndrome.

Anatomy

Three areas of potential compression:

1. *Scalene triangle*: at the thoracic outlet, a *triangle* formed by the scalenus anticus in front, the first rib at the base, and the scalenus medius behind.

2. *Costoclavicular space*: space between the clavicle and first rib.

3. *Pectoralis minor space*: under the pectoralis minor tendon and the coracoid process.

Only the brachial plexus and subclavian artery traverse the first one, whereas all the three structures (including subclavian vein) course through the other two areas.

Angulation or stretching of the neuro-vascular bundles may occur due to factors related to

- (i) ribs
- (ii) muscles and
- (iii) others.

i) Rib factors

A) CERVICAL RIB: Arising from the seventh cervical transverse process, found in 0.5% of population and commoner in females and on the right side and bilateral in 25%, though one side more developed than the other. Three types of cervical rib are found:

1) Complete rib, articulating anteriorly with first rib (scaleni may be attached to it) or

rarely to the manubrium sterni

2) Incomplete rib with the free end expanding to form a bony mass, often palpable in the supraclavicular region

3) The rib tapering to a point, and connected by a fibrous band to the scalene tubercule of the first rib

4) short tapering rib termed beaking of the rib (looks like a bird's beak).

B) BROAD FIRST RIB is self explanatory

(ii) Muscle factors: they narrow the interscalene space

1) Wide/bulky scalenus anticus muscle
2) An additional scalene muscle
3) Unusual proximity of the insertions of the scalenus anticus and medius, narrowing the triangle.

(iii) Other factors

1. Congenital bands running between the muscles may compress neurovascular structures.
2. An abnormally long C-7 transverse process may cause symptoms.
3. Fractures of the clavicle or the first rib, with callus formation or malunion.

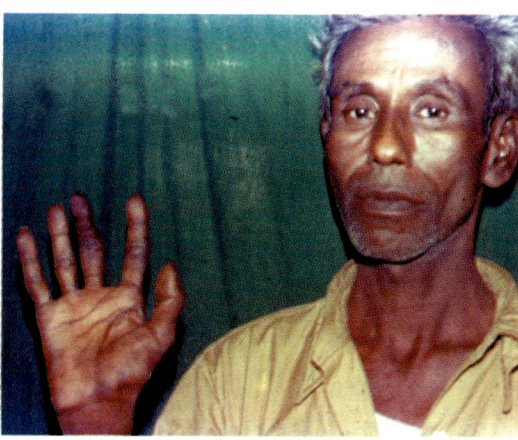

Fig. 78.1. Ischemia of middle finger and hypothenar atrophy due to cervical rib
(courtesy: Halsted Surgical Clinic, Chennai)

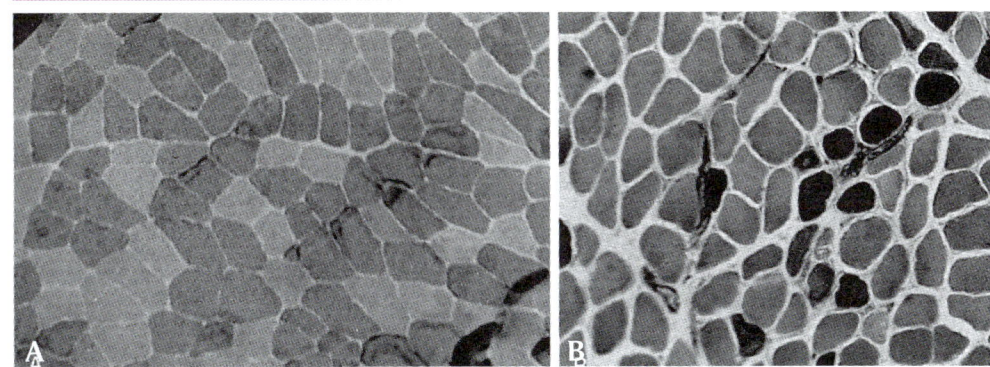

Fig. 78.2. Histology of scalene muscle
A. Normal with equal distribution of light and dark staining (type 1&2) fibers
B. Increase in type 1 fibers and connective tissue around each muscle fiber in TOS

4. Apical lung (Pancoast's) tumor.

5. Angulation of T-1 root: The first thoracic nerve becomes stretched or acutely angulated over the first rib, unless the brachial plexus is prefixed. *Wood Jones' law*, which states that one major congenital anomaly (fully formed cervical rib) is often associated with another major anomaly (prefixation of brachial plexus), is invoked to explain why predominant vascular symptoms are seen when a fully developed rib is found and more neurological symptoms on the side of less developed rib.

(6) Cervico-thoracic scoliosis may put the neurovascular bundles on stretch.

Pathology

Muscles: In the absence of a cervical rib, muscle pathology plays a major role and main pathology seems to be related to some bygone trauma or repetitive stretch at occupation. Following injury, microhematomas form in the muscle leading to fibrosis and transformation of type 2 by type 1 muscle fibres.

Types of skeletal muscle fibres:

Type 1: Slow twitch, fatigue resistant (red), oxidative

Type 2-A: Fast twitch, fatigue resistant (red), oxidative

Type 2-B: Fast twitch, fatigue prone (white), glycolytic.

Normally types 1 and 2 (light and dark staining respectively) are equally distributed (50/50), whereas in TAO the type 2 fibres are gradually replaced by type 1 fibres (75/25), with considerable increase of connective tissue around each fibre.

Brachial plexus

Humural head

Glenoid cavity

First rib

Fig. 78.3. Scheme of hyperabduction compression

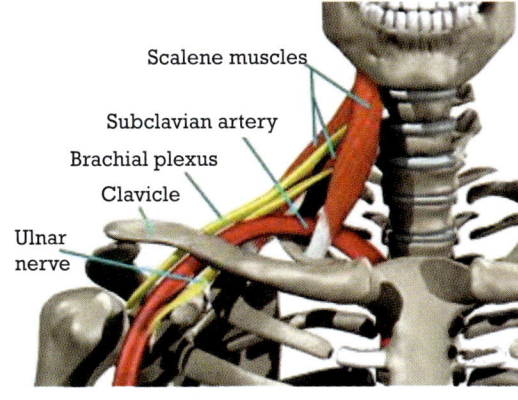

Scalene muscles

Subclavian artery

Brachial plexus

Clavicle

Ulnar nerve

Fig. 78.4. Anatomy of root of neck

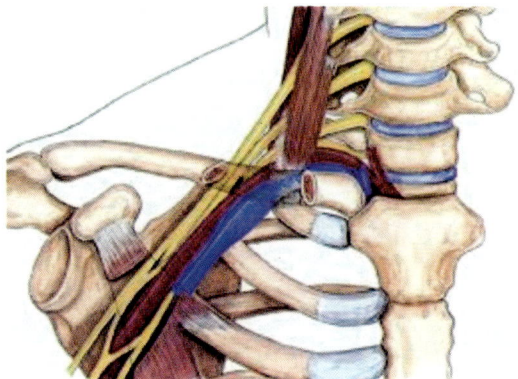

Fig. 78.5. Anatomy of root of neck
(clavicle removed)

Artery: Angulation or partial occlusion of the subclavian artery occurs with upper limb 'claudication', pallor, coldness, numbness and paresthesia as early vascular symptoms. Narrowing of lumen is followed by *post-stenotic dilatation*, within which thrombus may form. This often gets fragmented, throwing showers of emboli distally, initially producing secondary Raynaud's disease, and ultimately frank ischemia and sometimes gangrene of the tips of the fingers. Ulnar artery being the larger branch of and more in line with the brachial, little and ring fingers are often involved, in any embolic process of upper extremity. Rarely, retrograde propagation of thrombus may involve the origin of the vertebral artery (or common carotid on the right) causing cerebral embolism (TIA).

The exact mechanism of formation of post-stenotic dilatation is not clear; most popular explanation is that the vasa-vasora supplying the subclavian artery immediately adjacent to the rib, are damaged, producing ischemic weakness of the arterial wall. The turbulence of the blood flow, generating eddy currents, might be a contributory factor.

Nerve plexus: Sensory disturbances along the distribution of C8 and T1 (lower trunk) fibres are the earliest, followed by motor involvement and wasting of small muscles of the hand (T1). Vasomotor instability due to sympathetic irritation may cause Raynaud's phenomenon (secondary Raynaud's disease) of the limb.

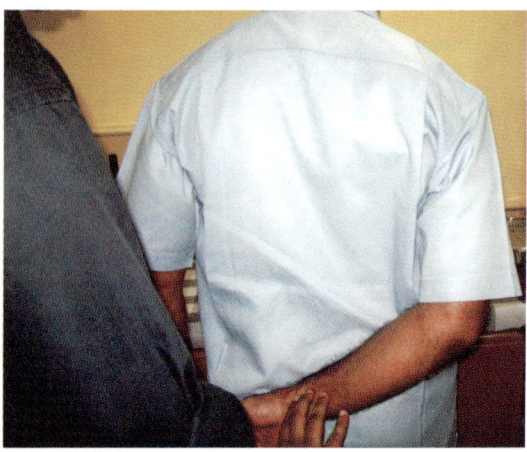

Fig. 78.6. Costoclavicular maneuver
(Dorsum of the hand touching the opposite sacroiliac joint)
(courtesy: Halsted Surgical Clinic, Chennai)

Vein: Rarely venous obstruction may occur, due to subclavian venous compression or thrombosis, with development of edema or secondary varicosities.

Symptoms

They may be neurological, vasomotor and vascular:

1. Pain or tingling and numbness along the ulnar side of the hand and forearm
2. Weakness of the small muscles of hand and fine digital movements
3. Coldness of fingers with blanching and blushing, when exposed to cold (Raynaud's syndrome or secondary Raynaud's disease)
4. Digital ulceration, pregangrene and gangrene
5. Venous edema and cyanosis

Since the sympathetic fibres accompany the

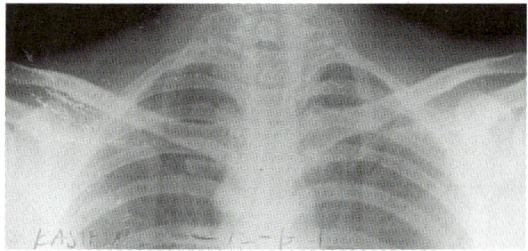

Fig. 78.7. Bilateral cervical ribs
(courtesy: Halsted Surgical Clinic, Chennai)

lower trunk, vasomotor symptoms may indicate neurologic compression.

Occipital headache may be seen due to referral through the cervical plexus from scalene muscles.

Symptoms appear around puberty when sagging of shoulder girdles occur. An interesting observation is that in bilateral cervical ribs, the patient is often less symptomatic in the side, on which the rib is more developed (see above for Wood Jones principle).

Signs

a) Difference in pulses of the upper extremities
b) Palpable bony hard mass (end of rib) in the supraclavicular or aneurysm in the infraclavicular or axillary space.
c) Pallor on elevation of arm and features of chronic ischemia (atrophy of skin, brittle nails, digital ulceration).
d) Adson's maneuver: The radial pulse becomes feeble when the patient turns his head towards the affected side and takes a deep inspiration. This puts stretch on the scalenus anticus and exaggerates compression. This test is not very sensitive, hence not as reliable as once believed and may be positive in some normal individuals.
e) Hyperabduction maneuver (Halsted): When the patient hyperabducts the arm on the affected side, the pectoralis minor tendon com-

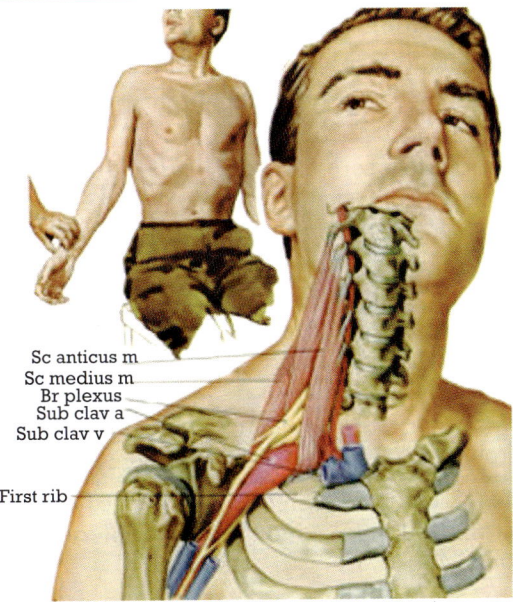

Sc anticus m
Sc medius m
Br plexus
Sub clav a
Sub clav v

First rib

Fig. 78.9. The mechanism of Adson's maneuver

presses the artery and can bring on symptoms by reduction or total obliteration of radial pulse. The angle at which this occurs may indicate the degree of compression. A modification of this, elevated arm stress test (EAST), described by Ross, is by rapidly closing and opening the fist in a limb elevated by 90^0, reproducing the symptoms.
f) Costo-clavicular maneuver: This is done by bringing the wrist behind the trunk, to reach the opposite sacroiliac joint, which depresses the clavicle and narrows the space between it and the first rib, causing compression.
g) Auscultation may reveal a supraclavicular or axillary bruit.
h) Sensory deficit of fine touch, vibration, pain and temperature may be present along the medial aspect of the forearm, hand and medial two fingers.
i) Motor deficit of the intrinsic muscles of the hand (T-1 innervated) may be found, in cases with significant nerve compression.

The tests for weakness of ulnar nerve, such as grasping a card placed between the fingers (for interossei) or Froment's sign (for adductor pollicis) may be positive.

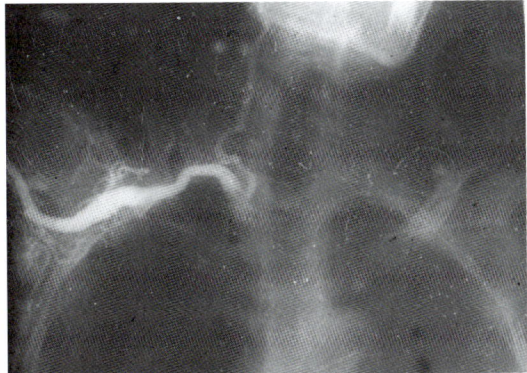

Fig. 78.8. Subclavian angiogram in a case of cervical rib showing post-stenotic aneurysm
(courtesy: Dr C R S Reddy, Chennai)

Differential diagnosis

If the neurological features are predominant, the following diseases may mimic/coexist with TOS:

1. cervical spondylosis
2. cervical cord compression (SOL) including syringomyelia
3. Pancoast's tumor of the apex of the lung
4. primary/secondary Raynaud's disease
5. brachial neuralgia
6. carpal tunnel syndrome
7. Hansen's disease
8. tardy ulnar palsy
9. Other rarer conditions to be differentiated from TAO are:

Tennis elbow or Golfer's elbow, due to fibrositis around lateral and medial epicondyles respectively:

Acromioclavicular impingement syndrome

Cuboid/Guyon's tunnel syndrome
Tendinitis of shoulder rotator cuff or biceps brachii muscle

Investigations

1. Comparing both brachial blood pressures, will identify if there is any significant occlusion of subclavian/axillary/brachial arterial segments, justifying further studies in that direction.

2. X-ray neck/chest will show a cervical rib, fracture callus, narrowed intervertebral foramina, apical lung tumor and cervicodorsal scoliosis. *Cervical rib is identified by the transverse process of C-7, which runs downwards and outwards, as against that of T-1, running upwards and outwards, all four forming a rhomboid.*

3. Duplex imaging or USG helps to confirm post-stenotic aneurysm and thrombus.

4. MRI is the single most useful investigation. It will rule out cervical cord/spine disease and can help localize compression of the brachial plexus/subclavian artery, delineate an aneurysm, rendering invasive investigations unnecessary.

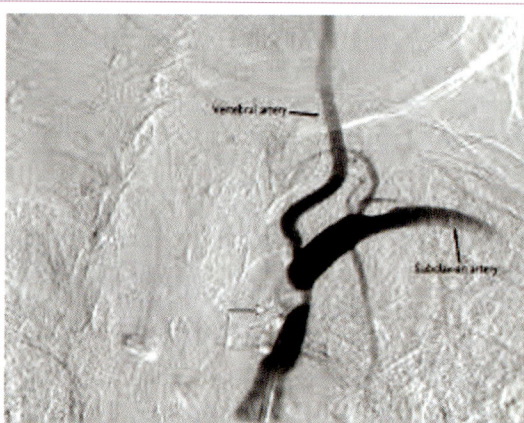

Fig. 78.10. DSA left subclavian artery showing proximal stenosis and steal phenomenon

5. Arteriogram is mainly indicated to exclude thrombus within an aneurysm or if critical occlusion of proximal vessels is suspected, requiring reconstruction, otherwise it is not absolutely essential. The type of angiogram, such as conventional, DSA or MR or isotopic, angiogram (vide supra), may be selected as described.

6. Myelogram, being an invasive procedure, is rarely done nowadays, to localize cord/root compression; this has been largely replaced by CT/MRI.

7. EMG and nerve conduction studies will confirm neural compression but not very reliable, may be helpful to exclude other conditions. Since there is more of sensory involvement, the EMG may be normal; nerve conduction velocity (NCV) and somatosensory- evoked potential (SSEP) may be more helpful

8. Ascending venogram may be useful in diagnosing venous thrombosis. Dynamic venography with compressive maneuvers may be more informative.

Treatment

1. *Conservative*: this should be tried first for patients with neurological or vasomotor manifestations, consisting of reassurance, weight reduction, analgesics/muscle relaxants and physiotherapy to strengthen the levators of the shoulder girdle. Alteration in ergonomics at work might be beneficial, Avoiding lifting heavy

weights is beneficial. Neck stretching and posture exercises and training in abdominal breathing may be helpful. This may help in about 75% of patients, but if the symptoms persist after adequate trial, surgery is advisable, before vascular complications develop.

2. *Operative*: A thorough decompression of the throracic outlet is carried out, under general anesthesia. The arm is pulled down and tied to the table, to open up the neck spaces on that side, with face turned to the opposite side. The main steps of surgery include:

a) Scalenotomy (division of the scalenus anticus tendon) is an integral part of any surgery for TOS.

b) If cervical rib is present, it should be excised extraperiosteally, to prevent bony regrowth from the periosteum

c) First rib removal was advocated to decompress the base of the scalene triangle on the principle that it forms the 'common denominator' in any compression in that region, if a cervical rib is absent (Clagett), but it has no universal acceptance and is rarely done.

d) Pectoralis minor tenotomy, if hyperabduction test is positive and scalenotomy has not given the desired result.

e) Division of all fibrous bands in the root of neck, to adequately decompress the neurovascular structures

f) If Raynaud's syndrome is present, a dorsal sympathectomy (D-1,2,3) may be added, after the parietal pleura is lifted from the posterior chest wall, through the same supraclavicular incision.

g) If significant poststenotic aneurysmal changes are seen in the subclavian artery, it should be resected and replaced by a vein or synthetic (PTFE) graft. Minimal dilatation (less than twice the diameter of the native vessel) is left alone as progression is unlikely, if the compression is relieved.

h) If subclavian thrombosis is present a thromboendarterectomy is performed, through a longitudinal arteriotomy.

i) Rarely, excision of part of the clavicle is required, if it is found to be responsible for the compression.

Excision of cervical rib is performed through one of the following approaches:

i) Supraclavicular route (Henley) is the commonest:

Incision: An inch above the clavicle, from lateral border of the SCM to the anterior border of trapezius. The scalenus anterior is exposed after retraction of SCM and dividing the inferior belly of omohyoid muscle. The phrenic nerve is seen coursing on the surface of the scalenus anticus, as soon as the pad of fat over the muscle is pushed away. This is protected and entire muscular and tendinous portions of the scalene is divided piecemeal. Complete exposure of the subclavian artery is an indication that the scalenus anticus muscle is totally divided. Sometimes, a part of the scalenus medius also may have to be divided after downward retraction of the brachial plexus. Constant attention has to be paid to the brachial plexus, since one of the trunks may run parallel to these muscles vulnerable for injury and undue traction on the plexus may produce troublesome postoperative neuralgia/neurapraxia/axonotmesis. The cervical rib is dissected free of its muscular attachments, but not the periosteum, disarticulated at the costotransverse joint or divided as posteriorly as possible and excised extraperiosteally (with the periosteum), to prevent regeneration of bone.

II) Trans-axillary route (Roos): This is preferred if the first rib is to be resected, but access to subclavian artery is difficult. The scalene triangle is approached from the base of the axilla, by a transverse incision and the first rib is exposed. Scalenotomy is done from below, before the cervical/first rib is resected. Pleural injury is a little more commoner with this approach but it is not serious if identified and intercostal drainage (ICD) of the pleural space is employed as necessary.

III) Trans-clavicular approach (least popular), by resecting the middle third of clavicle, allows wide exposure of the supraclavicular and axillary regions, but preferred only if the supraclavicular access is insufficient or if the compression is caused by the callus/malunion of clavicular fracture.

An anterolateral thoracic approach has been described, but not generally preferred due to additional morbidity of thoracotomy.

Advantages of cervical approach

Surgeons feel more at home in the neck
Scalenotomy is easier
Easy to access cervical rib
Sympathectomy carried out readily
Easy to identify anomalies, bands etc
Less chance of vessel injury and if it should occur, it can be easily handled

Advantages of axillary approach

Excision of the anterior end of 1st rib for venous TOS
Recurrence after cervical surgery
Note: If no cervical rib is found, only scalenotomy is performed, any fibrous bands present at the outlet, should be meticulously divided and the subclavian artery fully skeletonized.

Dorsal sympathectomy (D-1,2,3) is indicated along with decompression procedures, only if there are vasomotor or vascular complications, with obvious or impending tissue necrosis. It is also expressed as cervico-dorsal sympathectomy, whenever cervical (supraclavicular) approach is employed, other routes being axillary, posterior thoracic (extrapleural) and thoracoscopic. The significance of division of *nerve of Kuntz* (a grey ramus from T-2 ganglion to T-1 nerve root) is debatable.

Asymptomatic cervical rib: It is not unusual to detect either fully formed or rudimentary cervical rib during routine skiagrams, in patients who are otherwise asymptomatic. Careful evaluation must be done to see if they have any symptoms/signs attributable to the accessory rib, if so, surgery should be advised, before more troublesome vascular complications supervene. *Totally asymptomatic rib may be left alone and followed* up, on the presumption that the abnormal anatomy is well adjusted to the structures in the vicinity. The patient should be reassured that it is a harmless congenital anomaly, but to report immediately if any symptoms develop.

Patients are often treated for 'recurrent whitlows' and 'atypical Hansen's disease' for several years before the extra rib is found and excised. The unwise practice of advising the patients presenting with typical symptoms, against surgery, under the pretext of avoiding a 'complicated' operation, should be discouraged.

Complications of surgery for TOS

1) Phrenic nerve injury, during scalenotomy

2) Avulsion of the thyrocervical trunk from the subclavian artery, while retracting the subclavian artery downwards

3) Injury to pleura, producing pneumo or hemothorax, requiring intercostal drainage (ICD) of the chest. If not identified and treated promptly, this may lead to troublesome postoperative pulmonary complications.

4) Intractable brachial neuralgia/neuropraxia/axonotmesis, due to retraction of the plexus, while approaching the cervical/first rib, which may take several weeks to resolve. Very soft rubber slings should be used to lift/retract the plexus, to minimize this common complication.

5) Injury to brachial plexus, during scalenotomy, as occasionally one of its trunks may take a parallel course and lie in close proximity of the scalenus anticus muscle.

6) Injury to lymphatics, thoracic duct on the left and mediastinal/subclavian/jugular lymph ducts on the right, as they enter into the brachiocephalic venous confluence. Lymph cyst may form in the wound postoperatively, which may open and discharge through the suture line, producing lymphorrhea. Usually it is a self-limiting problem, if attention is paid towards the prevention of secondary infection.

While dissecting the scalene pad of fat, dividing

it as far laterally as possible and pushing the pad medially towards internal jugular vein will protect the lymphatics accompanying the vein.

If lymph collection in the wound has occurred, aspiration under strict aseptic conditions, once or twice may be necessary.

7. Horner's syndrome is a very common, but innocuous complication following dorsal sympathecctomy, due to injury to inferior cervical ganglion. It consists of unilateral ptosis, enophthalmos, miosis, anhidrosis of head and neck and loss of spinociliary reflex. Surgically induced disorder needs no treatment, as it recovers within a few weeks.

Recent advance

Intra-scalene injection of botulinum toxin (Botox) under USG/CT guide, in place of scalenotomy, is under evaluation.

79 Upper Limb Ischemia

Symptomatic UPPER LIMB ISCHEMIA is much less common than that of lower limb, probably because of liberal collaterals and less work done by the upper limbs. An embolus from the heart and aortic arch rarely lodges in the upper limb arteries, in view of the angle of their origin from the aorta, whereas common iliac arteries are terminal branches, almost in line with the aorta. Right upper limb is more often involved than the left, attributable to the origin of brachiocephalic (innominate) artery in line with ascending aorta. However a special group of diseases termed thoracic outlet compression syndrome, are peculiar to the upper limb, forming a sizeable percentage of causes of upper limb pain/ischemia, by their neurovascular manifestations.

Common causes of upper limb ischemia may be listed here:

1. Thoracic outlet (or inlet) compression syndrome (TOS), see chapter 78.

2. Vasculitis
   a) allergic or toxic
   b) autoimmune (SLE, scleroderma, polyarteritis, giant cell arteritis etc)
   c) nonspecific aorto-arteritis (NAA)
   d) thromboangiitis obliterans (Buerger's disease)

3. Atherosclerosis, including subclavian steal syndrome

4. Thrombo-embolism (acute)

5. Raynaud's syndrome
   a) Primary Raynaud's disease (rare)
   b) Raynaud's phenomenon (secondary Raynaud's disease)

6. Occupational disorders
   a) vibration-induced injury
   b) hypothenar hammer syndrome (rare)

7. Hematological disorders and dysproteinemias

8. Volkmann's ischemic contracture (see chapter 62)

Clinical evaluation

Careful history, physicial examination, including the state of peripheral pulses, bruit in the neck or axilla, evidence of impending/frank tissue necrosis, usually of finger tips, has to be performed. Associated visceral ischemia has to be looked for, in generalized arterial disease or transient cerebral ischemic attacks (TIAs) in carotid occlusion and subclavial steal syndrome.

Pulsations of upper limb arteries

The subclavian artery, as it arches over the first rib, lies just above the level of medial half of the clavicle, behind the clavicular head of SCM. Since it is deep to the scalenus anticus muscle, normally it may be just palpable in thin individuals with sagging shoulders, but in obese patient with short neck, it may not be felt, unless it is lifted by an accessory (cervical) rib.

The axillary artery is virtually surrounded by the major nerves arising from the brachial plexus. Its distal or third part, below the pectoralis minor tendon, is readily palpable against the upper humerus, just below the anterior axillary fold, between coracobrachiasis and the long head of triceps brachii.

The brachial artery is superficial throughout, lying between the biceps and triceps muscles and can be palpated against the humerus in its upper part and the capsule of the elbow joint, in the lower part. In an abducted arm, its course may be marked by a line drawn from a point anterior to the posterior axillary fold to the front of elbow joint, medial to the tendon of biceps brachii. The artery going under its aponeurosis, beyond this point, it has a deep course in the cubital fossa, divides into its terminal branches, ulnar (larger and more in line with the parent) and radial, about 5cm

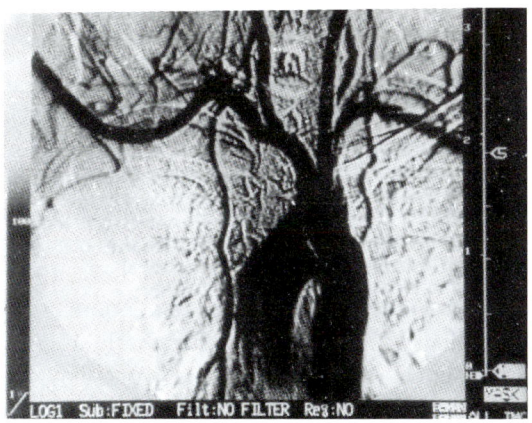

Fig. 79.1. DSA of aortic arch showing kinked subclavian arteries due to bilateral cervical ribs
(courtesy: Halsted Surgical Clinic, Chennai)

below the elbow joint (at the level of neck of radius) and not clinically palpable.

The ulnar artery has a straight course in the lower third of forearm, indicated by a line drawn from the front of medial epicondyle to just lateral to the pisiform bone at the wrist, with forearm in full supination. It lies over the flexor digitorum profundis, between the flexor carpi ulnaris medially and flexor digitorum sublimis laterally, where it can be palpated at about 4cm above the wrist.

The radial artery is the most common pulse felt during physical examination, against the distal radius, over the flexor pollicis longus and pronator quadratus muscles, lateral to the long flexor tendons, about an inch above the wrist. It passes under the tendons of abductor pollicis longus and extensor pollicis brevis, to enter the triangular depression behind the radial styloid, known as 'anatomical snuff box', where it can be felt. In the first interosseous space, it passes between the two heads of the first interosseous muscle, to reach the palm and form the deep palmar arch.

The digital braches to the thumb and index finger may be palpated in the first dorsal interosseous space, against their metacarpal bones.

Allen's test is designed to identify occlusion of one of the two arteries at the wrist. The patient is asked to clench the fist tight and the forearm just above the wrist is grasped firmly, occluding the vessels. The patient is asked to open the hand after 30sec., when the palm becomes pale white. Then the pressure on the radial artery is released; if the palm color returns to normal, it means that the radial artery is patent. The entire process is repeated, but this time releasing the pressure on the ulnar artery first, to identify its patency.

Investigations

Routine studies such as hematology and serum chemistry to exclude diabetes mellitus, dyslipidemia, dysproteinemia, coagulopathy, should be done.

Specific investigations

a) Skiagram of chest and neck, to exclude cervical rib/spondylosis

b) Venous filling time, which is the time taken for veins to appear, after an elevated limb is lowered, gives a rough index of severity of ischemia. Normal up to 15sec. and >30sec.is considered critical.

c) Segmental arterial pressures, comparing with opposite side, will exclude major vessel occlusion.

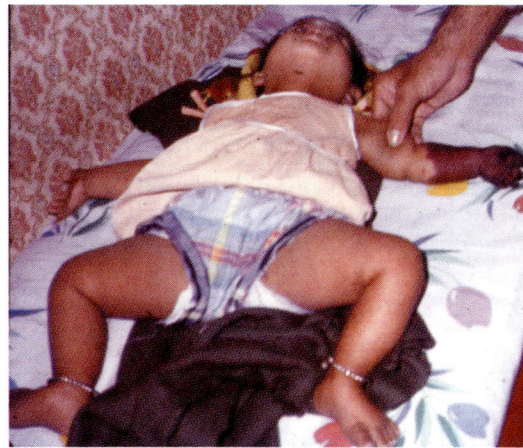

Fig. 79.2. Gangrene of hand and forearm due to inadvertant intra-arterial injection of an anticonvulsant drug to a child
(courtesy: Halsted Surgical clinic, Chennai)

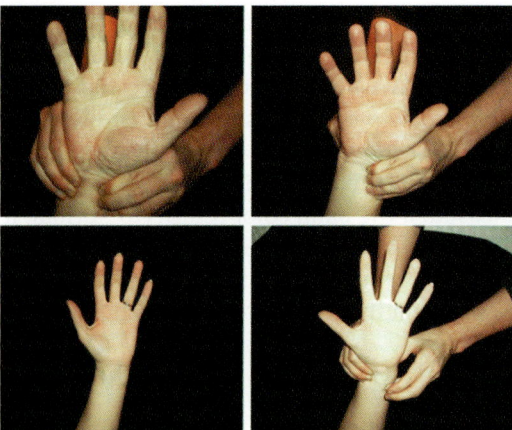

Fig. 79.3. Allen's test. Compression of both radial and ulnar arteries till the palm blanches, followed by release of one of them. The procedure is repeated, this time releasing the other artery

d) Transcutaneous oxygen tension (TcPO$_2$), a noninvasive study, to give baseline partial oxygen tension and also to assess progress after therapy.

e) Doppler/duplex imaging of major vessels

f) ECG and echocardiogram, if embolism is suspected

g) Angiogram, conventional, CT or DSA

Management

This mainly depends on the clinical presentation, whether acute or chronic.

Acute arterial occlusion: This is due to thromboembolic process, the usual sources of emboli being chambers/valves of heart, atherosclerotic plaques from aortic arch and aneurysms. Microemboli occur due to precipitation of cryoglobulins or cold agglutinins, on exposure to low temperatures. They may be also seen in thoracic outlet compression with or without a post-stenotic dilatation. In the management of acute arterial occlusion, it is important to identify if it occurred in a healthy vessel or it was an acute-on-chronic occlusion, because immediate surgical intervention is indicated and highly rewarding only in the former. (see chapter 77)

Accidental intra-arterial injection

A rare but disastrous cause of acute ischemia of hand/fingers is an *accidental* intra-arterial

(brachial) injection of a drug, meant to be given intravenously, such as anticonvulsants, thiopentone etc. It is also encountered among drug addicts. The basic problems in such cases are thrombosis and vasospasm of the distal arterial tree, complementing each other, quickly resulting in tissue necrosis. An urgent Doppler study will clinch the diagnosis, but an angiogram in that situation is not essential and may consume precious time, delaying intervention.

Immediately the hand/fingers become blue, cold and painful, the pulses at the wrist may be absent. If it is identified, when the needle is still inside the artery, an unlikely event, injection of heparin and papaverine through the same needle should be done. If needle has been withdrawn before realizing the misadventure, urgent exploration of the vessel should be done, confirming the diagnosis by a Doppler/Duplex study. Anticoagulant/ anti-platelet/hemorrheological agents should be started immediately on suspicion, to be continued for about 72 hours after surgery.

Procrastination invariably ends in catastrophic tissue loss in such situations. Arteriotomy, Fogarty thrombectomy and infusion with lignocaine/papaverine (for vasodilatation), urokinase/streptokinase (for dissolving distal microthrombi), if necessary supplemented by a stellate (sympathetic) block, are the essential limb-saving steps of the procedure.

Intraoperative post-procedure angiogram is very useful, to identify any residual disease, before conclusion. As a prophylaxis, it is wise to avoid using median cubital or basilic veins, coursing in close relation to the brachial artery, for intravenous injections, particularly in urgent situations.

In **chronic occlusion,** there is sufficient time for detailed investigations, to arrive at a definite diagnosis and to study the extent of the disease. If there is a major/medium sized vessel occlusion with a good distal run-off, some form of reconstructive procedure may be done (vide infra). If the disease is confined to distal small vessels, unsuitable for direct arterial surgery, only indirect procedures, such as dorsal preganglionic

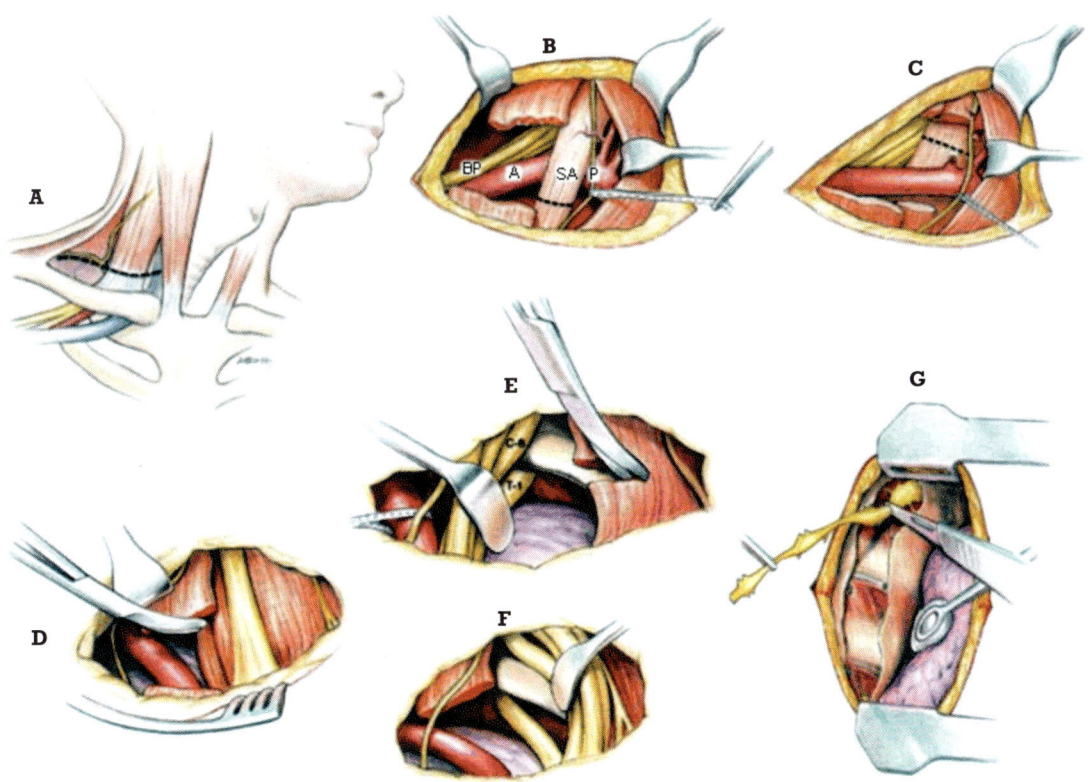

Fig. 79.4. Dorsal sympathectomy - Supraclavicular approach
A. Supraclavicular incision
B. division of scalenus anticus muscle (scelenotomy)
C. anterior retraction of subclavian artery
D-F. retraction of lung with pleura **G.** removal of D-1, 2 & 3 sypathetic ganglia
(**A**: subclavian artery; **BP**: brachial plexus; **P**: phrenic nerve; **SA**: scalenus anticus muscle)

sympathectomy (see chapter 78) may be done, excising D1-3 ganglia, complemented by standard medical treatment. This improves collateral flow, relieves any vasospastic component, enough to promote neovascularization.

Empirical scalenotomy and sympathetic ganglionectomy have a definite place in patients coming with nonhealing ischemic ulcers or minimal tissue necrosis, in whom the etiology of ischemia is unclear, after having excluded correctable organic diseases.

Management of specific conditions

1. Thoracic outlet compression syndrome (see chapter 78)
2. Atherosclerosis: Stenosis of the origin of the subclavian artery is a common condition, producing an interesting condition called *subclavian steal syndrome*, comprising symptoms of upper limb 'claudication' or ischemia, delayed low volume radial pulse on that side, with attacks of transient ischemic attacks (TIAs), which is more common on the left side.

Due to occlusion of the subclavian artery, proximal to the origin of the vertebral; as the pressure in the distal subclavian is so low, there is reversal of flow in the vertebral, drawing blood from the *circle of Willis*, to nourish the upper limb. Patients present either with attacks of TIA or features of upper limb ischemia, sometimes with gangrene of the tips of the fingers. Weak delayed

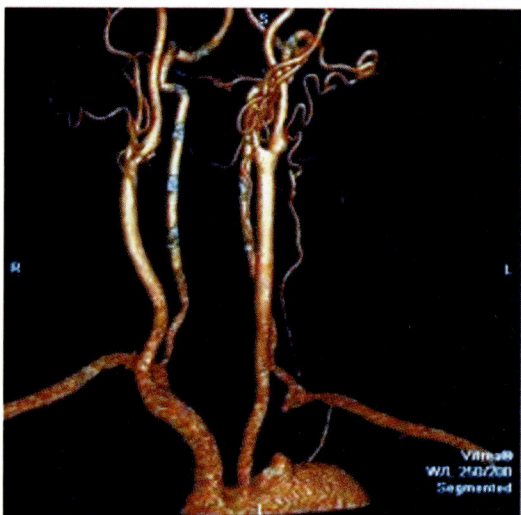

Fig. 79.5. CT angiogram of aortic arch showing proximal left subclavian stenosis with flow reversal in vertebral artery

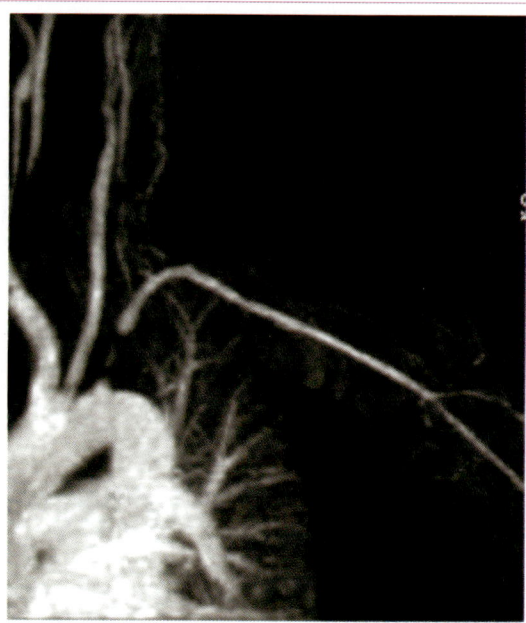

Fig. 79.6. CT angiogram of aortic arch showing proximal left subclavian stenosis with steal phenomenon

radial pulse, with attacks of TIA is so typical, that the diagnosis may be made in the office. Syncopal attacks sometimes induced by exercise of the affected arm is a typical feature, to be confirmed by a cine aortogram, to fix the site of occlusion and trace the flow pattern in the subclavian and its branches, especially the vertebral.

Surgery is definitive in established cases, either by endarterectomy, aortosubclavian bypass or percutaneous transluminal angioplasty (PTA), by dilating the stenotic segments with a balloon catheter (Gruntzig).

3. Thromboembolism: described earlier

4. Raynaud's syndrome (secondary Raynaud's disease) is more common than primary Raynaud's disease in India. This phenomenon, considered to be due to instability of the vasomotor system, is associated with the following diseases:

a) vasculitis, such as Buerger's disease or systemic collagen vascular diseases

b) occupational, in those using rapid vibrating drills or using the hypothenar eminence for hammering objects (hypothenar hammer syndrome).

c) dysproteinemia (e.g. cryoglobulinemia)

d) thoracic outlet compression syndrome

e) bleomycin toxicity

f) CREST syndrome: It is an autoimmune disorder, considered to be a type of scleroderma, associated with **c**alcinosis, **R**aynaud's phenomenon, **e**sophageal dysmotility, **s**clerodactyly and **t**elangiectasia.

In conditions associated with vasospasm, such as Raynaud's disease (primary and secondary), drugs like nifedipine (calcium channel blocker), prostaglandin E1 (vasodilator and antiplatelet agent) and ketanserin (5-hydroxytryptamine antagonist) have been found to be beneficial to some extent.

Role of sympathectomy: Notwithstanding the controversy existing with regards to the efficacy of sympathetic ganglionectomy, the consensus still is in its favour, whenever direct arterial surgery is not feasible in an ischemic limb, provided there are no objections, such as diabetes mellitus, age >50 and gross tissue necrosis. In diabetics, there is already autonomic neuropathy and in those >50, the sclerotic vessels are unlikely to obey the autonomic commands. For the technique of dorsal sympathectomy, (see chapter 78).

Sympathetic block (syn: stellate block) is sometimes done with phenol, alcohol or bupivacaine, in acute conditions such as frost bite, accidental intra-arterial injection of drugs or allergic/toxic vasculitis with impending digital ischemia. A needle is introduced about an inch below and lateral to the carotid (Chassaignac) tubercle of the C-6 transverse process, medial to the carotid pulsations, to hit the transverse process of D-1, where the stellate ganglion (confluence of inferior cervical and first dorsal sympathetic ganglia) is located. After ascertaining that the needle tip is not in a vessel, about 10-20ml of the drug is injected, to see the limb becoming warm within a few minutes, if it is effective. Development of Horner's syndrome immediately after the procedure confirms the injection at the right place.

Intra-arterial reserpine/guanethidine

In patients who develop symptoms of recurrent ischemia, after sympathectomy or in those unsuitable for surgery, slow injection of diluted reserpine (Serpasil) or guanethidine (Ismelin) into the proximal artery (brachial for digital ischemia), has given relief of symptoms for several months. Besides prolonged vasodilation, reserpine depletes the tissue stores of catacholamines, by blocking the entry of biogenic amines such as norepinephrine, dopamine and serotonin into the storage vesicles of adrenegic receptors, from their cytoplasm, essentially producing 'sympathectomy effect'. Guanethidine blocks release of stored norepinephrine, producing similar effect. These injections, however, not freely available now.

Management of upper limb ischemia

Brachial pressure on that side would be very low; duplex/color Doppler may provide necessary information to plan treatment, thus avoiding an invasive angiogram. Endarterectomy, aorto-subclavian bypass or more recently, minimally invasive PTA, are the surgical options. Since the right subclavian arises from innominate, almost in the neck, thoracotomy is not needed, but on the left, access to its origin can be achieved only by left anterolateral thoracotomy. Most of these patients have a good distal run-off; hence the results of revascularization procedures are excellent.

Amputations in the upper limb

Unlike in the lower limb, there are no 'sites of election' for choosing the levels of amputation in the upper limb, since the lowest level that heals is the best, saving every inch of the extremity, for functional advantage. If most of the forearm is retained, it may be made very useful functionally, by splitting it between the two bones (Krukenberg operation), to carry on many routine functions of the hand, including writing or picking up a tiny object from the floor etc. Following amputations, both cosmetic and functional types of prostheses are available and the appliance technology is so advanced, with computerized controls, that even a fore-quadrant amputee may be able to drive a motor vehicle comfortably, appropriate commands provided by the movements of the opposite shoulder girdle. (see chapter 130 on Amputation).

80 Vascular Anomalies

There is some confusion regarding their nature and nomenclature in the literature, but the recent trend appears to be to classify them based upon the endothelial turnover.

Accordingly they may be broadly divided into:

a) infantile hemangiomas: with endothelial hyperplasia and high turnover;

b) arteriovenous malformations: with normal endothelial turnover, which may be of either low or high flow anomalies;

c) predominantly venous lesions, including dysplasias and cavernous malformations, with normal endothelial turnover.

INFANTILE HEMANGIOMA

Hemangiomas are actually hamartomatous vascular malformations (hamartos: fault or missing the aim), involving the venous system and not true neoplasms, though this concept is being contested recently, considering them as benign neoplasms. They are usually seen in infants and children, with female preponderance (5:1), growing with them for a year or two, showing spontaneous regression thereafter, most of them totally disappearing by the age of ten. The earlier classification into cavernous and capillary types is not in much use now. It is also known as *iceberg* lesion, since most of the malformation is buried in deeper planes, only a small fraction is seen on the surface.

Clinical features

A painless circumscribed raspberry-like swelling, elevated over the skin or mucous membrane, in a new born is typical. Soft, compressible swelling with local warmth is seen, common in females (5:1), usual sites being face, back, scalp and extremities. The color and absence of transillumination differentiate this from a lymphangioma. If located in deeper planes, bluish or purple hue of the overlying skin, associated with other features described, provide the clue to diagnosis. Liver and oral cavity, including tongue form the common extracutaneous sites of this lesion.

Differential diagnosis

Includes other vascular lesions, such as lymphangioma, port-wine stain, high flow AVM, venous aneurysm, neurofibroma and when the hemangioma is infected, pyogenic granuloma has to be excluded.

Investigations

There are no specific investigations to diagnose surface hemangiomas, but imaging modalities, such as USG/CT/MRI, are useful for visceral lesions. Isotope studies, to identify pooling of blood in the lesion, to differentiate from other SOLs, are rarely needed, for diagnosis.

Treatment

Therapeutic intervention is helpful to hasten resolution and to prevent complications, as well as for those interfering with bodily functions, such as vision,

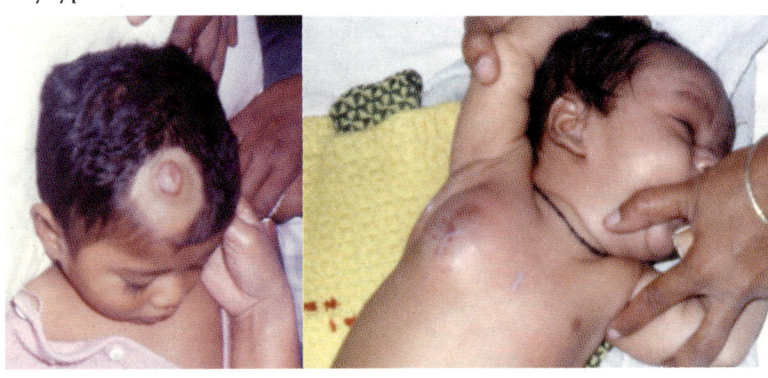

Fig. 80.1 & 80.2. Hemangioma scalp and pectoral regions in children
(courtesy: Dr C J Reddy, Gudur, AP)

feeding, urination etc. Surgery is least preferred, as it may be formidable and often results in incomplete excision. Visceral hemangiomas (e.g. liver) are harmless and are best left alone, but their potential for bleeding into peritoneal cavity (hemoperitoneum) or biliary tract (hemobilia), following blunt injuries should be remembered.

1. Medical therapy with high dose corticosteroids and interferon-alfa-2a have been tried, but are probably more useful in arresting the growth of rapidly enlarging lesions.

2. Sclerotherapy with 3% sodium tetradecylsulfate (STD/Thrombovar)), 3% polidocanol (Ethoxysclerol) or boiling aqua is found to be very effective and less mutilating. Given into and around the lesion (to obliterate feeding channels), under short general anesthesia, at 4-6week intervals, usually for 4-6 sittings (depending upon the size), by which time, most of the lesion, if not entirely, may be expected to regress.

3. Surgery is done for strictly localized disease or for residual lesion/disfigurement following sclerotherapy, which 'firms up' the lesion, facilitating excision

4. Laser excision following a few sittings of sclerotherapy is currently the most popular form of treatment.

Complications

Ulceration, bleeding and infection are the usual complications, besides physical and cosmetic considerations; malignant change into angiosarcoma, is very rare.

Kasabach-Merritt syndrome, a type of consumption coagulopathy, is seen in extensive hemangiomatous lesions, owing to platelet trapping within the lesion, leading to thrombocytopenia and purpura.

Sturge-Weber syndrome consists of port-wine stain of face, hemangiomas of leptomeninges and choroids, often associated with contralateral hemiplegia, mental retardation, epilepsy and glaucoma.

Other vascular malformations

Capillary malformations

Typically bright red (*port wine stain*) macular or maculopapular lesion is present on the lip, usually since birth, with a high tendency for spontaneous regression. Thus reassurance of the anxious parents with masterly inactivity and watchful expectancy is recommended along with camouflauging lipstick. If total regression has not occurred in the preschool age or if recurrent infection/bleeding complicate, Laser photocoagulation/excision may be done. The wavelength of the Nd-YAG laser is 1064 mm. and is selectively absorbed by the blood in the hemangioma delivering maximum energy into the lesion.

Telengiectasia

These are really very tiny vascular malformations, always asymptomatic but for the cosmetic effect, and scattered per orally in conditions like

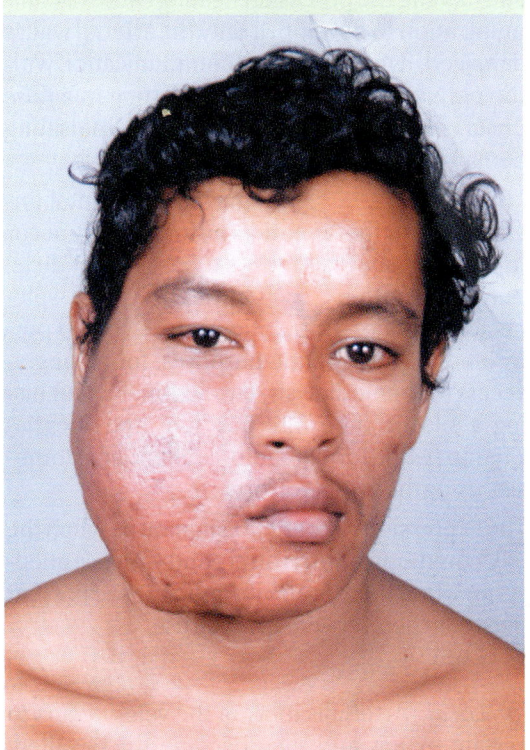

Fig. 80.3. Cavernous hemangioma, cheek (courtesy: Lifeline Hospitals, Chennai)

Osler Rendu Weber Syndrome or Peutz-Jegher`s syndrome. The treatment of choice is photo-thermolysis of the lesion using pulsed dye laser.

ARTERIOVENOUS FISTULA/MALFORMATION (AVF/AVM)

Definition: This is a high flow lesion, wherein there is an abnormal communication between an artery and an adjacent vein. This could be congenital or acquired, the latter may be.traumatic or iatrogenic (iatros: physician).

Etiology

(1) Congenital AVM are direct shunts between artery and vein, may occur in any part of the body most commonly in leg, arm or scalp. The embryonic vascular system initially consists of interlacing blood spaces in the primitive mesenchyme, which subsequently *zonalize* into arterial, capillary and venous areas. The AVMs are thought to be the result of persistence of primitive connections. Depending on the stage at which this failure occurs, they may range from just above capillary level to large arterial channels, termed *micro* or *macrofistula*, respectively.

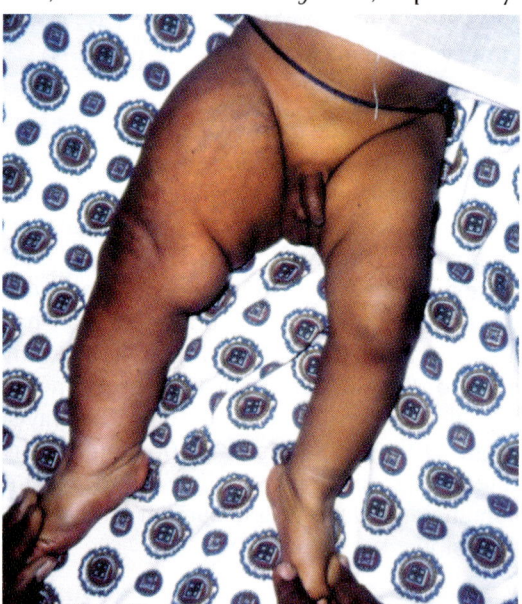

Fig. 80.4. Congenital AVM of right lower limb with soft tissue hypertrophy (courtesy: Halsted Surgical Clinic, Chennai)

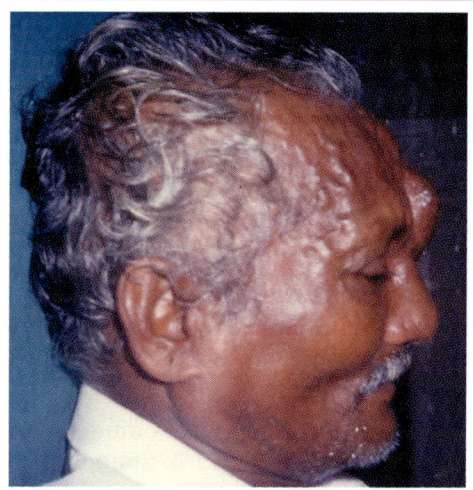

Fig. 80.5. Extensive AVM involving face and scalp, following blunt injury (courtesy: Halsted Surgical Clinic, Chennai)

(2) Acquired AVM is usually secondary to a penetrating or blunt injury of the vessels, both artery and its vein; the process of healing causes a communication to develop. If only the arterial wall is damaged, it may develop a communication with the perivascular hematoma, resulting in a *false aneurysm* (syn: traumatic aneurysm, pulsating hematoma).

(3) Iatrogenic AV fistula may be accidental (inadvertent) or therapeutic. The former may occur following mass ligation of a vascular pedicle, during operations, such as nephrectomy, splenectomy, major amputations etc. It is also performed for therapeutic purposes, for an angio-access for hemodialysis, e.g. Scribner shunt (using a silastic tube interposition) and Brescia-Cimino fistula (direct radio-cephalic anastomosis), using the vessels of forearm.

The expressions like aneurysmal varix, when the A-V communication is direct and varicose aneurysm, when there is an intermediate sac present between them, are not in much use.

Effects

a) Local: 'Arterialisation' of the veins occurs to certain extent and they become thick-walled, dilated, tortuous, and pulsatile. The collaterals also increase in size and number, raising the

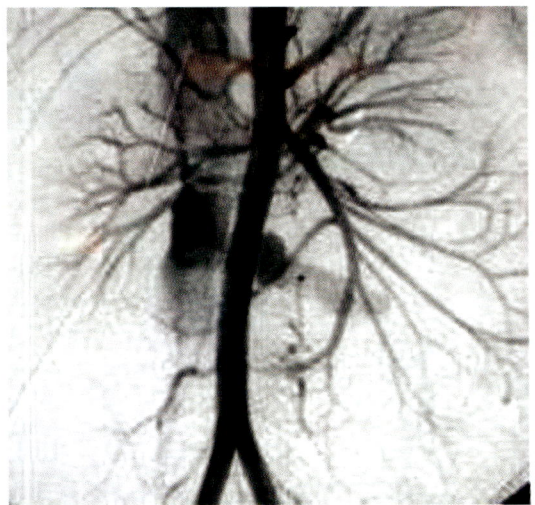

Fig. 80.6. Aortocaval fistula following blunt injury. IVC is seen in the arterial phase of the aortogram

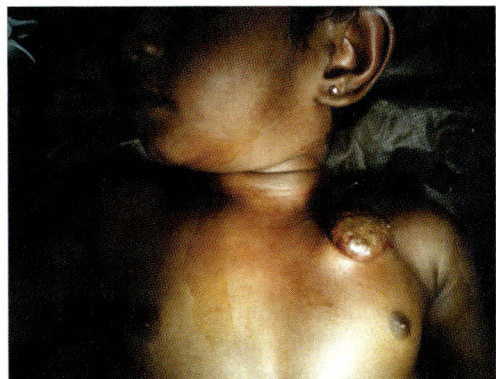

Fig. 80.7. Cavernous hemangioma of chest wall (courtesy: Halsted Surgical Clinic, Chennai)

local temperature. If this occurs before the eiphyseal fusion, there may be local gigantism.

b) Distal: as short circuiting of arterial blood (*steal phenomenon*) occurs, leading to oxygen desaturation, distal ischemia may be seen producing muscle wasting, ulcers or gangrene.

c) Circulatory system: Increase in pulse rate and cardiac output with wide pulse pressure is typically seen, an example for hyperdynamic (or hyperkinetic) state of circulation (syn: collapsing, water-hammer or Corrigan pulse). Tachycardia occurs due to increased venous return to the heart, leading eventually to cardiomegaly, left ventricular hypertrophy and high output cardiac failure.

Signs

1. Pulsatile swelling
2. Dilated collaterals with increased local temperature
3. Scar, in traumatic or iatrogenic cases
4. Prominent pulsatile and often varicose superficial veins (secondary varicosities)
5. A thrill and a bruit of machinery character may be present.
6. The skin is warmer proximally, but the temperature may drop to subnormal, as the limb is traced distally

7. Features of chronic ischemia of the peripheral part of the limb (loss of hair, reduction in subcutaneous and muscle mass, brittle grooved nails, ulcerations and digital gangrene)
8. Increased bone length in congenital AVM or if acquired before epiphyseal fusion (local gigantism)
9. *Branham's* (or Nicolodani's) *sign:* compression of the artery proximal to the fistula will produce reduction in heart rate, by reducing venous return to heart (Bainbridge reflex).
10. Hyperdynamic pulse, with wide pulse pressure
11. Harvey's sign: a venous segment is emptied by milking it by two fingers and distal finger is released; rapid filling of that segment indicates significant AVM

Some of these findings (1, 3, 5 & 6) may be lacking in congenital microfistulae.

Clinical types

Localized: usually traumatic or iatrogenic, eminently suitable for surgical intervention.

Diffuse: usually congenital, the communications are multiple, wide spread both in breadth and depth. Surgery is formidable and hazardous and better avoided.

Plexiform aneurysm (syn: cirsoid aneurysm) is a congenital AVM, in which diffuse pulsatile arteries and arterialised veins, feeling like a bag of pulsating worms, are seen commonly over scalp or forehead.

Investigations

Doppler study and *Duplex* imaging are non-invasive.studies, to confirm and delineate the AV communications.

Angiography: Three types of angiography are used to study AVM.

(i) *Conventional:* not only demonstrates the AVM but quantifies the shunt. Serial filming by cine-angio is very useful, to study the flow pattern. Therapeutic embolization, followed by post-embolization angiographic evaluation, can be done at the same time. Normal angiogram has arterial, capillary (tissue) and venous phases; in AVM, venous filling is seen in arterial phase itself.

(ii) *Isotope* (^{99m}Tc) *angiogram* is preferred in evaluating children with congenital AVM.

(iii) *Digital subtraction angio-gram* (DSA) and *MR Angiogram* (MRA) are newer and more satisfactory methods of assessing an AVM.

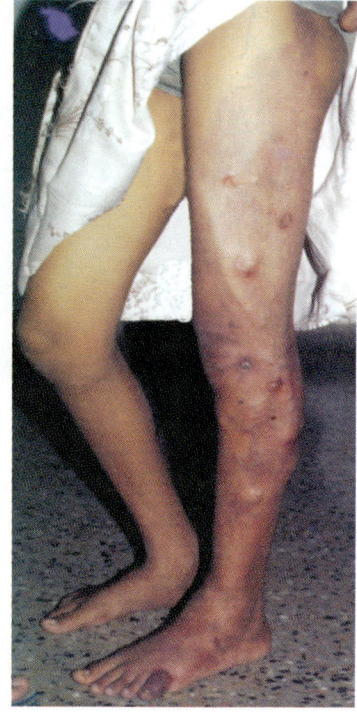

Fig. 80.11.
18 year old girl with Klippel-Trenaunay syndrome. Note the prominent vein of Giacomini and hypertrophy of the little toe.
(courtesy: Halsted Surgical Clinic, Chennai)

Treatment

Congenital lesions: These are usually static and can be left alone. Elastic support, drugs to improve venous tone (diosmin, dobesilate, troxirutin etc) and antiedema therapy may palliate them. If there is recurrent bleeding or if the deformity is severe, selective arterial embolization (therapeutic) with autologous muscle, clot (thromboplastin), silastic pellets, polystyrene coils or rapidly polymerizing acrylic compound, is advised. Direct infiltration of sclerosants at multiple sittings is another alternative, but may turn out to be a cumbersome exercise. Surgical intervention is done as a last resort for complications like infection, disabling hemorrhage or frank gangrene. Amputation of gangrenous part of the limb is associated with significant bleeding. Troublesome secondary varicose veins, generally having bizarre distribution, may be excised/stripped, to prevent cuta-

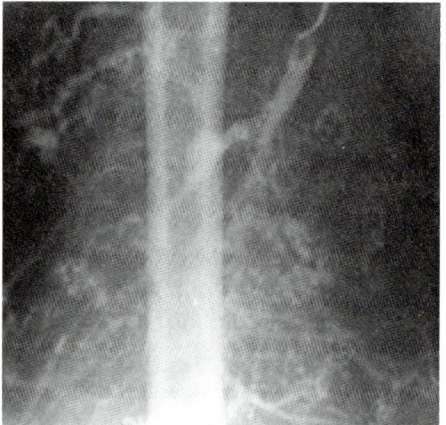

Fig. 80.8. Traumatic AVM of thigh treated by therapeutic embolization, angiogram showing venous blush

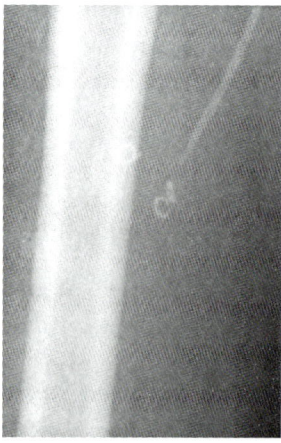

80.9. Silastic pellets are being deployed

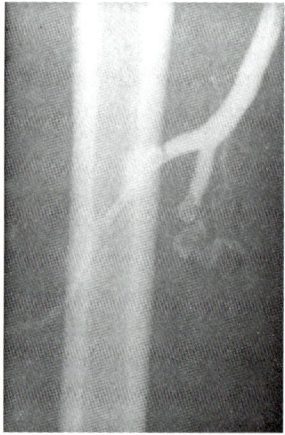

80.10. Post-embolization angiogram

(courtesy: Dr V Balaji, Chennai)

neous complications of venous hypertension.

Acquired AVF: These are ideally treated by surgery because they are strictly localized and progessive. Preliminary angiographic evaluation is essential.

1. Reconstruction with removal of the intervening sac, and repair of the artery, if necessary replacing with a vein/dacron/PTFE graft, is the treatment of choice. The involved vein may be sacrificed, if it can not be salvaged.

2. In small vessel lesions where reconstruction is difficult, quadruple ligation of the involved artery and vein above and below the lesion, may be more expedient.

3. Percutaneous trans-catheter embolization, either as the sole therapy or as a preoperative adjunct, definitely has a role, in reducing.complications and blood loss during surgery.

4. A covered endovascular stent may be deployed percutaneously to shut off the A-V communication.

Several syndromes have been associated with AVMs; the most common one is the *Klippel-Trenaunay syndrome*, which is a specific complex of vascular malformation, involving mainly capillaries and veins of one or more limbs. Secondary varicose veins of unusual distribution, capillary port-wine patches, limb/toe hypertrophy and lymphatic abnormalities are typically seen in children and young adults, usually brought for ugly veins, pigmentation, recurrent bleeding or local tissue hypertrophy. As already indicated, palliative surgery to excise the troublesome veins may be necessary, if conservative therapy has not given physical and emotional comfort. Occasional nonexistence of the deep venous system in these patients, should

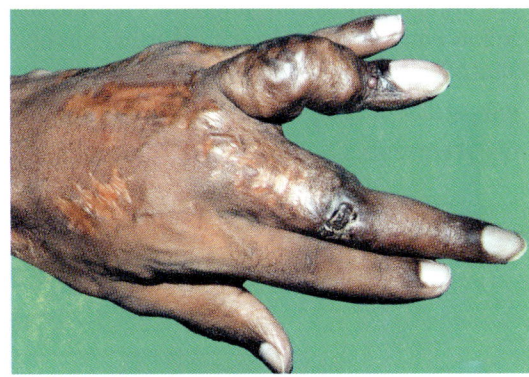

Fig. 80.12. Recurrent AVM of hand and fingers with ulceration
(courtesy: Halsted Surgical Clinic, Chennai)

	Feature	Hemangioma	AVM
1	Nature	Neoplasm/hamartoma	Congenital anomaly
2	Age	30% at birth	90% at birth
3	Sex	F:M:: 5:1	Equal
4	Endothelial proliferation	Present	Absent
5	Growth in tissue culture	Present	Absent
6	Cellular stroma	Present	Absent
7	Mast cells	Abundant	Absent
8	Spontaneous involution	Present	Absent
9	Venous engorgement/pulsation	Absent	Usally present
10	Hyperdynamic circulation	Absent	Present
11	Branham sign	Absent	Present
12	Distal ischemia of limb	Absent	Present
13	Thrombocytopenia	May be seen	Not common
14	Sclerotherpay	Suitable	Unsuitable
15	Therapeutic embolization	Not possible	Possible

Table-80.1: Differences between hemangioma and AVM

be borne in mind, while dealing with superficial system.

Complications

(i) cosmetic.

(ii) skin pigmentation, eczema, ulceration and bleeding.

(iii) secondary varicosities and their complications.

(iv) increased limb/toe length, resulting in limp/disfigurement.

(v) distal ischemia and gangrene. This may also follow embolization, if a critical artery has been shut off, by a therapeutic misadventure.

(vi) cardiac decompensation.

(vii) recurrence.

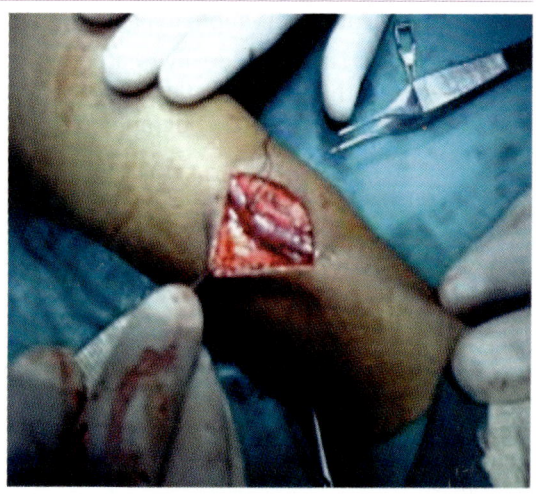

Fig. 80.14. End-to-side AVF in the distal forearm completed

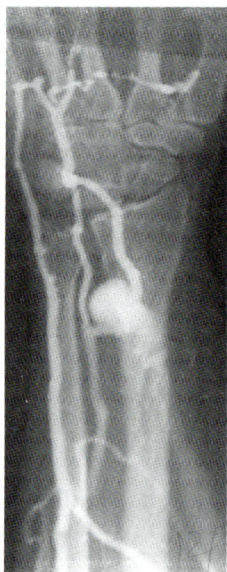

Fig. 80.13.
AV Fistula, of forearm, showing a venous aneurysm in angiogram (courtesy: Halsted Surgical Clinic, Chennai)

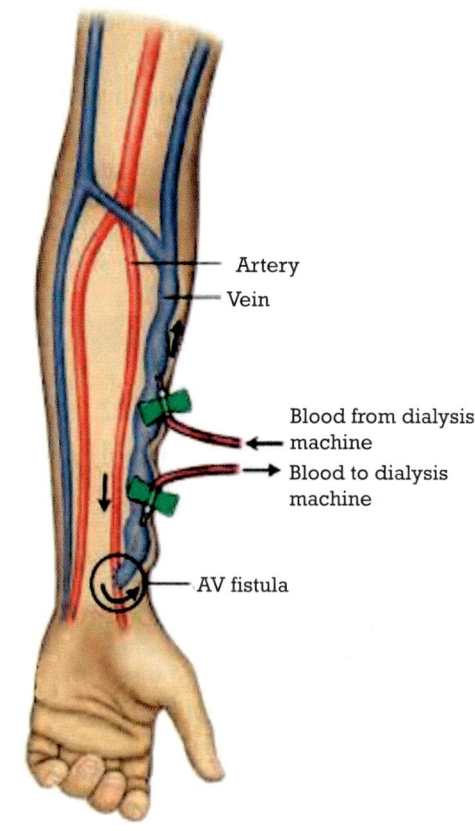

Fig. 80.15. Radio-cephalic AVF created for hemodialysis (Brescia-Cimino fistula)

81 Arterial Aneurysm

(Aneurysma: widening)

Definition: An ANEURYSM is a localized dilatation of a blood vessel. It is classified in several ways, depending upon whether it has all three layers or not, by its shape and by the etiology.

Depending upon layers of the wall

i) *true* aneurysm, containing all coats of the vessel wall;

ii) *false* or traumatic aneurysm, which does not contain all layers.

Depending upon its shape

i) *fusiform* or spindle-shapped is the commonest variety

ii) *saccular* aneurysm develops when a part of circumference expands to one side, rest being normal

iii) *dissecting* aneurysm is due to intimal injury, seen often in hypertensive patients, where the vessel wall is split, lifting the inner layer (intima and part of media) to occlude the lumen totally or partially. The false lumen may reopen distally by another intimal tear, allowing flow of blood into the vessel or it may rupture externally, causing massive hemorrhage. Thoracic aorta is the commonest region involved, with acute presentation closely mimicking cardiac infarction. Besides atherosclerosis, other degenerative diseases of vessel wall, such as cystic medial necrosis may also produce dissection.

Depending upon the etiology

1) *Congenital*

i) congenital aneurysm, due to defective elastic lamina, is often seen in the circle of Willis (Berry) and rarely other vessels. Another favor-

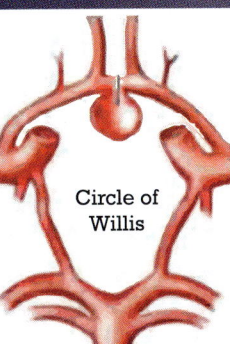

Fig. 81.1. Congenital aneurysm (Berry) of the anterior communicating artery

Circle of Willis

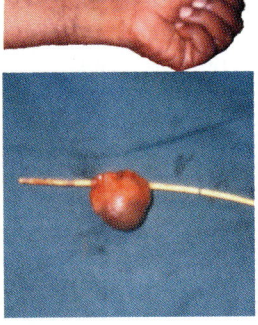

Fig. 81.2. Radial artery aneurysm and resected specimen
courtesy: Halsted Surgical Clinic, Chennai

ite site is the splenic artery, which may go undetected till it ruptures (artery of abdominal apoplexy). Berry aneurysm is located commonly in relation to the anterior communicating branch of anterior cerebral; when it ruptures life threatening subarachnoid or intracerebral hemorrhage may occur.

ii) arteriovenous malformation may result in an aneurysm. Cirsoid aneurysm is a pulsating mass due to an AVM, with serpentine arteries and vessels around it, seen often over the scalp.

iii) some diseases are associated with congenital aneurysm of aorta, e.g. Marfan's syndrome or coarctation.

2) *Acquired* may be traumatic, degenerative, infective and due to a collagen disorder.

i) **traumatic** (syn: false aneurysm, pulsating hematoma) is due to a penetrating or blunt injury of the vessel wall. A hematoma is formed initially, communicating with the vessel lumen through a small rent, and hence pulsatile, which slowly expands into various tissue planes, with irregular outline and no arterial wall covering, the cavity just surrounded by compressed soft tissue.

ii) **degenerative** type is the most common, atherosclerosis being the predominant preexisting disease. Seen more in elderly males, it may occur in any artery, but common sites are, thoracic/abdominal aorta, popliteal and radial arteries.

The pathogenesis of aneurysmal dilatation in atherosclerosis is defective intima and most of the media, due to loss of elastin in the wall, which is considered to be a result of imbalance between two enzymes

471

controlling its metabolism; elastase (for degradation) and α-antitrypsin (for antidegradation).

The physical change in the aortic diameter can occur secondary to trauma, infection, an intrinsic defect in the protein construction of the aortic wall, or due to progressive destruction of aortic proteins by enzymes. After initial dilatation, it gradually expands by the principle of *Laplace*, by which the circumferential stress is related to intraluminal pressure and radius of the vessel, where as the the rupture of an aneurysm occurs when the tangential stress over the the wall exceeds the tensile strength of any point of the vessel. Copper deficiency appears to have some relation to the develoment of arterial aneurysms, by its effect on elastin metabolism.

Splenic artery aneurysm has a special predilection for females (4:1) and the highest incidence is seen in multiparous women. Excessive blood flow through the artery due to increased splenic arterio-venous shunting during pregnancy is considered to be the contributory factor, besides preexisting structural abnormalities (fibrodysplasia) inherent to splenic artery, so also for the high incidence of rupture of those aneurysm (artery of abdominal apoplexy). Similar phenomenon is seen in portal hypertension and splenomegaly, due to torrential (hyperkinetic) blood flow in the artery, which increases its diameter. Rupture of this aneurysm into the lesser sack is known to produce a hemorrhagic pseudocyst.

Other types of degenerative aneurysms are *post-stenotic dilatation* of subclavian artery in cervical rib, capillary microaneurysms of retinal vessels seen in diabetics and a rare disease seen in South African Negros, developing aortic aneurysm in children due to mucoid degeneration of

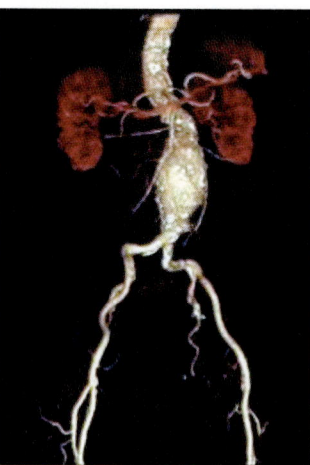
Fig. 81.3. CT aortography - infrarenal aortic fusiform aneurysm

tunica media. The pathogenesis of post-stenotic aneurysm is not clear; injury to vasavasorum, supplying the artery immediately distal to the rib, causing ischemic damage to the vessel wall, is one explanation. As they occur distal to coarctation of aorta and aortic/pulmonary stenosis, increased lateral pressure on the wall due to eddy currents generated due to stenosis (Bernoulli's theorem) is an alternate hypothesis, accounting for initial dilatation; once dilated they progressively enlarge as per Laplace's law.

iii) **infective:** they are mycotic, syphilitic or tuberculous

Mycotic aneurysms are due to bacterial infection (not fungal contrary to the name) and can occur in any artery in the body, as part of a pyemic process, e.g. in subacute bacterial endocarditis, within an abscess cavity and rarely in collagen disorders such as polyarteritis nodosa.

Syphilitic aneurysm due to endarteritis of vasa vasorum may occur, commonly seen in thoracic aorta, often presenting as a pulsatile swelling eroding the sternum, rarely seen nowadays. *Microaneurysms* (of Rasmussen) develop within

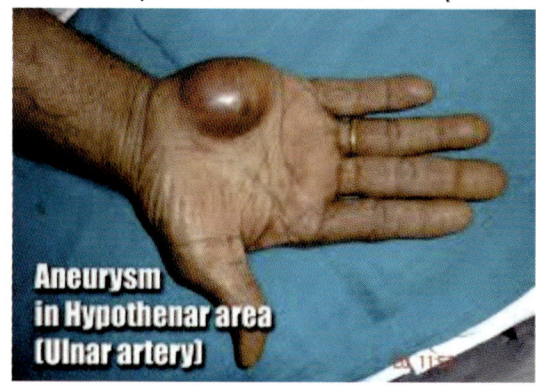
Fig. 81.4. Traumatic aneurysm of ulnar artery. Patient is a carpenter, uses his hand as a hammer

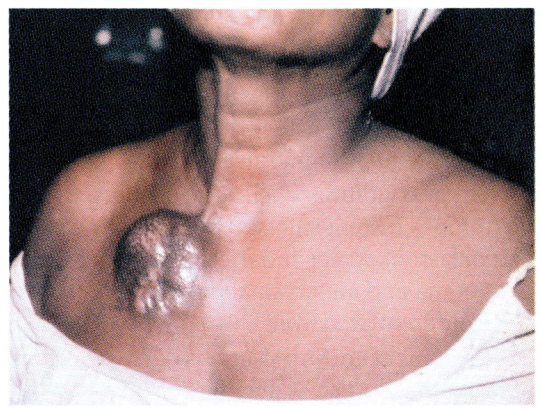

Fig. 81.5. Aneurysm of aortic arch, eroding the sternum
(courtesy: Lifeline Hospitals, Chennai)

a tuberculous abscess in the lung, may leak and cause recurrent troublesome hemoptysis.

iv) **collagen diseases** Marfan's syndrome, Ehlers Danlos syndrome

Complications of an aneurysm (occur in 95% in 5 years):

a) leak or hemorrhage
b) erosion into adjacent bony structures
c) thromboembolic manifestations, from the fragmented intramural laminated clot
d) pressure on sensory nerves in the vicinity
e) venous obstruction
f) pressure on adjacent viscera, such as esophagus causing dysphagia

g) internal fistula, e.g. aorto-enteric fistula, producing massive gastrointestinal bleeding, commonest site being the 3rd part of duodenum.

h) infection, which may be the cause or an effect of an aneurysm

i) rarely, the lumen may be totally obliterated by a thrombus and spontaneous 'cure' may be observed, more so in a saccular type.

Clinical features

i) an aneurysm may be asymptomatic, detected during routine examination

ii) pain is a very common symptom, generally signifies some complication, and it may be dull (erosion), acute (leak) or referred (pressure on adjacent nerves).

iii) mass, usually showing expansile pulsations, is characteristic

iv) evidence of distal ischemia due to embolic phenomenon

v) external pressure on the accompanying vein, may produce stasis related problems, such as edema, pigmentation, ulceration, large collaterals and thromboembolism

vi) infection is a very difficult complication causing septicemia, pyemia and tendency to rupture.

vii) dysphagia, hemoptysis and massive hematemesis, as mentioned above

	Feature	Expansile Pulse	Transmitted Pulse
1.	Consistency	Soft/compressible	Firm/hard
2.	Two finger/match stick test (not reliable for deep-seated mass)	They move apart	Negative
3.	Compression of proximal artery (not possible in abdomen)	The swelling becomes soft and fills up slowly	No change
4.	Knee-elbow position	No change	Pulsation may cease
5.	Movements with respiration	Absent	May move
6.	Intrinsic mobility	Absent	May be present
7.	Evidence of distal ischemia	May be seen	Absent

Table-81.1: Differences between expansile and transmitted pulse of an abdominal mass

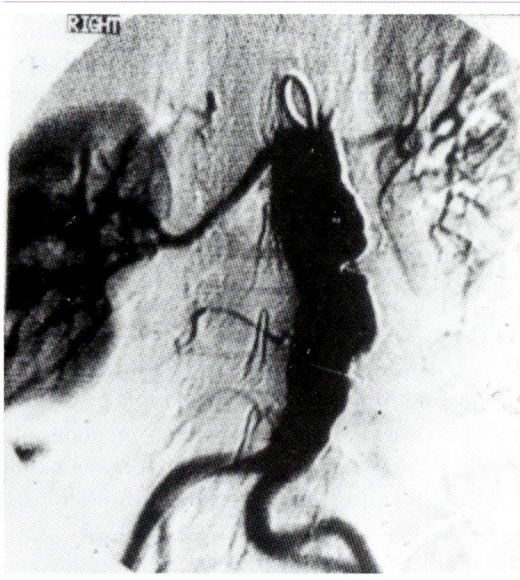

Fig. 81.6. DSA of abdominal aorta showing a fusiform aneurysm. Right renal artery is also seen (courtesy: Halsted Surgical Clinic, Chennai)

Signs: A compressible swelling over the course of an artery, exhibiting expansile pulsations, movable across the axis of the vessel, is an aneurysm, until proved otherwise. A thrill and bruit may be appreciated, usually immediately distal to the sac. Similar swellings may be evident in other parts of the body.

It has been observed that AAA grows 3mm in size every year till it reaches a diameter of 5cm and later 5mm per year.

Sign of tracheal tug

This is seen in the aneurysm of arch of aorta, impinging on the left main bronchus. The patient is asked to swallow, when the larynx moves up. With two fingers, it is fixed in that level and not allowed to come down; a pulsatile tug is appreciated by the fingers, as the aneurysmal pulsations are transmitted through the tracheobronchial apparatus to the larynx.

Differential diagnosis

1) Transmitted pulsations by an SOL sitting over the main artery. Two finger/match stick test may be useful for a superficial lesion but not in a deep-seated mass, where several layers of soft tissue are interposed between it and the exam-

ining fingers.

2) Large vessel coursing over a mass, as external carotid over a carotid body tumor

3) A serpentine artery, usually carotid or innominate, may mimic an aneurysm

4) Other conditions such as an abscess, vascular tumors (osteogenic sarcoma or a vascular osteoclastoma), secondaries from renal cell carcinoma and aneurysmal bone cyst etc. have to be differentiated from an aneurysm.

5) Prominent aortic pulsations due to exaggerated lumbar lordosis, may be mistaken for an aneurysm

Investigations

Routine investigations include blood/urine examination, serology for syphilis, chest/abdominal skiagram for soft tissue shadow and bony erosion (calcification of wall of aortic aneurysm may be seen in a lateral view). Investigations to assess the fitness for anesthesia and surgery, of course are necessary.

Specific investigations

Duplex imaging, USG/CT scan for better delineation

Angiography to see the extent, state of proximal/distal vessels, evidence of distal embolism

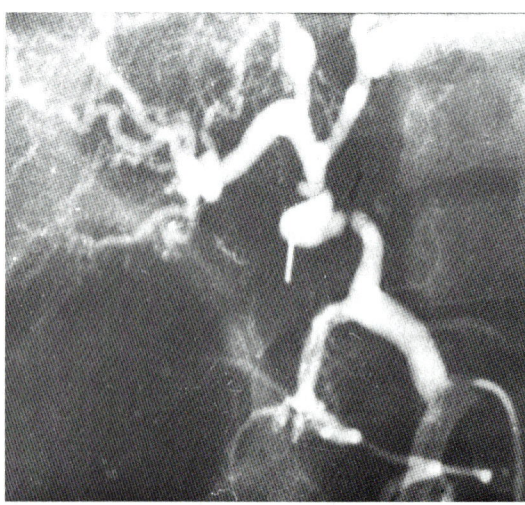

Fig. 81.7. Hepatic angiogram after liver transplantation. False aneurysm at the site of hepaticarterial anastomosis (courtesy: Prof Mohamed Rela, Global Hospitals, Chennai)

etc. Because of intramural thrombus, it always under-estimates the size of an aneurysm, but coupled with CT, accurate size may be assessed. Angiogram also outlines an AVM, if present.

If mycotic aneurysm is suspected, appropriate imaging/microbiological studies are required to identify the source and nature of infection.

Treatment: Surgery in some form, is the definitive treatment.

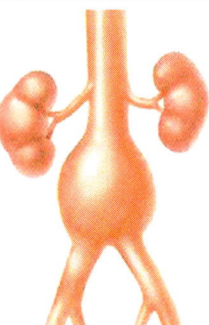

Fig.81.8.Infrarenal abdominalaortic aneurysm

Indications

1) if the life expectancy of the patient is >5years, since 95% of them produce some complication or other within 5years of diagnosis.

2) if its diameter is twice that of the native artery bearing the aneurysm, due to a high risk of rupture

3) development of complications

They may be broadly classified into open and endovascular procedures:

Open operations

1) *Ligations* are more of historical interest, and rarely done nowadays. Various levels of ligation, such as proximal (Hunter and Anel), distal (Brasdor and Wardrop)) and both sides (Antylus) have been described.

2) *Endoaneurysmorrhaphy*, by introducing coils of wire into the sac to obliterate the lumen, has also become obsolete.

3) *Wrapping* the aneurysm, to prevent expansion and rupture, with fascia lata, PTFE, prolene etc, may be life saving, in situations where excision is difficult and risky. Going around an adherent aneurysm may occasionally be equally tedious and hazardous.

4) *Aneurysmectomy* (Matas) may be done for saccular types, lateral defect in the vessel sutured with fine nonabsorbable material or repaired with a patch graft.

5) *Exclusion bypass* is sometimes necessary, by proximal/distal ligation and bypass grafting either with vein or a synthetic conduit.

6) *Excision* and direct anastomosis is possible if there is tortuous and redundant artery adjacent to the aneurysm, which is healthy enough for direct end-to-end suturing.

7) Excision of the aneurysm and *replacement* of vessel with a suitable graft, is the modern standard treatment. If the disease involves a bifurcation, as in distal aorta, a 'Y' graft is used, suturing the stem to the aorta and limbs to the iliac arteries.

Endovascular procedures

1) Percutaneous *intraluminal stenting*, to exclude the dilated segment from the blood stream is becoming increasingly popular.

2) Another novel day-care procedure is

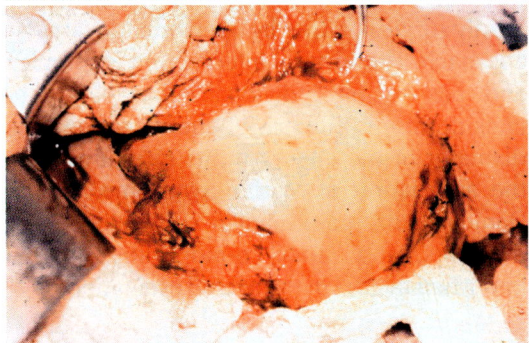

Fig. 81.9. Abdominal aortic aneurysm

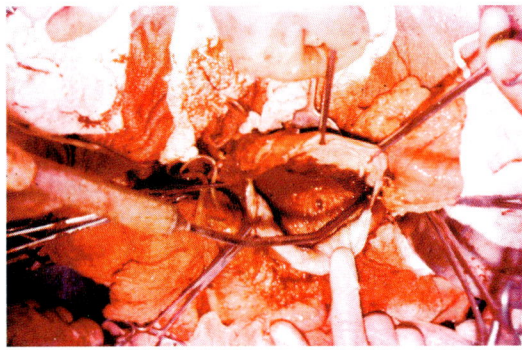

Fig. 81.10. Sac opened after proximal/distal clamping (courtesy: Halsted Surgical Clinic, Chennai)

percutaneous transluminal *balloon obliteration* of sac, done for tiny inaccessible vessels, such as Berry aneurysm. A catheter with a detachable balloon is negotiated into the aneurysmal sac and the catheter is withdrawn, deploying the inflated balloon, to permanently obliterate the sac, thus avoiding life-threatening rupture.

ABDOMINAL AORTIC ANEURYSM

Abdominal aortic aneurysm (AAA) is the most common type of aortic aneurysms. One reason for this is that elastin, the principal tension-bearing protein present in the wall of the aorta, is reduced in its abdominal segment as compared to the thoracic region (nearer the heart). Another reason is that the abdominal aorta does not possess vasa vasorum, hindering repair. Most are *true aneurysms* that involve all three layers (tunica intima, media and adventitia), and are generally asymptomatic before rupture.

An AAA may remain asymptomatic indefinitely. There is a large risk of rupture once the size has reached 5 cm (twice the diameter of the native vessel), though some of them may swell to over 15 cm in diameter before rupturing. Uncomplicated AAA may present as a large, pulsatile mass above the umbilicus. A bruit may be heard from the turbulent flow in a severe atherosclerotic aneurysm or if thrombosis occurs. Unfortunately, however, rupture is usually the first hint of AAA. Once an aneurysm has ruptured, it presents with a classic triad of *pain-hypotension-mass*.

The diagnosis of an abdominal aortic aneurysm can be confirmed at the bedside by the use of ultrasound. Rupture could be indicated by the presence of free fluid in potential abdominal spaces, such as Morison's pouch, the splenorenal space (between the spleen and left kidney), subdiaphragmatic (under the diaphragm) and pelvic spaces. A contrast-enhanced abdominal CT (CECT) scan is confirmatory.

Only 10-25% of patients survive rupture due to high perioperative mortality. The physical change in the aortic diameter can occur secondary to trauma, infection, an intrinsic defect in the protein construction of the aortic wall, or due to progressive destruction of aortic proteins by enzymes. The annual mortality from ruptured AAA in the USA alone is about 15,000. Another important complication of AAA is the formation of a thrombus in the aneurysm. The prevalence of AAAs increases with age, with an average age of 65-70 at the time of diagnosis. AAAs have been attributed to atherosclerosis, though other factors are involved in their formation.

Medical therapy

Medical therapy of aortic aneurysms involves strict blood pressure control. This does not treat the aortic aneurysm per se, but control of hypertension may decrease the rate of expansion and risk of rupture.

Prevention

Attention to patient's general blood pressure, smoking and cholesterol risks helps reduce the risk on an individual basis. There have been proposals to introduce ultrasound scans as a screening tool for those most at risk: men over the age of 65. Non-selective β-blocker, propranolol and antibiotics such as tetracyclines or doxycycline are currently being investigated to prevent progression of aortic aneurysm, when detected early, due to their matrix metalloproteinase (MMP) inhibitor and collagen stabilizing properties.

The definitive treatment for an aortic aneurysm is only surgical, either by open or endovascular approach. The surgical intervention is complex and has to be individualized, taking into consideration the risk/benefit ratio. The diameter of the aneurysm, its rate of growth, the association of Marfan syndrome, Ehlers-Danlos syndrome or similar connective tissue disorders, and other co-morbidities are all important factors in the overall evaluation.

Open surgery

Open surgery typically involves dissection of

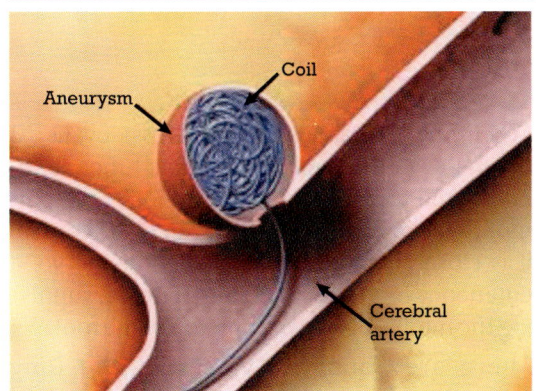

Fig. 81.11 Endoaneurysmorrhaphy using a coil to obliterate an intracranial aneurysm (historical interest)

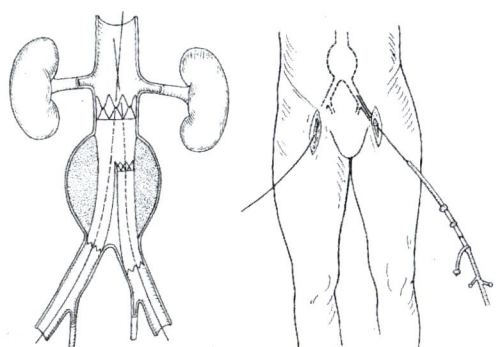

Fig. 81.12. Endovascular prosthetic stenting of AAA

the dilated portion of the aorta and insertion of a synthetic (Dacron or PTFE) prosthesis. Once the tube is sewn into the proximal and distal portions of the aorta, the aneurysmal sac is closed around the artificial tube. Instead of suturing the tube ends, use of rigid and expandable by nitinol wireframe, can be simpler and expedient. They may be effectively ("water-tight" seal) inserted into the vascular lumina and permanently fixed by external sutures.

Endovascular therapy: See chapter 84 on endovascular surgery.

Complications of surgery for abdominal aortic aneurysm (AAA)

1. primary and reactionary *hemorrhage*
2. *renal failure*, may occur even if the aorta is cross-clamped below the renal arteries, but is a serious complication of suprarenal clamping (renal tolerance to ischemia at 37° C is 30min. which may be prolonged by hypothermia or intraoperative perfusion methods)
3. *declamping hypotension*, as the aortic clamp is released, redistributing the cardiac output to the entire body

4. *distal embolization and 'trash foot'*
5. *ischemic damage* to colon, if the inferior mesenteric artery is ligated. This may not occur if the other two (celiac and superior mesenteric) arteries are normal.
6. complications of *anesthesia*
7. anastomotic false aneurysm or internal (aorto-enteric) fistula may occur.
8. graft infection
9. Cross clamping of the aorta and its branches during surgery, may lead to inadequate blood supply to the spinal cord, resulting in neurological deficits. Preoperative cerebrospinal fluid drainage (CSFD), when performed under experienced supervision, reduces the risk of ischemic spinal cord injury, as evidenced by randomized trials, by increasing the perfusion pressure to the spinal cord.

Recent advances

Long term use of non-selective β-blocker, propranolol and doxycycline (by its property of inhibiting matrix metalloproteinases-MMP) is being tried to discourage growth of aneurysms, when detected in early stages.

82 Varicose Veins

This is a penalty man pays for acquiring the vertical (bipedal) posture in the process of evolution. Varicose veins are dilated, tortuous and elongated veins and occur at the following common sites in the body:

1. superficial venous system of the limbs
2. gastroesophageal varices in portal hypertension
3. anorectal veins in hemorrhoids
4. spermatic (testicular) veins and pampiniform plexus in varicocele
5. ovarian, vulval and fundal (uterine) varicosities

Only lower limb varices will be discussed in this chapter.

VARICOSE VEINS OF LOWER LIMB

Anatomy: Venous drainage of the lower limb is by

(1) deep veins,
(2) superficial veins and
(3) perforating or communicating veins connecting the above two.

DEEP VEINS: They correspond to the main arteries viz. common, superficial and profunda femoral, popliteal, anterior and posterior tibial and peroneal veins. There are numerous valves in these veins directing the blood upwards, to prevent reflux. Incompetency of these valves results in ambulant venous hypertension. There is a huge venous lake in the calf muscles (soleal plexus) devoid of valves, known as *peripheral heart* (pump) and venous return from this plexus occurs during calf muscle contractions.

SUPERFICIAL VEINS

(i) Long saphenous vein: This is the longest vein in the body, beginning in front of the medial malleolus as the continuation of dorsal venous arch (medial marginal vein) of the foot. It runs upwards and backwards and enters the thigh from postero-medial aspect of the knee to end in the saphenous opening (fossa ovalis), 3 cm below and lateral to the pubic tubercle, to pierce the cribriform fascia and join the common femoral vein. In its infragenicular course, it is closely related to the saphenous nerve, a cutaneous branch of the femoral nerve, supplying the medial part of the dorsum of the foot.

There are about 20 valves in the long saphenous vein out of which the majority are below knee. The constant and most important valve is located at the sapheno-femoral junction (SFJ).

Tributaries

1. At the ankle from the sole of the foot through the dorsal venous arch

2. In the leg, one or two veins connecting the short saphenous vein

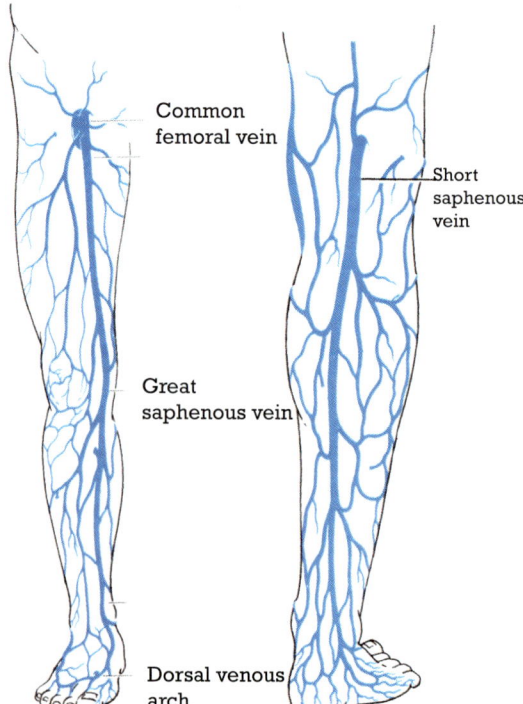

Common femoral vein

Short saphenous vein

Great saphenous vein

Dorsal venous arch

Fig. 82.1. Long and short saphenous venous systems of right leg

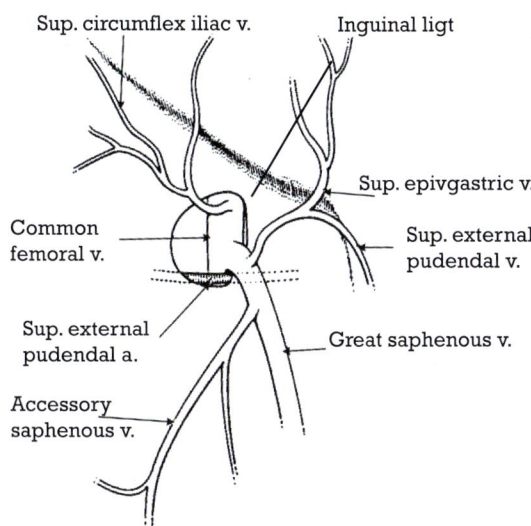

Fig. 82.2. Right sapheno-femoral junction showing tributaries

3. In the thigh, an anterolateral and posteromedial tributaries (the latter sometimes called the accessory saphenous vein) join the long saphenous, just below its termination. At the saphenous opening there are four constant tributaries

(1) superficial epigastric
(2) superficial external pudendal
(3) superficial circumflex iliac
(4) accessory saphenous vein

It is important that these tributaries are adequately disconnected by flush ligation of the sapheno-femoral junction, during surgery for long saphenous varicosities.

(ii) *Short saphenous vein:* Beginning behind the lateral malleolus as the continuation of the lateral marginal vein of the foot, it courses along the lateral border of the tendo Achilles reaching the midline of the back of the calf, perforates the deep fascia at a variable point in the lower part of the popliteal fossa to join the popliteal vein, about 3-7 cm above the level of the knee. The vein is accompanied by the sural nerve, which supplies the skin of the lateral aspect of the dorsum of the foot and the little toe. It has about 10 valves, the most constant and impor-

tant one being at the sapheno-popliteal junction (SPJ).

Vein of Giacomini is sometimes seen in front of the thigh, communicating long and short saphenous veins.

PERFORATOR OR COMMUNICATING VEINS

By piercing the deep fascia, they connect the superficial to deep system, possessing valves directing the flow towards the deep veins. There are about a dozen perforators for the long saphenous, four in the thigh and six in the leg and two at the ankle and about four for the short saphenous, two in the leg and two at the ankle. Except those at the level of the malleoli, their position is rather inconsistent. They are generally classified as those in upper and mid thigh, upper middle and lower leg and at the malleoli. The mid thigh perforators are named after *Dodd*; the upper leg, also known as soleal perforators after *Boyd*; those in the lower leg after *Cockett* and the ankle perforators at the *gaiter* (a shoe that extends upto the lower leg) area after *May* or *Kuster*. Obviously by their potential to exert maximum hydrostatic pres-

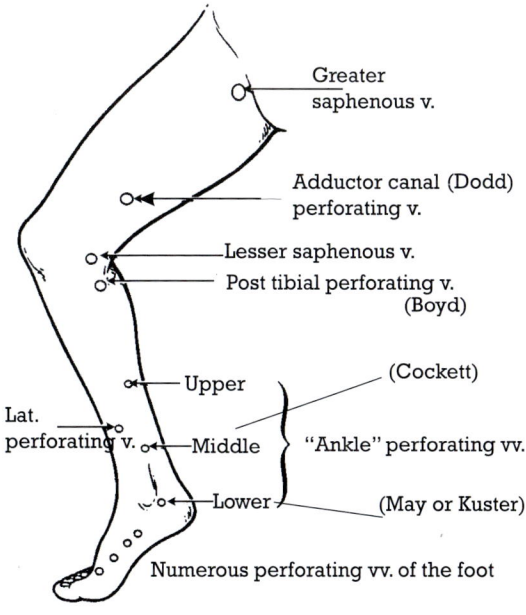

Fig. 82.3. Location of perforators in the lower limb

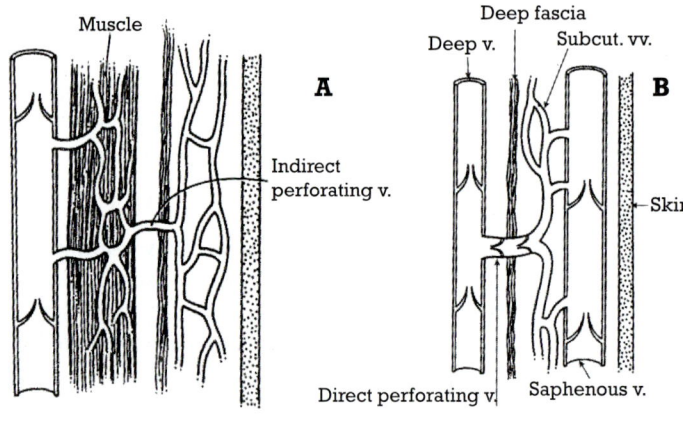

Fig. 82.4. Indirect & direct perforators

sure on the cutaneous venous circulation, the latter two groups in relation to the long saphenous system (those in lower leg and at the ankle) are of profound pathological significance and responsible for the classical sites of venous ulcer.

Indirect perforators seen mostly in the upper leg, join intermediary venous channels under the fascia, which in turn drain into the deep system. *Direct* perforators leave the superficial veins, pierce the fascia and join the deep system, without any relay channels. *There are perforators in the foot, but allowing the blood flow in reverse direction, from the sole to the dorsum of the foot (deep to superficial).*

Physiology of venous circulation: The blood is propelled in the veins towards the heart by:

1. negative intrathoracic pressure
2. gravity
3. peripheral muscle pump
4. propelling force from the arterial pressure
5. Competent valves

Etiology of varicose veins

Incompetency of the valves in a superficial venous system and the perforators is the fundamental

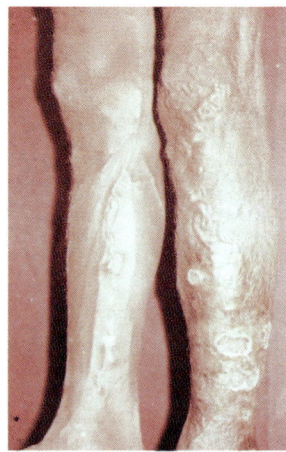

Fig. 82.5. Varicose veins of legs
(courtesy: Halsted Surgical Clinic, Chennai)

defect, leading to venous varicosities. They may be primary (idiopathic) or secondary due to an identifiable cause.

The causes of primary varicose veins

1. *Heredity:* inherent weakness of venous valves due to collagen defect or increased lysosomal activity in the vessel wall

2. *Erect posture:* constant hydrostatic pressure, on unsupported veins

3. *Hormonal*: quite often varicose veins appear during pregnancy for this reason. Increased flow through hypogastric veins may also contribute to venous hypertension of the lower limb

s in pregnancy

4. *Anatomical:* All venous diseases of lower limbs are more common on the left, because the venous pressure in the left lower limb is always higher than in the right, for the following reasons:

a) The left common iliac vein joins the IVC at an angle, whereas the right one is almost in line with it.

b) The right common iliac artery crosses in front of the left common iliac vein, immediately after aortic bifurcation, compressing the vein against the pelvic brim (May-Thurner syndrome).

c) The loaded, mobile sigmoid colon exerts pressure over the pelvic veins on the left, there is no such factor on the right.

The causes of secondary varicose veins

(1) deep vein disease (DVD).
(2) space occupying lesions (SOL) exerting pressure over deep veins, such as a pelvic/retroperitoneal tumor, pregnancy or aneurysm of an artery.

Pregnancy and varicose veins

It is interesting to know that they start developing varicosities from the first trimester, long before the uterus exerts 'SOL' effect, which may be relevant only after 20 weeks. It is considered to be due to the effect of progesterone from corpus luteum, which reduces venous tone and increases venous distensibility. Under the hormonal influence, they may also develop telangiectasia. Similar effect may be seen in the premenstrual period for the same reason. Another contributory factor is the increased venous return from the gravid uterus, leading to high pelvic venous pressure.

(3) arterio-venous malformation (AVM) or fistula (AVF)

CEAP classification of varicose veins

(Clinical, Etiological, Anatomical & Pathophysiological)

C0: No visible of palpable varicose veins
C1: Telangiectasia (<1mm dia) or reticular veins (<4mm dia)
C2: Varicose veins (>4mm dia)
C3: Edema
C4: Pigmentation
C5: Healed ulcers and scars
C6: Active ulceration with fibrosis
Ec: Congenital
Ep: Primary or idiopathic
Es: Secondary, DVT, SOL, AVM, trauma etc
A: Location of VV: GSV or SSV and Foot, Calf, Thigh, Deep veins
P:Pr: With reflux &

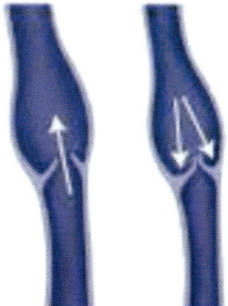 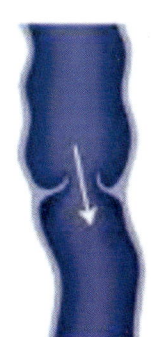

Fig. 82.6. Normal venous valve   Fig. 82.7. Incompetent valve in varicose vein

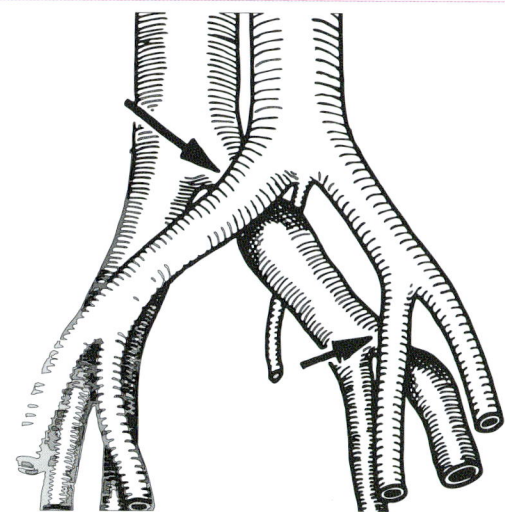

Fig. 82.8. Right common iliac artery crossing the left common iliac vein and left hypogastric artery crossing the left external iliac vein (May-Thurner syndrome). Arrows indicate points of compression

Po: with obstruction
Ankle flare: corona phlebectatica

Problems of open surgery: neovascularization, leading to recurrent varicosities

Symptoms

1. tired and aching sensation in the leg
2. pain in grossly dilated veins or perforators
3. cosmesis (often the presenting feature in women)
4. swelling of the foot/ankle/leg
5. pigmentation of the skin
6. dermatitis and eczema
7. ulceration
8. superficial thrombophlebitis or deep vein thrombosis (phlebothrombosis)
9. bleeding

Signs

Prominent veins especially when the patient stands up. Skin in the lower part may be pigmented, edematous, eczematous or ulcerated. It should be noted that persistent edema of the leg is the hallmark of deep venous disease; pure superficial venous disease rarely produces edema. The swelling is always more towards the end of the day, reducing to minimum at night, due to recumbency. A swelling may be seen at the sapheno-femoral junction (saphena varix). There may be a cough impulse over the tortuous veins.

It is important to know that there are three routes by which blood can reach the superficial veins, so that the clinical tests designed in this context, can be intelligently interpreted.

(1) normal venous return from capillaries and venules

(2) incompetent perforators with reflux

(3) sapheno-femoral/sapheno-popliteal incompetence with reflux

Normally only (1) is operating, whereas in patients with varicose veins, (1)+(2), (1)+(3) or (1)+(2)+(3) may be present. The following clinical tests are necessary for routine evaluation, which are designed to identify the competence or otherwise of the latter two (2 & 3) factors. It is important to rule out deep vein thrombosis, since stripping of the only functional superficial venous channels may be hazardous.

(1) **Brodie-Trendelenburg test:** This is performed in two steps as follows-

Step 1: The leg is elevated to empty the veins, the SFJ or SPJ is occluded by the thumb and the patient is asked to stand up. Normally there will be slow filling of the veins (from normal venous return). If there is faster filling, it implies reflux of blood from deep to superficial veins through incompetent perforators.

Step 2: The procedure is repeated and the thumb is released as soon as the patient stands up. If there is incompetence of the SFJ or SPJ valve, there will be rapid filling of the vein from above, faster than that seen in step 1. If those valves are normal, same rate of filling will be observed as in step 1.

(2) **Perthes' test:** An Esmarch bandage is applied over the entire leg from below and the patient is asked to walk. If the deep veins are totally occluded (without any recanalization) patient will not tolerate and will experience severe discomfort, cautioning the surgeon against overzealous stripping of the superficial veins.

(3) **Modified Perthes' test:** A tourniquet is applied at the highest point of the thigh, patient is asked to walk; normally some distension of veins is noticed but if the varicose veins appear to be over-distended, it denotes incompetent perforators.

(4) **Pratt's test:** is yet another modification of Perthes' test, not commonly employed.

(5) **Multiple tourniquet test:** By applying tourniquet at four levels (upper and lower thigh and upper and lower leg) and asking the patient to walk; depending upon the levels of incompetent perforators, those segments of saphenous vein get over distended.

(6) **Fegan's palpation:** Patient in standing position, the course of the saphenous vein is palpated to identify defects in deep fascia, approximately locating the incompetent and dilated perforators, which should be marked, just before surgery.

(7) **Schwartz test:** Patient in standing position, the saphenous vein is tapped at its lower end, the impulse can be appreciated by another finger kept over the saphenous opening and vice versa indicating incompetence of its valves. Normally impulse may be transmitted upwards but never downwards.

(8) **Morrissey's** (Cruveilhier's) **sign:** A thrill is felt over the saphenous opening on coughing if there is reflux of blood into the superficial system due to incompetent valve. In severe cases, cough impulse may be appreciated as low as knee or calf.

Venous aneurysm is localized dilatation of a vein, seen in any region, most commonly in lower limbs and highest incidence observed in the popliteal vein. They are considered congenital, though trauma has been blamed when it develops in superficial veins. Soft compressible swelling in the course of a vein, disappearing on elevating the part (usually the limb) is typical. It is vulnerable to rupture, bleeding and known to cause thromboembolic manifestations.

Generally they are asymptomatic and detected during routine screening in cases of pulmonary

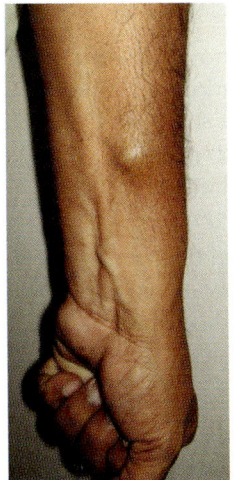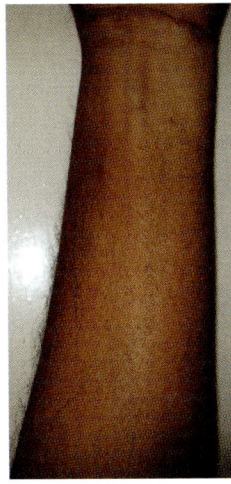

Fig. 82.9. Venous aneurysm of left forearm
It typically appears when the limb is lowered to
dependency and disappears on elevation
(courtesy: Halsted Surgical Clinic, Chennai)

embolism. They may be fusiform or saccular, and the latter is more prone to develop clots in the sac. The treatment of uncomplicated asymptomatic venous aneurysm is debatable, probably requiring only periodic surveillance with Duplex imaging, but those causing symptoms should be excised. Tangential excision may be sufficient in saccular type, but resection and ligation (smaller veins) or replacement with a vein graft is needed for fusiform dilatation. Long term anticoagulation is indicated in all symptomatic cases.

Complications of varicose veins

They occur mostly over the lower leg and ankle (gaiter area), due to the highest hydrostatic pressure exerted in erect posture by the lower most perforators in the leg, on the superficial venous system, influencing the cutaneous micro-circulation.

(1) *Thrombophlebitis:* This term is restricted only to superficial veins and appears as a painful, red and indurated segment of the affected vein. The treatment consists of elevating the leg, applying elastic bandage and use of antibiotics, antiplatelet, anticoagulant and NSAIDs. External applications of NSAIDs also are used for immediate symptomatic relief. External

injury and therapeutic injection of sclerosants are the other causes of superficial thrombophlebitis. Saphenous cut down in the leg has highest incidence of thrombophlebitis, hence it should be avoided, except in dire emergencies. Least incidence appears to be in the subclavian and jugular veins in the neck, which are preferred for prolonged venous cannulation, for total parenteral nutrition (TPN) or hemodialysis.

(2) *Pigmentation:* Extensive hemosiderin deposition in the perivenous tissue due to breakdown of RBC, migrated out of capillaries due to increased venous pressure, causes brownish black pigmentation. This defies any local treatment until the underlying venous disease is treated appropriately.

(3) *Dermatitis* and *eczema:* The pathogenesis is the same as above, but sometimes due to allergy to external applicants. Besides treating the venous disease, local treatment with steroids and/or zinc oxide, may help ameliorate the symptoms.

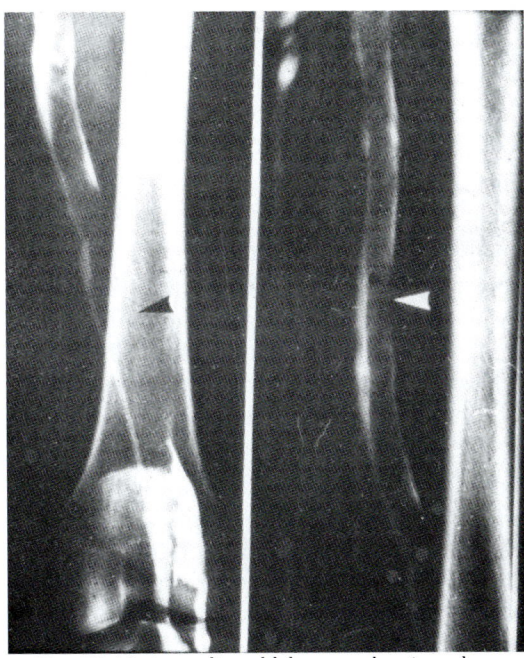

Fig. 82.10. Ascending phlebogram showing a long
thrombus in the superficial femoral vein
(courtesy: Halsted Surgical Clinic, Chennai)

(4) *Lipodermatosclerosis* (LDS): Chronic venous hypertension, due to deep vein dysfunction, sometimes results in this condition, which is a combination of brawny edema, atrophic and pigmented skin. Narrow ankle and lower leg with swollen calf bears the shape of an 'inverted champagne bottle'. Except treating the underlying venous disorder on its merits, no specific therapy is helpful.

(5) *Ankle flare* (corona phebectatica): In some patients with chronic ambulant venous hypertension, swelling and dilatation of veins near ankle develop, known as ankle flare. Compression bandage may be palliative but treating the underlying venous disease is curative.

(6) *Hemorrhage*: may be external or internal; the former is more common following a trivial injury of the thinned out skin over a vein. Prompt elevation of foot with compression should control venous bleeding.

(7) *Periostitis:* This is usually seen if there is a long standing ulcer over the medial surface of the tibia penetrating into the periosteum producing a reaction. Frank osteomyelitis is rare.

(8) *Calcification:* of dystrophic nature may occur in long standing varicose veins, by itself requiring no special treatment.

(9) *Equinus* deformity: results from the patient trying to walk on the ball of the foot to avoid pain, producing contracture of the calf muscles. If it is persistent and troublesome even after treating the venous problem, lengthening of the Achilles tendon may be necessary.

(10) *Malignant* transformation: Chronic nonhealing ulcer may predispose to SCC (Marjolin's ulcer). Because of the extensive fibrosis of the base involving neural and lymphatic channels, they are painless and slow to metastasize to the regional nodes, hence carry better prognosis. It is treated like SCC elsewhere.

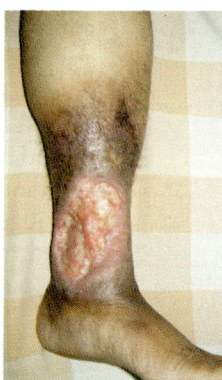

Fig. 82.11. Lipodermatosclerosis with extensive ulceration (Courtesy: Halsted Surgical Clinic,

11) Deep venous dysfunction (DVD) and chronic venous insufficiency (postphlebitic syndrome): It must be realised that pure superficial venous disease does not produce venous insufficiency of the limb. The usual sequence of events are:

(i) thrombosis of deep veins (DVT), produced by stasis of blood, hypercoagulability and intimal damage (*Virchow's triad*). All the three may not exist in every case.

(ii) propagation of thrombus

(iii) recanalization of thrombus, which may take several weeks to months

(iv) in the process, destruction of venous valves occurs, leading to reflux and stasis

(v) failure of peripheral (soleal) pump

(vi) venous hypertension and insufficiency

(vii) stasis problems of skin and subcutaneous

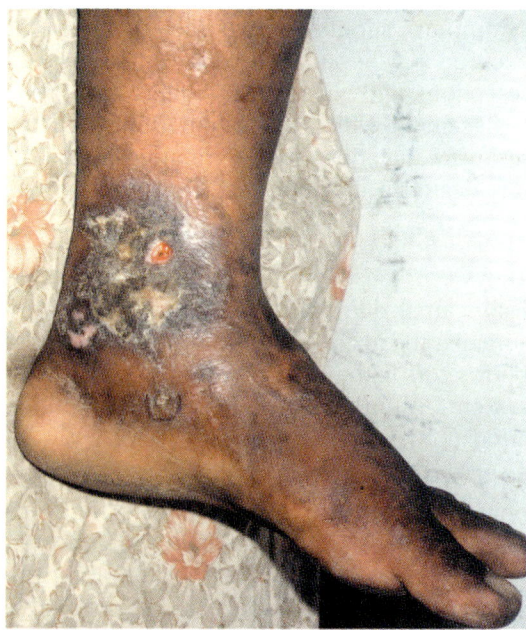

Fig. 82.12. Dermatitis and ulceration over medial malleolus (long saphenous disease) (courtesy: Prof M Raghuram, Chennai)

484

tissue, due to extravesated blood components

Extreme degree of acute DVT, known as phlegmasia alba/cerulea dolens is described later.

In countries where it is very common in the postoperative period, *Homan's* sign is a very useful bedside test to identify acute DVT. Sudden passive dorsiflexion of ankle elicits pain in the calf. Direct squeezing of the calf muscles also produces pain (*Moses'* sign), but it should be emphasized that these signs are useful only in *acute* and not in chronic venous disease. The current recommendation is against such vigorous maneuvers as they may serve to release clots into the circulation (and may send the patient to Moses!)

Thrombophilia (thrombos: clot, philein: to love), a condition with high predilection for thrombosis, is seen in several clinical situations, such as:

Congenital causes

i) deficiency of antithrombin-III, an autosomal dominant trait

ii) deficiency of protein-C or protein-S; these are vitamin K-dependent inhibitors of the procoagulant system, transmitted by an autosomal dominant trait.

iii) dysfibrinogenemias

iv) antiphospholipid antibody or lupus anticoagulant factor (anticardiolipin syndrome), it may be also acquired.

v) homocystinemia, an inborn error of sulfur aminoacid metabolism (vide supra)

vi) factor-V Leiden gene defect or activated protein-C resistance

vii) prothrombin 20210-A is a mutant prothrombin gene, associated with elevated prothrombin levels of blood.

If the patient is on anticoagulants, they should be temporarily discontinued before performing the tests designed for conditions 1 to 4 but not for the other conditions (5-7).

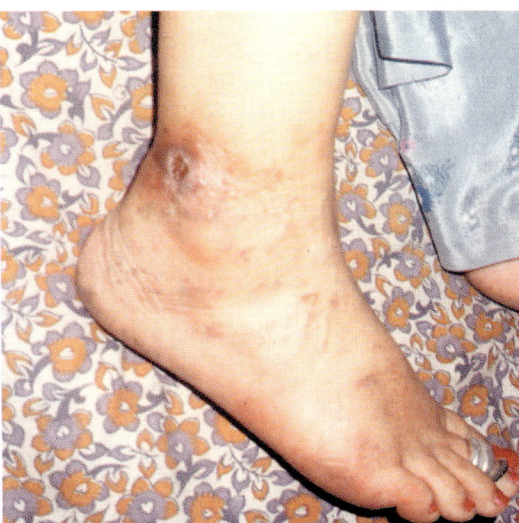

Fig. 82.13. Pigmentation and ulceration over lateral malleolus (short saphenous disease) (courtesy: Prof M Raghuram, Chennai)

Acquired causes

i) obesity

ii) pregnancy/puerperium

iii) postoperative/post-trauma states

iv) dyslipidemias, diabetes mellitus, states of hemoconcentration

v) polycythemia, nephrotic syndrome, inflammatory bowel diseases

vi) prolonged immobilization (orthopedic/neurological diseases)

vii) varicose veins

viii) hormones: high dose estrogens and contraceptives

ix) visceral malignancies (Trousseau's sign - migrating thrombophlebitis)

x) chlamydeal infection

(12) Venous ulcer: This is a general term used for an ulcer developing due to venous disease; if the patient has varicose veins, it may be specifically termed varicose ulcer. The basic pathology behind all skin complications of venous disease, is cutaneous venous hypertension. According to the *fibrin-cuff hypothesis*, fibrinogen is driven out of the venules, and acts as a barrier to the diffusion of oxygen and other nutrients into the tissues, leading to atrophy of the overlying skin

Anterior   Posterior

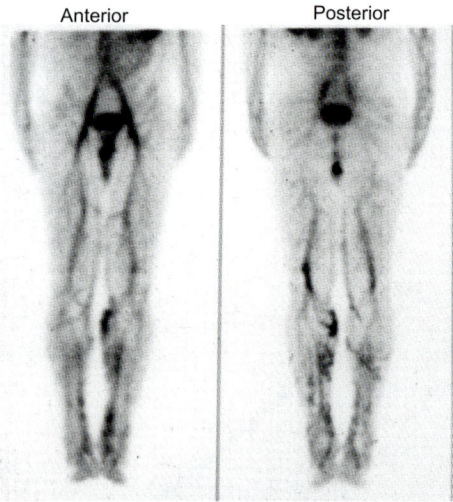

Fig. 82.14. Scintiscan of venous system showing varicosities and stasis on the left side
(courtesy: Halsted Surgical Clinic, Chennai)

which breaks down following some trivial injury, such as a nail scratch, forming an ulcer. Alternatively (*white cell hypothesis*), it has been suggested that polymorphonuclear leukocytes are driven out of the capillaries owing to endothelial injury; these excite a perivascular inflammatory reaction, leading to fibrosis and impede oxygen diffusion. If there is considerable fibrosis of the ulcer base, it interferes with wound contraction and results in an *unstable* scar even if the ulcer heals, only to break down for some flimsy reason, during 'unprotected' ambulation.

Treatment (Bisgaard's regime)

(a) Absolute rest and elevation of legs by an angle of 10-15 degrees.

(b) Elastic support by crepe bandage is most popular but least effective, but custom-made pressure-gradient elastic stockings or Unna paste boot is preferred Unna developed a gauze bandage, impregnated with zinc oxide, glycerine, gelatin and water, for application over clean ulcers, to promote healing, which can be changed once a week. Within a few minutes of application, it sets and develops leathery texture, providing a comfortable compression, but allowing some ankle movement. Optimally, a pressure-gradient of *30mm Hg* is required for the elastic compression; 50mm in the foot, 40mm at ankle, 30mm at midcalf and 20mm at knee level.

(c) Computer-programmed pneumatic compression devices are found to be very useful, to reduce venous and lymphatic edema, for short term application.

(d) Passive and active moments of the ankle

(e) Antibiotics, if there is obvious evidence of infection

(f) Antiplatelet therapy: Asprin and thrombaxane-A2 receptor antagonist (fetroban)

(g) anticoagulant/antiedema therapy

(h) Ulcer dressing with hypertonic saline, hydrogen peroxide or EUSOL (Edinburgh University solution)

(i) General attention to weight, smoking, diabetes etc.

(j) Excision of the ulcer with its base and split skin grafting may be necessary in some refractory cases.

(k) Patient is taught to live with the disease, by a 'new way of life'; he is advised against standing on his feet without elastic support, to keep the legs elevated as much as possible and avoid hobbies and sports which might injure the leg.

(13) Pulmonary embolism (vide infra)

Investigations of venous disease

1. Doppler recording and *duplex* imaging: Maps the veins, identifies incompetent perforators and valves and confirms deep vein patency.

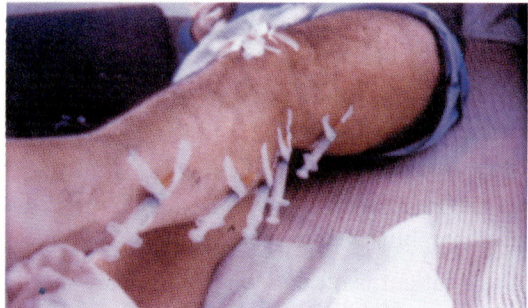

Fig. 82.15. Sclerotherapy by multiple syringes along the course of tortuous vein
(courtesy: Dr K Sureshkumar, Chennai)

2. Ascending phlebogram: This is not routinely done but only if the non-invasive investigations mentioned above do not give necessary information for treatment or if surgery on deep veins is contemplated (as in recurrent pulmonary embolism). It may be done either by injecting the contrast into the dorsal venous arch (transvenous) and applying a tourniquet just above the ankle forcing the contrast into the deep system or into the calcaneum directly (transosseous). Though the latter is superior, the fear of osteomyelitis of calcaneum, makes it less popular. The x-ray table is tilted head-up by 45°. before injecting the contrast to slow down the venous flow, to improve the resolution and the leg is medially rotated to avoid deep veins overlapping the tibia. If the contrast appears in the superficial veins above the tourniquet, it signifies incompetent perforators. A thrombus is seen as a linear filling defect within a major vein.
3. Thermography, xerography, plethysmography are rarely used routinely.
4. Ambulatory foot vein pressure, to assess the calf pump function
5. Isotope scan using radioactive fibrino-gen can detect even a small thrombus but is rarely necessary after the advent of non-invasive modalities of investigation.
6. Venodynamic study with ^{99m}Tc, to quantify venous insufficiency of leg as well as to determine the benefit following subfascial ligation of perforators (RB Rutherford, CMK Reddy et al)

7. It is important to exclude associated arterial disease, which might influence the management and ultimate outcome.

Treatment

1. Medical therapy
(i) Attention to weight, diabetes and abstinence from smoking
(ii) Diosmins (natural or synthetic) are micronized flavonoid agents (Venex), increase venous tone and decrease capillary permeability; hence discourage the migration of blood cells into the interstitial space, which is responsible for pigmentation, dermatitis, etc.
(iii) Calcium dobesilate (Dobium) also has a similar action, besides inhibiting platelet/erythrocyte aggregation and promoting release of tissue plasminogen activator (TPA), thus increasing fibrinolytic activity. However, it does not interfere with the normal clotting functions of the blood.
iv) other venotonic drugs: Troxerutin - hydroxy rutosides (Oxerute)

2. Sclerotherapy and compression (Fegan)

Indications

a. localized minimal varicose veins
b. for recurrent varicose veins
c. patient unsuitable for standard anesthesia/operation

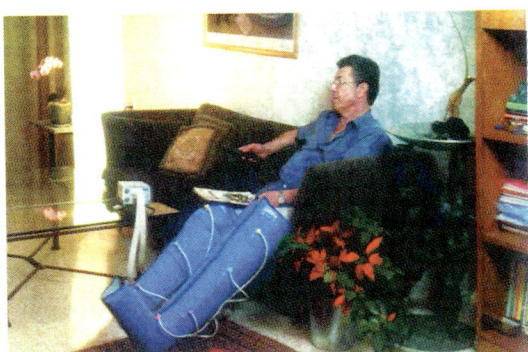

Fig. 82.16. DVT – Prophylaxis by intermittant graded pneumatic compression (ambulatory) (courtesy: Halsted Surgical Clinic, Chennai)

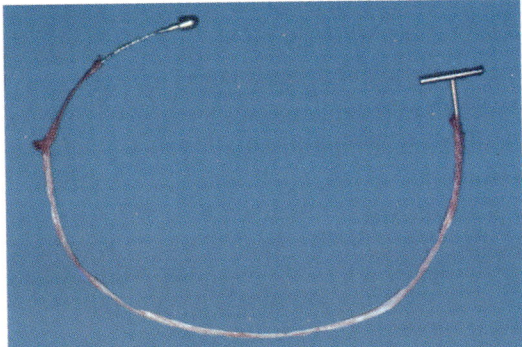

Fig. 82.17. Entire length of long saphenous vein retrieved by Myer's stripper (courtesy: Halsted Surgical Clinic, Chennai)

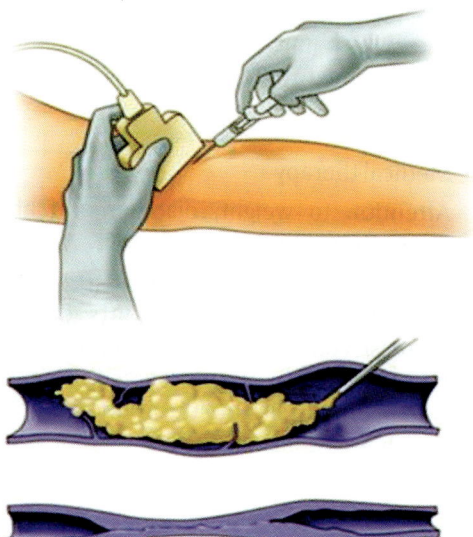

Fig. 82.18. Ultrasound-guided foam sclerotherapy, resulting in obliteration of a varicose vein

Procedure

Hypertonic (24%) saline, 3% sodium tetra-decylsulphate (STD-Thrombovar) 5% ethanolamine oleate or 3% polidocanol (Ethoxysclerol) is injected into the emptied vein (by elevation and compression the leg) and elastic bandage applied.

Contraindication: deep vein thrombosis

Complications

(i) necrosis of overlying skin and ulceration

(ii) spread of thrombotic process into the deep venous system

(3) **Operative treatment**

Indication for surgery: 3-Cs
Complaints (symptoms)
Cosmesis

Complications

PROCEDURES

(i) Simple high ligation at SFJ or SPJ
(ii) Ligation and stripping (Trendelenburg)
(iii) Ligation and multiple avulsions (syn: multiple cosmetic

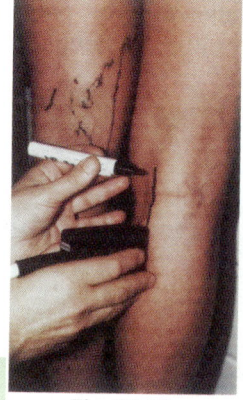

Fig. 82.19.
Preoperative marking the varicosities (courtesy: Halsted Surgical Clinic, Chennai)

phlebectomies of Rivlin)
(iv) Subfascial ligation of perforators (Cockett and Dodd). When combined with ligation of the superficial/common femoral vein (to prevent embolism), it is called Linton's operation, in the USA.
(v) Venous bypass
(vi) Valvuloplasty

(I) Simple ligation of long/short saphenous vein is rarely performed nowadays. By a small incision placed over the saphenous opening, approximately 2-3 cms medial to the common femoral pulsation, the termination of the long saphenous vein is identified along with the tributaries mentioned and ligated flush with the common femoral vein. The short saphenous vein also, if involved, is similarly ligated flush with the popliteal vein. This procedure is inferior to stripping, in terms of cosmesis/ cure, but has the advantage of retaining the veins, to be used as bypass conduits for the treatment of coronary/peripheral arterial occlusions, at a later date. It is, however, questionable if the 'varicose' veins, with weak, attenuated walls can serve as arterial channels at all.

(ii) Ligation and stripping: Before giving anesthesia, with the patient standing, all the varicose veins are marked by the surgeon, using indelible ink or a sterile hypodermic needle. This step is important, since most of these varicose veins may not be visible in the supine position and might be overlooked during surgery. Tilting the operating table head-down (Trendelenburg position) helps to reduce the venous bleeding during surgery. The long/ short saphenous vein is exposed at the highest and lowest points (sapheno-femoral/ sapheno-popliteal junction and in front of medial malleolus/behind lateral malleolus respectively) by making appropriate incisions. A Myer's (or Babcock's) vein stripper is introduced from the lower end and negotiated to reach the upper end, where it is brought out by a small venotomy. By a silk ligature, the end of vein in the groin is secured to the stripper, for which an olive of about 8mm is screwed in place. The whole stretch of the vein is stripped, by applying traction on the ankle end of the stripper, after dividing the vein beyond the entry and exit points of the stripper. Application of an elastic bandage to the leg or external manual pressure along the course of the vein, before pulling on the stripper, considerably reduces subcutaneous bleeding and hematoma formation.

Any other islands of varicosities not in line with the main vein, including those in the foot, are excised by multiple incisions, as necessary. Meticulous attention to all the tributaries in the groin is important, if simple high ligation is to be carried out, but may not be so if the entire vein is being stripped.

In cases of primary varicose veins, with a normal deep venous system, once the main vein is totally stripped, the incompetent perforators lose their pathological significance, by themselves requiring no further treatment. During isolation and stripping, the accompanying nerves (saphenous and sural) have to be protected, lest troublesome paresthesia/anesthesia

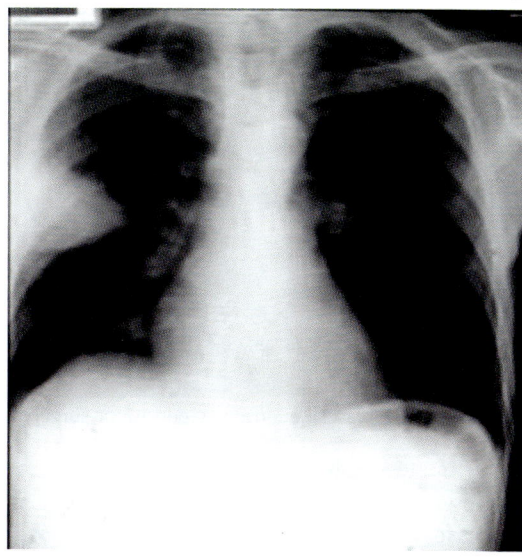

Fig. 82.21.. Typical wedge-shaped peripheral shadow in the right mid zone due to pulmonary embolism

may develop. The debate regarding the direction in which the stripper should be pulled (towards the groin or foot) is probably unwarranted, as it does not matter one way or the other. Most surgeons prefer to pull towards the foot for convenience and the incidence of injury to the saphenous nerve (a point in favour of pull-

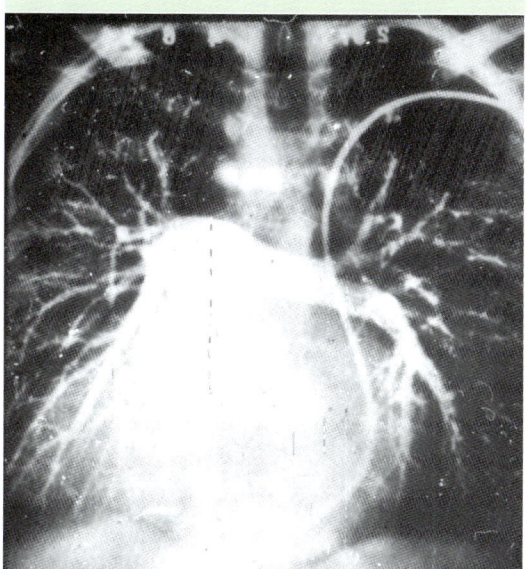

Fig. 82.20. Normal pulmonary angiogram
(courtesy: Dr P J Reddy, Texas, USA)

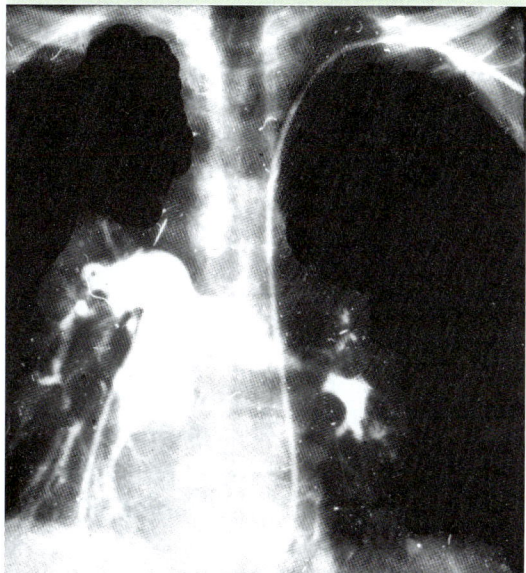

82.22. Massive bilateral pulmonary embolism

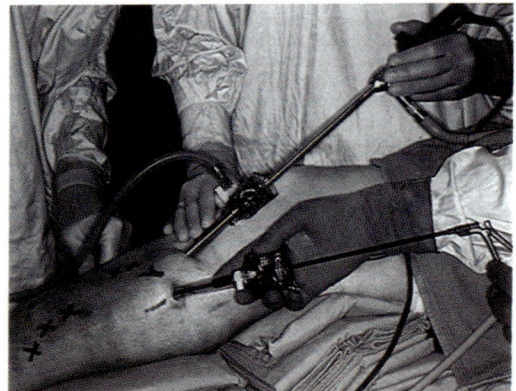

Fig. 82.23. Subfascial endoscopic perforator surgery (SEPS)
(courtesy: Halsted Surgical Clinic, Chennai)

ing towards the groin) is not much different, in any case.

The idea of some surgeons, to strip only the supragenicular segment of long saphenous vein, does not address the venostatic pathology nor cosmetic problems in the leg, hence not universally acceptable.

Recently stripping by *inversion* or *invagination* is gaining popularity, as it causes less bleeding and trauma to the adjacent tissues. Using a metal pin-stripper of Oesch, which has a small head, the entire inverted saphenous vein can be retrieved. The procedure banks on the tensile strength of the vein and if it snaps during traction, the remaining vein has to be carefully recovered by an olive-ended retriever.

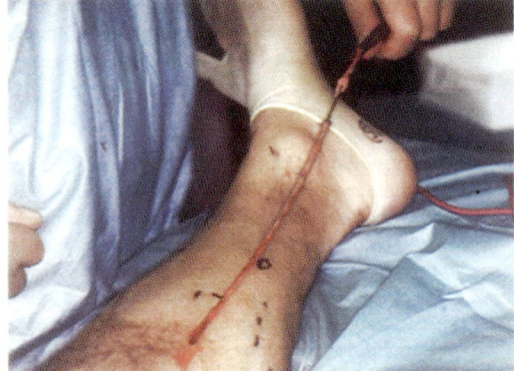

Fig. 82.24. Retrieving the saphenous vein using a Pin Stripper (Oesch)
(courtesy: Halsted Surgical Clinic, Chennai)

(iii) Rivlin described a simplified procedure wherein multiple tiny incisions are made over the bulging veins, which are grasped by mosquito forceps and either ligated or avulsed. This is generally suitable for recurrent varicosities appearing after stripping the main vein, without deep vein disease.

(iv) *Subfascial ligation* (Cockett and Dodd) of direct and indirect perforators is performed by a long incision made parallel to the main superficial vein, which is taken down through the fascia. These communicating veins can easily be identified, as the fascia is lifted towards the superficial vein. Recently, to avoid complications of a long incision, this operation is being done by an endoscope, passed through a button-hole incision, known as subfascial endoscopic perforator surgery (SEPS) of Hauer.

The ability to accurately mark out the incompetent perforators, has prompted the introduction of minimally invasive surgery for them. The main disadvantages of this procedure are: cost, expertise and in LSD, due to dense fibrosis, it is technically difficult to get sufficient subfascial 'lift-off' in order to get adequate vision of the perforators.

This operation is essentially performed when there is significant dysfunction of the deep venous system, resulting in failure of the 'peripheral pump'. By preventing deep venous blood refluxing into the superficial system, ligating the perforators would considerably improve the efficiency of the 'peripheral pump'. This has been adequately demonstrated by isotope studies, which have quantified the venous insufficiency of the limb as well as documented the benefits following surgery.

(v) *Venous bypass*, for deep vein occlusion, using long saphenous/basilic vein, has been tried.

Palma procedure is done for iliac vein occulsion, in which long saphenous vein on the normal side is disconnected at knee level and swung to anastomose to the opposite femoral vein, below the point of occlusion (crossover vein bypass).

May-Husni procedure is anastamosing long saphenous to popliteal vein, to bypass an occluded femoral vein

(vi) *Valvuloplasty* or interposition vein grafting has been practised in some centers, but not yet become popular in the hands of the average surgeon.

vii) Endovenous procedures:

a) Endovenous laser therapy (EVLT): Endoluminal application of Laser energy causes non-thrombotic occlusion of the vein, by endothelial thermal injury (at temperatures between 300 to 1000 C, generated by 10-14 Watts, delivering about 60-80 Joules of energy per cm of vein), leading to collagen contraction and fibrosis

Tumescent local anesthesia is commonly employed for the procedure, by perivenous injection of a mixture of local anesthetic, soda bicarbonate and cold saline, under USG-guide, to form an anesthetic cushion around the vein to be ablated. The advantages of this type of anesthesia are: it provides sufficient anesthesia during and immediately after the procedure, it absorbs heat from the vein wall, sparing the surrounding tissue from thermal injury and lastly, it compresses the vein to some extent, for efficient obliteration.

Drawbacks:

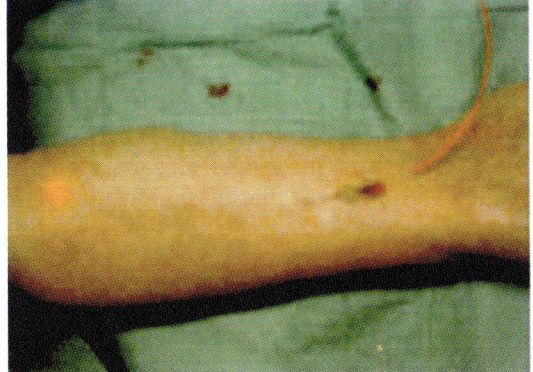

Fig. 82.25. LASER endovenous sclerotherapy (Note the illumination at the tip of LASER fibre)
(courtesy: Halsted Surgical Clinic, Chennai)

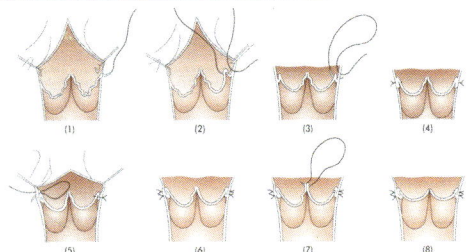

Fig. 82.26. Valvuloplasty of deep veins
(courtesy: Halsted Surgical Clinic, Chennai)

1 notwithstanding the claims made, there is considerable pain for a few days, after the procedure
2. ecchymosis
3. hematoma
4. thermal burn of skin and subcutaneous tissue
5. injury to the accompanying nerves
6. difficulty in canulating tortuous veins
7. possibility of DVT
8. cost & expertise

b) Radiofrequency ablation (RFA): This is a process by which electrical energy is converted into heat to denature the collagen and cause fibrosis. The technique is the same as EVLT, a heated probe (85-120 C) is used instead of laser. The procedure has the same drawbacks as EVLT, however overall complication rate is found to be lesser (8%) than EVLT (20%).

c) Foam sclerotherapy: liquid sclerosant has been used for over a century for varicosities, but using foam is a novel concept. The foam is 'home-made' in the office by Tessari technique, using polidocanol or STD. Using a 3-way stopcock, about 4 ml of sclerosant and 15 ml of air are taken into separate syringes and by to and fro movements foam is created and injected into the vein under USG guide. The initial concern about the risk of air embolism and DVT appeared to very minimal in actual experience, if no more than 20 ml of foam is injected in one sitting. The limb should be elevated during the procedure to empty the veins and compression bandage applied immediately after. It is very cheap, can be repeated as often as necessary, no anesthesia

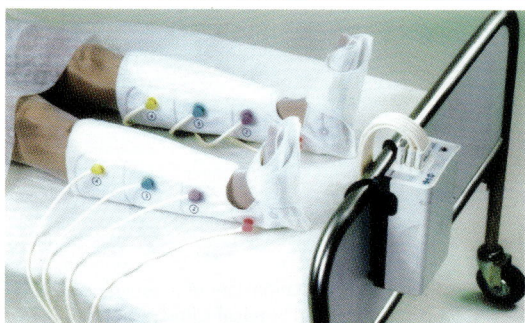

Fig. 82.27. DVT Prophylaxis by intermittent graded pneumatic compression
(courtesy: Halsted Surgical Clinic, Chennai)

required and no injury to adjacent structures, but requires elastic compression bandage for a few weeks, for optimal results.

d)   Steam sclerotherapy (Milleret): Boiling water is pressurized at 600 atmospheres converting into a hyperheated steam and allowed to flow into the vein through a canula, causing coagulation necrosis of vessel wall and obliteration. It is very cheap and appears to be suitable for use in developing countries, though the procedure and equipment need to be standardized.

ACUTE MASSIVE DEEP VEIN THROMBOSIS

Phlegmasia alba dolens (swollen white leg) is a result of acute iliofemoral phlebothrombosis, associated with lymphatic obstruction. Usually encountered in the bed-ridden or after confinement, the process of thrombosis starts in the soleal venous plexus and rapidly propagates proximally. Sudden onset of swelling of the whole limb upto the groin associated with pain and fever, limb becoming cooler than its fellow (initially it may be warmer) is typical of this condition. If untreated, it may become chronic, leading to venous insufficiency of the limb and aching on walking, known as venous claudication.

Phlegmasia cerulea dolens (swollen blue leg) is a more severe variant of the white leg, due to massive iliofemoral thrombosis, often presenting initially as white leg. The limb soon becomes deeply cyanotic with marked swelling, more below the knee, and associated with a continuous bursting type of pain. The limb feels tense and firm, and the initial warmth is replaced by a cold limb. Extensive venous gangrene may develop if this condition is untreated, often mimicking arterial insufficiency. The sequence of events, supported by Doppler findings in a massively swollen limb, clinches the diagnosis.

The coagulation profile, serum homocystine (and other biochemical risk factors indicated) estimation and duplex imaging of the venous/arterial tree, should be done, besides routine studies, while initiating treatment.

D-dimer is a degradation product of fibrin complex, elevated in conditions associated with intravascular thrombosis, especially DVT. It is 85% sensitive, credited to be of 95% negative predictive value in the diagnosis of DVT. False positivity may be observed in pregnancy, postop/postpartum state, advanced malignancy, sepsis and collagen disorders.

Venous thrombectomy, earlier popularized by Haller, has been totally replaced by thrombolysis with plasminogen activators (streptokinase, urokinase, tissue plasminogen activator etc). These fibrinolytic agents may be given IV, or by an indwelling catheter, directly into the clot. Appropriate antibiotics, heparinisation, elevation, elastic support and antiedema/antiplatelet therapy, are essential adjuvants to thrombolytic therapy. Aggressive management of these two conditions will be highly rewarding in reversing the process, especially if initiated within 48 hours of the onset of illness, impending tissue necrosis can be avoided or further loss of tissue can be prevented, if gangrene has already set in. The longterm care of these patients is similar to that of any postphlebitic syndrome.

DVT Prophylaxis

Fundamental concern in preventing DVT is to prevent its dreadful complication, pulmonary embolism, which forms an important cause of hospital death (up to 10%) following major surgery. This may be routinely indicated in a group of patients considered high risk for

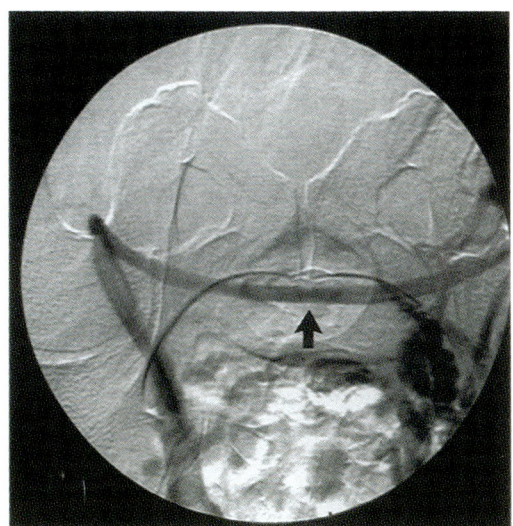

Fig. 82.28. Postoperative venogram through left com fem vein showing crossover venous bypass using right long saphenous vein
(courtesy: Halsted Surgical Clinic, Chennai)

developing venous thrombosis, such as those undergoing surgery for orthopedic, neurologic, peripheral vascular (arterial & venous) diseases, major thoracic, abdominal and pelvic surgery, multiple organ injury, advanced malignancy, obesity, consumers of tobacco, patients with congestive cardiac disease, diabetes, dyslipidemia, thrombophilia, blood dyscrasias, prolonged immobilization, age >40 and of course those with previous history of venous thromboembolism. Elderly individuals who undertake long air travels, particularly with very little freedom for leg movements (in economy class) have also higher incidence of DVT.

Commonly used modalities may be mechanical and pharmacological. Mechanical: perioperative use of pressure-gradient elastic stockings and intermittent sequential pneumatic leg compression, have been found to reduce the incidence of DVT.

Pharmacological: oral anticoagulation, low dose regular (unfractionated) heparin, low molecular-weight (fractionated) heparin (LMWH). Oral drugs have to be started 3-4 days before surgery, where as heparin may be started

few hours before, though some prefer to start soon after surgery, for fear of increased operative bleeding and risk of postoperative hematoma formation. Nowadays, LMWH is preferred because of once (or twice) a day administration, virtually no monitoring required and has fewer bleeding complications.

The role of pharmacological prophylaxis in pregnancy and delivery is controversial and many obstetricians prefer to use only mechanical devices. However, LMWH may be safely used in venous thromboembolism during pregnancy, since it does not cross the placental barrier.

In view of the reported higher incidence of venous thromboembolism even after the patient has been discharged from the hospital, it is advisable to continue the prophylaxis for few weeks, especially in high risk category.

PULMONARY EMBOLISM (PE): is an important cause of death in the postoperative period, accounting for over 10% of fatalities after major surgery, and detected in about 4% of autopsies of postoperative deaths. For reasons not clear, its incidence is much less in Asian countries, compared to the west.

Mortality of PE, untreated: 50% and when expediently treated it drops to 10%

Etiology and risk factors

(I) Deep vein thrombosis(DVT) of lower limb and pelvis is the most important causative fac-

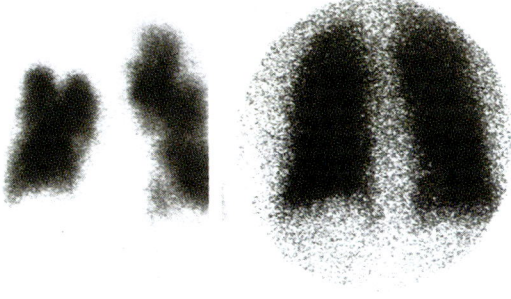

Fig. 82.29. Pulmonary scintiscans; **A:** ^{99m} Tc perfusion scan; **B:** ^{133} Xe ventilation scan
(courtesy: Halsted Surgical Clinic, Chennai)

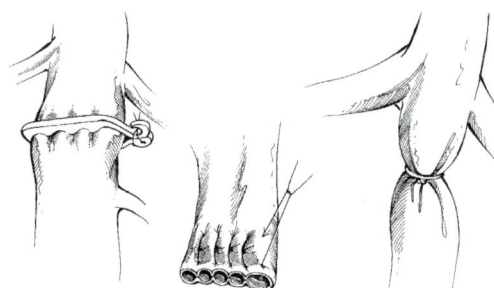

Fig. 82.30. Prevention of pulmonary embolism by IVC plication or ligation
(courtesy: Halsted Surgical Clinic, Chennai)

tor. The risk factors for PE, therefore, are in large measure the risk factors for DVT. They include:

1. prolonged immobilization
2. obesity
3. tobacco consumption
4. hypercoagulable states
5. elderly
6. advanced malignancy
7. congestive cardiac failure
8. major fractures/amputations
9. estrogen therapy etc.

(ii) Hypercoagulable state is observed in patients of multiple injuries, major surgery, following delivery and those with high serum homocystine levels (see thrombophilia). Orthopedic and vascular surgery are notorious for highest incidence of PE.

Differences between arterial and venous ulcer in the leg: A patient with a varicose ulcer may also have absent pedal pulses, when it becomes very important to decide if the ulcer is venous or arterial in origin.

Pathophysiology

Its pulmonary effects are rapid shallow breathing with increased minute ventilation and deadspace ventilation. Constriction of' the terminal bronchiole typically occurs, probably mediated by humoral factors. Effect on the CVS is increased pulmonary arterial pressure and pulmonary resistance, but if less than 50% of pulmonary vasculature is occluded, such changes may not be obvious. Intrapulmonary reflexes release humoral factors leading to vasoconstriction of entire pulmonary arterioles of both lungs, further rising the pulmonary resistance. Opening of intrapulmonary vascular shunts may be another contributory factor to decrease perfusion.

Pulmonary infarction occurs only in about 10% of cases of PE, owing to dual blood supply (pulmonary and bronchial vessels).

Clinical features

Acute chest pain (pleuritic type), dyspnea, cough and rusty expectoration are the classical traid of symptoms, but present only in 20% of cases. However, in a high risk patient, they alert the clinician regarding PE. Evidence of deep venous disease in the legs is present only in a small group of patients. Tachypnea and central type of cyanosis are present, with features of pulmonary hypertension. Clinically three degrees may be identified, the mildest forms probably often go unrecognized, and treated as atelectasis or pneumonitis, whereas the major PE may not reach a hospital or allow effective therapy to be instituted; they are rapidly fatal. Most of the clinical picture described refers to the intermediary group, which survive and produce sufficient morbidity, allowing for investigations and treatment.

Differential diagnosis

Cardiac infarction, atelectasis, pneumonitis, mediastinitis etc

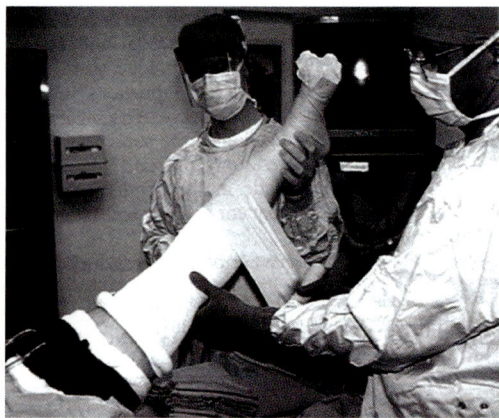

Fig. 82.31. Compression bandage after the vein stripping operation
(courtesy: Halsted Surgical Clinic, Chennai)

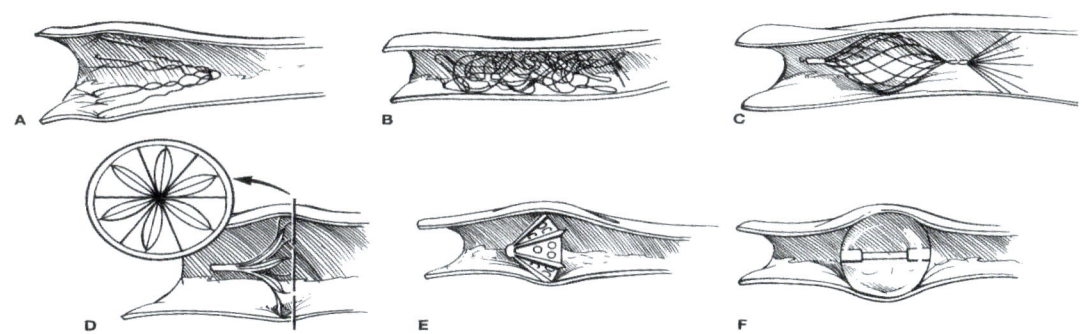

Fig. 82.32. Endoluminal venacaval filters **A:** Greenfield Filter; **B:** Bird's Nest Filter; **C:** Gunther Filter; **D:** Amplatz Filter; **E:** Mobin-Uddin Filter; **F:** Hunter Balloon

Investigations

A chest skiagram (peripheral wedge shadow), Westermark's sign: Dilatation of pulmonary artery proximal to the embolus and collapse distal to it

Hampton's sign: Triangular or rounded pleural-based infiltrate, usually adjacent to hilum, with the apex towards the hilum

ECG (right ventricular strain), arterial blood gases-ABG, ventilation/perfusion scan-V/Q scan, which shows ventilation-perfusion mismatch.

Serum enzymes such as, LDH, CPK, transaminases are helpful, but perfusion scan of the lung and pulmonary angiogram are clinching. Contrast-enhanced CT (CECT) or multidetector CT (MDCT) may be a useful noninvasive diagnostic tool. Identification of deep vein disease of the leg or pelvis (by Doppler or Duplex) is corroborative.

Treatment

Medical - Anticoagulation (heparinization) thrombolytic therapy and ventilatory support constitute the main stay of therapy.

Surgical - Pulmonary embolectomy (Trendelenburg's operation) done earlier in some sophisticated centers, has largely been replaced by fibrinolytic therapy. Even in those centers carrying it, there had always been a dilemma, that the patient should be ill enough to warrant it and well enough to tolerate it, a narrow window indeed.

Prevention of PE: In patients who are throwing repeated emboli, in spite of adequate anticoagulation, interruption of IVC either by ligation or plication may be considered, since most of them originate from the pelvic/leg veins. Similarly common femoral vein interruption was recommended (Linton) to discourage embolization from a particular leg. Plication implies converting the lumen into several small passages either by external clips or by endoluminal filtering devices, positioned through a percutaneous catheter.

Fat and air embolism are described in chapter 79.

Recent advances

Catheter-directed ultrasound accelerated thrombolysis (CUAT) for deep vein thrombosis is being attempted in some centres, to hasten resolution of DVT.

Percutaneous catheter embolectomy is a minimally invasive procedure, becoming popular, replacing open embolectomy.

83 Some Rules of Thumb in Vascular Surgery

CONGENITAL

1. Surgery is least preferred and is the last resort in hemangioma
2. Surgery is not only difficult but may be hazardous in congenital AVM

VASCULAR INJURY

3. Impaired peripheral pulse, expanding hematoma and circulatory instability indicate major vascular injury
4. Synthetic grafts are to be avoided in dirty wounds
5. Repair of vascular injury is not helpful, if associated fracture in the vicinity is not stabilized

ACUTE ARTERIAL OCCLUSION

6. Since circumstances of patients vary, there is no 'golden period' for thromboembolectomy in acute occlusions, but earlier the better
7. Procrastination is disastrous in accidental intra-arterial injection of drugs
8. Acute occlusion has to be distinguished from acute-on-chronic type, before considering thromboembolectomy, since it may not help in the latter
9. While managing embolism, a source of emboli, such as silent cardiac infarction, should be investigated and simultaneously treated
10. Underlying thrombophilia has to be excluded by appropriate investigations, including homocystine assay

CHRONIC ARTERIAL OCCLUSION

11. All occlusive diseases are more common in smokers, except nonspecific aortoarteritis (NAA) and collagen vascular diseases
12. At least some pathology of blood vessels due to smoking is reversible, if there is total abstinence from tobacco in any form

13. The relationship of smoking with vascular diseases is incontroversial.
14. Thromboangiitis obliterans (TAO) commonly affects the lower limbs, whereas Raynaud's disease/ phenomenon afflicts the upper limbs
15. Synthetic grafts are not ideal for infragenicular reconstructions or where a graft has to cross a joint
16. A patient being asymptomatic is not a certain indication of graft patency, following a bypass procedure
17. In end-stage arterial occlusive disease, resulting in gangrene, anything distal to a below-knee amputation does not heal
18. Distal vessel disease and early tissue necrosis are typical of TAO
19. Bilateral, episodic upper limb involvement in women is typical of Raynaud's disease
20. Dyslipidemia is not present in all patients of atherosclerosis; but if present, it influences the outcome
21. Angiogram is like a road map; it is necessary only if direct arterial surgery is indicated/ contemplated
22. Conventional peripheral angiogram over-estimates the occlusive lesion and fails to demonstrate a distal run-off, even when it is actually present (in about 25%)
23. Angiogram under-estimates the size of an aneurysm, due to thrombus partially filling the cavity
24. In arterial occlusions at two levels, the proximal one should be treated first, if both cannot be tackled at the same time
25. As most of the arterial occlusive diseases are systemic and progressive, any local reconstruction has to be considered as palliative

26. Gradual occlusion of an artery results in dry gangrene, whereas rapid occlusion of arterial and venous channels produces moist gangrene

27. Scalenotomy is an integral part of any surgery for thoracic outlet compression

28. Cervical rib should be excised even if it is minimally symptomatic, but may be left alone, if it is totally asymptomatic

29. Higher the level of arterial occlusion and lesser the tissue necrosis, greater the chances of having a distal run-off useful for reconstruction

SYMPATHECTOMY

30. Sympathectomy is generally ineffective in diabetics and those above 50

31. Sympathectomy is not a substitute for direct arterial surgery

32. Surgically induced Horner's syndrome is harmless, self-limiting and needs no treatment

33. There is no additional benefit by bilateral sympathectomy for unilateral ischemic disease

34. If one abstains from tobacco in any form, sympathectomy is curative in Buerger's disease (TAO)

35. There is no fool-proof method of predicting the efficacy of sympathectomy, except to 'do it and see', if there is no contraindication. Ankle/brachial index (ABI), >0.3 may be of some help

DIABETIC ANGIOPATHY

36. Development of microangiopathy in diabetics is more related to the duration than the severity of diabetes mellitus

37. In pure diabetic gangrene, peripheral pulses are well felt

38. Early excision of necrotic tissue should be done in diabetic gangrene, whereas 'wait and watch' is the rule in frost bite, since deeper tissue are usually uninvolved in the latter

39. Moist gangrene is a medical emergency both in terms of life and limb

40. A combination of smoking and diabetes is disastrous for leg circulation

41. Associated macroangiopathy in diabetes should be treated with suitable vascular reconstruction

ANEURYSM

42. Surgery is indicated in an arterial aneurysm, if its diameter is twice that of the native vessel and the life expectancy of the patient is over five years

43. Once diagnosed, an arterial aneurysm will produce some complication in about 95% of the patients in five years

VENOUS DISEASES

44. If a limb has both arterial and venous insufficiency, the former should be treated first

45. Thrombolytic agents have radically improved the outlook in massive pulmonary/peripheral thromboembolism and deep vein thrombosis

46. In unilateral limb edema, local venous/lymphatic/inflammatory causes have to be looked for, whereas in bilateral cases, systemic causes, such as cardiac, hepatic, renal, nutritional, hormonal etc. have to be considered

47. Superficial venous insufficiency rarely causes edema of the limb

48. If the deep venous system is otherwise normal, incompetent perforators lose their pathogenic significance, after stripping of superficial (varicose) veins

49. Since edema is the hallmark of deep vein dysfunction, deep vein disease may be reasonably excluded, if there is no history of edema

50. Embolic manifestation is rarely if ever, seen in superficial thrombophlebitis

51. Simple Trendelenburg stripping is curative in primary varicose veins of leg

52. Subfascial ligation of perforators (Cockett & Dodd) is indicated only if there is evidence of deep vein disease, to improve the function of the peripheral pump
53. Typically venous ulcers are around ankle, whereas arterial ulcers are at the tips of the toes
54. Thrombosis of superficial veins is called thrombophlebitis, whereas in the deep veins it is called phlebothrombosis

GENERAL

55. Knowing the principles of vascular surgery would make one, a good and expedient general surgeon
56. These 'rules of thumb' are to be applied in their proper context and spirit, and not to be considered as 'irrevocable doctrines'

	Feature	Arterial	Venous
1	Location	Tips of toes	Around the ankle
2	Claudication	Present	Absent
3	Pigmentation	Absent	Present
4	Dermatitis	Absent	Present
5	Edema	Absent	Present
6	Arterial pulses	Absent	Present
7	Varicose veins	Absent	May be seen
8	Local temperature	Cold	Warm
9	Pain relief by	Dependency	Elevation
10	Trophic ulcer	Present	Absent
11	Elastic support	Does not help	Helps
12	Gangrene	Common	Rare

Table-83.1: Differences between an arterial and a venous ulcer

84 Endovascular Surgery

ndovascular surgery is a branch of vascular surgery which involves treatment of peripheral vascular disease by minimally invasive methods. Though both arterial and venous diseases are managed by these methods, conventionally it refers to management of arterial diseases.

The history of endovascular surgery dates back to 1953, when Seldinger developed a technique where a percutaneous trans-femoral arterial entry was made through a needle for angiographic procedures. Today this technique is being widely used to treat most of the vascular diseases through minimal intervention.

The main advantages of endovascular procedures, as in any minimal access surgery, are short hospital stay and minimal morbidity and mortality which can be performed in high risk patients.

The disadvantages are, they are relatively more expensive, not suitable for all lesions, need for reinterventions, requires special training and more importantly the long term results are not comparable to open surgical procedures.

With accumulating experience and technological advances, virtually all large and medium-sized vessels are brought under the purview of endovascular surgery. The commonest lesions which are being treated by percutaneous procedure are coronary, iliac/femoral occlusive disease, abdominal and thoracic aneurysmal diseases, forming the bulk of endovascular procedures performed worldwide. The other areas include popliteal, infra-popliteal, subclavian, renal and carotid occlusions.

The basis of endovascular procedures are catheters, balloons and stents. Today, due to improvement in technology we

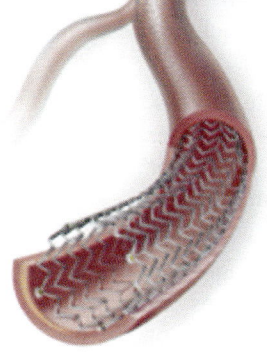

Fig. 84.1. Bare metallic stent

have different types, shapes and sizes of catheters, balloons and stents which make the procedures less morbid and offer better long term results, thereby expanding their applications.

Initial evaluation

It is important before formulating a revascularisation plan, to distinguish between significant and non significant lesions. Measurement of segmental pressures during DSA may be useful. Pressure gradients of 10-20mmHg are borderline and may not be critical, but >30mm are always significant. In addition noninvasive studies like pulse volume recordings provide important clues to hemodynamic significance of stenosis. Duplex ultrasound provides excellent information about patients with single level disease but not very useful with multilevel occlusive disease.

Selection of procedures

Understanding the natural history of the disease in the context of the patient's history and physical examination as well as evaluation of serious co-morbidities, are essential. Those with gross necrosis of the foot and who are non-ambulatory are better treated by apropriate amputation rather than revascularization. Patients, who are poor surgical candidates, compromised target vessel and nonavailability of optimal venous conduits are naturally the best candidates for endovascular interventions.

Access site

The commonest access site is common femoral artery but other sites like radial, brachial, axillary and popliteal arteries may also be used. The common femoral artery is the most convenient and safest site, which can be accessed both in antegrade and retrograde

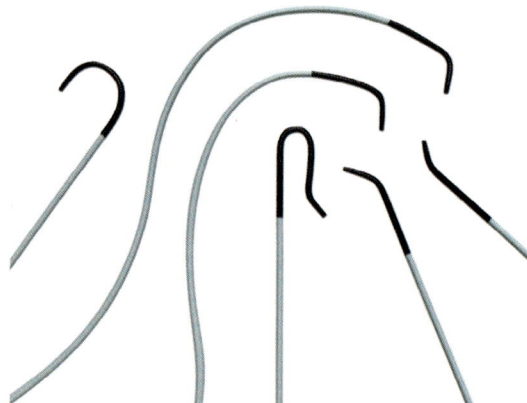

Fig. 84.2 Different types of catheter tips

fashion. From this site therapeutic intervention on the contralateral iliac, femoral and popliteal arteries can be performed. The arterial puncture high in CFA may predispose to retroperitoneal bleeding, whereas very low puncture carry a higher incidence of arteriovenous fistula, hematoma and pseudoaneurysm formation. The puncture of an artery with narrow calibre and low flow can be challenging, when a Doppler-guided entry may be very helpful.

Guide wires, catheters, balloons and stents

Many types of wires are available for intervention. Stainless steel wires which are normally used, have high negotiability but deform easily. But nitinol wires improve flexibility and shape retention. These wires usually have 'J' tip at their entry to avoid intimal dissection. Hydrophilic wires which have slippery coating are available, which facilitate easy passage across difficult occlusions.

Appropriate sheaths provide stable access, minimal blood loss and improve catheter manipulation. Long sheaths are used for contralateral work. Smaller size sheath is used for upper limb access.

Pigtail catheters are used for diagnostic angiography. There are different types of catheters available according to the shape of the artery to be entered. Trackability of these

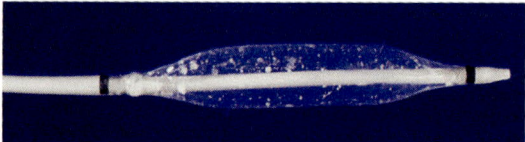

Fig. 84.3. Angioplasty balloon

catheters enables them to be advanced through tortuous anatomy without pulling the wire out of position.

Various types of balloons are used for dilating the narrowed artery. The basic principle of balloon angioplasty is to cause a controlled injury to the vessel wall which produces plaque fracture and medial and adventitial stretching. Sometimes, a limited dissection is created which is non flow-limiting. Disruption of intima leads onto intimal hyperplasia. Balloons are available in different diameter, length, strength, compliance profile and designing. Most balloons are made of polypropylene, polyethylene or nylon. Nylon balloons are noncompliant, puncture resistant and used for stent deployment and dilatation.

Special type of balloons are available for treating difficult lesions. Cryoballoons are used for cryoplasty which involves cooling of balloon to 10°C using liquid nitrous oxide for inflation. The theoretical advantage claimed of this technique is induction of smooth muscle apotopsis, thereby avoiding recoil and reducing

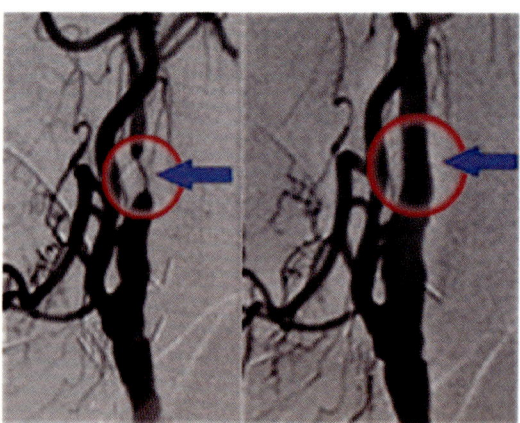

Fig. 84.4. Internal carotid artery occlusion (90%) treated by angioplasty and stenting (courtesy: Dr V Balaji, Chennai)

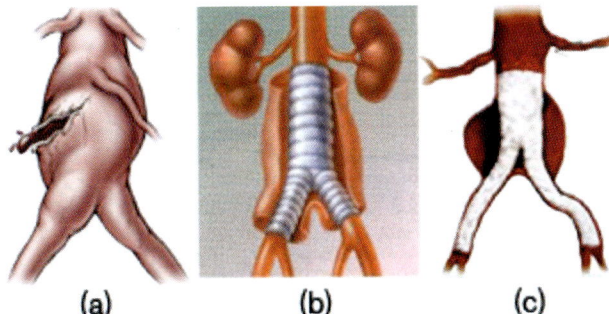

(a)   **(b)**   **(c)**

Fig. 84.5. (A) Infrarenal AAA (B) bifurcated graft in place (C) stent graft deployed percutaneously

the incidence of restenosis. However, this has not been substantiated in controlled trials.

Drug coated balloons deliver sirolimus or paclitaxel (antirestenotic drugs) locally during balloon angioplasty. This technique also claims less restenosis and hence better long term stent patency.

Stents are metallic tubes inserted inside the arteries to keep the vessel opened after an angioplasty. Two main types available are balloon expandable stents which is preloaded onto a balloon and deployed at the site of narrowing. Self expanding stents expand when exposed to body temperature inside the lumen of the vessel. Stents can be placed immediately after angioplasty (primary stenting) or with failed angioplasty (secondary stenting). Stent fracture is common in the treatment of long segments and those subjected to longitudinal bending and torsional forces such as popliteal artery. In general experience, the results of stenting are better in treating claudication rather than critical limb ischemia.

Drug eluting stents have been used in the management of peripheral arterial disease but the results are not encouraging as with coronary artery stenting (see chapter 77).

Two types of stents which are in common use are sirolimus-coated Smart nitinol stents (Cordis) and polymer free paclitaxel-coated Zilver stents (Cook). However, further experience is required to determine their benefits and the potential complications.

Covered stents have a graft material made of either Dacron or polytetrafluroethylene (PTFE) wrapping the metallic stent . This can be external or internal or both. This prevents restenosis by avoiding ingrowth of intima through the stent. However, the main indication for these stents is in treating aortic/peripheral aneurysms and AV fistulae. The basic principle of inserting the covered stent is exclusion of the aneurysm from the flow. This can be used in management of both pseudo or true aneurysms. Deploying these sophisticated prostheses has considerably reduced the morbidity and mortality in the management of high risk abdominal or thoracic aortic aneurysms.

The abdominal aneurysms stent graft (EVAR)

It is a modular graft consisting of one body and ipsilateral limb and another for contralateral limb. Extension grafts are available to cover extra length of aneurysms.

Areas where endovascular procedures are in common use

Arterial system

1. Fogarty thrombo-embolectomy
2. Percutaneous transluminal angioplasty and stenting for arterial stenosis

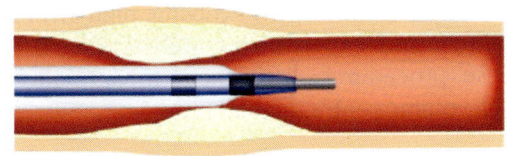

Fig. 84.6. Percutaneous balloon angioplasty

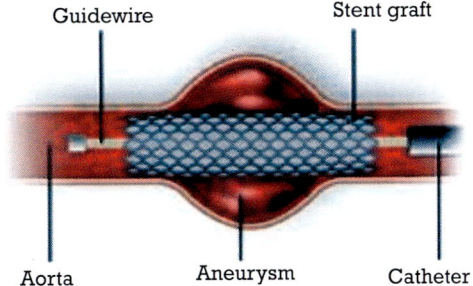

Fig. 84.7. Stright endoprosthesis for aortic aneurysm

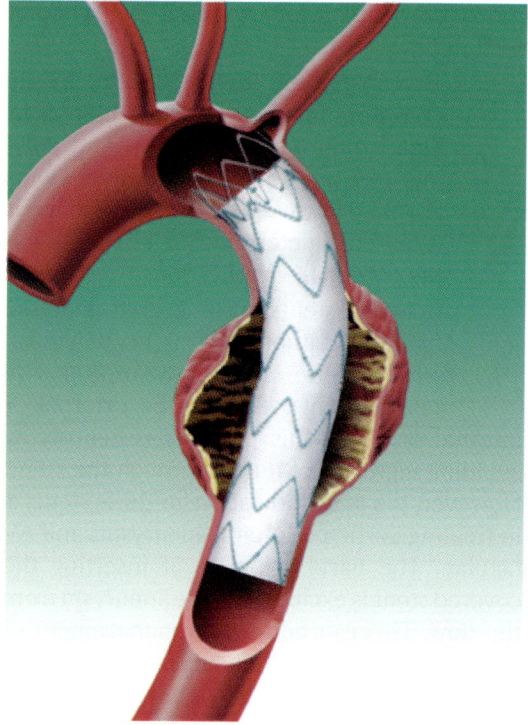

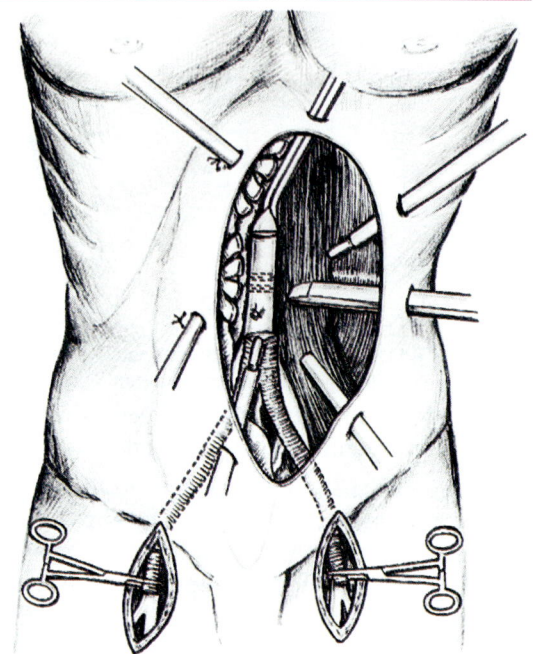

Fig. 84.9 Endoscopic retroperitoneal exposure for aorto-bifemoral bypass

Fig. 84.8 Endoprosthesis of descending thoracic aorta

3. Dilatation of coarctation of aorta

4. Aneurysm of major arteries (thoracic and abdominal aorta and iliac arteries)

5. Percutaneous aortic valvotomy or trans-catheter aortic valve implantation (TAVI)

6. Arterio-venous malformations

7. Angioscopic atherectomy

Venous diseases

Common applications for these procedures in the venous system, at the present time, are

1. Venacaval interruption devices (placation filters) to prevent pulmonary embolization

2. High IVC occlusions with or without Budd-Chiari syndrome

3. Trans-jugular intrahepatic portal systemic shunting (TIPSS) in portal hypertension

4. Valvulotomy of saphenous vein, for doing an 'in-situ' vein bypass for infragenicular arterial occlusions

5. Endoluminal management of varicose veins (Laser, RFA, thermal, foam sclerotherapy)

6. To deliver thrombolytic agents for DVT and pulmonary embolism

7. Arterio-venous fistula

Conclusion

There is increasing evidence coming up in favour of endovascular therapy for patients with critical limb ischemia. Technical advances in catheters, balloons, stents and pharmacotherapies allow application to a wider variety of clinical and anatomical problems. Covered or coated stents may be useful to provide higher long-term patency. As the newer technology is evolving, high level of training and expertise required for some of these procedures, limit them to specialized high volume centres in this field.

85 Postoperative Analgesia

Patients experience severe pain in the immediate postoperative period, but as it is a subjective feeling, measurement is always difficult. However, thoracotomy and laparotomy associated with painful breathing do permit direct measurement of FEV1 and PFR and their improvement with analgesia; otherwise, a (rough) linear analogue is used in which the patient makes a mark on a 10cm line, one end of which is marked as no pain and the other as the worst pain. The position of the mark on the line measures how much pain the patient is experiencing. This technique is known as visual analog scale (VAS) and is considered better than analgesimetry.

With the Cardiff palliator or Newcastle Interactive demand apparatus, operated by the patient himself by pressing a button to add a small increment of IV narcotic, pain can be analyzed quantitatively by the rate of administration of narcotic analgesic. This is called patient-controlled analgesia (PCA).

Pain, a common presenting feature of many disease processes, is usually associated with actual or impending tissue damage. Acute pain in a perioperative setting is defined as pain that is present in a surgical patient because of pre existing disease, surgical procedure or a combination of these. It is an unpleasant and inevitable component of the post surgical experience. An individual who undergoes surgery would probably consider it his/her right to obtain adequate relief of postoperative pain. Patients however continue to suffer silently because of a lack of a concerted effort on the part of the anesthesiologist and surgeon to offer relieve the pain. If one considers adequate pain relief to be a basic right of the patient, failure to relieve pain is tantamount to a moral and ethical lapse on the part of the doctor.

Recent years have witnessed an increasing interest in postoperative pain management. As a result, an increasing number of patients have become more medically informed and more likely to request specific and more effective modes of treatment.

The aim of postoperative pain treatment is to provide subjective comfort in addition to inhibiting trauma-induced nociceptive impulses in order to blunt autonomic and somatic reflex responses to pain and subsequently to enhance restoration of function by allowing the patient to breathe, cough and move about more easily.

Harmful cytokines and immunosuppressive peptides are released as part of the pain response, hence efficient analgesia naturally facilitates better clinical outcome.

Peculiarity of postoperative pain

Constant surgically-related pain, frequently described as aching in nature and ordinarily near the surgical site (basal pain).

Acute exacerbation of pain added to the basal pain and due to activities such as coughing, getting out of bed, physiotherapy, and dressing changes.

It is a self limiting condition.

Usually there is a progressive improvement over a relatively short period of time.

Unrelieved pain after surgery is often an unpleasant experience; fortunately is preven-

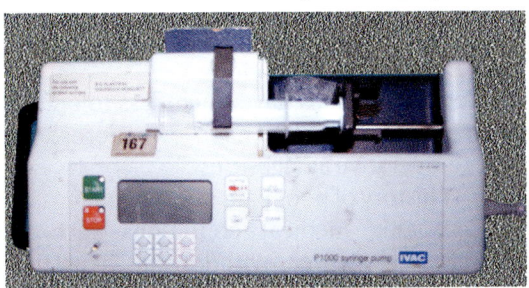

Fig. 85.1. Programmed pulsed injector
(courtesy: Lifeline Hospitals, Chennai)

table or controllable in a vast majority of cases.

Pain control may have a further benefit of improving clinical outcome by reducing the incidence of postoperative complications such as:

- myocardial infarction or ischemia
- risk of tachycardia and dysrhythmia
- impaired wound healing
- risk of atelectasis
- thromboembolic events
- peripheral vasoconstriction
- metabolic acidosis.

Clinical assessment of acute pain

Several pain scoring systems available include the categorical rating scale (CRS), where pain is rated as no pain, mild, moderate and severe pain. The visual analog scale (VAS) where the individual scores the pain on a 10 cm scale where the left anchor point is labelled 'no pain'and the right anchor point is labelled 'worst possible pain' or the verbal numerical rating scale (VNRS) where the patient estimates the pain as a number between 0 indicating 'no pain' and 10, indicating 'worst possible pain'.

Irrespective of the scoring system used,one must record postoperative pain both at rest and during specifically directed movement (chest physiotherapy for thoracotomies, passive knee movements following knee surgery etc). It should be recorded as frequently as every 5 minutes during the initial phase when bolus injections of intravenous opioids or epidural opioids, local anesthetics are being given in an incremental manner. Once adequate basal analgesia has been established, the frequency of assessment can be reduced to once every 2 hours during the first 24 to 48 hours and once every 4 hours thereafter.

In addition pain scores should be considered along with sedation scores and the traditional ward recordings of temperature, pulse rate, blood pressure and respiratory rate. These six observations constitute the minimum set of data to be recorded in the postoperative chart (with pain score and sedation score being given

the status of the 5th and 6th vital signs. Recording postoperative pain is one way of focusing the attention of all care givers to the presence of acute postoperative pain, and the consequent need for its effective management.

Management of acute postoperative pain

Management strategies for postoperative pain are aimed at reducing a patient's pain to a tolerable level. Complete abolition of pain should not be the objective and certainly not desirable. Though the traditional approach has been to begin pain therapy when surgery is complete the concept of 'preemptive analgesia' has become increasingly popular wherein antinociceptive treatment is started before the onset of pain. Such treatment prevents the establishment of altered central processing which normally amplifies postoperative pain by sensitizing the CNS to sensory input.

Just as 'balanced anesthetic techniques' are used to meet the intraoperative anesthetic needs of patients by making use of several agents 'balanced analgesia' uses several modalities of pain management to provide pain and stress free state, thereby promoting good postoperative outcome. Multimodal techniques of pain management involves administration of two or more drugs that act by different mechanisms via a single route (e.g. epidural opioids + local anesthetics + clonidine) for providing superior analgesic efficacy with reduced adverse effects (recommendation of the American Society of Anesthesiologists - ASA)

Factors influencing analgesic requirements

1. Age of the patient: elderly patients require smaller doses.
2. Gender: females have much less tolerance to narcotic analgesic and need lower doses.
3. Pre-operative analgesic use.
4. Past history of poor pain management.
5. Coexisting medical conditions such as substance abuse or withdrawal, hyperthyroidism, anxiety disorder, affective disorder, acid-peptic disease, hypertension, hepatic or renal impairments.

Jewels of Gyan - 85.1

Wong-Baker Faces - Pain Rating Scale

Visual analog scale (VAS) for children
All patients may experience some pain from cancer or cancer treatment. Only the patient knows it best, but may not be able to communicate it to the members of the health care team as well as to the family members.

Communicating the pain
Using a pain rating scale, like the one below, is helpful for young patients to

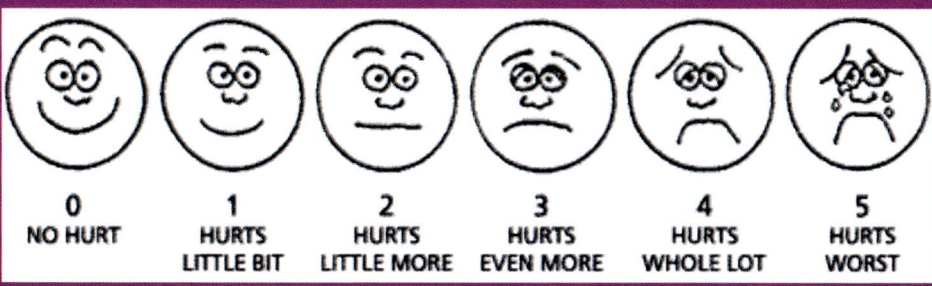

0	1	2	3	4	5
NO HURT	HURTS LITTLE BIT	HURTS LITTLE MORE	HURTS EVEN MORE	HURTS WHOLE LOT	HURTS WORST

The picture is self explanatory. The child has to choose the face that best describes the intensity of pain

6. Cultural factors and personality. (e.g. patients vary from being intolerant of any discomfort to surprising self-control or patients consider pain to be a normal part of life).

7. Preoperative patient education - appropriate preoperative education can improve expectations, compliance and ability to effectively interact with pain management techniques.

8. Site of operation: thoracic and upper abdominal operations are associated with the most severe pain.

9. Individual variation in response and pain threshold.

10. Attitude of the ward staff.

Pain management techniques

To ensure that pain management is done effectively, formal means must be developed and used within each institution to assess pain management practices and to obtain patient feedback to calibrate the adequacy of pain control.

Pre-emptive analgesic therapy

There is a lot of interest in controlling the "wind-up" phenomenon as related to postoperative pain. To this end the application of opioids, local anesthetic blocks and other analgesic modalities are being instituted and established before surgery in an attempt to decrease the intensity and duration of postoperative IDs

Pharmacological management of mild to moderate postoperative pain should begin, unless there is contraindication, for the use of NSAIDs, which decrease levels of inflammatory mediators generated at the site of tissue injury.

NSAIDs have several advantages over opioids. They do not have hemodynamic effects; do not cause respiratory depression, or slow gastric emptying or small bowel transit time. The pharmacy cost of some of them, however, is significantly greater than that of morphine, even by the oral route. IV parecoxib is very effective but expensive.

Numerical pain rating scale

You may experience some pain from cancer or cancer treatment. Only you know how much pain you have. You need to be able to describe your pain to your health care team as well as to your family or friends

Using a pain rating scale, like the one below is helpful in describing how much pain you are feeling.

No pain	Minimal pain	Moderate pain	Worst pain

0 1 2 3 4 5 6 7 8 9 10

Try to assign a number from 0 (zero) to 10 (ten) to your pain level. If you have no pain, use a 0.

As the number get higher, they stand for pain that is getting worse. A 10 means the pain is as bad as it can be.

Rating scale to describe the pain:

Feels at its worst

Feels most of the time

Feels at its least

Changes with treatment

Risks include increased bleeding, GI damage, renal impairment, exacerbation of aspirin-induced asthma, poor bone or wound healing, etc. Bone healing issues may be a contraindication in spinal fusion procedures. Additionally, NSAIDS are inadequate analgesics alone for severe pain; they seem best utilized in conjunction with other agents.

NSAIDs may cause significant renal impairment, particularly in patients with renal disease or decreased circulating blood volume, and may induce fluid retention, edema and hypertension. When systemic vasoconstriction occurs, local prostaglandin release causes renal vasodilatation, thus maintaining renal blood flow and glomerular filtration rate near normal. Usually these drugs are not prescribed for visceral pain.

Increased bleeding due to platelet inhibition is a risk when 'older' or non-selective cyclooxygenase (COX)-1 inhibitors (paracetamol,

indomethacin, piroxicam, meloxicam, diclo-fenac, aceclofenac etc.) are used periope-ratively. The new highly selective COX-2 inhibitors (e.g. rofecoxib, celecoxib, etoricoxib, zaltoprofen etc) inhibit prostaglandin synthesis without inhibition of platelet aggregation and with reduced renal and GI toxicity. In some studies perioperative bloodloss was actually reduced when highly-selective COX-2 inhibitors were administered preoperatively. Unfortunately, the increased risk of arterial thrombosis and myocardial infarction with long term use of Rofecoxib, forcing its withdrawal from the market. They may be ideal for short term use in the immediate peri-operative period (i.e. during surgery until acute haemostasis was secured).

Meloxicam has greater COX-2 than COX-1 inhibition, but in clinically adequate doses COX-1 inhibition is probable so bleeding may be a problem in some patients. No-study has conclusively evaluated significance of bleeding with perioperative meloxicam in humans.

Ketorolac and parecoxib can be administered intravenously. Ketorolac is very potent and predominantly affects COX-1, whereas parecoxib is a precursor of valdecoxib, a highly-selective COX-2 inhibitor.

Acetaminophen or paracetamol is commonly used as a mild analgesic in the peri-operative setting. It has no COX-1 or COX-2 activity, so does not affect platelet aggregation, nor does it provide peripheral anti-inflammatory activity. There is a definite possibility of severe hepatic impairment in overdose (deliberate or accidental). If the patient cannot tolerate oral medication, Perfalgan, an IV preparation, or alternative routes such as rectal administration can be used.

At present, one NSAID, ketorolac is approved in some countries for parenteral use along with IV paracetamol. The introduction of parenteral NSAIDs has increased the number of patients who can benefit from non opioid analgesic - especially those who are to receive nothing by mouth. Ketorolac administration reduced morphine requirements by 50% in patients recovering from abdominal surgery.

OPIOID DRUGS

For postoperative pain, the most commonly used opioid drugs are morphine, papaveretum, pethidine, codeine and methadone. Some actions are due to metabolites.

Opioids may be administered by a variety of routes:

ORAL OPIOIDS - e.g. oxycodone, codeine, tramadol, morphine. Medicines given by mouth cause less discomfort than injections, but they can work just as well. They are inexpensive, simple to give, but there may be a delay in pain relief. Short and long-duration presentations are available. Metabolic conversion of codeine to morphine (10%) and to codeine-6-glucuronide (80%), is necessary for its analgesic effect. This is subjected to considerable inter-patient variability and it can be an unreliable analgesic in some patients.

Tramadol, a central analgesic with low affinity for opioid receptors, has been used extensively in postoperative management. It has proven to be a very weak opioid with an analgesic potency roughly similar to pethidine that is due primarily to non-opioid actions. At low doses it potentiates opioid actions. Dependency liability is low. Little respiratory depression occurs unless given in large doses. Serotoninergic side-effects (confusion, disorientation, even dementia) can occur, and physicians need to be alert for the development of the serotonin syndrome. Nausea is common after IV administration.

INTRAMUSCULAR ADMINISTRATION

Opioids, particularly morphine sulphate, meperidine hydrochloride (pethidine) administered by the intramuscular, subcutaneous or IV route, have been the mainstay of postoperative analgesia. Meperidine (pethidine) is shorter acting, but is metabolized to active agents (norpethidine) that can precipitate seizures and therefore is not recommended for prolonged administration.

Opioids given by intermittent injection generally are not able to maintain steady analgesic plasma levels for 2 to 4 hours. Opioids are

Footnote: Cyclooxygenase (COX) is an enzyme, considered to be an important biomediator for the synthesis of prostaglandins, prostacycline and thromboxane, necessary for inflammation, pain mucosal integrity and platelet activity. Inhibition of COX by NSAIDs causes considerable reduction in inflammatory response and pain, but has the disadvantage of causing GI mucosal damage, platelet and renal dysfunction. They also retain fluid, causing edema and hypertension, thereby increasing the risk of cardiovascular events. The new generation of COX-2 inhibitors are highly selective in their action on inflammatory mediators, with minimal effects on mucosa, platelets and kidneys, hence safer in clinical practice.

often significantly under-dosed because of a widespread, dominant fear for patient safety.

Disadvantages of this technique:

IM injections are painful.

a steady blood concentration is difficult to sustain

there are prolonged intervals where the patient experiences pain

SUBCUTANEOUS INJECTIONS - May provide a very effective method of pain relief. The onset of pain relief occurs at about the same time as with the intramuscular route. The injection is less painful and the effect lasts longer.

Unless the dose and the timing are judged appropriately, there are still periods of unrelieved pain.

Transdermal drug delivery allows continuous parenteral administration of drug without the need for needles or infusion devices. Lipid soluble drugs like fentanyl are suitable. Trans-dermal fentanyl patches are available with different delivery rates ranging from 25 to 100 micrograms per hour. Currently available patches have a slow onset and offset of action and absorption continues for up to 72 hours while the patch is in place.

INTRAVENOUS ROUTE - Continuous intravenous infusions provide pain control as long as steady state concentrations are maintained above the minimum effective analgesic blood concentrations. Steady state concentrations are dependent on systemic clearance and this is related to hepatic blood flow.

Both pethidine and morphine are suitable drugs for continuous intravenous infusions but unless a loading dose is used, a steady state is not achieved for about 24 hrs. To avoid the side effects of a large bolus, a loading dose given as an infusion is preferable, always remembering that there is drug elimination during loading.

EPIDURAL OPIOID DRUGS - Drugs administered by these routes can reduce the dosage of opioid required for adequate pain

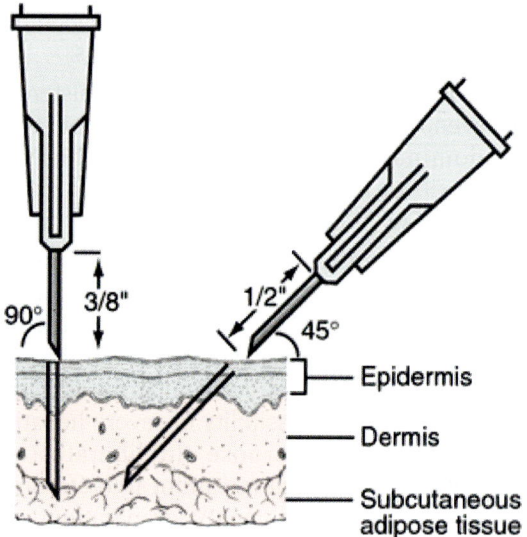

Fig. 85.2. Angles of needle insertion for administering a subcutaneous injection

relief, especially if administered in association with local anesthetics. There is no sensory loss, no muscle paresis and no autonomic blockade with opioid drugs administered by these routes.

With intrathecal injections there is a variation in the rate of onset of analgesia and its duration depending on whether the drug is lipophilic or hydrophilic and by transport within the cerebro-spinal fluid. Morphine is hydrophilic. When administered by the spinal routes it takes about 45 minutes to reach maximum effect and lasts for 8-12 hours. Pethidine, methadone and fentanyl being lipophilic act quickly, but the duration of action is short.

Of considerable concern is the risk of delayed respiratory depression which may occur up to 18 hrs after the opioid drug is injected. Very small intrathecal doses (less than 1mg of morphine, even less in the elderly) are considered safest, and post-administration monitoring must record respiratory rate at least hourly. Resuscitation facilities and trained staff must be available. The respiratory depression is reversed by naloxone.

The dose of morphine by the epidural route is about 5-10 times that of the intrathecal route.

Analgesic adjuvants

NMDA antagonists: ketamine, dextro-methorphan, magnesium and adenosine have been tried as analgesic adjuvants for postoperative pain management. These have been shown to inhibit the receptor-gated calcium currents that amplify neuronal firing. Ketamine has been shown to be a useful adjuvant when given as an IV bolus, continuous IV infusion (0.5-1.0mg/kg/hr) or epidural infusion (0.25 mg/kg/hr) without any adverse CNS effects.

α2 agonists: Low dose clonidine has proved to be a useful adjuvant analgesic when given neuraxially (150 mcgm intrathecally or 2-3 mcgm/kg epidurally) and in combination with peripheral nerve blocks (0.5mcgm/kg). Higher doses are associated with adverse effects such as sedation, bradycardia and hypotension and should be avoided.

Neostigmine: Intrathecal administration of 25-100 mcgm neostigmine has been associated with high incidence of nausea and vomiting, bradycardia, hypotension, sweating, agitation and distress. Hence it is not recommended for intrathecal use, but it is being investigated as an analgesic adjuvant for intra-articular and epidural use.

Naloxone, corticosteroids and gabapentine are other drugs are being investigated for use as analgesic adjuvants.

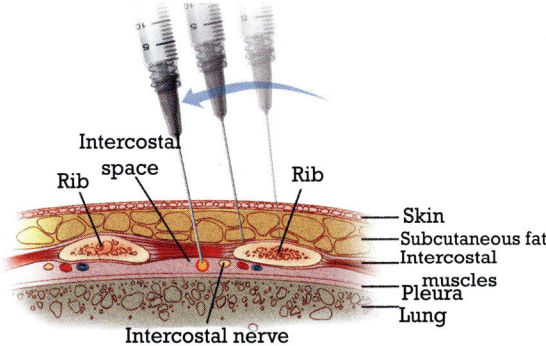

Fig. 85.3. Administration of intercostal block for postoperative analgesia
(courtesy: Lifeline Hospitals, Chennai)

Regional and local analgesia

Direct injection of local analgesic drugs close to peripheral nerves, major nerve trunks or nerve roots produces analgesia by blocking conduction of afferent impulses.

Neural blockade with neuraxial administration of local anesthetics and/or opioids has now been established as being an effective means of postoperative pain treatment. In some situations, such as major abdominal, ortho-pedic and thoracic surgery, it has been documented to provide superior pain relief to alternative techniques. Risks of epidural local anesthetics include hypotension, epidural abscess or hematoma, paraplegia, etc.

A number of peripheral nerve blocks are very useful in the PACU for the transitional period immediately following general anesthesia before the patient is fully awake and stable: intermittent or continuous paravertebral, intercostal, femoral nerve, brachial plexus block, and wound infiltration are the various techniques usually employed.

Relatively few side effects occur ordinarily, providing that these techniques are carefully managed by highly qualified staff.

Intrathecal block - Intrathecal local anesthesia provides analgesia during the postoperative period especially if long acting analgesic drugs such as bupivacaine are used. If opioid drugs are administered before the block wears off, very good pain relief is possible. Usually, to avoid PDPH, a small gauge pencil-point needle is used. Small diameter catheters have made it possible to use continuous spinal techniques but these have been associated with a high complication rates.

Epidural analgesia - This is a more useful technique for the relief of postoperative pain since an indwelling catheter can be used to maintain analgesia in the postoperative period. 'Top up' is done only by doctors and/or administered by programmed pump. Administration of drugs via a continuous

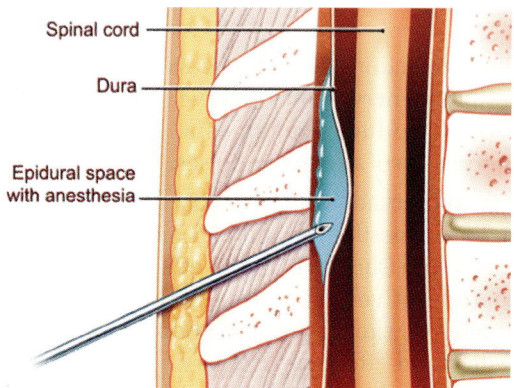

Spinal cord

Dura

Epidural space
with anesthesia

Fig. 85.4. Technique of epidural injection for postoperative analgesia
(courtesy: Lifeline Hospitals, Chennai)

infusion pump or via Infuser® Baxter (non-electric device) avoids fluctuations in the level of analgesia.

Intercostal block - This is performed at the angle of the rib where the intercostal nerves pass round the chest wall beneath the inferior border of the ribs. This carries a risk of creating pneumothorax. Multiple blocks are necessary and the high blood levels are reached. This is a particularly useful technique for pain relief in patients with chest injuries. Transversus abdominis plane (TAP) blocks with ultrasound guidance employed at the end of surgery is a very useful method for the relief of post operative pain for procedures like umbilical hernia repair, laparoscopic surgery, laparotomy etc.

Interpleural analgesia - is the percutaneous introduction of a catheter into the pleural space, placed at an interspace just below the level of the incision. Local anesthetic is introduced through the catheter into the pleural space. Analgesia occurs due to diffusion of local anesthetic to the intercostal nerves, sympathetic chain and direct action on pleural nerve endings. The results of several studies have varied from moderate to excellent analgesia to no analgesia and further work on defining the exact role of interpleural analgesia is currently underway.

Nerve blocks - Of particular benefit are the '3-in-1' block, the femoral nerve block, the sciatic nerve block for postoperative analgesia after lower limbs orthopedic procedures and the block of the dorsal nerve of the penis for pain relief following circumcision. Brachial plexus blocks are great for the upper limb Nowadays nerve blocks are performed under ultrasound or nerve stimulator guidance with a high degree of success and least complications.

Physical methods

Commonly used physical agents include applications of cold (cryoanalgesia for thoracotomy), massage, movement, Transcutaneous electrical nerve stimulation (TENS), and rest or immobilization. TENS may be effective in reducing pain and improving physical function. This is used with varying degrees of success in the management of postoperative pain. Evidence is accumulating that TENS acts by increasing CSF levels of β-endorphins, together with activating of the 'pain gate' by counter irritation.

Patient controlled analgesia (PCA) allows a patient to receive drugs on demand. A PCA pump administers drugs, usually intravenously, when the patient pushes a button. The physician is given the facility of fixing the intermittent injection dose (the dose received

DRUG	DOSAGE	
	Intravenous bolus	Intravenous infusion
Morphine	0.1- 0.2 mg/kg	20-30 mcgm/kg/hr
Pethidine	0.1-1 mg/kg	200-300mcgm/kg/hr
Fentanyl	1-5 mcgm/kg	0.5-2mcgm/kg/hr
Tramadol	0.5-1mgm/kg	0.1-0.2 mg/kg/hr

Table-85.1 The intravenous doses of the commonly used opiates

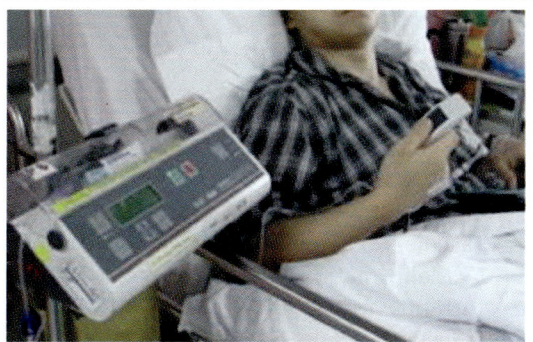

Fig. 85.5. Programmed patient-controlled analgesia (PCA) unit

when the patient pushes the button), the lockout interval (the minimal length of time that must elapse between consecutive doses), a limit to how much drug may be injected in a limited time (1-4 hours), a bolus dose to be administered by a nurse through the machine, and a basal rate (continuous infusion rate

without the need for patient or care givers intervention).

The equipment is expensive, and the technique may allow breakthrough pain on an intermittent basis because when the patient is asleep, the administration ceases. This can be overcome by a slow background infusion that is supplemented by a patient controlled additional dose. Adequate patient information and cooperation are essential for optimal results.

Patient education

Preparing patients in order to understand their responsibilities in pain management is important. To ensure that postoperative pain measurement is both valid and reliable, the staff should review the selected pain measurement scale or tool with the patient before surgery.

86 Neck Swellings

In a clinical context, the various swellings encountered may be classified into acute and chronic ones:

Acute swellings

Acute lymphadenitis, with or without suppuration

Inflamed thyroglossal cyst

Furuncle (boil) and carbuncle

Ludwig's angina: florid cellulitis of sublingual and submandibular spaces

Chronic swellings may be cystic, solid or pulsatile:

I) **Cystic swellings**
   - Sebaceous cyst
   - Cold abscess
   - Abscess of suppurated lymph nodes
   - Thyroglossal cyst
   - Branchial cyst
   - Dermoid cyst
   - Cystic hygroma or lymph cyst
   - Cystic tumors of thyroid, benign and malignant
   - Plunging ranula
   - Pharyngeal pouch
   - Laryngocele
   - Retention salivary cyst

ii) **Solid swellings**
   - Salivary gland swellings
   - Thyroid swellings, including tumors from thyroglossal cyst and ectopic thyroid
   - Lymph node swellings
   - Carotid body tumor
   - Cervical rib
   - Branchiogenic carcinoma
   - Thymic swellings
   - Sternomastoid tumor
   - Soft tissue tumors, benign or malignant including Pancoast tumor of the lung

iii) **Pulsatile swellings**
   - Aneurysm of carotid, subclavian, innominate and vertebral
   - Prominent subclavian pulse over a cervical rib
   - Carotid body tumor
   - Vascular toxic goiter
   - AV Malformation
   - Tortuous vessel
   - Transmitted pulse by a solid swellings.

Swellings common to any region: lipoma, neurofibroma, sebaceous cyst, hemangioma etc.

Note: Lymph nodes and cold abscess also may present in any area. Primary thyroid mass and secondaries in lymph nodes, especially metastatic papillary carcinoma, may be either solid or cystic

Laryngocele

A diverticulum from the laryngeal vestibule, located between the true and false vocal cords.

It may be congenital, but more often acquired, seen above the age of 50, related to occupations involving forced expiration, such as glassblowers or trumpet players and those with chronic cough. Initially it may be internal, within the laryngeal framework (not visible outside), but in due course it becomes external,

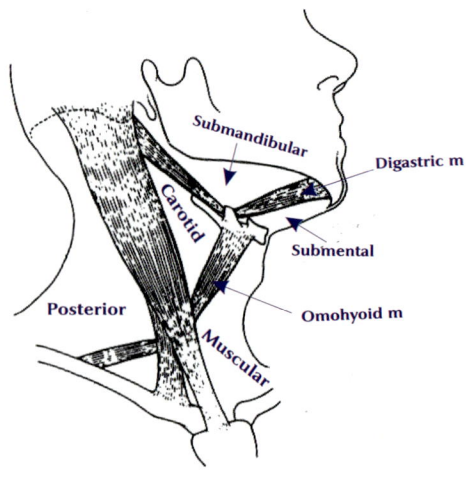

Fig. 86.1. Triangles of the neck

when it passes through the thyrohyoid membrane and presents as a soft, compressible, resonant mass on one side of the larynx, exhibiting cough impulse. It may also be brought out by Valsalva maneuver. Hoarseness of voice and recurrent infection may draw the attention of the patient towards the underlying disease.

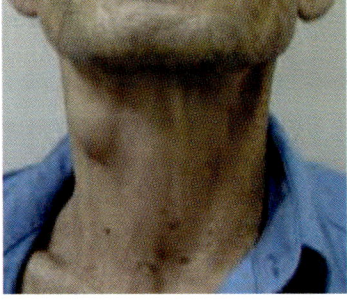

Fig. 86.2. Laryngocele, right side

children, not communicating with the laryngeal cavity. A pharyngeal diverticulum is located at a much lower level, in the posterior triangle, behind the SCM muscle.

A paralaryngeal air pocket may be seen in a plain skiagram and CT scan demonstrating the communicating pouch, confirms the diagnosis.

Differential diagnosis

It has to be differentiated from a saccular cyst of the larynx, which is a mucous cyst, seen more in

Treatment of large laryngocele is by excision, but smaller ones may be dealt by inversion with a purse-string suture around the neck of the diverticulum.

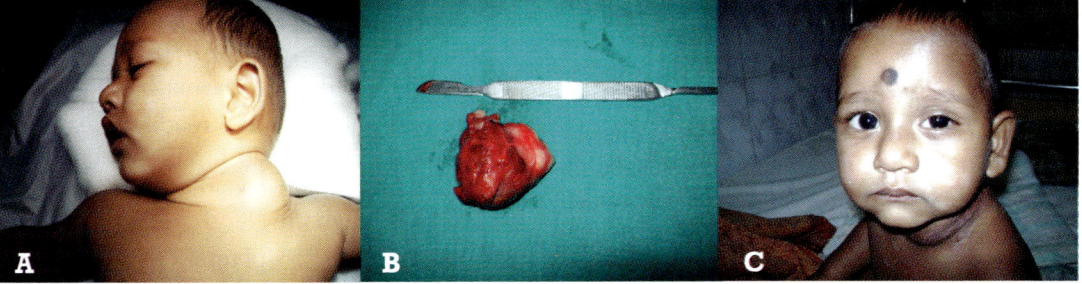

Fig. 86.3. A. 9 months old child with a large malignant schwannoma from the left cervical sympathetic chain
B. Capsulated tumor excised. **C.** Postoperative picture showing Horner's syndrome
(courtesy: Dr C M Kishore, Chennai)

Location	Solid	Cystic
Midline	Lymph nodes Thyroid isthmus	Thyroglossal cyst Dermoid Subhyoid bursitis Plunging ranula Laryngocele Cold abscess
Submandibular triangle	Salivary glands Lymph nodes	Salivary retention cyst
Carotid triangle	Lymph nodes Thyroid lobe Parathyroid Carotid body tumor Sternomastoid tumor	Branchial cyst Cold abscess Cystic hygroma Laryngocele Carotid aneurysm
Posterior triangle	Lymph nodes Cervical rib Pancoast tumor	Cystic hygroma Cold abscess Pharyngeal pouch Subclavian aneurysm Pneumatocele

Table-86.1 Neck swellings

87 Thyroid Gland

(Thyr : Red Indian shield, with a central handle)

Embryology: Exocrine in lower animals (larvae of lamprey fish); this probably explains the thyroglossal duct, which initially opens into the mouth, gets obliterated and becomes ductless (endocrine) in man, its opening represented by the foramen cecum of the tongue (cecum: blind). The fact that thyroxine is the only orally active natural hormone also supports this contention.

From the floor of the primitive pharynx, a diverticulum extends from the foramen cecum of tongue, into the neck, in front of the body of the hyoid (sometimes behind), called thyroglossal duct. The caudal end of this duct produces the main gland and its connection to the gland is represented by the pyramidal lobe, just to the left of the midline, over the isthmus. The bulk of the gland, however, is derived from the endoderm of the 4th pharyngeal pouch.

The calcitonin-producing parafollicular (C) cells are derived from the ultimobranchial body, an outgrowth from the fourth pharyngeal pouch as well as from the rudimentary fifth (APUD cells).

Physiology: Synthesis of thyroid hormones is dependent upon exogenous iodine, about 100mcgm/day, fish, milk, eggs and iodized salt being the principal sources. Iodides are absorbed from stomach and jejunum to get distributed throughout the extracellular space, but mostly concentrated in the thyroid gland by an active process, reaching a normal thyroid-serum ratio of 50:1, which may go as high as 500:1, in states of iodine deficiency or thyrotoxicosis.

Synthesis of thyroid hormones

a) active trapping and concentration of iodides in the follicular cells (by *dehalogenase*)

b) oxidation of iodide to iodine (by *peroxidase*)

c) linkage of iodine with tyrosine, to form monoiodotyrosine (MIT) and diiodotyrosine (DIT)

d) coupling of MIT and DIT, to form *tri-iodothyronine* (T_3) and *thyroxine* (T_4) (by *coupling enzyme*)

TSH stimulates iodine uptake by the gland, whereas a high dose of iodide blocks trapping as well as the proteolysis necessary for the release of thyroid hormone, thus being the fastest acting antithyroid drug. T_4 and T_3 are stored in the colloid of thyroid follicles, released into plasma to bind with carrier serum proteins, *thyroid hormone-binding globulin* (TBG) and prealbumin (TBPA). T_3 plasma binding is less secure and released more readily to enter tissue; hence it is biologically more active, but circulating plasma levels are much lower than T_4 (1:15). Though the gland produces both the hormones, about 75% of total T_3 is derived from peripheral conversion from T_4, implying that T_4 may actually be a *prohormone*. After tissue utilization, the hormones are deiodinated and the released iodine enters the metabolic pool. Residual hormones are conjugated with glucuronic acid and excreted through urine and bile. Significant amounts of T_3, T_4 and iodine may be present in milk during lactation.

The TSH is secreted by the anterior pituitary, under the influence of thyrotropin-releasing hormone (TRH) secreted by the hypothalamus, but both TSH and TRH are inhibited by high plasma levels of T_3 and T_4, in a homeostatic feedback loop. Iodine deficiency, either absolute or relative to demand, increases the goitrogenic effect of TSH.

Biochemistry: Thyroid hormones are essentially catabolic in action. They increase the glucose absorption from the gut, mobilize liver glycogen, promote gluconeogenesis (production of glucose from noncarbohydrate sources viz.

proteins and fats), increase appetite, gut motility, heart rate and sweating and decrease body weight and menstrual flow. Hence blood glucose, serum creatinine and urinary excretion of creatinine are elevated, whereas cholesterol levels are lowered in thyrotoxicosis.

Calcitonin (also called thyrocalcitonin) is a 32-amino acid linear polypeptide hormone that is produced in humans primarily by the parafollicular cells (also known as C-cells) of the thyroid, derived from APUD cells of neuroectodermal origin. It acts to reduce blood calcium (Ca^{2+}), opposing the effects of parathormone (PTH). Its importance in humans has not been well established, its function is not significant in the regulation of normal calcium homeostasis and in many ways, calcitonin counteracts PTH.

More specifically, calcitonin lowers blood Ca levels in two ways: it inhibits Ca absorption by the intestines and osteoclast activity in bones. it protects against calcium loss from skeleton during periods of calcium mobilization, such as pregnancy and lactation.

While calcitonin is the antipode of PTH in those actions, it is not dissimilar in its effect on electrolyte reabsorption from the kidneys, i.e. it inhibits phosphate reabsorption by the kidney tubules and decreases tubular reabsorption of Ca, leading to increased rates of its loss in urine.

Calcitonin is commercially produced from salmon fish and is used for the treatment of postmenopausal osteoporosis, hypercalcemia, Paget's disease, skeletal metastases, phantom limb pain and in the management of spinal stenosis. It is useful as a tumor marker for medullary thyroid carcinoma (MTC), which arises from the parafollicular (C) cells of thyroid.

Anatomy

The normal adult thyroid is a bilobed endocrine gland connected by an isthmus, wrapped around the proximal trachea, in front of the lower neck in the visceral compartment, deep to the investing fascia (and strap muscles). It weighs around 25gm and has a brownish color and firm consistency. The lobes are wedged between the trachea and carotid sheath; esophagus and prevertebral fascia/muscles forming the posteromedial and posterior relations respectively and the upper poles reaching as high as the middle of the thyroid cartilage. The isthmus, about 2cm broad, crosses the midline in front of the 2nd, 3rd and 4th tracheal rings. A small upward projection of gland from the isthmus, just to the left of the midline is known as the *pyramidal lobe*, which is sometimes attached to the hyoid bone by a fibrous band and occasionally muscle fibres, called *levator glandulae thyroideae*, both representing remnants of the *thyroglossal diverticulum*.

The gland is encased in a false capsule formed by the pretracheal fascia, a condensation of which, called the *suspensory ligament of Berry*, suspends it to the cricoid and thyroid cartilages. The gland with the false capsule is intimately wrapped around the trachea, often requiring sharp dissection to separate, during thyroidectomy. These two factors are responsible for the thyroid gland *moving up with deglutition*, an important clinical sign for identification. The true capsule is a thin fibrous layer, that sends

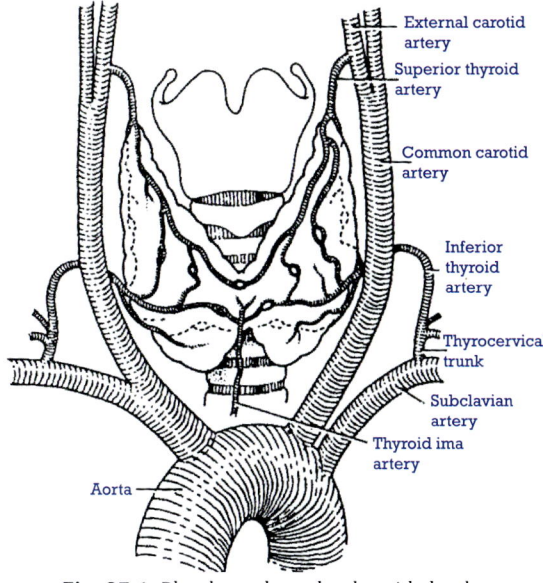

Fig. 87.1. Blood supply to the thyroid gland

External carotid artery
Superior thyroid artery
Common carotid artery
Inferior thyroid artery
Thyrocervical trunk
Subclavian artery
Thyroid ima artery
Aorta

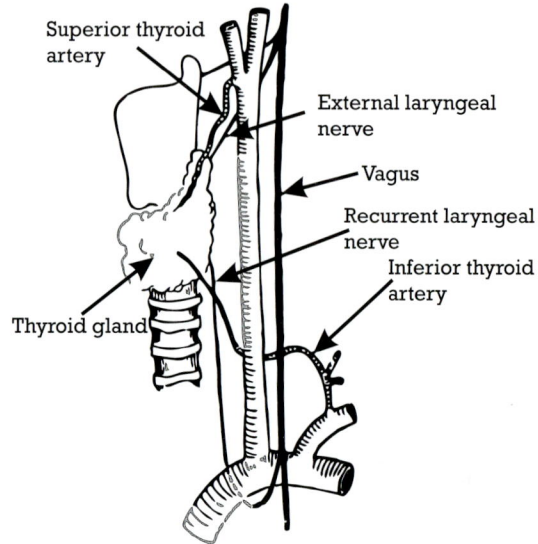

Fig. 87.2. Anatomy of left recurrent laryngeal nerve, inferior and superior thyroid arteries

septa into the gland substance, forming pseudo-lobules. The normal thyroid may be palpable in thin individuals, whereas even a moderately enlarged gland in an obese patient may elude an experienced clinician.

While exposing large goiters during surgery, it may be necessary to divide the strap muscles on one or both sides, which should be done as high as possible, since the nerve supply from ansa cervicalis (derived from hypoglossal and C1,2&3 roots) enter them from their lower end. This also explains the occipital headache the patients often get in the postoperative period, which follows division or traction on the strap muscles.

The four *parathyroid glands* are closely related to the thyroid, on its posterolateral aspect. The upper pair are usually constant in location, and situated in a more posterior plane at the level of the cricoid cartilage. The lower pair, variable in location, are placed at the lower poles of the lobes, in close proximity to the recurrent laryngeal nerves. Each one weighs around 50mg, with 4x4x4mm size; bearing a golden yellow color, they are often indistinguishable from fat lobules. But their darker hue, with 'grains of salt' on close inspection, are helpful in identification during surgery.

When ectopic, they may be placed anywhere from the mandible to the pericardium; the upper parathyroids may descend into the superior/anterior mediastinum; the inferior ones, into the superior/posterior mediastinum, but regardless of their placement, they invariably draw their blood supply from the inferior thy-

roid artery. In patients with an ectopic thyroid, the parathyroids may be normally placed, since their embryological origins are different.

Blood supply to the thyroid gland is profuse, by a pair of superior thyroid (from external carotid) and inferior thyroid arteries (from thyrocervical trunk of subclavian), running in close relation to superior and recurrent laryngeal nerves respectively. Occasionally a fifth one arising directly from the aortic arch or innominate artery, called *thyroidea ima*, may be present, to reach the isthmus from below. Three sets of veins, superior, middle and inferior thyroid veins drain the gland into internal jugular and left innominate veins.

Lymphatic drainage primarily goes into the upper, middle and lower deep cervical nodes. Other nodes, such as prelaryngeal (Delphian), pretracheal (in the suprasternal space of Burns) and paratracheal (along the recurrent nerves), may also assume importance while treating thyroid malignancies.

Superior and recurrent laryngeal nerves are described in chapter 98.

History in a thyroid swelling

i)   age, sex and place of living

ii)   family history of similar swelling

iii) where it started and rate of growth

iv)   any other swellings in the neck and else-where

v)   pressure symptoms: dyspnea (exertional or positional), dysphagia, dysphonia or stridor

vi)   appetite and weight: weight loss with incre-ased appetite is a feature of thyrotoxicosis

vii) easy fatiguability or irritability

viii) menstrual history: oligomenorrhea in hyperthyroid and menorrhagia in hypothy-roid states

ix)   palpitation, sweating and tremors

x)   prominent eye balls and visual distur-bances

xi)   pain: local and over long/skull bones

Physical examination

i) *inspection*: size, shape, location, surface, movement with deglutition, secondary skin changes, other swellings in the neck, anatomi-cal plane by contracting the SCM and strap mus-cles and stretching the deep fascia of the neck (effected by turning the face to the opposite side and depressing the chin against resistance for the muscles and passive lateral flexion of neck to the opposite side for fascia).

ii) *palpation*: confirm the inspection findings, consistency, warmth, tenderness, diffuse or asymmetrical, if nodular, solitary or multiple, ability to reach the lower pole, position of tra-chea (both are interrelated, if the lower pole can

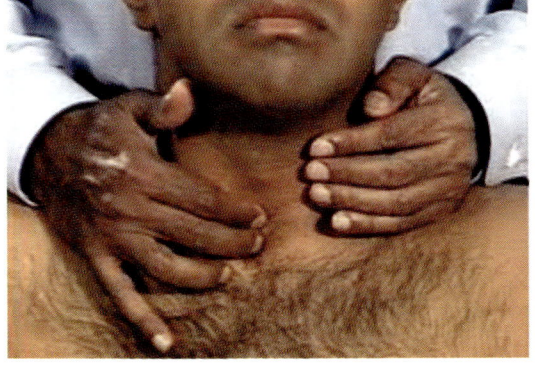

Fig. 87.3. Palpation of thyroid gland from behind

not be appreciated, because it is dipping behind the sternum, the tracheal position can not be palpated). Normal position of trachea is either in the midline or slightly to the right, due to the aortic arch displacing the carina. It should be realized that along with the larynx, the entire trachea and carina also move up during deglutition.

iii) *percussion* for widening of superior mediastinal dullness

iv) *auscultation* for bruit over the carotids for hyperdynamic flow and souffle over the gland for hypervascularity. Tracheal position can be precisely located by the bronchial (or cavern-ous) breath sounds heard over it.

v) examination of all groups of cervical *lymph nodes* should be systematically done

vi) Special maneuvers

1) *Pizzillo's method* of inspection is to make a minimally enlarged gland prominent, by asking the patient push the head backwards against his hands placed over the occiput.

2) *Lahey's method* of palpation: This is prefera-bly done from behind, hands of the exam-iner reaching the trachea from both sides, the trachea is gently pushed to one side, mak-ing any small nodules more conspicuous on that side, to be palpated by the other hand placed over that lobe. The procedure is repeated for palpating the other lobe.

3) *Berry's sign*: feeling for the common carotid pulse at the level of the cricoid cartilage: in benign swellings the carotids are simply displaced posterolaterally, whereas in advanced malignancies, the carotid pulse is not felt, if the tumor 'engulfs' the carotid sheath. (This is rarely positive even in estab-lished malignancies, and hence not reli-able).

4) *Kocher's sign*: This is a risky procedure, intended to identify unusual softening of tracheal rings, known as tracheomalacia, in which gentle pressure over the enlarged lateral lobe produces stridor.

vii) Examination of the eyes for *exophthalmos:* most of these signs are designed to identify sympathetic overactivity, differentiating from other causes of protrusion of eye balls, known as proptosis. (vide infra)

viii) In advanced malignancy, *Horner's syndrome*, due to the involvement of cervical sympathetic chain: ipsilateral ptosis, enophthalmos, anhydrosis, loss of ciliospinal reflex (pinching the skin over the neck produces dilatation of pupil) and miosis(more conspicuous during adaptation to darkness).

ix) systemic examination for tachycardia/ tachyarrhythmias, fine tremors, impaired tendon reflexes, evidence of metastatic disease

Goiter *is a swelling of the thyroid gland* (guttur: throat). While giving out the diagnosis of a thyroid swelling, three aspects have to be taken into consideration, anatomical, functional and pathological.

i) *anatomical:* diffuse, asymmetrical, multinodular (MNG) or solitary nodular goiter (SNG).

ii) *functional:* euthyroid, hypothyroid or hyperthyroid

iii) *pathological:* solid or cystic, inflammatory or neoplastic and benign or malignant

A working scheme for clinical diagnosis of thyroid swellings:

Clinical diagnosis of a goiter can be made mathematically, by identifying the following:

1) diffuse (symmetrical) or nodular (asymmetrical)
2) toxic or nontoxic
3) features of inflammation
4) features of malignancy

By considering (1) and (2), the goiters can be put into four groups, diffuse toxic, diffuse nontoxic, nodular nontoxic and nodular toxic.

1) *Diffuse toxic:* under this there is only one condition, diffuse toxic goiter (Graves' disease)

2) *Diffuse nontoxic:*
a) simple: physiological, endemic or diffuse colloid goiters
b) dyshormonogenic (genetic) goiter
c) inflammatory goiters (features of inflammation): acute, subacute and chronic thyroiditis, the latter may be Hashimoto's, Riedel's and rarely tuberculous thyroiditis
d) rarely an anaplastic carcinoma or a lymphoma may have this presentation

3) *Nodular nontoxic:* the nodule may be a solitary (SNG) or multiple (MNG)
a) solitary nodular goiter (clinically discrete mass), the following possibilities exist:
   i) colloid cyst
   ii) colloid nodule
   iii) focal thyroiditis
   iv) a dominant nodule in an MNG
   v) true neoplasms
       benign: adenoma
       malignant (features of malignancy): carcinoma
b) multinodular goiter: under this there is only one condition, bearing the same name, MNG

4) *Nodular toxic:* out of the above, only an adenoma or an MNG may become toxic, others (colloid cyst, colloid nodule, focal thyroiditis and carcinoma) have very little potential to become toxic.

Individual types

1) DYSHORMONOGENIC GOITER, (syn: familial goiter) a genetic defective synthesis of hormones, due to deficiency of certain enzymes, such as *dehalogenase* (trapping the inorganic iodide), *peroxidase* (oxidation of iodides to iodine) and *coupling enzyme* (coupling the iodotyrosines). Large diffuse goiter in children, often hypothyroid, not com-

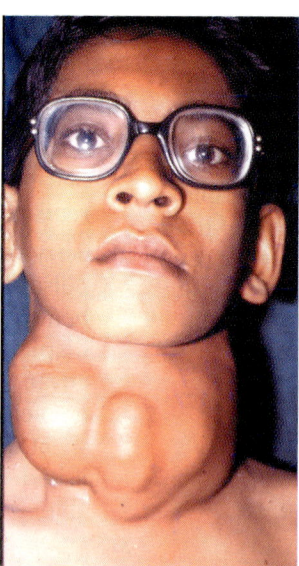

Fig. 87.4. Dyshormonogenic goiter
(courtesy: Prof S Vittal, Chennai)

ing from endemic belts is characteristic. The history of the parents or siblings suffering from a similar problem is corroborative. When associated with congenital deafness, it is known as *Pendred's syndrome*.

Differential diagnosis

Endemic and colloid goitres

Investigations

Thyroid profile to assess the hormonal status(low T_3 and T_4 with high TSH) should be done. Except histochemical studies, done only in very few centres, no specific clinching investigation is available.

Treatment

In minimal enlargements, hormone therapy (thyroxine 100mcg/day) may be tried initially. Surgery (subtotal excision) is done for cosmetic reasons or tracheal/esophageal compression, to be followed by life long thyroxine replacement.

2) SIMPLE GOITER, better called diffuse hyperplastic goiter, is the name given to thyroid enlargement, due to no fault of the gland, under the influence of TSH, which may be of endemic, physiological or colloid types.

a) Endemic goiter is seen in populations consuming a diet deficient in iodine, and in certain belts with low levels of iodine in drinking water, affecting almost all those living in such areas. Presentation and treatment is similar to genetic type, but these goiters are preventable by dietary iodine supplement. Statutory requirement of iodizing cooking salt has totally eliminated this disease in developed count-

ries. Typically there is dissociation of the values of two important investigations, i.e., normal or low levels of T_3 and T_4, but increased uptake of radioiodine (as seen in hyperthyroidism), due to a high affinity (or avidity) of the gland for iodine (iodine hungry). This phenomenon is seen in any disease associated with iodine deficiency, relative or absolute. Attributable to the influence of persistently high levels of TSH, these goiters are more prone to develop follicular carcinoma, in the long run.

b) Physiological goiter is better termed *stress-induced* goiter, since it is the result of increased demand of thyroid hormones, during periods of stress, either physiological (puberty, pregnancy, lactation etc) or pathological (a focus of chronic sepsis, such as tonsillitis or dental infection). Human chorionic gonadotrophin has TSH receptor stimulating property, which may explain goiter developing during pregnancy.

Commonly seen in females around puberty, it presents as a minimal diffuse firm enlargement of thyroid, in clinically euthyroid state. Serum levels of thyroid hormones are normal, with elevated TSH. Small dose of thyroxine (50-100mcg/day) will generally make the gland regress, but may have to be taken for over an year. Rarely it may fail to do so, transforming itself into a colloid type.

c) Colloid goiter is a distinct entity of unclear etiology, seen mostly in women in child-bearing age. It is considered to be due to a disturbance in the normal cyclical hyperplasia and involution process taking place in the gland, where it gets

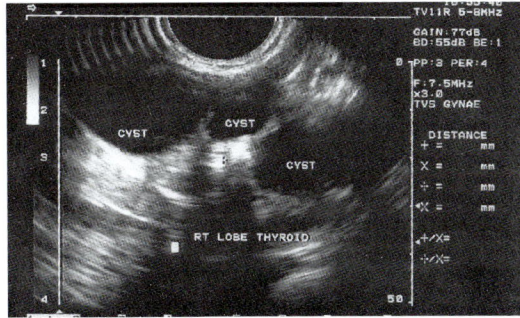

Fig. 87.5. USG of thyroid showing multiple colloid cysts
(courtesy: Halsted Surgical Clinic, Chennai)

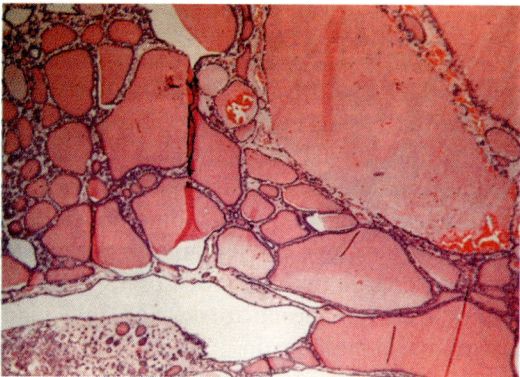

Fig. 87.6. Histology of colloid goiter
(courtesy: Histo Lab, Chennai)

arrested in a state of hyperplasia. If the pathology is of uniform nature, it results in *diffuse colloid goiter*, if it has patchy distribution, a *multinodular goiter* (MNG) develops and if the involvement is unifocal, a *solitary* colloid nodule (SNG) is the result. The subtle role played by increased TSH is also blamed in the etiology altering the mitotic cycle of the follicles. The patient is usually euthyroid and unlike stress (physiological) goiter, its response to medical therapy is poor.

Differential diagnosis

Stress-induced and inflammatory goiters.

Investigations

Hormone profile to assess the functional status and USG of neck to differentiate a diffuse from nodular variety and in the latter, whether single (SNG) or multiple (MNG) and solid or cystic.

Treatment: Hormone therapy is initially given to avoid even a remote chance of unnecessary surgery, which (subtotal thyroidectomy) is done mostly for cosmetic purpose, the other indications being pressure effects and fear of toxicity. Life long hormone replacement may be needed following surgery.

3) INFLAMMATORY GOITERS: They are acute, subacute and chronic thyroiditis

a) Acute thyroiditis is often viral or bacterial in etiology, presenting as an acute diffuse goiter, usually following an attack of respiratory infection. An autoimmune thyroiditis may also have an acute presentation. Fever, local pain, warmth and tenderness are present, sometimes associated with dysphagia. Occasionally it assumes an asymmetrical shape, due to suppuration and abscess formation in the gland substance. A course of antibiotics and NSAIDs may suffice, surgery required only to drain an abscess. If it cannot be differentiated from the subacute type, a short course of steroids should be given, as a therapeutic trial.

b) Subacute (de Quervain's) thyroiditis (syn: granulomatous thyroiditis) is considered mostly autoimmune, though it also often follows a recent upper respiratory infection or 'flu', thus incriminating viral infection also in its causation. A painful thyroid swelling of few weeks duration, associated with constitutional symptoms, is typical. A minimally enlarged warm, tender, firm gland is seen, usually without regional lymphadenopathy. There may be a transient hyperthyroidism, due to increased vascularity of the gland, that soon reverts to the euthyroid state.

Differential diagnosis

Acute and chronic thyroiditis

Investigations

Leukocytosis and elevated ESR may be present.

Thyroid antibodies may be present in some cases; thyroid hormone profile may initially show elevated T_3 and T_4, with low TSH level and ^{131}I uptake value, later becoming normal.

Treatment

Antibiotics and NSAIDs may relieve symptoms, but the sheet anchor of therapy is steroids, prednisolone 20-30mg/day, in divided doses, given for 4-8weeks. The resolution of the painful goiter is so dramatic, that it is often used as a 'therapeutic test', so that if it is not responding to steroid therapy, within 2-3 weeks, the diagnosis needs to be reviewed. These drugs may be tapered over a period of 4-8 weeks and stopped.

c) Chronic thyroiditis: These are Hashimoto's and Riedel's goiter and tuberculous thyroiditis.

I) Hashimoto's thyroiditis (syn: struma lymphomatosa, lymphadenoid goiter)This auto-immune disorder leads to gradual destruction of follicles with lymphoid infiltration and eventual fibrosis. It may be inherited as an autosomal dominant trait and is typically seen in postmenopausal women, with a firm or rubbery diffuse (occasionally localized) enlargement. It is known to predispose to non-Hodgkin's lymphoma (NHL) of the thyroid gland. *This disease is the commonest cause of adult hypothyroidism, all over the world.*

Clinical features

They present with tightness in the neck, thyromegaly and in longstanding cases, hypothyroidism, replacing an initial transient hyperfunction (Hashitoxicosis). *It may be stated that any long standing goiter of several years, but still in euthyroid state, is against the diagnosis of Hashimoto's disease.* A diffusely enlarged gland with a bosselated surface and some restriction of intrinsic mobility may be diagnostic. Minimal hepatosplenomegaly may be corroborative to the diagnosis of autoimmune disease. Features of tracheal/ esophageal compression may be present in large goiters, but recurrent laryngeal nerves are spared. Relentless enlargement of the gland, despite thyroxine/steroid therapy must alert the clinician to the possibility of lymphoma developing in such a gland.

Differential diagnosis

Diffuse colloid goiter, MNG, subacute thyroiditis, NHL etc.

Investigations

Antithyroglobulin antibodies (ATGA) and thyroid antimicrosomal antibodies (TAMA) may be found in serum, but not pathognomonic of this disease. FNAC not only clinches the diagnosis, but excludes a lymphoma, developing in Hashimoto's thyroiditis.

Treatment

Unless compressive symptoms or cosmetic considerations exist, hormone therapy is initiated, regression may be anticipated in early cases and in younger patients. Steroids are not indicated, in view of their unwanted effects from long term therapy. However a short course of steroid may be given for acute local manifestations, to provide symptomatic relief.

Indications for surgery are pressure effects, cosmesis and suspected malignancy. Subtotal or near total thyroidectomy has to be performed and hormone therapy continued for an indefinite period of time.

If NHL is diagnosed, it may be treated by radio/chemotherapy, on its merits and role of surgery is extremely limited.

ii) Riedel's thyroiditis
(syn: woody thyroid)

It is a rare inflammatory disease of unclear etiology, characterized by dense invasive fibrosis, extending beyond the gland, involving strap muscles, trachea, esophagus, carotid sheath etc., probably related to generalized fibrosclerosis, which causes a similar process in areas like retroperitoneum, mediastinum, lacrimal glands, bile ducts etc. The other explanation, that it is an autoimmune disease and may be the end stage of Hashimoto's disease, does not enjoy much patronage.

Clinical features
Progressive compressive symptoms, such as dyspnea, hoarseness, stridor or dysphagia, dominate the picture, with a moderate sized, hard, nontender, diffuse goiter, moving minimally with deglutition, but virtually without intrinsic mobility. Total destruction of the thyroid will lead to hypothyroidism in due course. Involvement of recurrent laryngeal nerves by fibrosis, will produce vocal cord palsy. Occasionally it may be associated with retroperitoneal fibrosis.

Differential diagnosis
1) anaplastic carcinoma (large, rapidly increasing irregular swelling, with early nodal and distant spread)

2) lymphoma of thyroid, which is of the non-Hodgkin's type

Investigations

Thyroid profile, to assess the functional status

Laryngoscopic examination to see the movement of the vocal cords

Chest/neck x-ray to see the tracheal compression or pulmonary secondaries (in Ca)

FNAC to exclude malignancy

Treatment

Medical: NSAIDs, steroids, tamoxifen citrate and stanozolol have all been tried with some success. Thyroxine replacement is necessary in the later stages.

Surgical: It is technically difficult, in view of loss of tissue planes and fibrous infiltration. Excision of isthmus (isthmusectomy), not only establishes the diagnosis, but divides the constricting thyroid tissue, allowing the lobes to fall apart. This is the safest and most popular procedure done. Sharp dissection may be needed to separate the gland from the trachea, carefully avoiding 'button-holing' it. Any attempt to identify the recurrent laryngeal nerves is unsafe and unwarranted.

iii) Tuberculous thyroiditis is a rare disease, associated with a diffuse tender goiter, regional lymphadenopathy, evidence of pulmonary tuberculosis and constitutional symptoms. Often a node biopsy clinches the diagnosis, supported by high ESR and immunological tests. Treatment is by anti-tuberculous chemotherapy for 6-9 months, depending upon the clinical response. Cold abscess may need aspiration/drainage under cover of drug therapy.

4) SOLITARY NODULAR GOITER (SNG) (syn: clinically discrete nodule)

The conditions clinically presenting as an SNG are:
a)   colloid nodule or cyst
b)   dominant nodule of an MNG
c)   focal thyroiditis
d)   true neoplasms
    l)   adenoma (commonest, 30% of SNGs)
    ii) carcinoma

a) Colloid nodule develops as a variant of diffuse colloid goiter (vide supra), with focal hyperplasia of follicles, and with accumulation of colloid it may become cystic. It may also develop from colloid degeneration of an adenoma. It is a painless nonfunctioning nodule, without appreciable rate of growth nor risk of toxicity/malignancy. After USG confirmation, hormone therapy may be safely tried, to see the response. A cyst may be aspirated and fluid sent for cytology, the gland being immediately palpated for any residual mass, which differentiates a simple from a neoplastic cyst. Surgery (hemithyroidectomy) is required, only if it shows enlargement, compression or cytological suspicion of malignancy.

b) Dominant nodule of MNG (see under MNG)

c) Focal thyroiditis usually develops into a unilateral swelling; the nodule may be indistinct, without a tendency to 'slip under the palpating finger', since the intrinsic mobility is restricted by inflammatory reaction. USG and FNAC may be useful to clinch the diagnosis and

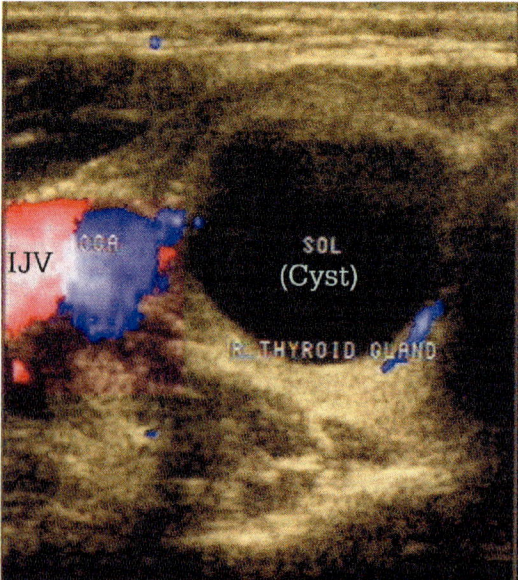

Fig. 87.7. Color scan (USG) of thyroid showing a large simple (colloid) cyst
(courtesy: Halsted Surgical Clinic, Chennai)

having excluded malignancy by cytology, treatment is only conservative.

d) ADENOMA is the commonest disease presenting as SNG, hence it may be given out as the provisional diagnosis, if no obvious features of malignancy are present, adding the other conditions under differential diagnosis.

Types of adenoma: *Follicular* adenoma (more common), which may be:

i)   embryonal (columns of cells, with little attempt to form follicles or colloid)

ii) fetal or microfollicular (with miniature follicles and scanty colloid)

iii) simple (resembles normal gland architecture)

iv) colloid or macrofollicular (excessive accumulation of colloid in dilated follicles)

v)   Hurthle-cell (large polygonal cells with abundant acidophilic cytoplasm, arranged in solid masses or columns, in the outer surface of the follicles, not unlike that seen in liver)

Papillary adenoma is much less common than follicular, with characteristic papillary processes wth delicate fronds of epithelium, which may be evident to close observation by naked eye. Most workers strongly feel that there is no such entity as a 'benign' papillary adenoma and they only represent highly differentiated carcinoma.

Investigations

Most of the controversies in relation to management of goiters, are centered around SNG, as it is the most common presentation of malignancy. The two primary objectives of investigations are to exclude malignancy and toxicity, priorities being guided by the clinical probabilities.

I)   *Sleeping pulse rate* should be the normal pulse rate. If necessary, mild sedation may be given to induce sleep, when anxiety-related tachycardia disappears, but organic reasons persist. Normal pulse rate reasonably excludes thyrotoxicosis, but persistent tachycardia is by no means diagnostic and its value is limited to assessing clinical improvement with treatment.

ii) *Biochemistry:* plasma sugar, cholesterol, creatinine and urinary creatinine, protein bound iodine (PBI), butanol extractable iodine (BEI), direct T_3/T_4/TSH radioimmunoassay. The TSH elevation is more sensitive to detect subclinical hypothyroidism, where T_3 and T_4 may be normal.

The thyroid hormones bound to proteins are not physiologically active and total T_3 and T_4 levels may not reflect the functional status of the gland. Resin uptake and free hormone (T_3 and T_4) index may be useful, to assess the functional activity, especially if there is serum protein abnormality.

iii) *Basal metabolic rate* (BMR) is based on the fact that oxygen consumption by an individual at basal conditions is proportionate to metabolic rate, per unit surface area. It is not very popular because it is difficult to bring the patient to the basal conditions prescribed, it is very cumbersome and false low values may be reported if the patient has perforated ear drums, because he also 'breathes through the ears' (normal range is -20% to +20%).

iv) ^{131}I uptake (normally 20-40% of isotope

T_3	T_4	TSH	^{131}I Uptake	Disease
Normal	Normal	High	High	Physiological goiter
Low	Low	High	Low	Primary hypothyroidism Dyshormonogenic goiter
Low	Low	High	High	Endemic goiter Iodine deficiency
High	High	Low	High	Thyrotoxicosis (primary & secondary)
High	Normal	Low	High	T_3 toxicosis
High	High	Low	Low	Toxic thyroiditis Factitious thyrotoxicosis

Table-87.1. Hormone levels and uptake values in various diseases of thyroid

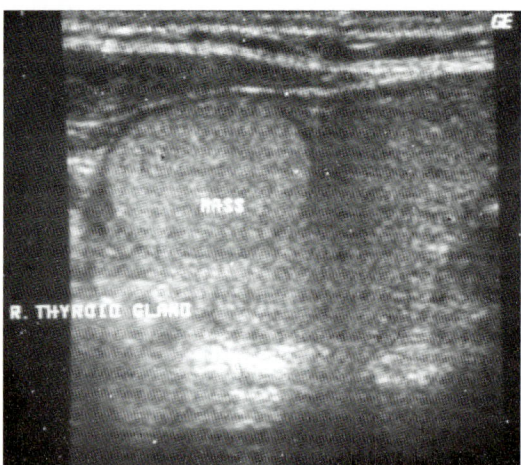

Fig. 87.8. USG of thyroid showing a discrete nodule (adenoma)
(courtesy: Halsted Surgical Clinic, Chennai)

pertechnetate, for their shorter half-life and lower radiation dose delivered to the gland. The half-life of ^{123}I is 13 hours and ^{99m}Tc is 6 hours. The radiation dose received by thyroid gland during ^{99m}Tc scanning has been calculated to be 1/10,000, compared to ^{131}I scanning.

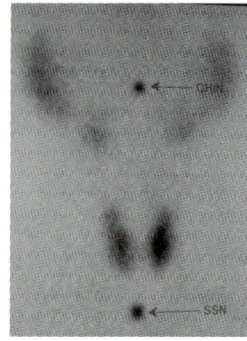

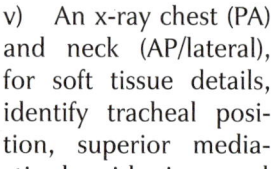

Fig. 87.10. ^{99m}Tc scintiscan of thyroid, showing a filling defect in the right upper pole. Note the isotope detected in the salivary glands.
(courtesy: Halsted Surgical Clinic, Chennai)

administered is taken up in 24hrs):This isotope with a half-life of 7 days, is given orally on the previous day and uptake by the gland is measured after 24hours. A scintiscan is also routinely done at the same time, to outline the gland including any retrosternal extension, to see areas of hypo and hyperactivity (cold and hot spots respectively), to detect ectopic gland tissue and functioning secondaries in the vicinity. As the diagnostic dose of isotope is in microcuries, radiation hazard is negligible, as against the therapeutic dose, which is in millicuries (thousand times), with considerable risk.

Other isotopes preferred in some centres for thyroid scanning are ^{123}I and ^{99m}Tc -

v) An x-ray chest (PA) and neck (AP/lateral), for soft tissue details, identify tracheal position, superior mediastinal widening and pulmonary/pleural/nodal/skeletal secondaries. In large adenomas the trachea may be grossly displaced to opposite side, precariously compressed, assuming the shape of a sword (*scabbard trachea*).

vi) USG/CT/MRI scan: these are very useful to detect nonpalpable nodules, to differentiate simple and neoplastic cysts, detect preclinical cervical lymph nodes, retrosternal extension, tracheal infiltration etc. MRI is very useful in assessing recurrent disease, to distinguish tumor from scar tissue.

vii) Biopsy: whenever the diagnosis of malignancy is under active consideration, establish-

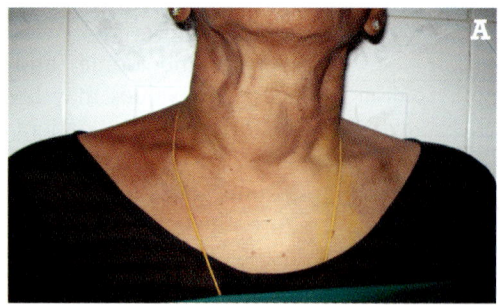

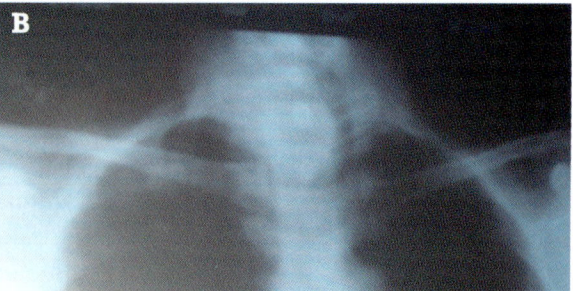

Fig. 87.9. A. Large adenoma, right lobe of thyroid
B. Chest x-ray showing grossly deviated tracheal shadow (to left)
(scabbard trachea)

ing tissue diagnosis is crucial to management. Several types of biopsies are available, to choose from:

1) *needle biopsy* : Fine needle aspiration cytology (FNAC), drill and wide-bore (Trucut) needle biopsy. If the nodule is over 3cm diameter, wide-bore needle biopsy is preferable to FNAC. One important limitation of needle biopsy is with follicular carcinoma, since it is diagnosed only by vascular/capsular invasion; this is not made out in cytology specimens and it is therefore not possible to clinch the issue with certainty. Detection of normal levels of thyroid peroxidase by immunohistochemistry in needle biopsy specimen is in favor of a benign lesion.

2) fluid *aspiration cytology* from a cyst
3) *open* or *wedge* biopsy
4) *excision* or enucleation biopsy (rarely done)
5) post-thyroidectomy biopsy

viii) Indirect laryngoscopy (IDL), to document mobility of vocal cords preoperatively, is of great medicolegal significance, besides its diagnostic value in malignancy and incidental neuropathy.

Treatment

Definitive treatment for an adenoma is surgery; medical therapy is indicated only if

(1) colloid nodule/cyst or other non-neoplastic conditions can not be excluded,

(2) very small, FNAC-negative lesions. Even if it does not regress, sometimes a few months of hormone therapy makes the patient 'earn' the operation. Hemithyroidectomy (excision of a lobe and isthmus) is the standard operation for an adenoma, though some aggressive oncologists advise total extirpation, under the pretext that the benign nature of an 'adenoma' cannot be inferred with certainty, despite all the available preoperative investigations. This approach has thankfully few protagonists, especially in this era charged with conservative/organ preserving philosophy.

Hemithyroidectomy vs lobectomy

Hemithyroidectomy (and not simple excision or lobectomy) is advocated for adenoma for sev-

eral reasons: firstly it has no true capsule, allowing tiny 'pseudopodia' of tumor to invade the adjacent gland, secondly in an unpleasant surprise event of the final biopsy reporting malignancy, a reoperation to remove the remaining lobe is not needed in the opinion of the large majority of surgeons (except in medullary carcinoma) and lastly, if the rest of the gland undergoes compensatory hypertrophy, swelling of the isthmus should not cause cosmetic problems.

An adenoma detected during routine ultrasound examination of neck (incidentaloma) should be kept under surveillance and treated on its merits.

e) CARCINOMA

No other malignancy shows such a wide range of biological behavior as thyroid carcinoma. At one end there is the highly differentiated cystic papillary carcinoma, occurring in women under 25, extremely slow growing, spreading only to cervical nodes, easily amenable to surgery and running a' benign' course. At the other extreme, there is the highly anaplastic tumor, with rapid growth, spreading by all modalities, with virtually no survivals after one year of diagnosis and considered an oncological disaster.

Histological types are:

A) *Differentiated*
   i) Papillary... 72% (20-40yrs) 'lateral aberrant thyroid'... 5% (metastatic papillary carcinoma in the nodes)

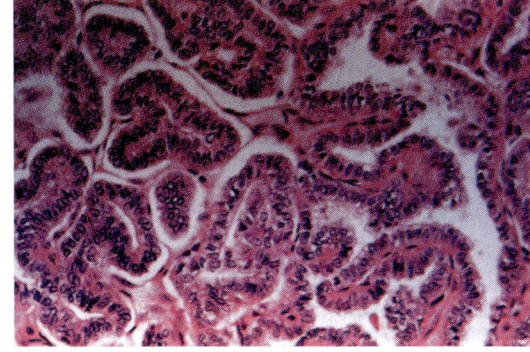

Fig. 87.11. Histology of papillary carcinoma
Thyroid
(courtesy: Histo Lab, Chennai)

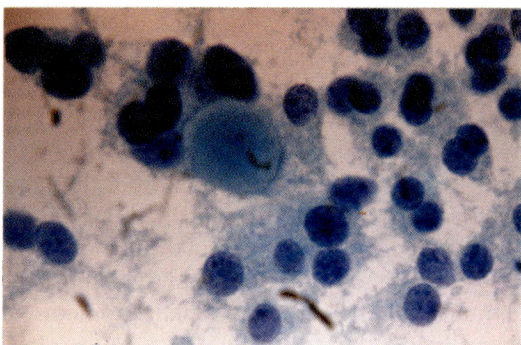

Fig. 87.12. FNAC of thyroid carcinoma
(courtesy: Histo Lab, Chennai)

ii) Follicular … 16% (30-50yrs)
  Hurthle-cell type … 4%
  Benign metastasizing goiter … rare
iii) Medullary … 3% (30-50yrs)

B) *Undifferentiated*
  Anaplastic… 8% (>50yrs)

C) *Lymphoma*…<1%(>50yrs) almost always an NHL (on Hashimoto's), but very rarely it may occur in patients <20, as a feature of Burkitt's tumor, prevalent in Africa and Guinea.

D) *Miscellaneous*… Epidermoid, metastatic carcinoma and fibrosarcoma are pathological curiosities.

Features of malignancy in a goiter

Presentation as nontoxic solitary nodule (except the anaplastic type, which rapidly spreads through the entire gland, and lymphoma), is typical. Other features are rapid rate of growth

(except papillary type), local pain, hard consistency, restricted mobility (intrinsic and with deglutition), early appearance of pressure symptoms (out of proportion to the size of the goiter), and evidence of regional/distant spread.

Plain x-ray may show stippled calcification (*psammoma bodies*) and tracheal compression. Scintiscan may reveal a cold nodule and functioning secondaries.

Appropriate biopsy will clinch the matter; however a 'negative' report in a needle biopsy cannot guarantee benignancy of a goiter.

The incidence of malignancy in solitary nodules in general is around 5% and jumps to 15-20%, in cold (nonfunctioning) nodules, whereas it is only <1% in functioning nodules, which implies that all solitary cold nodules should be either biopsied or resected. As in other lesions of the

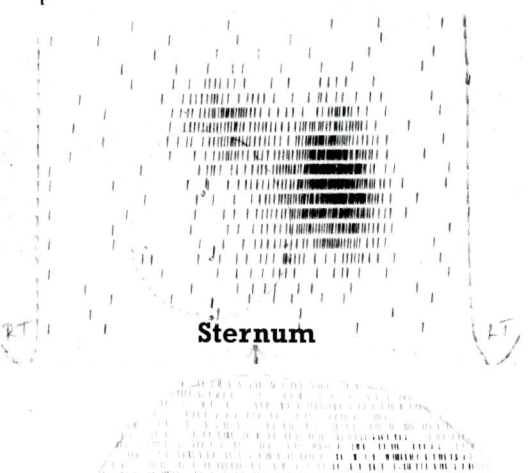

Sternum

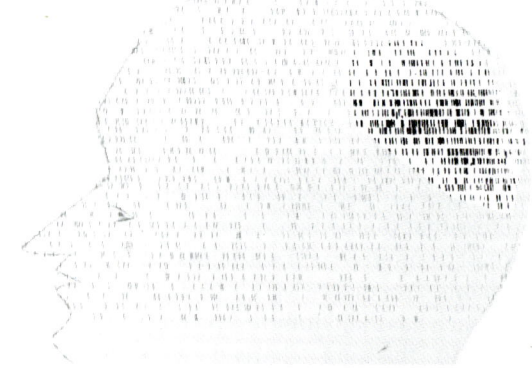

Fig. 87.13. ^{131}I scan of neck showing filling defect (carcinoma) in the right lobe
87.13. Metastatic tumor in the scalp concentrating iodine
(courtesy: Halsted Surgical Clinic, Chennai)

Jewels of Gyan - 87.2

Tumor - Hot & Cold

A question that often worries a student is why the primary tumor is cold and the secondaries are hot; it should be realized that it is only *relative to the surrounding tissue.* Since the normal thyroid gland concentrates iodine, the lesser active tumor area appears cold, whereas the iodine pickup by other parts of the body is so low, that the more active thyroid secondary appears hot.

thyroid, carcinoma has a female preponderance (3:1). The lymph nodal secondaries from papillary carcinoma have some special features: they may be occult, extremely slow growing (sometimes years), intracapsular, cystic, show bluish discoloration and do not significantly influence the prognosis.

Etiology

1) Age distribution (vide supra)

2) Sex: Female preponderance (3:1). An 'adenoma' in males has always to be viewed with suspicion.

3) Endemic goiters have a higher incidence of malignancy due to TSH influence

4) Radiation: This is historical; in the last century, certain benign diseases in the face and neck, such as acne, scrofuloderma, tuberculous cervical lymphadenitis, chronic tonsillitis, thymic enlargement etc. in children were treated by ionizing radiation, which was responsible for the development of cancers of thyroid decades later; however these were mostly well differentiated and carried good prognosis. Increased incidence of carcinoma in children exposed to radiation was noted after the nuclear bombing of Hiroshima and Nagasaki in Japan.

5) Benign lesions (adenoma usually predisposes to papillary and MNG to follicular type).

6) Multiple endocrine neoplasia syndromes, MEN-2A (Sipple) and 2B are associated with medullary thyroid carcinoma (MTC). Familial medullary thyroid carcinoma (FMTC) constitutes 10 to 20% of MTC.

7) Hashimoto's thyroiditis is known to predispose to lymphoma of thyroid

8) PTC may occasionally be familial, in association with Gardner's syndrome

Special investigations for malignancies

1) skiagram of chest and neck

2) laryngoscopic examination

3) USG/CT/MRI of neck to see the extent of local invasion

4) Scintiscan with ^{131}I, ^{123}I or ^{99m}Tc; a cold nodule has a higher incidence of malignancy. A cold solitary nodule has 20% chance of being malignant, whereas it is only <1% in a functional nodule. Iodine scintiscan also picks up functional secondaries, hence whole body scan is performed, if dissemination of differentiated cancer is suspected. Tc-labelled sestamibi is usefull for identifying MTC. Selenomethionine scan, earlier considered useful to detect active mitosis, has not been very reliable since not all thyroid cancers show rapid growth; this is no longer done.

5) tumor markers: thyroglobulin for papillary/follicular carcinoma
Calcitonin, CEA, serotonin and calcitonin gene-related peptide(CGRP) for MTC

6) needle biopsy or cytology of the thyroid nodule or a secondary deposit

Staging of thyroid carcinoma is done either by TNMG method or AGES (Mayo Clinic, USA): **a**ge, histological **g**rade, **e**xtrathyroid disease (loco-regional and distant) and **s**ize of the tumor.

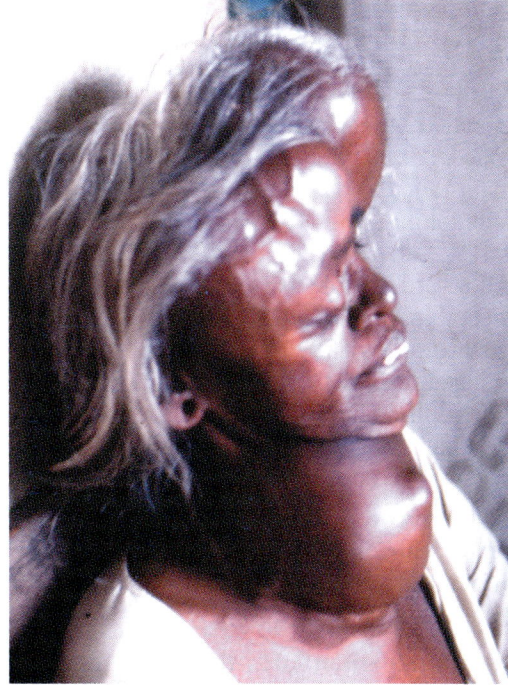

Fig. 87.14. Advanced follicular carcinoma with large skull secondaries (courtesy: Prof. S Vittal, Chennai)

Treatment

Total thyroidectomy is the treatment of choice, whenever possible, for differentiated thyroid cancers, but has limited value in anaplastic carcinoma and lymphoma. The term *near-total* thyroidectomy has been coined, to remind an over-zealous surgeon to leave behind a few grams of thyroid tissue posteriorly, necessary to preserve parathyroids and their blood supply, in the interests of avoiding metabolic crippling.

Lymph nodes : The most common site of lymph node involvement is in the central compartment (level 6), the jugular lymph node chains (levels 2-4) are the next most common sites of cervical node involvement.

In PTC, there appears to be some advantage in removing paratracheal nodes, situated along the ipsilateral recurrent laryngeal nerve, even though they are not grossly involved, at the time of initial surgery.

It should be realized that as in the neck, levels of nodes is only for anatomic description, but not indicative of stage of the disease.

RaI (^{131}I) ablation therapy : Patients with medullary, anaplastic, and most Hurthle cell cancers do not benefit from this therapy. Once metastatic thyroid cancer becomes resistant to radioiodine, the 10-year survival drops to <15%. A promising new development for follow-up thyroid scanning is the use of recombinant human TSH as opposed to thyroid hormone withdrawal to increase the endogenous TSH levels. The optimal level of TSH suppression for treating PTC, is to bring it to <0.5 mU/L in high risk patients and <1 mU/L in low risk group (normal TSH level : 0.3 to 5.0)

With chemotherapy and targeted therapy occasional objective responses have been documented, their protocols are being evaluated.

The management of individual tumors

PAPILLARY THYROID CARCINOMA (PTC), which includes mixed papillary follicular tumor, is fortunately the most common and least malignant of all. Occurring in younger ages (20-40), it spreads mainly by direct invasion or lymphatics and almost never beyond the neck. A characteristic fibrovascular stroma with calcification (psammoma bodies) may be present. The differentiation may be so high that it closely resembles normal thyroid, extraglandular spread being the only clue to its real nature. Another distinctive feature of this tumor is the presence of optically clear large nuclei with a pale staining 'ground-glass' appearance, known as 'Orphan Annie eye nuclei". Cervical lymph nodal deposits are notorious for their slow growth and extreme differentiation, justifying the earlier misnomer, *lateral aberrant thyroid*, much against any embryological explanation, now known as papillary microcarcinoma (PMC). Well differentiated PTC enjoys over 80% 10-year cure rate. There is no place for 'prophylactic' node dissection, but enlarged cervical nodes are treated by functional modified block dissection. The earlier practiced node (berry) picking operation, is no longer acceptable and is to be discarded. Late nodal recurrence is to be expected which may be considerably reduced by postoperative adjuvant RaI ablative therapy, to address micrometastases. With low diagnostic sensitivity, thyroglobulin as a tumor marker is useful for detecting tumor recurrence, during follow up of differentiated tumors.

Prognostic factors: AGES scale: younger age, with well differentiated tumor, without extraglandular spread and a small primary lesion, confer the best prognosis. This is the only thyroid tumor with established hormone (TSH) dependency; hence they should receive suppressive doses of thyroxine (0.2-0.3mg/day), for an indefinite period of time, following histologic confirmation of the type of tumor. A tall cell variant of PTC appears to carry slightly unfavorable prognosis.

FOLLICULAR THYROID CARCINOMA (FTC) (syn: alveolar carcinoma) is more aggressive and takes up more iodine than the papillary type.

Feature	Papillary	Follicular	Medullary	Anaplastic
Incidence	60%	15%	5%	10%
Age	20-40yrs	30-50yrs	30-50yrs	>50yrs
Clinical presentation	Goiter with neck nodes	Goiter with bone mets	Not specific	Goiter with fixity, stridor
Rate of growth	Slow	Moderate	Moderate	Rapid
Spread	Lymphatics	Blood stream	Blood stream	All modalities
Microscopy	Orphan Annie eye nuclei Psommoma bodies	Angio invasion Capsular invasion	Amyloid stroma	Poorly differented
Hormone dependency	Often (TSH)	No	No	No
Genetic tendency	No	No	Yes (autosome-10)	No
Tumor markers	Thyroglobulin	Thyroglobulin	Calcitonin, CEA serotonin, CGRP	None
Ral therapy	Effective	Effective	No effect	No effect
Prognosis	Excellent	Good	Good	Dismal

CEA: carcinoembryonic antigen CGRP: calcitonin gene-related peptide
Table-87.2. Features of various types of thyroid malignancies

Occurring between 30-50years, it spreads mostly by the blood stream, to lungs and bones. It is often difficult to distinguish it from an adenoma, unless capsular and vascular invasion is identified on histology. Total body isotope scan or positron emission tomography (PET) CT scan is necessary to detect distant spread before surgery, but their affinity to pick up iodine is enhanced by prior extirpation of the normal gland, a principle utilized in postoperative adjuvant Ral therapy (radioisotopic ablation of disseminated disease).

MEDULLARY THYROID CARCINOMA (MTC) or HYALINE CARCINOMA belongs to *APUD tumors* (amine precursor uptake and decarboxylation), arising from calcitonin-producing parafollicular (C) cells, with a distinct familial tendency in about 10-20% of cases (FMTC). In association with parathyroid tumor/ hyperplasia and pheochromocytoma, it constitutes *MEN-2A (Sipple) syndrome and 2B* (in addition to 2A,

ganglioneuromatosis, mucosal neuromas and megacolon), hence the need to screen for the other two as a routine, is obvious. With the same age group as the follicular type, it is moderately aggressive, known for its multicentric origin and spreads by all routes. It secretes mostly calcitonin, a parathormone antagonist, which is used as a tumor marker, but also many other peptides, such as carcinoembryonic antigen (CEA), histaminase, calcitonin gene related peptide (CGRP), serotonin and prostaglandins-E_2 and F_2, which are used in immunohistochemistry for tissue diagnosis. Due to ectopic production of ACTH as a paraneoplastic manifestation, occasional features of Cushing's syndrome may be seen. However, sporadic (non-familial) cases constitute 80% of MTC.

Postive family history, finding a nontoxic solitary thyroid nodule, elevated calcitonin and CEA and FNAC of the nodule are helpful in the diagnosis of MTC. The first degree relatives of the patient have to be screened by tumor markers (if necessary by *provoking* with calcium or pentagastrin) and if positive, close surveillance is mandatory. Autosome-10 is identified to be carrying the gene responsible for MTC (Ret proto-oncogene); hence it is now possible to screen the family members and children at risk, so that the appropriate follow up may be done. An aggressive group believes that total thyroidectomy for those with elevated calcitonin, is indicated as 'prophylaxis', which sounds logical but not practical. Radioiodine scan is useless in MTC, since it does not concentrate iodine. The scintiscans of choice are, ^{99m}Tc-labeled sestamibi (this is also useful to image parathyroids) and Indium-labeled octreotide.

Treatment

Total thyroidectomy with nodal dissection of the *central* compartment (triangle between both internal jugular veins and aero-digestive structures) is the treatment of choice, even if nodes are not clinically involved. If the excised nodes are microscopically positive or there is obvious involvement of lateral nodes, a standard radical neck dissection, on one or both sides, should be performed. There is no place for hormone or chemotherapy and MTC is poorly radiosensitive.

ANAPLASTIC OR UNDIFFERENTIATED THYROID CARCINOMA (ATC): This is the worst of all, with virtually no one-year survivals, after diagnosis. It is of two types, *small-cell type*, histologically mimicking NHL, and carrying a slightly better prognosis, and the *giant-cell type*, the most virulent of all thyroid tumors, microscopically resembling anaplastic fibrosarcoma. It spreads by all modalities, quickly causing local pressure symptoms. As surgery of any kind has not been shown to influence the ultimate outcome, many prefer not to operate, if a preoperative diagnosis of anaplastic tumor is made.

Mutation of P53 gene is present in most of the cases of anaplastic carcinoma. Mucomycin is found to block the specific proto-oncogene and the tumor growth.

LYMPHOMA: As mentioned, it is almost always an NHL and occurs commonly in the backdrop of Hashimoto's thyroiditis in patients >40, and as a feature of Burkitt's lymphoma, in patients <20. It is treated by radio/chemotherapy as for NHL, role of surgery is limited to establishing the diagnosis (biopsy). Prognosis of this disease is excellent, with >80% cure rate.

Histological surprise: There is considerable controversy regarding the management of a patient, who has undergone hemithyroidectomy for a 'benign nodule', wherein the final pathology report reveals malignancy. Needless to say, it largely depends on the cell type: some broad guidelines are given here:

Regardless of the cell type, all patients have to be re-examined clinically and by imaging modalities, to establish the stage of disease, before further treatment can be planned.

Jewels of Gyan - 87.3

Multiple Endocrine Neoplasia (MEN) Syndromes (APUD system)

MEN-1 (Wermer) : Tumor/hyperplasia of parathyroid, pituitary and pancreatic islets

MEN-2A (Sipple) : Tumor/hyperplasia of parathyroid, medullary thyroid carcinoma and pheochromocytoma, due to defective chromosome-10

MEN-2B : In addition to 2A, ganglioneuromatosis, mucosal neuromas and megacolon.

Carney's complex is a multiple neoplasia syndrome, comprising of myxomatous neoplasms (cardiac, endocrine, cutaneous and neural) and a host of pigmented lesions of skin and mucosae, including a rarely occurring epitheloid blue nevus.

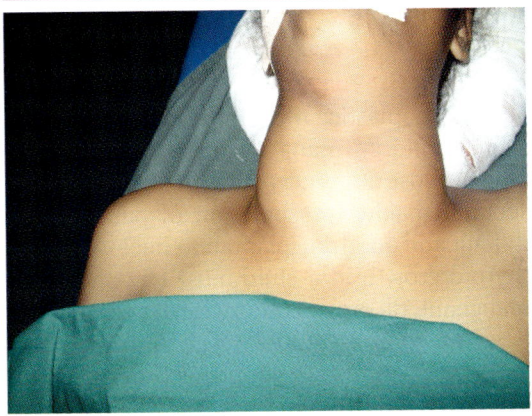

Fig. 87.15. Diffuse toxic goiter
(Graves' disease)

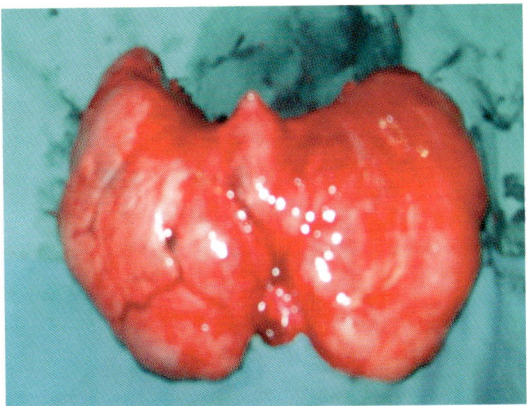

Fig. 87.16. Surgical specimen of subtotal thyroidectomy
(courtesy: Laxmi Hospital, Kakinada)

i) papillary carcinoma: if no cervical nodes are detected clinically or by ultrasonography, no further surgery is necessary, except RaI ablation suppressive dose (0.2-0.3mg/day) of thyroxine and close follow up, by periodic thyroglobulin (tumor marker) assay. Recurrent disease may appear either in the remaining lobe, ipsilateral or contralateral cervical lymph nodes. If it is in the remaining lobe, completion thyroidectomy is indicated. If the nodes on the same side are involved, a functional neck dissection has to be done. If the recurrence is in the nodes on the opposite side, completion thyroidectomy and node excision will be necessary. Advocates of a more aggressive approach by carrying out completion total thyroidectomy, on receiving the biopsy report, give multicentricity of the tumor as the reason, but the fact that most recurrences are seen in the nodes and not in the residual gland, does not support this view. Furthermore, there is no evidence that total thyroidectomy has any advantage over limited surgery in the long run, but certainly has a greater incidence of laryngeal nerve and parathyroid morbidity.

ii) follicular carcinoma: in addition to the above, a whole body ^{131}I screening is necessary to detect occult spread and if necessary, radioisotopic ablation may be done, to hit the remote targets with 'guided missiles'. Completion thyroidectomy, to facilitate isotope trapping by the secondaries has been advised;

however its benefit has to be extrapolated against the morbidity of another surgery (physical and emotional) and parathyroid crippling, in a given case. With advances in nuclear medicine, it is possible to initially saturate the normal thyroid with iodine and administer another dose to hit the secondaries, thus obviating reoperation.

iii) medullary carcinoma (MTC): In addition to general evaluation, calcitonin (tumor marker) screening should be done on the patient, as well as for the first degree relatives. As part of the MEN syndrome, tumors of other endocrine glands, such as parathyroid and adrenal medulla (pheochromocytoma) have to be excluded before further treatment can be chalked out. In view of its well documented multicentric nature, completion thyroidectomy is clearly indicated for MTC along with nodal dissection, if they are involved. It has no affinity to iodine; hence isotope therapy or hormone suppression treatment have no place. However, external radiation to the neck may be given for locally advanced tumors if the cancer clearance has been less than ideal, during surgery.

iv) anaplastic carcinoma : The role of surgery being limited, in terms of improving survival, the wisdom of operating in the first place itself is questionable, much less reoperation. After a quick general assessment and a PET scan (for

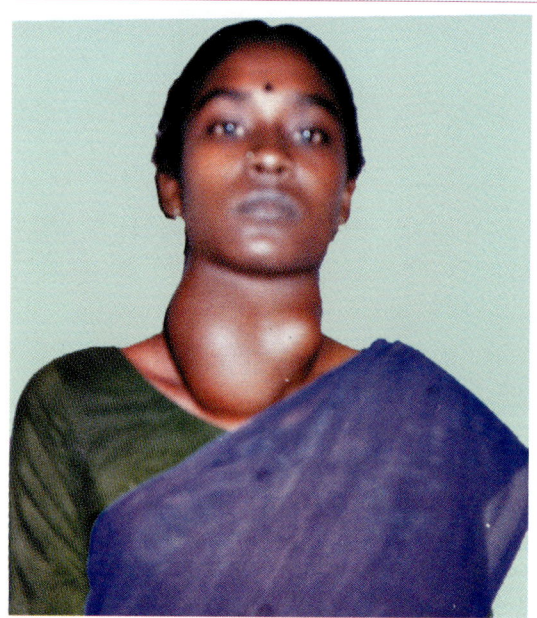

Fig. 87.17. Multinodular goiter
(courtesy: Halsted Surgical Clinic, Chennai)

staging, since the tumor does not pick up iodine), external radiotherapy should be immediately started, from the third day onwards (even before suture removal), with a hope of discouraging tumor resurgence, followed by chemotherapy in desperation.

THYROID CARCINOMA IN CHILDREN

Except anaplastic, the other cancers may be seen in children, managed in the same way as in adults. Most of them require central node dissection, making preservation of parathyroids diffcult and autotransplantation necessary. Any thyroid growth in a child must be considered malignant, till proved otherwise. However they have a favorable outlook, even with extensive metastasis, as they respond well to adequate surgery and RaI therapy.

MULTINODULAR GOITER (MNG)

As already stated, it is a variant of diffuse colloid goiter; hence the same etiology is applicable. It may also present clinically as SNG with a dominant nodule, rest being impalpable. The MNG has a very low potential to develop malignancy (usually follicular type), though some recent reports show significant incidence (upto 5%), These often become toxic, due to autonomous hyperactivity of internodular tissue, called secondary thyrotoxicosis or toxic MNG (Plummer's disease). Some genetic predisposition through chromosome 14q has been identified.

	Feature	Primary thyrotoxicosis	Secondary thyrotoxicosis
1.	Sequence of events	Toxic symptoms and swelling Appear simultaneously	Toxicity develops in a pre-existing goiter
2.	Age incidence	20-40 yrs	35-50 yrs
3.	Surface of goiter	Smooth and diffuse	Asymmetrical and nodular
4.	Neck bruit	Usually present	Absent
5.	Predominant symptoms	CNS	CVS
6.	Exophthalmos	Often present	Never
7.	Pretibial myxedema	Often present	Never
8.	Myopathy	Proximal type	None
9.	Response to medical therapy	Excellent, surgery may be needed, in only about 50%	Only to control toxicity. Surgery is necessary for cure
10.	TRAb (antibodies)	Present	Absent

Table-87.3. Differences between primary and secondary thyrotoxicosis

Clinical features

Bilateral thyroid swelling in an otherwise asymptomatic patient is the usual presentation. If features of hyperthyroidism develop, it is secondary type, with predominant CVS manifestations (vide infra). Multiple firm (sometimes cystic) nodules of varying size are felt, distributed in both lobes, without features of malignancy. If any of the nodules exhibits hard consistency, unusual growth, early pressure symptoms or palpable lymph nodes, malignancy has to be suspected and an attempt to establish tissue diagnosis should be made.

Investigations

To exclude toxicity and malignancy, other routine investigations to assess for anesthesia and surgery, including an IDL. It is important to realize that the nodules in MNG are always cold in ^{131}I scan, hence not helpful in differentiating benign and malignant nodules.

Treatment

Minimal goiter may be tried on thyroxine therapy for a few months, as for a SNG, to see if it regresses, or at least to make the patient 'earn' the operation. Indications for surgery are pressure symptoms, cosmetic considerations and risk of toxicity. *Subtotal thyroidectomy*, removing 5/6th of the gland, including all the nodule-bearing tissue, is the operation of choice. A misnomer for this operation, calling it a *partial thyroidectomy* should be avoided, since it is ambiguous and does not indicate the precise extent of the resection. If the nodules are confined to only one lobe, and the other lobe is normal by peroperative palpation, a hemithyroidectomy should suffice. Most of these patients require lifelong substitution hormone therapy, which is the reason why some surgeons prefer total to near total excision for an MNG, eliminating even a remote possibility of recurrence of the goiter.

HYPERTHYROIDISM – causes

i)   Primary thyrotoxicosis (syn: Graves' disease, diffuse toxic goiter, Basedow's disease)

ii)   Toxic MNG (syn: Plummer's disease, toxic nodular goiter). In this condition the internodular gland tissue and not the nodules, which is hyperfunctioning.

iii) Toxic adenoma (Goetsch's disease) Increased sensitivity of TSH receptors in adenomatous tissue has been implicated in hyperactivity and the remaining gland may undergo compensatory hypoplasia. (ii & iii constitute secondary thyrotoxicosis)

Iv) Inflammatory goiters, e.g. subacute thyroiditis and Hashitoxicosis (usually mild and transient)

v)   Factitious hyperthyroidism (syn: artificial or iatrogenic hyperthyrodism, Jod-Basedow disease) is due to over administration of iodine or thyroid hormones, usually during therapy for hyperplastic endemic goiters; it subsides on withdrawal of the drug, though rarely the hyperactivity of iodine-hungry gland may persist (jod: iodine)

vi) Ectopic hyperfunctioning thyroid tissue, such as lingual, mediastinal or ovarian

vii) Functioning malignant tumors (differentiated carcinoma, papillary or follicular), rare

viii) Recurrent (postoperative) thyrotoxicosis.

ix) T_3 toxicosis, is considered when a patient is clinically toxic, but hormone assay is within normal levels; only estimation of free T_3 will clinch the diagnosis.

x)   Drugs: amiodarone, an antiarrhythmic agent, contains iodine, may be a cause.

Features of toxicity in a patient with a goiter

Symptoms

Nervousness, irritability, easy fatiguability, increased appetite and thirst (polyphagia and polydypsia), excessive sweating, diarrhea, weight loss, intolerance to warmer climates, tremors, dyspnea, palpitation, oligo/amenorrhea and visual disturbances.

Signs

Evidence of recent weight loss, anxious staring look, tachyarrhythmias, collapsing pulse, wide pulse pressure, fine tremors of tongue and hands, brisk tendon reflexes, pretibial myxedema, warm clammy (wet) skin,

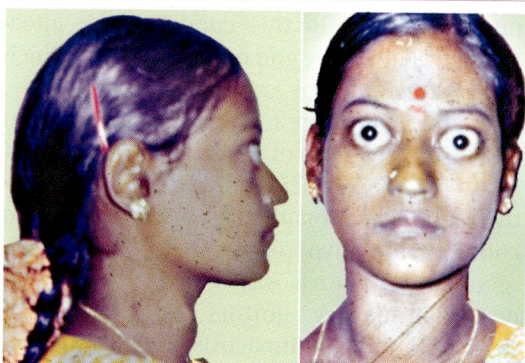

Fig. 87.18 & 87.19. Dysthyroid exophthalmos
(courtesy: Halsted Surgical Clinic, Chennai)

dermopathy and eye signs (only in primary), such as exophthalmos, chemosis, periorbital edema, visual disturbances etc.

The tremors of the hand may be so fine, that it may require placing a post card over the hand to detect them.

Thyrotoxicosis should be suspected under the following situations:

1)   behavioral problem or myopathy develops in a child,

2)   unexplained weight loss or diarrhea

3)   tachycardia or arrhythmia in elderly.

4)   Apathetic thyrotoxicosis : in elderly group, long standing thyrotoxicosis may produce behavioral changes such as depression, replacing the commonly encountered anxiety, but the diagnosis is made on other clinical criteria and laboratory data. This is a rare presentation with more pronounced wasting and cardiac manifestations.

Another useful feature is, malignancy and toxicity very rarely coexist, hence if the diagnosis of any one of them has been established, the probability of the other becomes remote. However a recent review of the subject appears to disagree with this, claiming that toxic goiter, particularly an adenoma, has some potential to harbor malignancy and recommends needle biopsy before definitive surgery, after controlling toxicity.

Wayne's clinical diagnostic index for thyrotoxicosis is based on all the symptoms and signs of thyrotoxicosis, to arrive at the probability of the diagnosis. Since the clinical diagnosis is generally made on those manifestations, it is considered redundant and not popular.

Extrathyroid manifestations

Pretibial myxedema
Proximal myopathy
Exophthalmos and ophthalmoplegia
Acropachy (clubbing of fingers and toes)
Tachyarrhythmias
Dupuytren contracture
Gynecomastia

Gynecomastia is a rare complication, due to activation of aromatase, an enzyme converting endogenous androgens to estrogens.

GRAVES' DISEASE

Etiology

This is the commonest form of thyrotoxicosis, mostly seen in the young, with a female preponderance (6:1). It is an autoimmune disease, with genetic predisposition, in which thyroid-stimulating immunoglobulins activate the TSH receptors in the follicular cells, to produce the hormones profusely. At one time, the globulin was thought to be long acting thyroid stimulant (LATS); now it is known that many more antibodies (immunoglobulins- IgG), collectively known as thyroid receptor antibodies (TRAb), are responsible for the disease. What initiates this antibody production is unclear and it may probably be due to defective suppressor T-lymphocytes, allowing helper T-cells to stimulate helper B-cell clones to produce TRAb. Alternately, it is suggested that an immune response is triggered by altered antigens on the surface of follicular cells. It may be assoicated with other autoimmune conditions, such as Addison's disease, myasthenia gravis, rheumatoid arthritis or pernicious anemia.

Clinical features

General features of toxicity have been described above. Locally, the gland is diffusely enlarged, soft and feels warm due to hypervascularity; sometimes a thrill is felt and soufflé is heard over the lateral lobes. Exophthalmos is present in most of the patients; other systemic manifestations are, pretibial myxedema, dermopathy (hair loss, nail changes), fine tremors of the tongue and hands, muscle wasting, weakness of the proximal group of muscles due to myasthenia-like picture and brisk deep tendon reflexes. *Pretibial myxedema* is thickening of the skin and subcutaneous tissues in the anterior aspect of the leg, due to deposition of mucopolysac-charides, seen in current or treated cases of primary thyrotoxicosis with exophth-almos, associated with elevated TRAb.

It is important to distinguish this from secondary thyrotoxicosis in a preexisting nodular goiter, since T_3, T_4 are elevated and TSH is reduced in both types.

The reason for predominant CNS symptoms in primary type is that its basic problem lies in the CNS (hypothalamo-hypophyseal axis), thyroid gland being only a target organ, whereas due to the peripheral effects of T_3 and T_4, more CVS manifestations are seen in the secondary type. Response to medical therapy is of clinical importance, so that the patient may be cautioned about the chances of requiring surgery for cure.

The anomalous nomenclature of primary and secondary merits explanation, since usually primary refers to originating from the organ and secondary means the organ is targeted by external influence, but here it is reversed. At the time these names were coined, the etiology of primary thyrotoxicosis was unknown (primary or idiopathic), while that of secondary was known to be due autonomous hyperactivity by an nodular goiter (secondary meaning due to a known reason). Though now we know the pathogenesis of primary disease, the nomenclature has not been changed.

Differential diagnosis

Other types of thyrotoxicosis, diffuse colloid goiter, MNG, Hashimoto's thyroiditis etc.

Investigations

Thyroid profile will reveal high T_3, T_4 and low TSH, due to negative feedback influence on pituitary, by the thyroid hormones. The significance of sleeping pulse rate and other biochemical tests have been described earlier. An USG of neck may be helpful, if the nodularity of the gland in doubt. Other studies including a biopsy are rarely needed.

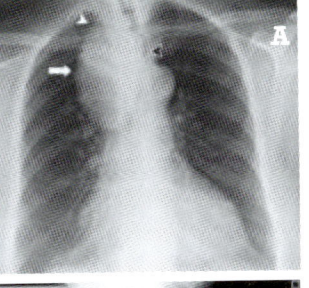

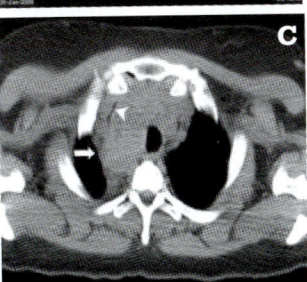

Fig. 87.21.
A. Chest x-ray showing a large retrosternal goiter with compressed trachea
B. Lateral view of the same
C. CT scan of the chest of the same patient

Treatment

Three standard modalities are medical, surgical and radioactive ablation.

Medical

i) General supportive therapy such as rest, tranquillization, high calorific diet, anabolic steroids, appetite stimulants etc.

ii) Specific *antithyroid drugs*: carbimazole (Neomercazole) and propylthiouracil, the former is commonly used, given orally 20-40mg/day in divided doses. Besides its antithyroid action by inhibiting organic binding of iodine and coupling of iodotyrosines, it is known to be an immunosuppressant, blocking TRAb production. Main untoward effect of this drug is on the bone marrow, inducing *granulo-cytopenia* (the term *agranulocyto-*

sis has to be discarded, as it may be mistaken to mean increased agranulocytes, instead of decreased granulocytes), which has to be periodically monitored and drug withdrawn promptly; if identified and acted in time, the effect on bone marrow is reversible. Other side effects are, skin rash, peripheral neuropathy and polyarteritis. These drugs cross placenta, to affect the fetal thyroid and are excreted in breast milk.

iii) *β-adrenergic blocking agents*: There are two types of adrenergic receptors, namely α and β. Actions mediated through α-receptors on CVS are, constriction of arterioles to increase BP and in high doses induce cardiac arrhythmias, whereas stimulation of β–receptors increase cardiac rate, force of contraction and conduction velocity.

Many of the symptoms in thyrotoxicosis are due to hyperdynamic peripheral adrenergic effects, which may be controlled by β-blockers like propranolol, pindolol, nadolol (non-selective) or metoprolol, atenolol and acebutol (selective). They also block peripheral conversion of T_4 to T_3 and adrenergically provoked tremors, hence induce faster symptomatic remission. Though propranolol (30-60mg/day in divided doses) is most popular (it is cheap and time-tested), it is nonselective, blocking both β-1 (located in CVS) and β-2 (located in bronchial and skeletal musculature) adrenergic receptors, hence can not be used in patients with bronchospastic disorder, whereas the (cardio) selective β-1 blockers, are devoid of this drawback, when given in proper doses.

As may be expected, occasionally the goiter may enlarge under medical therapy, due to iatrogenic hypothyroidism, which can be circumvented by giving thyroxine along with antithyroid drugs, the so-called 'block and replacement therapy'. It is not possible to predict which patient is likely to develop recurrent thyrotoxicosis, following remission with adequate (about 6 months) medical therapy, but some correlation may be obtained by the esti-mation of TRAb and human lymphocyte antigen (HLA) status.

Surgical therapy

The patient should be made euthyroid by medical therapy before surgery, to avoid a thyroid crisis or storm. Indications for surgery are

(1) large sized residual goiter and

(2) recurrent thyrotoxicosis after adequate medical therapy.

The preoperative parameters to ascertain the functional status of the thyroid are, patient's subjective improvement, weight gain, pulse rate and thyroid profile (T_3, T_4 and TSH) in blood. A 10-day course of *Lugol's iodine* (5% iodine in 10% potassium iodide) given orally, reduces vascularity of the gland, makes the gland firmer for easy handling during surgery and controls any overlooked subclinical toxicity. However, this 'routine' is not practiced any longer by many surgeons, who rely mainly on β-blockers, to serve a similar purpose. For reasons poorly understood, such an action of high dose iodine, in blocking the release of thyroglobulin into the system, is short-lived and lasts for about two weeks. But for this drawback, iodine would have been the primary drug of choice in the treatment of thyrotoxicosis. Use of a nonselective anticholinergic agent, like atropine, as a pre-anesthetic antisecretary drug is to be avoided, since it causes tachycardia, confusing with hyperthyroidism; instead, a selective M (muscarine)-3 antagonist, glycopyrrolate (Glyco-P), which has no significant effect on heart rate, is preferred for the purpose.

Subtotal thyroidectomy is the standard procedure for Graves' disease or toxic MNG (Plummer's disease). However while doing surgery for a nontoxic MNG, it should be aimed to retain as much of normal gland tissue as possible, to prevent hypothyroidism, whereas for a thyrotoxic gland, at least 7/8th of the gland should be excised, leaving not more than 3-5gm of tissue on either side, erring on removing more than less, since recurrent thyrotoxicosis poses a greater problem than hypothyroidism.

A standard collar crease incision is made, about 2" above the sternum, marked by an impression with a silk thread, to avoid obliquity. The skin flaps are raised (both above and below) including the platysma and a Joule's self-retaining retractor is positioned. The investing deep fascia is incised in the midline, separating strap muscles, to expose the gland, which is identified by the color and vascular plexus over it. The superior pole on one side is initially exposed, delivered and vessels ligated and divided as close to the pole as possible. While treating a benign disease, it does no harm if a rim of gland is left behind, with the upper vascular pedicle. Then the lobe is retracted medially, exposing the tracheo-esophageal groove, where the recurrent laryngeal nerve is seen crossing the inferior thyroid vascular pedicle, in the loose areolar tissue, entering the larynx behind the cricothyroid joint. The vascular pedicle is ligated in continuity, well away from the gland and the nerve gently teased away from the gland. Some veins at the lower pole of the gland and occasionally the ima artery in the inferior midline are clamped and divided, to free the lobe. Similar steps are followed for the other lobe and based on the distribution of disease in the gland, a decision has to be taken as to how much of gland substance on each side should be removed.

The parathyroids (at least one on each side) stuck to the thyroid tissue, are identified by their complexion and carefully protected. A continuous locking 'hemostatic' stitch for the remaining gland tissue, taking bites also in the peritracheal tissue, will fix the stumps to either side of the trachea. After proper hemostasis and positioning a drain (either corrugated plastic or vacuum type), for any sero-sanguinous collection, the wound is closed in layers. As a routine the anesthesiologist should inspect the vocal cords following extubation and record the findings in his notes, for future reference. For the first 12 hours, the patient is kept in propped up (Fowler's) position and liquid diet started after 6

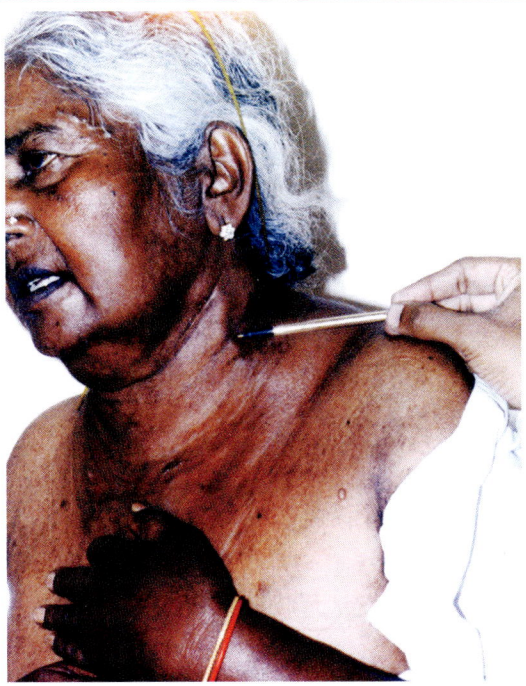

Fig. 87.20. Superior mediastinal compression due to a retrosternal goiter. Note edema of left upper limb and distended jugulars
(courtesy: Lifeline Hospitals, Chennai)

hours. The drain is removed after 48 and the skin sutures (or clips) after 96 hours.

Radioisotopic ablation therapy: Many nuclear physicians feel that there is no place for surgery in the management of thyrotoxicosis, but consensus is against such a 'blanket' approach and is in favor of individualization of cases for radioisotopic therapy. The prime indications are:

i)   recurrent thyrotoxicosis following surgery, where reoperation may be difficult and hazardous

ii)   when surgery is contraindicated because of cardiac or other problems, increasing morbidity and mortality of surgery

iii)   intolerance to drugs, hence unable to bring the patient to euthyroid state

The only *absolute* contraindications for radioisotopic therapy are *child bearing* age,

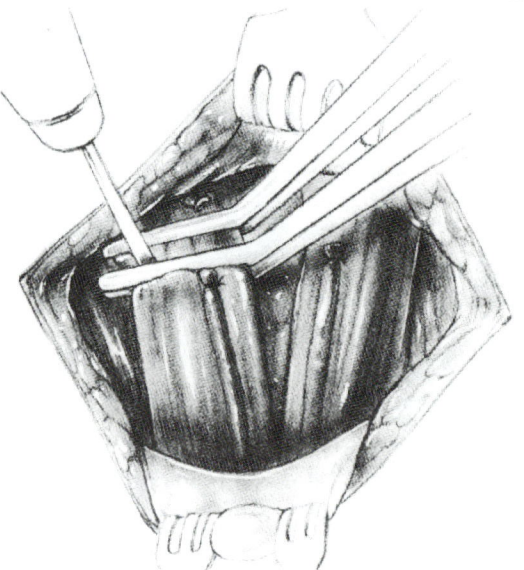

Fig. 87.22. Dividing the strap muscles as high as possible to retain their nerve supply

because of teratogenic potential and *lactation*, since the isotope passes into milk; other objections, such as carcinogenic potential on the thyroid, secondary radiation hazard for healthcare workers and permanent hypothyroidism etc. are *relative*. It takes about 12weeks for clinical return to euthyroid status, following administration of ^{131}I; hence it is important to continue medical therapy, until then. Surgery however, may be needed for a bulky goiter, whether diffuse or nodular, at some point of time, in most of the patients. Children treated with ^{131}I for Graves' disease, may develop hyperparathyroidism, later on.

Exophthalmos (syn: thyrotoxic or Graves' ophthalmopathy, dysthyroid exophthalmos): The pathogenesis of exophthalmos is not clear; once it was considered to be due to the influence of exophthalmos producing substance (EPS), an immunoglobulin, causing diffuse lymphocytic and fibroblastic infiltration in the retroorbital tissue, with formation of mucopolysaccharide, leading to edema and fibrosis. Probable cross-reaction of thyroid antigen and ocular muscle tissue is another suggestion for the ophthalmopathy.

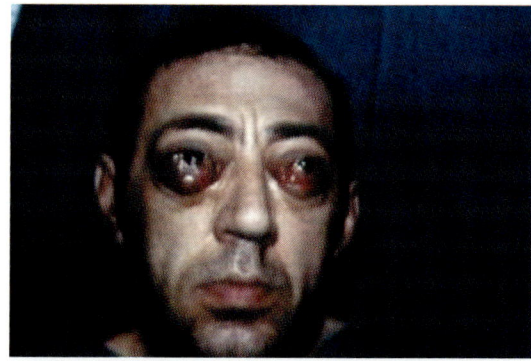

Fig. 87.23. Malignant exophthalmos

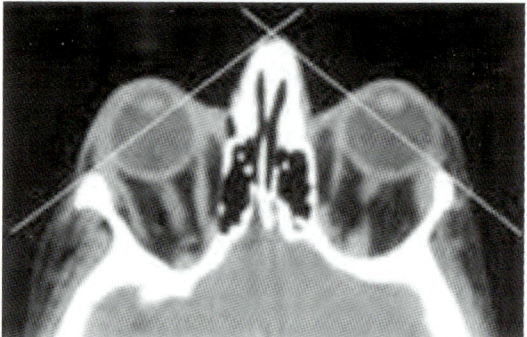

Fig. 87.24. CT scan of eye balls in exophthalmos

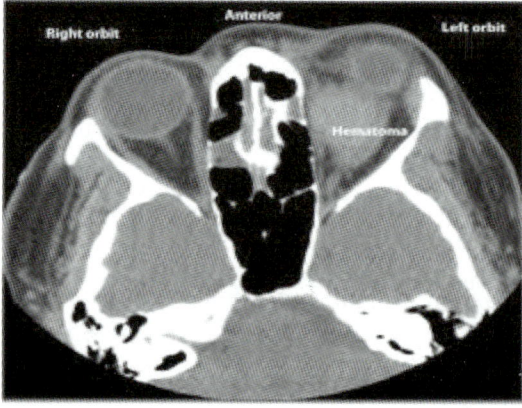

Fig. 87.25. Proptosis of left eye due to retroorbital hematoma

Pathology in exophthalmos in Graves' disease : Activated T-cell infiltrate retroorbital contents and stimulate fibroblasts leading to enlargement of extraocular muscles, cellular infiltration of retroorbital interstitial tissue, proliferation of orbital fat and connective tissue. Incidence of optic neuropathy is 5%.

Clinical signs of exophthalmos

1) Wide palpebral fissure (Dalrymple): sclera all around the cornea becomes visible.

2) Sign of lid lag (von Graefe): With the head fixed, the patient is asked to look down: the sclera above the cornea becomes visible, due to spasm of Muller's muscle (involuntary portion of levator palpebrae superioris), supplied by sympathetic.

3) Defective convergence of both eyes (Moebius): the normal convergence distance is <30cm. but a patient with exophthalmos gets diplopia even for objects farther than 30cm. This is due to a myasthenia-like phenomenon, known as thyrotoxic ophthalmoplegia.

4) Staring look and infrequent blinking (Stellwag): due to sympathetic overactivity (blinking is involuntary whereas winking is voluntary, especially if directed at the opposite sex !)

5) Absence of forehead wrinkling, when the patient looks up (Joffroy): this is because the normal reflex elevation of eye brows, to enlarge the field of vision, is abolished, as it is no longer needed for the protruded eye balls.

6) Tangential examination of the eye balls from the top (Naffziger), to see the extent of protrusion

Exophthalmometry (Hertel), using the principle of vernier calipers, is the most accurate method to document the magnitude of the displacement of eye balls and to assess improvement.

Normal protrusion of cornea over orbital margin: 16 - 21mm. Abnormal protrusion: >22mm or >2mm difference between the two eyes

Investigations: USG/CT/MRI/biopsy

Treatment of exophthalmos is best done in a three tier method. Majority (>90%) of them do not require separate treatment, as the protrusion of the eye balls recedes, when the toxicity is controlled. There is a belief that total thyroidectomy alleviates the ocular problem, more than subtotal, but solid proof to that effect is lacking. Because of persistence or worsening of the condition, about 5-10% of them require specific therapy, with the addition of thyroxine, systemic steroids (prednisolone), eye drops with steroids or β-blockers, elevation and antiedema therapy. There is a rare third group, in whom, in spite of the above mentioned therapy, the condition progresses, leading to chemosis, exposure keratitis and optic neuropathy, with deterioration of vision, called *malignant exophthalmos*. This requires more aggressive treatment, such as lateral tarsorrhaphy (to prevent exposure keratits), retroorbital radiation and surgical decompression, before permanent loss of vision occurs. The latter surgery may be accomplished either by the temporal (Naffziger) or frontal (Rowbotham) approach.

Feature	Exophthalmos	Proptosis
Etiology	Endocrinological usually dysthyroid	Non-endocrinological tumor, inflammation, hemorrhage, AVM, dermoid, Wagener's granulomatosis etc
Bilaterality	Common	Rare
Onset	Insidious	May be acute
Progression	Progressive	May be recurrent
Compressibility	Never	May be (in hemangioma, lymphangioma. varices, A-V malformations etc)
Eye signs related to sympathetic hyperactivity	Present	Absent
Treatment	Mostly medical	Mostly surgical

Table-87.4. Differences between exophthalmos and proptosis

Proptosis is a general term used for any protrusion of eye ball, but conventionally it is applied to non-endocrinal causes, whereas exophthalmos refers to endocrinal reasons, particularly in hyperthyroidism (Graves' disease), hence it is also called dysthyroid ophthalmopathy.

RETROSTERNAL GOITER (syn: intrathoracic or mediastinal goiter)

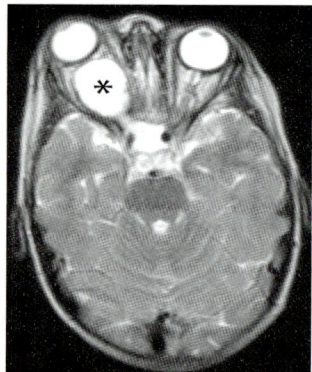

Fig. 87.26. Proptosis of left eye due to retrobulbar policytic astrocytoma

Very rarely they are from ectopic thyroid tissue in the chest (primary type), but usually they arise from the lower poles of the lobes of the thyroid (secondary type), negative intrathoracic pressure drawing them into the superior mediastinum. It may pop in and out of the chest, during coughing, sneezing or straining, when it is called *plunging goiter*. They usually draw blood supply from the inferior thyroid vessels and may be single (SNG) or associated with more nodules in the gland in the neck (MNG). When the lower border of the goiter is not appreciated on deglutition, the diagnosis is 'intrathoracic' goiter; if it is clearly made out it is known as 'plunging' goiter.

Clinical features

They may be asymptomatic or may have features of tracheal compression of varying degrees. Patients are often treated for 'asthma' for a considerable period of time, before the actual diagnosis is made. If there is recurrent laryngeal nerve involvement by its pressure, it is always on the left side, since the right nerve does not have an intrathoracic course. Often they are on only one side of the trachea, and when large, produce gravitational pressure whenever the patient lies on the other side, rather typical of this goiter. Engorgement of neck veins may be seen, sometimes exaggerated by hyperabduction of both arms, typically nonpulsatile, due to pressure on innominate veins or rarely superior vena cava (Pemberton's sign). Inability to appreciate the lower pole of

the lobe on that side and widening of superior mediastinal dullness are supportive of the diagnosis.

Investigations

Chest x-ray (soft tissue shadow, tracheal deviation and calcification of the goiter), CT or scintiscan of thyroid are useful in detecting and delineating an intrathoracic goiter, as well as mediastinal lymphadenopathy. IDL for vocal cord movements and a flexible bronchoscopy for evidence of tracheal infiltration, have to be done, if a malignant nodule is suspected. These investigations influence the approach to be adopted during surgery, particularly the need for sternotomy, depending upon the size, configuration, relation to vital structures and malignant potential.

Treatment

In the vast majority of cases, intrathoracic goiter can easily be digitally 'shelled out' during thyroidectomy through the cervical incision. Invasive malignancy and true ectopic intrathoracic goiter (which draws blood supply from within the chest), form the main indications for median sternotomy. In large *benign* goiters, sometimes the capsule may be deliberately broken and the contents scooped out, to facilitate delivery of the mass, to avoid a sternotomy.

　　1% rule
　　1% of goiters are intrathoracic
　　1% of them are malignant and
　　1% of the retrosternal goiters may require sternotomy for excision

LINGUAL THYROID

Embryology : The thyroglossal diverticulum fails to descend into the neck and the thyroid tissue develops at the foramen cecum of the tongue.

A rounded swelling over the tongue in the midline due to the development of the thyroid gland at the foramen cecum; it is most often the only thyroid tissue present, the condition being known as *cervical athyriosis* (no thyroid in the neck). This is more common in females and noticed around puberty, probably due to physiological hyperplasia, with the symptoms of dysphagia, recurrent bleeding from ulceration or impaired speech. Most of them are euthyroid; rarely hypothyroidism is observed.

Differential diagnosis

Hamartoma, dermoid cyst and thyroid neoplasms

Investigations

On careful palpation, the thyroid lobes may be missing, making the tracheal rings conspicuously palpable. A scintiscan clinches the diagnosis and also confirms the absence of thyroid in the normal place.

Treatment: If not very troublesome, hormone therapy (as for physiological goiter) may be given for a few months; about 75% of them regress enough to become 'asymptomatic'. The remaining require excision, ideally using cryo or laser technique. A frozen section of the excised specimen should be carried out, to exclude a neoplasm, before autotransplantation of the fragmented gland tissue in muscle (SCM or

Management of Primary Thyrotoxicosis (Graves' disease)			
	Medical	**Surgery**	**Ral therapy**
	Antithyroid β-blockers	Subtotal thyroidectomy	0.3-0.5 milli Curies/gm tissue
	Anabolic steroids Anxiolytic agents	Near total thyroidectomy	Approx 20-50 milli Curies (1000 μCu = 1 milli Curie)
Advantages	No surgery	Permanent cure	No surgery
	No risk	No systemic effects	No drugs
Disadvantages	Prolonged therapy	Morbidity and mortality	Teratogenic potential
	Granulocytopenia	Storm & other complications	Permanent hypothyroidism
	Low compliance	Recurrence	Exacerbation of arrhythmias
	Relapses	Expertise needed	Slow acting (takes 12 weeks)
Indications	Patient unwilling for surgery	Young patients fit for surgery	After child-bearing age
	To postpone surgery	Large goiter	Recurrence after surgery
	Recurrence after surgery	Retrosternal goiter	Thyrocardiac patients
		Pregnancy	Small sized goiter
		Children	Intolerance to drugs (hence patient cannot be made euthyroid before surgery)
Contra-indications	Intolerance to drugs	Serious co-morbidities	Child-bearing age
	Poor compliance	Recurrence after surgery	Children
	Suspected malignancy	Lack of expertise	Retrosternal goiter

Table-87.5

flexor muscles of the forearm) may be considered. A hypothyroid state with elevated TSH, increases the prospects of survival of the implanted tissue, *Halsted's law* states that transplanted endocrine tissue survives better if the individual is deficient in that hormone, due to favorable trophic influences.

Complications of thyroid surgery

1) Hemorrhage, which may be primary or reactionary (slipped ligature?). More than the blood loss, pressure built up in a closed space, may cause tracheal compression and acute respiratory distress. Immediate reopening of the wound (in the ward itself) and evacuation of the hematoma should be done; the patient is then shifted to the operating room for exploration, hemostasis and closure.

2) Respiratory obstruction may be due to laryngeal edema from traumatic intubation, wound hematoma (as already described) or *tracheomalacia*. The latter term is used to denote softening of the tracheal rings in long-standing large goiters; there is a tendency for tracheal collapse when the supporting gland is excised. Recurrent nerve injury does not result in immediate airway problems, unless associated with edema or neurapraxia. Immediate reintubation of trachea tackles the crisis and buys time for proper assessment and management, particularly when evacuation of hematoma fails to relieve airway obstruction. If tracheomalacia is anticipated (in long standing large goiters), the endotracheal tube may be left in for 24-48hrs, by which time the tissues around the trachea condense to give the necessary support.

3) Laryngeal nerve injuries, have occurred even in experienced hands and the patients should be forewarned about such a possibility and its consequences, short and long term. Identifying the recurrent nerves in the tracheo-esophageal groove, ligating the superior pedicle close to and inferior pedicle as far away from the gland as possible are the standard technical precautions against injuring the nerves. Mandatory

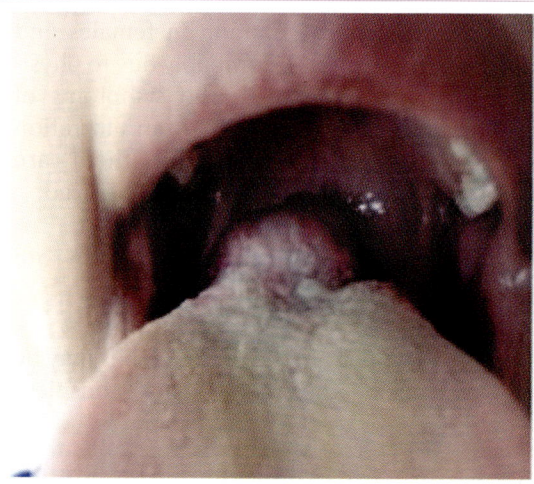

Fig. 87.27. Lingual thyroid

identification of the recurrent nerve during surgery has reduced the incidence dramatically; most of the time they have transient palsy (neurapraxia), caused by handling of the nerve, or the usage of monopolar diathermy in the vicinity of nerves which recovers within a few weeks. If the division of recurrent nerve was identified during surgery, fine perineural anastomosis with 8-0 prolene sutures may be attempted. Unilateral palsy may be asymptomatic and can be managed with speech therapy, but bilateral palsy is more troublesome, requiring lateral fixation of the cords or arytenoids (arytenoidopexy). Currently laser posterior cordectomy is the preferred treatment for this complication. Anomalous course of the nerves are described in chapter 96.

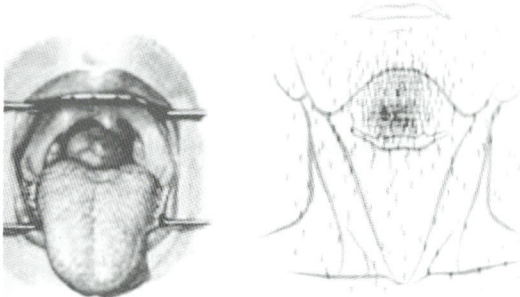

Fig. 87.28. Lingual thyroid.[131]I scan shows cervical athyriosis

4) *Hypoparathyroidism* is also a largely preventable complication, more related to injury/ischemia than actual removal of all four parathyroids. The symptoms may appear anywhere from the immediate postoperative period to several weeks, but the earlier they manifest, the longer they may last. It is called *hypocalcemic tetany*, perioral tingling and numbness being the earliest symptoms, followed by neuromuscular excitability, carpopedal spasm and rarely laryngeal spasm, which may be life threatening. *Chvostek's sign* (tapping the preauricular region over the facial nerve causes twitching of the facial muscles on that side) and *Trousseau's sign*, production of carpopedal spasm (acute flexion of the metacarpo-phalangeal and extension of the interphalangeal joints, the socalled *main de accoucheur*, also called *obstetrician's hand*), by inflating the sphygmomanometer, above the brachial systolic pressure for 3 minutes, are the classical signs elicited in acute hypoparathyroidism. After collecting a blood sample for calcium estimation, 10% Calcium gluconate should be given intravenously, which immediately relieves the symptoms. Subsequently intramuscular or oral calcium and vitamin-D or its active metabolite, dihydroxycholecalciferol (to increase absorption of calcium and phosphorus from the gut), has to be continued for some time, on a trial and error basis. Most often symptoms subside within a few days to weeks, as the glands regenerate; permanent hypoparathyroidism and need for parathormone replacement are extremely rare.

5) *Hypothyroidism* and recurrent *hyperthyroidism* are self explanatory, the former is easier to manage (with thyroxine supplement) than the latter (requiring radio-iodine ablation). Deficiency of calcitonin has no pathological/clinical significance.

6) Thyroid crisis or storm, fortunately is a rarity nowadays, thanks to effective antithyroid and β-blocking drugs available. It is a form of acute hyperthyroidism, due to sudden release

---

Jewels of Gyan - 87.2

Why do thyroid swellings move up during deglutition?

1. The pretracheal fascia, forming a false capsule of the gland is intimately attached to the thyroid cartilage
2. The gland is closely attached to the trachea
3. The ligament of Berry, (pretracheal fascia condensation) lifts the thyroid gland along with the larynx

Does the trachea move up during deglutition?
Of course, yes.

---

of thyroid hormones into circulation, with secondary effects of increased catecholamines, explaining the whole spectrum of clinical features, such as extreme tachycardia, hypertension, hyperthermia, delirium, dehydration, high output cardiac failure, pulmonary edema etc. ultimately leading to coma. This usually occurs during surgery, while the gland is being manipulated (hence it is first noticed by the anesthesiologist), or in the immediate postoperative period. It can also occur rarely during non-thyroid surgery in a thyrotoxic patient, as a result of infection, such as pneumonitis or pharyngitis and following ^{131}I therapy for thyrotoxicosis.

Treatment

Adequate preoperative preparation to bring the patient to euthyroid status and 10-day therapy with Lugol's iodine, has virtually eliminated this complication in recent times. Once recognized during surgery, handling of the gland should be stopped and intense therapy initiated to counter various manifestations, with the following agents given parenterally:

i) I.V. potassium iodide, to block the release of T_3 and T_4 into circulation

ii) antipyretics and hypothermia to bring down temperature

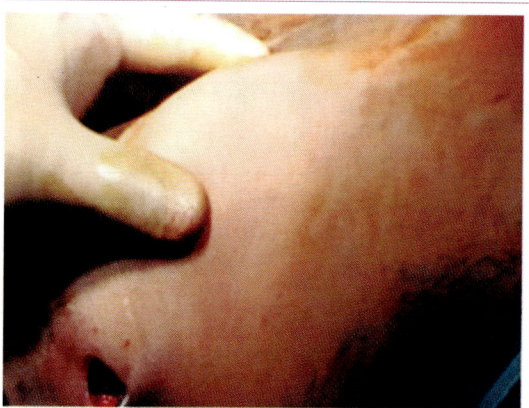

Fig. 87.29. Endoscopic thyroidectomy. A balloon dilatation is used to develop tissue planes (courtesy: Lifeline Hospitals, Chennai)

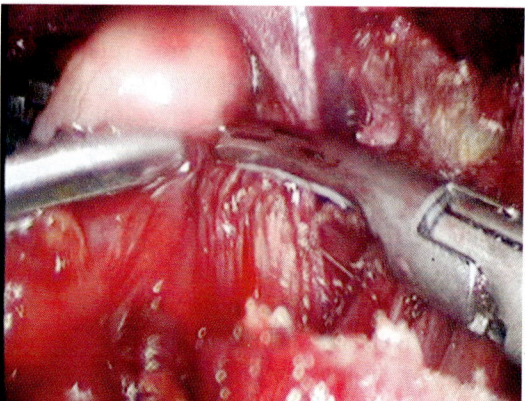

Fig. 87.30. Endoscopic hemithyroidectomy for an adenoma (courtesy: Lifeline Hospitals, Chennai)

iii) α/β-blockers to bring down blood pressure and pulse rate

iv) guanethidine and reserpine to deplete the tissue reserves of catacholamines

v) corticosteroids to prevent peripheral failure and to help lower body temperature

vi) digoxine, theophyllin and frusemide, to treat cardiac failure and pulmonary edema

vii) sedation if necessary

Usually thyroid surgery may be completed without any problem, once the 'storm' has subsided and the drug therapy tailored according to the requirement. Prognosis is excellent if prompt therapy is instituted, for this potentially fatal complication.

7. *Scar hypertrophy*, occurs more often at the stab wound, made for the drain. This may be prevented to a large extent by placing a skin stitch for the drain wound, which is tied after the removal of drain (48hrs). This facilitates wound healing by primary intention. Further there is tendency for this scar to migrate down on to the presternal region and vulnerable for keloid formation.

Injection of depo-steroids into the scars may discourage hypertrophy (see chapter 25)

8. *Tracheal* or *esophageal injury*, generally due to adherent goiter, often identified during surgery, may be repaired immediately. The endotracheal tube may be retained for 24-48hrs. if a significant leak is expected from the injured trachea. If esophagus is injured, it may be repaired by standard two-layer closure and the wound drained for 5 days; till such time, the patient is nourished through a nasogastric feeding tube.

9. Other complications are, wound infection, suture granuloma or sinus and those related to anesthesia.

Endoscopic thyroidectomy

As in other areas, endoscopic approach is being used to perform thyroidectomy for benign conditions, through three ports and the harmonic shears. A subfascial plane is developed under the strap muscles, to expose the pathology in the gland. An ultrasonic scalpel is used to disconnect the vessels and cut across the parenchyma, depending upon the extent of resection. The specimen is delivered through the 10mm suprasternal central port, which is also used to place a drain if necessary.

The procedure has a steep learning curve, but seems to demonstrate improved cosmesis with reduced postoperative pain and shortened hospital stay.

88 Thyroglossal Disease

THYROGLOSSAL CYST: Embryology: The thyroglossal tract extends from the *foramen cecum* of the tongue, coursing through the lingual musculature and in front of (sometimes behind) the body of the hyoid to reach the pyramidal lobe of the thyroid gland, just to the left of the midline. A cyst may develop in any part of the unobliterated tract, the most common position however being the subhyoid.

Natural fate of the thyroglossal tract

1. The cranial end of the tract, near the foramen cecum, may be the seat of a lingual thyroid. This is almost always associated with absence of thyroid in the neck (*cervical athyriosis*).

2. An ectopic thyroid gland may be located anywhere along the tract, due to imperfect descent of the gland into its normal place.

3. The infrahyoid part of the tract may persist as the levator glandulae thyroidea.

4. A thyroglossal cyst may develop, which is a tubulo-dermoid.

Pathology

The cyst contains mucoid material which may become turbid by accumulation of secretions or superadded infection. The lining of the cyst is usually ciliated columnar or squamous epithe-

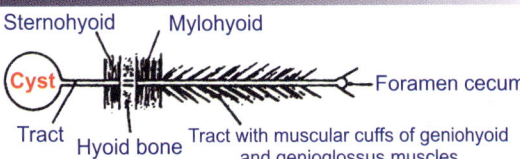
Fig. 88.2. Schematic diagram of thyroglossal duct

lium, with subepithelial lymphoid tissue, accounting for frequent infections. The glandular elements may persist, which may be the seat of an adenoma or carcinoma (papillary cystadenocarcinoma). It may rupture spontaneously or following surgical drainage of an infected cyst, resulting in thyroglossal sinus or fistula (which is *never congenital*).

Clinical features

More common in females and second decade of life, presenting as a painless, nontransilluminant, mobile, cystic swelling usually in the anterior midline of the neck (subhyoid region) or slightly to the left, placed under the strap muscles, which moves on deglutition as well as protrusion of the tongue, the latter feature being

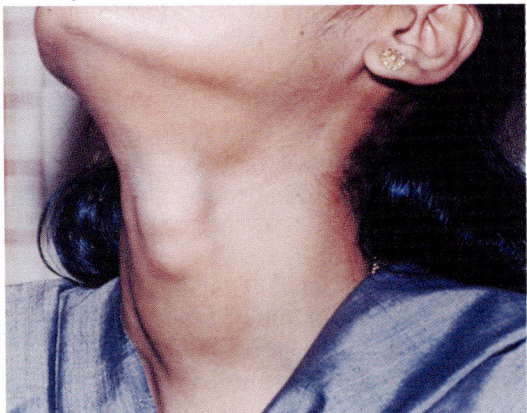
Fig. 88.1. Bilocular thyroglossal cyst
(courtesy: Lifeline Hospitals, Chennai)

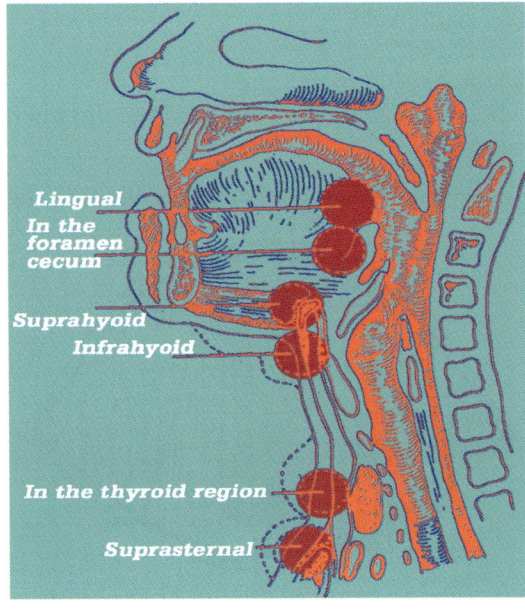
Fig. 88.3. Various locations of the thyroglossal cyst

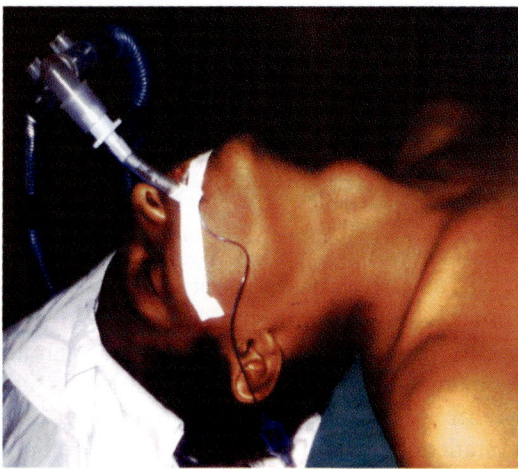

Fig. 88.4. Position on the operating table for excision of thyroglossal cyst
(courtesy: Halsted Surgical Clinic, Chennai)

virtually pathognomonic of the disease. While demonstrating this crucial sign, it is important to fix the lower jaw in the open-mouth position, to avoid its movements influencing the movements of the cyst. The various positions occupied by the cyst, in decreasing order of frequency, are

(i) subhyoid (65%)
(ii) thyroid
(iii) suprahyoid
(Iv) cricoid
(v) floor of the mouth and
(vi) intralingual, just beneath the foramen cecum.

The regional lymphnodes may be enlarged if the

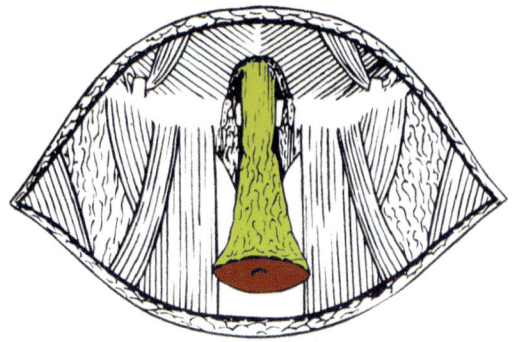

Fig. 88.5. Excision of thyroglossal sinus along with a part of the hyoid bone

cyst gets inflamed or undergoes malignant change; the latter is blissfully uncommon (incidence of malignancy: <1%).

Differential diagnosis

1. Sublingual dermoid
2. Subhyoid bursitis
3. Enlarged prelaryngeal (Delphian) lymph node
4. Ectopic (undescended) thyroid
5. Subcutaneous soft tissue benign tumors
6. Lymph cyst

Investigations

An USG to ascertain the cystic nature of the swelling and presence of thyroid gland in its place is important, besides routine investigations. If it is found to be solid, needle biopsy may be done, to identify the histology.

Complications

Infection, sinus/fistula formation and malignancy, have already been described, but rare.

Treatment

Total excision of the cyst including the thyroglossal tract, preferably up to the base of the tongue (Sistrunk's operation), is the definitive treatment. Access to the base of tongue is facilitated by the excision of the central portion of the body of the hyoid, a mandatory step, so as not to miss another cyst higher up leading to invariable recurrence. Surprisingly, no speech disability is seen following excision of the body of the hyoid.

THYROGLOSSAL FISTULA (or SINUS)

This is never congenital and follows a spontaneous rupture or inadvertent incision of an inflamed thyroglossal cyst. An incompletely excised cyst may also lead to a persistent sinus.

Pathology

The tract is lined by columnar epithelium internally and squamous epithelium near the external opening, discharging mucus and when infected it may be mucopurulent in nature.

Clinical features

If there is a history of preexisting thyroglossal

cyst which ruptured or was drained surgically, the diagnosis becomes obvious. The typical location of the external opening is in the lower anterior midline of the neck, guarded by a hood of skin with its concavity downwards. Indrawing of the external opening along with the surrounding skin during deglutition and protrusion of tongue is diagnostic.

Differential diagnosis

A branchial (cervical) sinus and sinus from tuberculous lymphadenitis are other common diseases that cause a similar sinus.

Investigations: No specific investigation is nec-

essary in typical cases, if doubt exists as to the nature of the sinus, either a contrast study (sinogram) or MRI may be considered. To confirm the presence of normal thyroid gland, ^{131}I or ^{99m}Tc scintiscan may be done.

Treatment

As in thyroglossal cyst, total excision of the tract along with its mouth, by multiple transverse incisions (Sistrunk) is the definitive treatment. A course of appropriate antibiotics may be given prior to surgery if there is infection. Histopathology of the excised track is essential, to exclude specific infection or malignancy.

89 Branchial Cyst

Histogenetic theory: Entrapment of the 1st or 2nd branchial cleft ectoderm in the depth, forming a cyst lined by respiratory or squamous epithelium, containing cholesterol crystals and generally located at the anterior border of the upper third of the SCM muscle.

Illingworth's theory: Inclusion of salivary epithelium in the upper deep cervical lymph nodes, subsequently undergoing cystic changes.(in contrast to Warthin's tumor, in which lymphatic tissue gets sequestrated within the salivary gland)

Pathology

Lining: Although usually lined by squamous epithelium, it can be lined by ciliated columnar epithelium, if arising from the internal branchial furrow.

Wall: Large amount of lymphoid tissue, hence it is prone to infection.

Contents: viscid, cheesy and rich in *cholesterol*.

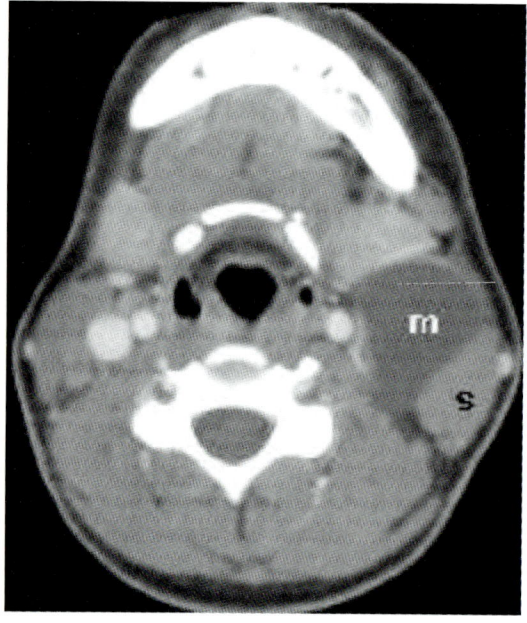

Fig. 89.1. CT scan of branchial cyst

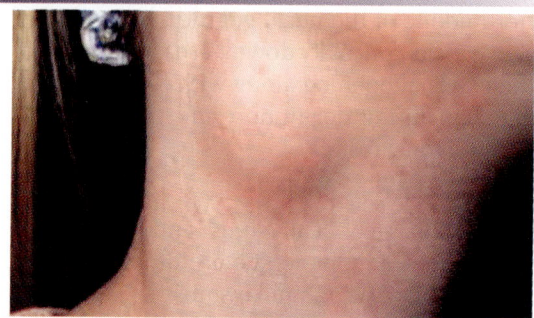

Fig.89.2. Branchial cyst, right side

Clinical features

Although congenital, it manifests around the 3rd decade of life (takes time for fluid to accumulate). A painless swelling in the upper part of the neck in the carotid triangle, is the classical presentation (note: branchial fistula presents in the lower part). If infected, a branchial cyst may mimic chronic specific or nonspecific lymphadenitis with abscess formation.

Round or oval swelling, deep to the investing fascia and the upper third of SCM (the muscle arises from the 2nd cervical myotome, hence the cyst will be deeper). It has a smooth surface, distinct edge, soft and cystic in consistency (sometimes tense, giving a firm feeling). The overlying skin is normal (unless infected), it is mobile in all axes, not transilluminant, cannot be compressed and aspiration yields cholesterol crystals, when examined under a microscope.

Differential diagnosis

I)   Cold abscess: Other nodes may be found, systemic features of Koch's disease my be

Jewels of Gyan - 89.1

Other cholesterol containing cysts

Dental
Dentigerous
Some thyroglossal cysts and
Cystic hygroma.

present. Aspiration reveals no cholesterol crystals, only sterile pus.

ii) Carotid body tumor: Solid swelling, with transmitted pulsations, may be bilateral.

iii) Cervical lymphadenopathy: usually multiple solid swellings

iv) Cystic hygroma: present since birth or early childhood, very soft, brilliantly translucent, located in the posterior triangle of neck, may attain very large size.

v) Plunging ranula: brilliantly transluscent, cross fluctuation can be elicited between the swelling in the neck and the floor of the mouth

vi) Other soft tissue benign tumors, such as fibrolipoma, fibromyx fibroma etc.

Investigations

USG/CT may delineate the relations to adjacent strctures. Aspiration or FNAC, if complications (such as infection or malignancy) are suspected, for appropriate studies. Any other tests are only to see the fitness for anesthesia and surgery.

Complications

I. Recurrent infection (lymphoid tissue in the wall)

ii. Inadvertent incision causes an acquired branchial sinus.

iii. *Branchiogenic carcinoma* is a rare complication and is usually an SCC. Variable consistency and regional lymphadenopathy should alert the clinician of this probability, which can be diagnosed by an USG, confirmed by FNAC and treated like SCC elsewhere. Often, this is diagnosed only after excision, by routine histopathology. In view of its critical location in the neck in close relation to vital structures, reoperation may not be practical, except for excision of enlarged nodes, hence adjuvant radio/chemotherapy is the preferred alternative.

Treatment

The treatment is excision of the entire cyst under general anesthesia by a transverse incision over a skin crease. The spinal accessory nerve, running to the apex of the posterior triangle in a superficial plane, the internal jugular vein, hypoglossal and glossopharyngeal nerves situated deep to the cyst should be identified and protected.

90 Branchial Fistula and Sinus

Embryology: It is better termed persistent cervical sinus and is due to defective closure of the endocervical sinus of His (usually 1st and 2nd, but sometimes 3rd, 4th, 5th branchial clefts). When it is complete it is lined by *ciliated columnar* epithelium at the pharyngeal end and *stratified squamous* epithelium on the external side. 10% of them have a positive family history. The brachial arches are so named because they resemble gills of fish (branchia: gills).

Track: From its external opening, the fistula passes subcutaneously to the level of the upper border of the thyroid cartilage, where it pierces the deep cervical fascia and passes through the carotid fork, being deep to the external carotid and superficial to the internal carotid, it crosses superficial to the internal jugular vein, glossopharyngeal and hypoglossal nerves (3rd arch derivatives) and pierces the superior con-

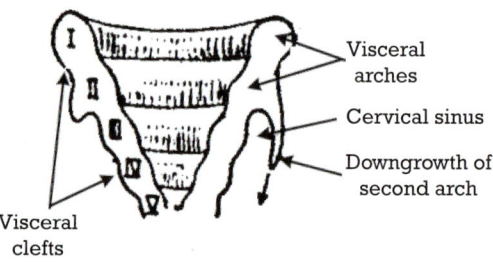

Visceral arches

Cervical sinus

Downgrowth of second arch

Visceral clefts

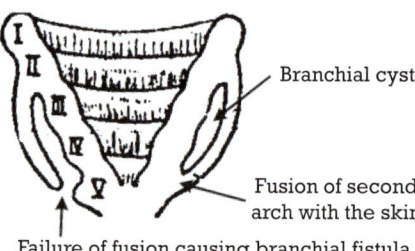

Branchial cyst

Fusion of second arch with the skin

Failure of fusion causing branchial fistula

Fig. 90.2. Formation of branchial sinus and cyst

strictor to emerge at the internal opening, on the posterior pillar of the fauces behind the tonsil. Position of its internal opening explains why the fistula sometimes makes its appearance following an attack of acute tonsillitis or tonsillectomy, due to its blockage.

Pathology

Lining: Stratified squamous or ciliated columnar, with lymphoid nodules sometimes seen subepithelially (accounting for frequent infection).

Complete fistula: The muscular coat sometimes is continuous externally with the platsyma and internally with the palatopharyngeus, accounting for puckering of the external opening on deglutition.

External opening may be marked by a skin tag or cartilage (branchial cartilage), derived from branchial arch mesenchyme.

Diagnosis

Commonly presents in the second decade, 30%

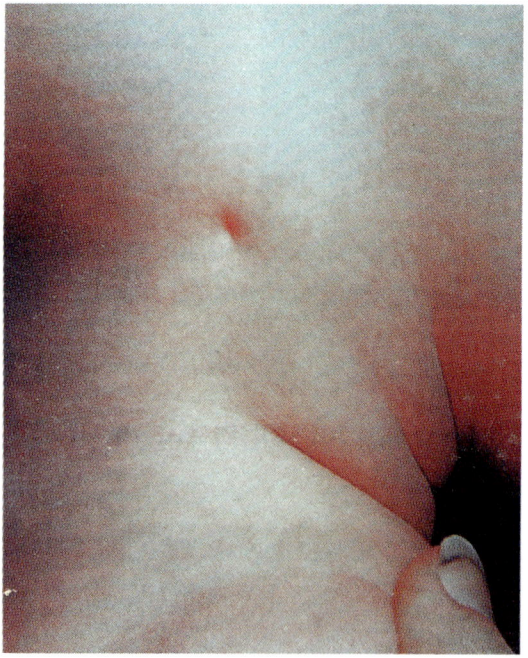

Fig. 90.1. External opening of a branchial sinus
(courtesy: Lifeline Hospitals, Chennai)

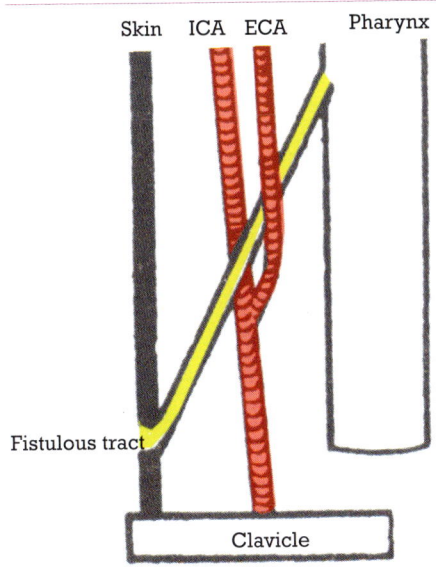

Fig. 90.3. Diagramatic representation of branchial fistula, coursing through the carotid fork

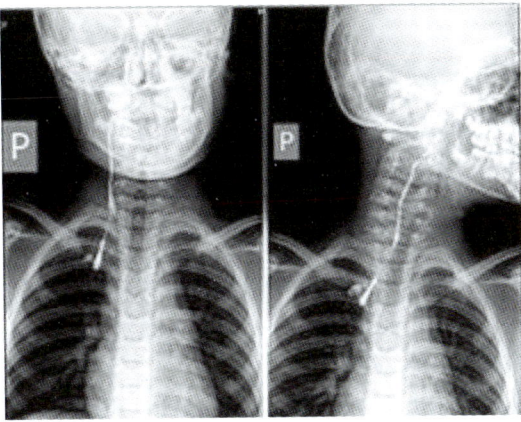

Fig. 90.4. Right branchial fistulogram (courtesy: Dr K R Reddy, Kakinada)

are bilateral. Indrawing of the skin at the external orifice during deglutition, is typical.

Differential diagnosis

Thyroglossal fistula (following inadvertent incision of a cyst) and tuberculous sinus.

Investigations: Sinogram, with contrast injected into the external opening through a polythene tube, will show the upper limit or internal communication of the track with the pharynx. A purse string suture is placed around the mouth, before injection, to prevent back spill. An MRI is very useful, in identifying its relations to adjacent structures, allowing expedient surgery.

Treatment

Excision of the entire track is recommended by multiple transverse incisions (after Small), to prevent recurrence.

Surgery

By an elliptical incision around the external opening, the track is dissected upwards, upto the upper border of the thyroid cartilage. A second incision is made at this level, to continue the dissection of the track through the carotid fork up to the pharyngeal wall. This is called the *step ladder* technique (Bailey). A ureteric catheter may be inserted into the track to aid dissection. Bilateral excision may be done at the same sitting, without much additional morbidity. Complete fistula, with pharyngeal opening is sometimes managed by combined cervical and oral approach.

91 Cystic Hygroma

(syn: hydrocele of neck, multiloculated lymph cyst of neck)

This is a large multiseptate cavernous lymphangioma of the neck, a congenital hamartomatous swelling, appearing in early infancy and childhood (rare after the age of three), first described by Wernher.

Embryology

Several lymph sacs develop during the formation of the embryo in various parts of the body. Two such large lymph sacs exist, one on each side of the neck, in relation to the internal jugular veins, known as jugular lymph sacs. Sequestration of a part of one of these sacs by the failure to establish communication with the rest of the lymphatic network, accounts for the formation of cystic hygroma. This condition is strongly associated with Turner's Syndrome, Down syndrome, trisomy-18 and Noonan Syndrome.

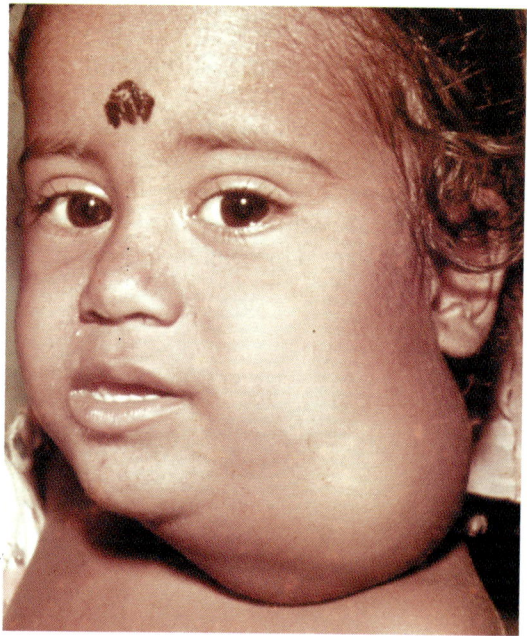

Fig. 91.1. Cystic hygroma
(courtesy: Prof T Dorairajan, Chennai)

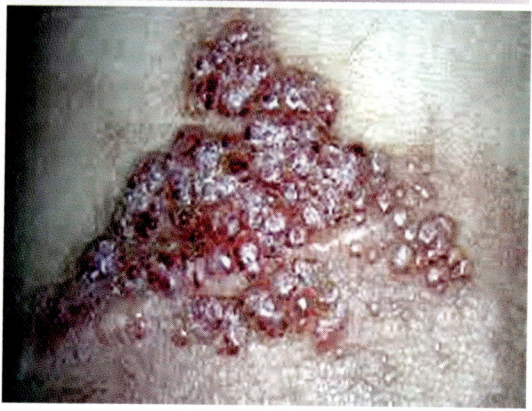

Fig. 91.2. Lymphangioma circumscripta

Pathology

The cyst with multiple loculi of different sizes, lined by a single epithelial layer and multiple septae dividing the space either completely or incompletely, is seen. The fluid is clear straw-colored lymph, hence the characteristic translucency.

Clinical features

A large hygroma in a fetus can sometimes obstruct the birth passages and produce dystocia. Usually the mother brings the child for a painless large soft swelling in the neck, which is smooth or bosselated, partially compressible and brilliantly transilluminant. Apart from the disfigurement, it is prone to secondary infection, which may cause constitutional symptoms, local pain, redness/warmth of the overlying skin and regional lymphadenopathy.

Position: usually in the posterior triangle of neck, but it may extend into the anterior triangle or into the superior mediastinum.

Anatomic plane: It is usually subfascial, but may extend into the intermuscular plane as well. It is partially compressible as the fluid often gets displaced from one locule into another. Less common sites are: cheek, axilla, groin, mediastinum and retroperitoneum.

Differential diagnosis

1)   Cavernous hemangioma: Surface is bluish, which is compressible and not transilluminant. They may be multiple.

2)   Branchial cyst: situated in the upper third of anterior border of SCM and not translucent.

Complications

1)   Extremely rapid growth rate may cause tracheal compression, producing upper airway obstruction, sometimes necessitating tracheostomy.

2)   Infection may supervene converting it into a large abscess and its systemic/local complications.

3)   Dystocia (dys: difficult; tokos: birth): When present in a fetus, in extreme cases, there may be obstruction to labor.

Investigations

No specific investigations are necessary, except for excluding hamartomas in other sites and for anesthetic evaluation. An USG/ CT scan may be helpful in delineating the topography of the lesion, but MRI is considered most useful investigation.

Treatment

Surgical removal is the treatment of choice, undertaken at an optimal age of 3 years. As a preoperative measure, a sclerosant, such as STD, ethoxysclerol or boiling aqua is injected into the cyst for a few sittings to fibrose the capsule and to facilitate excision later on. Many

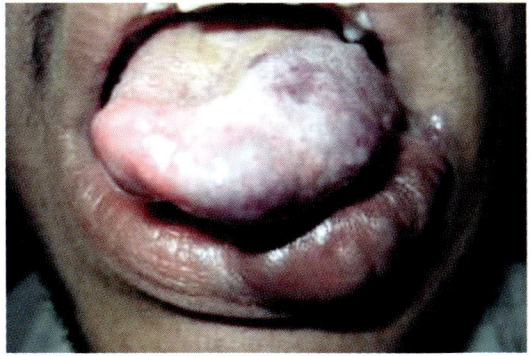

Fig. 91.3. Lymphangioma tongue and lower lip

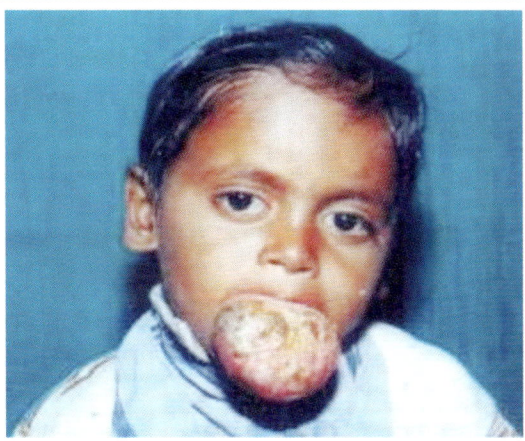

Fig. 91.4. Lymphangioma lower lip

surgeons feel this step is unnecessary, but employ intraoperative sclerotherapy, for residual lesions, which cannot be excised.

The surgery is undertaken through a long low transverse cervical incision and another smaller one higher up if necessary. The entire swelling should be carefully dissected out including the loculi and the 'pseudopodia' going into the intermuscular planes. Once adequately excised, recurrences are uncommon; residual/recurrent disease is best treated by sclerotherapy.

Newer modalities of treatment:

1.   Radiofrequency ablation (RFA)

2.   MRI-guided Laser-induced interstitial thermo (sclero) therapy.

Complications of surgery

i)   Injury to spinal accessory, vagus, jugular veins and cutaneous nerves.

ii)   Collection of blood/lymph under the flaps, which may be treated by aspiration under aseptic conditions.

iii)   Flap necrosis, chylous fistula, lymphorrhoea (or lymphorrhagia) and secondary hemorrhage.

Complications

1)   Airway compression as indicated.

2)   Infection may supervene converting it into a large abscess and its systemic/local complications.

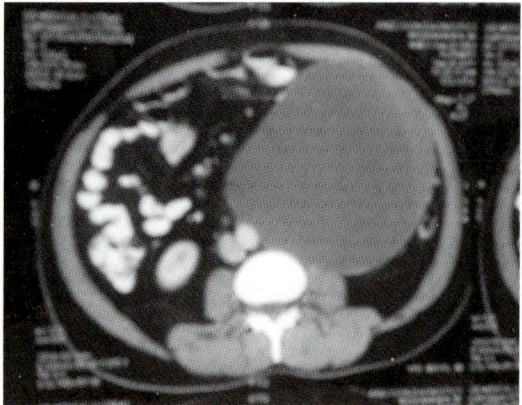

Fig. 91.5. CT scan of a large lymph cyst in the left upper retroperitoneum, displacing the aorta
(courtesy: Halsted Surgical Clinic, Chennai

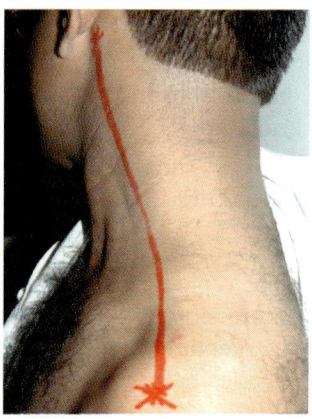

Fig. 91.6. The course of spinal accessory nerve is marked by a line drawn from the tip of the mastoid to the tip of the acromion
(courtesy: Lifeline Hospitals, Chennai

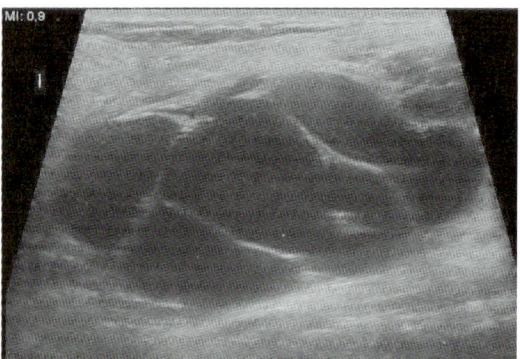

Fig. 91.7. Ultrasonogram of a 19-weeks fetus, showing cystic hygroma

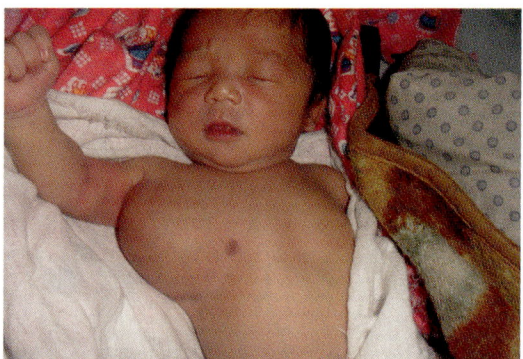

Fig. 91.8. Right axillary lymph cyst in a child

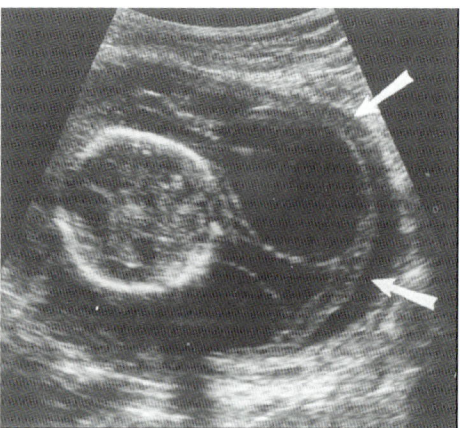

Fig. 91.9. Ultrasonogram of a cystic hygroma, showing loculations

(syn: chemodectoma, non-chromaffin paraganglioma, potato tumor)

Definition: This is a tumor arising from the cells of the carotid body, a chemoreceptor organ located at the common carotid bifurcation.

Embryology

The chief cells of the carotid body arise from the neural crest and migrate to their permanent location. They belong to the APUD family (amine precursor uptake and decarboxylation) like the adrenal medullary and pancreatic islet cells, a concept currently under debate.

Anatomy

Normal carotid body is less than 5mm in diameter, an inconspicuous, flattened brown nodule in the adventitia of the medial aspect of the bifurcation of the carotid or just below it. It is not encapsulated and consists of nests of two main types of cells

(1) chief (glomus type I) or epitheloid cells, which are large with pale cytoplasmic staining, containing granules of catecholamine.

(2) sustentacular cells (glomus type II) with long processes embracing capillaries. These two types of cells help in physiological feedback to the medulla oblongata about arterial pO_2, pCO_2 and pH, to modulate respiratory and cardiovascular functions. It is attached to the carotid fork, by a thin strand of adventitia, known as Meyer's ligament, which carries a tiny branch of the external carotid, supplying the carotid body and a twig from glossopharyngeal nerve.

Etiology

The observation that patients with chronic hypoxia (e.g. COPD), have enlargement (hyperplasia) of the carotid body and the higher incidence of these tumors in people living in high altitudes, points to the etiology of this tumor, in non-familial cases. They also have some familial occurrence, by an autosomal dominant trait (MEN syndrome), when a third of them may be bilateral, whereas only 5% of the non-familial (sporadic) tumors are bilateral. Carney's triad is the coexistence of neoplasms in young women, including malignant GIST of stomach, pulmonary chondroma and extra-adrenal paragangioma

Pathology

Three types of tumors are recognized namely, non-familial (85%), familial and functional hyperplasia. Macroscopically rubbery firm, well demarcated, on section shows a light tan or reddish color, with a homogeneous cut surface (hence called potato tumor) or spongy and vascular, akin to neuroblastoma and pheochromocytoma. The tumor contains masses of cells resembling chief cells, set in a fibrous stroma, surrounded by a capsule, with occasional nuclear pleomorphism. About 5% of these tumors may be endocrine-active, producing catecholamines, but not enough to be clinically significant. These capsulated, benign tumors are so closely adherent to carotids, that sacrificing part of the vessel wall may become necessary in order to accomplish total excision. Longstanding tumors show some tendency to become malignant, which is identified by their biological behavior (regional and rarely distant metastases) and not by tumor histology.

Histologically the typical pattern is one of nests of neoplastic chief cells, which are histochemically positive for neuroendocrine markers. About 3% of them behave in a malignant fashion and metastasize.

Other sites of chemodectomas:

(1) aortic body: at the origin of left coronary artery or the pulmonary arterial bifurcation

(2) glomus tumor of nail beds

(3) glomus jugulare, in the adventitia of the jugular bulb

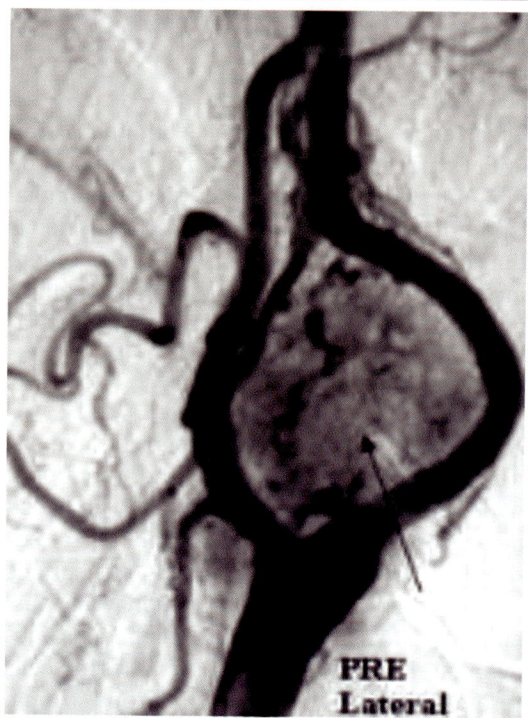

Fig. 92.1. Carotid body tumor splaying the carotid fork seen in the angiogram

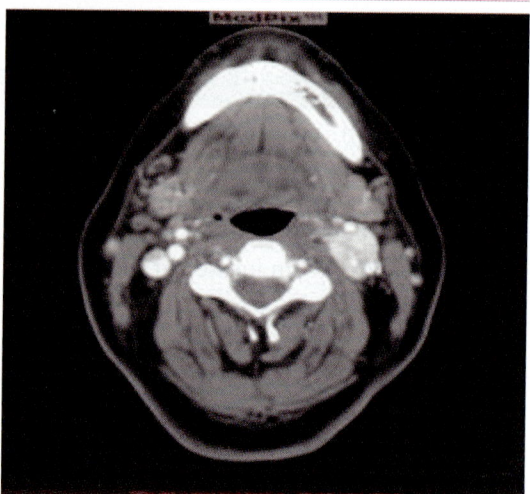

Fig. 92.2. CT scan showing carotid body tumor, after contrast injection

(4) glomus intravagale, associated with the ganglion nodosum of the vagus nerve

(5) paraganglion tympanicum along the tympanic branch of the glossopharyngeal nerve and rarely along the femoral artery in the femoral canal, in the mesentery and in the retroperitoneum.

Symptoms

Commonest presentation is an indolently growing painless lump in the carotid triangle of the neck, in a middle-aged individual (no sex predilection). Syncopal attacks due to transient cerebral ischemia (TIA) consequent to compression on the carotid artery may be present (this symptom may be reproducible by external pressure on the lump).

Hoarseness of voice due to recurrent laryngeal nerve pressure or dysphagia from direct compression, are rare, as also Horner's syndrome, unless the tumor is located on the deeper aspect of the carotids.

Involvement of cranial nerves (glossopharyngel, recurrent laryngeal, vagus, spinal accessory and hypoglossal) is seen in about 10% of cases.

Signs

Firm rounded or uneven (due to 'pseudopodia') lump is seen beneath the anterior border of the SCM at the level of the upper border of the thyroid cartilage. The overlying skin is normal, with some mobility horizontally but not vertically (Fontaine sign). Pulsation may occur, either transmitted from the underlying carotid artery or a displaced external carotid which becomes palpable. Rarely, increased vascularity may make the tumor pulsatile. Careful palpation of the contralateral side has to be done, as well as for regional nodal involvement, the latter should alert malignancy. Its association in MEN syndrome, as a familial disease, prompts screening for other endocrine tumors, such as carcinoid tumor, pheochromocytoma, medullary thyroid carcinoma (MTC), islet cell tumors of pancreas etc. not only in the patient, but also in the first degree relatives for such disorders if necessary.

Differential diagnosis

1. Tuberculous lymphadenitis
2. Metastatic lymph node
3. Carotid aneurysm

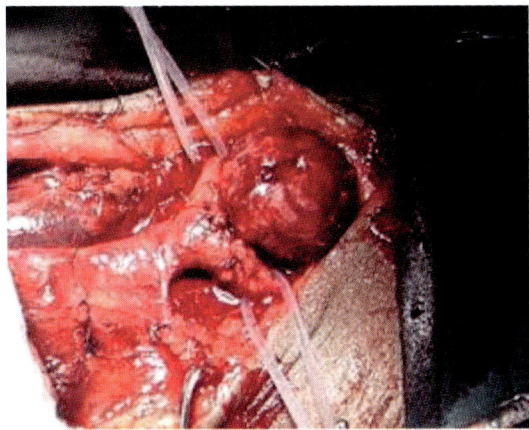

Fig. 92.3. Carotid body tumor being dissected from carotid fork

4. Branchial cyst
5. Paraganglioma from the cervical sympathetic chain
6. Other soft tissue tumors, such as lipoma, neurofibroma, fibromyxoma, etc.

Rares of carotid body tumor

It is a rare tumor
Rarely malignant
Rarely metastasizes
Rarely bilateral
Rarely done by a general surgeon (in view of its intimate relation to carotids)

Investigations

1) An USG will show a solid tumor at the carotid bifurcation, enlarged nodes etc.

2) Angiography or duplex imaging, reveals 'splaying' of the carotid fork and tumor neovascularity and helps to differentiate this tumor from a carotid aneurysm.

3) CT/MRI to delineate the relation to adjacent neurovascular structures.

4) Tumor markers for MTC (serum calcitonin), pheochromocytoma (urinary catacholamines and vanillyl mandelic acid-VMA), carcinoid (urinary 5-hydroxy indole acetic acid, 5-HIAA) etc.

5) Neither a needle nor an open biopsy should be performed, because (a) it is highly vascular, (b) risk of injuring carotid vessels and lastly (c) it cannot clinch malignancy in any event.

Treatment

(1) Surgery is the only option, as the tumor is not radio/chemosensitive. Exploration and meticulous dissection from the carotids has to be carried out to excise the tumor in toto.

(2) If it is large and inseparable from the vessels, it is excised along with the vessels and a venous or synthetic (Dacron/PTFE) graft is interposed between the common and the internal carotids so that cerebral circulation is restored, ignoring the external carotid artery. During the period of carotid clamping, an internal shunt (such as Javid shunt) is used to perfuse the brain, to prevent cerebral ischemia, particularly in the elderly. Hence this procedure is generally done by a vascular surgeon.

Classification of the tumor (Shambling) into three categories.

a. Small tumors easily removable
b. Partially surrounding the carotids
c. Totally engulfing the carotid vessels

(3) In the very elderly with a long history of tumor, it is best left alone, as the risk/benefit ratio is against such formidable surgery. Preoperative embolization may be useful in large tumors. Concomitant excision of bilateral tumors is undesirable.

(4) Adjuvant RT is advisable following resection, either total or subtotal, of a malignant carotid body tumor and palliative RT may be considered for those with difficult nonresectable malignant tumors and those who are unfit for surgery.

(Syn: Zenker's diverticulum)

Definition: Pharyngeal pouch or diverticulum is a protrusion of the mucosa through *Killian's dehiscence*, the weak area in the posterior pharyngeal wall between the oblique (thyropharyngeus) and the sphincter-like transverse fibres (cricopharyngeus) of the inferior constrictor muscle of pharynx.

Thyropharyngeus: The fibres of this part of the inferior constrictor are oblique in direction and take origin mainly from the oblique line of the thyroid cartilage, inserting into the posterior median fibrous raphe of the pharynx. The main nerve supply is by the pharyngeal branch of vagus and its main function is to propel food during deglutition.

Cricopharyngeus: The fibres of this part of the inferior constrictor arise from the side of the cricoid cartilage and pass backwards horizontally being continuous below with the circular fibres of the esophagus, this part of the inferior constrictor is supplied mainly by the recurrent laryngeal nerve. This surrounds the narrowest part of the pharynx, acting as a sphincter, which relaxes during swallowing. Failure of its relaxation will cause an increased pressure in the lower part of the pharynx and result in herniation of the pharyngeal mucosa, through the gap between the two components of the inferior constrictor.

Etiopathogenesis

This is a pulsion diverticulum, secondary to cricopharyngeal dysfunction attributable to esophageal dysmotility or incoordination.

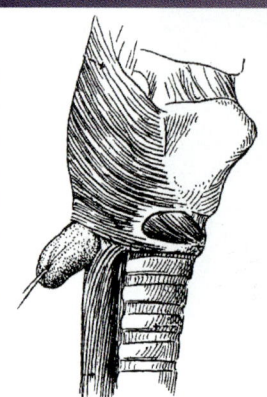

Fig. 93.1. Pharyngeal pouch

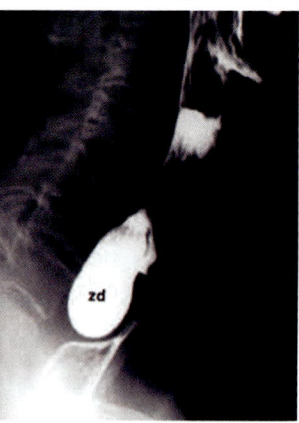

Fig. 93.2 Barium swallow - Zenker's diverticulum (courtesy: Laxmi Hospital, Kakinada)

It develops as a posterior midline mucosal out-pouching at the pharyngo-esophageal junction. As the posterior extension is limited by the spine, it enlarges to lie on one side (usually left), to appear behind the SCM muscle, in the posterior triangle.

Other predisposing factors

1. Gastroesophageal reflux disease (GERD) with hypertonic cricopharyngeal sphincter

2. Motility disorders of esophagus, such as achalasia or diffuse esophageal spasm.

Clinical features

Pharyngeal pouch usually appears as a soft, rounded, compressible swelling of about 5 cm. in the posterior triangle of neck, at about the level of cricoid, in elderly individuals. It is twice as common in men as in women, located deep to investing fascia; the edges may be illdefined, without fluctuation, transillumination or regional lymphadenopathy. In a clinical context, three stages of the diverticulum have been described:

1st stage: A small pouch, often detected only during barium swallow examination, directed posteriorly, usually in an asymptomatic patient or with minimal dysphagia.

2nd stage: It gets larger and becomes globular, still in the midline, with a tilt to one side. The patient complains of regurgitation of food and troublesome nocturnal cough or recurrent respiratory infections, due to aspiration.

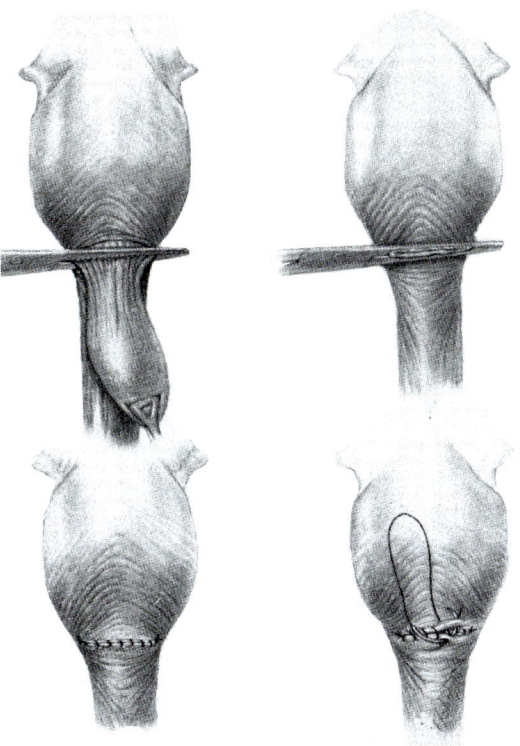

Fig. 93.3. Steps of excision of a pharyngeal diverticulum

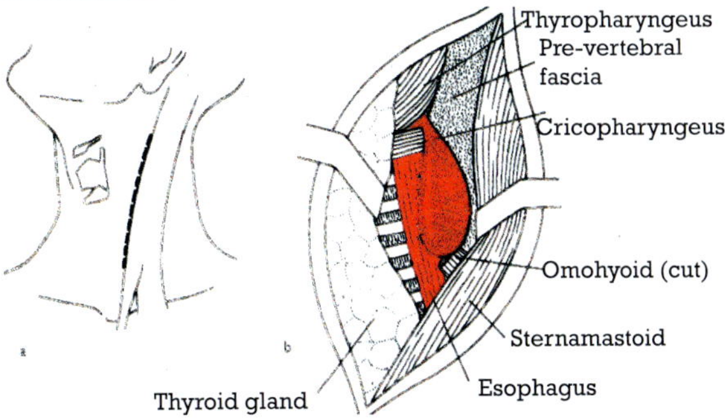

Fig. 93.4. Incision and exposure of pharyngeal diverticulum from the left side

(Labels on Fig. 93.4: Thyropharyngeus, Pre-vertebral fascia, Cricopharyngeus, Omohyoid (cut), Sternamastoid, Esophagus, Thyroid gland)

3rd stage: The diverticulum becomes bigger and pushed commonly to the left, with its dependent fundus seen in the posterior triangle. Besides the symptoms mentioned in the earlier stages, the patient presents with a soft swelling in the neck, expanding with a gurgle whenever liquids are consumed, associated with dysphagia and weight loss. Frank pulmonary suppuration may be seen, due to aspiration and poor nutritional status. Occasionally a cervical swelling may be absent, though the patient is symptomatic.

General examination reveals, depending upon the stage, an undernourished patient, with evidence of GERD or respiratory infection (or a lung abscess).

Complications

1. Aspiration pneumonitis, lung abscess, pulmonary atelectasis
2. Recurrent ulceration and bleeding (hematemesis)
3. Perforation, causing local cellulitis, abscess and rarely external (pharyngo-cutaneous) fistula.
4. Carcinoma (0.3%)

Investigations

1. Barium swallow - lateral films demonstrate the diverticulum better, outline its neck and any esophageal compression. It also identifies coexisting/predisposing esophageal motility disorders.

2. Endoscopy - this is neither essential nor safe, unless for tissue diagnosis if malignancy is suspected, since it carries a risk of perforation.

3. Esophageal manometry - this is not necessary for diagnosis except in motility disorders of esophagus.

4. pH monitoring - this is advisable in patients with GERD.

5. Chest x-ray - to rule out pulmonary complications.

6. CT/MRI scan of neck may define its topography as well as any local complications

Treatment

Surgery is indicated in second and third stages, but it is debatable in the first stage of the disease. As it is certainly going to expand with time, an aggressive approach is advocated by some, even if an early diverticulum is identified, unless the patient has a limited life expectancy or it is otherwise contraindicated.

Surgical approach is through an oblique cervical incision, along the anterior border of the SCM, in the midneck. The options are:

1. Cricopharyngeal myotomy, suitable for small, nondependent diverticula. This may be done alone or as adjunct to other procedures. This is similar to Heller's esophagocardio-myotomy for achalasia cardia.

2. Diverticulectomy: Using extreme caution, a preliminary endoscopy is done for proper orientation of anatomy and a nasogastric tube is passed, for identification of structures during surgery as well as for postoperative feeding.

3. Diverticulopexy may be done, by invaginating and plicating the pouch, suitable for early cases and certainly not for those complicated by infection and adhesions.

4. Endoscopic division of septum with stapling is sometimes resorted to, in a high risk elderly patient with large dependent diverticulum (Dohlmann's technique).

Postoperative complications

1. Infection usually due to sutureline leak at the pharyngeal wall, may lead to cellulitis or an abscess and even mediastinitis. Adequate perioperative antibiotic coverage is necessary, as it is a 'clean-contaminated' wound.

2. Fistula - this also is a result of leaked sutureline, more so if the two layers are not meticulously sutured while closing the neck of the pouch. It usually closes spontaneously, with a conservative approach (antibiotics, nasogastric feeding etc), provided the interim nutrition is maintained and there is no distal (esophageal) obstruction.

3. Recurrence may occur if it is incompletely excised or underlying esophageal dysmotility is overlooked.

94 Nutrition in Surgery

Normal daily requirements: Total 2000 Kcals per day, for an average adult, working to 30-40 Kcal/Kg body weight, depending upon the metabolic need. In hypercatabolic states, such as fever, sepsis or postoperative/post-traumatic states, the requirement may go upto 50Kcal/Kg/day. It is normally derived from carbohydrates (50%), proteins (30%) and fats (20%).

ALTERED BIOCHEMISTRY IN STRESS-INDUCED MALNUTRITION

The hypermetabolic state seen in stressful situations, increases resting energy expenditure. It is more of catabolism, triggered by various hormonal influences with loss of lean tissue, causing negative nitrogen balance. The counter-regulatory hormones, such as catacholamines, cortisol and glucagon (all of them have anti-insulin property) are elevated. Though the insulin levels are also elevated, there is relative insulin resistance, with a tendency for hyperglycemia and in diabetics, it makes the sugar levels labile and glycemic control difficult. Unless this trend of 'auto cannibalism' is aggressively reversed, continuous loss of protein leads to irreversible changes in various tissues, including immunological system, ultimately to death.

The basic difference between general community-related malnutrition and that occurs in stress-induced states, with altered physiology and biochemistry, has to be appreciated and physician should be highly sensitive to the effects of inadequate nutrition on various normal processes necessary for healing and early recovery from stress, trauma or sepsis.

Basic energy expenditure (BEE) depends on the age, gender, physiological activity and hypermetabolic states, such as stress, sepsis etc. which averages to 25Kcal/kg/day. The formula proposed by Harris and Benedict is too complicated for routine clinical application and is found to overestimate the calorific requirements in hospilized patients.

The *total energy expenditure* (TEE) may be calculated by multiplying BEE with the *stress factor*, as indicated below:

Minor surgery	1.1
Major surgery/injury	1.3
Infection	1.3
Gross sepsis	1.8
Major burns	2.0

EFFECTS OF MALNUTRITION

1. Increased morbidity due to delayed wound healing (external and internal), increased risk of infection, pulmonary complications and impaired immunity
2. Prolonged hospitalization with its attendant complications
3. Increased convalescence time
4. Altered quality of life
5. Immediate and late mortality

CLINICAL ASSESSMENT OF NUTRITIONAL STATUS

Three main factors are very useful in assessing the nutritional status of a hospitalized patient, though none of them offer early warning signals, to enable prevention:

1. Loss of weight

The anthropometric measurements such as weight, thickness of triceps skin fold, mid-arm muscle circumference, as compared to standard charts available, for grading purposes. 5% reduction in there parameters over a month or 10% over a longer period are considered significant

2. Plasma proteins

Among the serum proteins, albumin (<3gm%), pre-albumin and transferrin levels are routinely used in clinical practice. Albumin has a half-life of 21 days, for transferrin it is 7 days and for

Parameter	Severe	Moderate	Mild	Half-life
Albumin (gm%)	<2.5	2.5-3.0	3.0-3.5	21 days
Transferrin (mg%)	<160	160-190	190-220	7days
TLC	<900	900-1500	1500-1800	

Table-94.1. Stratification of nutritional status based on the common markers

prealbumin, 3 days. Hence the latter two are better markers in acute conditions.

3. Transferrin: it is a β-globulin that transports iron in plasma, with a half-life of 7-10 days, which gives an advantage over albumin as a nutritional marker. Transferrin levels (normal: 250-300mg%) respond to the iron status; increasing in iron deficiency and decreasing in states of iron overload. Hence its values have to be correlated with the iron levels.

4. Total lymphocyte count (TLC) is arrived by multiplying the total WBC count with %age of lymphocytes (normal: 2-3000) and levels <1,800 are significant.

With high index of suspicion, even apparently healthy-looking patients have to be critically evaluated within a few days of hospitalization for major trauma, infection, organ dysfunction or malignancy, to initiate appropriate remedial steps immediately, without waiting for the classical biochemical changes to appear.

Besides the above mentioned findings, systematic clinical examination for skin, mucosal and hair changes, sclera discoloration, features of dehydration, impaired hepatic, cardiac, renal and cerebral functions, have to be done on periodic basis. Specific laboratory studies for hematological, hepatic, renal functions, electrolytes, cholesterol, magnesium, calcium, phosphate levels have to be regularly monitored. This is also known as micro-nutritional assessment (MNA)

As a general rule, the GI tract should be used as frequently and completely as possible. However, repeated attempts to feed enterally for patients who have intermittent episodes of ileus or intolerance to the feeds, are not advisable and parenteral nutrition is a better choice. It may be necessary to use more than one type of enteral nutrition or a combination of enteral and parenteral feedings.

Enteral nutrition is also used in patients with a normally functioning GI tract who cannot eat enough.

It may be given:

1. orally.

2. via nasoenteric soft silastic fine bore tube with continuous slow infusion. Such tubes are tolerated well even for 2 months with few complications. The large bore nasogastric tube should be avoided since it is poorly tolerated and associated with aspiration and other pulmonary complications.

3. via tube enterostomies.

4. via continuous rectal infusion (rarely done).

Enteral diets are relatively inexpensive. They maintain intestinal mucosal intergrity and reduces bacterial translocation. There are three types: blenderised diets, partially hydrolysed and elemental diets. Complications are related to diet hyperosmolarity.

Parenteral nutrition is the treatment of choice in the absence of a normally functioning GI tract

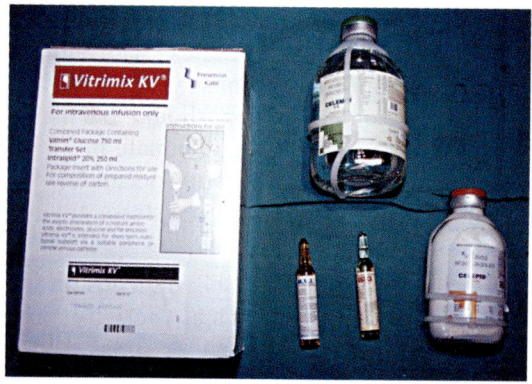

Fig. 94.1. Some of the TPN solutions

and in rapidly progressive catabolic states.

In addition to standard central IV hyper-alimentation there are other easier to administer and safer forms of parenteral nutrition which can be used for patients with lesser nutritional needs. These include the infusion of aminoacids alone or in combination with fat emulsions by either peripheral or central vein.

Total parenteral nutrition (TPN)

Principles of TPN: It may be discussed under:

(A) indications,
(B) techniques and
(C) complications

A) Indications

1)   in patients who cannot ingest food as a result of anorexia, neurological disorders, intracranial surgery, central nervous system trauma and coma, multiple injuries especially maxillofacial, head and neck fractures.

2)   in patients with malfunctioning gastrointestinal tract due to:

short-bowel syndrome secondary to massive small bowel resection.

enteroenteric, enterocolic, entero-vesical or enterocutaneous fistulae.

Intestinal obstruction.

paralytic ileus.

Crohn's disease and ulcerative colitis.

3)   hypercatabolic patients with major diseases, fever of more than 38°C, tachycardia and increased respiratory rate and urea production rate of more than 20g/24h, as seen in:

a)   severe trauma and major fractures.

b)   extensive burns.

c)   selected patients on chemotherapy or radiotherapy particularly for gastrointestinal tumors.

d)   infants with major gastrointestinal anomalies or who fail to thrive because of gastrointestinal insufficiency from short-bowel syndrome, malabsorption, enzyme deficiency, meconium ileus or idiopathic diarrhea.

B)   Techniques of administration

Either the internal jugular or subclavian vein may be used as the access line. The latter is more preferred, as the infraclavicular hollow comfortably houses the CVP apparatus and the neck movements are not interfered with. Central venous cannulation should be done aseptically, using a subcutaneous tunnel, before puncturing the vein, to reduce transmigration of bacteria from skin. A chest skiagram is mandatory after the percutaneous venous cannulation, to exclude pneumo/hemothorax (commoner in subclavian than in IJV). If a triple-lumen cannula is used, simultaneous CVP recording may be possible, in hemodynamically unstable patients. Subsequent management of the central venous catheter involves strict aseptic precautions and nursing protocol.

The available solutions are

1)   Dextrose or fructose, 10% or 20% as 500 or 1000ml bottles
2)   Aminoacids, 7Gm or 14Gm per litre as 500ml bottles
3)   Emulsified fat, 10Gm or 20Gm% as 500ml bottles
4)   Combination of the above

Administration of TPN

The above solutions are combined judiciously and administered to patients, keeping the following basic rules in mind:

i)   20% Dextrose or fructose solutions are irritant to veins, and cause thrombophlebitis.

ii)   20% lipid solution is also a strong irritant and heparin is needed to buffer it's effect on the vein wall.

iii) Except in very septic and malnourished patients, fat solutions can be avoided if the TPN support is only for a few days.

iv) In order to prevent excess breakdown of indigenous muscle protein, the nitrogen/ calorie ratio should be maintained at 1:160, i.e., 10gms of nitrogen should be provided for every 1600 Kcal infused.

v) Multivitamins and trace elements should always be added.

vi) Monitoring of these patients should be done, as several electrolyte and osmotic complications may occur (vide infra). Thus daily monitoring of serum urea and electrolytes, and biweekly monitoring of trace elements and complete blood counts are recommended. Other investigations are performed based on clinical suspicion, e.g. hypophosphatema or hyponatremia. Liver function tests should be done twice weekly in all patients on TPN (see below).

C) Complications

They may be complications of access (1 to 7) or related to the infusion (8 to 15). The former are sequel to the central venous cannulation.

1) pneumothorax

2) accidental arterial cannulation

3) thrombosis, embolization or false aneurysm. Covering with low dose LMWH has been shown to reduce thromboembolic complications

4) central line sepsis

A daily spike of temperature in every patient with a central line should invoke the possibility of central line sepsis unless proved otherwise. In such cases the line should be changed and the catheter tip sent for Gm stain, culture and sensitivity.

5) osteomyelitis of clavicle

6) hemothorax

7) proximal migration of detached venous cannula.

8) overfeeding is a increasingly recognized complications of nutritional support.

9) prolonged hypervitaminosis (especialy fat soluble) is also a harmful misadventure

10) fluid overload

11) prolonged (>4 weeks) TPN may lead to disuse atrophy of the intestinal mucosa.

12) the other complications of TPN mostly stem from osmotic and electrolyte changes in the internal milieu as a result of the TPN. Thus, hypo/hypernatremia, hypo/hyperkalemia, hypomagnesemia and hypophosphatemia can occur, giving rise to a perplexing set of clinical syndromes. Prompt recognition, confirmation by blood values and correction by changing the infusate, are essential for optimal results.

13) a fat embolism-like syndrome with pulmonary insufficiency is known to occur with infusions of large volume of fat, which can be corrected by withdrawing the solution, heparinization and general support.

14) abnormal LFTs, hepatic cholestasis and steatosis are very commonly seen in the background of the TPN. Sepsis, hypoxia, hypophosphatemia with decreased production of hepatotrophic factors have all been implicated in the production of this syndrome. Fortunately spontaneous resolution occurs in most cases.

15) TPN psychosis refers to the mental dysequilibrium that many of these patients exhibit due to a combination of several factors including low cerebral perfusion, sepsis, and electrolyte disturbance. Apart from close monitoring of all the parameters and appropriate counseling, no specific treatment is required for this syndrome.

95 Breast

Embryology: The breast is a modified apocrine (apo: from; krino: separate) sweat gland, peculiar to mammals. Ectodermal ridges are seen from the axilla to the groin on either side, the so called milk lines. Only the pectoral portion stays in humans, while the rest disappears. The upper part becomes the axillary tail (of Spence). Hair and sweat glands regress over the breasts and sebaceous glands develop fully only over the areolae (Montgomery's tubercles).

At about the 15th week, the breast tissue paradoxically is highly sensitive to testosterone, as a result of which condensation of mesenchyme around the epithelial stalks occur, leading to rupture and attenuation of the ductal system, whereas normal mammary development takes place in females due to the absence of androgens. At birth, under the influence of maternal estrogens and fetal prolactin, a thin serous fluid is secreted for a few weeks in both sexes, known as colostrum (witch's milk). The mammary tissue may remain quiescent for a few years, but later starts growing to reach the final size in the 3rd decade of life, usually at the birth of the first child.

Anatomy

It lies in the subcutaneous plane over the pectoral region, base extending from midline to anterior or midaxillary line and 2nd to 6th ribs, nipple approximately situated at the level of the 4th intercostal space. It overlies the pectoralis major, serratus anterior and to some extent the rectus sheath and external oblique muscle, but is separated from them by a condensation of superficial fascia (akin to Scarpa's fascia over the abdomen), called pectoral fascia. A small extension in the upper outer quadrant, reaching the medial wall of axilla, is known as the axillary tail of Spence, which is often poorly connected with the ductal system. Its clinical significance lies in that swellings arising from this tail, may be readily mistaken for lymph

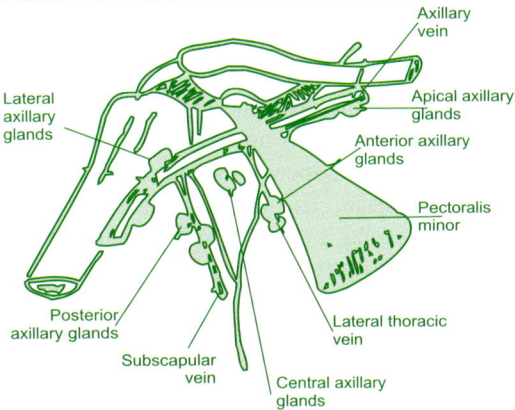

Fig. 95.1. Axillary anatomy

nodes. The axillary tail enters the axilla through an opening in the pectoral fasica, known as foramen of Langer, at the level of 3rd interspace.

About 20 lactiferous ducts converge radially to open on the nipple, a cylindrical projection on the summit of the breast, which is surrounded by circular pigmented skin, called the areola. Sebaceous glands under the areola form small elevations, known as Montgomery tubercles. Fibrous septa running between the skin and pectoral fascia (suspensory ligaments of Cooper), through the mammary tissue help to maintain the shape in young breasts and their atrophy in elderly accounts for sagging of the breasts. These septa also explain skin tethering in early malignancy and the orange peel (peau d' orange) appearance in diseases that produce cutaneous lymphedema.

Axilla

It is a pyramidal space wedged between the upper arm and the side of the chest and ceases to exist when the arm is hyper-abducted. It is limited by anterior and posterior folds, communicating above with the supraclavicular fossa, through the apex, which transmits the neurovascular and lymphatic structures. The anterior wall is fomed by pectoralis major, minor, subclavius and clavipectoral fascia. The posterior wall extends lower and is formed by subscapularis, teres major and latissimus dorsi. The lateral wall is the narrowest, since the anterior and posterior walls converge to the lips of the bicipital groove, this is formed by the upper humerus, coracobrachialis, biceps muscles and the axillary neurovascular structures. Medially it is bounded by the upper five ribs and the intercostals and upper digitation of the serratus anterior muscle. The floor is formed by the axillary fascia, bridging from fascia over serratus anterior to the deep fascia of arm. The action of pectoralis major is adduction and internal rotation of the shoulder, the former is employed to put the muscle to contraction, to detect fixity of a breast mass.

Lymphatic drainage of breast is of great clinical significance, outer quadrants predominantly draining into axillary and inner quadrants into internal mammary group of nodes on the same side. However when these channels are blocked, alternate drainage may take place, into supraclavicular nodes, opposite breast (and axilla), peritoneal cavity and liver via rectus sheath and falciform ligament. The lymphatics of nipple and areola drain into subareolar *plexus* of Sappey, before they reach the regional nodes. The axillary lymph nodes numbering around 50, are grouped as follows:

1.   anterior or pectoral group, located under the anterior axillary fold

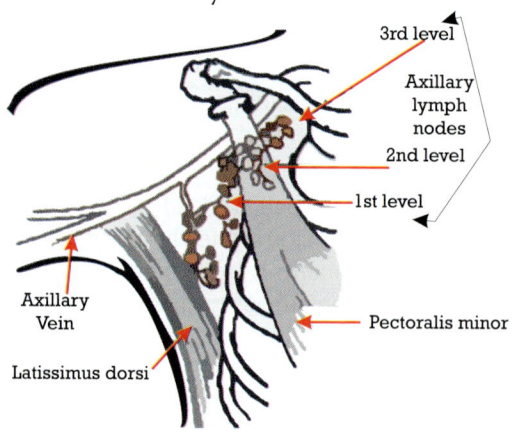

Fig. 95.2. levels of axillary lymph nodes

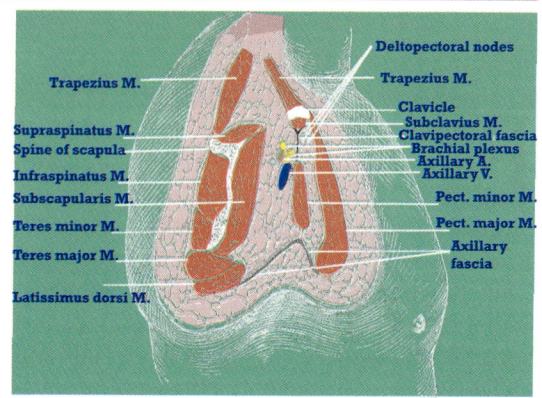

95.3. Axilla-sagittal section

2.   posterior or subscapular group, located in the postero-medial wall of axilla, in relation to the posterior fold.

3.   lateral group, along the axillary vessels

4.   central group, situated in the floor of axilla and the central pad of fat

5.   apical group, which form the junction between axillary and supraclavicular chains (similar to the node of Cloquet in the femoral canal)

6.   deltopectoral group located above/ medial to the pectoralis minor, in relation to clavi-pectoral fascia

7.   interpectoral group, located between pectoralis major and minor muscles

8.   Rotter's nodes, subpectoral group, in relation to chest wall.

Levels of axillary lymph nodes depending upon their relation to pectoralis minor (corresponding to the 3 parts of axillary artery)

Level 1:   below the pectoralis minor muscle (3rd part of axillary artery)

Level 2:   behind the pectoralis minor (2nd part of axillary artery)

Level 3:   above the pectoralis minor (1st part of axillary artery)

It should be realized that as in the neck, level of nodes is only for anatomic description, but not indicative of stage of the disease.

Anomalies of breast

One or both breasts may be hypoplastic due to underdevelopment of the lactiferous apparatus or grossly hypertrophied and pendulous (gigantomastia).

Amastia - absence of breast, may be seen in Turner syndrome and congenital adrenal hyperplasia or tumors. Absence of a breast, sternocostal head of pectoralis major muscle, syndactylism and nephropathy is known as Poland's syndrome

Athelia - absence of nipple

Polymastia or polythelia - Supernumerary breasts or nipples might develop along the milk line, most often in the inframammary regions, due to incomplete involution of the mammary ridge (milk line).

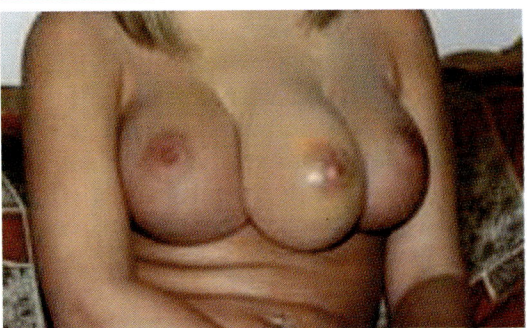

Fig. 95.4. Polymastia

BENIGN LESIONS OF THE BREAST

ABSCESS

In relation to breast, it may be acute, chronic (antibioma) or retromammary, the latter one being usually a tuberculous cold abscess.

ACUTE ABSCESS

It is produced by strepto/staphylococci, gaining entry through the cracked nipple, commonly seen in lactating women. It may also be a result of acute mastitis, which has gone on to local suppuration or an infected cyst. Typical fever, local signs of inflammation with softening would provide the necessary clue, confirmed by USG or needling. There may be regional lymphadenopathy.

Under adequate antibiotic cover, the abscess is incised over the area of fluctuation and drained. If necessary another counter drain may be introduced at a dependent point for additional exit. Another cosmetically favorable option, is repeated aspirations with a wide-bore needle, under antibiotic cover, reserving incision for delayed or recurrent cases. This is very effective for infected galactocele or a lymph cyst.

CHRONIC ABSCESS

It is also known as antibioma, a short form for antibiotic-induced granuloma. It is the result of administering antibiotics for an abscess, without drainage. The signs of inflammation subside, pus may become sterile, the wall gets fibrosed and overlying cutaneous edema may give a peau d' orange appearance. These features associated with fixity of the mass to breast tissue and axillary lymphadenopathy, often make it clinically indistinguishable from carcinoma.

Needle aspiration/biopsy and USG are confirmatory. Treatment is by total excision in smaller lesions and subtotal excision (deroofing) for larger ones, under cover of appropriate antibiotics. The excised wall of the cavity should be subjected to histopathology, to exclude a degenerated tumor or specific infection, such as tuberculosis.

Feature	Antibioma	Fat necrosis	Carcinoma
Onset	As acute abscess	Trauma	Incidious
Anat plane	Mammary	Subcutaneous	Mammary
Peau d' orange	Sometimes	Never	Often
Consistence	Firm/hard	Firm	Hard
Intrinsic mobility	Absent	Present	Absent
Axillary nodes	Soft	Absent	Firm/hard
USG	Central cavity	Solid	Solid

Table-95.1. Differences between chronic abscess (antibioma), traumatic fat necrosis and carcinoma

TRAUMATIC FAT NECROSIS

It may be acute or subacute, follows blunt injuries to chest or breast, but as a rule, such history is wanting. The importance of this disease lies in its resemblence to scirrhous carcinoma. It presents commonly in fatty middle-aged women, as a hard subcutaneous mass, restricting the mobility of the overlying skin and the mass typically can be 'lifted away' from the breast tissue. History of trauma, absence of appreciable growth and its anatomic plane, provide the valuable clues to the diagnosis, but should be confirmed by mammography and needle or excision biopsy.

On section, chalky white necrotic fat may be seen, not unlike that seen in resolving acute pancreatitis. Microscopically granular histiocytes surround 'oil cells' of varying size are seen. Collagenous scarring may be seen in later stages of the disease. Simple local excision is sufficient for cure and for reassurance against a neoplasm.

FIBROADENOMA

Etiology

Like fibroadenosis, this is now considered to be an aberration of normal development and involution of the breast - ANDI (usually seen in 2nd and 3rd decades), though some pathologists still maintain that it is a benign neoplasm. The possible etiology is the hormonal influence on the developing permanent duct lobular unit.

Unlike carcinoma, these arise from an entire breast lobule rather than a single cell, but show estrogen sensitivity, undergoing involution at menopause. They generally stop growing beyond 3-4cm and very rarely, if at all, undergo malignant change.

Pathology

Depending upon the growth of the fibroadenoma in relation to the ducts, these lesions were earlier classified into pericanalicular (hard) and intracanalicular (soft) types. The latter was considered to have a high incidence of bilaterality with a slightly higher risk of malignancy. However this pathological classification is no longer used. Those cancers that are reported in fibroadenomas are now termed as chance occurrence cancers and they are seen only in women over 40. Fibroadenomas are now considered to be one end of the spectrum of development of normal breast tissue. They possess receptors for progesterone (PR) but not for estrogen (ER).

The lobular arrangement of mixed glandular and mesenchymal elements is maintained, with a well defined capsule, from which septa radiate into the tumor mass. Cut surface of a fibroadenoma is typically fleshy and turns convex, due to the tissue tension within the capsule, whereas it remains flat in a carcinoma. Microscopically, a mature differentiated breast lobular architecture is preserved. There is a very

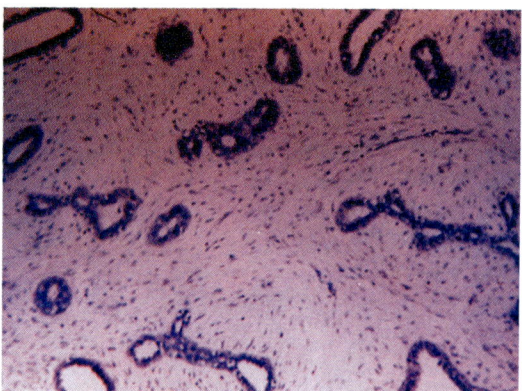

Fig. 95.5. Histology of fibroadenoma of breast (courtesy: Histo Lab, Chennai)

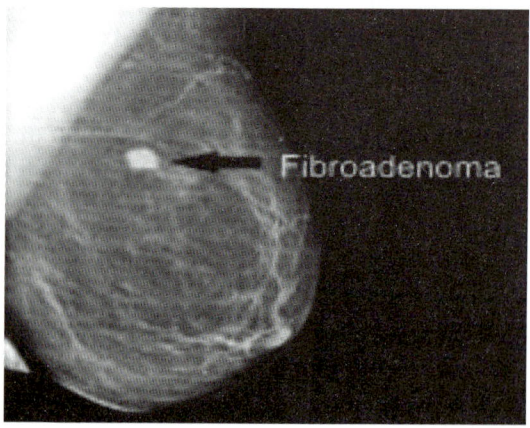

Fig. 95.6. Fibroadenoma in a mammogram

low potential (<0.3%) for malignant transformation (fibrosarcoma and lobular carcinoma), often being discovered by histopathology of a clinically 'benign' lump. Hyalinization, calcification, myxoid change, lactational foci, infarction and fibrocystic change all can occur in a fibroadenoma.

Lactating adenoma is a tubular tumor, representing an exaggerated physiological response to the excess estradiol levels in pregnancy. It contains tubular elements in a concentric manner, with minimal stroma and no lobular detail.

Clinical features

A painless slippery lump in a young woman is typical, examination reveals a smooth, rounded (sometimes uneven, due to 'pseudopodia'), discrete, nontender, firm mass, with free intrinsic mobility within the breast tissue (breast mouse), slipping under the palpating fingers. It has no fixity to either overlying skin or underlying pectoral fascia, nor regional lymphadenopathy.

Differential diagnosis

1) cyst in the breast (cystic, aspiration and ultrasound are conclusive, re-examination of the breast should be done immediately after aspiration, and if a residual mass is felt, it goes in favor of a neoplastic cyst).

2) carcinoma (hard consistency, fixity to the breast tissue and if extramammary invasion has occurred, to the skin and pectoral fascia/muscle or chest wall, with evidence of regional and distant spread)

3) hematoma (history of trauma, evidence of bruising of overlying skin and soft tissue)

4) traumatic fat necrosis (history of trauma may be present, no appreciable increase in size with time, located in the plane of subcutaneous fat, tethered to the skin,

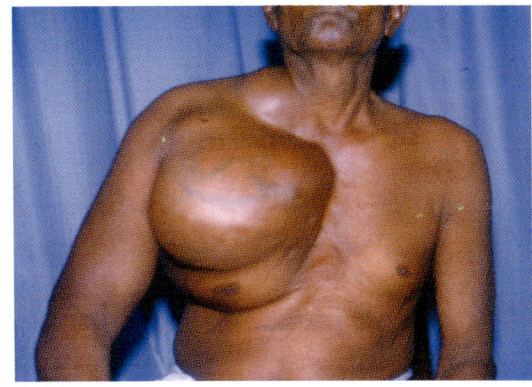

Fig. 95.8. Phyllodes tumor of breast
(courtesy: Dr K Sreekanth, Chennai)

the mass can be pinched or lifted away from the breast tissue, firm to hard in consistency, irregular borders. Diagnosis clinched by FNAC)

Investigations

When the presentation is typical, no specific investigations are necessary.

1) USG is reliable to make out the typical solid and well defined lump in the breast; it rules out a cyst and may pick up early malignant change, however, reliable early sonographic signs of malignancy are yet to be unequivocally defined. A color duplex imaging is a sensitive and useful adjunct in the assessment of small breast lumps, as it detects increased vascularity in malignancies.

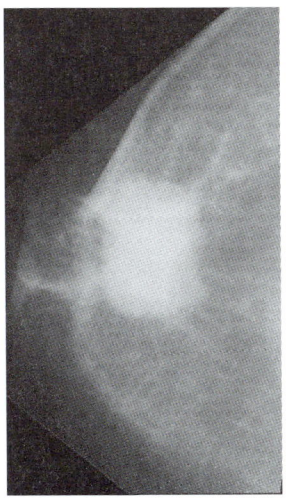

Fig. 95.7. Mammogram showing a carcinoma. (typical crab-like)
(courtesy: Halsted Surgical Clinic, Chennai)

2) mammography is insensitive in preclinical detection of malignancy in a fibroadenoma as the radio-density and micro-calcification commonly seen in benign lesions, may mask early radiological signs. Furthermore, the high density of breast tissue in young women (<30), dampens radiological resolution.

3) FNAC is the best option to reliably rule out malignancy, but employed only in atypical cases, with some suspicion of malignancy.

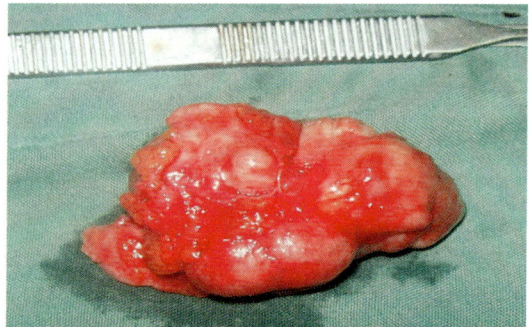

Fig. 95.9. Excised fibroadenoma with typical 'pseudopodia'

Treatment

Excision or enucleation of the fibroadenoma is the standard treatment, carried out through a cosmetically-placed, circumareolar or submammary incision (upper medial quadrant incisions should be avoided, to enable them to wear a low-necked jacket!). The tumor can be easily shelled out like a pea from a pod (intracapsular excision).

In recent years however, conservative management of fibroadenoma is being considered. Several studies have shown that small fibroadenomas when followed up over a period of time (2-4 years), gradually regress and even disappear. This, coupled with proven very low incidence of malignancy, has emboldened a conservative approach. However, before adopting this 'expectant' management, triple assessment of the lump, by USG, mammogram and FNAC, is mandatory to establish its benign nature. All scientific data aside, majority of women are still comfortable when the tumor is out and in the pathology department. Excision of the lump is done in a day-care set up, has minimal morbidity, offers complete pathological examination and high patient acceptability, with virtual cure.

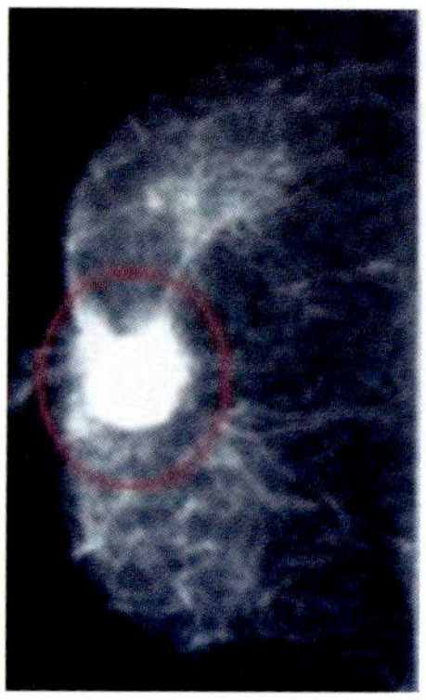

PHYLLODES TUMOR (syn: cystosarcoma phyllodes, giant fibroadenoma, serocystic disease of Brodie) (sarkos: flesh; phyllon: leaf)

Pathology

A rare fibroepithelial tumor of breast, first described by Muller. This is a benign tumor, which grows to very large proportions, with bimodal age incidence, occurring either in the 2nd or 5th decades. There is a high tendency for local recurrence and frank sarcomatous change.

Histologically, branching leaf-like papillary projections are seen in the tumor tissue invaginating into the cystic areas. This feature in combination with the fleshy appearance on cut section, is responsible for its name. They have a similar basic structure to the intracanalicular fibroadenomas but show a greater degree of stromal cellularity, without a true capsule. The connective tissue element is the essential feature to distinguish this tumor from fibroadenoma. Histological features of malignant change are, stromal overgrowth, high mitotic activity and infiltrating margins. In several large series, up to 9% of phyllodes tumors were classified as malignant with detectable hematogenous pulmonary, skeletal and visceral metastases.

Clinical features

They present as rapidly growing large tumors with an uneven or bosselated surface, but they always remain freely mobile under the stretched out skin and over pectoralis major. The huge protuberance produces appreciable asymmetry of the breasts and grows away from the chest wall, often causing pressure ulceration of skin. Some local warmth and engorged veins may be seen due to hypervascularity. A variable consistency (soft-cystic-firm) is not uncommon due to avascular necrosis of the tumor, outgrowing its blood supply.

Differential diagnosis

1) virginal hypertrophy of breast (usually bilateral, no distinct mass felt nor hyper-vascularity)

Fig. 95.10. Mammographic appearance of carcinoma

2) soft tissue sarcoma (may be practically indistinguishable except by

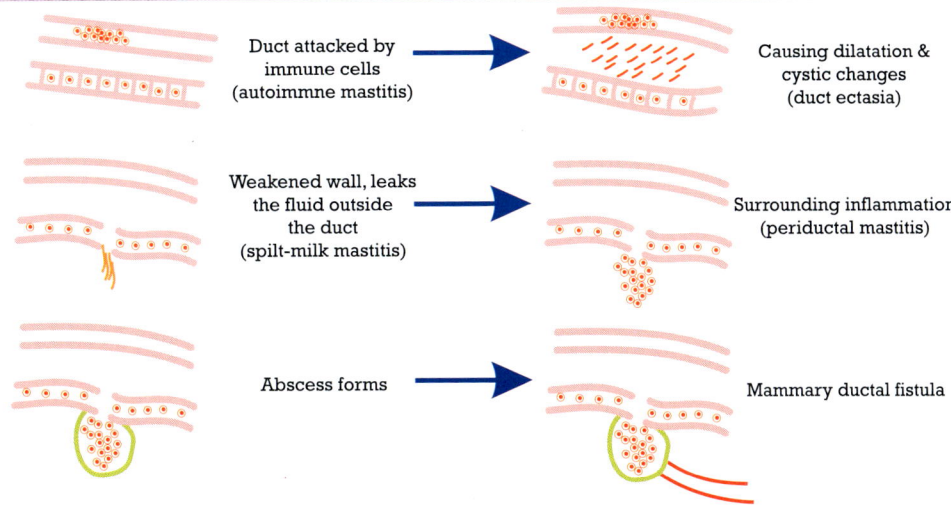

Fig. 95.11. Pathogenesis of mammary duct ectasia - the significance of its synonyms indicated

histopathology, unless evidences of local invasion and distant spread are present)

3) rapidly growing carcinoma, especially mastitis carcinomatosa (history of lactation, early fixity to chest wall, local signs of 'inflammation' and regional nodal involvement)

4) desmoid tumor is only a pathological curiosity, without clinical clues.

The index of clinical suspicion of malignancy should be high in elderly and those with positive family history.

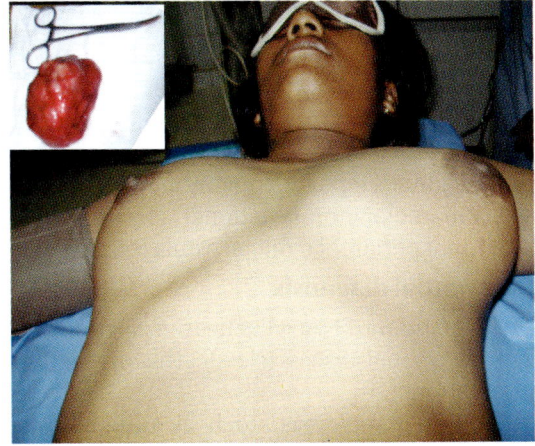

Fig. 95.12. Asymmetry of the left breast due to a giant fibroadenoma. Excised specimen is shown in the inset

Investigations

1) chest skiagram
2) USG of breast
3) mammography
4) wide-bore needle biopsy
5) if the biopsy shows malignancy, USG abdomen and skeletal survey for staging

Treatment

Adequate local surgery is required to safeguard against recurrence. Care is taken to exclude sarcomatous change with certainty, by serial histopathological sections. Simple excision has a recurrence rate of about 10%, hence some schools advocate total mastectomy, by a submammary incision (of Gaillard Thomas), preserving the areola and nipple for reconstruction, as the procedure of choice. Many reserve such a mutilative step for recurrent disease following adequate excision, for better patient compliance. In contrast to fibroadenomas, they do not have a true capsule, hence enucleation should never be done.

Adjuvant RT to pectoral region reduces the incidence of local recurance, following surgery for large tumors with narrow margin of resection. There is no place for chemotherapy, in treating phyllodes tumor.

Stage	Normal process	Abnormal process
Early reproductive period (15-25 yrs)	Lobule formation, stroma formation	Fibroadenoma juvenile hypertrophy
Mature reprod period (25-40 yrs)	Cyclical hormone influence on gland tissue & stroma	Exaggerated effects cyclical mastalgia
Involution period (35-55 yrs)	Lobule formation, stroma formation	Cystic disease, adenosis fibrosis
	Epithelial turnover	Epithelial hyperplasia
	Ductal involution	Ductectasia, periductal mastitis

Table-95.2. Aberration of normal development and involution (ANDI)

MAMMARY DUCT ECTASIA (syn: periductal mastitis, plasma cell mastitis, 'spilt-milk' mastitis, autoimmune mastitis, mastitis obliterans, granulomatous mastitis):

This is a perplexing clinical condition, as evident by its synonyms, where there is dilatation of all the ductal system associated with periductal inflammation, seen more in smokers. It appears that the basic defect is related to the mammary ducts especially the terminal or the subareolar ducts.

Etiology

Hormone-induced muscular relaxation and ductal dilation and an autoimmune periductal inflammation, with secondary anaerobic bacterial infection, have been suggested in the etiology. The high incidence of this disease in smoking women, has also raised the possibility of a

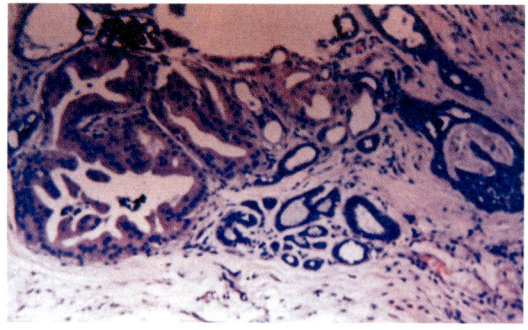

Fig. 95.13. Histology of fibrocystic disease of the breast
(courtesy: Histo Lab, Chennai)

nicotine-induced vasculitis with attenuation and dilatation of duct walls, which is the primary event in the disease.

Pathology

Classically there is dilatation of one or more subareolar ducts which are filled with its dark green or brown secretions. This fluid may set up a chronic plasma cell-rich (autoimmune?) inflammation of the surrounding tissue, resulting in a subareolar mass with progressive fibrosis and nipple retraction, which mimics carcinoma. An abscess may develop and when it is drained, a fistula formation may complicate the picture. The duct wall contains increased elastic tissue.

Clinical features

1) minor nipple discharge along with noncyclical mastalgia in early stages.
2) the mass may be firm to hard, without intrinsic mobility due to inflammatory fibrosis
3) regional lymphadenopathy may be present
4) subareolar non-lactational abscess and a persistent periareolar ductal fistula (rare)

Differential diagnosis

1) carcinoma (FNAC clinches the diagnosis)
2) lactational abscess (classical history, period of lactation)
3) other granulomas, such as tuberculosis, filariasis
4) fibroadenosis

Treatment

1) In view of the causal relationship, they should permanently refrain from tobacco abuse.

2) discharge from the nipple must be examined for occult blood and subjected to cytological examination

3) for the non-cyclical mastalgia especially localized areas of breast tenderness, a short course of antibiotics may help.

4) in non-lactating women some tender subareolar and peripheral breast lumps may be short-lived or persistent. FNAC will show subacute inflammation, often with foamy macrophages and endothelial histiocytes. If the fluid is purulent, surgical drainage may become necessary, under cover of appropriate antibiotics.

5) in women under 40, periareolar abscess may be related to a single duct disease, after the abscess drainage, limited duct excision and fistulectomy may be required.

6) If the abscess is extensive and multilocular, it must be drained and deroofed for adequate saucerization.

7) if troublesome duct discharge, recurrent inflammatory masses or recurrent major sepsis with fistula formation occur, a carefully performed major duct excision, after a course of antibiotics, is the procedure of choice (Urban's or Hadfield's procedure).

8) rapidly developing tender para-areolar breast cyst, when drained or aspirated, may result in a fistula. Excision of the cyst should be accompanied by removal of the diseased ducts and a segment of areola to prevent fistula formation.

9) blood stained discharge is rare in this disease although dark brown or green discharge is common. A cytological smear is obligatory. Any epithelial atypia requires major duct excision.

10) even after apparently adequate excision, in a small percentage of patients, sepsis and fistula may reappear. This is accounted for by a small proportion of patients who have extensive disease not only in the terminal subareolar ducts but even at the lobular level. Careful repeated excisions of all the affected ducts as and when septic complications supervene is necessary.

FIBROADENOSIS (syn: Reclus disease, fibrocystic disease, chronic cystic mastitis, mazoplasia, chronic interstitial mastitis, cystic mastopathy, ANDI)

This is considered to be an aberration of normal development and involution (ANDI), due to a disturbance in the cyclical hyperplasia/involution changes occurring in the breast, often bilateral. It is seen in the 3rd and 4th decades of life and is common in spinsters, nullipara and those who have not breast-fed their children. There appears to be some relation to consumption of coffee, tea and cola drinks, but no hard evidence is available against caffeine, methylxanthine or avitaminosis-E. The premenstrual accentuation of subjective or objective features favor a hormonal hypothesis, supported by the relief of symptoms by cyclical hormonal treatment, however their precise role is ill understood.

Pathology

Its pathogenesis is not clear and a wide range of processes occur, such as fibrosis, adenosis, epitheliosis, cystic changes and inflammation, in various proportions and combinations, justifying the confusion. The process starts with periductal fibrosis, probably secondary to estrogen stimulation, which causes irritation of the cells lining the ducts and increased epithelial proliferation (epitheliosis). Progressive epithelial clumping gives a gland-like appearance (adenosis) and obstruction to the ductal drainage causes cystic changes. Another histological feature is apocrine metaplasia, manifested by the cells near the blocked ducts. Solid and cystic lumps appear and regress, not necessarily correlating with the magnitude of symptoms experienced. When a single cyst gets enlarged, containing bluish blood pigments, it is called blue-domed cyst of Bloodgood. The premalignant potential of fibroadenosis is debatable and the

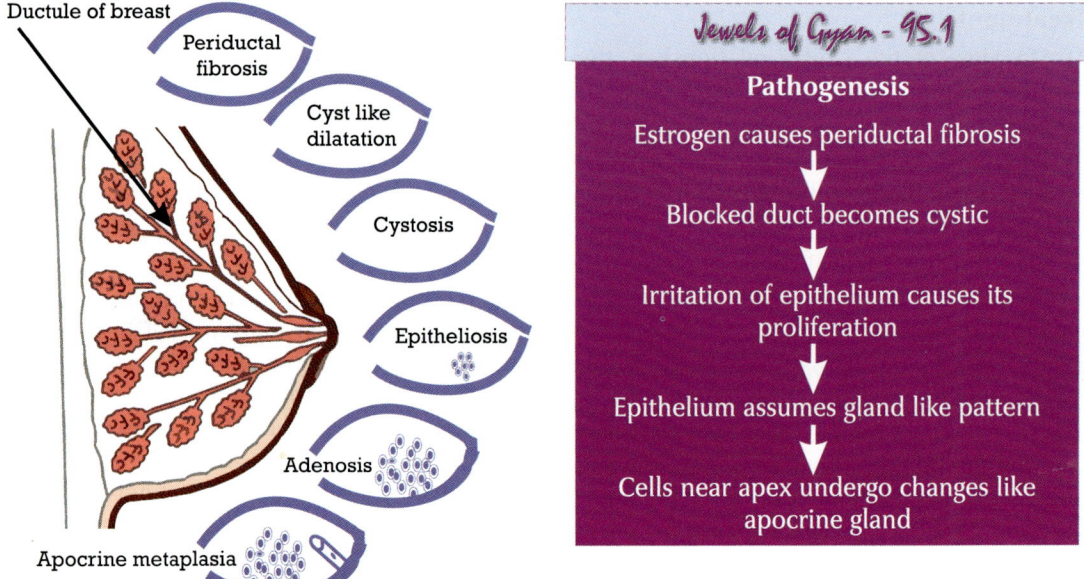

Fig. 95.14. Conventional pathological changes in fibroadenosis

higher incidence of malignancy seen in this disease may be related to the continued estrogen influence, which is the common denominator for both the diseases.

Clinical features

Cyclical perimenstrual mastalgia

(or mastodynia) in young women, is the typical presentation. Bilateral diffuse tenderness of the breasts with coarse nodularity appreciated by palpation with the flat of the hand (lubricated with soap), with or without definite nodules and serous nipple discharge, which may be multiductal and bilateral, almost clinches the diagnosis. The emotional undercurrents and frequent self examinations, created by 'cancer phobia' compound the symptomatology. There may be regional lymphadenopathy, usually small and insignificant, but enough to cause concern at times. Cardiff"s breast score, to quantitatively evaluate cyclical and noncyclical mastalgias and to correlate clinical progress, is sometimes needed.

CARDIFF BREAST PAIN SCORE (CBS)

This is to evaluate the magnitude of symptoms and efficacy of medical treatment for mastodynia, due to benign disorders of breast:

CB Score-1: Excellent response, totally free from pain

CB Score-2: Substantial relief with bearable discomfort

CB Score-3: Poor response, considerable pain persists

CB Score-4: No response at all; same pain persists

Differential diagnosis

a)   fibroadenoma
b)   other benign lesions of breast
c)   carcinoma
d)   costochondritis (Tietze's syndrome)

Investigations

USG, mammography and FNAC of a suspicious nodule are the investigations, done to reassure the patient. When the mass in question is small and indistinct, needle biopsy is best done under mammographic or ultrasound guidance, to increase the sensitivity. A chest skiagram may be done to exclude diseases of chest wall.

Treatment
Medical

a)   reassurance

b) analgesia with NSAIDs

c) anxiolytic agents

d) vitamin E and other antioxidants

e) danacrine sulfate (Danazol), antigona-dotrophic agent, very specific (commonest drug used)

f) oil of evening primrose (Primosa), which has polyunsaturated fatty acids (PUFA) and acts by influencing prostaglandin (PGE_1) metabolism

g) cyclical hormone (progesterone/estrogen) therapy

h) tamoxifen citrate (Oncomox), an anti-estrogen compound (not used much)

i) bromocriptine or cybergoline, prolactin antagonists (not used much)

Surgical

a) aspiration for a simple cyst may be curative (fluid cytology is essential)

b) excision biopsy of a suspicious nodule or cyst

c) wedge resection of breast, if a particular segment is the seat of recurrent problems

d) total mastectomy is rarely done, if at all, for fear of malignancy, either a biopsy showing pre-cancerous changes, or a strong positive family history. By a curved submammary incision (of Gaillard Thomas), the entire breast tissue is excised, preserving the nipple and areola, leaving a drain in the dead space. Appropriate reconstruction may be done at the same time or later.

DUCT PAPILLOMA

Solitary papilloma is a tiny tumor, located in larger lactiferous ducts in the periareolar region, whereas peripheral lesions may be multiple and blend with hyperplastic changes occurring in the lobular system.

Pathology

They are papillary epithelial outgrowths in a dilated ductal system, rarely larger than 5mm, with branching stroma covered by epithelium. With time, ulceration, fibrosis, features of atypical hyperplasia and ductal carcinoma in situ (DCIS), may develop, with high propensity towards invasive carcinoma.

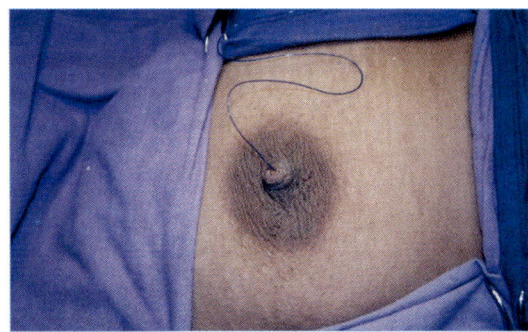

Fig. 95.15. Localization of a duct papilloma using a nylon bristle

Clinical features

Intraductal papilloma is the most common cause of sanguinous (bloody) nipple discharge and the clinical significance lies in that, its malignant counterpart is the next common disease producing the symptom. On careful examination, under magnification if necessary, the discharge is uniductal, from a single orifice. Occasionally the discharge may appear serous, but is chemically positive for occult blood. As benign lesions are usually small, a palpable mass is more in favour of malignancy, corroborated by the enlargement of regional nodes.

Investigations

I) if the discharge is serous, test for occult blood and exfoliated cells should be done

ii) ductogram may reveal a dilated duct with a filling defect. Occasionally a false positive report due to a blood clot, is possible. This is not routinely performed.

iii) mammogram will identify the mass, but may not be helpful in distinguishing benign from malignant lesions in the initial stage.

Treatment

Excision of the tumor with the involved duct, known as microdochectomy, is the procedure of choice. Under general anesthesia, the discharging duct is identified and its orifice dilated with a lachrymal dilator or a probe, which is held in place as a guide. A radially elliptical incision is made over the areola and the duct containing the probe, is excised up to its orifice. Identification of the tumor in the specimen has to be done by gross inspection and microscopy to ensure removal of the 'right' duct, before the patient can be considered cured. If invasive carcinoma is found, staging investigations, appropriate surgery and other modalities of treatment should follow.

Hadfield operation is done when the origin of nipple discharge is uncertain. A periareolar incision, covering half the circumference and cone excision of lactiferous sinuses and ducts for about 5cm from nipple, upto the pectoral fascia, is carried out. Since most of the papillomas will be located within that zone, it ensures removal of the culprit duct and sinus.

MONDOR'S DISEASE

It is superficial thrombophlebitis of the anterior chest wall and breast, presenting as a tender thrombosed vein, adjacent to breast, the so called string phlebitis. Its etiology is not clear, surgical procedure, infection, trauma by repetitive movements etc. have been responsible in initiating the condition. It is not associated with similar lesions in other parts of body and may be rarely bilateral.

Treatment

If the diagnosis is in doubt or it is associated with a mass underneath, it should be excised for biopsy. Otherwise it is self-limiting, requiring only expectant therapy, including antibiotics, antiplatelet/anticoagulant agents and local heat. Shoulder rest and breast support provide symptomatic relief, NSAIDs are reserved for unbearable discomfort.

BREAST CYSTS: classification:

1) non-neoplastic
a) lymph cyst
b) cysts of fibroadenosis, multiple (more common) or single, which is known as blue-domed cyst of Bloodgood.
c) galactocele (periareolar, dating from lactation)
d) abscess, acute, chronic or cold
e) hematoma
f) parasitic
2) neoplastic
a) benign: phyllodes tumor (serocystic disease of Brodie), microcysts of ANDI and cystadenoma
b) malignant: colloid or mucinous cystadenocarcinoma and cystic degeneration of sarcoma

Differential diagnosis

i) benign and solid tumors
ii) periductal mastitis (lesion behind the areola, often with nipple discharge, pain, tenderness and local warmth almost always present).

Investigations

USG, aspiration cytology/bacteriology and mammogram are helpful for planning the treatment, besides chest x-ray and other routine investigations.

Treatment

Aspiration is done early, which is both diagnostic and therapeutic. No further treatment is necessary if:

i) the fluid is not blood stained

	Color	Contents	Cause
1	Clear	Serous	Physiological, duct papilloma, duct Ectasia or use of contraceptive pills
2	Red	Blood	Duct papilloma or carcinoma
3	Green	Cellular debris	Fibroadenosis or duct ectasia
4	Yellow	Exudates	Fibroadenosis or abscess
5	White	Milk	Lactation or galactorrhea
6	Creamy	Paste-like	Duct ectasia

Table - 95.3. Types of nipple discharge

ii) post-aspiration palpation reveals no residual mass

iii) cyst does not refill

iv) fluid cytology reveals no malignant cells

Cysts which do not fulfil the above criteria, should be investigated further and excision for histopathology has to be considered, even if a slight possibility of a neoplasm exists.

NIPPLE DISCHARGE

It is significant, if it is seen occurring spontaneously in a non-lactating woman. It is expressed from the ductal system and should not be confused with any external disease, such as eczema, fistula, Paget's disease etc. producing discharge. Unilateral and uniductal discharge is more ominous, signifying an underlying tumor, than bilateral or multiductal.

Examination of the discharge should be done for occult blood, bacteriology and cytology.

Careful palpation for an underlying mass, regional lymphadenopathy and opposite breast has to be carried out. Mammography to exclude an SOL is necessary in all cases of uniductal discharge, more so, if it is blood-stained.

Treatment depends upon the cause, if blood-stained or persistent from a single duct, microdochectomy should be considered (see under duct papilloma).

GALACTORRHEA

It is secretion of milk in a women who is not lactating or nursing. Even profuse milk secretion in a lactating women is also referred as galactorrhea.

Causes

1. Psychological: Stress, stimulation of chest wall, breast or nipple

2. Endocrinal: Hyperprolactinemia due to pituitary adenoma (prolactinoma), compression of pituitary stalk and hypothyroidism

3. Drugs: H2 receptor blockers, PPIs, liquorice, methyl dopa, opiates, antipsychotics (by blocking the dopamine receptors, which regulate the release of prolactin), of which domperidone is notorious.

4. Diseases: herpes zoster, renal failure and granulomatous conditions

5. Paraneoplastic syndromes (non-pituitary secretion of prolactin) in malignancies

6. Idiopathic

Hyperprolactinemia may lead to osteoporosis and infertility in both genders, causing amenorrhea in women and oligospermia in men.

Treatment

If a cause can be identified, it should be treated appropriately or suspected drug withdrawn.

Antiprolactin agents, such as bromocriptine and cabergoline, may be given for a few weeks for a faster symptomatic relief.

CARCINOMA BREAST

There is no human disease which has evoked as much controversy in the world as the management of carcinoma breast and even today there are several areas of disagreement among the surgeons and oncologists.

Etiology
Geographical

Highest incidence is reported in Europe and North America, whereas it is much lower in India.

Hormonal

This is commonest in nullipara and those with an early age of menarche, late menopause (>50), late age at first child birth(>30) and prolonged use of contraceptive pills. All these factors point to a prolonged exposure to estrogens

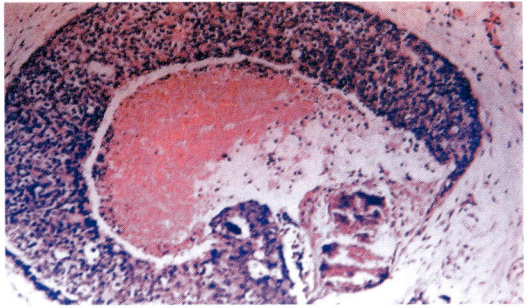

Fig. 95.16. Histology of ductal carcinoma-in-situ
(courtesy: Histo Lab, Chennai)

(especially if unopposed by progestogens) and constitute risk factors. Although there is a marginal increase in the incidence of breast cancer in women on hormone replacement therapy (HRT), it is generally accepted when given for the proper indication, the benefits outweigh the risks of such therapy. HRT with estrogens and progesterone is more harmful than estrogen alone. The protective role of breast feeding is being questioned now, particularly in postmenopausal cancers, but undoubtedly early first child birth (<20) and menopause (<45) either natural or surgically-induced, have an protective influence against malignancy. The higher incidence of breast cancer in dizygotic twins is related to the high levels of circulating maternal gonadotropins.

Obesity

In postmenopausal women obesity is associated with an increased risk of breast cancer. The ovaries lose their estrogenic activity a few years after menopause (about 3 yrs), when the estrogens are derived entirely from the aromatization of androgens, by an enzyme, aromatase, in the adipose tissue. Thus estrogen levels in postmenopausal women are positively correlated with body weight. Recently a link between obesity gene (FTO) and breast carcinoma has been identified

Diet

There is some evidence that there is a link with diets rich in phytoestrogens. A high fat consumption seems to predispose, probably through the obesity channel.

Benign diseases

Diseases such as fibroadenoma, fibroadenosis, duct ectasia, papilloma etc. have increased incidence of malignancy in the breast.

Family history: Women with a first degree relative with breast carcinoma carry a risk, 2-3 times that of general population.

Genetic

About 5% of breast cancers are genetic; mutation of an autosomal dominant gene seems to account for the development of cancer. The BRCA-I (the breast cancer gene) found on the long arm of chromosome-17 (17q) is implicated in some breast cancers and has been recently cloned. Some mutations in this gene cause it to lose its function of suppression of cell division. BRCA-I is also associated with 10-15% lifetime risk of ovarian cancer. Another breast cancer gene, BRCA-II has been identified on the long arm of chromosome-13 (13q) and is also associated with increased risk of developing breast and ovarian malignancies. In inherited breast cancer, other genetic defects also have been established, e.g. mutation or loss of heterozygosity of the p53 tumor suppressor gene on the short arm of chromosome 17 (17p). This occurs in Li-Fraumeni syndrome, in which there is an increased tendency to develop soft tissue sarcoma, breast cancer, melanoma etc. When associated with ovarian and colonic cancers, it is known as Lynch type-II syndrome. Those with ataxia-telangiectasia syndrome also have an increased risk of developing breast carcinoma, as also Cowden's disease (multiple hamartoma syndrome) due to defective tumor suppressor gene.

Patients carrying a genetically high risk require a close clinical surveillance i.e., physical examination every six months and mammography annually. The situation is further complicated by the data that exposure to radiation during mammography, may increase the oncogenic risk in mutation carriers. Prophylactic bilateral mastectomy, recommended by some in such cir-

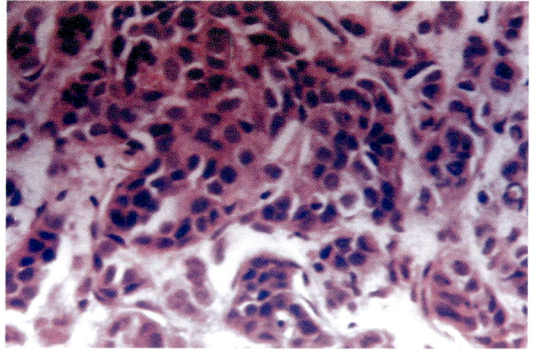

Fig. 95.17. Histology of invasive ductal carcinoma (courtesy: Histo Lab, Chennai)

cumstances, appears too aggressive and lacks universal approval at the present time.

Pathology

It is necessary to know whether the tumor is confined to the glandular component alone (carcinoma in situ or preinvasive) or whether stromal invasion has occurred (invasive carcinoma). The preinvasive carcinoma may be ductal or lobular type, ductal being commoner.

Spread

Carcinoma breast spreads by all modalities, but has special preference to lung, bones and liver. The paravertebral venous plexus (Bateson) is responsible for the preferential involvement of the axial skeleton.

Involvement of lymph nodes is not necessarily of chronological significance, but speaks more of the tumor potential to metastasize. Lymphatic spread from the inner quadrants of breast preferentially go to the internal mammary chain of nodes, sometimes even before axillary nodal involvement. From the lower quadrants, the lymphatics penetrate the rectus sheath, to join the parietal and intraperitoneal plexus, responsible for peritoneal spread, ascites, deposits in rectovaginal (Douglas) pouch and in premenopausal woman, Krukenberg tumor of ovary. Spread along the falciform ligament is the explanation for the liver secondaries and Sister Joseph nodules around the umbilicus. Obviously involvement of abdominal or thoracic viscera signifies advanced stage of the disease.

Mode of spread to the opposite axilla is through the crossover lymphatics from the internal mammary chain and retrograde spread to the axilla; hence it is considered as distant

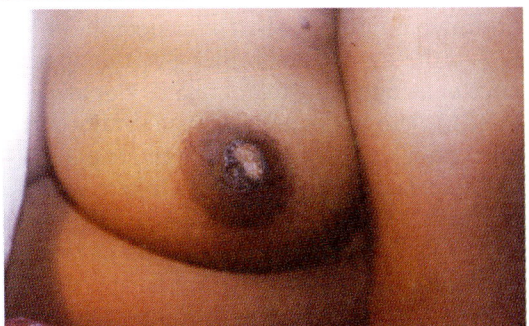

Fig. 95.18. Paget's disease of breast (courtesy: Dr K Sreekanth, Chennai)

metastasis. In such situation, the possibility of another primary in the opposite breast also has to be considered.

PREINVASIVE CARCINOMA

DUCTAL CARCINOMA-IN-SITU (DCIS)

Broder's definition of DCIS still holds good, as the transformation of epithelial cells of any duct in the body into malignant cells, which however remains in the same normal anatomic position without having breached the basement membrane. In the premammography era, DCIS was rarely diagnosed clinically. It presented as discharge from the nipple or in later stages as Paget's disease of the nipple, with a palpable mass, but with the advent of mammography there has been a big surge in the detection of DCIS. It is however not logical to adopt the same course of treatment for symptomatic and asymptomatic (mammographically detected) DCIS. The commonest mammographic findings are calcifications (which originate from intraductal debris), necrotic tumor cells in the ductal epithelium and other tumor cell secretions. 10% may present as soft tissue abnormalities, as in an invasive carcinoma.

The degree of cellular atypia and the presence of necrosis are the main features that delineate the grades of malignancy. For example a high grade lesion like comedo DCIS displays

	Feature	Paget's disease	Eczema
1.	Age	Menopausal	Child-bearing
2.	Bilaterality	No	Common
3.	Vesicles	No	Yes
4.	Mass underneath	May be present	Absent
5.	Response to therapy	No effect	Cures

Table-95.4. Differences between Paget's disease and eczema of nipple

both atypia and necrosis. It is the necrotic debris within the ductal lumen that give the appearance of a comedone (black head). The low and intermediate grades of DCIS, such as cribriform, micropapillary, papillary and circinate patterns, are associated with atypical cytology without necrosis. Multiple areas of rounded spaces within a stratified ductal epithelium characterize the cribriform pattern, giving an appearance of a sieve. In papillary type, the duct is filled with complex papillary folds; this has to be distinguished from a benign papilloma. The treatment of DCIS is controversial (vide infra).

LOBULAR CARCINOMA-IN-SITU (LCIS)

This has no characteristic clinical features and is sometimes found incidentally in mastectomy specimens. Its main properties are its high bilaterality (40%), multicentricity (70%) and high risk (ten times greater than controls) of the subsequent development of invasive carcinoma in one or both breasts.

The duration required for the development of invasive carcinoma from LCIS may be >10 years, but these lesions (LCIS and DCIS) require close monitoring by half yearly clinical examination and annual mammography. The advent of mammography has made surveillance of these patients more comfortable and reassuring, but it is important that they are enlisted for a life time screening program, because with the passage of time the anxiety becomes less; but unfortunately the risk becomes more !

INVASIVE CARCINOMA

When stromal invasion is detectable, the tumors come under this category. By far the commonest variety is the invasive ductal carcinoma of nonspecific type referred to as NOS (not otherwise specified). This forms >80% of all carcinomas of the breast, in which no specific pattern is recognized. All the special subtypes form the remaining, such as tubular, mucinous, medullary and invasive lobular, which tend to be better differentiated and have a better prognosis than the NOS. This implies that most ductal carcinomas are undifferentiated and

cannot be easily classified morphologically. The tumor cells may be in groups, cords or glands. The amount of stroma ranges from none to abundant and its appearance from cellular to densely fibrous. In some of the cases of abundant stroma, it may be difficult to identify the tumor (earlier called atrophic scirrhous type). The Bloom and Richardson grading, to determine the degree of aggressiveness of the tumor, is based on:

a) the tendency of cells to form tubules
b) the pleomorphism of the nucleoli
c) frequency of hyperchromatic nuclei

Other histological types of invasive carcinoma:

Tubular carcinoma representing about 3-5% of invasive carcinomas shows the tumor cells differentiated into tubular pattern. In its pure form, it rarely metastasizes. No further therapy is required if these tumors are excised with a 2 cm margin of normal tissue in all dimensions.

Cribriform carcinoma (vide supra for histopathology) is another tumor that behaves biologically similar to tubular carcinoma.

Mucinous colloid carcinoma, in which pools of extracellular mucin are found in with an embedded aggregates of tumor cells. This comprises 2-4% of invasive carcinoma, usually presents in older women and carries an excellent prognosis.

Medullary carcinoma has solid sheets of large cells, associated with a lymphocytic reaction.

Lobular carcinoma tends to be multifocal and often bilateral.

PAGET'S DISEASE OF BREAST

This type of breast carcinoma presents as a chronic eczema-like lesion of the nipple/ areola with nipple discharge. Upto 50% of the patients have a palpable breast lump. It is seen in association with noninvasive ductal carcinoma, which in due course turns invasive and may be limited to the ducts just beneath the nipple or sometimes beyond. Microscopically, it is characterized by the presence of large, ovoid (Paget) cells with abundant, clear, pale-staining cytoplasm

Prognosis		Explanation

Prognosis — Good

Papillary

Cells thrown into papillary folds

Not so good — Cribriform

Tubes and ducts going through spaces of cells

Bad — Solid

Completely filling duct

Worse — Comedo

Filling duct and oozing out through cut edges

Normal Duct

Ductal carcinoma in situ

Invasive breast cancer

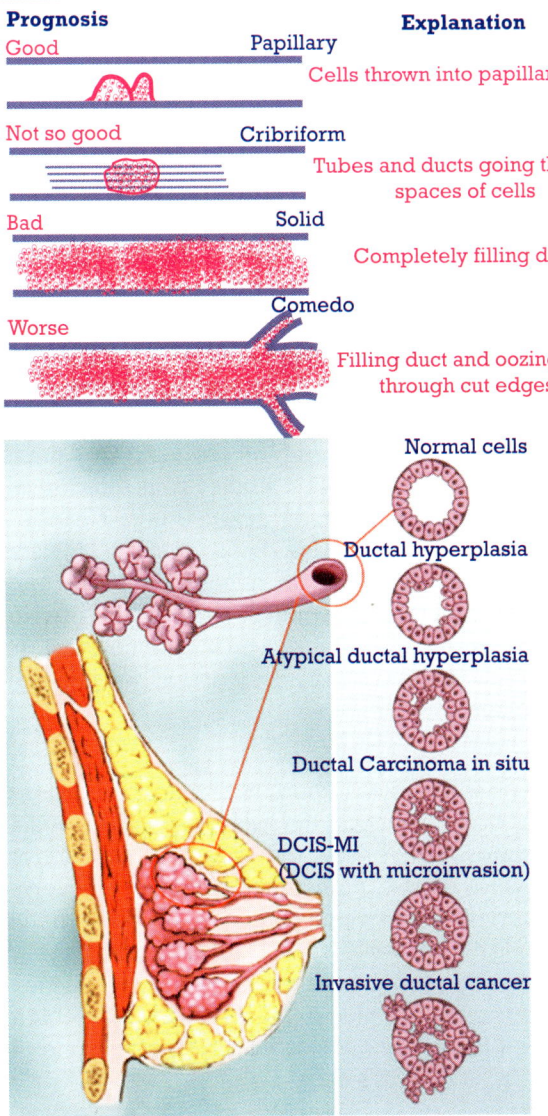

Normal cells

Ductal hyperplasia

Atypical ductal hyperplasia

Ductal Carcinoma in situ

DCIS-MI
(DCIS with microinvasion)

Invasive ductal cancer

Fig. 95.19. Types of DCIS

in the Malpighian layer of epidermis. If 'eczema' is not responding to conventional therapy within a few weeks, skin biopsy must be done, as the prognosis is excellent, if treated before a mass is clinically felt, by wide local excision or mastectomy. With a palpable mass, it is treated as per the guidelines given for other invasive malignancies of breast.

INFLAMMATORY CARCINOMA (syn: mastitis carcinomatosa, acute lactating carcinoma)

It is a distinct clinical rather than pathological entity, fortunately rare and usually seen in pregnant or lactating women, accounting for <2% of breast cancers. Its occurrence in women who are neither pregnant nor lactating has generated confusion about the etiology of the disease. Clinically local signs of 'inflammation' of the breast are characteristic, with engorged veins running over it and regional lymphadenopathy.

The histological findings may be nonspecific but the typical feature is the invasion of dermal lymphatics by the malignant cells. High vascularity and profuse lymphatics of the lactating breast are responsible for early extramammary spread of the disease and the worst prognosis. Due to the associated erythema, peau d' orange, 'cellulitis', with or without a palpable mass, its clinical differentiation from acute mastitis may be delayed, further contributing to the dismal outlook, about a third of them harbouring skeletal metastases at the time of presentation. High grade NHL of the breast may also occur during pregnancy or lactation, confusing the clinical picture.

Absence of fever, leukocytosis or anticipated response to antibiotics generally provide clues, but confirmation is only by generous biopsy of skin, subcutaneous tissue and parenchyma. After routine and specific studies for diagnosis and staging, multimodal treatment has to be instituted. It consists of several cycles of neoadjuvant chemotherapy, which usually cause substantial tumor regression (because of the high mitotic rate), mastectomy &/or radiation, followed by additional chemo/hormone therapy ('sandwich' method), which has been shown to improve disease control and quality of life.

There is no place for breast conservative surgery and radical procedures have not shown any survival advantage. Majority of these tumors are ER and PR negative, but the positive cases respond well to hormonal therapy and carry better prognosis. In view of the aggressive nature of the cancer, Trastuzumab (Herceptin) therapy may also be considered if there is Her2 expression. Termination of pregnancy has not been shown to be beneficial, however it may be considered to facilitate chemo/radiotherapy, provided the child is not very precious.

Prognostic factors in breast cancer

Tumor size

Large tumors have a significantly worse prognosis; all the other factors obviously contribute to the metastatic potential of a given tumor. The recurrence rate is significantly higher for a larger tumor, and the relapse free survival significantly lower. From the excised specimen assessing the degree of invasive component of the breast is a better predictor of its biological behavior than the total tumor size.

Tumor type

A pure mucinous or papillary type has a significantly better prognosis than a comedo carcinoma or a NOS type.

Tumor grade

The Bloom and Richardson classification grades the histological and nuclear changes of the tumor with grade III being poorly differentiated and grade I being well differentiated. This positively correlates with 5-year survival.

Cell kinetics and ploidy

The most significant predictor for loco-regional relapse of carcinoma breast is cellular proliferation i.e., measuring the percentage of cells dividing at any given point of time and also the degree of cell division (which is shown by the nuclear grade). Measurement of the rate of tumor cell division and the quantity of DNA (ploidy) in each cell helps to predict the course of node negative cancer. The mitotic index (number of mitotic figures/10 HPF) has predictive value for prognosis, with a distinctive advantage if it is <10 figures.

The DNA index and the 'S' phase fraction measurement by flow cytometry are quick and reliable methods of quantifying the growth characteristics of the tumor and serve as good predictors of survival and recurrence. The main impact of cell kinetic studies is in the clinical management of node negative breast cancer. The high 'S' phase fraction and aneuploidy are features that indicate a poor prognosis and adjuvant therapy would be strongly indicated in this group of patients, even if node negative, as these tumors have a higher risk of loco-regional recurrence.

Nodal status

The single most important prognostic indicator of breast cancer is the ipsilateral axillary nodal status, with 4 being the 'magic' number, above which there is dramatic reduction of long term survival. The overall prognosis is good for node negative disease, with 75% disease-free 10-year survival, provided the other prognostic factors are favorable (vide supra), but it drops to 50%, if <4 nodes are microscopically involved, and to

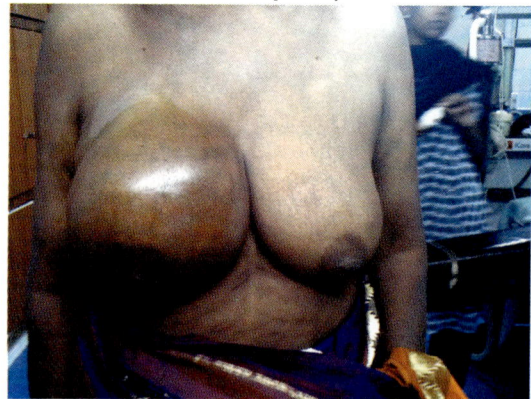

Fig. 95.20. Inflammatory carcinoma right breast

25% if >4 nodes are positive. As may be expected, lymphatic or vascular invasion has also been shown to be a poor prognostic factor.

Nodal involvement in the contralateral axilla is considered as distant metastatic disease and hence indicates Manchester stage-IV and TNM stage-M1. If this is the only finding upstaging the disease to stage-IV and materially altering the course of events, it has to be established beyond doubt, by either needle or excision biopsy. It would be disastrous to deny the patient the benefit of curative therapy, if the contralateral node is ultimately proved to be nonmalignant.

Hormone receptor status

Identification of the estrogen (ER) and progesterone receptors (PR) in the tumor cells by immunohistochemistry (IHC) is helpful in the prognosis and to predict the response to hormone therapy. When a high level of these receptors is found, it often indicates that the tumor is slow growing and the prognosis consequently better, with 90% probability of the tumor responding to endocrine manipulation.

The reasons for better prognosis in ER/PR positive patients are:

1. they are generally well differentiated and slow growing tumors

2. it is considered to be an index of cellular synthetic functions, influenced by alteration of hormonal milieu

3. high probability of the additional weapon (of hormonal therapy) against the tumor being effective. Recently aromatase receptors (AR) are also discovered in breast carcinoma.

Newer prognostic factors

The newer markers that have been identified are growth factors that are important in the transformation from hyperplasia to neoplasia.

Her 2 neu (earlier called c-erb 2)

HER: Human epidermal growth factor receptor-2, is a tyrosinekinase receptor, which plays a major role in normal cell growth.

Over expression of Her 2 neu (an oncogene) has been correlated with more aggressive cancer. Even in node negative women with over expression of Her 2, there is a strong correlation with early recurrence. In future it may be possible to identify those with increased levels of Her 2, with other risk factors like positive axillary nodes and to consider more aggressive treatment like higher doses of chemotherapy, autologous bone marrow transplantation (BMT) and the use of Her 2 antibodies (Trastuzumab or Herceptin).

Though initial detection is done by IHC, gene amplification is to be verified by florescence-in-situ hybridation (FISH) technique, to exclude false positive reporting.

Cathepsin-D

Cathepsins are a family of enzymes that cleave the interior bonds of various proteins. Normal breast tissue contains very little cathepsin-D, but high levels are seen in breast cancer tissue. The higher the cathepsin-D levels the shorter the disease free interval and over all survival.

P-53

Over expression of the tumor suppressor gene p-53 has been found to correlate with aggressive behavior of the tumor. This also reduces radio/chemosensitivity of the tumor, affecting the ultimate prognosis.

Tumor staging
Manchester staging

Stage I: tumor confined to the breast, no nodes, no metastasis (T1/2/3:N0:M0)

Stage II: mobile ipsilateral axillary nodes (T1/2/3:N1:M0)

Stage III: tumor fixed to pectoral fascia/muscle, skin involved beyond the area of tumor, axillary nodes fixed to each other or to chest wall, supraclavicular/internal mammary nodes are involved (T1/2/3/4: N1/2/3: M0). It should be realized that in this stage, the disease is confined to the breast and its immediate vicinity, in other words, within the radiation zone (see under treatment).

Stage IV: tumor fixed to chest wall, distant

Low	Moderate	High
Early menarche, late menopause	Minimal radiation	Heavy radiation
Nulliparous	Opp breast was treated for Ca	DCIS
Age > 35 at first child birth	Mammographic dense breast	LCIS
Postmenopausal obesity, alcohol consumption, hormone replacement therapy (HRT)	Family history	Strong family history

Table-95.5. Rating of risk for developing breast carcinoma

metastasis, including contralateral axillary nodes and recurrent disease (T-any:N-any:M1).

For purposes of treatment, all inner quadrant tumors are considered as minimum stage-III, in view of the high incidence of involvement of the internal mammary chain. It should be realized that clinical staging, before investigations, is only cursory and definitive staging for purposes of treatment or prognostication, can be arrived only after all the relevant investigations.

As can be appreciated from the Manchester staging, there are too many variables, which make comparison of results of one center from the other difficult, hence it has been largely replaced by TNM staging. Its main virtue, however, is to orient to treatment, in terms of four stages, since various combinations and permutations of TNM staging may be too cumbersome to interpolate.

TNM staging

T: tumor size T1: <2cm; T2: 2-5cm; T3: 5-10cm and T4: >10cm

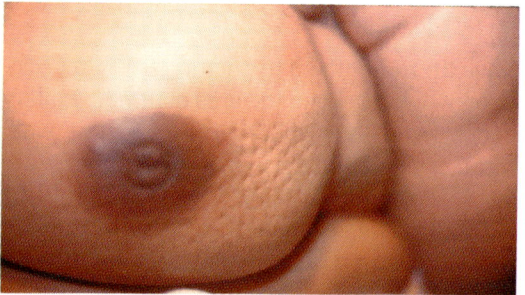

Fig. 95.21. Peau d' orange appearance of infiltrating breast carcinoma
(courtesy: Dr K Sreekanth, Chennai)

N: nodes - N1: mobile, discrete ipsilateral axillary nodes; N2: nodes fixed to each other or to the chest wall and N3: supraclavicular/ internal mammary nodes involved

M: metastasis - Mx: uninvestigated for secondaries; M0: no metastatic disease and M1: distant metastases present, including opposite breast/axilla/supraclavicular/internal mammary areas.

TNMG staging

Elston has proposed a prognostic index (Nottingham prognostic index) in which tumor stage and histological grade are combined. This stratifies patients into low, intermediate and high risk for recurrence. Tumors <1cm are unlikely to recur, those between 1-2cm with poorly differentiated (grade III) carcinomas have a relative risk of recurrence of 20%, about twice the risk of moderately differentiated carcinoma of the same size.

History

Positive family history to identify any first degree relatives, the age at which they developed cancer and the outcome, ages at menarche, at first child birth, at menopause (if attained) and if she breast-fed the children, have to be noted. Use of hormone preparations, such as HRT or contraceptive pills and, if the patient had undergone surgical menopause, the age at the time of surgery and if the ovaries were removed, are important.

History of any underlying benign breast disease, nipple discharge, secondary changes over the mass (if so, whether they were spontaneous or followed some external applications), similar masses in axillae or elsewhere, exposure to ionizing radiation for malignant disease in childhood or adolescence, particularly for Hodgkin's disease (sometimes the pectoral region is included in the field of radiotherapy), have to be recorded.

Physical examination

A safe dictum has to be remembered: all lumps in the breast are malignant, until proved otherwise, especially if the patient is postmenopausal. Physical examination of the breast is performed in the supine and upright positions, with arms by the side and hyperabducted. If the breast tissue is pulled up to a higher position than the opposite breast on hyperabduction of arms, it implies that the breast mass is probably fixed to the pectoral fascia/muscle. Distortion, asymmetry, retraction of nipple or the skin over the mass; secondary changes, such as peau d' orange, ulceration, fungation etc., Should be looked for. The size, location, surface, mobility and consistency (fluctuation and transillumination as necessary) of the mass are recorded. It is important to use the flat surface of the straightened fingers, to palpate the breast, the sensitivity further enhanced by lubricating with soap. The typical carcinomatous mass is painless, solitary, discrete, stony hard, irregular, without intrinsic mobility (within the breast tissue) and with or without fixity to the skin, pectoral fascia/muscle or chest wall. The upper outer quadrant is the common site for carcinoma and a mass in relation to the axillary tail of Spence is likely to be mistaken for a lymph node

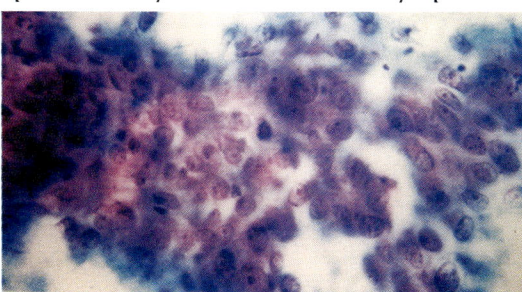

Fig. 95.22. FNAC smear of breast carcinoma (courtesy: Lifeline Hospitals, Chennai)

(level-1).

An early sign of skin fixity is dimpling or retraction. Later, due to blockage of subdermal lymphatics, cutaneous lymphedema develops with the typical orange peel appearance due to tiny pits created by the ligaments of Cooper which run between the skin and breast tissue. This is known as peau d' orange (peau: skin), not pathognomonic of cancer as it may be seen in inflammatory lesions such as an abscess or a granuloma. Fixity to pectoral fascia is identified by restriction of mobility of the mass, when the fascia is put under stretch by hyperabduction of the shoulder. Fixity to pectoral muscles is identified by examining the mass with the muscles put to contraction by adduction against resistance. Fixity to the rib cage is detected by the breast not falling forwards in the stooping position and total lack of mobility of the mass. Bilateral masses are seen in <1% of cases of malignancy, hence when the disease is bilateral, the probability of them being benign is more. The axillae and supraclavicular fossae are then examined systematically for nodal enlargement, and if present, their location, number, size, consistency, fixity (to each other and to chest wall) and pressure effects over the limb have to be noted.

Systemic examination of chest, abdomen, long bones and spine, including a pelvic/rectal examination has to be performed. In the chest, involvement of

(a) lung parenchyma,
(b) pleurae,
(c) lymph nodes and
(d) bony cage, have to be looked for.

In the abdomen, involvement of

(a) liver,
(b) peritoneum and
(c) pelvic organs/pouch of Douglas are to be evaluated, including Krukenberg's tumor of the ovaries.

Breast self examination (BSE)

This is a simple and expedient procedure to help early detection of a breast mass, which every woman should be taught, since, statistically,

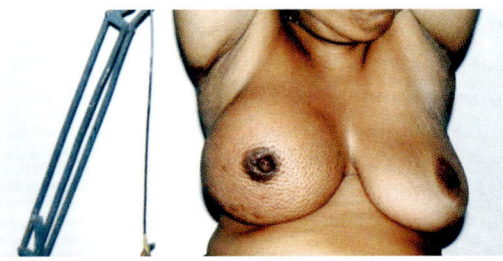

Fig. 95.23. Inspection of the breast with arms hyperabducted. Note elevation on the affected side, indicating fixity of the mass to pectoral fascia. The typical peau d'orange appearance is also seen

>90% of breast cancers are first discovered by the patients themselves.

Standing in front of a mirror, both the breasts should be compared (palpated quadrant-wise, including the axillae and supraclavicular so with arms elevated) and systematically paregions.

Though it seems probable to bring down the overall mortality from breast cancer if more women practiced periodic BSE, convincing proof for such long term protection is wanting . Of course, whenever an abnormality during BSE is detected, appropriate medical examination and necessary investigations should promptly follow.

Differential diagnosis

a) benign lesions of breast: fibroadenoma, fibroadenosis, phyllodes tumor, plasma cell mastitis etc
b) granulomatous conditions: chronic abscess, tuberculosis, filariasis etc
c) traumatic fat necrosis
d) cystic conditions of breast: galactocele,

cyst of fibroadenosis, cold abscess etc
d) sarcoma of breast
e) secondary malignant deposit.

Investigations

Besides routine studies of blood, urine and a chest x-ray, an USG helps to differentiate between a solid and cystic mass, a simple and a neoplastic cyst and if it is encapsulated. It may also pick up other clinically impalpable masses in the breast or axilla, as an adjunct to mammography. A carcinoma is characterized by its irregular, indistinct and sometimes jagged margins, generally having hypo or anechoic internal pattern. The USG is however not useful for routine breast cancer screening because of its inability to detect microcalcification. Thermography and ductal lavage are some of the recent additions to the investigations. CA-15.3 as a tumor marker for carcinoma breast is under evaluation.

Mammography is a very important investigation for a patient with a solid dominant mass. Its primary purpose is to image the entire breast tissue on either side for nonpalpable masses apart from corroborating the features of a solid dominant mass. It is not recommended as an initial investigation in women under 30, because cancer is rare in this group and the diagnostic pitfalls due to the hyperdense breast parenchyma, unless there is high index of suspicion. Apart from a soft tissue mass, it shows the microcalcification (fine punctate and stippled) of intra-ductal epithelium. In young women, ^{99m}Tc-labeled sestamibi scintiscan of

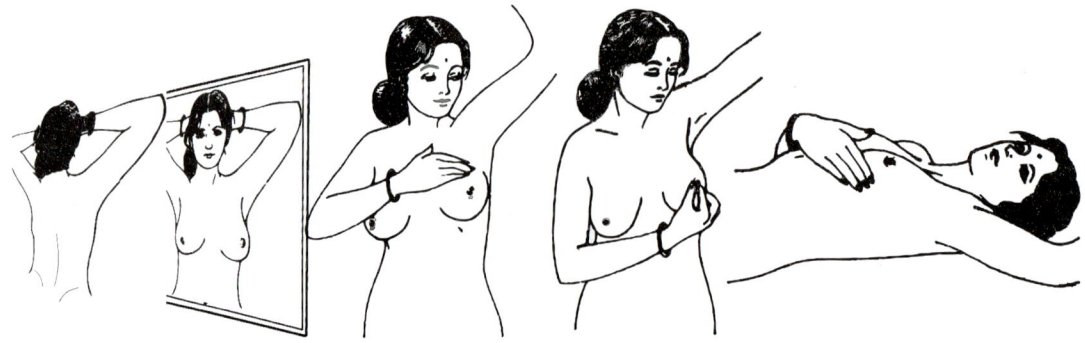

Fig. 95.24. Breast self examination

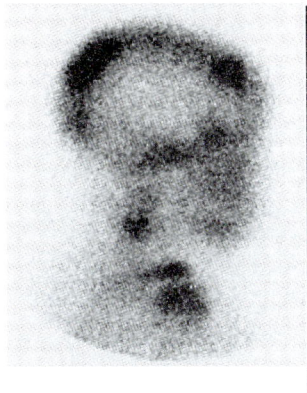

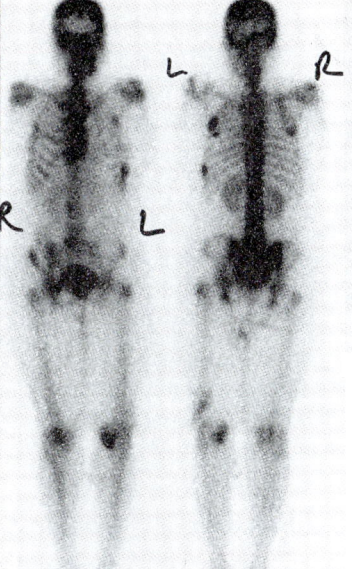

Anterior   *Posterior*

Fig. 95.25.
Whole body skeletal scintiscan (^{99m}Tc), showing multiple second-aries (courtesy: Halsted Surgical Clinic, Chennai)

breasts may be more valuable than conventional mammography.

Types of calcification
Benign

a) small round pearl-like, in a rosette-like distribution, due to calcification within the dilated terminal ductal lobular units (TDLU).

b) 'cup and saucer':corresponding to ' milk of calcium' sedimenting within the microcytes.

Malignant

a) thin linear and branching calcifications (casting) represent tumor debris within the ductal system.

b) small, sharp dense tightly grouped 'crushed stones' appearance is typical but not pathognomonic, as it may be seen in sclerosing adenosis.

Magnetic resonance mammography (MRM) scores over the conventional mammography in patients who have had previous breast surgery, with parenchymal scarring, as well as in young women with mammogra-phically dense breast, obscuring a small focus of malignancy. The

higher cost and limited availability are the only draw backs with this investigation.

FNAC is a simple and relatively painless procedure, with a specificity of 98% and sensitivity of 80%. However several passages of the needle through the lesion are necessary to obtain a satisfactory sample. False positive rate is negligible but false negative rate may be as high as 20%, because of sampling error and problems of interpretation. Stereo-tactic core biopsy, magnification mammography, preliminary placement of hooked wire under mammographic control for accurate localization of nonpalpable masses, MRI etc. are some of the means of improving the accuracy of needle biopsy. Ductography has been attempted to localize lesions in cases of uniductal nipple discharge, complementary to mammography.

Any mass remaining after aspiration of a cyst should be excised. Negative findings of FNAC in the presence of a clinically suspicious mass should not preclude further diagnostic work up such as core or open biopsy.

Core biopsy, using a cutting type of wide bore (Tru-cut) needle to retrieve a cylindrical sample of breast mass (10-20mm long and 1-2mm dia.), provided the lesion is >2.5cm, is preferred by many, as it improves sensitivity considerably, besides providing tissue for grading and ER/PR/Her-2 studies. Using immunocyto-chemical assay (ICA), a qualitative study of

Triple assessment

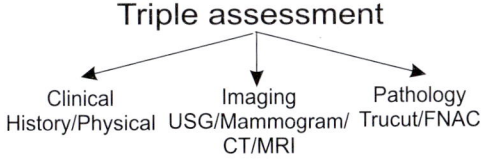

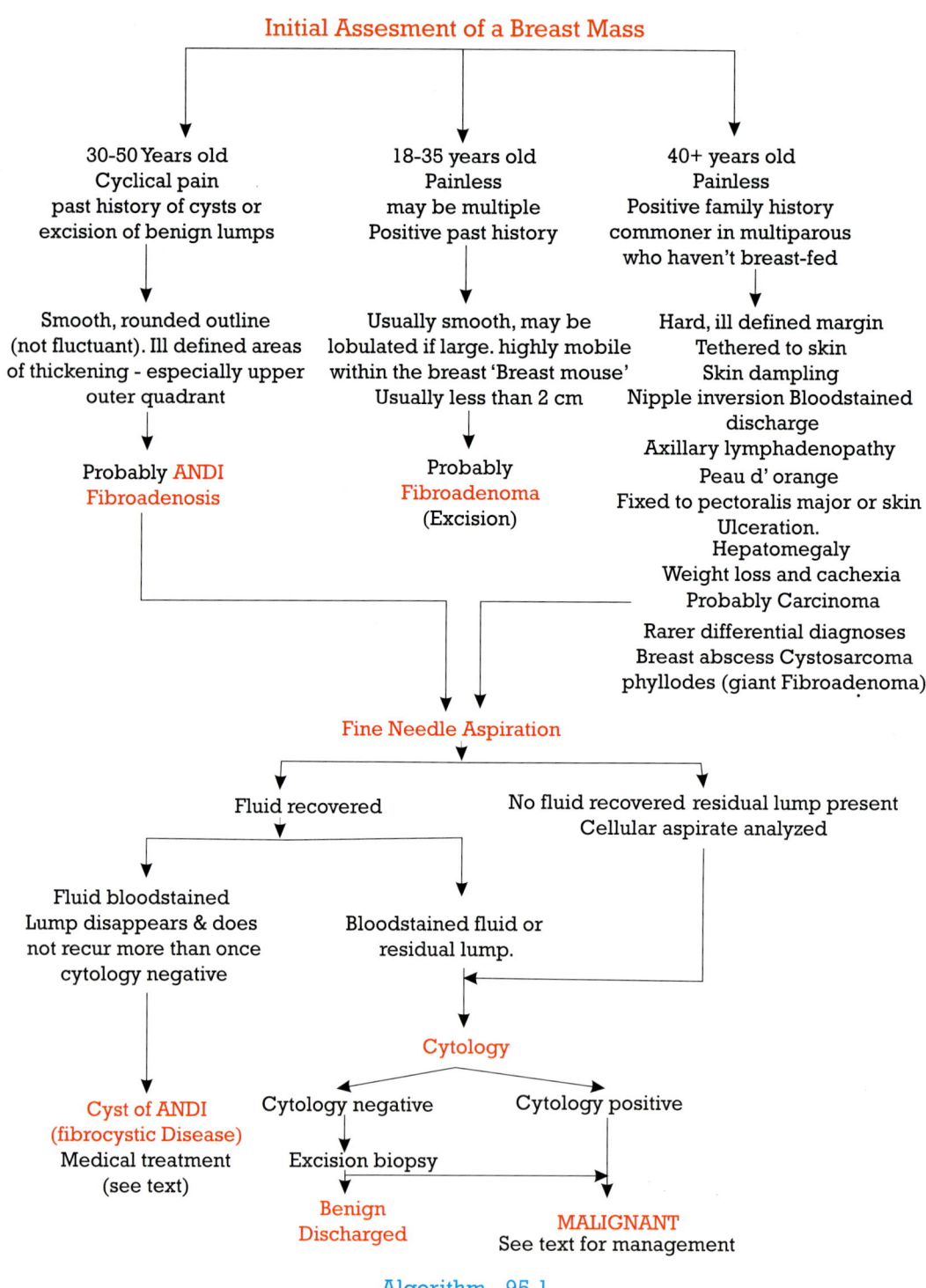

Initial Assesment of a Breast Mass

30-50 Years old
Cyclical pain
past history of cysts or
excision of benign lumps

18-35 years old
Painless
may be multiple
Positive past history

40+ years old
Painless
Positive family history
commoner in multiparous
who haven't breast-fed

Smooth, rounded outline
(not fluctuant). Ill defined areas
of thickening - especially upper
outer quadrant

Usually smooth, may be
lobulated if large. highly mobile
within the breast 'Breast mouse'
Usually less than 2 cm

Hard, ill defined margin
Tethered to skin
Skin dampling
Nipple inversion Bloodstained
discharge
Axillary lymphadenopathy
Peau d' orange
Fixed to pectoralis major or skin
Ulceration.
Hepatomegaly
Weight loss and cachexia
Probably Carcinoma

Probably ANDI
Fibroadenosis

Probably
Fibroadenoma
(Excision)

Rarer differential diagnoses
Breast abscess Cystosarcoma
phyllodes (giant Fibroadenoma)

Fine Needle Aspiration

Fluid recovered

No fluid recovered residual lump present
Cellular aspirate analyzed

Fluid bloodstained
Lump disappears & does
not recur more than once
cytology negative

Bloodstained fluid or
residual lump.

Cytology

Cytology negative   Cytology positive

Cyst of ANDI
(fibrocystic Disease)
Medical treatment
(see text)

Excision biopsy

Benign
Discharged

MALIGNANT
See text for management

Algorithm - 95.1

ER/PR may be done with minute amounts of tumor tissue (obtained by Tru-cut needle).

Open surgical biopsy

Open surgical biopsy is the most reliable method for obtaining a specific diagnosis of a breast lump or a suspicious area discovered mammographically, which can be done under local or general anesthesia. For clinically nonpalpable lesions, preoperative needle localization and a hooked wire positioning by imaging devices are very useful, in improving the yield. In ductal carcinoma in situ (DCIS), the extent of the calcification to the margin of the specimen may suggest that there is a residual tumor in the breast, when further resection is indicated. A post-excision mammography may be done if necessary to ensure complete removal of the abnormal tissue.

Excision biopsies for palpable or non-palpable breast lesions should produce a single intact specimen and not in piece meal. Histologically negative margins, at times, do not guarantee complete removal of the lesion because ductal carcinoma in situ may grow in a discontinous fashion. Approximately 20% of women with early breast cancer undergoing conservative surgery and radiation for invasive ductal carcinoma have an extensive intraductal component (EIC). This group has an increased risk of disease recurrence in the breast. The minimum margin required for even for 'lumpectomy' is 1-2cm of normal tissue beyond the gross edge of the tumor.

Role of frozen section examination

Frozen section examination is generally unsatisfactory for breast disease, because atypical ductal hyperplasia and small foci of ductal carcinoma-in-situ or even micro-invasive carcinoma are difficult to interpret due to freezing artifacts. A safer approach under such circumstances is to subject a part of the specimen for frozen section (retaining the rest for regular paraffin study) and to give credit only for a positive report, to decide course of action during the initial surgery.

Mastectomy being a mutilative procedure, when in doubt, it is wise to wait for the paraffin section report. There appears to be no significant difference in the overall results between one stage or two stage procedure, provided the tumor tissue is not cut into while carrying out excision, in the latter.

^{99m}Tc skeletal scan is a very important investigation, since it is highly sensitive (95%) in detecting bone secondaries, but unfortunately its specificity is only 75%, since other degenerative diseases of bones and joints may show false positive readings.

PET-CT scan has emerged as a very useful single investigation in recent times, since it can replace several studies, such as CT abdomen, chest, neck and brain, skeletal scintiscan and bone marrow scan.

Bone marrow study, if there is hematological abnormality

Screening mammography

Screening mammogram is employed to evaluate healthy women with no symptoms to detect early signs of malignancy. The baseline screening also provides a record of normal breast image, against which any changes can be compared later. The diagnosis of breast cancer, however, is clinched only by biopsy and not by imaging. The current recommendation is to do a mammograpm every year after 40 in the high risk group and for the rest, after 50, until the age of 65, or for life, if the patient so desires.

The high risk group consists of:
1. strong positive family history
2. opposite breast following mastectomy for malignancy on one side
3. obese women
4. those on hormone therapy
5. those undergone local excision for pre-invasive disease
6. fibroadenosis
7. other risk factors described earlier

Triple assessment (of breast diseases) by clinical, imaging and pathology (TACIP):

Primary objective in any breast disease is to exclude malignancy and it is done comfortably (>95%) by the three modalities mentioned. Dedicated mammographic units employ low voltage and high amperage x-rays, for better penetration and resolution.

Management of early breast cancer

As one can understand from the tumor biology, nearly 2/3 of tumor life is preclinical, hence it is very difficult to define what precisely constitutes early cancer. For practical purposes, Manchester stages-I and II are considered early enough to aim for a curative form of treatment.

This can be divided into management of invasive carcinoma and management of in-situ carcinoma. It is prudent to mention at this point that the shift has swung completely from radical mastectomy introduced by Halsted almost a century ago, in which the pectoral muscles were completely removed and Patey's modification, which spares pectoralis major, in favor of wide local excision (quadrantectomy) with axillary dissection. More and more extensive resections, such as Urban's extended radical mastectomy, have not stood the test of time, in terms of translating into improved survival.

Management of invasive carcinoma

Breast conserving surgery of Veronasi (QUART: QUadrantectomy, Axillary dissection and RT) is becoming the standard treatment for all women with stage I and II breast cancer and it is as effective as mastectomy, provided a wide local excision (i.e., 1-2 cm of margin around the tumor) is performed, followed by adjuvant RT. Preoperative mammographic evaluation to rule out multicentric tumor and biopsy to exclude histological features such as EIC (extensive intraductal component), is mandatory. If a patient has EIC, either wider resection or mastectomy may be necessary. Following RT, the use of chemo/ hormone therapy is logical as per the standard protocol to conquer the disease, considered one of the largest killers in women. The benefits and risks of mastectomy vs breast conservation should be discussed in every case, considering the following:

(a) the long term survival
(b) local recurrence
(c) cosmetic outcome
(d) psychological adjustment

(e) sexual adaptation
(f) functional compliance

Absolute contraindications for breast conservation:

1. pregnancy
2. size >5cm or multicentric tumor
3. diffuse microcalcification
4. persistent positive margins
5. collagen vascular diseases

Relative contraindications

1. the ratio of size of tumor/size of the breast not suitable for acceptable cosmesis
2. positive BRCA-1 or 2 mutation
3. subareolar (central) tumor

Technique of breast conservative surgery

An elliptical skin incision, along the Langer's lines, is made encircling the tumor, which is excised with 1-2cm rim of normal tissue. The breast tissue is not re-approximated and skin is closed with drainage. Clips are used to outline the margins of the defect to plan radiation therapy. A separate incision is made for the axillary nodal dissection, excising all the involved nodes up to the apex. For invasive tumors under 1 cm size and with a favorable histological type (i.e., tubular mucinous or papillary) removal of level-1 nodes is adequate and for staging purposes, removal up to level II is needed, but excision of level III nodes is advised only when encompassing obvious disease. As soon as the surgical wound has healed adequately, RT should begin, usually within 2-4 weeks after surgery.

After completion of radiotherapy for the entire breast, an additional 1000-2000 cgy is applied to the tumor bed, usually with interstitial implantation. This boost is omitted in those treated with more extensive resection and with clear negative resected margins.

ONCOPLASTIC SURGERY

Breast, face and bone are some of the areas, where plastic reconstruction of the resultant defect after surgery for malignancies (oncoplastic surgery) has been popularly applied. In breast it may be:

1. breast conservative surgery
2. immediate or delayed reconstruction

3. previously operated patients may also be offered

The choice of oncoplastic surgery depends upon a number of factors, including the extent of resection, location of tumor, age of patient and expertise available. However, the primary objective of cancer cure, should not be lost sight of and basic principles of cancer clearance and postoperative surveillance cannot be compromised, while planning oncoplastic procedures, either to improve the appearance or function.

Recent data shows marginally higher rate of reoperation for those undergone breast conservative surgery, than standard mastectomy, for invasive cancer.

Management of carcinoma-in-situ (CIS)

Most of the ductal CIS are identified mammographically by the microcalcifications. This requires surgical localization by the needle hook method (vide supra). The needle hook is inserted under image intensification and the

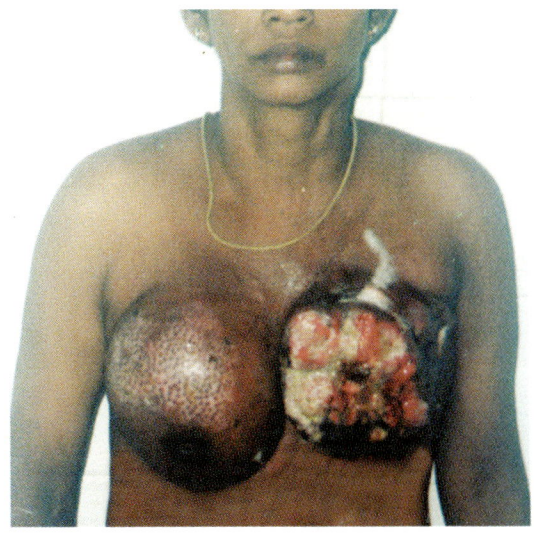

Fig. 95.27. Bilateral advanced breast cancers (courtesy: Prof M Raghuram, Chennai)

patient is taken to the operation room. The incision should be closest to the tip of wire to achieve the best cosmetic result, and the specimen is removed in one piece. Often, for good cosmesis, the biopsy cavity is allowed to fill up with serum. No drains are inserted and the skin is closed with a subcuticular suture. Specimen radiography should be done to determine if the lesion has been properly excised and the following factors are looked into to assess the risk of recurrence and the need for further surgery:

1. the nuclear grade and tumor necrosis
2. adequacy of clearance
3. multicentricity
4. postoperative mammogram

There is no place for adjuvant radio/chemo/hormone therapy in CIS.

Therapeutic strategy in carcinoma breast

No disease of man is subjected to so much controversy all over the world as breast carcinoma, and despite improved follow up and free exchange of statistics from various centers involved in clinical studies, there is a lack of unanimity in several areas. For purposes of easy assimilation, generally accepted guidelines of management are given here:

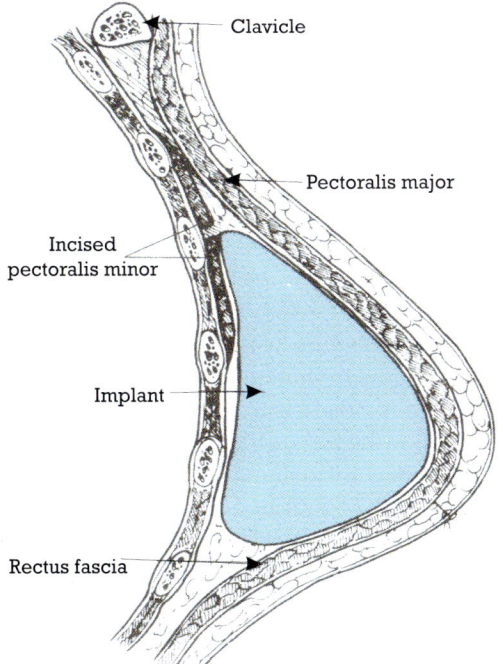

Clavicle

Pectoralis major

Incised pectoralis minor

Implant

Rectus fascia

Fig. 95.26. Retropectoral placement of a silicone prosthesis

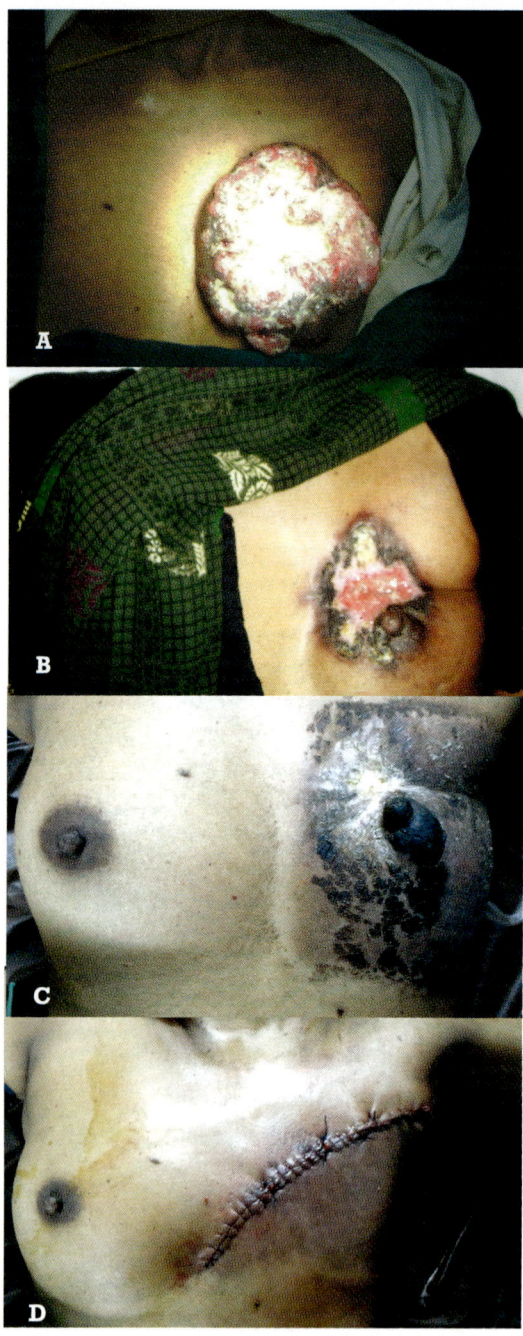

Fig. 95.28
A. advanced fungating carcinoma left breast; B. after neoadjuvant chemo/radiation therapy; C. final result after chemo/raditation; D. salvage total mastectomy performed
(courtesy: Dr K R Reddy, Kakinada)

Stages I and II are considered early diseases, and curative therapy is the aim; stages III and IV are considered advanced diseases, where palliative treatment is offered. Surgery and radiation are local forms of therapy, whereas chemo and hormone therapy are systemic forms of therapy.

For stages I and II:

Both forms of local therapy and one of the systemic forms of therapy, saving the other for future (recurrence).

For stages III and IV:

Role of surgery:

(a) establishing the diagnosis (biopsy),
(b) debulking (cytoreduction) and
(c) palliative or toilet mastectomy.

Role of RT: In stage III, as the disease is confined to 'radiation zone', radical RT may still be attempted, but in stage IV, it is only palliative; e.g. spine secondaries producing paraplegia.

Both forms of systemic therapy are given, as there is little reason to save for the future. At this context it should be reiterated that inner quadrant tumors, which have high potential for internal mammary nodal involvement, are to be treated as minimum stage III and no radical surgery is recommended.

Surgery

The standard Halsted's radical mastectomy lost popularity as early as late 60s, as it provided no additional advantage over lesser procedures. It has many drawbacks such as:

extensive procedure, with more blood loss
interference with shoulder functions
cosmetically unattractive, due to infraclavicular hollowing
poor prospects of mammary reconstruction
more chances of injuring axillary vessels, nerves to latissimus dorsi and serratus anterior muscles
increased incidence of edema of arm.

Such an extensive axillary dissection is unnecessary for inner quadrant tumors, which have a high predilection to spread to the internal mammary chain. It is interesting to note that Halsted's original description was to remove

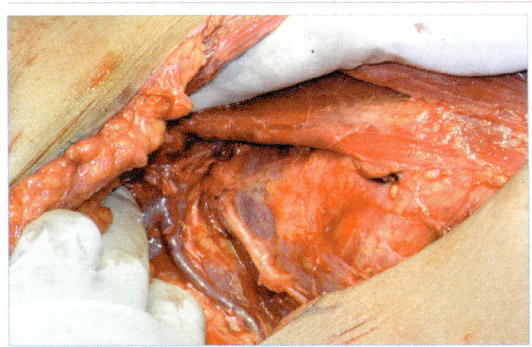

Fig. 95.29. Final appearance after Patey's modification of radical mastectomy, preserving pectoralis major muscle

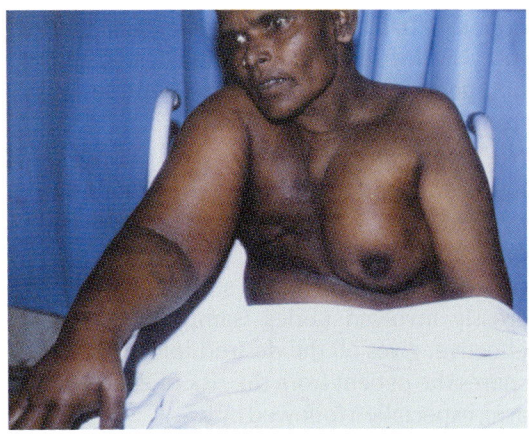

Fig. 95.30. Chest wall infiltration and edema of arm in advanced recurrent carcinoma of right breast (courtesy: Dr K Sreekanth, Chennai)

only the breast and pectoralis major muscle first (minor muscle was not removed) and axillary dissection done later. Additional removal of pectoralis minor and the axilla-first method was popularized by Meyer, but the name (Halsted's radical) could not be changed (William Halsted was probably too influential!). The advantage of the axilla-first approach is to carry out nodal dissection, preserving important neurovascular structures while the field is relatively bloodless, very similar to cystic duct-first method while doing cholecystectomy.

More extensive Urban's extended radical mastectomy (including internal mammary nodes), Dahl-Iversen's inclusion of supraclavicular nodes and lesser modifications such as Patey's mastectomy (preserving pectoralis major, but removing pectoralis minor, for better access to the axilla and deltopectoral nodes) have all been given up, replaced by simple (total) mastectomy and axillary node sampling or excision.

Jewels of Gyan - 95.3

Evolution of Surgery for Ca breast

Earlier: Total mastectomy (TM)
1894: Halsted - Radical mastectomy (RM) retaining pect minor (breast-first)
1894: Meyer - Radical mastectomy including pect minor (standard – axilla-first)
1948: Mc Whirter – Total mastectomy and RT
1949: Patey – Modified radical mastectomy (MRM) retaining pect major
1952: Urban – Extended radical mastectomy (ERM) including internal mammary nodes
Dahl-Iversen- Radical mastectomy including supraclavicular nodes
1952: West – Bilateral adrenalectomy
1955: Luft-Hypophysectomy
1956: Treves – Bilateral oophorectomy
1960: Crile – Total mastectomy only
1970: Freeman - Nipple-sparing or Areola-sparing mastectomy (NSM or ASM)
1972: Greening – Partial mastectomy and axillary dissection (no RT)
1976: Zucali – Neoadjuvant therapy and salvage mastectomy
1977: Cabanas & Morton – Sentinel node concept for axillary dissection
1982: Veronesi – Quadrantectomy, axillary dissection and RT (QUART)
1999: Hartmann – Bilateral prophylactic mastectomy for BRCA-I & II
2001: Harness – Oncoplastic breast surgery

Popularly used term, 'modified radical mastectomy' (MRM) is to be discouraged, since it does not specify the exact procedure, which may vary from surgeon to surgeon.

Node sampling vs dissection (or clearance): It has been found that excising the axillary nodes by itself has no favorable effect on survival, but only provides debulking, proper staging and prognostication. Hence simple removal of grossly involved nodes (sampling) is equally effective, gives all the desired information and spares the patient from the risk of edema of the arm, especially if followed by RT.

Technique of mastectomy: Under general anesthesia, with arm on the affected side semiabducted, either by an oblique (Halsted) or transverse elliptical incision (Stewart), encircling the tumor and the areola (and of course, the biopsy site), skin flaps are raised, till the edges of breast tissue are seen. The outer flap is dissected superiorly to enter the axilla for direct palpation of nodal enlargement. All the palpable nodes, upto the apex, including the deltopectoral group are dissected out at the initial stage, before the breast is removed including the pectoral fascia, in a proper plane, coagulating the muscle perforators by electrocautery. The breast and the axillary nodes (if any) are removed preferably in one piece. Skin flaps are brought together by 'far and near' tension sutures, before normal closure in layers. An ambulatory vacuum drain (Redivac) is left in situ for 48 hrs to prevent lymph collection.

In addition to this, in radical mastectomy, both the pectoral muscles and entire axillary pad of fat bearing the nodes are removed, skeletonizing the axillary vessels, preserving the nerves to

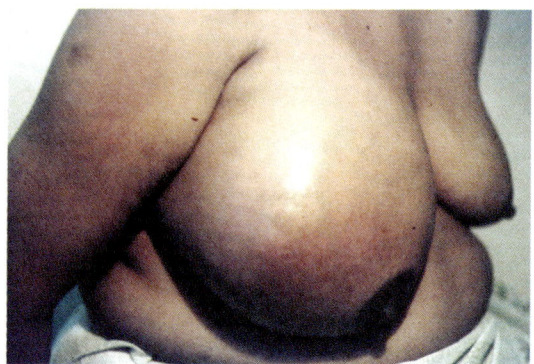

Fig. 95.31. Sarcoma breast
(courtesy: Dr K Sreekanth, Hyderabad)

latissimus dorsi and serratus anterior (long thoracic nerve of Bell) and if possible intercosto-brachial nerve (derived from 2nd intercostal), a cutaneous nerve to medial aspect of arm.

It should be realized that adequate cancer clearance is more important than primary wound closure and there should be no hesitation to remove more skin and resort to split skin graft, if necessary, to cover the wound. To control the temptation of the surgeon to manage primary closure 'somehow', teachers of earlier generations observed that mastectomy should be done by two surgeons, one carrying out resection and the other doing the closure, so that the first is not bothered about how the second is going to close, explicitly driving home the proper message to junior surgeons.

Sentinel node concept (Cabanas & Morton): In diseases such as melanoma, penile and breast carcinomas, when there is lymphatic spread, the first node to be involved (also the most proximal) is known as the sentinel node. For penis, it is usually the most medial of the superficial horizontal inguinal group and for breast it is the

Feature	Secondary	Second primary
Time of occurrence	Within 18 months	Usually after
Common location	Inner quadrants	Upper outer quadrant
Histology	Same	May or may not be same
Evidence of dissemination	Usually present	Usually absent
Treatment	Local excision	Standard surgery
Prognosis	Unfavourable	Favourable

Table-95.6: Differences between a secondary and a second primary in the opposite breast

node adjacent to the axillary tail, belonging to the anteromedial axillary group. It may be identified by injecting either a dye or a radioisotope around the tumor and locating by dissection or scintiprobe, during surgery, and is excised for biopsy. There are no false positives, but false negatives (10%) may be seen, if the lymphatics are blocked and alternate channels established for drainage, circumventing the sentinel node. As on date, its status is more investigational than for clinical application (see in melanoma), done only in a few centres.

Complications of breast and axilla surgery

1. injury to axillary vessels, long thoracic nerve, nerve to latissimus dorsi or intercostobrachial nerve.
2. skin flap necrosis
3. lymph collection under the flaps and lymphorrhea (see chapter 33)
4. lymphedema of upper limb (late): see chapter 33.
5. limitation of shoulder movements

Radiotherapy (RT): This was popularized by Mc Whirter, with the aim of avoiding tedious pectoral/axillary dissection, substituting simple (total) mastectomy for Halsted's radical procedure, followed by radiotherapy, claiming comparable results. It is given as curative therapy in stages I and II, may be in stage III and for palliation in stage IV disease. About 6-8000r is given in 6-8weeks, covering the ipsilateral pectoral, axillary, supraclavicular and internal mammary regions. The main problems with RT are edema of arm, radiation pneumonitis leading to pulmonary fibrosis and rarely injury to myocardium.

Management of advanced breast cancer

Advanced breast cancer may be defined as a stage of the disease for which no prospect of cure can be reasonably anticipated, i.e., beyond T2:N2:M0 or Manchester stage III as well as recurrent disease. Any new symptom in a patient with a previous diagnosis of carcinoma breast demands a critical work up. The natural history of untreated breast cancer is extremely variable. The disease may pursue an indolent course with slow local progress and late occur-

rence of metastasis. At the other extreme, the disease may be explosive, relentless with rapid progression and early death.

Generally patients with skeletal metastasis have a better survival rate compared to those with visceral spread. The mandatory investigations for a patient with an advanced breast cancer are full blood count, liver function tests including alkaline phosphatase, serum calcium, USG of abdomen, chest radiograph and an isotope bone scan. If possible, a PET-CT scan can replace the entire battery of imaging studies.

The objectives of hospice treatment in advanced breast cancer are dictated by the facts that cure is an unrealistic expectation and the primary aim is palliation of symptoms due to local/systemic disease, relief of pain, anxiety and provide emotional support (Zimmerman). Life or function threatening deposits should be identified and measured clinically, radiologically and biochemically and the same parameters may be used to determine response to a particular line of treatment. The response may be divided into four categories:

Complete response - there is disappearance of evidence of tumor

Partial response - reduction of measured lesion is >50%

Stable disease - reduction of measured lesion is <50%

Progressive disease - increase in measured lesion by <25%

Local treatment

For a locally advanced, ulcerated, bleeding and foul smelling breast cancer with metastases, a toilet (palliative) mastectomy is done, often requiring skin grafting for cover. While doing mastectomy for debulking or palliation, there is absolutely no logic in carrying out axillary dissection, as it increases morbidity without additional benefit. In the case of a lesion fixed to the chest wall, where surgery is not technically feasible, palliative radio/ chemotherapy may be considered. Alternately, if the patient can tolerate, neoadjuvant chemotherapy may be given to down-stage the disease, making it resectable.

Systemic therapy

Whether to use hormonal and chemotherapy, synchronously or sequentially is controversial. Advocates of the former, base their modality on the assumption that different clones of cells are affected and so there is a high response rate, whereas the proponents of sequential treatment feel that the entire ammunition against breast cancer should not be used in the first round. In general, hormonal therapy has fewer side effects than chemotherapy and is preferred in ER/PR positive group, particularly with skeletal metastases. The role of Herceptin in Her-2 positive patients has been discussed earlier.

Chemotherapy appears to be more effective and better tolerated by premenopausal patients, compared to postmenopausal group.

Hormonal therapy

About 90% of ER/PR positive and 10% of ER/PR negative tumors are hormone dependent. Hence the rationale in offering hormone therapy is obvious. It may be simplified as follows:

Premenopausal women (upto 3 years after menopause): Ovarian ablation and tamoxifen, to counter extra-ovarian source of estrogen, for about 3 years.

Postmenopausal women: Since the estrogenic activity of ovaries ceases, only tamoxifen administration is sufficient. In a perimenopausal woman, who has had surgical menopause earlier, the estrogenic status may be identified by a simple vaginal cytology (increased glycogen content, fern formation etc) or by more sophisticated biochemical androgen/estrogen ratio.

Therapeutic role of tamoxifen

Tamoxifen is an antagonist of the estrogen receptor in breast tissue via its active metabolite, hydroxytamoxifen. In other tissues such as the endometrium, it behaves as an agonist, hence tamoxifen may be characterized as a mixed agonist/antagonist. It has a half-life of 5-7 days and been the standard endocrine (anti-estrogen) therapy for hormone receptor-positive breast cancer in premenopausal women, while aromatase inhibitors are preferred for postmenopausal women.

Cells of some breast cancers require estrogen to grow. Estrogen binds to and activates the ER in these cells. Tamoxifen is metabolized into compounds that also bind to the ER but do not activate it. Because of this competitive antagonism, tamoxifen acts like a key broken off in the lock that prevents any other key from being inserted, preventing estrogen from binding to its receptor. Hence breast cancer cell growth is blocked.

Tamoxifen is currently used for the treatment of both early and advanced ER+ve breast cancer in pre and postmenopausal women. Additionally, it is the most common agent used in the hormone treatment for male breast cancer. It is also advocated for the prevention of breast cancer in high risk women, e.g. against cancer in the contralateral breast), though the concept has not gained wide popularity.

Tamoxifen is used with some benefit in the management of desmoid tumor. Other anti-estrogen compounds in use: raloxifene and anastrozole are found to be equally effective against breast cancer, but with lesser risk of developing uterine cancers and thromboembolic complications.

Non-oncological uses of tamoxifen

1. Infertility: It is used to treat infertility in women with anovulatory disorders.
2. Retroperitoneal fibrosis
3. It is used to prevent estrogen-related gynecomastia, including in sex offenders undergoing temporary chemical castration
4. Bipolar disorders: Tamoxifen has been shown to be effective in the treatment of mania in patients with bipolar disorder by blocking proteinkinase-C (PKC), an enzyme that regulates neuronal activity in the brain. It is believed PKC is overactive during the mania in bipolar patients.
5. Riedel's thyroiditis.

Adverse effects

1. Endometrial cancer: Tamoxifen is a selective estrogen receptor modulator. Even though it is an antagonist in breast tissue it acts as partial agonist on the endometrium and has been linked to endometrial cancer in some women. This risk appears to be related to the duration of its use, hence it is generally withdrawn after 3-5 years

2. On bones: a beneficial side effect of tamoxifen is that it prevents bone loss by acting as an estrogen receptor agonist (i.e., mimicking the effects of estrogen). Therefore, by inhibiting osteoclasts, it prevents osteoporosis, contrary to logical belief that it would act as an estrogen receptor antagonist in all tissue, including bone, and therefore it was feared that it would contribute to osteoporosis. The surprise finding lead to the new concept of selective estrogen receptor modulators (SERMs). However, tamoxifen appears to promote bone loss in premenopausal women, who continue to menstruate after adjuvant chemotherapy. Tamoxifen has been shown to increase the possibility of premature bone fusion and should be used with caution in growing age.

3, On cardiovascular and metabolic: Tamoxifen treatment of postmenopausal women is associated with beneficial effects on serum lipid profiles. However, longterm data from clinical trials have failed to demonstrate a cardioprotective effect. For some women, tamoxifen can cause a rapid increase in triglyceride concentration in the blood. In addition there is an increased risk of thromboembolism especially during and immediately after major surgery or periods of immobility. Tamoxifen is also known to cause fatty liver (nonalcoholic steatohepatosis- NASH).

4. On central nervous system: Tamoxifen treated breast cancer patients show evidence of reduced cognition and semantic memory scores, but found to be less severe compared with those treated with anastrozole (an aromatase inhibitor). A significant number of tamoxifen treated breast cancer patients experience a reduction of libido.

5. Drug interaction with some psychotropic agents may reduce the pharmacological effects of tamoxifen.

Therapeutic role of letrozole

Letrozole is an oral nonsteroidal aromatase inhibitor for the treatment of hormone responsive breast cancer after surgery, in postmenopausal women. Estrogens are produced by the conversion of androgens through the activity of the aromatase enzyme, which then bind to estrogen receptors, stimulating cell division. Letrozole prevents the aromatase from producing estrogens by competitive, reversible binding to the heme of its cytochrome P450 unit. The action is specific and does not interfere with the production of mineralo or glucocorticosteroids.

Letrozole is more effective in postmenopausal women, in whom estrogen is produced predominantly in peripheral tissues (i.e. in adipose tissue and a number of sites in the brain). Since in premenopausal women, the main source of estrogen is from the ovaries and not the peripheral tissues, letrozole is ineffective.

Non-oncological uses of letrozole

1. For ovarian stimulation in the treatment of infertility (in females) and in non-obstructive oligo/azospermia (in males)

2. In the treatment of endometriosis

3. Pre-treatment for termination of pregnancy, in association of mesoprostol (prostaglandin)

4. Used by body builders and athletes, to counter the side effects of anabolic steroids (e.g. gynecomastia)

5. Its property of delaying epiphyseal fusion in long bones, is utilized in the treatment of children with short stature, as an adjunct to growth hormone therapy

Adverse effects

The most common side effects are sweating, hot flushes, arthralgia and fatigue.

Features of hypoestrogenism leading to osteoporosis, hence longterm use of letrozole is generally accompanied by anti-osteoporosis medications such as bisphosphonates. It is also contraindicated during pregnancy and lactation. It is considerably more expensive than tamoxifen, hence used only in specific indications.

Hormonal manipulation for breast carcinoma

1. Ovarian ablation (surgery or radiation)
2. Antiestrogens (tamoxifen)
3. Progestogens (medroxyprogesterone)
4. Aromatase inhibitors (aminoglutethimide, letrozole, raloxifene and anastrozole)
5. Goserelin - luteinizing hormone/releasing hormone (LH/RH) agonist acts as chemical castration
6. Major endocrine ablation (MEA) therapy-bilateral adrenalectomy or hypophysectomy: after the advent of chemical endocrine ablation therapy, MEA therapy (which is associated with several metabolic drawbacks) has been virtually abandoned.

Chemotherapy

I line CMF or CAF (cyclophosphamide, methotrexate/adriamycin, 5-fluorouracil)
II line Taxoids (paclitaxel, docetaxel)
III line vinca alkaloids (vinorelbine)

Edema of the arm

This is usually a lymphedema, a very troublesome complication of breast carcinoma and may be due to:
1. Tumor infiltration producing lymphatic obstruction
2. surgical removal of lymphatics (elephantiasis chirurgens)
3. radiation fibrosis

Highest incidence is seen when RT is given following axillary block dissection, as done in standard radical mastectomy and probably one of the main reasons for the ill reputation suffered by Halsted's operation.

Lymphangiosarcoma (Stewart-Treves syndrome) is a rare complication of lymphedema, following axillary surgery/RT for breast malignancy, responsible for rapid deterioration of health.

Treatment

As it is often seen in advanced/recurrent malignancy, the treatment is largely palliative. General measures, such as elevation, elastic support, antiedema (diuretic), anti-fibroblastic (stanozolol) and steroid therapy may be routinely employed. Specific treatment depends upon the cause. It is to be planned according to the merits of the situation, avoiding unrewarding adventurism or lymphatic reconstructive procedures.

Cancer-en-cuirasse (cuirasse: breast plate worn by soldiers) is another terminal event due to diffuse infiltration of the chest wall by cancer and is usually associated with edema and limitation of movements of arm; this is commonly seen in recurrent carcinoma, especially following RT. Appropriate combination of chemo/hormone therapy, depending upon the general condition, may palliate the distressed patients but certainly, cure is far fetched.

Specific complications

Hypercalcemia

Treated by pamidronate or alendronate. Rarely if the serum calcium level does not come down with pamidronate, steroids or calcitonin may be used. Bisphosphonates may be prescribed to prevent hypercalcemia due to osseous metastases.

Endometrial carcinoma

Longterm use of tamoxifen may be associated with a higher incidence of endometrial carcinoma, hence it is ideally withdrawn after 3 years.

Leucoerythroblastic anemia

Due to infiltration of bone marrow by the cancer cells, a leucoerythroblastic anemia develops and is treated by blood and platelet transfusions and androgens.

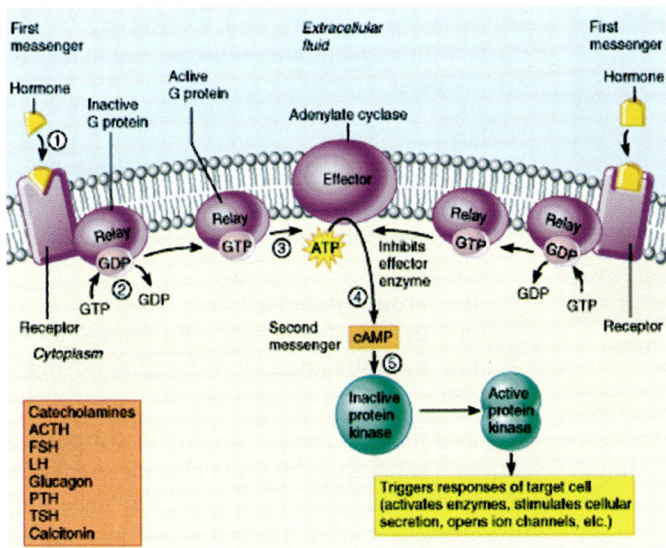

Fig. 95.32. Hormone receptor complex

Cord compression

This is a true oncological emergency. Any patient with weakness of legs and bladder and bowel disturbances should be evaluated with CT scan and the cord compression should be relieved immediately by RT or surgery.

Cerebral metastasis

Treatment of choice is by radiotherapy. Diuretics, dexamethasone, mannitol or oral glycerol decrease the raised intracranial tension and reduce vomiting and headache.

Pleural effusion

This has better prognosis than lymphangitis carcinomatosa. Treatment is by intercostal drainage (ICD) by a wide bore tube and systemic treatment. Intrapleural chemotherapy has not been very useful, but chemical or surgical pleurodesis may be considered to prevent troublesome reaccumulation of fluid.

Follow up surveillance

Regular history and physical examination should be done every 4-6 months. Mammography is also recommended of the contralateral breast and earlier mammograms should be available to compare with the follow up mammograms. Magnification mammography is one of the techniques to augment sensitivity in detecting small foci of residual malignant calcification in the postoperative breast.

Bilateral cancers of breast

When malignant masses are detected in both breasts, either synchronously or metachrono-usly (in the contralateral breast, after six months following mastectomy), a moot question often comes up as to whether it is a secondary or a second primary.

Sarcoma breast

It is a rare tumor, usually the spindle-cell type of fibrosarcoma, occasionally arising from an intra-canalicular fibroadenoma or a phyllodes tumor. It may also follow several years after irradiation for some other disease like lymphoma. It occurs in younger women and shows faster growth, compared to carcinoma, at times histologically resembling medullary carcinoma. Hematogenous spread to lungs and bones is seen early, regional lymph nodes are involved late.

After confirming the diagnosis either by a wide bore (Tru-cut) needle or open (wedge) biopsy, it is treated by total mastectomy and postoperative RT/chemotherapy. There is no place for breast conservative surgery (QUART) and in view of early blood spread, the prognosis is worse than carcinoma.

Postmastectomy breast reconstruction

This is ideally done in those women, in whom 'reasonable cure' can be anticipated following the multimodal therapy and who can understand its short/long-term implications and possible complications. With the advent of sophisticated imaging modalities, the fear of delayed detection of local recurrence following reconstruction, appears to be theoretical. Though many patients prefer immediate restoration of shape and size, the wisdom of the surgeon in a given set up, may dictate to do it at a later stage after being assured of no residual disease, hav-

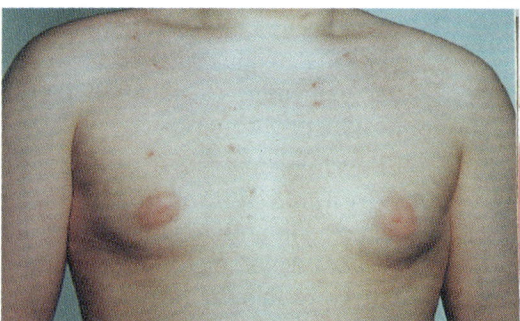

Fig. 95.33. Bilateral gynecomastia in a man of 16
(courtesy: Lifeline Hospitals, Chennai)

ing gone through the 'run of the mill' of various forms of therapy. Needless to say, in this context, that any form of esthetic surgery should not compromise the relentless war against cancer, at any stage.

Technically it may be done by autologous or synthetic (alloplastic) material. The former comprises the use of myocutaneous flaps, such as latissimus dorsi or TRAM (transverse rectus abdominis myocutaneous) flap and the alloplastic method involves the use of tissue expanders and prosthetic implants. The nipple reconstruction, either from local dermal flap or graft from the contralateral nipple is generally delayed for 6-8 weeks.

In view of the high failure rate of the TRAM flap due to ischemic necrosis, especially in smokers, use of tissue expanders has gained popularity for mammary reconstruction.

GYNECOMASTIA

It is the abnormal hypertrophy of mammary tissue in a male, resembling female breast.

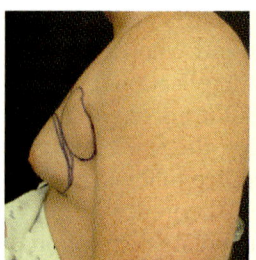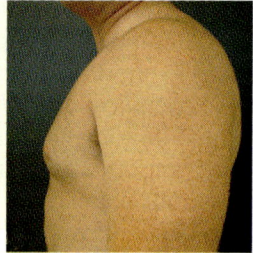

Fig. 95.34. Gynecomastia-before and after reduction by liposuction
(courtesy: Lifeline Hospitals, Chennai)

There is hypertrophy and elongation of the ducts with considerable fibrosis. The acini are not involved.

Causes

1) physiological: occurs in three age groups:

   (a) in infants due to circulating maternal estrogens, which generally regress within a few months,

   (b) around puberty and

   (c) in elderly, around climacteric, both due to imbalance of estrogen/androgen ratio.

2) metabolic causes: cirrhosis (impaired estrogen catabolism by liver), chronic renal failure (disturbed hypophysis-testicular axis) and thyrotoxicosis (due to increased aromatase activity, which converts testosterone to estrogen)

3) drugs: estrogen administration for prostatic carcinoma, digitalis, spironolactone, cimetidine, methyldopa, ketoconazole, captopril, tricyclic antidepressants, chemotherapy for testicular tumors etc

4) tumors: feminizing tumors of testes, tumors of adrenal cortex producing testosterone, which is converted into estrogen, paraneoplastic syndromes seen in bronchogenic carcinoma or pancreatic tumors (producing gonadotrophins) and hepatic tumors, producing aromatase.

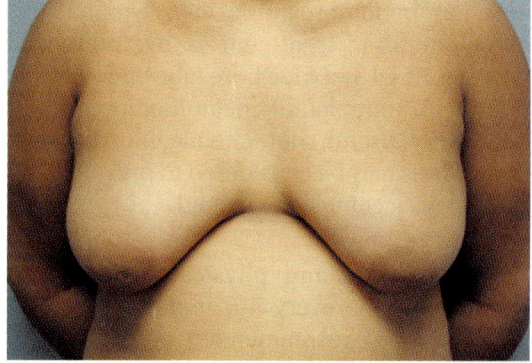

Fig. 95.35. Gynecomastia - a complication of cirrhosis of liver
(courtesy: Halsted Surgical Clinic, Chennai)

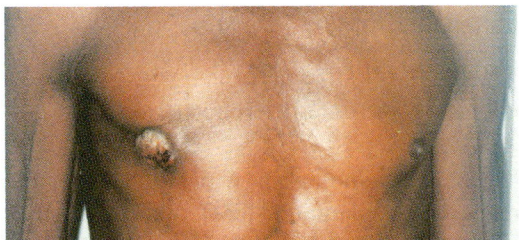

Fig. 95.36. Carcinoma male breast
(courtesy: Dr K Sureshkumar, Chennai)

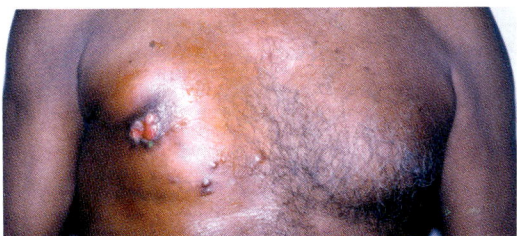

Fig. 95.37. Advanced carcinoma male breast, with
satellite nodules
(courtesy: Dr K Sreekanth, Chennai)

5) hypogonadism: cryptorchism, anorchism, mumps, Hansen's disease, trauma or surgical removal, Klinefelter's syndrome (44-XXY), intersex etc.

6) idiopathic.

To remember the important causes (MASTIA)
M-malignant tumor (teratoma or paraneoplastic syndrome)
A-atrophy testis (injury, infection, undescended testis, surgical removal)
S-sex chromosal disorders
T-therapy (drugs)
I-idiopathic
A-alcohol (cirrhosis liver).

Clinical features

There is painless insidious breast enlargement, either unilateral or bilateral. In the latter situation, diffuse deposition of fat due to obesity has to be differentiated. Mammary tissue can be palpated as a slightly tender mass, slipping under the fingers. Thorough examination to detect any cause indicated above should be done, with special reference to the testicular size and evidence of cirrhosis. The incidence of malignancy is higher in gynecomastia than in normal male breasts.

Investigations aimed at detecting underlying disease, especially endocrinopathy and chromosomal defects have to be done in appropriate cases. Since in a large majority of young men it is idiopathic, elaborate and expensive investigations are unwarranted, as a routine.

ER, PR, AR (aromatase) and AgR (androgen receptors) may be detected in male breast tissue, but only PR is considered important in the etiology and treatment.

Treatment

If a cause can be identified, it should be treated, to see the response. Danacrine sulfate, a gonadotrophic antagonist, tamoxifen citrate, an antiestrogen compound and cabergoline, an antiprolactin agent may be helpful given early in the course, on an empirical basis. Surgery is definitive and preferred in larger swellings and in emotionally disturbed young subjects, consisting of total excision of mammary tissue, by a semilunar incision under the areola (subareolar mastectomy of Webster), with excellent physical and esthetic results.

LIPOSUCTION

This is a minimally invasive technique done for gynecomastia under general anesthesia, employing a special suction device introduced subcutaneously through a 5mm incision and aspirating the entire fat and mammary tissue in the pectoral region. Preliminary injection of saline (with adrenaline) into the subcutaneous fat facilitates the procedure, followed by compression dressings, to prevent lymphatic collection in the 'dead space' created. Occasionally, a small subareolar incision is also required to excise residual firm, fibrous mammary tissue, which cannot be aspirated.

CARCINOMA OF THE MALE BREAST

The incidence is <1% of cases of carcinoma of the breast. It may develop under the background of gynecomastia or estrogen administration, usually in men >50 yrs. Klinefelter syndrome (44+XXY), testicular feminizing syndromes and irradiation are associated with a high incidence of carcinoma male breast. It presents as a painless mass, which quickly ulcerates and infiltrates the pectoral muscles. In view of the smaller size of the breast, extramammary spread occurs more readily than in females; hence carries a worse prognosis. Histologically it tends to be an infiltrating duct cell carcinoma, further contributing to the unfavourable outlook.

Clinical staging, investigations and principles of therapy are more or less identical to female disease, but they seem to respond better to orchidectomy than do females (to oophorectomy). Tamoxifen is also useful in ER+ve patients. Adequate clearance invariably amounts to 'mastectomy' and removing part of the pectoral muscles.

Recent advances

Radioactive strontium has been tried in skeletal secondaries.

High dose chemotherapy with autologous bone marrow transplantation (BMT) and colony stimulating factors, is being tried in some centers with promising results, in otherwise hopeless cases.

Increase of matrix metalloproteinase (MMP) expression and activity correlates with early tumor dissemination. This supports the role of MMP inhibitors (Betastatin) in the management of breast cancer.

96 Cranial Nerves

Only some aspects of surgical importance of the cranial nerves are considered here.

Olfactory nerve (first)

Disruption of the olfactory fibres may occur during head injury and cause anosmia on the corresponding side. In bilateral injury there is total *anosmia*.

Parasmia is perversion of sense of smell, e.g. offensive substances seem to have a pleasant odor and vice versa.

Optic nerve (second)

From retina, fibres of optic nerve pass back to the optic chiasm, where the fibres from the inner (nasal) half of each retina, catering temporal field, descussate, whilst those from outer (temporal) side, representing the nasal field, remain on the same side. Each optic tract originating from the chiasm, pass through the geniculate body, optic radiation to project into occipital cortex. It therefore consists of fibres from outer retina of same side and inner retina of the opposite side.

The optic nerve may be involved by gliomas or compressed by meningiomas. It may also be damaged by contusions/fractures involving the optic foramina. The optic chiasma may be compressed by pituitary tumors, producing bitemporal hemianopia. In lesions of optic nerve, the afferent pathway is affected, hence consensual papillary reflex (beaming the light into the opposite eye) is brisker than the direct reflex (focusing the light into the affected eye).

Oculomotor nerve (third)

It supplies all the external ocular muscles including levator palpebrae superioris, except superior oblique and lateral rectus and also carries parasympathetic fibers to the pupillary constrictors. Ptosis, fixed dilated pupil and loss of accommodation are typically seen following its palsy.

Oculomotor nerves are involved by tumors, trauma involving spheniodal fissure or orbit and aneurysms. The uncal herniation due to increased pressure in the supratentorial compartment, in head injury may result in a dilated pupil due to parasympathetic paralysis (Kernohan's notch). Painless third nerve palsy is a characteristic sign of posterior communicating artery aneurysm.

The *Argyll Robertson pupil* described classically in neurosyphilis, is a small, irregular pupil which reacts to accommodation (ARP-accomodation reflex preserved) but not to direct/consensual light (PRA-pupillary reflex absent). In *Horner's syndrome*, miosis and ptosis, due to paralysis of the cervical sympathetic chain are essential components.

Hutchinson's pupil is described in head injuries, with progressive cerebral compression. As the 3rd nerve is being pressed against the tentorium, initially the ipsilateral pupil is constricted (irritation of parasympathetic), while the contralateral one is normal, followed by dilated ipsilateral (paralysis of parasympathetic) and constricted opposite pupil and finaly as the SOL expands further, the compression paralyses both, making them dilate and unreactive. Fixed dilated pupils are considered as one of the features of 'brain death', while making a crucial decision to discontinue cardiopulmonary resuscitation (CPR), in a patient who has suffered protracted cerebral hypoxia.

Trochlear nerve (fourth)

It supplies the superior oblique muscle, which rotates the eye downwards in adducted position. It is rarely involved alone; diplopia and deficient movement of the eye in a downward and inward direction may be observed.

Trigeminal nerve (fifth)

It supplies sensations to entire half of face, including anterior scalp, conjunctiva, cornea, jaws, palate up to the tonsils and motor supply to muscles of mastication.

In injury to the sensory root there is anesthesia of the face on the side of the lesion, insensibility of the conjunctiva, dryness of the nose and diminished secretion of the lacrimal and salivary glands, with neurotrophic keratitis. Impaired palatal reflex may be seen. The motor component is incorporated in the mandibular division, to supply the muscles of mastication. It can be tested by asking the patient to clench the jaw, when the masseter and temporalis muscles are seen firming up. When the mouth is opened, there will be deviation of the jaw to the affected side, due to the unopposed action of lateral pterygoid muscle on the normal side.

The trigeminal nerve is often the seat of *neuralgia*, in which second (maxillary) and third (mandibular) divisions are more commonly affected. Pain in their distribution, is characteristically shooting or burning in nature. It may occur spontaneously or in response to stimulation of trigger points by light touch, chewing, swallowing, talking, brushing the teeth or by cold wind.

Tumors (epidermoid cyst, meningioma, angioma and acoustic neuroma) account for 5% of the cases.

Management involves CT/MRI scan to exclude a cerebellopontine angle lesion. A thorough dental evaluation is essential, as the pain originating from the dental roots may mimic neuralgia. Initial treatment with carbamazepine 200 mg t.i.d. with addition of phenytoin 100mg t.i.d. and anxiolytic/analgesic agents, if necessary, may be effective.

When drugs do not control the pain, destruction of the *Gasserian ganglion* by injection of absolute alcohol or phenol or direct section of the sensory root by stereotactic method or radiofrequency ablation (RFA) may be necessary.

Abducent nerve (sixth)

It supplies the lateral rectus muscle, which deviates the eye externally. Due to its long intracranial course, this nerve is often involved in fractures of the base of the skull and basal meningitis, resulting in internal or convergent squint

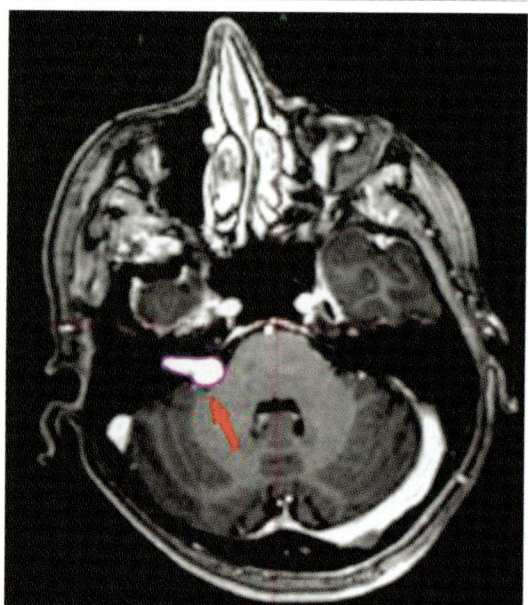

Fig. 96.1. CT scan showing acoustic neuroma (red pointer)

(due to paralysis of lateral rectus muscle). Because of its position, any rise in intracranial pressure may cause its palsy (false localization sign).

Facial nerve (seventh)

It is the motor nerve to muscles of facial expression, platysma, stapedius and posterior belly of digastric muscle and carries chorda tympani (carrying taste fibers from anterior 2/3 of tongue) for some distance. In clinical practice the motor loss is the most important lesion of the seventh cranial nerve, which may be either upper motor neurone (UMN) or lower motor nerurone (LMN) type, depending upon the level of lesion.

UMN lesions: The lesions above the facial nucleus in the pons produce paralysis of the muscles of the lower half of the face only because the upper facial muscles (forehead and eyebrow) enjoy bilateral innervation. The patient is able to wrinkle the forehead or close the eye but will not be able to blow whistle or say 'EE', properly.

LMN lesions: These include lesions of the facial nucleus or below, but for a surgeon, intrapetrous and extra-cranial portions are important. In this type the entire half of the face on that side is affected.

The intraosseous part (within the petrous temporal bone) of the facial nerve may be injured by fractures of the base of skull or middle cranial fossa, or during operations on the middle ear and mastoid antrum.

The extra cranial part of facial nerve may be injured or deliberately sacrificed during surgery for the parotid tumors.

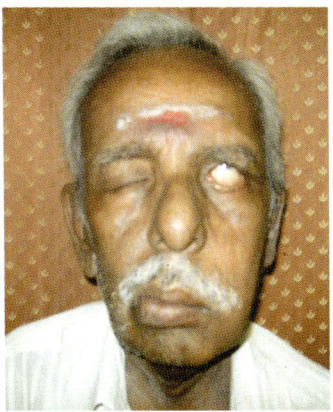

Fig. 96.2. Left facial palsy with Bell's phenomenon

Malignant parotid tumors involve the facial nerve early and its paralysis is an important clinical marker for the diagnosis. The nerve is commonly involved by Bell's palsy and follows exposure to cold or drought. More than 70% recover completely in few months. Rarely it may be involved in herpes zoster (Ramsay-Hunt syndrome).

Bell's phenomenon: The eye ball rolls upwards during attempted forced closure of eye. This is a normal reflex which is preserved in LMN type of facial paralysis and becomes conspicuous since the patient is unable to close the eye lid.

Branches of the facial nerve may be damaged by ill-placed incisions on the face and neck (marginal mandibular branch in submandibular salivary gland surgery) and occasionally by a broken wind screen. The paralysed face is flat and expressionless. The eye fails to close, the forehead does not wrinkle, the angle of the mouth droops and food collects in the oral vestibule. All facial expressions in response to emotion are lost on the affected side and failure to close the lids may result in exposure (neuroparalytic) keratitis.

Treatment

The damaged facial nerve should be repaired or grafted promptly. The replacement of lost facial nerve by interposing either a sural nerve or lateral cutaneous nerve of the thigh has been advised. Alternatively a hypoglossal-facial anas-

tomosis, a crossed facial repair or other plastic surgical techniques may be used to improve the resting state of the face.

The treatment after a long established facial nerve paralysis is by static or dynamic suspension of the eyelids, cheek and angle of mouth using fasia lata strips or temporalis slings. Newer techniques include muscle transfer employing the muscles of mastication, which are supplied by the mandibular branch of the trigeminal.

Vestibulocochlear nerve (eighth)

It carries information from the vestibular apparatus and the organ of Corti. The surgical significance of the eighth cranial nerve is that it may be involved in fracture of the middle cranial fossa or a tumor (acoustic neuroma). This may initially produce tinnitus and high frequency hearing loss. CT/MRI may be useful in diagnosing these tumors of the cerebellopontine angle region.

Glossopharyngeal nerve (ninth)

The motor supply of the ninth cranial nerve is to the stylopharyngeus muscle, which cannot be tested alone clinically. But it may be tested together with the vagus, by eliciting the palatal reflex. The patient is asked to say 'aah' or the back of pharynx is tickled, to see the contraction of soft palate. The afferent is 9th and the efferent is the 10th nerve. In unilateral palsy, it may be seen deviating to the opposite side. It is affected by fractures of the skull base or by brain stem pathology involving the lower cranial nerve roots. Glossopharyngeal neuralgia which is a rare condition resulting in severe pain in the region of the tonsil or deep in the ear, may be a presenting feature in carcinoma of the posterior third of tongue and the oropharynx.

Vagus nerve (tenth)

It is called so because of its widespread distribution in the body. It originates in the medulla oblongata and enters the neck via the jugular foramen (along with 9th and 11th cranial nerves). It carries both motor and sensory fibres the vagus nerve has two sensory ganglia, a superior one situated on the nerve within the jugular foramen and an inferior one (ganglion nodosum) which lies on the nerve below the foramen. The cranial root of the 11th nerve (accessory nerve) joins the vagus at this level in the neck.

The superior laryngeal nerve arises from the inferior ganglia and divides into a larger internal and a smaller external laryngeal branches. The *internal* branch enters the larynx through the thyrohyoid membrane and supplies sensory fibres to the epiglottis and larygeal mucosa, above the vocal cords. In many instances the internal branch also innervates the arytenoid muscles (arytaina: ladle, jug or pitcher) which are important in phonation, because they cause approximation of the posterior portions of the vocal cords.

The *external* branch descends in the neck accompanied by superior thyroid artery, passes deep to the thyroid gland and after giving a branch to the inferior constrictor muscle of the pharynx, innervates the cricothyroid muscle, a tensor of vocal cords. Paralysis of the cricothyroid causes the voice to be weak, unable to generate a high pitch, and gets easily fatigued. Injury to external laryngeal is common, due to its proximity to superior thyroid artery; it can be avoided by ligating the skeletonized artery, close to the upper pole of the thyroid gland. High mass ligation of the superior thyroid 'pedicle' is not acceptable for this reason.

The recurrent (inferior) laryngeal nerve has a different course on either side. On the *right*, the nerve emerges from the vagus as it crosses anterior to the subclavian artery, encircles the artery and ascends with a medial inclination into the neck to seek its position in the tracheoesphageal groove, postero-medial to the thyroid lobe. On the *left*, it originates from the vagus as it crosses infront of the the aortic arch, encircles the aorta lateral to the *ligamentum arteriosum* and

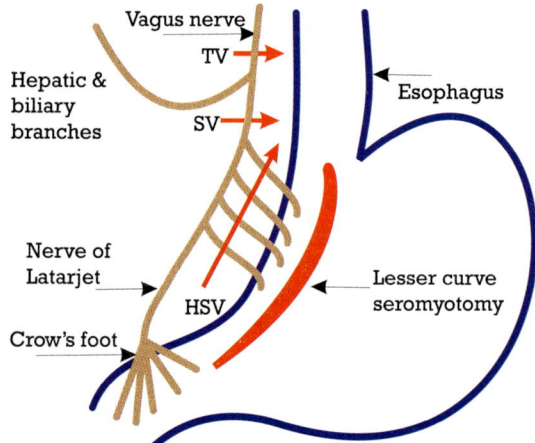

Fig. 96.3. Types of vagotomy for acid-peptic disease TV: truncal vagotomy; SV: selective vagotomy; HSV: highly selective vagotomy

ascends in the neck behind the origin of the left common carotid, in a vertical course, to reach the tracheoesophageal groove. Both nerves cross the inferior thyroid arteries, and run behind the cricothyroid joints, to enter the larynx under cover of the inferior constrictor muscle. The variable relationship of this nerve to the inferior thyroid artery is very important to the surgeon, it may pass deep to the artery (75%), superficial (16%), in between its branches (7%) or take an intraglandular course (2%).

On rare occasions, invariably on the right side, the inferior laryngeal nerve is 'non-recurrent' arising from the vagus in the neck and coming medially towards the tracheoesphageal groove in a relatively close relationship to the inferior thyroid artery or cephalad to it. This is usually associated with anomalies of aortic arch and great vessels. Whenever during routine search for the recurrent nerve, it is not found in its normal location, either intraglandular course or non-recurrence (right side) has to be suspected especially so in a patient with major cardiovascular anomalies. Sometimes the nerve divides before disappearing under the inferior constrictor muscle and the medial branch may be injured inadvertently while mobilizing the lobe. The pharyngeal (medial) branches of recurrent laryngeal nerve communicate with the branches of superior laryngeal nerve, forming the 'loop of Galen' which is vulnerable to injury during the dissection of the superior thyroid pedicle.

The recurrent laryngeal nerve provides sensations to the larynx below the vocal cords and is the motor nerve to all the intrinsic muscles of the larynx, except the cricothyroid. It also innervates part of the inferior constrictor muscle, during its intramuscular course. From the foregone discussion, it is evident that the recurrent laryngeal nerve is the main concern during thyroid surgery. The surgeons should be grateful to nature for placing the nerve so vulnerable that patients requiring thyroid surgery are 'sincerely' referred to them, lest all general practitioners start doing thyroidectomies!

A complete recurrent laryngeal nerve palsy results in paralysis of both adductors and abductors of the corresponding vocal cord, which thereby adopts a neutral (cadaveric) position. Unilateral vocal cord palsy may be asymptomatic, since the opposite fellow compensates effectively, but more often there is some hoarseness and the typical non-occlusive (bovine) cough. Partial recurrent laryngeal nerve palsy has a predilection for the abductors leading to adduction of the vocal cord on the affected side. In bilateral cases, stridor may be seen requiring arytenoidopexy or tracheostomy. It is important to realize that up to 40% of unilateral recurrent nerve palsies are idiopathic, but may remain asymptomatic due to compensation by its opposite nerve, and hence the need to record laryngoscopic findings before thyroid surgery is obvious.

Semon's law states that in all progressive *organic* lesions of the center and trunks of laryngeal nerves, the fibres supplying the abductor muscles of vocal cord are first involved followed by adductors and recover in reverse order, i.e. first adductors and then the abductors. It implies that isolated adductor palsy is more likely to be *functional* than organic. This phenomenon may be due to the distribution of the fibres supplying those muscles within the nerves and their differ-

ent chronaxies, resulting in varying susceptibility. The phylogenetic explanation for this is more interesting, that the muscles that develop early during evolution, are the last to lose function, after total denervation. The adductors being the first laryngeal muscles to evolve (gills), they retain their function for a few more days, bringing the cords to approximation even after total denervation of the cords, during which period airway should be maintained by intubation. However this is only transient, the cords assuming neutral (cadaveric) position within 2-3 days.

Stridor in bilateral recurrent laryngeal nerve palsy is due to action of cricothyroid (tensor of vocal cords), bringing the cords to midline

In the neck the vagus also gives afferent supply to the carotid body and cervical cardiac branches to join the cardiac plexus. In mediastinal causes of recurrent nerve palsy, such as esophageal, bronchogenic malignancies or aortic arch aneurysm, it is always the left nerve that is involved, since the right one has no intrathoracic course.

In the thorax, it gives cardiac, esophageal and tracheal branches and finally forms the esophageal plexus, with its opposite fellow, behind the esophagus. From this plexus, anterior and posterior *vagal trunks* emerge, to enter the abdomen through the esophageal opening of the diaphragm, when they are also called *gastric nerves*. This position is due to the rotation of stomach, the **l**eft becoming **a**nterior and **r**ight goes to lie **p**osterior (LARP) at the lower end of the esophagus.

Their abdominal course is extremely important to the surgeon in the management of acid-peptic diseases. The anterior one, smaller of the two, descends in the anterior leaf of lesser (gastrohepatic) omentum, giving gastric and hepatobiliary branches. At about the incisura of the stomach, it is known as the *nerve of Latarjet*, and divides into its terminal branches like a 'crow-foot', supplying the anterior aspect of prepyloric antrum and pyloric sphincter. The posterior nerve runs in the posterior leaf of lesser omentum, giving gastric and splanchnic branches (the latter joining the splanchnic plexus, to supply the pancreas and gut upto the distal third of transverse colon, derived from midgut). It also divides at about incisura, into 'crow-foot', to supply the posterior aspect of prepyloric antrum and pyloric sphincter. Both gastric nerves stimulate acid (HCl) secretion from the parietal cells of the fundus and body and help gastric emptying, by contracting the gastric muscles and relaxing the pyloric sphincter.

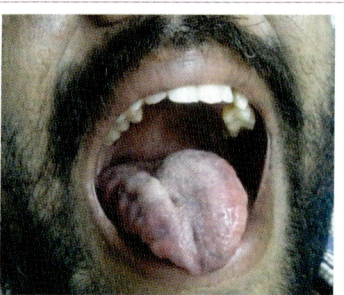

Fig. 96.4. Lingual hemiatrophy due to right hypoglossal palsy (courtesy: Laxmi Hospital, Kakinada)

Various types of **vagotomy** have been developed to reduce the neurogenic influences on gastric secretions, either by dividing the entire trunks as they enter the abdomen (truncal vagotomy), only gastric branches including the crow's foot, retaining the hepatobiliary and splanchnic supply (selective vagotomy) and the recent addition, where only proximal gastric branches to parietal cells are divided, preserving also the nerves of Latarjet and their crow's foot branches (highly selective or parietal cell vagotomy-PCV). In the former two types, the gastric emptying is affected and hence some drainage procedure, such as pyloroplasty or gastrojejunostomy should always follow those operations. In the last type however pyloric functions are unaffected and no drainage operation required, which is considered to be its main advantage over the others.

Other variations of PCV, sparing the anterior crow's foot, are:

(i) posterior truncal vagotomy and anterior (lesser curve) seromyotomy and

(ii) posterior truncal vagotomy and anterior (lesser curve) linear gastrectomy, using staplers. These are based on the observation that innervation of the anterior pylorus is sufficient for normal gastric emptying.

Accessory nerve (eleventh)

It has two roots, spinal and cranial. This is the nerve to the SCM and the upper part of the trapezius. It may be damaged by fractures of base of skull, but it is more commonly affected in its upper cervical course particularly as it passes through the apex of the posterior triangle during lymph node biopsy. It is important to remember that the nerve runs in a line drawn from tip of mastoid to tip of acromion, with the face turned to the opposite side (see Fig. 91.9).

Division of the nerve in the anterior triangle will produce paralysis of the SCM muscle, although in a third of the cases, there is an adequate supply from the second and third cervical roots to prevent a complete paralysis. If damage occurs in the posterior triangle the supply to trapezius alone will be affected, resulting in drooping of the shoulder and wasting of the trapezius with winging of scapula. Inability to shrug the shoulder differentiates this from the winging due to paralysis of serratus anterior.

Hypoglossal nerve (twelfth)

This is the motor nerve to the tongue and damage to this nerve results in wasting, weakness (lingual hemiatrophy) and fasciculations on the affected side and on protrusion, the tongue deviates towards the side of the lesion. Though the 12th nerve may be involved by intracranial pathology it is not affected by fractures of the base of the skull. It may be injured distally, during operations such as excision of the submandibular salivary gland or lymph nodes, sublingual dermoid, carotid body tumor, branchial sinus or cyst.

97 Peripheral Nerves

Classification of nerve injuries: (after Seddon)

(i) neurapraxia (apraxia: absence of action), the anatomy of the nerve is intact, but there is transient dysfunction,

(ii) axonotmesis (tmesis: cutting apart), where the axons have been disrupted but the sheaths are intact and

(iii) neurotmesis, where the nerve is totally divided. Another classification is into *degenerative* and *non-degenerative* injuries, depending upon whether the injury is lethal or sublethal, resulting in degeneration or otherwise of the distal neurone. Loss of sudomotor and vasomotor functions, evident in a week or two, is indicative of degenerative injury.

Non-degenerative lesions correspond to neurapraxia, produce short-term conduction blocks; these are seen following application of tourniquet and handling/retraction of the nerves during surgery such as brachial plexus during decompression of thoracic outlet.

Degenerative lesions correspond to axonotmesis and neurotmesis and are due to the more protracted and extensive injuries, such as traction, fractures, tight POP, crushing the nerve or total division. In axonotmesis, the recovery takes place by regeneration of distal axon, starting from the end organ towards the site of injury, at a rate of 1mm per day, which may be assessed by *Tinel's sign*; gentle tapping along the distal course of the nerve, from the site of injury elicits paresthesia, once the point of regeneration is reached. Neurotmesis has no chance of recovery, unless surgical repair is carried out.

Wallerian degeneration occurs in response to peripheral nerve injury, occurring in a retrograde direction (towards the spinal cord) until the next node of Ranvier. There is loss of myelin sheath, which is replaced by glial cells, macrophages and fibroblasts. This is followed by regeneration, starting from the same node, extending towards the point of injury. By electrical stimulation, there is a typical *reaction of degeneration*, starting by the 4th day following division and gets fully established in two weeks. No response to Faradic, but weak Galvanic response, with reversal of polarity is seen, i.e., anodal closing current (ACC) is more than cathodal closing current (KCC); normally it is the opposite.

After denervation, the muscle bulk reduces without a change in fiber count. Within a week progressive interstitial fibrosis sets in, which can be delayed by passive exercises. If the motor endplates are not reinner-vated within 18 months, the muscle loses its function permanently.
Endoneurium: sheath around individual axon
Perineurium: sheath around each fasciculus
Epineurium: sheath around a nerve trunk

The results of repair depends on several factors:

(i) injury type and level
(ii) associated soft tissue and bone injury
(iii) timing of repair

SUNDERLAND	SEDDON	NATURE OF INJURY
I	Neurapraxia	Conduction block, No loss of structural continuity
II	Axonotmesis	Axon severed, endoneurial tube intact
III		Endoneurial tube severed
IV		Only Epineurium intact
V	Neurotmesis	Loss of continuity of epi and endoneurium

Table. 97.1. - Classification of nerve injuries Sunderland and Seddon)

(iv) technique of repair
(v) type of nerve
(vi) age of patient and
(vii) patient's motivation and compliance. Clean cut injury of a nerve at a distal level, without much associated injuries, (pure sensory or motor) for which primary fascicular microsuturing done has been done in a well motivated, cooperative, young patient, offers the best results of repair.

Technique: The nerve repair may be primary (3-4 hours), delayed primary (4-5 days) or secondary (5-6

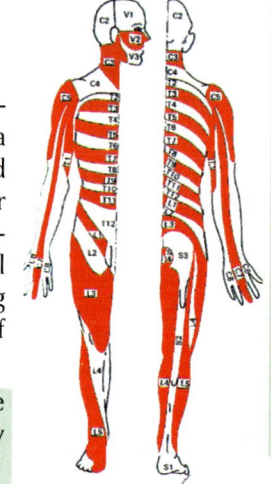

Fig. 97.2 Somatic innervation of spinal segments

weeks), which may be either direct anastomosis or nerve grafting. It should be done under magnification, using microsutures, approximating the perineurium of individual fasciculi (fascicular suture), without tension. Finally the epineurium, which surrounds the entire nerve, should be sutured, to restore original anatomy. Repairs are protected by appropriately relaxed joint immobilization for 3-4 weeks, following which physiotherapy and motor/sensory re-education are begun.

Neuromas: They are not tumors, but represent normal physiological response to injury. The cleaner the injury, the lesser is the risk of neuroma formation, their sensory component contributing to pain. Amputation neuroma should be prevented by dividing the nerve with a 'sharp' scalpel, as high in the wound as possible and should never be crushed. Since those close to surface become symptomatic, some tissue padding should be provided around a divided nerve, particularly in the fingers, to prevent painful neuroma formation.

Treatment of a neuroma is difficult and challenging, as evident by the innumerable surgical methods described for it, with no single method enjoying universal patronage. Meticulous dissection and transposition into deeper planes creating some soft tissue cushions around, is the

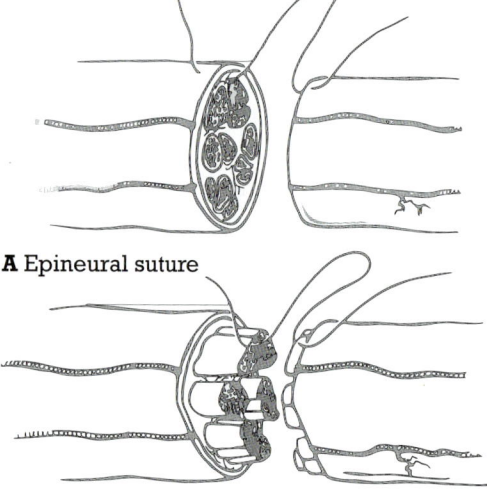

A Epineural suture

B Group fascicular

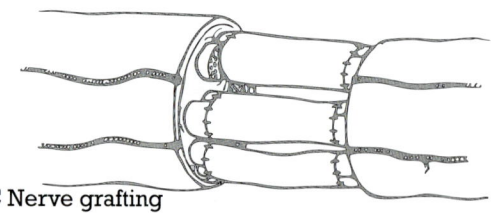

C Nerve grafting

Fig. 97.1. Techniques of nerve repair
A. direct epineural suture using surface vessels for alignment
B. Group fascicular repair
C. Nerve grafting using multiple strands of donor nerve to bridge defect

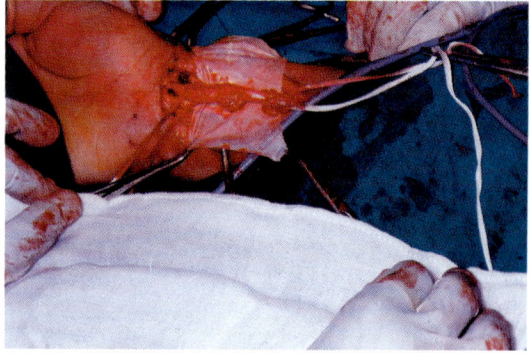

Fig. 97.3. Traumatic neuroma, median nerve (courtesy: Lifeline Hospitals, Chennai)

most popular approach, for anastomotic neuromas.

Motor testing: six grades of power are described, besides testing for muscle wasting, abnormal movements and reflexes, in relation to the affected nerve. In areas such as hand, with dual nerve supply, the signs may be more subtle and confusing.

0: no contraction
1: flicker
2: active movement perpendicular to gravity
3: movement against gravity
4: movement against gravity and some resistance
5: normal power

Sensory testing: is done by cotton wool for light touch and sterile needle for pain sensations, outlining the areas of impaired sensations, eliminating visual perception by asking the patient to close eyes, after explaining the procedure.

INDIVIDUAL NERVES
Cervical plexus

a) the spinal accessory nerve (C-2,3,4), supplies the SCM (C-2,3) and trepezius (C-3,4) muscles, the former escapes, if the nerve is injured in the posterior triangle. It runs just underneath the investing fascia, easily vulnerable for injury during biopsy of nodes in the posterior triangle. It is well to remember the surface marking for it, a line joining the angle of mandible to the tip of shoulder, before incising the deep fascia of neck. Winging of scapula, wasting of trapezius and inability to shrug the shoulder on that side are the features of spinal accessory nerve lesions.

b) Phrenic nerve (C-3,4,5) arising in the neck, travels infront of scalenus anticus muscle, to reach the thorax. It runs on either side of the

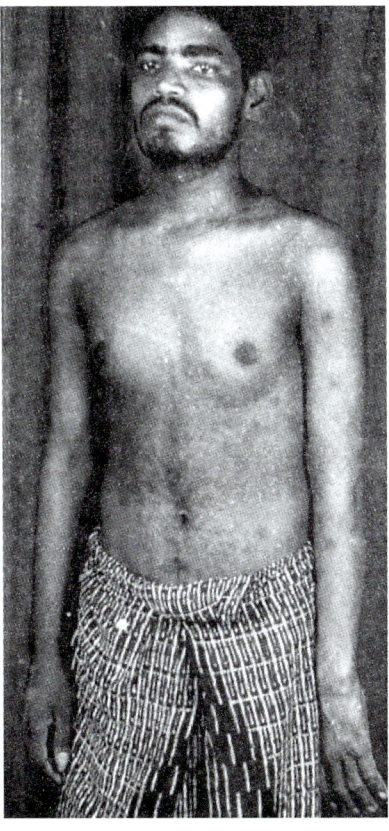

Fig. 97.4. Typical posture of Erb's palsy (policeman receiving tip) due to a tumor pressing on the upper trunk (courtesy: Lifeline Hospitals, Chennai)

pericardium, to the under surface of the diaphragm, right one passing through the hiatus for IVC and the left piercing the muscular portion, immediately adjacent to the pericardium, to innervate its hemi diaphragm, by dividing into three branches, anterior, lateral and posterior. It is sensory to the diaphragm, mediastinal pleura, fibrous pericardium, parietal layer of serous pericardium and the central portions of diaphragmatic pleura and peritoneum.

The pain originating from the diaphragm is referred to the tip of the shoulder (C-4), the basis for *Kehr sign* in ruptured spleen, pain felt around the left shoulder. To avoid injury to its branches, incision on the diaphragm should be round the periphery or radiating from the points of their entry into the abdomen.

Sensory distribution

Tactile localization, discrimination, pain, temperature, pressure, position and vibration

Upper limb

Ulnar: medial half of hand and medial 1½ fingers (front and back)

Median: lateral half hand on palmar side and lateral 3½ fingers (front and back) except back of thumb

Radial: lateral half of dorsum of hand and back of thumb

Lower limb

Common peroneal (common fibular or lateral politeal): lateral aspect of calf and entire dorsum of foot, except first interdigital (web) space

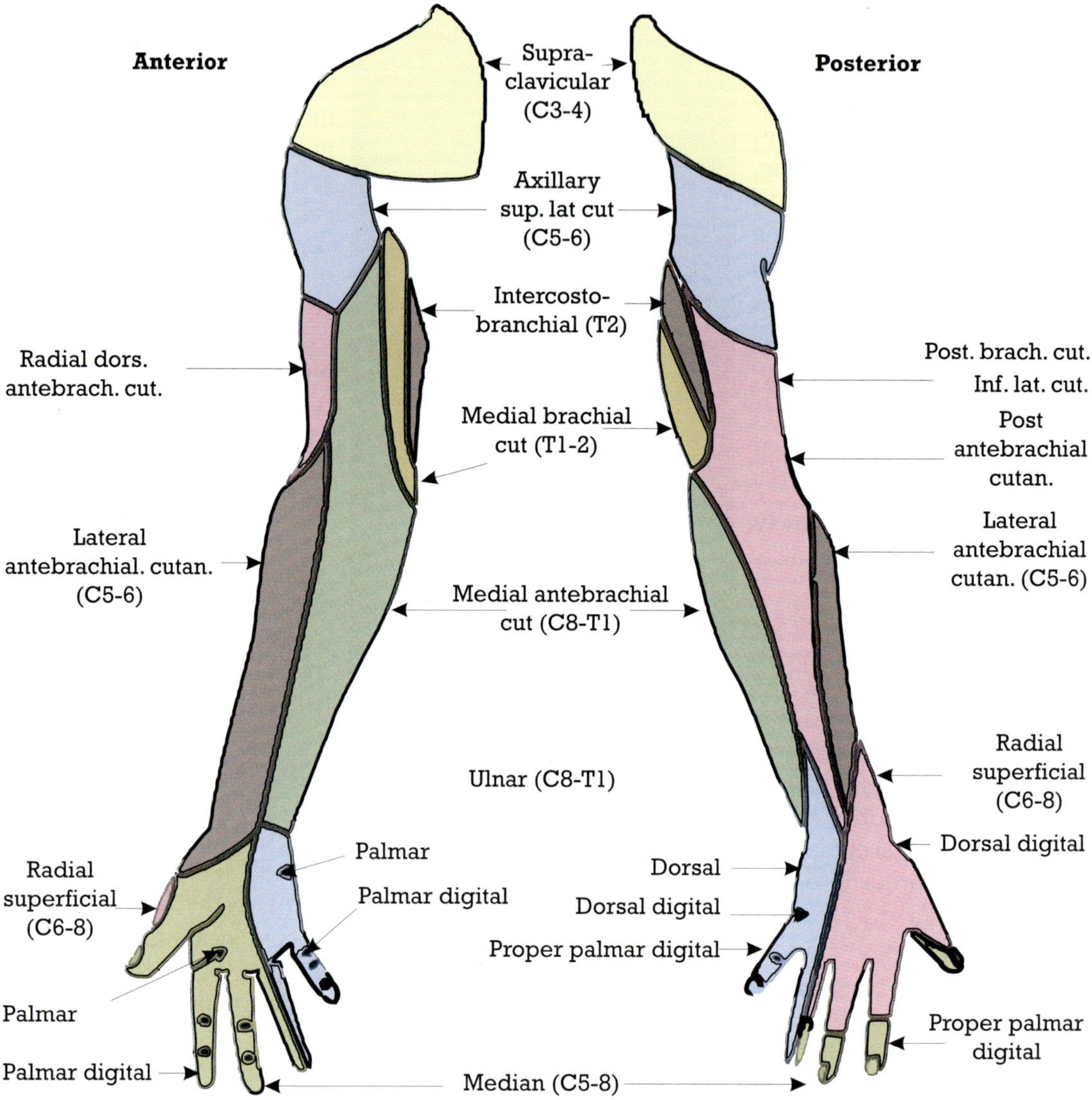

Anterior

Posterior

Supra-clavicular (C3-4)

Axillary sup. lat cut (C5-6)

Intercosto-branchial (T2)

Radial dors. antebrach. cut.

Medial brachial cut (T1-2)

Post. brach. cut.
Inf. lat. cut.

Post antebrachial cutan.

Lateral antebrachial. cutan. (C5-6)

Medial antebrachial cut (C8-T1)

Lateral antebrachial cutan. (C5-6)

Ulnar (C8-T1)

Radial superficial (C6-8)

Dorsal digital

Palmar

Radial superficial (C6-8)

Palmar digital

Dorsal

Dorsal digital

Proper palmar digital

Palmar

Proper palmar digital

Palmar digital

Median (C5-8)

Fig. 97.5. Cutaneous innervation of the upper limb

Tibial (medial politeal): plantar aspect of foot, except lateral border and toes

Musculocutaneous: lateral aspect of leg, entire dorsum of foot and toes, except first webspace

Deep peroneal or deep fibular: provides sensations to the first interdigital space. It is also known as 'nervus hesitans', because it hesitates

to cross the anterior tibial artery in the midleg, but never crosses and stays lateral to it.

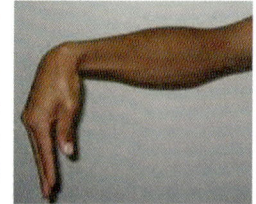

Fig. 97.6. Wrist drop

Sural: lateral border of foot (dorsal and plantar aspects)

Saphenous: Medial aspect of leg and dorsum of proximal foot

Brachial plexus: can be injured by penetrating injuries of neck, avulsed during dystocia or palsy may be seen in thoracic outlet compression or Pancoast tumor.

Nerve	Muscle involved	Maneuver	Result
Axillary nerve (C5, 6)	Deltoid	Extend shoulder against resistance	Not possible
Radial nerve (C5,6,7,8, T-1)	Brachioradialis	Flexion of elbow in semiprone position against resistance	No contraction felt muscle doesn't stand out
	Extensors of wrist	Arm extend, pronate forearm	Wrist drop
	Ext. digitorum	With MP joints flexed, extend the fingers	Not possible
	Ext. pollicis longus	Flex the IP joint of thumb against resistance	Not possible
Median nerve (C5,6,7,8, T-1)	Flex digitorum sublimis/profundus (lateral half)	Clasping both hands Ochsner's clasping sign	Affected index finger remains straight (pointing finger)
	Abd pollicis brevis	With hand placed flat on table on its dorsum, patient lifts thumb right angles to the palm	Not possible
	Opponens pollicis	Touch the bases of other fingers with the tip of thumb (sometimes this can be done by vicarious movement of add pollicis, supplied by ulnar nerver	Not possible
Ulnar nerve (C-8, T-1)	Flex carpi ulnaris	Flex wrist against resistance	Hand deviates outwards
	Palmar interossei	Adduction of fingers holding a card between them	Not possible
	Dorsal interossei	Abduction of fingers	Not possible
	Interossei & lumbricals	Extend fingers with MP joints extended	Not possible
	1st palm interosseous & add pollicis	Grasp book between thumb and other fingers (Froment's sign)	IP Joint goes into flexion
Com. Peroneal (lat pop) nerve (L-4,5, S-1,2)	Dorsiflexors of ankle	Attempt dorsiflexion of foot (foot drop)	Not possible
Tibial (medial pop) nerve (L-4, 5, S-1,2,3)	Plantar flexors of foot	Plantar flex ankle against resistance	Not Possible (talepes calcaneovalgus)
Same at ankle level	Small muscles of foot		High-arched or claw foot (pes cavus)

Table 97.2-Tests for nerve lesions in the limbs

Certain important nerve lesions are described here.

a) Erb's palsy: is the traction injury to C-5,6 roots (upper trunk), due to forced lateral flexion of neck (to the opposite side) and depression of shoulder, limb typically adducted, internally rotated at shoulder, extended at elbow and flexed at wrist, assuming the so called 'waiter's tip' position. This attitude used to be called the 'police man receiving tip', but has been discarded, probably because the policemen now take tips with extended arms.

b) Klumpke's palsy: is the lesion of C-8, T-1 roots (lower trunk), resulting from forced traction of abducted shoulder, as happens during delivery or grabbing a support, while falling from a height. The intrinsic muscles of hand are mainly affected, with impaired sensations over the medial forearm and hand. If the T-1 root is injured before giving the rami communicans to the sympathetic chain, Horner's syndrome may be seen, but not in distal lesions.

c) Axillary nerve (C-5,6) may be injured from fracture of surgical neck of humerus or scapula and sometimes by misplaced intramuscular injection. There is deltoid palsy and wasting with loss of sensation around its insertion (regimental patch).

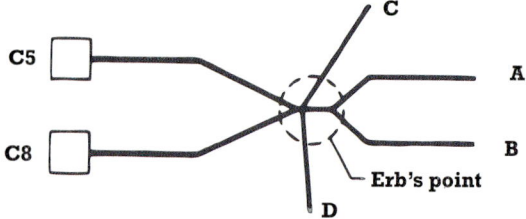

Fig. 97.8. Erb's point at upper trunk of brachial plexus A & B: The divisions of the upper trunk; C: Suprascapular nerve; D: Nerve to subclavius

d) Long thoracic nerve of Bell (C-5,6,7), supplying the serratus anterior, may be injured during heavy lifting or axillary surgery. The muscle helps to push the scapula forwards, *winging of scapula* is seen when it is paralyzed, while the patient pushes against a wall, with outstretched hands, but the shrugging of shoulder is retained, to differentiate from winging due to trapezius palsy.

e) Radial nerve (refer chapter 112)
f) Median nerve (refer chapter 113)
g) Ulnar nerve (refer chapter 114)

Lumbar plexus

a) Iliohypogastric and ilioinguinal nerves (L-1) lie in relation to quadratus lumborum, run forwards and downwards between transversus and internal oblique, supplying the conjoint tendon, rectus muscle. The ilioinguinal nerve traverses the inguinal canal and emerges through the external ring, to supply the skin over the femoral region, root of penis and anterior third of scrotum. The importance of these nerves is that they may be injured during operations requiring incisions in their line, such as appendectomy by McBurney incision, lumbar sympathectomy, surgery on kidneys, ureters and bladder, drainage of psoas abscess, sigmoid colostomy and low transverse (Pfannensteil) incision etc. This may predispose to the development of an inguinal hernia, due to weakness of the conjoint tendon. The distribution of these nerves explain the pain arising from the kidney or ureter (T-12,L-1) is classically referred from *loin to groin*.

b) genitofemoral nerve (L-1,2), Immediately after its origin, it runs in front of the psoas major

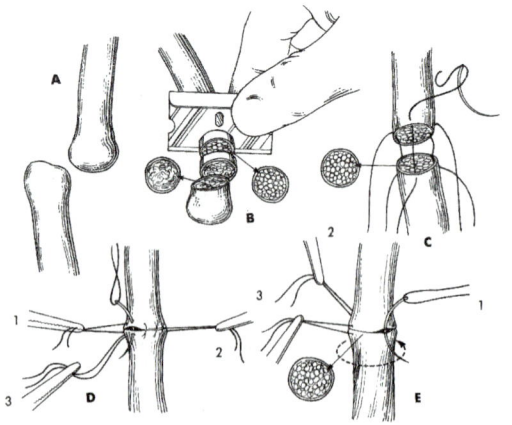

Fig. 97.7. Nerve repair
A. Divided nerve with neuroma; B. Sectioning the nerve till healthy; C. Epineural suturing; D.&E. Tying the sutures for approximation

muscle, to enter the inguinal canal in close relation to the external iliac artery and divides into femoral and genital branches. The femoral part (L-1) supplies a handsbreadth of skin below the inguinal ligament and the genital part (L-2) supplies spermatic cord, tunica vaginalis and motor to cremaster muscle. In females the genital branch is very slender, supplying round ligament and anterior labial skin.

c) femoral nerve (L-2,3,4) injuries are rare, which may be due to penetrating or missile wounds, retraction in hip surgery and an SOL, such as retroperitoneal hematoma or tumor. It supplies the quadriceps femoris muscle, when it is affected, the stability of the knee and the knee jerk are lost. Wasting of anterior thigh muscles and inability to extend the knee are present.

d) lateral cutaneous nerve of thigh (L-2,3) may be entrapped in the fibers of inguinal ligament, just medial to the anterior superior iliac spine, causing typical tingling and hyperesthesia of the upper lateral thigh, aggravated by exercise, known as *meralgia paresthetica*. If symptomatic treatment is not effective, decompression or rarely division of the nerve may be necessary.

Sacral plexus

a) sciatic (ischiatic) nerve (L-4,5, S-1,2,3) arises from the sacral plexus, leaves the pelvis through the sciatic notch, to reach the gluteal region and enters the posterior compartment of the thigh, under cover of gluteus maximus muscle. It may be injured in fracture dislocations of pelvis, misplaced intramuscular injection or persistent pressure by faulty sitting posture. It has two components, posterior tibial and common peroneal nerves. At the origin, the fibres of the latter are located centrifugally in the sciatic nerve, whereas those of the former are in the centripetal part of the nerve, which explains the frequent involvement of the common peroneal component, in superficial/partial injuries to sciatic nerve in the thigh. It divides usually just above the popliteal fossa, but the level can be variable, very rarely they may arise separately from the sacral plexus. In the thigh it supplies the

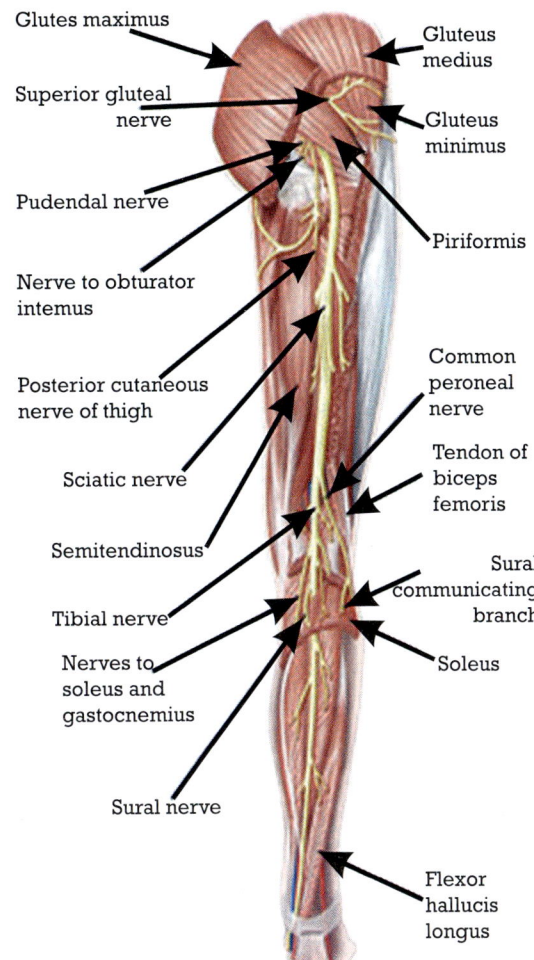

Fig. 97.9. Course and distribution of the sciatic nerve

knee flexors, which may be spared in injuries at knee level.

Sciatica is not a disease but a symptom complex consisting of radicular type of pain in the entire leg, caused by nerve root compression by a herniated disc, tumor, abscess, granuloma or an osteophyte. It may also be due to peripheral nerve compression by hematoma, tumor or an abscess. Inflammatory diseases of nerves, alcoholic/diabetic/syphilitic/herpetic neuropathy, collagen disorders, lead poisoning etc. may also produce this symptom. Typically pain radiates from the lumbar spine or gluteal region to the foot, and is aggravated by coughing, sneezing or

Joint	Movement	Segments	Movement	Segment
Shoulder	Abduction	C-5	Adduction	C-6,7
Elbow	Flexion	C-5,6	Extension	C-7,8
Forearm	Supination	C-6	Pronation	C-7,8
Wrist	Flexion	C-6,7	Extension	C-6,7
Fingers	Flexion Adduction	C-7,8 T-1	Extension Abduction	C-7,8 T-1
Hip	Flexion	L-2,3	Extension	L-4,5
Knee	Extension	L-2,3	Flexion	L-5, S-1
Ankle	Dorsiflexion	L-4,5	Plantar flexion	S-1,2
Subtalar	Eversion	L-4	Inversion	L-5, S-1
Toes	Extension	L-5, S-2	Flexion	S-1,2

Table-97.3. The segmental innervations for movements of joints (myotomes)

stooping forwards. All of which increase the disc pressure. Pain of root compression or irritation may also be elicited by *straight leg raising* (SLR), which is made worse by dorsiflexion of foot (*Lasegue's sign*); both maneuvers exert traction on nerve roots, through the sciatic nerve. Depending upon the level, tendon reflexes may be abolished (knee jerk- L-4 and ankle jerk-S-1) and weakness of extensor hallucis longus (EHL), innervated by deep peroneal nerve (L-5,S-1) may be present.

b) common peroneal nerve (L4,5, S-1,2) is the smaller of the two branches from the popliteal fossa; it reaches the anterolateral compartment by hooking around the neck of fibula, to supply the dorsiflexors/evertors of ankle and extensors of toes. It is highly vulnerable to injury as it goes around the fibular neck, in fractures, lacerations or tight plaster casts. It is also involved very often in Hansen's disease and palpating a thickened nerve against the neck of fibula is a diagnostic point. Its superficial location makes it a convenient point for nerve block, for surgery on the foot. Loss of dorsiflexion of ankle, known as *foot drop* is typical of this palsy leading to slapping gait, with most of the pressure borne by the lateral side, due to unopposed action of the evertors. It provides sensations to the medial half of dorsum and first interdigital space of the foot.

c) tibial nerve (L-4,5, S-1,2,3) is the larger of the two and is injured less often, it supplies mus cles of the calf and intrinsic muscles of the foot. In lesions of the tibial nerve, there is loss of plantar flexion and inability to stand on the toes. The foot assumes a calcaneo-valgus position, by the unopposed action of dorsiflexors of ankle and evertors of subtalar joint. There is loss of ankle jerk and sensations over the lateral half of the leg and foot.

In lesions at the ankle level, the small muscles of foot are involved and by the unopposed action of long flexor of toes and dorsiflexors of foot, it produces a high-arched or claw foot (pes cavus).

Clinical examination of a peripheral nerve lesion (applicable to all)

History

i) injury, recent/old, is very important; nature of injury and details of initial treatment given, including obstetric history for a newborn.

ii) intramuscular injections given in the deltoid and gluteal region

iii) past history of diabetes, Hansen's disease, malunion of a fracture etc.

iv) personal history of smoking, alcohol etc

v) occupational, such as working with lead or arsenic

Local examination

i) attitude, deformity and gait

ii) site of injury, location of scar, presence of a neuroma, free mobility of scar over the underlying fascia/muscles or nerve thickening in Hansen's disease

iii) motor system: nutrition, power, tone, abnormal movements and tendon reflexes

iv) sensory system: touch (light/gross), pain (superficial/deep), temperature, vibration and joint position

v) trophic changes of skin and nails

vi) special signs and tests for individual nerves, described above

Investigations

i) routine studies for diabetes, syphilis etc.

ii) skin/nasal smear for AFB (Hansen's)

iii) electrophysiological studies: electrical responses, EMG and nerve conduction studies

iv) X-ray for fracture malunion or callus

v) CT/MRI to exclude SOL in spinal canal or outside, causing nerve compression

The neurological manifestations of carpal tunnel syndrome and thoracic outlet syndrome (TOS) are described in chapters 65 and 78.

The spinal segments don't innervate individual muscles, but group of muscles carrying out particular movement of a joint, known as myotomes.

The basic principles of muscular innervations are:

1. Most muscles are supplied equally by two adjacent spinal segments. Some muscles in upper limb are unisegmental

2. Muscles sharing common primary action on a joint, irresepective of their anatomical location, are all supplied by same segment(s)

3. All their opponents, sharing the opposite action, are likewise supplied by same segment(s), usually in numerical sequence with the former

AUTONOMIC NERVOUS SYSTEM

Autonomous nervous system (ANS) is concerned with the innervations of viscera, glands, blood vessels and non-striated muscles. The peripheral autonomic system comprises of the sympathetic (thoracolumbar outflow) and the parasympathetic (craniosacral outflow) systems, under the control of central autonomic centres in the brain stem, hypothalamus and cerebral cortex. Though physiologically they may be considered opposite forces, often they are complimentary to each other, since one system will collapse if the other is absent, as may be understood by the principle of a 'see-saw'.

Efferent system

All autonomic efferent fibres are interrupted in their course by a synapse in the peripheral ganglion. The preganglionic fibres arising from CNS are medullated, while the postganglionic fibres are non-medullated.

In the sympathetic nervous system (SNS), the preganglionic fibres are the axons of nerve cells in the lateral column of grey matter of all thoracic and upper two lumbar segments of the spinal cord. They synapse with the nerve cells in:

a) paravertebral sympathetic plexus

b) collateral ganglia

c) adrenal medulla

In the parasympathetic nervous system (PNS), the preganglionic cranial fibres arise from Edinger-Westphal (3rd nerve), salivary (7th & 9th nerves), ambiguus and dorsal motor (10th nerve) nuclei in the brain stem. The sacral preganglionic fibres arise in the grey matter of the spinal cord from the 2nd to 4th sacral segments. The preganglionic fibres synapse with ganglia nearer the structures innervated (than to the CNS) and the ganglia dispersed in the walls of the viscera themselves. In the SNS, the preganglionic fibres are usually short and synapse with many postganglionic nerves, giving their discharge a widespread effect. In contrast, the PNS preganglionic fibres are very long and synapse with only a few postganglionic neurons, giving their discharges a more limited effect.

Afferent system

Some of the autonomic reflexes are:

a) Visceral reflexes which do not reach the level of consciousness, eg: breathing

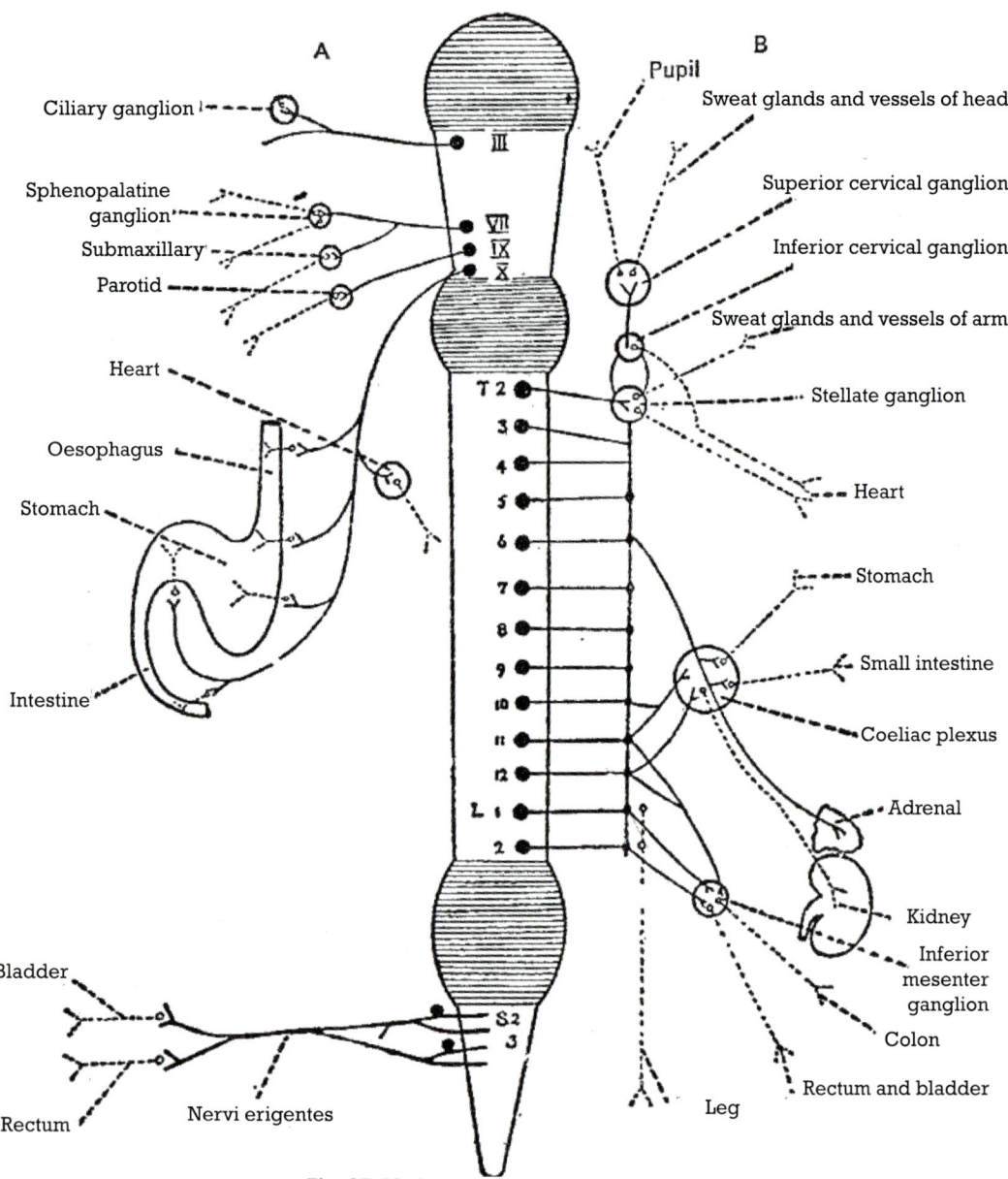

A

B

Pupil

Ciliary ganglion

Sweat glands and vessels of head

III

Superior cervical ganglion

Sphenopalatine
ganglion

Inferior cervical ganglion

VII
IX
X

Submaxillary

Parotid

Sweat glands and vessels of arm

Heart

Stellate ganglion

T 2

Oesophagus

3

4

Heart

Stomach

5

6

Stomach

7

8

9

Small intestine

10

Intestine

11

Coeliac plexus

12

L 1

Adrenal

2

Kidney

Inferior
mesenter
ganglion

Bladder

S2
3

Colon

Nervi erigentes

Rectum and bladder

Leg

Rectum

Fig. 97.10. Autonomic nervous system

b) Vascular reflexes such as those from carotid sinus, responding to arterial pressure

c) Organic visceral sensations such as hunger, visceral distension or ischemia

d) Visceral pain which is poorly localized, often referred to some other somatic structure deriving innervations from the same spinal segment (s). The pain arising from parietal layer of serous membranes, such as parietal peritoneum is directly transmitted in the somatic nervous system and is accurately localized.

Neuro-transmittor substances

SNS: Preganglionic nerve endings: acetylcholine

Postganglionic nerve endings: noradrenaline (except those to sweat glands, for which it is acetylcholine)

PNS: Acetylcholine (for all)

THE SYMPATHETIC NERVOUS SYSTEM

This is the system concerned with 'fright, fight and flight' and becomes a part of the general adaptation syndome (GAS). They arise from T1 to L2 spinal segments, leaving through the anterior roots of corresponding spinal nerves, upto the point beyond the junction of posterior roots and leave the spinal nerve as white rami communicans (myelinated), to join the sympathetic chain. After the synapse, they leave the ganglia as grey rami communicans (non-myelinated) to join the peripheral nerves. Due to developmental fusion, the number of ganglia is less than the spinal segments; with only 3 cervical, 11 dorsal, 4 lumbar and 4 sacral ganglia.

Contributions by the SNS

Cervical: cervical plexus, 9th, 10th & 12th cranial nerves, jugular bulb, larynx, pharyx, carotid body, skin over the upper limb, half of head & neck, iris of the eye, thyroid & parathyroid glands, salivary glands, cardiac branches

Cervical sympathetic chain is actually derived from T-1 root, but anatomically located in the neck, supplying the involuntary fibers (*Muller's muscle*) of levator palpebrae superioris and dilator muscles of pupil. Lesions of the chain produce Horner's syndrome (vide supra).

Thoracic: All the spinal nerves, pulmonary, cardiac plexus and 3 splanchnic nerves. The greater splanchnic nerve (T-5 to10) joins celiac plexus, the lesser splanchnic nerve (T-9&10) joins the aortorenal ganglion and the lowest splanchnic nerve (T-11) joins the renal plexus.

Lumbar: Here the chain is placed retroperitoneally in the groove between the psoas major and aorta (left) or IVC (right), in close relation to genotifemoral nerve and the ureter and crossed by lumbar vessels. It

supplies celiac, intermesenteric and superior hypogastric plexuses and the lumbar plexus of spinal nerves.

Pelvic: this part is situated in front of sacrum, medial to sacral foramina, converging below to form the ganglion impar, in the anterior aspect of coccyx. They supply the sacral and coccygeal nerves and inferior hypogastric plexus.

Effects of sympathectomy

In sympathectomized areas, there is loss of sweating (anhidrosis), cutaneous vasodilatation and muscular vasoconstriction and it is preeminently indicated to treat hyperhidrosis and vasospastic disorders, such as Raynaud's and Buerger's diseases. It may be ideally employed to treat nonhealing skin ulcers but not claudication.

THE PARASYMPATHETIC SYSTEM

It is mainly secretomotor to viscera and controls the cardiopulmonary activities, but has little influence on the skin, trunk and limbs.

Contributions by the PNS

Cranial: supplies all 4 cranial ganglia, namely the ciliary (to ocular muscles), sphenopalatine (to lachrymal glands), submandibular (to submandibular and sublingual salivary glands) and otic (to parotid gland) ganglia. The vagus (10th cranial) nerve arises from the dorsal nucleus and nucleus ambiguus, has widespread distribution (as the name implies), destined for cardiac, pulmonary, esophageal, and through the celiac plexuses, to the abdominal viscera. These fibres are relayed in small ganglia lying in the walls of the individual viscera.

Sacral: derived from S-2, 3 and sometimes 4 segments, forming the pelvic splanchnic nerve (nervi erigentes), to join the inferior hypogastric plexus to supply the pelvic viscera and penile vessels. Damage to these nerves in males during pelvic surgery, may cause erectile dysfunction.

CLINICAL TESTS FOR THE FUNCTIONS OF ANS

1. Pupillary reflexes for light and accommodation: SNS dilates and PNS contracts

2. Orthostatic hypotension: Normally there will be no significant fall of BP (<10), if the posture is abruptly changed from supine to erect. A fall of >20mm of systolic pressure is indicative of autonomic disturbance.

3. Deep breathing test: normally after doing 6-8 maximum deep breathing, the pulse rate drops by >15/min, if the autonomic functions are intact.

4. Hand grip test: Normally the diastolic blood pressure rises by >15mm, if sustained tight hand grip is maintained for 5min.

5. Valsalva test: The patient blows into sphygmomanometer, to maintain the pressure over 40mm, for about 15 seconds. Normally the pulse rate drops significantly, whereas in autonomic disturbance, there will no bradycardia seen, after the test.

6. Urinary bladder (detrusor) functions may be evaluated by urodynamic studies

7. Insulin test meal (Hollander's test): The principle that hypoglycemia (<50mg%) induces gastric hypersecretion, mediated through vagal stimulation, has been used in this test. It is done following alleged trunkal vagotomy, to check if it has been completely done. Soluble insulin is administered to bring the blood glucose level to <50 and measure the volume and acid content of the gastric secretions by nasogastric aspirations. Neither vagotomy nor the Hollander's test are commonly done nowadays, after the advent of proton pump inhibitors in the management of acid-peptic disease.

Disorders of ANS

They cause complex syndromes involving more than one system, mainly in relation to:

Blood pressure (especially postural disturbances)

Cardiac, pulmonary and sudomotor activity

Erectile dysfunction

Bowel motility (achalasia cardia, diabetic enteropathy, Hirschprung's disease etc)

They may be associated with other diseases such as Parkinson's disease, viral infections, autoimmune disorders (Guillain-Barre) etc

Certain drugs may induce dysfunction of ANS (e.g. calcium channel blockers, β-blockers, diuretics, opiates, ethanol, sildenafil, psychotropic agents).

Group	Myelinated	Diameter	Conduction velocity	Distribution
A	Yes	Large (13-20μm)	80-120 m/sec	Affer/effer peripheral nerves
B	Yes	Medium (5-8μm)	4-25 m/sec	Preganglionic ANS
C	No	Small (0.2-1.5μm)	0.5-2 m/sec	Postganglionic ANS

Table 97.4 – Types of nerve fibers (velocity depends on the size and presence of myelin sheath)

98 Lasers in Surgery

(LASER: **L**ight **a**mplification by **s**timulated **e**mission of **r**adiation)

The emission of a LASER beam first successfully achieved using a synthetic ruby by Maiman in 1960, was one of the greatest discoveries of the last century. Unlike ordinary light, a laser beam is coherent, monochromatic, focusable and directable. Since 1961, when the ruby laser was first used to photocoagulate a detached retina, laser medicine has become firmly established, with successful applications in many clinical specialties and basic research, including general surgery, neurosurgery, otolaryngology, gynecology, cosmetic surgery and other fields.

The first clinically significant application of the Nd:YAG laser to surgery was by Peter Kiefhaber in West Germany to control massive gastrointestinal bleeding in humans. In 1978, Hofstetter and Rothenberger tried coagulation of tumors of the bladder wall, transmitting the laser beam through an optical fiber inserted via cystoscope.

A low energy laser has a power output of less than 100mW and an energy density of less than 50mW/cm^2.

Properties of laser

1) the light of laser is collimated, i.e. parallel beam with minimal divergence. This allows a

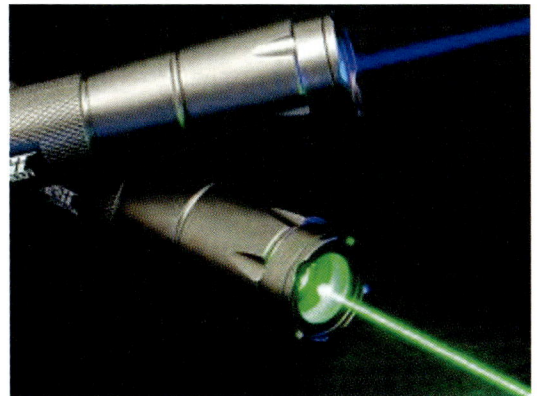

Fig. 98.1. Monochromatic coherent light of laser

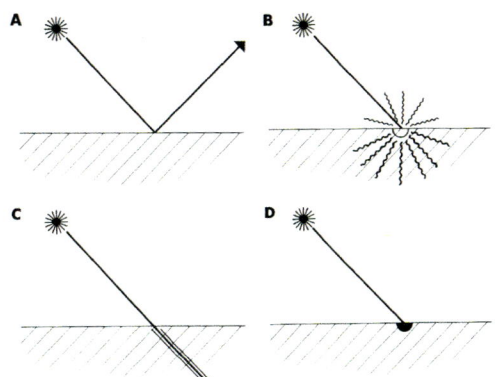

Fig. 98.2. Laser tissue interaction
A. Reflection; **B.** Scattering; **C.** Transmission; **D.** Absorption

high irradiance of tissue in a given unit area.

2) lasers are monochromatic. Thus depending upon the activation of specific chemical, a desirable wavelength is achieved with its therapeutic effects.

3) spatial coherence of the photon particles of laser give precise and predictable effects on target tissues

For the generation of a laser beam three components are essential:

1) the lasing medium, the particles of which finally form the beam

2) a power or pump source, which acts on the lasing medium

3) an optical cavity or resonator, within which the photons undergo continuous internal reflection

The lasing medium may be solid (ruby), liquid (rhodamine) or gas (CO_2). The power source energizes the lasing medium within the resonator, which is a vacuum tube with a totally reflective mirror at one end and a partially reflective mirror with a central tiny aperture at the other end, through which the laser beam exits.

The atoms of the lasing medium are excited from the resting phase by the effect of a power source. When they return to the ground state, release of photons occurs; these are reflected to and fro by the mirrors. Soon all the photons acquire the same wavelength and the other properties mentioned above and exit the resonator as the laser beam.

Classification

1) continuous wave laser
2) pulsed laser
3) either of the above may be Q-switched (wherein a shutter mechanism is used to close the aperture and build up tremendous pressure within the resonator, to produce a high energy

Laser	Color	Wavelength (nm)
Excimer	Ultra violet	
ArF		193
KrCl		222
KrF		248
XeCl		308
XeF		351
Helium–Cadmium		325
Argon	Blue	488
	Green	515
Frequency-doubled YAG (KTP)	Green	532
Krypton	Green	531
	Yellow	568
	Red	647
Dye Laser	Variable with dyes Red	632
	Yellow	577-585
Gold vapor	Red	628
Helium neon	Red	632
Ruby	Deep red	694
ND:YAG	Infrared	1064
		1318
Holmium YAG	Infrared	2100
Erbium YAG	Infrared	2900
Carbon dioxide	Infrared	10,600

Table-98.1. Description of laser color and wavelength

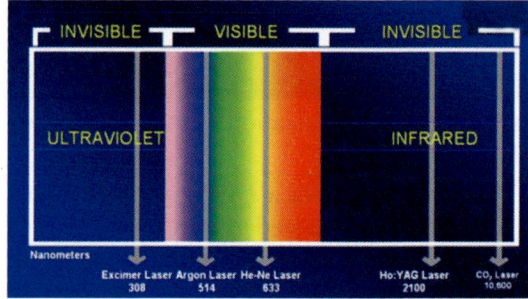

Fig. 98.3. Electromagnetic spectrum of light and laser

burst of photons, on letting open the aperture. The lasers are also classified depending upon their safety into 1 to 4, 1 being the safest and 4, the most hazardous; unfortunately most medical lasers come under the latter category.

Clinical applications of lasers

1) Therapeutic effects

a) *Photo-thermal:* it is used obtain photo-coagulation. CO_2 laser is used for cutting tissue, as it is absorbed by tissue water at 0.2mm depth. Nd:YAG (Neodymium: Yttrium-Aluminium-Garnet) laser is effective in coagulation and shrinking blood vessels, hence used in gastrointestinal bleeding (see below).

Argon laser is used to photocoagulate diseased vessels etc. in retinal disorders

b) *Photo-chemical:* A classic example is photodynamic therapy (PDT). The scientific basis of this treatment is prior administration of a photosensitizer, such as hematopor-phyrin derivative(HpD) or tetracyclines, which is taken up by dysplastic or neoplastic tissues only. The use of a selective laser then destroys the target tissues by producing toxic singlet oxygen radicals within these tissues. This is used in nonresectable bronchial/esophageal/ bladder malignancies and is now coming to the fore in the management of *Barrett's esophagus*. The main disadvantage of PDT is persistence of HpD in the body for weeks, precluding exposure to sun light, for fear of inducing burns.

c) *Photo-ablative:* The ablative effects are used with the Argon fluoride laser for band keratopathy and to refashion corneal curvature in refractive errors.

d) *Photo-mechanical:* The high intensity pulses developed in the Q-switched Nd:Yag laser are used in the contact mode to fragment CBD/ ureteric calculi and also for capsulotomy and iridotomy.

2) Stimulation of healing

Low power laser of Helium-Neon or Gallium arsenide is used to increase vascularity and fibroblastic activity in nonhealing wounds, as also for the relief of chronic musculoskeletal pains.

3) Diagnosis: Laser light within the ultraviolet range is combined with endoscopy and a chemical agent, like aminolevulinic acid (ALA), to detect foci of dysplasia or carcinoma-in-situ, in GI tract, bronchus and bladder. This is known as *fluorescence endoscopy.*

4) Optical alignment: The visible range laser light is used for patient positioning in radiotherapy and for accurate localization in stereotactic surgery. It is also used as a light guide for the photocoagulation probes of Nd:YAG.

Many of the medical lasers were developed in Japan, including the world's smallest portable CO_2 laser scalpel of 10 W, and nontoxic halide fibers to deliver the CO_2 laser beam, were developed as well as the widely used contact Nd:YAG laser.

Some recent applications of laser

Microvascular anastomosis by CO_2 laser (*laser welding*).

Choledocholithotripsy by contact Nd:YAG laser

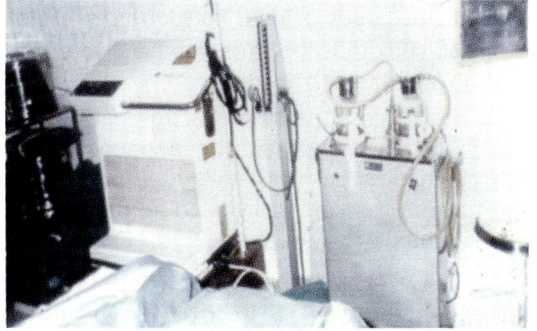

Fig. 98.4. Laser unit
(courtesy: Lifeline Hospitals, Chennai)

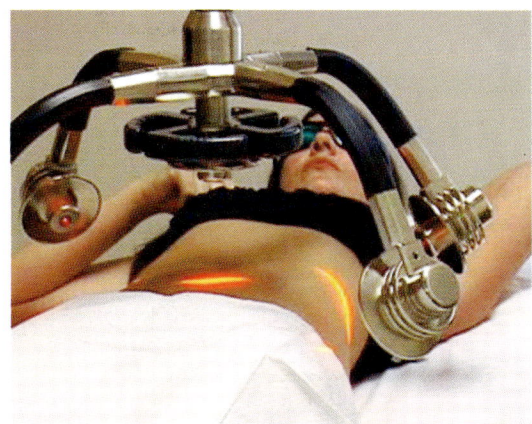

Fig. 98.5. Zerona laser lipolysis unit

with new ceramic probes.

Ureterolithotripsy by contact Nd:YAG laser with new ceramic probes.

Pain relief by semiconductor laser.

Laser endoscopy treatment for ectopic pregnancy.

Selective vagotomy by CO_2 laser.

Laser lipolysis

The process is easy and painless. The patient simply lies down and allows the Zerona laser to shine down on the skin. Since it is a cold laser, the patient will feel no pain, but the fat cells underneath the skin are disrupted by the laser and begin to emulsify. The fat cells leak out their contents, which is then naturally expelled from the body. This treatment is repeated for several sessions over a period of a few weeks.

Today, the Nd:YAG laser has become a standard instrument in general surgery, complementing

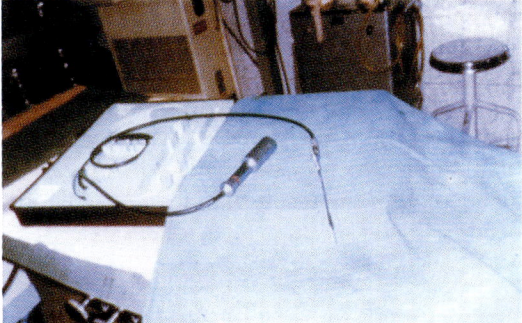

Fig. 98.6. Light channel assembly with the fibreoptic endoscope

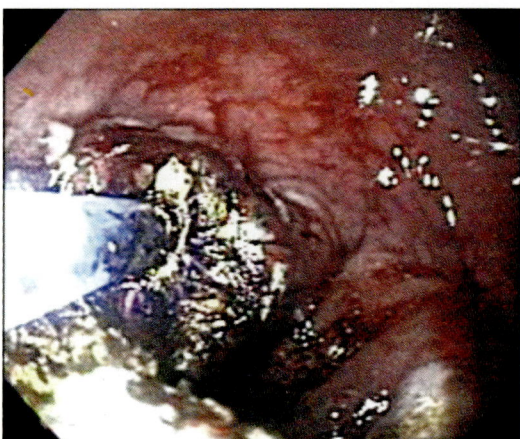

Fig. 98.7. Laser vaporization of lower esophageal polypoid tumor. The tip of endoscope is seen (courtesy: Lifeline Hospitals, Chennai)

the CO_2, which originally dominated the field. Its applications extend to bronchology, gastroenterology, dermatology, gynecology, ophthalmology, neurosurgery, urology, and vascular surgery. There is probably no part of the human body that cannot be surgically treated in an effective manner by the Nd:YAG laser in one form or another.

Effects of Nd:YAG laser beam on tissue

The effects at the surface of the tissue are, for the most part, influenced by the power density applied on irradiation. The focused Nd:YAG laser beam, 1064nm, power density and approximately 10kw/cm^2, ruptures the tissue surface and leads to a wide, conical coagulation lesion.

The main advantage of the Nd:YAG laser is the possibility of coagulating without vaporization. If carbonization occurs on the surface, absorption increases and the tissue is vaporized. If the surface of the tissue is cooled with water, the blanching effect is delayed, carbonization avoided, with the result that deep coagulation occurs.

Instrumentation for endoscopic application

In gastroenterology all routine diagnostic instruments are used without any modification. The light guide is passed directly through the working channel and can be advanced distally as far as desired.

The noncontact application of the Nd:YAG laser in gastroenterology is suitable for stanching bleedings from esophageal varices, ulcers, and Mallory-Weiss tears. The treatment of tumors in the upper and lower gastrointestinal tract, palliative elimination of stenosing tumors, curative radiation of sessile neoplastic polyps and benign intestinal and esophageal stenoses, are additional indications, which are rapidly becoming more important than hemostasis.

For treating tumors in the genitourinary system, such as multicentric tumors or colonizing tumors of the urethral, vesical, and ureteral mucosa, and tumors in the pyelo-calyceal area, several endoscopic laser instruments are available.

Owing to the homogeneous coagulation effect, the Nd:YAG laser is also successfully applied in tubal surgery in the gynecologic field. The laparoscopic sterilization by partial coagulation of the oviducts improves the chances of future recanalization. The laparoscope insert is equipped with distal forceps to ensure a permanent obturation of the ovular tuba. The gas-cooled light guide is combined with the forceps insert. The forceps are so constructed that the laser beam always remains within the branches. This prevents damage to the surrounding tissue.

For laparoscopic application of the Nd:YAG laser in gynecology, such as in the treatment of endometriosis, the laser light guide with a coaxial gas flow can be adapted to the routine operation laparoscopes using a special laser insert. The distal flexibility permits exact and safe irradiation of the area to be treated.

A laser laryngoscope/tracheoscope operate on the same principles as the bronchoscopes described previously. Distal illumination and the flexible gas-cooled light guide allow optimal, targeted irradiation.

Instrumentation for open surgery

For operations that have to be performed under microscopic control, hand applicators of various designs have been developed that permit free, 3-dimensional working. Both gas-cooled and liquid-flushed systems are used. The small, 3mm, diameter of these instruments, does not impair vision. In addition to the standard shapes, hand applicators with flexible tubes enable the surgeon to reach otherwise inaccessible regions.

Contact probes

Contact laser probes are designed to serve four general medical functions: cutting, vaporization, coagulation, and delivery of interstitial irradiation. Each of these functions results from the induction of a thermal effect of given intensity in a certain tissue volume. Cutting requires intense, highly localized heat to vaporize small tissue volumes rapidly, creating a controlled incision with little damage to adjacent areas. For vaporization of fairly large tissue volumes, an intense but broader thermal effect is needed, whereas coagulation requires milder temperatures in yet larger volumes.

Clinical applications in GI bleeding

Bleeding gastric and duodenal ulcers with a visible vessel.

Initially the flat probe is applied circumferentially around the rim of the ulcer. Subsequently, the probe can be applied directly to the vessel for final coagulation and coaptation. If the probe sticks to the vessel, the laser power is set too high, producing vaporization of tissue, then the power should be adjusted down (under 10 W), and with the laser activated, the probe can be gently disengaged from the tissue.

Bleeding erosions

They often have several punctate bleeding points from arteriolar and capillary vessels at the edges or in the base of the erosion. Using the flat probe, these can be directly photo-coagulated. If there is a diffuse ooze, the Z-shooting technique is used. With laser power on, the probe is moved back and forth over the tissue surface in a zigzag fashion. This coagulates the vessels feeding into the bleeding area. The bleeding points within the triangular areas are then directly treated.

Bleeding Mallory-Weiss tear

The flat probe is applied around the bleeding site, which coagulates the blood vessels supplying the bleeding point. Once bleeding has diminished, the bleeding point itself can be coagulated.

Lower GI bleeding

Although there are many causes of lower GI bleeding, angiodysplasia is the condition for which the Nd:YAG laser, particularly when used in conjunction with contact probes, has demonstrated clear advantages.

Contact photocoagulation with the flat probe is performed circumferentially around the angiodysplastic lesion in an attempt to seal off the feeding vessels. Immediately upon coagulation and coaptation of the feeding vessels, bleeding stops.

More recently a hollow cylindrical contact probe at low power is being evaluated. The probe is used only with coaxial saline to prevent air embolization. The thermal effect simulates the noncontact high-powered laser, producing an effect on tissue at greater depth, but with the added advantage of coaptation. This endoprobe may be especially useful in the very actively bleeding visible vessel, such as arterial spurters.

Contact laser photocoagulation combines the coagulating properties of the Nd:YAG laser with the tactile feedback and coaptive features of the contact endoprobe. It provides safe, rapid and effective hemostasis. Accurately targeted low power Nd:YAG laser energy causes less surface damage and lateral necrosis than other thermal techniques, yet offers a controlled penetrating thermal effect. Moreover, with a single versatile instrument, one has the ability not only to coagulate, but to cut and vaporize for other pathologic conditions.

Advanced and recurrent cancer

Use of the laser for local radical cure is an effective conservative therapy for early cancers. However, the laser can also increase longevity by palliating the symptoms of patients with advanced and recurrent cancer, who complain of bleeding, pain, or exudation, by laser luminization and laser hemostasis of hollow viscus malignancies.

Interstitial laser hyperthermic ablation (laser induced interstitial thermotherapy)

prolonged heating of tumour cells to 45 to 55°c leads to cell death.

It uses diode (or) Nd:YAG laser either by percutaneous placement of the probe or by laparoscopy.

Ear, nose and throat

for tonsillar dissection

Excision of vocal cord (singer's) nodules

laryngeal papilloma excision with CO_2 laser

proliferating hemangiomas treated with Nd: YAG or KTP laser.

Varicose veins

endovenous laser therapy (EVLT) uses a laser probe placed under USG-guidance into the varicose veins and the laser pulse causes endothelial damage and causes obliteration of the lumen.

Dermatology

'Tunable dye lasers' where an organic dye is used as the lasing medium possible to treat portwine stain and superficial vascular malformations.

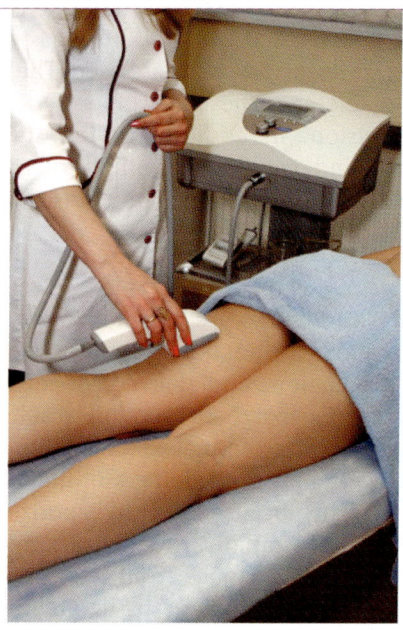

Fig. 98.8. Laser application in cosmetology

Ruby lasers are used to remove tattoos.

CO_2 laser used for removal of warts, syringomas and epidermal nevi, also treats facial wrinkling and chronic sun damaged skin.

Urology

KTP/Holmium laser is used in the resection of prostate in benign hyperplasia, causes minimal postoperative bleeding.

Disintegration of ureteric stone by mounting laser probe on to ureteroscopes.

(syn: Minimally invasive, Key hole, Pin hole, Laparoscopic, Endoscopic surgery)

Introduced by gynecologists for diagnostic pelvic examination, endoscopic surgery has quickly spread to the entire world, throwing its tentacles in virtually every field of surgery. The driving force generated by the public demand, supported by the innovative equipment, including endostaplers, created by the biomedical engineering industry has also helped to find new applications for this technique. Successful procedure requires good hand-eye coordination, thorough understanding of the various gadgets, energy generating sources and their ergonomics. Functioning of all the gadgets has to be verified before each procedure, to avoid 'trouble-shooting' during surgery and ideally technicians trained to expediently handle such problems as they arise, should be available. Reorientation of anatomy is essential for the laparoscopic surgeon, in areas such as groin hernia, since various important relations and landmarks have to be realized, in 'different angles'.

The main advantages of minimally invasive surgery are:

1. Small, cosmetically esthetic incisions
2. Minimal pain or discomfort
3. Short hospital stay
4. Early return to work

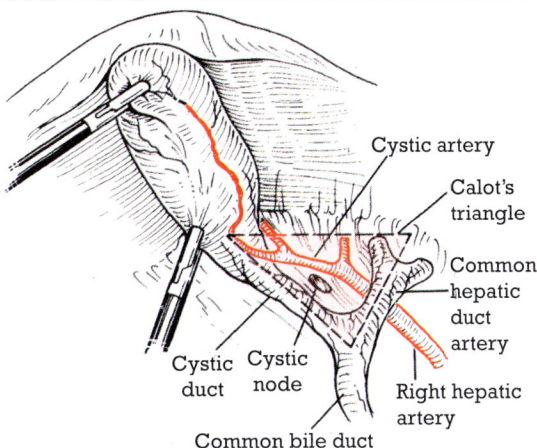

Fig. 99.2. Calot's triangle formed by cystic duct, common hepatic duct and under surface of the liver

5. Minimal wound complications
6. Reduced postoperative adhesions due to minimal bowel handling
7. Early return of bowel function, obviating the need for gastric decompression
8. Due to reduced systemic inflammatory response (sis), there may be immunological advantage
9. Facility to record the procedure for future review.

Contraindications (relative and absolute) for laparoscopic surgery:

1. Generalized peritonitis
2. Clotting abnormalities

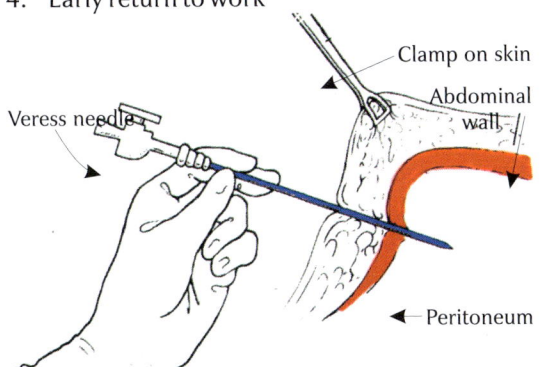

Fig. 99.1. Creating pneumoperitoneum using Veress needle

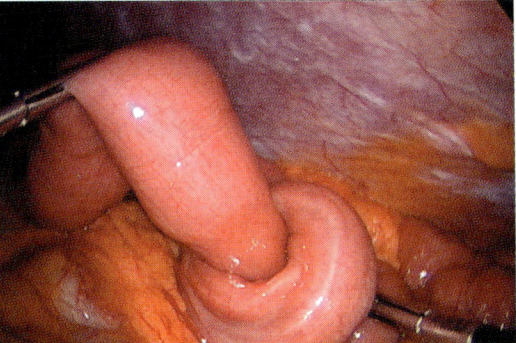

Fig. 99.3. Laparoscopic reduction of ileo-ileal intussusception

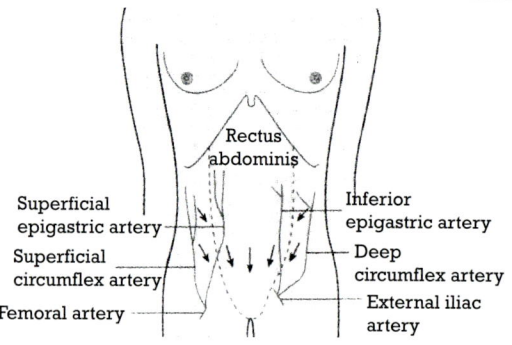

Fig. 99.4. Port selection over the abdominal wall to avoid main vessels

3. High risk for general anesthesia
4. Compromised cardiac function and intolerance to pneumoperitoneum
5. Abdominal aortic aneurysm
6. Pregnancy
7. Anticipated multiple adhesions
8. Patient refusal
9. Lack of expertise.

The components of equipment

Optical system: cold light source transmitted through fibreoptic cable, camera and high resolution video monitors. The visual angle of laparoscope, straight (0°) versus angled (30 or 45°), is a matter of personal choice, many prefer the latter for better maneuverability of field of vision. Currently Xenon light source is popularly used for better color resolution.

Insufflation (sufflare: to blow) system to create artificial pneumoperitoneum, including Veress needle or Hasson cannula, high pressure source of gas with controlled delivery, usually CO_2.

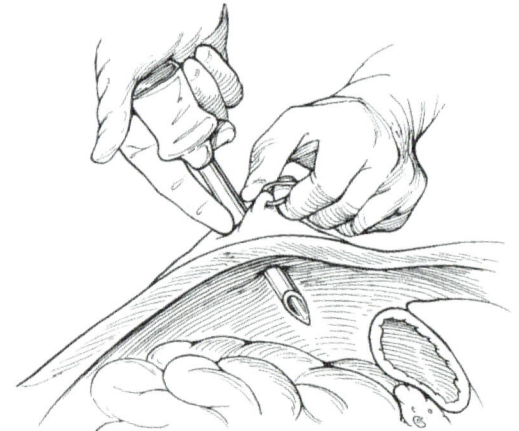

Fig. 99.5. Introduction of first (umbilical) port

Ports and hand instruments

The ports vary in diameter, from 3mm to 20mm, depending on the instrument used. (refer table 99.1).

Hand instruments: Parallel to open surgical instruments, they come in all sizes, shapes and patterns. The commonly used ones are :

Maryland's dissector (curved, non-ratcheted)
Duckbill dissector (straight, non-ratcheted)
Graspers (toothed & non-toothed)
Right-angled grasper
Fan retractor & spatula
Hook dissector
Bipolar diathermy grasper
Harmonic probes
Knot pusher (plastic or metal)
Needle holders (standard & Endostitch)
Robotic instruments (see Fig. 1.17)

Irrigation and suction system

Energy sources such as Diathermy (monopolar

PORT SIZE	INSTRUMENTS
3mm	grasper/dissector
5mm	grasper/dissector/retractor/telescope/suction/irrigation/harmonic probe
10mm	telescope/clip applicator/crocodile grasper/suction/specimen retrieval
12mm	endostapler (white, gray, blue & gold)/ morcellator
15mm	endostapler (green)/endobag/specimen retrieval
20mm	SILS (single incision laparoscopic surgery) port

Table 99.1 - Laparoscopic ports

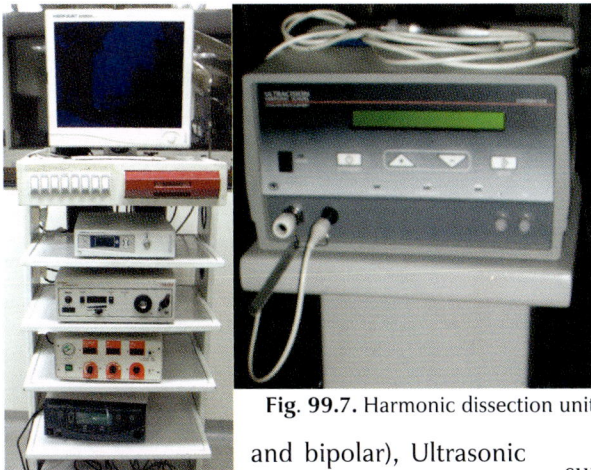

Fig. 99.6. Laparoscopy unit

Fig. 99.7. Harmonic dissection unit

and bipolar), Ultrasonic (Harmonic) shears, Ligasure diathermy, Laser, Monopolar floating ball, Cavitron Ultrasonic Aspirator (CUSA), Radiofrequency (RF) probe etc.

Endoclips, loops, sutures, staplers and morcellators

PATIENT PREPARATION

Adequate patient counseling has to be done with reference to the probable complications, the risk of conversion etc. The pros and cons of open versus endoscopic surgery have to be thoroughly discussed, to arrive at a consensus in favor of the latter. Besides routine preoperative assessment, elderly patients should also have evaluation of cardiac and pulmonary functions, since their tolerance to pneumoperitoneum, hypercapnea and hypoxia may be less. Six hours of starvation and nasogastric aspiration is necessary for gastric

decompression. Lower abdominal procedures (and all extensive operations with expected hemodynamic impact) should have an indwelling urinary catheter. Monitoring devices should include pulsoximetry and end tidal CO_2 measurement. Appropriate prophylactic IV bactericidal antibiotic may be started at the time of induction of anesthesia.

OPERATION ROOM SETUP

The position of patient and placement of various components depend on the planned procedure and anticipated surgical maneuvers. Unlike in open surgery, the restricted freedom for the surgeon to move around, by the placement of ports has to be visualized. For most of the routine procedures, such as chole-cystectomy, appendectomy, inguinal hernia repair, the surgeon stands on the left of the patient, while the assistant stands on the right, with the monitors either at the headend or footend, depending on whether the procedure is upper or lower abdominal or pelvic. For some advanced procedures such as anti-reflux or bariatric surgery, the patient is placed in semi-lithotomy position and surgeon stands in between the thighs of patient.

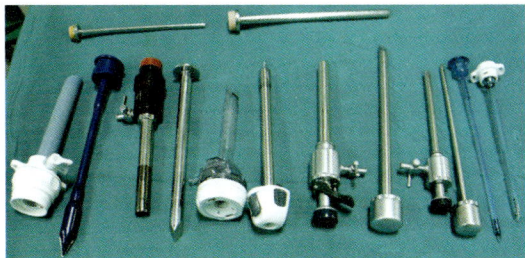

Fig. 99.8. Laparoscopic ports

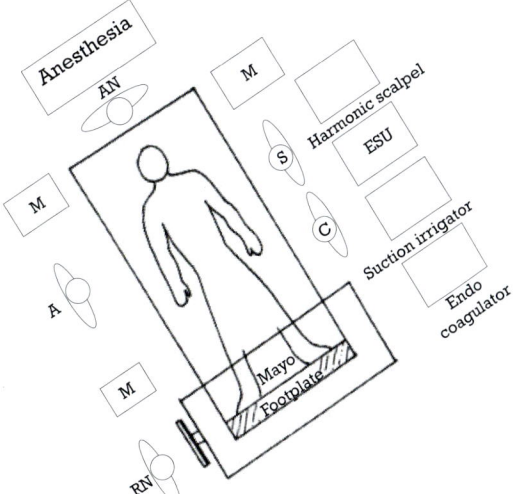

Fig. 99.9. Operation room setup for laparoscopic cholecystectomy

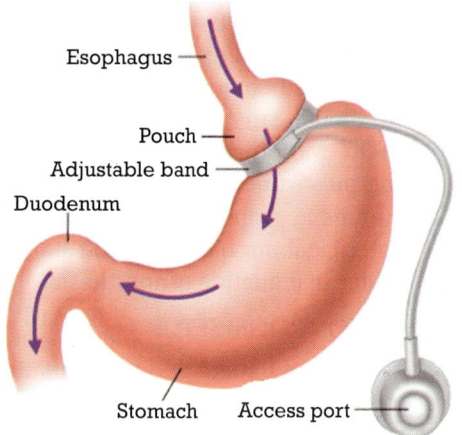

Fig. 99.10. Bariatric surgery - adjustable gastric band

CREATION OF PNEUMOPERITONEUM

Creation of pneumoperitoneum and introduction of first (usually the umbilical, since both skin and peritoneum are adherent to fascia at that point) port are of paramount importance; there are two standard methods, the closed (conventional) technique with Veress needle or open (under vision), using Hasson cannula. Obviously in patients who had earlier abdominal surgery and anticipated bowel or omental adhesions, the latter is preferred.

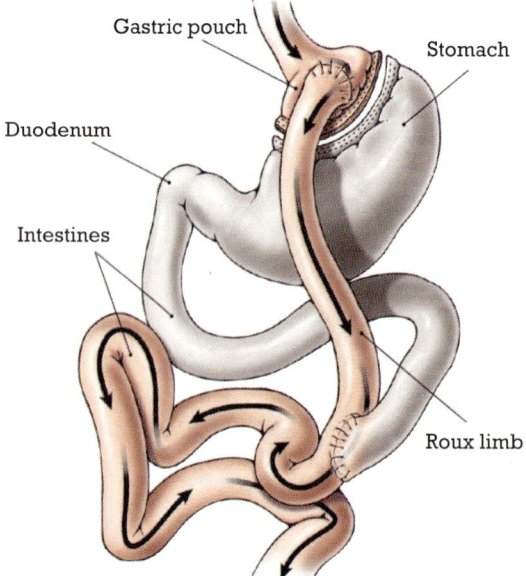

Fig. 99.11. Bariatric surgery - gastric bypass
(Roux-en-Y)

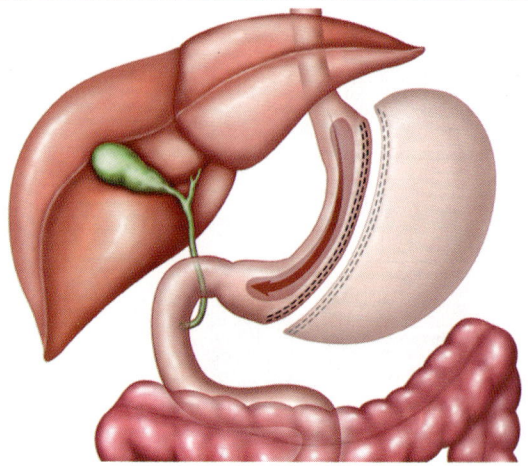

Fig. 99.12. Bariatric surgery - gastric sleeve resection

Some surgeons routinely employ the open method, as a matter of additional safety. Placement of other ports is done under vision, with virtually no risk of internal injury.

Generally gas pressure is maintained between 12 to 15mm Hg. Fall in gas pressure may be due to insufficient gas source (cylinder), to leak in the system and sometimes due to over use of suction in the peritoneal cavity. The last may be prevented by ensuring the suction tip is fully immersed in fluid to be aspirated and minimal gas is sucked out. Abnormally raised pressure may be due to inadequate muscle relaxation (true) or externally compressed or kinked gas conduits (apparent).

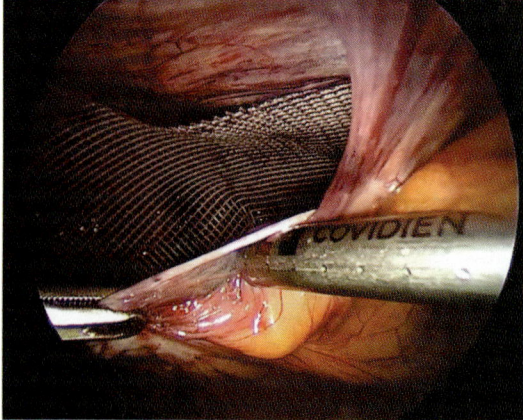

Fig. 99.13. Laparoscopic mesh repair of groin hernia
(courtesy: Lifeline Hopitals, Chennai)

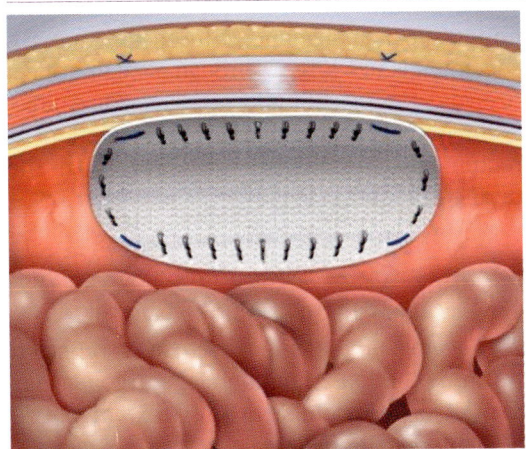

Fig. 99.14. Laparoscopic ventral hernioplasty (mesh)

Maintaining low pressure pneumoperitoneum (8-10mm) is preferred in elderly and those with compromised cardio-pulmonary functions and is also shown to have a low incidence of referred shoulder pain (caused by the stretch of diaphragm).

ERGONOMETRIC CONSIDERATONS

Placement of ports should be so planned to derive maximum ergonomic advantage and ideally at least 6" apart, to prevent the instruments crossing each other while being used. It is preferable that the surgeon becomes skilful in use both hands with equal efficiency (ambidexterous), including handling instruments, placement of endosutures and knots.

DISSECTION AND HEMOSTASIS

Even minimal bleeding obscures vision, due to absorption of photons by the hemoglobin, hence meticulous hemostasis as the surgery progresses, is vital in critical areas, which may be accomplished by diathermy of ultrasonic (harmonic) device. The monopolar diathermy, in which current passes through the tissues, has to be used with extreme caution in proximity of important structures. The entire uninsulated portion of the tip of the energy probe has to be kept in sight, to avoid it coming in contact with structures not intended for it. There is no doubt that the availability of wide spectrum of technology in energy generation in the recent

times, has made advanced endoscopic procedures easier and less time-consuming, and brought in more and more procedures under the purview of minimal access surgery. Even a trivial bleeding may appear frightening due to magnification of the image and is usually controlled with simple pressure, preferably with a piece of dry gauze, for a few minutes.

ENDOSUTURING AND STAPLING

It is advisable that every laparoscopic surgeon be familiar with endoscopic suturing, since the ability to place one or two sutures to repair some minor mishap, would avoid conversion, during any procedure. Jaw-to-jaw crossover type of needle holders (Endostitch) and skill for instrument tying are very handy for endosuturing. Pretied sutures (Endoloop), preferably with chromic catgut, are used in areas such as cystic duct, appendix or a major bleeder. The grasper goes through the preformed loop and grasps the tissue to be ligated; the knot of the sliding loop is then pushed to secure it over the tissue and excess suture material is cut and removed.

The staples available for open suturing, are now available for endoscopic use, through 12mm port, which may be for extra or intracorporeal application. With lesser incidence of anastomotic leaks, when properly used, the surgery

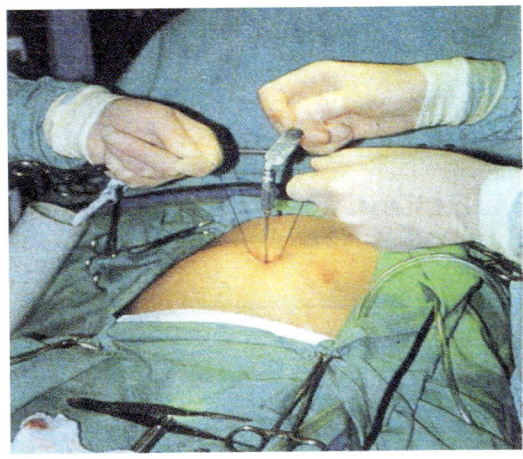

Fig. 99.15. Droplet test to verify intraperitoneal placement of Veress needle

on hollow viscera has become much simpler and expedient, with the use of staplers and they have become integral part of advanced laparoscopic or thoracoscopic surgery.

RETRIEVAL OF RESECTED SPECIMEN

Most of the resected organs (e.g.appendix, gallbladder, ovarian cyst, biopsy specimen etc) may be conveniently removed through the 10mm port, but special methods have to be employed for larger organs (e.g.: spleen, pancreas, stomach, colon, kidney etc).

1. Bert bag: the specimen is manipulated into a bag with purse-string and removed, commonly used for the gallbladder

2. Removing in piece-meal: after aspirating the fluid from a benign ovarian cyst, the sac is cut into several pieces and removed. Often the stones in the gallbladder are initially removed with an 'ovum' forceps, before it is puled out through the epigastric port incision.

3. Morcellator: benign solid organs (e.g.spleen, uterine fibroid etc) may be removed by the use of powerful grinding and suction devices converting them into soft pulp

4. Through natural orifice: the uterus is conveniently removed per vagina, after completing the vaginal component of surgery

5. Through a mini laparotomy: larger organs (e.g. stomach, spleen, kidney, adrenal, colon etc) require a small incisional opening for removal. If a bowel anastomosis is necessary, the same incision is used for carrying it out extraco rporeally. Further , it is

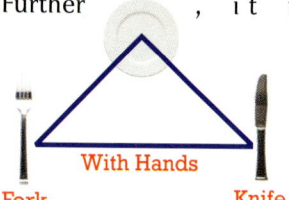

With Hands

Fork   Knife

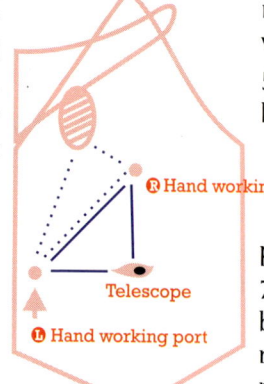

Ⓡ Hand working port

Telescope

Ⓛ Hand working port

Fig. 99.16. Priniciples of Optical Triangle

important in malignancies to ensure that the specimen is not forced through a small orifice, to avoid tumor spill and seedling. Of course, following an abdominoperineal resection of rectum, the specimen is removed through the perineal wound.

Other intra and postoperative problems peculiar to laparoscopic surgery

1. Trocar and thermal injuries to bowel

2. Fogging of the optics, requiring repeated warming the lens. Commercial anti-fog agents may lessen the problem to a large extent, but do not eliminate it.

3. Trocar site bleeding has to be routinely checked at the time of conclusion and necessary steps taken to arrest it. A Foley's catheter is introduced through the port wound, fully inflated and traction applied, to jam the balloon against the inner opening for a few minutes, to stop bleeding.

4. Pneumoperitonem related complications:
a) Interference with venous return
b) Hypercarbia/hypoxia/metabolic acidosis
c) Respiratory embarrassment
d) Gas embolism
e) Capnothorax (gas entering the pleural cavity through a defect in the diaphragm, or while dissecting at the esophageal hiatus).

The tolerance to the effects of pneumoperitoneum is less in elderly or those with compromised cardiac functions, hence advocated with great caution.

5. Coagulopathy may be more difficult to handle endoscopically

6. Port site hernia is a possibility, more often seen from 10mm ports in the lower abdomen, unless the fascia is properly closed after the procedure.

7. Port site seedling of cancer may occur if the biopsy or resected specimen of cancer is retrieved through the trocar site, leading to recurrence. This can be prevented by a mini laparotomy made to deliver the cancer-bearing surgical specimen.

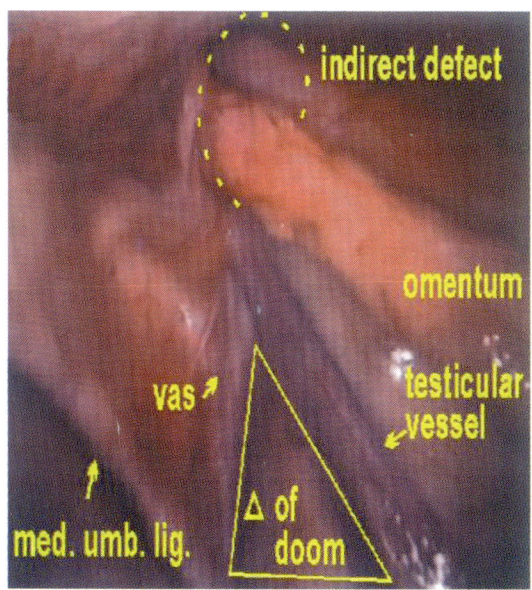

Fig. 99.17. Laproscopic anatomy of the groin - the triangle of doom

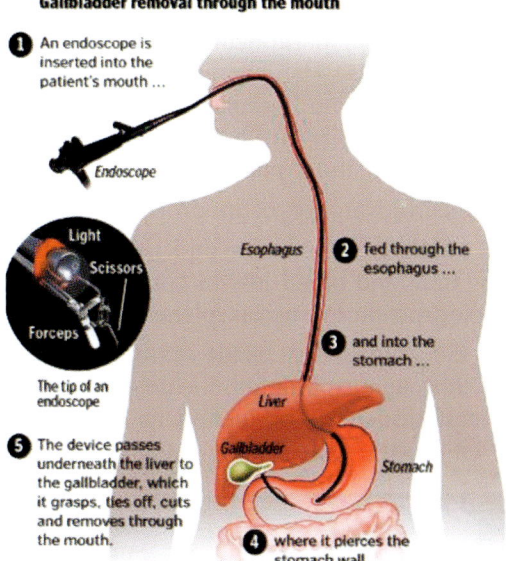

Gallbladder removal through the mouth

1 An endoscope is inserted into the patient's mouth ...

2 fed through the esophagus ...

3 and into the stomach ...

4 where it pierces the stomach wall.

5 The device passes underneath the liver to the gallbladder, which it grasps, ties off, cuts and removes through the mouth.

Fig. 99.19. Routes of access for NOTES cholecystectomy

8. With the advent of 'daycare' surgery, too early discharge from the hospital may lead to some delay in detecting certain complications, generally seen after 24 hours, such as postoperative ileus, bowel perforation, bile leak, anastomotic dehiscence, DVT, cardiac infarction and stroke. These issues have to be discussed in detail with the patient's family and appropriate guidelines given to them, preferably in writing, as to the warning symptoms requiring immediate attention.

9. Equipment failure is a preventable reason for conversion. Laparoscopic procedure being highly gadget-dependent, routine check of all the components and availability of trained technician during the procedure, would mostly eliminate this contingency.

NEW INNOVATIONS

HANDOSCOPIC SURGERY

This was introduced by Meyer et al (1998), is a hybrid procedure employed in complex abdominal procedures, in which through a mini laparotomy hand of the surgeon (or assistant) is invaginated into the abdomen, for expediency

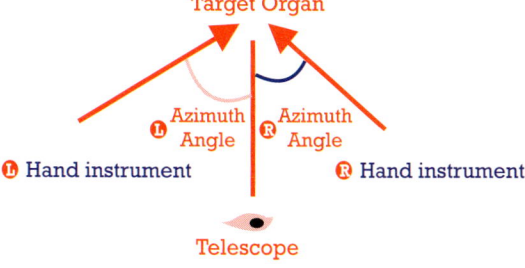

Fig. 99.18. Ergonomics in minimal access surgery

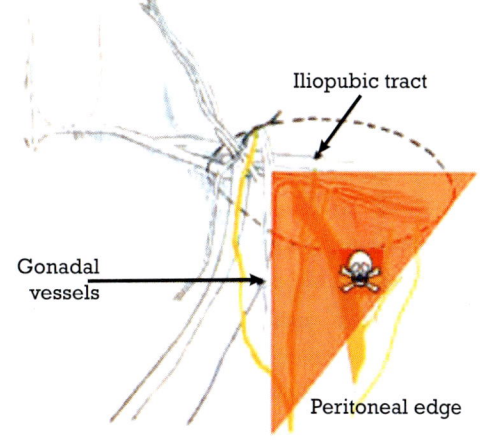

Fig. 99.20. Laproscopic anatomy of the groin - the triangle of pain

and efficiency in laparoscopic procedures. A special pneumoperitoneum protecting sleeve device (Lap disc, Hand Port system, Gel Port or Dexterity Pneumo Sleeve) is used to seal off the peritoneal cavity from leak, while freely allowing the hand to move about.

The main advantages of this procedure are:

1. improves expediency and reduces operating time and blood loss in complex laparoscopic procedures, such as splenectomy

2. the all important tactile sensation is useful for thorough exploration, including search for metastatic deposits or splenunculi

3. the mini laparotomy made for hand

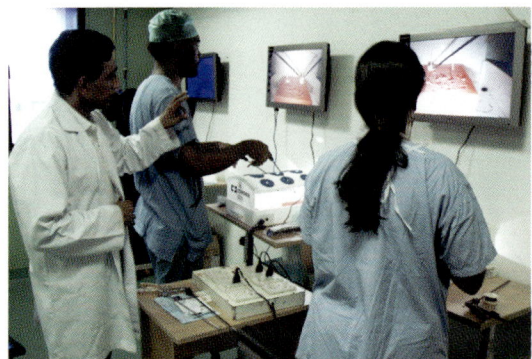

Fig. 99.23. A virtual module for hands-on training in laproscopic surgery

insertion, is also used to deliver the surgical specimen

4. enables endoscopic approach for diseases, which hitherto were considered not possible

5. multiple bowel adhesions may be conveniently released.

Some of the common applications for this procedure at present are:

Splenectomy
Colectomy for malignancy
Gastrectomy for malignancy
Esophagectomy
Hepatic resection
Pancreatic surgery

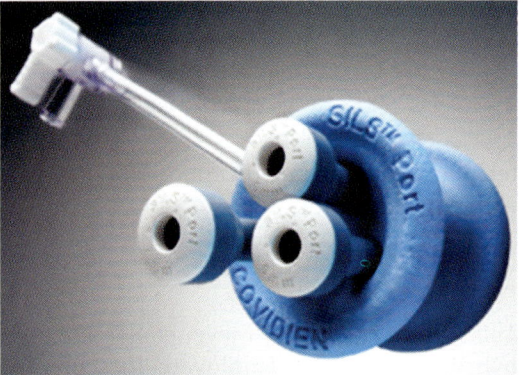

Fig. 99.21. A SILS 3-in-1 port (Covidien)

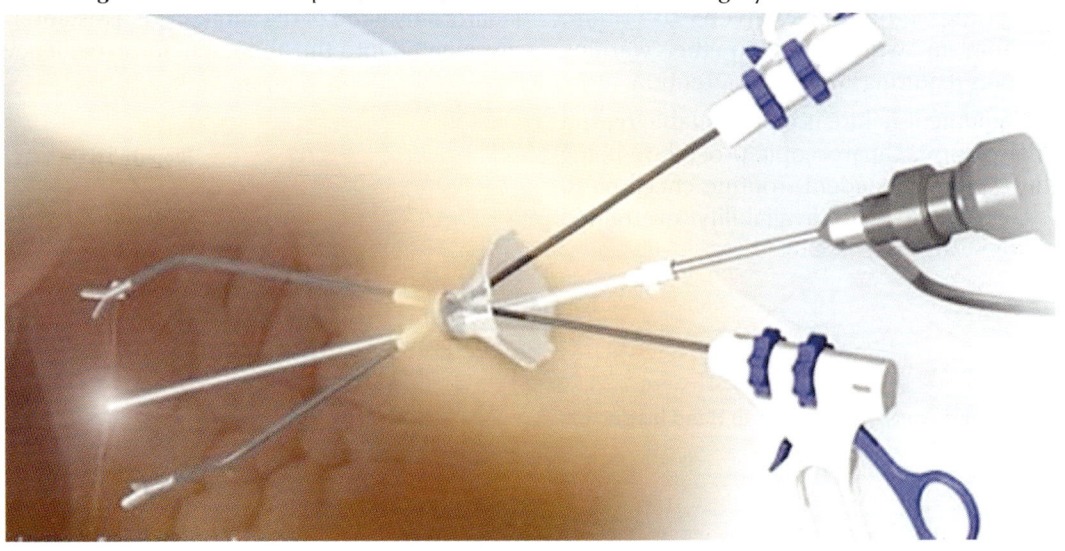

Fig. 99.22. The angled instruments and 3-in-1 port of SILS (Covidien)

Bariatric surgery

Surgery on morbidly obese patients

The main drawback of the procedure is failure to maintain effective pneumoperitoneum, due to inability to achieve 'air-tight' situation around the forearm by the available devices.

NATURAL ORIFICE TRANSLUMINAL ENDOSCOPIC SURGERY (NOTES)

Orginally described by Anthony Kalloo in USA, after animal experiments, now being used in humans. In this, the internal surgery is performed by specially designed endoscopes passed through natural orifices, to avoid external incision or somatic pain, hence requiring no anesthesia. The debate exists whether NOTES should be performed by medical gastroenterologist (who is more familiar with endoscopic interventions) or by his surgical counterpart (who is more competent to handle complications or conversions, as may be required). At present it belongs to both, but whenever it is done by the former, it is preferable that the latter stands by the procedure or at least immediately available for assistance.

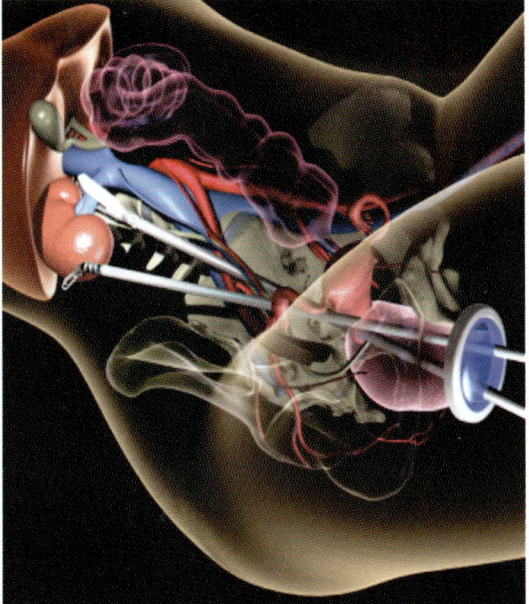

Fig. 99.24. Cholecystectomy by NOTES (transvaginal)

Common routes of entry are oral (trans-gastric), vagina, rectum or urethra (trans-vesical). Vaginal route is currently most preferred, since it allows straight access to upper abdominal structures and the posterior fornix of vaginal may be directly closed after the procedure. The trans-vesical route has the advantage that the small rent in the fundus of bladder need not be closed after the procedure, it will spontaneously seal off, if the bladder is kept empty for a few days by an indwelling catheter. The trans-rectal approach is least preferred due to high risk of peritoneal contamination.

The scope has to be passed through a tiny hole made in the stomach, to enter the peritoneal cavity to carry out the required procedure. The main drawbacks of this technique are:

1. Since the light source, hand instruments are placed parallelly close to each other, without 'triangulating' advantage, it poses technical challenge.

2. If the perforation made intentionally in the stomach (or other viscera) is not properly closed after withdrawing the scope, it may lead to a leak and its complications.

3. Since before opening, we cannot see the outside the bowel, the enterotomy may be wrongly placed (e.g. into the lesser sac instead of general peritoneal cavity)

4. The dilemma whether the procedure be done by a medical or surgical gastroenterologist.

SINGLE INCISION LAPAROSCOPIC SURGERY (SILS) syn: Single port access surgery (SPAS) or One port umbilical surgery (OPUS)

This utilizes a single umbilical 20mm incision, through which a port with 3 entry access points is positioned. The ultimate scar merges with the umbilicus, leaving no appreciable mark. Special right-angled instruments are required to get some triangulating and ergonomic advantage. Though there is only one external incision, there is no recovery advantage over the standard (multiport) surgery and has a steep learning curve.

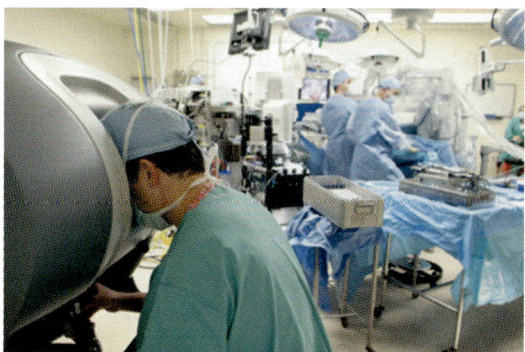

Fig. 99.25. Robotics surgery - the surgeon working on the console

ROBOTIC SURGERY

With the advances made in computer and robotic technology, now it is possible to perform minimal access surgery using human-slave manipulators. Currently two surgical telemanipulators are available: da Vinci system and Zeus system.

The da Vinci robotic system consists of 3 components, a surgeon console with an integrated 3-D visual stereo display, a robotic manipulator with 3 cart-mounted arms (for the camera and 2 instruments) and a vision cart. Unique laparoscopic instrument tips, called Endo-Wrist instruments, provide articulated movements, matching the human wrist, electronically controlled to provide the hand-eye orientation and natural operative maneuverability. The precision of movements is so high that this technic finds place in areas such as cardiac, pediatric or microsurgery. After the initial learning curve, the surgeon gets so used to perform robotic surgery that he often finds it uncomfortable doing open conventional procedures ! With the help of robotics, now it is possible to perform surgery in remote areas, such as war front, with the surgeon operating the console system from his chamber (telesurgery).

SOME OF THE PROCEDURES DONE BY MIS

Gastrointestinal

*Appendectomy
*Cholecystectomy, CBD exploration
Vagotomy
Gastric/Bowel resection or bypass
Anti-reflux procedures
Bariatric surgery
Rectopexy for prolapse
Pancreatic resection
Hepatic resection
Splenectomy
Cancer surgery
*Adhesiolysis
*Diagnostic/staging procedure

Gynecology

*Hysterectomy (lap-assisted vaginal hysterectomy - LAVH)
*Salpingo-oopherectomy
*Ovarian cyst excision
*Myomectomy
*Ventrifixation of uterus
Ectopic gestation
*Tubal ligation

Retroperitoneum

Nephrectomy
Hydronephrosis reconstruction (pyeloplasty)
Adrenal tumors
Lumbar sympathectomy
*Clipping of spermatic veins (for varicocele)
Undescended testis

Thoracic

Esophagectomy
Heller's cardiomyotomy

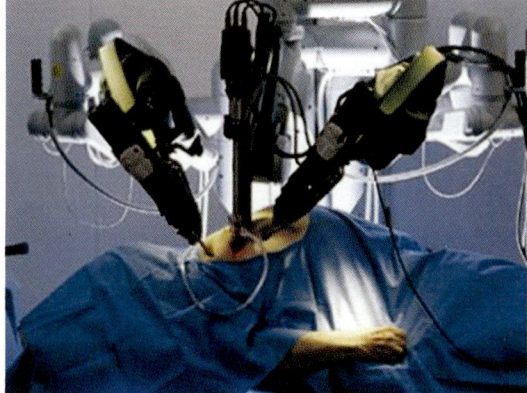

Fig. 99.26. Robotics laparoscopic surgery

Danger Zones in Laparoscopic Groin Surgery

1. Triangle of doom - between the vas deferens and gonodal vessels. Application of monopolar diathermy may lead to thrombosis of iliac vein

2. Triangle of pain - between iliopubic tract and gonodal vessels. The genitofemoral and lateral cutaneous nerve of the thigh traverse this zone

3. Circle of death (corona mortis) the area of Cooper and Gimbernat's ligaments - high risk zone for injuring abnormal obturator artery

Thoracic sympathectomy
CABG/cardiac valve surgery
*Lung biopsy

*Hernia surgery

Inguinal/femoral/umbilical/ventral/obturator hernia

Orthopedic surgery

*Arthroscopy, diagnostic and therapeutic

Knee, hip, ankle, shoulder, elbow, wrist etc

> Meniscectomy
> Synovectomy
> Loose body extraction
> Repair of torn ligament
> Biopsy

Spine surgery

ENT Surgery

*Paranasal diseases (functional endoscopic sinus surgery FESS)
*Trans-sphenoidal hypophysectomy
Surgery for CSF rhinorrhea

Ophthalmology

Dacryocysto-rhinostomy

Orbital decompression

Miscellaneous

Thyroidectomy
Endovascular surgery
Perforator vein surgery (SEPS)
Lymphadenectomy (axillary, mediastinal, retroperitoneal and ilio-inguinal)
Prostatectomy

MIS in emergencies

Evaluation of 'acute abdomen'
*Hollow viscus perforation
Trauma (abdominal and thoracic)

CONCLUSION

Fully realizing the potential and the limitations of endoscopic surgery, one should be familiar with open procedures, before embarking on these operations. Conversion to open operation need not be considered as failure or incompetence, but to be regarded as life-saving decision in the best interest of the patient in a given circumstance and speaks well of the wisdom of the surgeon. Advanced laparoscopic procedures with high incidence of complications, should be attempted only after one becomes proficient in routine procedures and developed certain level of dexterity of handling instruments.

edical Ethics deals with the moral principles which guide members of medical profession in their dealings with each other, their patients, the community and the State. Medical Etiquette refers to the conventions and courtesies observed between the colleagues and other members of medical profession, while discharging their professional obligations.

As an outcome of request from the society and consumer organizations, the Medical Councils, both at the National and State level, have formed strict guidelines to the professional conduct, coming into effect the day one joins the profession, either as a graduate medical student or as a registered practitioner (which includes postgraduate training period). However the legal responsibility of overseeing the professional conduct and performance of a graduate medical student (before registration with the Council) rests with the qualified teachers and supervisors.

Jewels of Gyan - 100.1

The medical curriculum has three ingredients

1. to assimilate various facts and figures of medical science

2. to acquire various skills required in the execution of diagnostic and therapeutic procedures on a patient

3. nurturing the proper attitude towards the patient.

Needless to say, it is only for the third ingredient, the medical graduate is respectfully called as a 'doctor', instead of titling as B.Sc. (Medicine).

There may be many instances where high moral and ethical values are expected in medical profession, only some of the examples of ideal professional conduct, their breach attracting the punitive action by the Medical Council, are given here:

1. exercise reasonable degree of knowledge, skill and care in profession

2. update professional knowledge by attending regular CME programs, in his chosen area of speciality

3. obtain a valid informed consent, before carrying out an invasive diagnostic procedure, treatment or surgery

4. provide relevant medical records and discharge summaries to patients on request, within a reasonable period

5. maintain all in-patient records for at least 3 years and those of MLCs permanently

6. should maintain free communication, transparency in dealing with patients and explain the various therapeutic options to the patient/relatives and involve them to the extent possible in making decision, before proceeding with the treatment

7. avoid improper conduct, including adultery, with patient or his/her family members

8. no conviction by a Court of Law for offences involving moral turpitude

9. do not issue a false, improper or misleading certificate, in connection with sick benefit, insurance claim, attendance in Court of Law or public services

10. do not withhold from the Health authorities, information of notifiable diseases or statistical data

11. no abortion to be performed without proper medical indication or for gender preference of the fetus (genocide)

12. respect the rule of secrecy or confidentiality of medical information, except to the Court of Law or Insurance Company. This includes even the findings at autopsy

13. do not refuse to provide emergency life-saving treatment required, without a valid reason

14. scheduled drugs should not be supplied, without proper license and protocol laid down by the state

15. no dichotomy (sharing the fees with a referring doctor, including offering or accepting commission or kick-back)

16. do not employ touts or agents to procure patients

17. do not put up unusually large name boards, with any material to attract clients

18. do not advertise, except starting or interruption of practice or change of address

19. do not employ unqualified medical or paramedical staff to perform the duties

20. no association with medical/surgical manufacturing firms, including accepting any kind of gift through their representatives

21. should not write an illegible or coded prescription, avoid prescription on phone

22. do not run a medical shop

23. do not refuse medical services on racial, religious or community grounds

24. do not discharge duties in an inebriated condition (alcohol or drugs)

25. do not use red cross emblem, except by the members or institutions of army medical services

26. do not practice secret or magic remedies, not in accordance with science and pharmacopeia

27. do not conduct experiments potentially hazardous to life on patients without their informed consent and the approval of the Ethical Committee of the hospital

28. do not practice euthanasia (in countries where it is not legal)

29. do not perform organ transplantation with commercial interest

30. basically a doctor, as a member of a noble profession, is expected to maintain certain level of dignity and decorum, befitting the profession, should be a law-abiding citizen, be familiar with the statutory requirements related to medical practice and act judiciously, not only while discharging his professional duties, but also in normal life.

Though many of the subjects mentioned above are obvious and logical, it is a pity that the delicate doctor-patient relationship is constantly under strain and scrutiny in the present context, since some members of the profession do not respect the moral/ethical code. And that a small number of 'black sheep' bring discredit to the entire profession, spoil the public image of a doctor, undermining the excellent work done by the vast majority of the members, in the true spirit of service and sacrifice. The phenomenon of corporate hospitals, as 'everything under one roof', has several advantages, but utmost vigilance has to be exercised by the profession, so as not to lose sight of the principles of empathy and personalized care.

EVIDENCE-BASED MEDICINE

EBM or evidence-based practice (EBP) aims to apply the best available evidence gained from the scientific methods to clinical decision making. It seeks to assess the strength of evidence of the risks and benefits of treatments (including lack of treatment) and diagnostic tests. Evidence quality can range from meta-analyses and systematic reviews of double-blind, placebo-controlled clinical trials at the top end, down to conventional wisdom and anecdotal experience at the bottom.

Evidence-based individual decision (EBID) making is evidence-based medicine as practiced by the individual health care provider. There is concern that current evidence-based medicine focuses excessively on EBID.

Limitations

Although evidence-based medicine is being regarded as the 'gold standard' for clinical

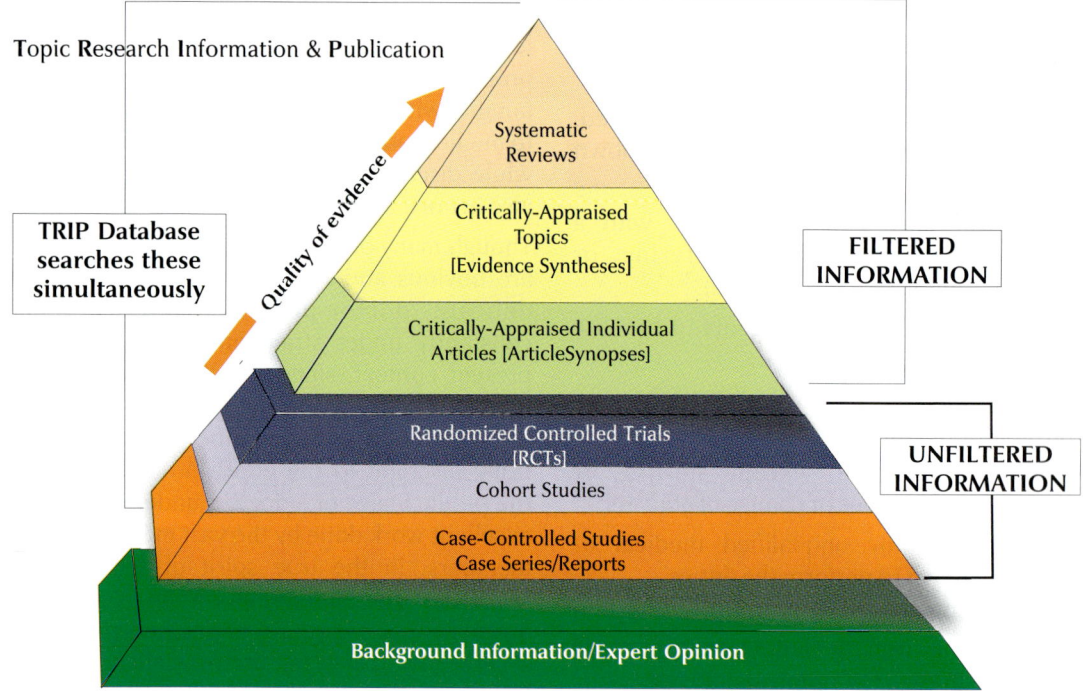

Topic Research Information & Publication

Fig.100.1. Levels of scientific evidence for clinical application

practice there are a number of limitations and criticisms of its use.

Ethical objections

In some cases, such as in open-heart surgery or neurosurgery, conducting randomized, placebo-controlled trials is commonly considered to be unethical, although observational studies may address these problems to some degree. It may be difficult to get a clearance by the Ethical Committee, if there is unacceptable (or undetermined) risk to patients in any wing of the study, either by omission or commission.

For example, an older generic statin drug had been shown to reduce mortality, but a newer and much more expensive statin drug was found to lower cholesterol more effectively. However, evidence came to light about safety concerns with the new drug which caused some insurers to stop supporting, since it was found to cause glucose intolerance, even though marketing approval was not withdrawn. Some

people are willing to take their chances to gamble their health on the success of new drugs or old drugs in new situations which may not yet have been fully tested in clinical trials. However the third party payers (TPP) are reluctant to accept such treatments, preferring instead to take the safer route of awaiting the results of clinical testing and leaving the funding of such trials to the manufacturer or researcher.

Publication bias

It is recognised that not all evidence available in the literature is transparent and reliable, which can limit the effectiveness of any approach and hence efforts to eliminate publication bias and retrieval bias is required. The practitioner has to be highly vigilant to filter the right ones from the biased lot and to develop the wisdom to know the difference, by scrutinizing the methodology and statistical significance of each publication.

Retrospective studies, inability to randomize or failure to publish trials which yielded negative results are the most obvious gaps and moves to register all trials at the outset, and then to pursue their results, are underway. Changes in publication methods, particularly related to the Web, should reduce the difficulty of obtaining publication for a paper on a trial that concludes it did not prove anything new, including its starting hypothesis.

Systems to stratify evidence by quality have been developed, such as this one shown below to rank evidence about the effectiveness of treatment or screening:

Level I: Evidence obtained from at least one properly designed randomized controlled trial.

Recommendation: Good scientific evidence suggests that the benefits of the clinical service substantially outweigh the potential risks. Clinicians should discuss the service with eligible patients.

Level II-A: Evidence obtained from well-designed controlled trials without randomization.

Recommendation: At least fair scientific evidence suggests that the benefits of the clinical service outweighs the potential risks. Clinicians should discuss the service with eligible patients.

Level II-B: Evidence obtained from well-designed cohort or case-control analytic studies, preferably from more than one center or research group.

Recommendation: At least fair scientific evidence suggests that there are benefits provided by the clinical service, but the balance between benefits and risks are too close for making general recommendations. Clinicians need not offer it unless there are individual considerations.

Level II-C: Evidence obtained from multiple time series with or without the intervention. Dramatic results in uncontrolled trials might also be regarded as this type of evidence.

Recommendation: At least fair scientific evidence suggests that the risks of the clinical service outweighs potential benefits. Clinicians should not routinely offer the service to asymptomatic patients

Level III: Opinions of respected authorities, based on clinical experience, descriptive studies, or reports of expert committees.

Recommendation: Scientific evidence is lacking, of poor quality, or conflicting, such that the risk versus benefit balance cannot be assessed. Clinicians should help patients understand the uncertainty surrounding the clinical service.

In conclusion, EBM is the application of evidence in medical practice in a 4-tier fashion:

1. a fact which is true and has been proven to be true; it has to be made the 'standard of care' or continued if already in clinical application

2. a fact which may be true but not sufficiently proven yet; it needs to be further studied scientifically to generate level I evidence, so that it could become 'standard of care'

3. a fact which has been proven false or unsafe; it should be promptly eliminated from the current practice

4. a fact which is likely to be false, but is yet unproven; it is a potential source of danger and has to be rejected or if already in practice, should be quickly discarded. This poses considerable risk to the patients subjecting themselves to 'research' and extreme caution has to be exercised while formulating the methodology for study, both by the researchers and those overseeing the ethical aspects, to avoid unacceptable damage, which may occur before the final proof of its ineffectiveness or potential risk is established.

It should be realized that too much of the socalled 'good and safe' practice of the past had crumbled when scrutinized through the eyes of EBM. A safe surgeon should not only be versatile in anatomical dissection during surgery but also be proficient in sorting out available scientific data by proper intellectual dissection into 'good, bad and ugly'.

SURGICAL AUDIT

Every doctor cares more for his reputation than his efficiency' - **E A Codman**

It matters how the patient feels after the treatment rather than what the doctor feels about the outcome nor what he thinks the patient ought to feel.

Definition: The systematic and objective analysis of quality of medicare, including diagnostic and therapeutic procedures, optimal utilization of resources, untoward incidences, unanticipated morbidity, quality of life after treatment and of course, the final outcome.

It serves not only to review ones overall results, but also comparative analysis of those of colleagues and national data base, with a sole aim of plugging the deficiencies, improving performance and planning future strategies, rather than pointing an accusing finger to any one nor paving way for litigations. The end point of this elaborate and sometimes embarrassing exercise is to be able to answer the two fundamental questions: 'are we doing the right thing ?' and 'are we doing the things right ?'

There are two types of audit; medical and clinical. Medical audit is the assessment by peer review of medical care provided by a physician. The clinical audit is a multidisciplinary assessment of the total care provided to the patient by the healthcare personnel.

The following guidelines were proposed for the audit system:

Purpose: should be educational relevant to patient care

Control: should be by clinical peers with voluntary participation

Resources: should be inexpensive and accessible

Standards: should be set locally by participating physicians

Methods: must be non-threatening, simple, interesting, objective and reproducible

Records: should contain adequate clinical information necessary to arrive useful inferences and be easily retrievable

In the implementation of Medical audit, three basic steps have to be followed:

Structure or methodology of collection of various relevant data

Processing the methods adopted, interpolating against the results

Evaluating the outcome or end result, including the quality of life and patient satisfaction

These steps have any meaning only if suggestions to improve the existing set up could be generated and when implemented, they lead to ultimate improvement of outcome.

To illustrate the benefit of simple auditing the OR scheduling in an institution, the following facts emerged from the data analysis:

1. 40% of listed cases started late

2. In 80% it was due to late arrival of patient to the OR.

3. 15% of cases were due to the unexpected delay by the previous surgeon in completing the operation on time

4. There was more than 15min cleaning interval between cases in 50% of cases

5. 75% of times, scheduled cases were cancelled for want of OR time

6. Reasons for cancellations were, overscheduling, overrunning time by 'slow' surgeons and intrusion of emergencies into the elective list

The study concluded that if these factors could be corrected, it would lead to 25% more utilization of the OR, without extending working hours.

In UK, National Confidential Enquiry into Perioperative Deaths (NCEPOD) was started in 1986 and detailed retrospective analysis of all mortalities within 30 days of surgery was carried out by two independent specialists (surgeon and anesthesiologist)

The following aspects were analyzed and the results were sent to the surgeons:

1. appropriateness of preoperative preparation

2. appropriateness of the operation

3. appropriateness of grade of surgeon
4. soundness and the infrastructure of the Institution
5. functioning of equipment
6. failure of human skill and service
7. adverse drug reaction
8. competence and application of knowledge
9. level of concern and empathy
10. probability of fatigue, leading to physical/mental impairment
11. level of supervision
12. honesty in recording the events

The survey also concluded that the hospital monthly meetings to review morbidity and mortality were not organized well, leading to poor attendance and involvement

Conclusion: Scientific knowledge is never complete, hence perfect practice can never be expected, but we have to untiringly keep trying to reach the target. The audit process provides us systematic method of self analysis, opportunity to correct and to improve performance, to the point of reaching near perfection, before somebody (e.g. professional forum, litigant or his lawyer) points out our deficiencies.

It takes profound determination by the physician to adopt evidence-based protocols at all times, overriding strong personal beliefs and convictions.

'Doing surgery without an audit is like playing cricket without keeping a score' - **H B Devlin**

Introduction - Ever since the first clinical application of ether to general anesthesia by Morton (1846), the field of anesthesia has come a long way, the ancsthesiologist today is involved in many different areas of patient care including surgical anesthesia, critical care, acute and chronic pain management, labor analgesia, cardiopulmonary resuscitation, and emergency intubation. In the operating room (OR), the anesthesiologists are called upon to provide a wide variety of care to patients of all ages, including premature neonates with life threatening congenital abnormalities and chronically ill geriatric patients. Surgical anesthesia includes monitored anesthesia care (MAC), regional anesthesia, and general anesthesia. We will briefly touch on each of these aspects.

Local anesthesia

Mode of action of nerve block

The impulse in a nerve fibre is transmitted by progressive opening of sodium (Na) channels across the cell membrane, leading to sudden influx of Na. Local anesthetic agents block the sodium channel, thereby arresting the nerve impulse.

Local anesthesia is given by infiltration of the anesthetic agent into the area of incision. The addition of 1/2,50,000 adrenaline solution to them is used to minimize bleeding and also to prolong their action, by delaying absorption. (this dilution may be obtained by adding 0.25ml of 1/1000 solution of adrenaline to about 60 ml of local anesthetic agent). Higher concentration or more than 500mcgm of total dose of adrenaline is not safe.

Lignocaine: it is the most popular agent used as 0.5-1.0% solution. It acts in a few minutes and lasts for 30-60 minutes. It is also used for nerve blocks (1-2%) and topical anesthesia (4%). Maximum safe dose is 3.5mg/kg (plain) which may be doubled if adrenaline is added.

Prilocaine: it is less toxic and less potent and used mostly for topical (4%) and nerve blocks (2-3%). Maximum safe dose is 5mg/kg and methemoglobinemia and cyanosis may result from overdose, which is treated by I.V administration of 1% methylene blue solution (1mg/kg).

Bupivacaine: it is more toxic and more potent and slow acting. It is used as 0.25-0.5% solution, acts for about 2-4 hours and the maximum safe dose is around 2mg/kg.

Monitored anesthesia care

Monitored anesthesia care (MAC) is requested to supplement local anesthesia. Anesthesiologists usually participate for one of two reasons. One is that some patients or procedures require more potent sedative drugs. The other is that some acutely or chronically ill patients require close monitoring and hemodynamic or respiratory support.

Field-block anesthesia

Areas, such as penis, finger, cervical or inguinal regions etc. may be effectively blocked by infil-

Agent	Onset of action	Safe dose/kg	Max dose	Duration of action
Lignocaine plain	Rapid	3.5mg	250mg	30-60min
Lignocaine+epinephrine		7.0mg	500mg	60-120min
Prilocaine plain	Medium	5.0mg	350mg	90-120min
Prilocaine+ epinephrine		7.5mg	500mg	120-240min
Bupivacaine plain	Slow	2.0mg	175mg	120-240min
Bupivacaine+ epinephrine		3.0mg	225mg	180-420min

Table - 101.1 Local anesthetic agents in common use

trating the agent into the sensory nerves supplying the agent into the sensory nerves supplying the operative field. Entire upper or lower limb may be blocked (see below), for patients unsuitable for standard anesthesia.

However, while carrying out penile or digital blocks, adrenaline *should not* be added for fear of inducing protracted vasoconstriction and irreversible ischemia.

Regional anesthesia

Regional anesthesia is useful for operations on the upper and lower extremities, pelvis, and lower abdomen. Patients can remain awake and, if needed, intravenous (I.V) sedation can be used to supplement blocks. Regional anesthesia avoids general anesthesia, but not without its own inherent risks.

Upper extremity

Operations on the upper extremity are well suited for regional blocks. Nerves in the lower arm (ulnar, median, or radial) can be blocked individually, but more commonly the entire brachial plexus is blocked proximally. Four common approaches to the brachial plexus include axillary, supraclavicular, infraclavicular and interscalene blocks. The procedure earlier done utilizing blind landmark guided techniques are increasingly replaced by either nerve stimulator-guided or ultrasound-guided techniques.

The main complications seen with these blocks are nerve damage (very rare) and systemic local anesthetic toxicity (more common) from either overdose or accidental intravascular injection. An additional complication seen with blocks in the neck (especially supraclavicular) or intercostal is pneumothorax.

Bier's block (modified by McHomes)

This technique of intravenous regional anesthesia involves inflating a tourniquet around the upper arm and injecting a dilute solution of local anesthetic into the venous system of the exsanguinated hand or forearm; the local anesthetic diffuses to anesthetize the arm distal to the tourniquet. The potential hazard of sudden release of the anesthetic agent into the circulation, if there is sudden release of the tourniquet, has made this procedure unpopular.

Lower extremity

By individually blocking the sciatic and femoral nerves the entire leg below the knee can be anesthetized. This is especially useful for below-knee amputations on critically ill patients who are at high risk for other types of anesthesia. This technique is not useful for operations above-knee because the obturator and lateral femoral cutaneous nerves also needed to be blocked, as also for pain associated with the use of a tourniquet around the thigh. Blocking the popliteal nerves is useful for operations on the heel and is easy to perform. Another common technique is the

---

Jewels of Gyan – 101.1

Some pharmacological blockades in medicine

Neurotransmitter blockage – psychotropic agents and muscle relaxants

Ca^{++} channel blockage – relax blood vessels, including coronaries, lower BP

K^+ channel blockage – antiarrhythmic agents (amiodarone, bretylium, procainamide)

Na^+ channel blockage – local anesthetic agents

H_1 receptor blockage – antihistamin agents

H_2 receptor blockage – gastric antisecretory agents

α-adrenergic receptor blockage – peripheral vasodilatation, lowers BP, relaxes internal vesical sphincter

β-adrenergic receptor blockage – slows heart rate, causes bronchospasm

Parasympathetic blockade - Anticholinergic and antisecretory agents

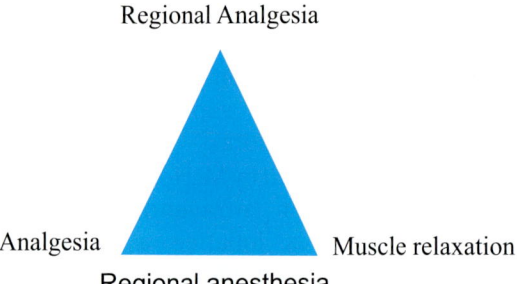

Regional Analgesia

Analgesia — Muscle relaxation

Regional anesthesia

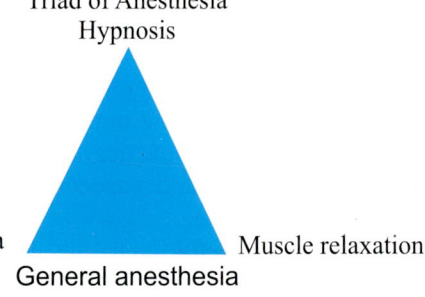

Triad of Anesthesia
Hypnosis

Analgesia — Muscle relaxation

General anesthesia

ankle block, which anesthetizes the entire foot by blocking five individual nerves at the level of the ankle.

3-in-1 block: the lumbar plexus is sandwiched between the psoas sheath and quadratus lumborum and here 3 nerves (femoral, lateral femoral cutaneous and obturator nerves) may be effectively blocked by injecting into this plane, about an inch lateral to the femoral pulse, just below the inguinal ligament.

Complications of local anesthesia
Neurotoxicity
Cardiotoxicity (intravascular injection)
Anaphylaxis (safer to give a test dose)
Risk of spreading the local infection (cellulitis)
Nerve injury (usually neurapraxia)
Methemoglobinemia and hypoxia
Related to adrenaline (when used)

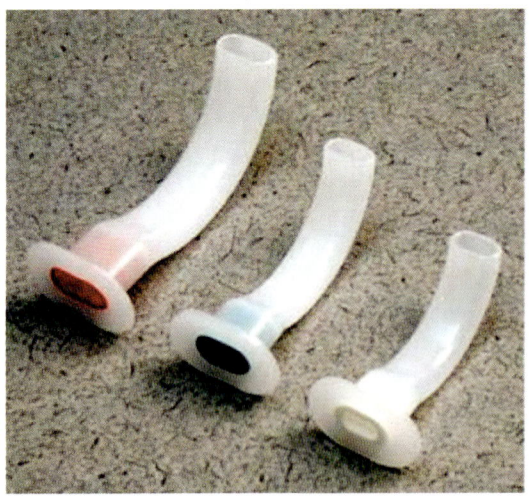

Fig. 101.1. Airway to prevent tongue falling back

Tachyarrhythmias
Protracted vasoconstriction, as indicated

Spinal anesthesia
Spinal anesthesia or subarachnoid block (SAB) is useful for operations on the lower abdomen, pelvis, or lower extremities. It is performed by advancing a small needle (usually 25 or 27 G.) through the dura into the cerebrospinal fluid (CSF) in the lower lumbar area and injecting a small dose of local anesthetic. This leads to sensory, motor and autonomic blockade below the level of the block. A hyperbaric solution (more dense than CSF) is used to control the level by adjusting the position of the patient. By a slight tilt of the patient head-down for a few minutes, higher level of anesthesia, even up to epigastrium (D-8), can be achieved.

The motor block may be noted at the level of injection, whereas sensory block affects two segments higher and sympathetic block two segments higher than the sensory block.

Saddle-block is to give SAB in sitting position and allow the heavy anesthetic agent gravitate to the end of CSF column (S-1 level), involving only sacral segments (cauda equina), thereby producing anesthesia of the perineum, like the area of a saddle. This is highly useful for perineal, vaginal, anorectal surgery, with very minimal vasomotor effects, applicable for elderly.

Complications of SAB
1. Hypotension (autonomic block). Higher the block, more the risk of hypotension, least in saddle block. It may be corrected by adequate hydration and use of sympathomimetic agents, such as ephedrine, mephenteramine or

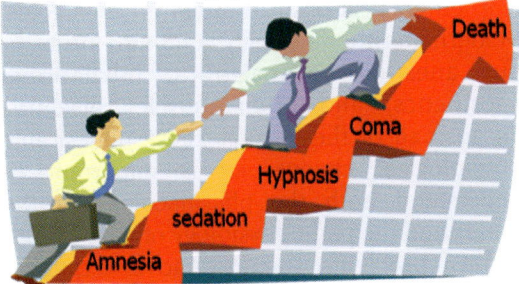

Hypnosis

Death

Coma

Hypnosis

sedation

Amnesia

Awake

dopamine. Left untreated, it may lead to profound hypotension (spinal shock).

The vasodilatation in the lower part of the body and compensatory vasoconstriction of the upper part of the body earns the name "pink trousers and blue jacket" phenomenon.

2. Excessive cephalad spread leading to respiratory insufficiency. It needs ventilatory support, till the anesthetic wares out (about an hour for lidocaine and up to 3 hours for bupivacaine)

3. Post-lumbar puncture headache (PLPH) more common with larger needles and in younger patients. This is thought to be mainly due to the leak of CSF through the needle hole and probably related to fluid shift into CSF space, due to osmotic changes

This is prevented/treated by adequate hydra-tion and infusion of hyperosmolar solution, such as 20% manitol or 10% dextrose.

4. Retention of urine is commonly seen following spinal anesthesia, especially in elderly and those with prostatic enlargements

5. Infection, leading to meningitis

6. Bleeding into spinal canal, common in those with coagulopathy or on anticoagulant therapy

7. Injury to spinal cord, more in children, in whom the conus medullaris is at a lower level

Epidural anesthesia

Lumbar epidural anesthesia (LEA) produces autonomic sensory and motor blockade similar to that produced by SAB. The difference is that the needle is placed in the epidural space and does not enter the cerebrospinal fluid. Proper placement of the needle is ascertained by injecting air, which should go without much resistance. A catheter is then threaded through the needle for about four centimeters beyond the needle in the epidural space and the needle is withdrawn. The indwelling catheter permits slow injection of the local anesthetic and makes repeat injections possible. In comparison to SAB, LEA produces less abrupt hemodynamic changes, provides the possibility of prolonged epidural drug administration and avoids PLPH (unless the dura is punctured accidentally).

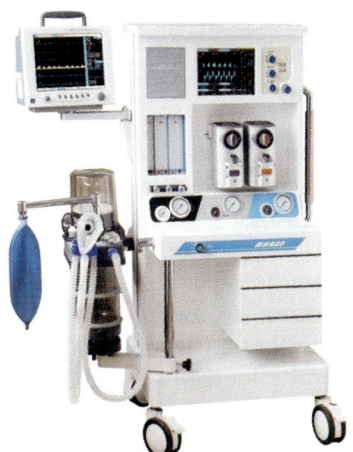
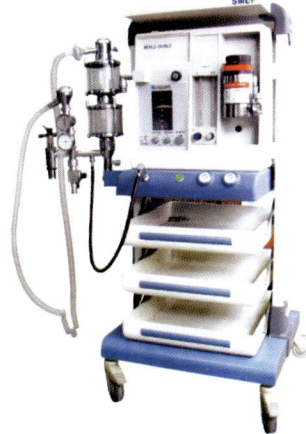
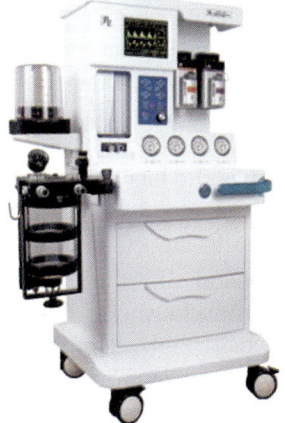

Fig. 101.2. Boyle's apparatus different models

Another benefit is that epidural opioids can be added to provide postoperative pain relief at the spinal level (opiate receptors) while reducing the side effects of systemic narcotics (especially respiratory depression). The complications of LEA are basically the same as those for SAB; however; if the subarachnoid space is accidentally punctured by the larger epidural needle the likelihood of PLPH is greater than for SAB. The disadvantages of LEA are that it takes longer to perform and take effect than SAB and the block is not usually as dense. Another complication which is much more likely with LEA is accidental intravascular injection and local anesthetic toxicity (see Fig. 85.4).

Anesthetic toxicity

When used for regional anesthesia, the toxicity of local anesthetics is dependent upon the site of injection and the speed of absorption. The main symptoms seen with local anesthetic toxicity are related to CNS and CVS. The symptoms that are usually seen with either an overdose or inadvertent intravascular injection are numbness of the tongue or lips, light-headedness, tinnitus or visual disturbances. The signs of toxicity can progress to slurred speech, irrational conversation, and grand mal seizures. With higher doses of local anesthetic, cardiovascular collapse may ensue. The primary treatment is oxygen, airway and cardiovascular support. If a seizure does not terminate spontaneously, a benzodiazepine (e.g. midazolam) or thiopental may be given. Always aspirate before injecting local anesthetics and know the toxic dose of the drug being used. It is mandatory that the necessary drugs and facilities for emergency resuscitation are immediately available.

General anesthesia

General anesthesia is a reversible state of unconsciousness, the mechanisms of which remain poorly defined.

The components of general anesthesia consist of amnesia, analgesia, inhibition of noxious reflexes, and skeletal muscle relaxation. At one time, a high dose of a single inhalational agent (e.g. ether) was used to attain all four goals. Modern anesthesia usually combines intravenous anesthetics, analgesics, inhalational anesthetics, and often muscle relaxants. Because all of these drugs cause undesirable physiological changes, it is important to understand both the pharmacology of the agents and the pathophysiology of the patient's medical problems. The major adverse changes associated with anesthetic drugs are loss of adequate airway, respiratory and cardio-vascular depression, leading to hypoxia (with possible CNS damage), hypotension, cardiac arrest, and aspiration of acidic gastric contents (which can lead to severe pulmonary damage). Dental damage is more frequent but less severe. Anesthesiologist is also responsible for managing complications of intraoperative positioning, administration of I.V fluids, blood, hemodynamic support and monitoring.

Induction

Induction or the "take-off" for a general anesthetic, is one of the most critical periods. More serious complications occur during induction than at any other time of the anesthesia. During this brief, intense interval, the patient must be rendered unconscious, the airway secured, ventilation begun, the cardiovascular system stabilized, and the patient positioned for surgery. There are several different ways of inducing general anesthesia depending upon the patient and the type of surgery to be performed.

Inhalation induction

In the early days of ether and chloroform anesthesia, induction consisted of having the patient breathe the anesthetic from a mask while the anesthesiologist gradually assumed maintenance of the airway. Induction was often turbulent and hazardous because patients progressed slowly from an awake state to a surgical level of anesthesia (stage 3). Patients would spend several minutes in stage 2 (the excitement stage), gets agitated, combative and difficult to restrain. During this hazardous interval, patients are at risk for laryngospasm, vomiting and aspiration. Although modern inhalational agents induce anesthesia more rapidly and safely, they are currently reserved for induction of children, in selected adult patients and some patients in whom the airway may be difficult to secure. Children rapidly progress through stage 2, and post-induction placement of I.V line avoids the trauma of insertion in struggling children.

Intravenous induction

Intravenous induction is used commonly in elective adult cases. The patient is first preoxygenated with 100% oxygen to wash out nitrogen (79% of room air) from the lungs and to provide the patient with a reservoir of oxygen should mask ventilation or intubation be difficult. A rapidly acting, intravenous induction agent is then administered. Commonly used induction agents include thiopental (an ultrashort-acting barbiturate), propofol, ketamine, etomidate, diazepam, midazolam, or opioids (e.g. fentanyl, sufentanil, or alfentanil). Each of these agents, in sufficient doses, can quickly render patients unconscious and apneic. The anesthesiologist then assures the ability to manually ventilate the patient using a mask. If mask ventilation is satisfactory, the patient is administered a neuromuscular blocker, such as succinylcholine (a depolarizing relaxant) or a nondepolarizing agent. After the patient is adequately relaxed, endotracheal intubation is performed, which maintains a patent airway and limits the possibility of gastric aspiration. The anesthesia is then continued using intravenous agents, nitrous oxide, volatile anesthetic agents, or more commonly, a combination of the above. The important drawback to intravenous induction is that endotracheal intubation may be performed while the patient is 'light', thereby precipitating hypertension, tachycardia, or bronchospasm and the spontaneous ventilation is abolished without certainty that manual ventilation can be accomplished. Adjuvant agents, e.g. lidocaine and opioids, may be used to blunt reflex responses to intubation.

Preoperative airway evaluation reduces the risky situation of the patient being abruptly rendered "unable to ventilate and unable to intubate."

Maintenance of the airway by face mask, a skill that comes with experience, is probably more difficult to master than intubation. There are several techniques which can be used to keep the tongue from falling against the posterior wall of the pharynx and occluding the airway. The mandible can be manipulated, and an oral or nasal airway can be inserted. If the procedure is brief and there are no contraindications, the procedure can be completed using a face mask.

If an endotracheal intubation is not possible, the use of a laryngeal mask airway (LMA) is an alternative, which maintains airway patency and permits gentle ventilatory assistance, though it does not totally protect against aspiration of gastric contents. The remainder of the anesthesia is maintained with a volatile anesthetic agent with or without supplemental nitrous oxide and intravenous drugs.

Rapid sequence induction

Rapid sequence induction (RSI) is used for patients who are at high risk for acid aspiration. This includes those who had recently eaten, obese patients, patients with symptomatic gastroesophageal reflux, obstetric patients or those with a bowel obstruction. All emergency patients are considered 'full stomach', because it is often not known when they last ate, and pain or injury itself may delay gastric emptying. The concept of RSI is to pass as quickly as possible from the awake state to the anesthetized, in an endotracheally intubated state. This is done by first preoxygenating the patient, then giving thiopental (or another intravenous induction agent) together with succinylcholine, waiting 60 seconds and intubating the trachea. During the onset of the action of the drugs, pressure is held on the cricoid cartilage (Sellick's maneuver) to help prevent passive regurgitation of the gastric contents into the pharynx. The risk of these techniques is that the

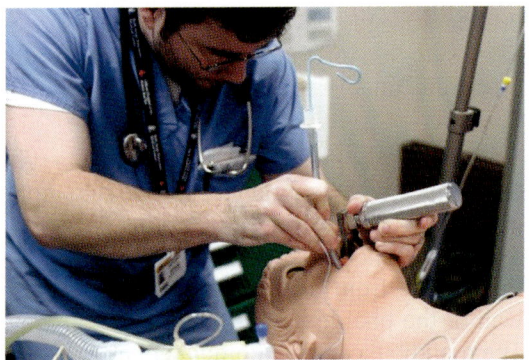

Fig. 101.3. Training endotracheal intubation

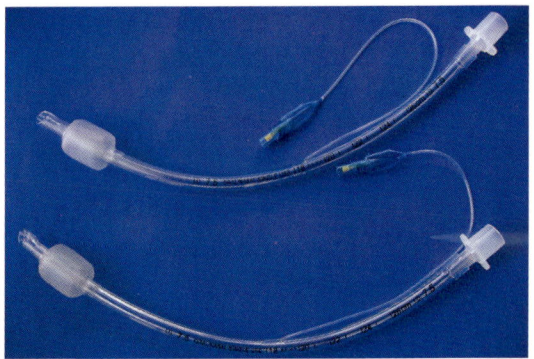

Fig. 101.5. Cuffed endotracheal tubes

anesthesiologist gives a paralyzing dose of muscle relaxant without knowing whether the mask ventilation is possible. If intubation cannot be performed successfully, and if mask ventilation proves unsatisfactory, hypoxia and its sequella, including arrhythmias and cardiac arrest, may be anticipated.

Awake intubation

In some patients it is not safe to induce anesthesia without first securing the airway; in such patients an awake intubation is required. Indications for awake intubation include inadequate mouth opening, facial trauma, known or suspected cervical spine injury (cannot safely flex or extend the neck), and lesions in the upper airway. It is usually accomplished by the "blind" nasal route or by direct visualization using fiberoptic bronchoscope and a Magill's forceps. In the blind nasal approach, the larynx is not directly visualized. The endotracheal tube is inserted through the nose and guided into the trachea by

listening to the patient's breath sounds through the tube. The fiberoptic intubation is performed by passing an endotracheal tube through the nose or mouth initially into the pharynx. The bronchoscope is then passed through the tube, visualizing the larynx and the trachea and threading the tube into the trachea under vision.

Inhalational anesthetic agents

These are among the few drugs which are administered by the inhalation route. Since inhalational agents undergo limited metabolism, their excretion is largely dependent on ventilation. The advantage of these drugs is that all, with the exception of nitrous oxide, have the properties of a complete anesthetic. That is, they can provide amnesia, analgesia, inhibition of noxious reflexes, and skeletal muscle relaxation if used in sufficient

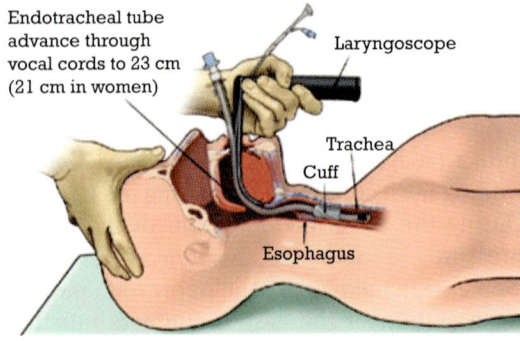

Endotracheal tube advance through vocal cords to 23 cm (21 cm in women)

Laryngoscope

Trachea

Cuff

Esophagus

Fig. 101.4. Endotracheal intubation

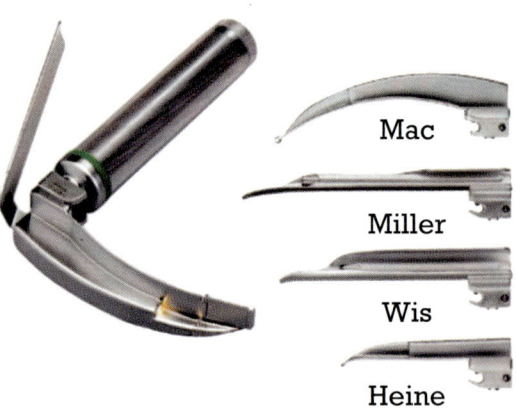

Mac

Miller

Wis

Heine

Fig. 101.6. Laryngoscope with different blades

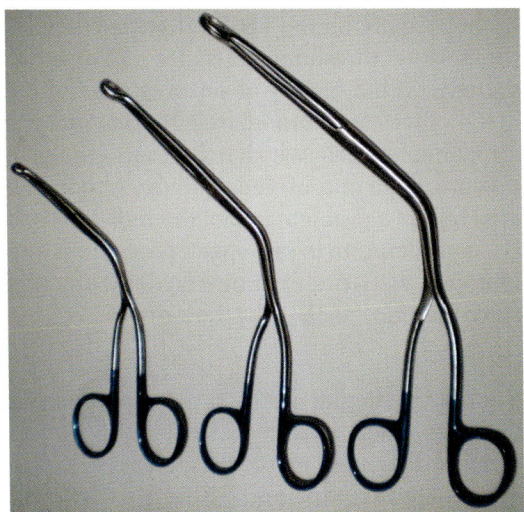

Fig. 101.7. Megill's forceps used for nasotracheal intubation

doses. The disadvantage of the volatile agents (all inhalational agents except nitrous oxide) is that they cause profound respiratory and cardiovascular depression. For the inhaled drugs, potency is commonly referred to as the minimum alveolar concentration (MAC) of the anesthetic. This is the alveolar concentration of anesthetic at the atmospheric pressure that prevents movement in 50% of patients in response to a painful stimulus (i.e., incision). Another critical physical characteristic of inhalation agents is the blood/gas solubility coefficient. The higher the B/G solubility coefficient, the more slowly the agent is taken up or eliminated; the lower the coefficient the more rapidly the agent is taken up or eliminated. For example, the B/G solubility coefficient of diethyl ether is approximately 13. Therefore, induction and emergence with ether occurred slowly. Halothane, with a B/G solubility coefficient of 2.3, greatly accelerated the speed at which patients could be anesthetized and awakened Enflurane and isoflurane were slightly faster. Nitrous oxide, with a B/G solubility coefficient of approximately 0.47, until recently was the only nonflammable inhalation agent that permitted very rapid uptake and elimination. However, two recently

available agents, desflurane and sevoflurane, have B/G solubility coefficients of 0.42 and 0.65, respectively. These represent the first highly potent, nonflammable agents with the potential for such rapid uptake and elimination.

Nitrous oxide

This gas only provides partial anesthesia at atmospheric pressure (MAC-104%). Because it has only minimal effects on respiration and hemodynamics, it is often combined with one of the potent volatile agents in order to limit the side effects of the second agent, to reduce the cost of potent agents, and to facilitate rapid induction and emergence with more soluble agents. Nitrous oxide is not used in the presence of closed air spaces such as pneumothorax, small bowel obstruction, middle ear surgery, or retinal surgery in which an intraocular gas bubble is created, because nitrous oxide can increase the volume or pressure of these spaces. This occurs because nitrous oxide is 30 times more soluble than nitrogen and diffuses into the space faster than nitrogen can diffuse out.

Halothane

Halothane, the oldest of the currently used potent volatile agents, causes minimal irritation to the trachea and bronchial tree, especially useful for inhalation inductions and is the least expensive of the potent volatile agents. Because it sensitizes the heart to the arrhythmogenic

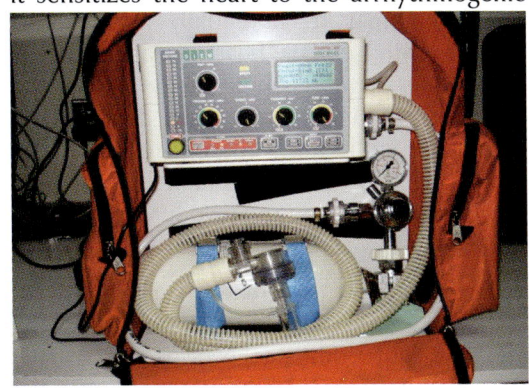

Fig. 101.8. Portable mechanical ventilator

effects of catecholamines, it is avoided when the surgeon plans to use relatively large amounts of subcutaneous epinephrine (plastic and oral surgery) or when the patient is receiving intravenous catecholamines.

Halothane has also been associated with a rare form of fulminant hepatitis which presents as postoperative fever and jaundice and may be indistinguishable from viral hepatitis. The incidence, about 1/35,000, is thought to be due to metabolites of halothane. This appears to be dependent upon the pre-existing liver disease or the degree of hypoxia of the liver.

Halothane is not, however, a direct hepato-toxin (in contrast to chloroform) and it does not cause liver damage in lower animals even at extremely high concentrations. The youngest case of halothane hepatitis was reported in an eight year old child, so it is safe to use it repeatedly in children under 8. In adults. It has been noted that the incidence of hepatitis is increased sevenfold if halothane is repeated within 3 months. As a matter of safety and for medicolegal reasons, its use should be avoided in cases where there is a potential for postoperative liver problems (trauma, history of viral hepatitis, liver surgery), or if the patient has taken enzyme-inducing drugs, such as phenobarbital, isoniazid etc. Halothane usually causes bradycardia and like other potent agents, decreases blood pressure by both cardiac depression and vasodilatation. Cardiac depression may be potentially beneficial in patients with ischemic heart disease, but may precipitate acute decompensation in patients with severe left ventricular dysfunction. Halothane is the most potent bronchodilator among the volatile agents, namely enflurane, isoflurane, desfiurane and sevoflurane.

Enflurane

Enflurane causes the greatest degree of both respiratory and cardiac depression of all the volatile agents, though the heart rate usually remains unaffected. Because enflurane is the only inhalational agent that causes "spike and dome" activity on the EEG and actually lowers the seizure threshold, it is not preferred in patients with a history of seizures. One of the metabolites of enflurane, free fluoride ion, is a direct nephrotoxin which may result (rarely) in polyuric (high output) renal failure. Although it may not be a problem in healthy individuals, it is a consideration in prolonged procedures and in those with pre-existing renal dysfunction since fluoride is cleared by the kidneys.

Isoflurane

Isoflurane is similar in structure to enflurane, as both are ether derivatives. It typically causes tachycardia which markedly increases cardiac oxygen consumption; therefore careful observation of the heart rate is necessary when it is used in patients with coronary artery disease. In concentrations of 1.0 MAC or less, isoflurane causes very little increase in cerebral blood flow and intracranial pressure (ICP) and depresses cerebral metabolic activity, more than halothane or enflurane. Thus, isoflurane is often used for intracranial surgery.

Desflurane

Desflurane is a potent inhalational agent that is rapidly taken up and eliminated. Because of its high volatility, it is administered from a heated, pressurized vaporizer. As the vapor is pungent, it is unsuitable for mask induction. In addition, when the inspired concentration is changed rapidly, tachycardia and hypertension may occur.

Sevoflurane

Sevoflurane is a potent inhalational agent that is taken up and eliminated nearly as rapidly as desfiurane and nitrous oxide. Because its vapor pressure is similar to that of conventional inhalational agents, it can be administered through a standard vaporizer. Pleasant to inhale, sevoflurane is quite suitable for mask induction, especially in children. Because the vapor is insoluble, emergence is rapid, it is well suited for outpatient surgery and mask induction of patients with potentially difficult airways. Although in many respects sevoflurane resembles an ideal anesthetic, it has several problems. The compound is extremely expensive. Secondly, it is metabolized to both fluoride and 'compound-A'. Increased fluoride levels appears to be only a minor problem, because it is rapidly eliminated. Compound-A is released by the reaction between sevoflurane and CO_2 absorbers (soda lime and baralyme), and is considered nephrotoxic. Again, the renal toxicity of compound-A appears to be theoretical and not clinically important, since it has been administered to millions of people in Japan, where it was first introduced, without evidence of renal toxicity.

Intravenous agents

These drugs are used for induction and occasionally for maintenance of anesthesia. Their advantage is the quick onset of action, but once given they are not easily eliminated and some, in larger doses, may cause delayed awakening. Elimination is dependent on the functions of liver and kidney.

Thiopental

This induction agent has a long record of safety since its introduction in the 1940's and is still a common induction agent used today. Its action is very short-lived because of redistribution out of the CNS into the bloodstream, hence it is an ideal agent for induction. However, the metabolism in the liver is slow, hence large doses may lead to prolonged somnolence. Thiopental causes significant vasodilatation and cardiac depression and is therefore avoided or given in reduced doses to hypovolemic patients (shock, trauma etc.) and in those with congestive heart failure.

Benzodiazepines

Diazepam (Valium) and midazolam (Versed) are often used for induction because they have minimal cardiovascular effects and are useful in patients with heart disease. The major difference between the two is that midazolam is much shorter acting (half-life of 2 hours as against 20 hours for diazepam).

Etomidate

Etomidate is an imidazole compound that is used as an alternative for induction of patients with cardiovascular disease. Like the benzodiazepines it produces very little change in hemodynamics. Its major drawbacks are pain on injection and abnormal muscular movements (myoclonus). In large doses for prolonged infusion (i.e., sedation of ICU patients) it may cause adrenal suppression.

Ketamine

Ketamine, chemically related to phencyclidine, produces a dissociative state of anesthesia. It is the only I.V induction agent that increases sympathetic outflow and in normal patients increases blood pressure and heart rate.

Advantages of ketamine

It is the drug of choice for hypovolemic patients (shock, trauma, etc.) because it causes the least fall in blood pressure of all the induction agents. It can be used as the sole maintenance anesthetic for superficial operations, because it produces profound analgesia and amnesia. It has no effect on pharyngeal reflexes, hence can be safely given in an emergency, where the patient may not be on empty stomach.It is especially useful for burn surgery because it tends to keep stable hemodynamics even in the presence of blood loss.

Drawbacks of ketamine

It causes direct cardiac depression which is often evident in patients with high preanes-thetic sympathetic tone. It is avoided in patients with coronary disease (tachycardia may induce ischemia) and in head injuries, since it increases ICP, the only I.V. agent to do so.

It is also not useful, for abdominal or delicate surgery because it produces no muscular relaxation, does not control visceral pain and patient often has a tendency to move. Another drawback is emergence delirium and bad dreams, especially when disturbed during recovery period which may be prevented by supplemental benzodiazepines or volatile agents.

Dose of ketamine: I.V up to 2mg/kg; IM up to 6mg/kg.

Propofol

Propofol is a short-acting induction agent that is associated with smooth, nausea-free emergence. Small doses also are useful for short-term sedation during brief procedures such as retrobulbar or peribulbar blocks in ophthalmology. The primary limitations of propofol are pain on injection and fall in blood pressure. The latter precludes use in patients who may be hypovolemic or in frank shock.

Narcotics

Narcotics are used in small doses to supplement volatile agents (balanced anesthesia) or in larger doses in combination with nitrous oxide and muscle relaxants, the so-called 'nitrous-narcotic' technique. Their advantages are that they produce profound analgesia and minimal cardiac depression. Their disadvantages are profound respiratory depression and poor amnesia when used alone. Morphine and meperidine are inexpensive and longer-acting agents that are sometimes used. More commonly the newer, short-acting opioids fentanyl (Sublimaze), sufentanil (Sufenta), and alfentanil (Alfenta) are used because they are more rapidly metabolized. Fentanyl is less expensive than the others.

Muscle relaxants

Succinylcholine

Succinylcholine (scoline) is a short-acting depolarizing muscle relaxant that is used for intubation. Because the duration of action is only five minutes, a patient who cannot be successfully intubated can be ventilated by mask for a short time until spontaneous respiration resumes. The side effects of succinylcholine are bradycardia, especially in children, and hyperkalemia in patients with bums, paraplegia, quadriplegia, and massive trauma. When combined with a volatile agent, it is also implicated in triggering malignant hyperthermia (MH) in susceptible individuals. It is therefore avoided in patients with a family history of MH or those with muscular dystrophy. Some anesthesiologists avoid succinylcholine in children, because it is a depolarizing agent and causes visible muscle fasciculations, it has been implicated in causing postoperative muscle pain. This can be reduced by pretreatment with a small dose of a nondepolarizing agent.

Non-depolarizing relaxants

The nondepolarizing relaxants are used when succinylcholine is contraindicated or when intraoperative relaxation is required such as in intra-abdominal procedures or mobilization of a joint. The longer-acting drugs pancuronium, d-tubocurare, and metocurine are useful for longer operations, while atracurium, vecuronium, mivacurium and rocuronium are used for shorter procedures. Knowledge of their individual side effects and route of metabolism play a major role in their selection by the anesthesiologist. The relaxant can be reversed at the end with an anticholinesterase (neostigmine or edrophonium), but atropine or glycopyrrolate must be included to counteract the muscarinic effects of the anticholinesterase.

Preoperative evaluation

Introduction

A detailed history and physical examination as done by the anesthesiologist is primarily focused on the airway, cardiovascular and pulmonary systems. However, significant problems in other organ systems are also scrutinized. For example, has the patient ever had a general anesthetic and were there any problems? Is the patient allergic to any drugs or is the patient currently on any medications? Family history is important for identifying patients with atypical pseudo-cholinesterase management. Malignant hyperthermia is transmitted as an autosomal dominant trait, hence it is very important to ask a patient about the first degree relatives who might have had high fever after an anesthetic.

Also of equal importance is evaluation of the airway. A significant proportion of anesthesia-related risk involves airway management and preoperative assesment will avoid unanticipated difficulties.

Organ systems of importance:

Cardiovascular

Pulmonary

Renal/GI/Neuro/Endocrine/Hematologic

Other anesthesia-specific concerns

In emergent situations, when time does not permit a full and detailed evaluation, the following mnemonic (AMPLE) is helpful in remembering what to ask for:

A: allergy/airway

M: medications

P: past medical history

L: last meal

E: event - what happened?

ASA Physical status classification system

Classification system adopted by the American Society of Anesthesiologists (ASA) for assessing preoperative physical status

I.   Normal healthy patient

II. Patient with mild systemic disease

III. Patient with severe systemic disease

IV. Patient with severe systemic disease that is

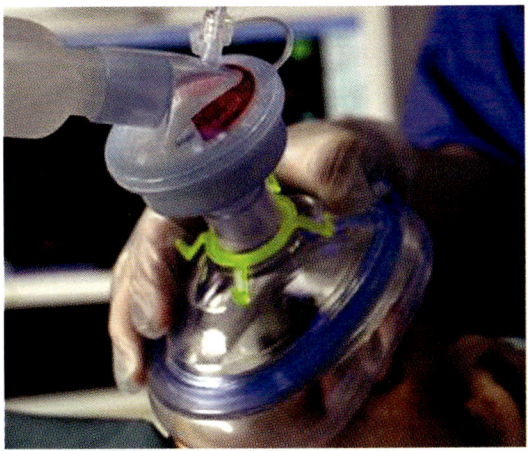

Fig. 101.9. Noninvasive ventilation using an air-tight mask

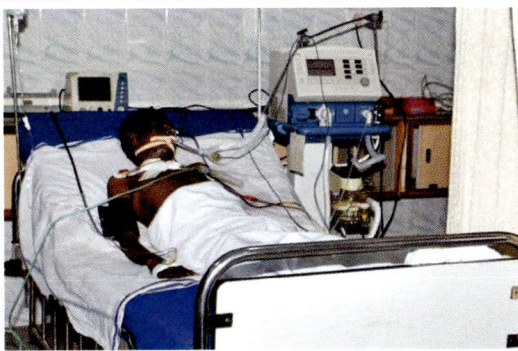

Fig. 101.10. Invasive ventilation with endotracheal intubation in an ICU

a constant threat to life

V. Moribund patient who is not expected to survive without the operation

VI. Brain-dead patient whose organs are being removed for transplantation

The addition of an 'E' indicates emergency surgery

Monitoring the anesthetized patients

Monitoring of anesthetized patients is designed to collect data that reflect:

(1) physiologic homeostasis, allowing prompt recognition of adverse changes

(2) responses to therapeutic interventions

(3) proper functioning of anesthetic equipment.

Monitoring may provide an early warning of adverse changes or trends before irreversible damage occurs, but the most important monitor in the operating room is the vigilant anesthesiologist, who continuously obtains subjective and objective inputs from the anesthetized patient. Subjective monitoring depends on the anesthesiologist's senses (visual, tactile, auditory) and experience. This is enhanced by the use of monitoring equipment designed to provide objective data relevant to the anesthetized patient's wellbeing and the integrity of the anesthesia system. Human vigilance is neither unlimited nor infallible, thus the importance of using monitors beyond the subjective inputs.

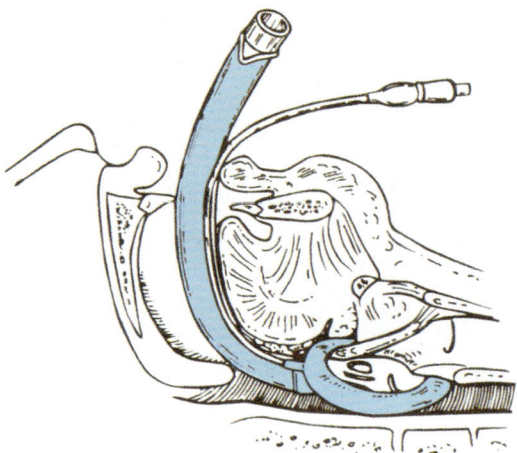
Fig. 101.11. Laryngeal mask closing the glottis

The ASA has adopted standards for basic intraoperative monitoring. They encourage or mandate the use of pulse oximetry, capnography, an oxygen analyzer, a disconnect alarm and a visual display electrocardiogram (ECG) in all patients under anesthesia. Additionally blood pressure and heart rate must be evaluated at least every 5 minutes. Depending on the patient's medical condition and the complexity of surgery, intraoperative monitoring may be expanded to include more technologically sophisticated and often invasive monitors. The inherent risks in the use of invasive monitors, must be weighed against the potential benefits in employing them on an individual basis.

Postoperative period

The Post Anesthesia Care Unit (PACU), also called postop recovery room, is where patients in transition between their anesthetized states toward their normal state are monitored. They may have been rendered unconscious, had their breathing and blood pressure controlled, or had major neural conduction block with a spinal or epidural anesthetic. Postoperative course is considered in the preop and intraop period in a variety of ways. Should a nerve block be placed for postop pain control? Has the patient had significant nausea after previous anesthesia and should he receive prophylactic medication? Will invasive monitoring be necessary to assess postoperative course (e.g. CVP, Swan-Ganz catheter).

Despite the best efforts, a number of complications are possible in the recovery period and must be watched for and promptly attended to. They include:

1. failure to awaken
2. cannot or will not breathe
3. hypertension or hypotension
4. abnormal cardiac rhythm
5. renal dysfunction
6. metabolic derangements
7. co-existing disease
8. temperature derangements
9. nausea and vomiting
10. airway obstruction.

Once discharge criteria are met, the patient may be shifted out from the PACU to their floor bed or to a day surgery unit.

GUIDELINES FOR DISCHARGE EVALUATION FROM A PACU

1. General condition: oriented to time, place, and surgical procedure

2. Responds to verbal input and follows simple instructions

3. Acceptable color without cyanosis, mottling or pallor

4. Adequate muscular strength and mobility for minimal self-care

5. Absence or control of specific acute surgical complications (e.g. bleeding, edema, neurologic weakness and low volume pulse)

6. Suitable control of nausea and emesis

7. Destination unit appropriate for patient's status

8. The blood pressure within ±20% of resting preoperative value

9. Heart rate and rhythm relatively constant for at least 30 min

10. Resolution of any new dysrhythmia

11. Acceptable intravascular volume status

12. Any suspicion of myocardial ischemia rectified

13. Ventilation and oxygenation: ventilatory rate greater than 10, less than 30 breaths/min

14. Forced vital capacity approximately twice tidal volume

15. Adequate ability to cough and clear secretions

16. Qualitatively acceptable respiratory excusions

17. Airway maintenance: protective reflexes (swallow, gag etc.) are intact

18. Absence of stridor, retraction, or partial obstruction

19. No further need for artificial airway support

20. Control of pain: ability to localize and identify intensity of surgical pain

21. Adequate analgesia, at least 15 min since last opioid

22. Safe, appropriate orders for post discharge analgesics

23. Renal function: urine output 30-60 ml/hr (catheterized patients)

24. Appropriate color and appearance of urine, evaluation of hematuria

25. Follow-up orders to measure renal output if spontaneous voiding has not occurred

26. Metabolic/laboratory: acceptable hematocrit level in view of hydration, volume deficit and potential for future losses

27. Suitable control of blood glucose

28. Appropriate electrolyte homeostasis

29. Evaluation of chest radiograph, ECG, and other tests as appropriate

30. Ambulatory patients: ability to ambulate without dizziness, hypotension or support

Not all criteria will be satisfied on all occasions by every patient, especially if discharge is to a critical care unit. Clinical judgment must always supersede established guidelines if the patient's condition is less than optimal in a

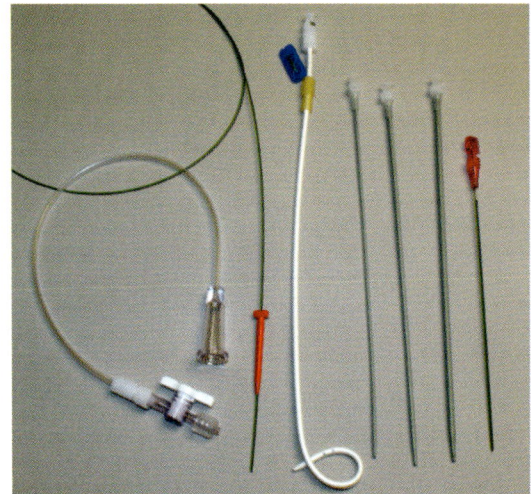

Fig.101.12. Cook's retrograde tracheal intubation guidewire

given area. Whenever doubt exists about diagnosis or patient safety, discharge should be deferred.

Retrograde tracheal intubation

There are some situations where the laryngeal inlet cannot be visualized normally through the mouth, such as severe trismus, oral/pharyngeal tumors, temporomandibular ankylosis etc.

Technic: Using a special intubation kit (Cook), a guidewire is passed by puncturing the trachea percutaneously, under local anesthesia, just below the cricoid ring, to go through the glottis and reach the oral cavity. An endotracheal tube is then 'rail-roaded' into the trachea over the guidewire and the wire withdrawn.

One lung ventilation (OLV)

During certain procedures, such as thoracic surgery, thoracoscopic operations on lung or esophagus, it becomes necessary to keep the lung collapsed to facilitate exposure. During this period, the other lung has to be adequately ventilated, using a double-lumened endotracheal tube, with tracheal and bronchial cuffs, for maintaining air-tight control for positive pressure breathing.

Central venous pressure (CVP)

Also known as right atrial pressure (RAP), is an

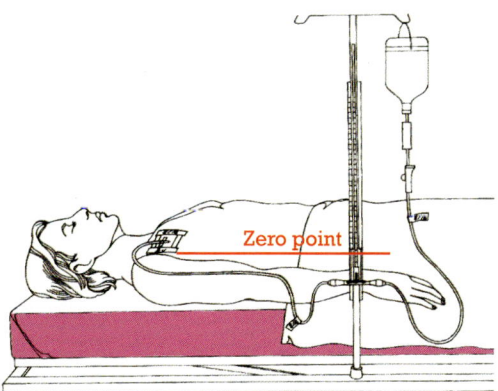

Fig. 101.13. Central venous pressure monitoring setup

index of the amount of blood returning to the right atrium and the ability of the heart to pump it into the arterial system. It has been estimated that about 70% of blood volume is in the venous system and any changes in the volume is initially reflected in the venous pressure, before the alteration of arterial pressure. A central vein is defined as the vein in continuity with the right atrium without any valves interposed; i.e., essentially the vena cavae and possibly their main tributaries.

The setup: A catheter is introduced percutaneously into the SVC (more common) or IVC and is connected to a manometer and an infusion set, through a 3-way hookup, as shown in the fig. 101.13. Right internal jugular vein in the neck or subclavian vein under the clavicle are the preferred points for SVC access. Common femoral vein at the groin may be used for IVC access. A long peripheral venous catheter introduced at the elbow, its tip placed in SVC, may also be used for the purpose. The 'zero-point is fixed at the level of right atrium (level of midaxillary line in a patient lying flat). Periodic measurements of CVP are made to monitor the fluid load vs cardiac output (normal is 8-15cm of water), thereby liberal fluid infusion may be given without fear of overload.

Situations where the CVP is high

Circulatory overload (hypervolemia)

Cardiac failure
Tension pneumothorax
Massive pleural effusion
Cardiac tamponade
Valsalva maneuver

Situations where the CVP is low

Hypovolemia
Deep inspiration
Increase venous compliance

The initial enthusiasm of using the CVP in intensive care units (in early 70s) has been

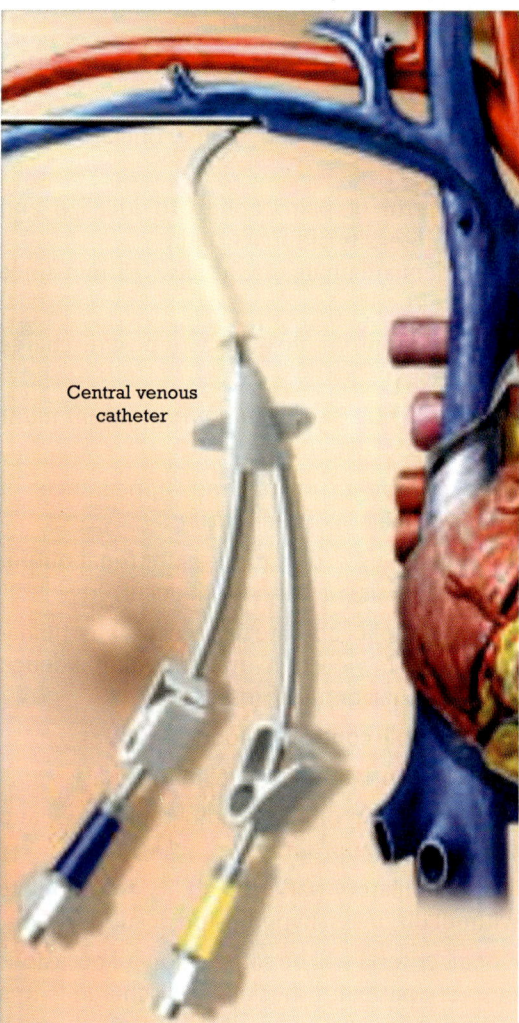

Fig. 101.14. CVP catheter introduced through right subclavian vein

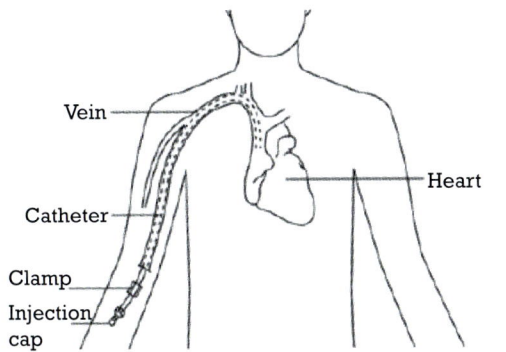

Fig. 101.15. A long peripheral venous catheter, pushed into SVC, for CVP monitoring

replaced by measuring pulmonary capillary wedge pressure (PCWP), using a Swan-Ganz catheter, which is considered to be more sensitive to hemodynamic changes. However, by virtue of its simplicity, CVP monitoring is still useful in not-so-critical situations. The central venous catheter may also be used to infuse hypertonic solutions and for TPN administration.

Complications of central venous cannulation

1.   Arterial puncture and hematoma
2.   Pneumothorax
3.   Air embolism
4.   Cardiac arrhythmia, if the catheter is advanced too far into the cardiac chamber. It should not be introduced beyond 15 cm from the point of entry into the jugular vein.
5.   Sepsis
6.   Venous thromboembolism

Medical imaging is the technique and process employed to create images of the human body (or parts and function thereof) for clinical application. It is a method by which images of internal tissues can be generated non-invasively, by means of observed signals. Although imaging of removed body parts can also be performed for medical reasons, it becomes part of pathological examination. Measurement and techniques which are not primarily designed to produce images, such as electroencephalography (EEG), magnetoencephalography (MEG), electrocardiography (ECG) etc. but which produce data represented as maps (i.e., containing positional or electrical information), may also considered as medical imaging.

The discovery of x-rays by Wilheim Conrad Rontgen in 1895 has opened a new era of diagnostic imaging in medicine.

In the clinical context, imaging by 'invisible light' is generally equated to radiology. 'Visible light' medical imaging involves digital video or still pictures that can be seen without special processing or equipment. As a field of scientific investigation, medical imaging constitutes a subdiscipline of biomedical engineering, research and development of which has greatly contributed to the growth of diagnostic and therapeutic imaging in the recent decades.

DIAGNOSTIC IMAGING

Two main forms of radiographic images are in medical imaging; projection radiology (static) and fluoroscopy (dynamic), the latter being useful in catheter guidance. These 2-D techniques are still in wide use despite the advent of 3-D tomography (CT), due to their low cost, high resolution and lower radiation dosages.

Fluoroscopy produces real-time images of internal structures, employing constant input of x-rays, at a lower dose rate. Earlier used image receptor, to convert the radiation into images, later gave way to an Image Amplifier, a large vacuum tube with a receiving end coated with cesium iodide and a mirror at the opposite end, eventually the mirror has been replaced by TV camera and monitor.

Projectional radiographs, commonly referred to as x-rays, may be plain pictures or employing radio-opaque contrast media, such as barium, iothalamate (Conray), gadolinium or sometimes air, to study the internal anatomy.

It has to be realized that about 0.02mSv of radiation is received while undergoing a plain x-ray and the dose received while doing a CT scan is equal to 400 x-rays.

Projection imaging

As already indicated the object to be imaged is brought as close to the plate as possible, as shown in some examples here :

Chest: PA view, to delineate the cardiac silhouette and great vessels.

AP view to visualize the posterior mediastinum, esophagus or dorsal spine.

It is of great value not only for routine health screening, but also in the evaluation of malignancies. In suspected malignancy, involvement of four areas have to be looked for in a chest skiagram:

1. pulmonary parenchyma (coin shadows or consolidation)
2. pleura (effusion)
3. lymph nodes (hilar or mediastinal)
4. bony structures (ribs, sternum, clavicle and vertebrae).

Abdomen: AP view, to see the retroperitoneal structures, such as aorta, pancreas, kidneys or ureters. Radioopaque calculi in urinary, biliary tract or pancreas may be visualized. A gallstone may be confused with right renal calculus, but lateral view will show the former anterior to the vertebral column.

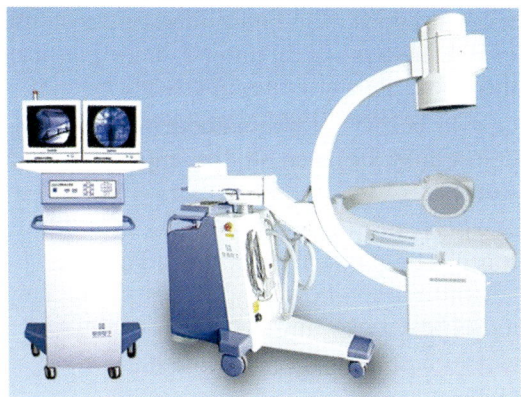

Fig. 102.1. X-ray machine with C-arm

Paranasal sinuses or facial bones: PA view

Some of the special studies are described here:

C-arm X-Ray unit

This system, so named because of its overall appearance, is used where greater positional flexibility in the examination process is needed, such as ortho, neuro or cardiac imaging. Modern C-arm equipment is a versatile gadget with the following components and special features:

Components

X-ray source
X-ray image intensifier (XRII), which converts x-rays into visible image
Tilt table for appropriate positioning of patient
Fluoroscopic exposure and program control
Post processing software
Viewing monitors

Special features

Real time viewing
Remote control keyboard
Contrast correction
Zoom and freezing image
Digital subtraction

Applications

Peripheral/cerebral angiography studies
Interventional procedures such as TIPS, transjugular liver biopsy, vascular stenting and embolization
Cardiac catheterization and coronary interventions
Orthopedic and neurological procedures

Digital Radiography

This is a form of x-ray imaging, where digital sensors are used instead of traditional photographic films. Advantages include time efficiency through bypassing chemical processing and ability to review immediately, digitally enhance, transfer or store images and involves less radiation. This is essentially filmless x-ray imaging, by digital technology, using a special image capture device, store it in a retrievable file, for interpretation and saved as part of patient's medical record. Besides improved expediency and quality of imaging, its potential to reduce the cost of processing and storage of films is the main motivating factor for the hospitals to quickly adopt digital x-ray technology.

Barium swallow: it is a picture taken while the patient is swallowing the barium, to visualize the pharynx and esophagus. The barium used is thicker than that used for Barium meal, to delay the esophageal transit time of the contrast, hence generally both the studies are not done together.

Indications: dysphagia and suspected Ca or benign causes of obstruction

Motility disorders, including achalasia cardia

Assessment of cardiac (left atrial) enlargement or SOL of superior/posterior mediastinum

Pharyngeal diverticulum

If tracheo-esophageal fistula or esophageal perforation is suspected, water soluble contrast, such as meglumine diatrizoate (Gastrograffin) is preferred.

Findings: Malignancy: persistent irregular filling defect, with proximal/distal shouldering and minimal proximal dilatation

Benign stricture: long segment narrowing without mucosal irregularity

Achalasia cardia: gross dilatation and sometimes elongation of esophagus, with typical 'rat-tailed' deformity

Scleroderma: dilatation, impaired peristalsis with gastro-esophageal reflux.

Barium meal series: It is a study of GI tract, usually stomach and beyond, sometimes up to the colon, depending upon the indication. If intestinal obstruction or perforation is suspected, Gastrograffin is used instead of barium sulfate, for fear of precipitating obstruction or causing barium peritonitis. Pictures are taken at regular intervals, usually 5, 30, 60 min, 3 and 6 hrs after ingestion of contrast, concluding the study after the pathology is identified.

Gastrografin sometimes has a therapeutic value, in relieving the obstruction, by its osmotic effect.

Indications: lesions of upper GI tract, such as peptic ulcer, malignancy, pyloroduodenal obstruction, pseudocyst of pancreas and diseases of small bowel. It is not very sensitive to detect causes of upper GI bleeding, where endoscopy is much preferred, which also facilitates therapeutic intervention.

Findings:

Uncomplicated **duodenal ulcer:** crater in proximal duodenum, with radiating mucosal folds or deformed duodenal cap

Complicated by stenosis: dilated stomach with giant waves, delayed emptying, non-visualization of duodenal cap. The typical mottling (honey-combing) may be seen in the stomach due to retained food particles and there may be secondary gastric ulcer in the body.

Gastric ulcer: ulcer crater (niche), usually over the lesser curve and a notch in the opposite greater curve, due to spasm of the circular muscle fibres of stomach. Ulcer over the greater curve, larger than 3cm, likely to be malignant.

Malignancy: depending upon the location in the stomach. At GE junction, there may be esophageal obstruction due to the persistent irregular mass. In the body, only a mass or a large ulcer may be seen. At the pylorus, it may have features of gastric outlet obstruction mentioned, except the gastric dilatation may not be as great as in benign disease. In diffuse infiltrating type of carcinoma (linitis plastica), the gastric peristalsis may be absent.

Gastric bezoars: Large smooth mobile filling defect may be seen in the antrum/body of stomach

Barium enema

It is a retrograde study of the large bowel, by administration of contrast through the rectum. It may be done by single or double contrast.

Indications: Change in bowel habit
Melena
Mass suspected to be arising from colon
Subacute large gut obstruction
IBD, tuberculosis, Crohn's disease of colon, colonic diverticulosis
Gastrocolic fistula, intussusception.

Contraindications

Toxic megacolon
Pseudomembranous colitis
Colonic perforation.

Findings:

Tuberculosis: see chapter 18 on abdominal tuberculosis

Idiopathic ulcerative colitis: Disease starts from rectum and progresses towards terminal ileum
loss of haustral pattern (pipe stem colon)
Fine granular mucosal surface, due to pseudo-polypi and ulceration
Strictures and malignancy may supervene.

Crohn's disease (granulomatous colitis) : multiple ulcerations

Thickening and distortion valvulae conniventes (in the terminal ileum)

Strictures with skipped lesions (string sign of Cantor)

Cobblestone pattern of bowel and fistula formation.

Malignancy: circumferential or eccentric mass with narrow lumen
There may be hold up (partial obstruction) of barium proximal to the lesion
Mucosal ulcerations

Benign polyp: may be single or multiple
Rounded filling defect; may be sessile or pedunculated

Entire colon may be studded in familial polyposis coli (FPC)

Intussusception: sudden cut off of barium with 'pincer' or 'meniscus' sign

It should not be done if bowel gangrene is suspected

Diverticulosis: situated more in the left colon

Multiple out pouching of mucosa, with saw-tooth appearance

Residual barium seen in the pouches after the evacuation of barium

Fistula (into urinary bladder or vagina) may be seen

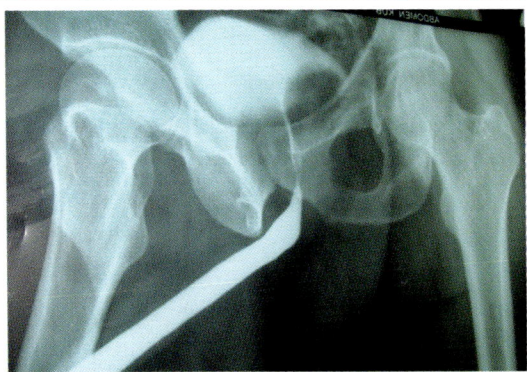

Fig. 102.3. Normal ascending urethrogram

Strictures may be seen, due to mass formation.

Urography

Urethrography or cysto-urethrography, may be done retrograde injection via urethra (ascending cysto-urethrogram- ACU) or by intravenous injection of contrast, to study the urodynamics of micturition, including the presence of vesico-ureteric reflux, called micturating cysto-urethrogram (MCU).

Excretion urography or intravenous urography (IVU) is a time-honored imaging modality of upper (pelvi-calyceal system) and lower urinary tract

Antegrade pyelography is injection of contrast through a nephrostomy or pyelostomy tube to see the distal anatomy.

Retrograde pyelography is to inject contrast through a ureteric catheter introduced into the renal pelvis via cystoscopic examination, to study the pelvi-calyceal system.

Renography is referred to nuclear imaging (scintiscan) of kidneys, to identify and quantitate their differential function.

Special contrast studies

Fistulography (to outline a bowel, branchial, periurethral or perianal fistula

Sialography (through either Stenson's or Wharton's duct)

Spleno-portography (in portal hypertension).

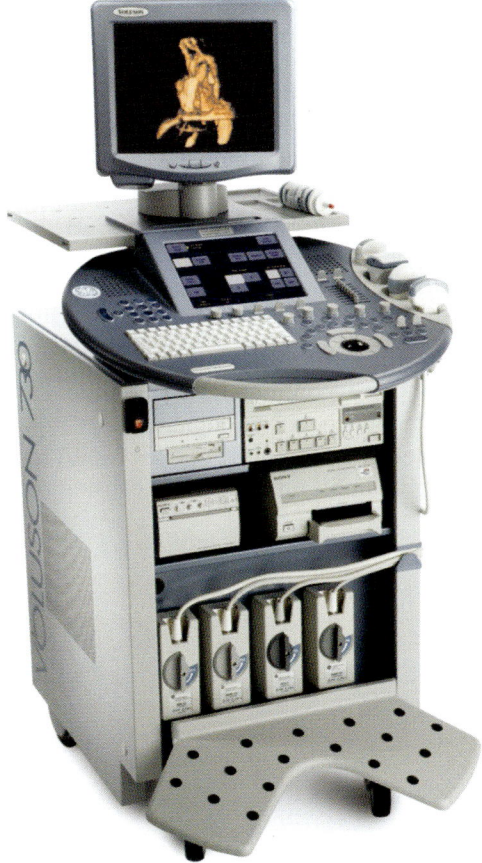

Fig. 102.2. 4D Ultrasonographic machine

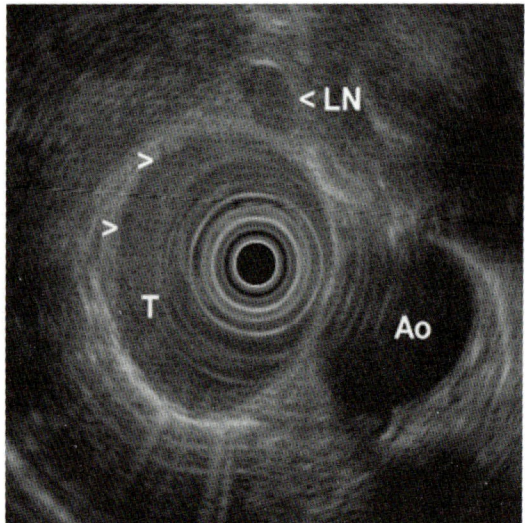

Fig. 102.4. Radial EUS in a patient with a T3N1 esophagus cancer. The tumor (T) has invaded through the muscularis propria (arrowheads) and is therefore staged as T3. A clear plane of separation between tumor ands aorta (Ao) exists and a 5 mm lymph node (LN) with features suspicious of malignancy is also seen.

Oral cholecystography (Graham Cole), before and after fat meal, to see the concentrating, contracting functions and filling defects in the GB (not done nowadays, replaced by USG).

Cholangiography (PTC, ERCP, I.V or peroperative cholangiography, MRCP etc)

Myelography (to demonstrate intraspinal lesions, such as prolapsed intervertebral disc, hematoma or a tumor. After the advent of CT/MRI, this study is rarely done.

Bronchography is done by instilling a contrast (Lipoidol, Iohexol or Visciodol) into the trachea to study the bronchial tree

Phlebography (see chapter 82).

Angiography (arteriography) or aortography (see chapter 77).

ULTRASONOGRAPHY (USG)

Medical ultrasonography uses high frequency broadband sound waves in the megahertz range that are reflected by tissue to a varying degrees to produce 3-D images and probably is the most common imaging modality in day-to-

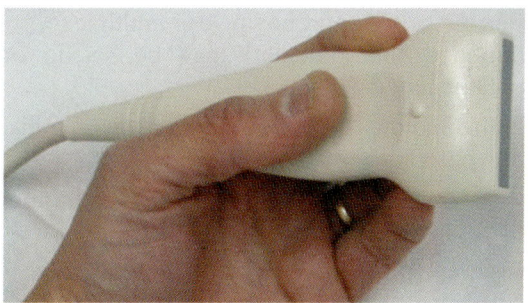

Fig. 102.5. Linear Array Transducer

day clinical use today, for the following reasons:

1. availability
2. portability
3. cost-effective
4. fast learning curve
5. devoid of use of ionizing radiation
6. low cost of maintenance of equipment

With improved expertise, its applications have widened to virtually every branch of medicine. However for optimal sonographic resolution, there should be no gas in the medium, hence not ideally suited for imaging thoracic cavity, hollow gas-filled abdominal viscera or those structures overlapped by them. Another innovation for better resolution is endo-ultrasound, such as trans-esophageal, trans-gastric, trans-vaginal, trans-rectal, intravascular ultrasound (IVUS). USG is also not suitable to image bony lesions.

Being a very common imaging modality in clinical practice, more detailed description is warranted. Ultrasound produces sound waves that are beamed into the body causing return

Jewels of Gyan - 102.1

Frequency of Sound Waves

Frequency of sound waves is measured as Hertz units (earlier called cycles per sec.)
KHz: 1,000 Hz
MHZ: 1,000 KHz or 1,000,000 Hz
Normal audible range: 20 Hz to 20 KHz
Medical Ultrasound: 2 MHz to 18 MHz

echoes that are recorded to 'visualize' structures beneath the skin. The ability to measure different echoes reflected from a variety of tissues allows a shadow picture to be constructed. The technology is especially accurate at seeing the interface between solid and fluid filled spaces, very similar to the principle of *sonar* on boats to see the bottom of the ocean.

In physics, the term 'ultrasound' applies to all sound waves with a frequency above the audible range of human hearing. The frequencies used in medical ultrasound are typically between 2 and 18 MHz.

Lower frequencies produce less resolution but image deeper into the body. Higher frequency sound waves have a smaller wavelength and thus are capable of reflecting or scattering from smaller structures. Higher frequency sound waves also have a larger attenuation coefficient and thus are more readily absorbed in tissue, limiting the depth of penetration of the sound wave into the body. Sonographers typically use a hand-held piezoelectric probe (called a transducer) that is placed directly on and moved over the patient.

The creation of an image from sound is done in three steps - producing a sound wave, receiving and interpreting the echoes. Typically solid structures in an USG are seen white, whereas fluid (gas or liquid) creates a black image.

Modes of sonography

Several different modes of ultrasound are used in medical imaging. These are:

A-mode: A-mode is the simplest type of ultrasound. A single transducer scans a line through the body with the echoes plotted on screen as a function of depth. Therapeutic ultrasound aimed at a specific tumor or calculus is also A-mode, to allow for pinpoint accurate focus of the destructive wave energy.

B-mode (B - brightness): In this ultrasound, a linear array of transducers simultaneously scans a plane through the body that can be viewed as a two-dimensional image on screen.

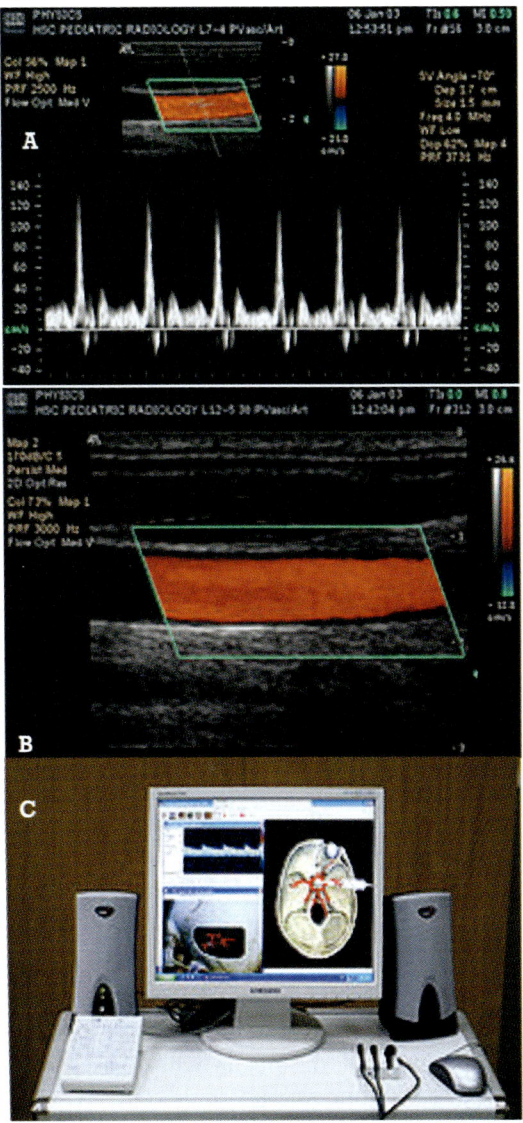

Fig. 102.6. **A.** Spectral Doppler of carotid artery **B.** Color Doppler of common carotid artery **C.** Computer-enhanced intracranial Doppler

C-mode: Here the image is formed in a plane normal to a B-mode image. A gate that selects data from a specific depth from an A-mode line is used; then the transducer is moved in the 2D plane to sample the entire region at this fixed depth. When the transducer traverses the area in a spiral, an area of 100 cm^2 can be scanned in around 10 seconds.

M-mode (M - motion): Ultrasound pulses are emitted in quick succession - each time, either an A-mode or B-mode image is taken. Over time, this is analogous to recording a video in ultrasound. As the organ boundaries that produce reflections move relative to the probe, this can be used to determine the velocity of specific organ structures.

Doppler mode: This mode makes use of the Doppler effect in measuring and visualizing blood flow

Color Doppler: Velocity information is presented as a color-coded overlay on top of a B-mode image

Continuous Doppler: Doppler information is sampled along a line through the body, and all velocities detected at each time point is presented (on a time line)

Pulsed wave (PW) **Doppler**: Doppler information is sampled from only a small sample volume (defined in 2D image), and presented on a timeline

Duplex: a common name for the simultaneous presentation of 2D and (usually) PW doppler information. (using modern ultrasound machines color doppler is almost always also used, hence the alternative name Triplex)

Pulse inversion mode: In this mode two successive pulses with opposite sign are emitted and then subtracted from each other. This implies that any linearly responding constituent will disappear while gases with non-linear compressibility stands out.

Harmonic mode: In this mode a deep penetrating fundamental frequency is emitted into the body and a harmonic overtone is detected. In this way depth penetration can be gained with improved lateral resolution.

Doppler sonography

Spectral Doppler of common carotid artery.
Color Doppler of common carotid artery.
Computer-enhanced transcranial doppler.

Contrast-enhanced ultrasound

The use of microbubble contrast media in medical sonography to improve ultrasound signal backscatter is known as contrast-enhanced ultrasound. This technique is currently used in echocardiography, and may have future applications in molecular imaging and drug delivery.

Compression ultrasonography

Compression ultrasonography is a technique used for diagnosing deep vein thrombosis and combines ultrasonography of the deep veins with venous compression. The technique can be used on deep veins of the upper and lower extremities, with some laboratories limiting the examination to the common femoral and popliteal veins, whereas others extend it to the calf, including the soleal veins.

Compression ultrasonography in B-mode has both high sensitivity and specificity for detecting proximal deep vein thrombosis in symptomatic patients (sensitivity: 90 to 100% and the specificity: 95 to 100%).

Drawbacks of USG

Sonographic devices have trouble penetrating bone. For example, sonography of the adult brain is of very limited value, though innovations are being made in transcranial ultrasonography.

Sonography performs very poorly when there is a gas between the transducer and the organ of interest, due to the extreme differences in acoustic impedance. For example, overlying gas in the gastrointestinal tract often makes ultrasound scanning of the pancreas difficult, and lung imaging is less than ideal, except for demarcating pleural effusion.

Even in the absence of bone or air, the depth penetration of ultrasound may be limited depending on the frequency of imaging, causing difficulties in visualizing structures deep in the body, especially in obese patients.

This is operator-dependent; a high level of skill and experience is needed to acquire good quality images and make accurate interpretation.

Tomography

Linear tomography is the most basic form of

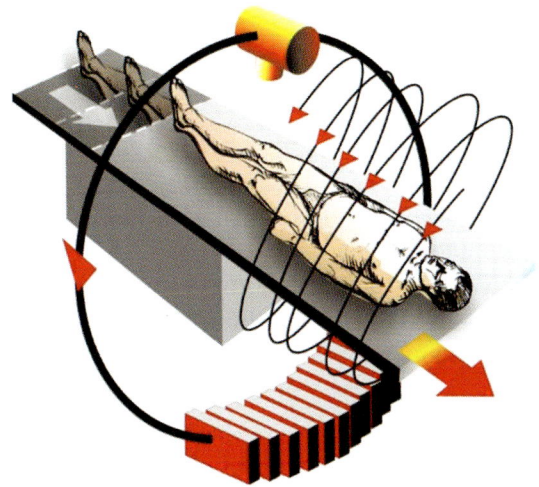

Fig. 102.7. Scheme of spiral CT

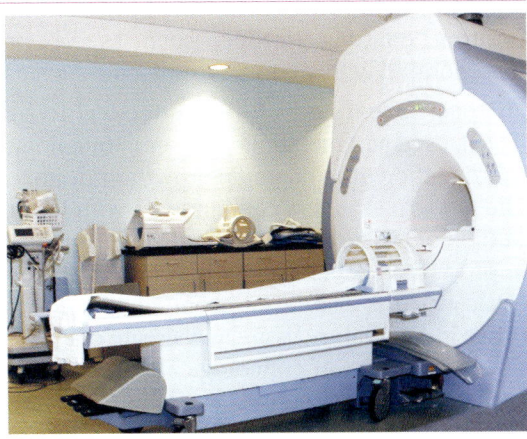

Fig. 102.8. MRI scanner

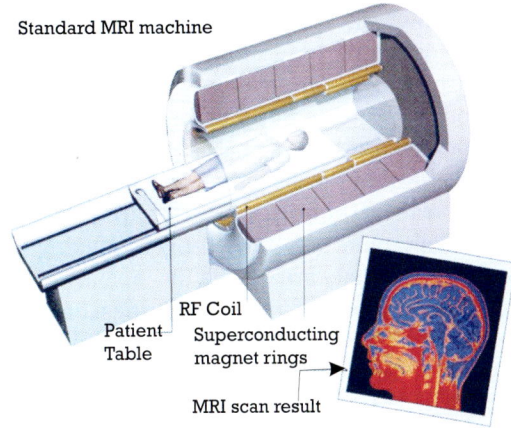

Standard MRI machine

RF Coil

Patient Table

Superconducting magnet rings

MRI scan result

Fig. 102.9. Scheme of MRI scanner

radiology, to serially image in single plane in 'slices' and arrive at 3-D orientation of the imaged object. Many advances were made in this technique, of which orthopantomography (OPG) and computed axial tomography (CAT or CT) are notable. The invention of CT by Hounsfield in 1971, may be considered as important landmark in the medical imaging technology, which has further advanced to multi-slice modality, by developing machines capable of taking 64, 128 or 256 slices in a second, shortening the scanning time, minimizing the radiation dose and eliminating the blurring effect on resolution due to physiological movements such a cardiac and respiratory activities (movement artifact). It is also useful in pediatrics or dealing with uncooperative or restless patients, since the required period of 'no movement' during exposure is very short. Injection of contrast (iodine containing) is used to improve tissue differentiation and diagnostic accuracy.

The density of the tissue as seen in a CT scan is measured in *Hounsfield units* (HU)

Water:	0 HU
Air:	-1000 HU
Fat:	-50 to 100 HU
CSF:	+3 HU
Clotted blood:	+60 to 80 HU

White matter:	+22 to 32 HU
Gray matter:	+36 to 46 HU
Bone:	+100 to 1000 HU

Helical (Spiral) CT

A spiral CT scan (also known as helical CT) is a new specialized CT technique that involves continuous movement of the patient through the scanner with the ability to scan faster with higher definition, but generating less noise. The spiral CT allows greater visualization of blood vessels and internal viscera in abdominal and thoracic cavities. This form may be particularly useful in the rapid evaluation a patient with multiple injuries.

Positron emission tomography (PET)

It is a molecular imaging, where a short-lived

positron emitting isotope, such as ^{18}F, is incorporated with an organic molecule such as glucose, creating ^{18}F-fluorodeoxyglucose (FDG), used as a metabolic marker in oncology, utilizing the virtue of rapid growth of tumors. The modern scanners combine PET with CT or MRI, to optimize the image reconstruction and improve the spatial orientation. However, the FDG, which is also taken up by metabolically active inflammatory tissue may create diagnostic difficulties in oncological evaluation. Further the information available may be suboptimal in poorly controlled diabetics.

Magnetic resonance imaging (MRI)

Also known as nuclear magnetic resonance (NMR) imaging uses powerful magnets to polarize and excite hydrogen nuclei (single photon) in water molecules in human tissue, producing detectable signals, which is spatially coded, resulting in images. The MRI machine emits radiofrequency (RF) pulses that specifically bind only to hydrogen, making its protons in that area spin in a particular direction, known as 'resonance', measured as Tesla units. These measurable signals collected through an RF antenna, producing 3-D images.

Differences between CT and MRI

1. Since MRI does not use ionizing radiation (x-rays), there is no radiation hazard to the patient or the technician handling the machine, unlike in CT.
2. The MRI is based on magnetic properties of the tissue, different resolution of isodense tissues makes it superior in terms of soft tissue contrasting than CT, which is a density-based imaging.
3. In MRI, however, there is a distinct health hazard associated with tissue heating from exposure to RF field in the presence of implanted metallic devices, such as pacemakers, orthopedic plates etc. limiting the scanning options.
4. CT scan is cheaper than MRI. Both are contraindicated during the first trimester of pregnancy.

Thermography

Commonly employed in breast, it utilizes the principle of higher metabolic activity and vascularity in both precancerous or cancerous tissues, leading to raised local surface temperature, often an earliest sign of malignancy. This is detected only by extremely sensitive infrared cameras and sophisticated computers, to identify and analyze the temperature variations, aiding diagnosis.

INTERVENTIONAL RADIOLOGY

The role of radiology has expanded from simple diagnostic imaging to sophisticated therapeutic interventions in virtually every branch of medicine. It may be for non-vascular or vascular indications.

Non-vascular

1. **Biopsy** or aspiration under image guidance

USG or CT are most commonly used modalities for these relatively simple daycare procedures. Biopsy from abdominal solid viscera, lymph nodes in inaccessible locations may be obtained using either fine or core needle, as appropriate. The availability of coaxial Trucut needle has made the procedure expedient and faster. Trans-jugular route is another option for liver biopsy, in the presence of coagulopathy or gross ascites.

Catheter drainage of hepatic, sub diaphragmatic or splenic abscess, may be performed.

Contraindications: Bleeding diathesis, critical vascular structures in the needle pathway, gross ascites for liver biopsy

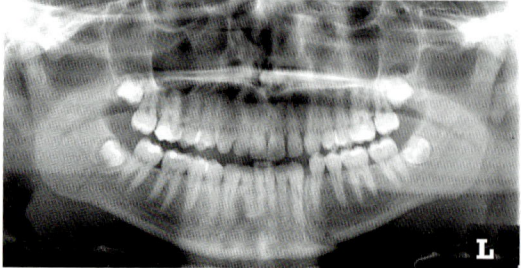

Fig. 102.10. Orthopantomogram (OPG) showing fracture left mandibular body
(courtesy: Dr Taritha Ram, Chennai)

2. **Hepatobiliary**: Endoscopic retrograde cholangio-pancreaticogram (ERCP), percutaneous transhepatic cholangiogram (PTC) and percutaneous transhepatic bilary drainage (PTBD)

3. **Urinary**: percutaneous nephrolithotomy (PCNL), percutaneous nephrostomy

4. Other procedures: catheter drainage of pseudocyst of pancreas, reduction of multiple pregnancy, retrieval of ovum or zygote in assisted reproductive technology (ART)

Vascular

1. **Percutaneous transluminal angioplasty** (PTA) and stenting

2. **Therapeutic embolization** to reduce vascularity of tumors before surgery or definitive treatment for arterio-venous malformations (AVM), aneurysms or gastrointestinal bleeding

3. **Deploying prosthetic stents** for aneurysm or AV fistula

4. **Transjugular intrahepatic portosystemic shunt** (TIPSS) or liver biopsy

5. Placement of **venacaval filter**s to prevent pulmonary embolization

6. **Chemo-embolization** by selective catheterization, to deliver maximum dose of drug to the tumor tissue

7. **Transcatheter thrombolysis**, in thrombotic episodes

8. **Deploying devices** to close atrial septal defect (ASD), ventricular septal defect (VSD) or patent ductus arteriosus (PDA)

Other **therapeutic applications** of USG

Therapeutic applications use ultrasound to bring heat or agitation into the body. Therefore much higher energies are used than in diagnostic ultrasound. In many cases the range of frequencies used are also very different.

It is sometimes used to clean teeth in dental hygiene. It may be used to generate regional heating and mechanical changes in biological tissue, e.g. in occupational therapy, physical therapy and cancer treatment. However the use of ultrasound in the treatment of musculoskeletal conditions has fallen out of favor.

Focused ultrasound may be used to break up kidney stones by lithotripsy.

It may be used for cataract treatment by phacoemulsification.

Additional physiological effects of low-intensity ultrasound have recently been discovered, e.g. its ability to stimulate bone-growth and its potential to disrupt the blood-brain barrier for drug delivery.

It is procoagulant at 5-12 MHz and may be used to control internal bleeding.

Nuclear Medicine

Also known as Molecular medicine, it encompasses both diagnostic and therapeutic application of certain properties of isotopes and energetic particles emitted from radioactive material, utilizing certain physiological

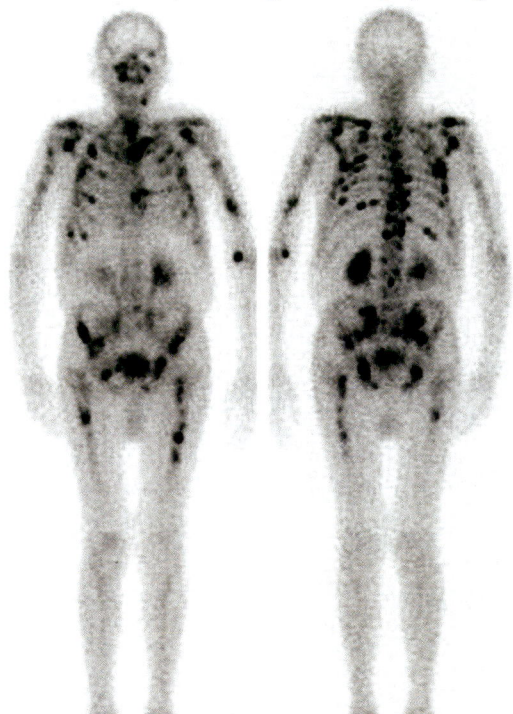

Fig. 102.11. ^{99m}Tc skeletal scan showing multiple metastatic lesions

properties of the target tissue. Gamma cameras are used in scintigraphy (diagnostic mapping of an isotope) such as single-photon emission computed tomography (SPECT) and positron emission tomography (PET), to detect biological activity that may be peculiar to certain pathological tissues. For instance, [123]I (half life of 13 hours) or [131]I (half life of 8 days), which is preferentially absorbed by thyroid tissue, is administered to a patient, captured by the gamma camera, creating a count and a 2-D image of the radio-pharmaceuticals, outlining the areas of normal and abnormal activity. This process of emitting gamma rays due to natural decaying of the isotope, essentially converts the human body into a source of radioactivity. It is mainly used in neurology and cardiology, at the present time.

Technitium[99m] (^{99m}Tc), with a half-life of 6 hours, is the most widely used radioisotope in medicine now, which is commercially generated from Molybdenum[99] (half life of 66 hours). [99m]Tc is ideally suited, since its half life is long enough to allow diagnostic imaging and short enough to minimize radiation dose. There are over 30 commercially available radio-pharmaceuticals based on ^{99m}Tc, used for functional imaging of organs such as brain, myocardium, thyroid, salivary glands, lungs, liver, spleen, gallbladder, Meckel's diverticulum, GI bleeding. kidneys, skeleton, sentinel lymph node, neuroendocrine tumors and many more.

The other applications of nuclear medicine

Thyrotoxicosis, differentiated thyroid cancers (^{131}I) and gastro-esophageal reflux disease (GERD), with ^{99m}Tc-Sulfur colloid.

Hepatobiliary (Bulida) scan, can be performed

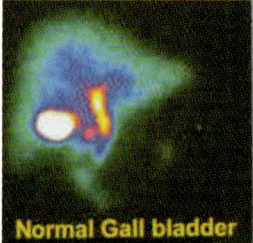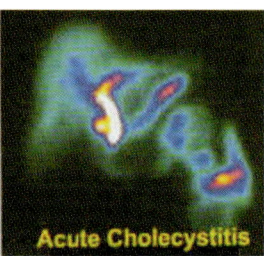

Normal Gall bladder   **Acute Cholecystitis**

Fig. 102.12. Bulida scan identifying gallbladder disease

in the presence of liver dysfunction with high levels of serum bilirubin, by using ^{99m}Tc-mebrofenin, to study the function of liver, gallbladder and anatomy of biliary tree. The ejection fraction of the gallbladder may also be assessed by giving fatty meal (normal >65%), to quantify biliary dyskinesia (motility disorder of gallbladder). Another agent used is ^{99m}Tc-labelled hepatic iminodiacetic acid known as HIDA scan.

Neuroendocrine tumors (APUD) can be imaged by ^{99m}Tc-Sestamibi or ^{99m}Tc-Tetrofosmin.

Conclusion

With the plethora of imaging modalities available, the physician has to exercise profound wisdom to choose the right one at the right place, to make the methodology in arriving at the diagnosis safe, expedient and cost-effective, realizing the virtues and limitations of each modality. Needless to say that simple, non-invasive and less expensive investigations have to be done initially and go to the next step only if these are not providing sufficient information for the management. As this edition is being printed, there can be no wonder, if more isotopes are introduced in medicine, more diseases are brought under the purview of diagnosis by scintiscans and treatment by targeted drug delivery (guided missile) concept.

Even in this era of high-tech diagnostic armamentarium, there is still a place for arriving at a clinical diagnosis, for the following reasons:

1. Shortlist the differential diagnosis

2. Minimize the investigations, thereby saving time and expense

3. Derive emotional satisfaction to the clinician and make him expedient and cost-effective

4. Boost patient's satisfaction and confidence, by detailed systematic physical examination

As in any disease, eliciting a detailed history and performing a thorough physical examination may provide valuable clues to the diagnosis. This chapter is aimed at senior students who are expected to possess basic skills of clinical examination, knowledge of pathophysiology of abdominal diseases and their clinico-pathological correlation.

HISTORY

Age: congenital anomalies, e.g. malrotation of gut, hamartomas are common in children. Congenital hypertrophic pyloric stenosis is a neonatal disease, commonly seen in the first born male child. Though it is common belief that malignancies are diseases of the elderly, there is a definite shift to the younger age group in the recent times, e.g. gastric, rectal cancers are seen even in 3rd decade of life.

Sex: Diseases of biliary tract, breast and desmoid tumors have a female predilection. Related to smoking and alcoholism, Indian males are more prone to acid-peptic disease, pancreatic disease, vascular disorders, pulmonary disorders and inflammatory bowel diseases.

Residence: Biliary tract disease are prevalent in North India, whereas due to dietary habits, acid-peptic disease is seen more in the South.

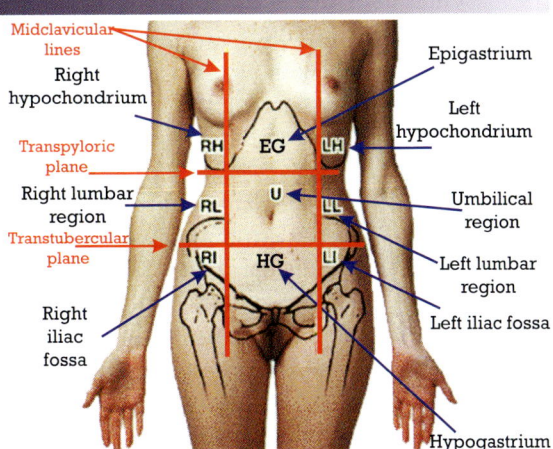

Fig. 103.1. Regions of abdomen for descriptive purposes

Hydatid disease is endemic in certain districts of Tamil Nadu. Cholangiocarcinoma seems to favor the geographic area of the Ganges basin.

About the mass

Mode of onset and duration: Insidious onset of a painless swelling is likely to be neoplastic, whereas short duration, acute onset with pain is in favor of inflammatory swelling.

Site: There are two issues here, viz: place of onset and current site. For e.g. a suprapubic swelling that subsequently occupies the lumbar area is more likely to be of pelvic origin. One should also consider all the structures in a given quadrant when evaluating a mass.

Similar swellings elsewhere: a classic example is multiple lipomas or neurofibromas in the abdominal wall, alerting the clinician to the possibility of a large relatively immobile mass being a retroperitoneal tumor (liposarcoma or neurofibrosarcoma).

Associated symptoms

Pain: learning the details of pain may offer valuable clue to the diagnosis.

Duration is long in benign conditions (e.g. hydatid cyst or ileocecal tuberculosis), whereas it may be short in malignancies.

Site is obviously a very important information to determine the most likely organ from which the mass may be arising

Aggravating or relieving factors: Food or beverage relieves pain in uncomplicated duodenal ulcer, whereas they aggravate symptoms in gastritis, gastric outlet or bowel obstruction, sometimes relieved by vomiting.

Character: It may be mild burning (e.g. hyperacidity), severe gripping (pancreatic, peptic ulcer, appendicular pain) or colicky (biliary, intestinal, ureteric or appendicular).

Radiation and referral of pain

Pain radiates from the site of origin to another region, e.g. pain from intervertebral disc protrusion is also felt along the entire course of the compressed nerve root, or pain from posterior abdominal structures, such as pancreas or abdominal aorta may radiate to back.

Referred pain implies pain occurring at a site far away from the site of origin, e.g. pain from the diaphragm (visceral nerve phrenic) is referred to the tip of shoulder, through C-4 somatic dermatome. Similarly pain originating from foregut (D-7,8), midgut (D-9,10) and hindgut (D-11,12) is referred to corresponding dermatomes over epigastrium, umbilical region and hypogastrium respectively.

Symptoms related to GI Tract

Regurgitation and vomiting: Essential difference between the two is that the regurgitant comes from esophagus, whereas vomitus comes from the stomach and is an important symptom of gastroduodenal and proximal gut obstruction.

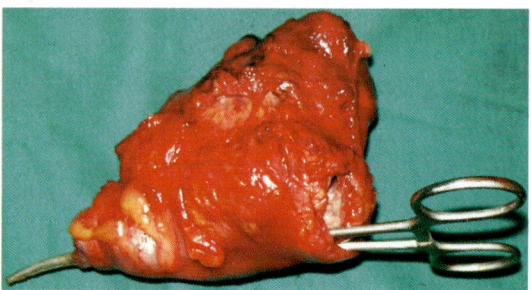

Fig.103.02. Sigmoid resection for a large GIST

Flatulent dyspepsia: This is eructation of swallowed air, with or without an organic disease. Biliary dyspepsia is intolerance to fatty foods, since fat is a cholagogue (makes gall-bladder expel bile into the gut) by the action of cholecystokinin released from duodenum. Acid eructations have two components acidity and reflux of gas and are typically seen in stenosed chronic duodenal ulcer, or obstructing growth in the gastric outlet.

Presence of ball rolling movements is characteristic of gastroduodenal and occasionally bowel obstruction. It is generally indicative of benign disease, with slow process of developing obstruction, but may be seen rarely in slow growing malignancy.

Abdominal distension may be localized or generalized (vide infra)

Jaundice due to extrahepatic biliary obstruction is also called 'surgical' jaundice, whereas the rest may be considered 'medical'. Earlier classification of hemolytic, hepatocellular and obstructive has been replaced by conjugated or unconjugated types of jaundice.

Hematemesis and melena indicate an ulcerated lesion bleeding into the bowel lumen, e.g. hemorrhaging gastric or small bowel tumor.

Bowel habit: Alteration of bowel habit is typical in distal bowel disease and in malignancy it worsens progressively. It may be also seen in proximal (high)

Table-103.1

Feature	Regurgitation	Vomiting
Origin	Esophagus	Stomach
Nature	Organic	Organic or functional
Preceding nausea	Absent	Present
Character	Mouthfuls	May be projectile
Dysphagia	Present	Absent
Timing with food	Immediate	After sometime
VGP	Absent	May be present
Features of gastric dilatation	Absent	May be present

obstructions due to reduced food intake. Alternating diarrhea and constipation is indicative of subacute (or incomplete) bowel obstruction, classically described in tuberculous strictures of bowel.

Symptoms related to GU Tract

Loin pain or fullness

Dysuria, frequency

Prostatism

Hematuria

Intermittent polyuria (Dietl's crisis)

Recurrent colics, typically radiating from loin to groin.

Retroperitoneum: It extends from the diaphragm to the pelvic floor, housing several structures, such as lymph nodes, parts of duodenum, pancreas, major vessels, adrenals, kidneys, ureters, sympathetic chains, presacral nerve plexus, distal rectum, vertebral column (upto coccyx), lymphatics, fat etc.

Constitutional symptoms: fever, reduced appetite, weight loss

PAST HISTORY

Previous major illness or surgery and other treatments received. Perusing the histo-pathology of tissue removed at previous surgery is important, to decide its relation to the present problem.

PERSONAL HISTORY

Life style, tobacco consumption (smoking, tobacco chewing, snuff, jarda etc) alcohol intake, hobbies etc. This may include current medications the patient is on.

FAMILY HISTORY

Acid-peptic disease, malignancies, inflammatory bowel diseases, colonic diverticulosis, multiple endocrine tumors, certain goiters etc may run in families.

PHYSICAL EXAMINATION

GENERAL SURVEY, (attitude, nutritional/hydration status, anemia, cyanosis, jaundice, clubbing of fingers, generalized edema or lymphadenopathy etc) including vital functions (pulse, respirations, blood pressure and temperature), for details see chapter 1.

Abdominal Examination: standard protocol for any local examination (inspection, palpation, percussion, auscultation, measurements and regional lymph nodes) has to be followed. Of course, no abdominal examination is complete without appropriate PV or PR examination.

INSPECTION

Normal contour of abdomen is flat (not scaphoid as commonly mistaken). In thin emaciated individuals, it is drawn inwards, assuming the shape of a boat, and hence termed scaphoid. It appears convex when there is generalized distension, in the following conditions (5-Fs):

Fat (obesity) due to parietal and intra-abdominal fat

Fluid (ascites, large ovarian, mesenteric cyst or pseudocyst of pancreas)

Feces (constipation or bowel obstruction)

Flatus (ileus, bowel obstruction or pneumo-peritoneum).

Fetus (in later weeks of pregnancy)

Movements of abdominal wall with respiration: In local peritonitis the part of the abdominal wall overlying the inflammatory process becomes immobile and rigid, by nature's attempt to give rest to the area, thereby minimizing the spread of disease. The entire anterior abdominal wall becomes immobile in general peritonitis and develops what is commonly known as board-like rigidity. Paradoxical movements may be seen in areas devoid of innervation (e.g. a phantom hernia in anterior poliomyelitis, divarication of recti, Malgaigne bulgings or sometimes following a subcostal incision) where part of the abdominal wall becomes flail, reversing its normal in and out (antero-posterior) movements.

Position and appearance of umbilicus

Normal umbilicus is slightly retracted and inverted. It may get everted to a variable degree in gross ascites and gets deeply inverted (tucked) in obesity

Its position may vary with intra-abdominal pathology

Tanyol's sign: An SOL in the upper abdomen (large pseudocyst of pancreas, gross hepatomegaly or splenomegaly), may displace the umbilicus down and lower abdominal or pelvic masses (including gravid uterus), push it upwards

In large loin swellings (renal or splenic), it may be displaced to the opposite side

Exomphalos minor or major: partial or total persistence of midgut in the umbilical cord (failure to return), causing herniation, seen in newborn

Gastroschisis: loops of bowel herniate through a defect in the abdominal wall, to the right of midline, without any coverings, due to insufficient development

An umbilical or paraumbilical hernia may be present

Enteroteratoma (syn: umbilical adenoma, polyp or raspberry tumor) is due to the prolapse of mucosa from the unobliterated vitello-intestinal duct, which bleeds on touch

Umbilical granuloma: protruding granulation tissue from umbilical sepsis, which bleeds on touch

Endometrioma: periodic swelling, pain and bleeding synchronizing with menstrual cycles

Acquired fistula: any abdominal sepsis, (including that due to a retained swab) may track externally through the umbilicus

Enteric fistula: this is due to patency of the entire intra-abdominal portion of the vitello-intestinal duct

Urinary fistula: patent urachus, connecting the fundus of urinary bladder

Omphalolith (syn: umbilical calculus) may develop due to poor hygiene, by collection of desquamated epithelium and other debris. It is a frequent finding in elderly obese patients and except for an indication of local hygiene, it has no clinical significance

A fibroma or primary carcinoma may develop (rare)

Secondary carcinomatous deposits (Sister Joseph's nodules) usually from stomach, colon, breast or ovary, seen as satellite nodules around umbilicus

Omphalitis of newborn is due to infection of the umbilical stump

An abscess may develop in relation to umbilicus

Pilonidal sinus: a tuft of hair is seen projecting from the sinus, usually associated with purulent discharge due to secondary infection

Engorged veins over anterior abdominal wall, their location and direction of flow:

In SVC obstruction, the direction of flow is downwards, both above and below the umbilicus.

They are seen in portal hypertension or IVC, common/external iliac vein obstruction

In portal hypertension, they radiate from centre, with flow away from umbilicus (caput Medusae)

In IVC obstruction, the veins are vertically placed, more towards flanks, with the flow from below upwards. In iliac vein occlusion, they are unilateral.

Note: Above the umbilicus, the direction of flow may be the same in both conditions, whereas below the umbilicus, it is reversed.

It is important that the engorged veins are observed when the patient is in a standing posture

HARVEY'S TEST is to detect the direction of blood flow in a superficial vein.

Place two fingers close together over a distended vein. Move one finger away over the vein, to empty that segment of vein (gets collapsed). Lift the second finger to see if blood flows in to fill the segment, which indicates the flow towards the first finger. Repeat the test in the other direction to confirm the inference

VISIBLE PERISTALSIS

In thin individuals, in the emaciated or due to thinned out abdominal wall (as in divarication of recti or large hernia), peristalsis of small bowel may be visible, without actual bowel pathology.

In other situations, it implies mechanical obstruction to a hollow viscus.

The direction of the waves may be of help to know the level of obstruction:

Left to right in the upper abdomen (gastric outlet), right to left in the upper or mid abdomen (colonic) and step-ladder pattern in the mid abdomen (small bowel).

External genitalia and hernial sites

Visible mass: if there is a visible mass, it should be examined like any mass, in the order of location, size, shape, surface, borders, pulsation, movements with respiration, anatomic plain, change in position with posture, secondary skin changes etc.

Deep-seated swelling, such as abdominal masses are never discrete (by inspection). If an abdominal mass has a discrete border, it is likely to be a parietal mass.

Identifying the anatomical plane of the mass is very helpful in short listing the probabilities. It may be parietal or intra-abdominal, the latter in turn may be properitoneal, intra or retroperitoneal.

Properitoneal plane is between the parietal muscles and anterior peritoneum, in which the fundus of the urinary bladder, remnants of urachus and vitellointestinal duct lie.

A mass visible but not palpable is likely to be a distended hollow viscus, e.g. stomach or sigmoid colon.

Movement with respiration (vide infra)

ABDOMINAL PULSATIONS

Visible epigastric pulsations, present normally, due to cardiac movements transmitted through the diaphragm, are not palpable. They are best appreciated by observing the anterior abdominal wall tangentially.

However, if they are palpable, there are abnormal and generally implies that there is an SOL between the palpating hand and the aorta. When palpable, see if it is moving with

respirations. If so, they may be transmitted, because aorta and its main branches are retroperitoneal and immobile.

Being away from the aorta, hepatic, splenic or renal swellings usually do not exhibit transmitted pulsations.

CULLEN SIGN

Bluish ecchymotic discoloration around the umbilicus noticed in retroperitoneal hemorrhage, typically described in hemorrhagic pancreatitis, due to the diffusion of blood pigments (methemalbumin from digested blood).

Cullen was an Obstetrician, who described the sign in ruptured tubal gestation.

GREY TURNER SIGN is the similar discoloration seen around the flanks.

These signs may also be seen in any retroperitoneal hemorrhage, such as blunt abdominal trauma, leaking aortic aneurysm and may take about 24-48 hours to appear.

PALPATION

Abdominal palpation has to be done from the right side of the patient, unless the clinician is *left-handed*. Occasionally, while examining a moderately enlarged spleen, finger insinuation test is more conveniently performed from the left side, by hooking all 4 fingers of the left hand, under the left costal margin. In cold environment, it is friendly to warm up the examining hand by rubbing against the other, before placing it over the abdomen of the patient.

Abdominal wall rigidity is involuntary, muscle guarding is voluntary reflex action against fear of being hurt, during palpation and also indicates underlying inflammation.

Palpation is generally done in 3 stages.

1. light palpation,
2. deep palpation
3. palpation during deep breathing and special methods of palpating individual organs, including dipping method if there is gross ascites.

Use of both the hands, placed one over the other, has the advantage of the top one being useful to exert pressure and the bottom one to appreciate the findings.

Nicholson's maneuver: Exerting pressure over the lower sternum with left hand during abdominal palpation, restricts thoracic movements and forces the patient to resort to abdominal respirations. This is rarely employed.

Palpable mass: If there is a palpable mass, it should be examined like any mass, in order of confirmation of inspection findings (location, size, shape and anatomic plane), warmth, tenderness, consistency, borders, pulsations etc. Additional findings for an abdominal mass include, movements with respiration and posture, bimanual palpation and ballotability. Special methods of palpation of masses arising from individual organs and detection of free peritoneal fluid are described below:

PALPATING LIVER

Start palpating from the right iliac fossa, inching towards the liver, as the patient is taking normal breaths. When the lower border of the liver is reached, move the hand down by about 2", then ask the patient to take a deep breath, to see the magnitude of liver excursions with respirations.

Then palpate the entire lower border, surface and if the fingers could be insinuated under the rib cage. If it is very large, check for bimanual palpability in the right loin.

Unless grossly enlarged, generally liver masses don't exhibit transmitted pulsations.

If there is gross ascites, palpate by employing 'dipping' method.

Note: Liver may be normally palpable up to the age of 3 years, later recedes under the rib cage, due to differential growth.

PALPATING SPLEEN

Contrary to general belief, the spleen is located quite behind, in the posterior axillary line. By virtue of its intimate relation to diaphragm , it moves freely with respiration and the suspending peritoneal folds direct the enlargement towards right iliac fossa, with a characteristic notch at its lower medial border.

It would be helpful to examine the patient with slight right lateral tilt, when palpating minimally enlarged spleen. When it is grossly enlarged, it is bimanually palpable, but never exhibits pulsations nor allows finger insinuation between it and the rib cage. Some prefer to do the finger insinuation from the left of the patient.

If there is gross ascites, palpate by employing the 'dipping' method.

Special maneuvers in difficult situations:

To "borrow" extra skin for finger insinuation, the left hand is used to slide down the skin over the lower chest, while palpating spleen (or liver).

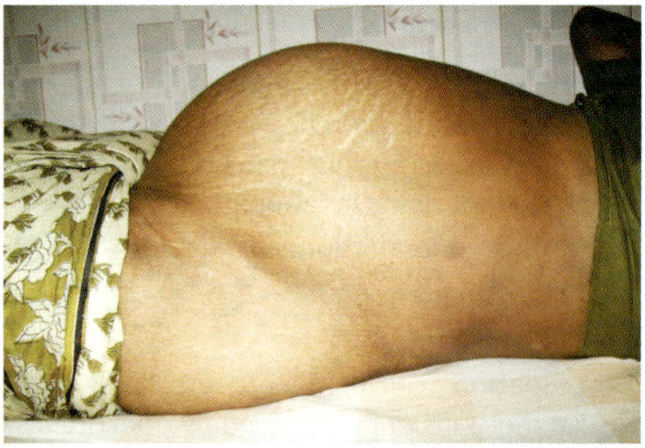

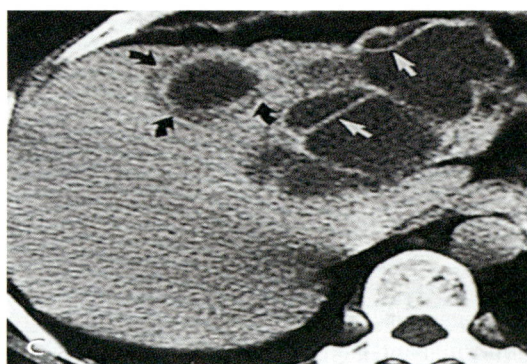

Fig. 103.3. Massive splenomegaly, occupying most of the abdomen in Gaucher's disease

Fig. 103.4. CT abdomen showing multilocular hydatid cyst of liver

Lifting the spleen by the left hand placed behind, makes it easily palpable by the right (anterior) hand.

PALPATING KIDNEY (see bimanual palpability and bellotability below)

MALLET-GUY'S SIGN of pancreatic disease

It is not possible to palpate the normal pancreas, unless it is swollen or has a large cyst or tumor. The patient is placed in right lateral position, with flexed hips and knees and perform deep palpation in epigastrium and left hypochondrium

Tenderness may be elicited in inflammatory conditions of pancreas

BALLANCE'S SIGN

It is seen in rupture of spleen with hemoperitoneum and a large perisplenic hamatoma. Fixed dullness over the splenic area and left loin (due to large hematoma) and shifting dullness over the rest of the abdomen, including right loin (due to free hemoperitoneum) are considered typical. The blood in the peritoneal cavity does not clot readily due to the fibrinolytic activity of the peritoneal fluid.

An enlarged and pathological spleen ruptures more readily, than a normal spleen

Consistency: Identify if the swelling is soft,

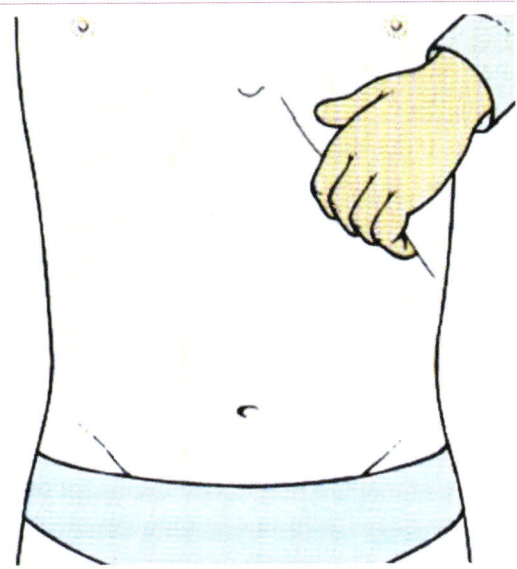

Fig. 103.6. Hooking the fingers under left costal margin (standing on the left of patient)

cystic, firm or hard or does it have a variable consistence (cystic tumors). If it is cystic, look for fluctuation and fluid thrill within the swelling, which may be appreciated if it is large and tense. Mass pitting on pressure may be a dermoid or fecal mass.

Mobility: Several aspects of mobility of the mass have to be examined

Movement with respirations: There are three degrees of movement with respirations: free movement, restricted movement and no movement.

By virtue of their proximity to the diaphragm, most of the upper abdominal structures such as liver, gallbladder or spleen, move *freely* with respirations.

Masses related to kidney, adrenal, lesser sac, stomach (including the 1st part of duodenum), flexures of colon and perigastric lymph nodes (epiploic groups) may exhibit *restricted* mobility

Whereas retroperitoneal structures, such as pancreas, paraaortic lymph nodes, abdominal aortic aneurysm (AAA), 2nd, 3rd and 4th parts of duodenum as well as lower abdominal and pelvic masses *do not move* with respirations.

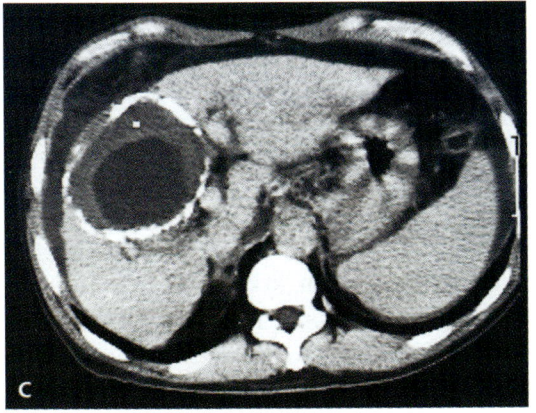

Fig. 103.5. CT abdomen showing calcified ectocyst of a long standing hydatid of liver

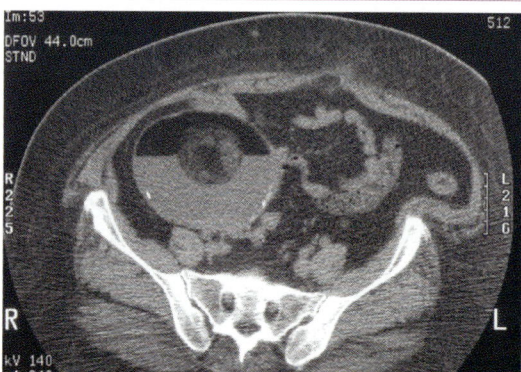

Fig. 103.7. Large dermoid cyst of right ovary

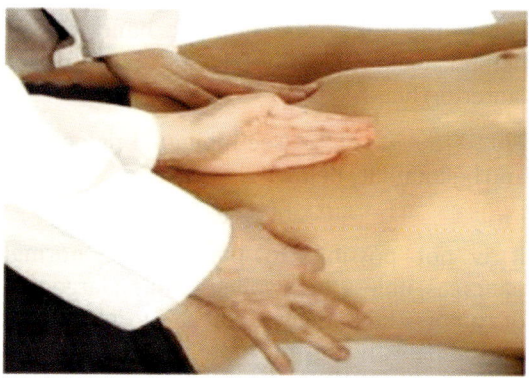

Fig. 103.8. Method of eliciting fluid thrill

Change of position with posture: supine, erect, stooping or knee-elbow.

Intrinsic mobility indicates movement independent of surrounding structures either in some or in all directions.

Bimanual palpability is an important feature of a loin mass which enjoys some intrinsic mobility. Though typically renal masses are bimanually palpable, it may also be appreciated in masses in relation to ascending/descending colon, head/tail of pancreas, part of enlarged liver/gallbladder/spleen (extending into loin), omental or other retroperitoneal masses which are not fixed by inflammatory or neoplastic process. It is also important to know which (anterior or posterior) hand appreciates the mass better, to determine the plane of the swelling in relation to the abdominal cavity.

It is not possible to perform this maneuver in any other area of the abdomen (except loins), because of intervening bony structures (this is the reason why two horizontal lines are drawn; at the level of the 12th rib above and highest point of the iliac crest below). Place both hands on anterior and posterior aspects of the mass and by applying pressure by alternating hands. If it could be made to move antero-posteriorly, the extent of it has to be noted. This method is also used to palpate a pelvic mass, including fetal head.

Ballotability (ballot: to toss around) is a more difficult sign to elicit and it is possible only in masses with their diameter lesser than the AP diameter of abdomen, since the mass pushed by one hand (usually posterior one) has to float in the abdomen to reach the other hand. It may also be elicited in a floating fetal head, a not-too-big ovarian cyst or a plunging uterine fibroid, during pelvic examination. It is difficult to explain why a ballotable renal swelling with considerable intrinsic mobility does not fall forwards by its own weight, in knee-elbow position !

It is inappropriate to attempt this maneuver if the swelling is visible by inspection, generally indicating that the mass is larger than the abdominal diameter

Feature	Ascites	Ovarian Cyst
Location	Diffuse	Lower abdomen
Umbilicus	Central	Displaced upwards
Epigastrium	Dull	Resonant
Flanks	Dull	Resonant
Shifting dullness	Present	Absent
Bimanual exam	Negative	May be palpable
Aortic pulsations	Absent	May be transmitted
CA–125	Normal	Elevated in cancer

Table-103.2. Differences between ascites and large ovarian cyst
Caution: both conditions may coexist in ovarian malignancy

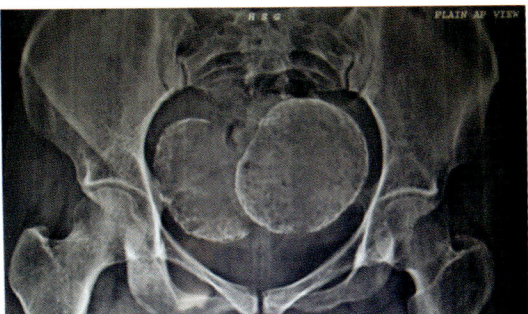

Fig. 103.9. Plain skiagram of pelvis showing two large calcified uterine fibroids

Yielding is typically seen in parietal/preperitoneal masses and those in the anterior abdominal cavity, such as edge of liver or gallbladder.

Moulding is appreciated in fecal concretions in the colon and dermoid cyst of ovary

Floating indicates the mass just moves around without much effort, as seen in renal, ovarian or omental masses in tuberculous of malignant ascites.

Head or leg raising sign (Carnett's): During these maneuvers, the abdominal muscles go into involuntary contraction, to stabilize the thoracic cage (and dorsal spine) and pelvis respectively, due to bow-stringing effect. A swelling that decreases in size with this maneuver is very likely to be intra-abdominal. If it remains unchanged, it is probably parietal in origin, e.g. irreducible ventral hernia, rectus hematoma or desmoid tumor.

Exaggerated lumbar lordosis may be mistaken for a mass in the umbilical region and prominent aortic pulsations for an aneurysm, which may be verified by passing a hand behind the lumbar spine.

SIGNE De DANCE

Feeling of emptiness of right iliac fossa, in ileocolic/colocolic intussusception or ileo-cecal tuberculosis, when the cecum is pulled up.

Sometimes a depression (hollowness) may be noted in the anterior abdominal wall, over the right iliac fossa, for the same reason.

HEPATO-JUGULAR REFLEX (or REFLUX)

In states of enlarged congestive liver disorders (particularly in right heart failure), jugular distension may be noted on applying pressure over the liver.

This is due to reflux of blood from the liver into IVC, right atrium, SVC and jugulars.

This was originally described by Pasteur in tricuspid regurgitation, but also observed in congestive heart failure. It may also be seen in normal individuals; hence not considered a very reliable sign of heart failure.

ASCITES

Presence of free fluid provides a very important clue to the diagnosis. While large volume (>2000ml) of ascites gives fluid thrill, smaller volumes (1000-1500ml) may be detected by shifting dullness and by puddle sign if the collection is very minimal (120-200ml).

FLUID THRILL

Keep a ruler (or blade of the hand) over the midline, to eliminate transmitted impulse through the skin. Give a gentle finger tap over one loin and appreciate the wave (thrill) reaching the hand placed over the opposite loin and repeat it in reverse direction.

Large cystic swellings occupying most of the abdomen (ovarian cyst, pancreatic pseudocyst or grossly distended urinary bladder) may produce a similar thrill, but the shifting dullness will be absent in such cases; in fact there will be dullness in the centre but resonance in the periphery of the abdomen, due to displaced gas-filled bowel, by the mass. Further, in a tense ovarian or mesenteric cyst, transmitted pulse from the abdominal aorta may be appreciated.

Shifting dullness and puddle sign are described under percussion.

In suspected case of intra-abdominal malignancy, a systematic search of secondary deposits has to be performed, in the following sites:

Liver (vide infra)

Left supraclavicular (Virchow) nodes

Para aortic nodes

Axillary nodes (parietal involvement above the umbilicus)

Ilioinguinal nodes (parietal involvement below the umbilicus)

Krukenberg's tumor (PV) in ovaries of premenopausal women

Blumer's shelf (PR) in the rectovaginal (Douglas) or restovesical pouch

Sister Joseph's nodules, around the umbilicus

Peritoneal spread causing ascites and nodules

Distant sites by hematogenous or lymphogenous spread.

SISTER JOSEPH'S NODULES

It is a late sign of abdominal malignancy, usually from stomach, pancreas, colon, ovary or rarely from breast. Lymphogenous metastatic subcutaneous nodules are seen around the umbilicus.

SAUSAGE SIGN IN INTUSSUSCEPTION

In infants, a soft sausage-shaped mass of ileoileal intussusception may be palpable in the umbilical region, becoming firm synchronizing with attacks of colicky pain (peristalsis of small bowel).

In adults, the mass may be felt in different areas, depending upon the type of intussusception.

The tip of the mass can sometimes be palpated per rectum (resembling cervix uteri by PV), in distal colocolic intussusception.

RULER SIGN

In moderate ascites, when the patient is in supine position, a ruler may be placed vertically over the abdomen, to touch the xiphoid, umbilicus and the pubic symphysis.

In cases of a large pseudocyst of pancreas, mesenteric or ovarian cyst, it will not be possible for the ruler to touch all the 3 points, so also if the ascites is very tense.

An alternative method is to place the ruler transversely at the level of umbilicus. The middle of the ruler is seen prominent in ovarian/mesenteric cyst, whereas the ends are more prominent in ascites.

KNEE-ELBOW POSITION

This position is employed in several situations, but it is an unpleasant position for the sick and elderly and may be resorted to only if the same information cannot be gained through other methods of examination.

1. to see if a swelling is falling forwards away from the posterior abdominal wall (intraperitoneal or properitoneal swellings)

2. if the pulsations of a mass diminish (transmitted pulsation)

3. to detect minimal free fluid (puddle sign) by percussion

4. Sometimes for doing digital rectal examination.

KNEE-CHEST POSITION

This position is also very inconvenient to the patient. Sometimes it is used to perform digital rectal examination or a rigid proctosigmoidoscopy.

SIM'S (LEFT LATERAL) POSITION

This is more comfortable to the patient and is a very popular position for rectal examination, procto-sigmoidoscopic examination. The right hip and knee are flexed to maximum, while keeping the left leg straight.

VALSALVA MANEUVER

This is forced expiration against closed glottis, increasing intrathoracic, intraabdominal and intracranial tensions. This in a way, precedes cough reflex and has many applications:

To demonstrate an external hernia, laryngocele, hiatal hernia (during fluoroscopy), cystocele or rectocele or put the lateral or posterior abdominal muscles to contraction (since head or leg rising only causes contraction of the anterior muscles).

While removing an intercostal (chest) drain, to prevent air entry into the pleural cavity, as the tube with multiple holes is being withdrawn.

PERCUSSION

Liver dullness and its span: Normally the upper border of liver is appreciated in the 4th space in the midclavicular line and the lower border is barely felt under the rib cage. Normal vertical span of the liver in the anterior axillary line is around 15 cms.

When an upper abdominal mass is dull to percussion, it has to be noted if it is continuous with hepatic or splenic dullness.

SHIFTING DULLNESS

This is a very useful sign when moderate amount of free fluid in the abdomen. Patient in supine position, start percussing from the umbilicus towards loin to find dullness. Fixing the pleximeter finger over the area of dullness, rotate the patient to the opposite side and percuss to find the dullness disappearing.

Repeat the test on the opposite side.

PUDDLE SIGN

With patient in knee-elbow position, start percussing from the loins to umbilical region; as the umbilicus is approached, dullness may be appreciated, if there is 'puddling' of peritoneal fluid (puddle: a small pool or lake).

Retreat percussing away from umbilicus, observe the resonance reappearing.

Renal angles obliteration of the normal resonance implies a solid mass in the renal fossa.

BLATIN'S SIGN

Hydatid thrill or fremitus (Blatin's sign) is elicited to determine floating daughter cysts in the mother cyst, by placing 3 fingers over the cyst and percussing over the middle, a thrill is appreciated by the other 2 fingers, due to the floating solid elements in the cyst. This phenomenon of recoil is dampened by the thick consistence of fluid due to rupture of daughter cysts, which is so common that this sign is rarely useful. (mother and daughter are inappropriate terms, since the nematode is a hermaphrodite)

CASTELL'S SIGN

Dullness over the left subcostal region in the

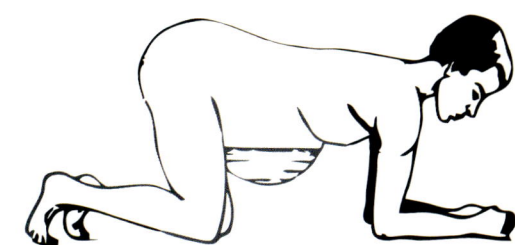

Fig. 103.10. Minimal fluid puddling near the umbilicus in knee-elbow position, identified by percussion (puddle sign)

mid and anterior axillary lines, on deep inspiration, due to minimally enlarged spleen coming down, which becomes resonant on expiration.

The point of intersection of subcostal and mid axillary lines is called Castell's point.

AUSCULTATION

Over a normal abdomen low pitched infrequent gurgles may be heard

Mechanical small bowel obstruction - high pitched frequent sounds (borborygmi), synchronizing with colicky pain

Sometimes gurgling sound of fluid flowing through a stenotic segment may be heard

Incomplete bowel obstruction: periodic, prolonged, loud gurgle, may be audible without stethoscope

Paralytic ileus occasional distant faint sounds

Peritonitis: totally silent (grave yard silence). Heart sounds may be heard over the abdomen

KENAWAY'S SIGN

Venous hum heard by auscultation over an enlarged spleen in portal hypertension or Egyptian splenomegaly

This may also be heard in the epigastrium, more so on deep inspiration, due to the compression of the spleen, causing engorgement of splenic vein.

CRUVELHIER-BAUMGARTEN'S SIGN

Continuous venous hum over the superficial veins of the anterior abdominal wall around the umbilicus in portal hypertension with extensive porta-azygos shunting.

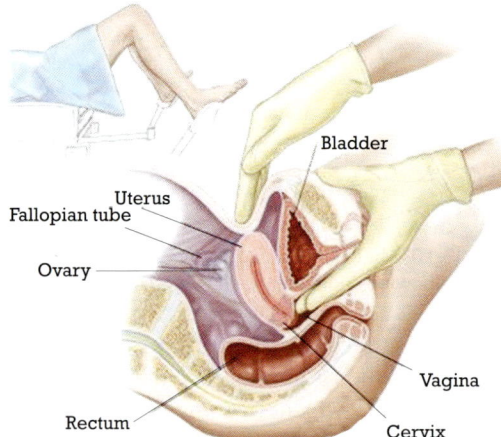

Fig. 103.11. Anteverted uterus - cervix pointing backwards and finger first touches the anterior lip

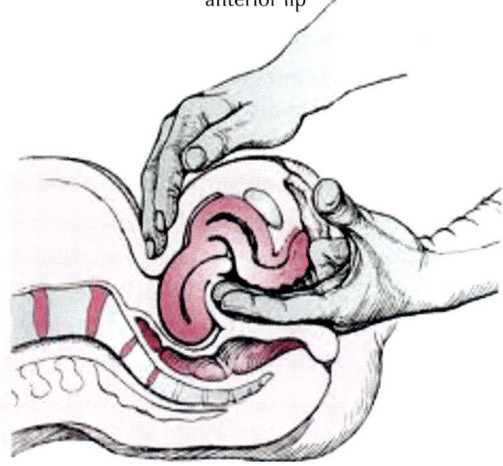

Fig. 103.12. Retroverted uterus - cervix pointing forwards and finger first touches the posterior lip

SUCCUSSION SPLASH OVER THE ABDOMEN

To demonstrate gastric stasis due to outlet obstruction

A minimum gap of 2-3 hrs after meals or liquids should be allowed before performing this test

Patient in supine position, place the stethoscope over the epigastrium and give a rigorous shake of the trunk.

A water splashing sound is appreciated, if there is considerable fluid remaining in the dilated stomach.

This test may also be positive in grossly dilated small bowel in intestinal obstruction and over the chest in hydropneumothorax.

AUSCULTO-PERCUSSION (or AUSCULTO-SCRATCHING)

This is to demonstrate gastric dilatation, by outlining its surface boundaries.

Place the stethoscope over the epigastrium and run a finger scratching the abdominal wall radiating from the stethoscope in various directions, marking the points where the audibility of the scratch sound diminushes, indicating the extent of dilated gas-filled stomach.

By joining the points marked, the gastric size and borders may be outlined.

BAID SIGN

To identify the anteriorly displaced stomach in a pseudocyst of pancreas which may be just lying under the anterior abdominal wall, a nasogastric tube is inserted into the stomach, which can sometimes be felt by palpation or appreciated by auscultation (as air is injected), in the epigastrium or umbilical region.

Note: In any large space-occupying lesion (SOL), behind the stomach, such a retroperitoneal lymph nodes, aortic aneurysm etc. this sign may be appreciated.

DIGITAL VAGINAL EXAMINATION (PV)

It may be done in several positions. Lithotomy (most common), left lateral or Sim's, supine and knee-chest positions. No abdominal examination in females is complete without PV and should be done before PR.

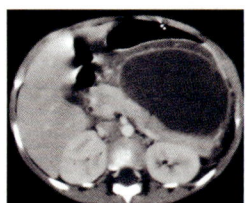

Fig.103.13. CT scan of pseudocyst of pancreas, displacing the stomach anteriorly (courtesy : Dr C M Kishor, Chennai)

Patient must be asked to empty the urinary bladder before commencing pelvic examination. After wearing a glove, well lubricated two fingers (index and middle) of the right hand are gently introduced into the introitus, to reach the fornices. If the cervix is pointing backwards and the fingers first encounter the anterior lip of the cervix, it denotes anteverted (normal) uterus.

Conversely in retroversion, the cervix points anteriorly and the finger first touches the posterior lip of cervix.

Check for consistence of cervix (firm normally, soft in pregnancy and friable with bleeding to touch in malignancy).

Presence of uterine descent (elongated cervix), cystocele or rectocele, (sliding hernia) in the anterior and posterior vaginal walls, have to be noted.

BIMANUAL PELVIC EXAMINATION

It may be done through vagina (common) or rectum in virgin females or in males.

During vaginal/rectal examination by the fingers of right hand, with the fingers of the left hand dipping into the hypogastrium, any tenderness or abnormal masses have to be identified.

The sensitivity of this examination improves with experience and decreases in obese or nulliparous patients.

DIGITAL RECTAL EXAMINATION (PR)

As vaginal examination, this may be done in several positions. Left lateral or Sim's (most common), supine, lithotomy and knee-chest positions. An abdominal examination never complete without PR.

External examination should be done for ulcers, fissures, warts, dermatitis, hemorrhoids, sinuses, growth etc.

A well lubricated right index finger is gently introduced into the anal orifice. Gentle massage over the anus for a few times before the actual entry, provides the much needed reassurance to the patient.

For esthetic and hygienic reasons, when both are required, PV should be done before doing PR.

As the anal canal is entered, the sphincteric tone (or spasm) has to be assessed. After ascertaining that no intrinsic or extrinsic

lesions exist, rotate the finger, the pulp facing anteriorly, to examine the prostate (or cervix uteri) and for Blumer's shelfing. Then rotate the finger in an orderly manner to feel all sides of rectum, including sacral hollow. If there is anal incontinence, ask the patient to tighten the sphincter around the finger, to judge its power.

In acute fissure, there may be severe pain due to sphincteric spasm, it is advisable either to avoid digital insinuation or to do it with gentle movement or still better, do it under anesthesia.

DIGITAL EXAMINATION OF PROSTATE

Note its size, tenderness, consistence, texture, median sulcus, asymmetry, mucosal fixity, seminal vesicles (above), membranous urethra (below) and collect urethral smear for examination after prostatic massage.

If prostatic malignancy is suspected, it is wise to draw a sample of blood before rectal examination, since digital massage of prostate may elevate the tumor markers in blood (acid phosphatase and PSA).

Stamey test is to perform urine microscopy before and after digital prostatic massage.

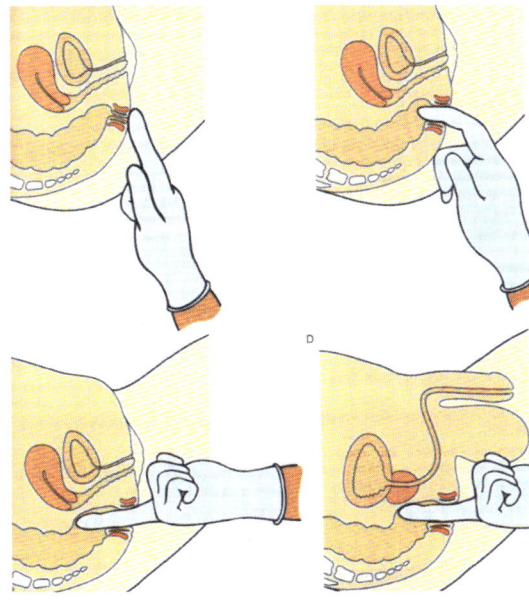

Fig. 103.14. Digital rectal examination

BLUMER'S SHELF

This is caused by trans-celomic secondary cancerous deposits in the recto-vaginal (Douglas) or recto-vesical pouch. A horizontal shelf-like extrinsic projection is felt in the anterior rectal wall, which denotes advanced stage of malignancy. This finding may also be seen in abdominal tuberculosis and sometimes in pelvic endometriosis.

The subject of ascites is dealt in the chapter 18, on abdominal tuberculosis.

PARIETAL SWELLINGS

Hernia

   True, interstitial and phantom

Soft tissue tumors

   Benign: lipoma, neurofibroma etc
   Malignant: desmoid, soft tissue sarcoma

Sebaceous cyst

   Hematoma of rectus sheath
   Sudden development of a painful swelling
   Abscess (pyogenic or cold)

Vitello-intestinal remnants
Urachal remnants
Hamartomas
Xiphoiditis

PHANTOM HERNIA

It is typically described in poliomyelitis, due to atrophy of the abdominal musculature caused by motor paralysis, in which, a part of the abdominal wall bulges while coughing or straining, resembling a hernia.

It is also seen in the right upper quadrant of the abdomen, as a sequel of a subcostal (Kocher's) incision, since it cuts across the line of intercostal nerves passing in that region, supplying the upper abdominal muscles. This is

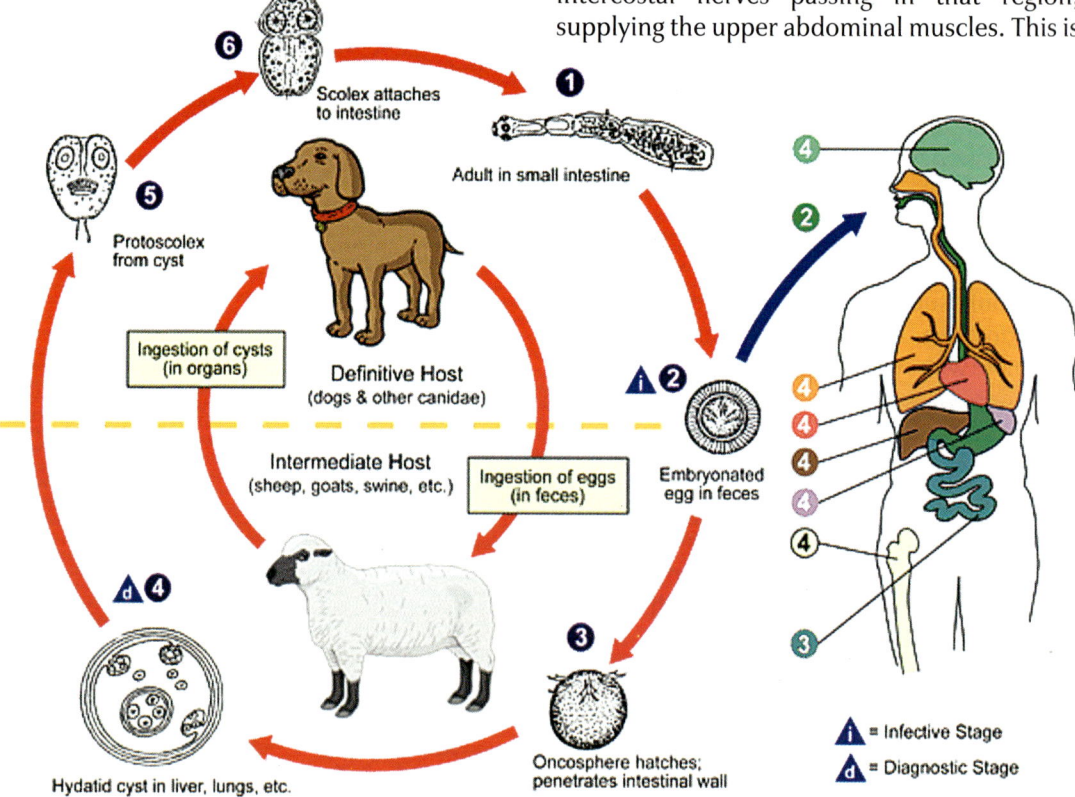

Fig. 103.15. Life cycle of Ecchinococcus granulosus
Definitive host: carnivorous animals; Intermediate host: sheep, goat, swine etc.
Man is an accidental (chance) intermediate host- various organs involved are shown

why many surgeons consider this incision unphysiological.

Malgaigne bulges (see chapter 47) in the inguinal region seen in elderly patients with poor muscle tone, divarication of recti abdominis, commonly seen in multiparous women and eventration of diaphragm due to phrenic nerve palsy are also examples of phantom hernia (see below).

DIVARICATION OF RECTI is due to attenuation of linea alba and adjacent rectus sheath,in which a linear midline bulge develops on coughing or head-raising, usually below the umbilicus, but which may extend up to the xiphoid. It is commonly seen in multiparous women, due to repeated stretch of the abdominal wall. Except for the appearance and its importance while placing an abdominal incision, it has no potential to strangulate.

FOTHERGILL'S SIGN

A mass which does not cross midline and does not alter its size by putting the abdominal muscles (especially rectus) to contraction, indicative of hematoma of rectus sheath. Irreducible or strangulated paramedian ventral hernia may also give similar findings

Masses presenting in various regions will be discussed here:

In HYPOCHONDRIUM, masses may be seen in relations to:

Liver/GB/Spleen
Colonic flexures
Stomach
Kidney/Adrenal
Pancreas
Lesser sac (left only)
Appendix (subhepatic)
Retroperitoneum.

Features of liver swelling

Mass in right hypochondrium/epigastrium/right loin

Moves freely with respiration

Lower border felt, sharp/rounded

Upper border goes under the rib cage, hence, digital insinuation not possible

There may be upward enlargement

Liver span is usually around 15cm in anterior axillary line in adults

Dull on percussion which is continuous with liver dullness

Surface may be smooth or nodular

Large swellings may be bimanually palpable

Hepatic Swellings may be classified as those involving only a part of the liver or entire liver

Entire liver involvement may be either smooth/uniform or irregular/ nodular

If a part of liver is involved, it may be Cyst (non-parasitic or parasitic).

Abscess

Riedel's lobe

Tumor

Primary

Secondary (more common).

If entire liver is involved and it is smooth and uniform

All the medical conditions come under this category

Hepatitis

Viral, bacterial, protozoal, spirochetal

Congestive liver

Cong heart failure, Budd-Chiari Syndrome

Early cirrhosis

Fatty infiltration: alcoholic and non-alcoholic steato-hepatosis (ASH & NASH)

Autoimmune disorders

Felty Syndrome

Hashimoto's disease

lymphoma/leukemia

Storage disorders

Gaucher's and Niemann-Pick's disease

Obstructive jaundice (only surgical condition in this group)

If entire liver involved and is irregular and nodular.

Multiple secondaries (most common)

Macronodular cirrhosis

Polycystic disease (non-parasitic or parasitic)

Multiple abscesses

If the liver massively enlarged

Multiple secondaries (melanoma or mucinous adenocarcinoma)

Polycystic disease

Hydatidosis

Storage disorders

Budd-Chiari syndrome (acute)

Polycystic disease of liver may be associated with polycystic kidneys and pancreas

Primary cancers going to liver

GIT: from lower third of esophagus to lower third of rectum (portal drainage)

GB, Pancreas

Breast

Lung

Melanoma

Right adrenal - Neuroblastoma (Pepper's tumor)

Right kidney (contiguous)

General dissemination

Courvoisier's law (rule) is a statement of probability.

In cases of extrahepatic biliary obstruction, if the gallbladder is palpable, it is likely to be due

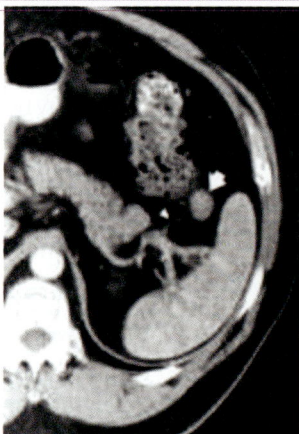

Fig. 103.16. Normal spleen in CT scan

to malignancy (the rationale being that a healthy uninflamed gall bladder is more likely to distend secondary to obstruction)

Exceptions to the rule:

A) With malignant obstructive jaundice and non palpable gallbladder

Klatskin tumor (proximal to cystic duct)

Previous cholecystectomy

Previous attacks of cholecystitis.

B) With palpable gallbladder and benign cause of obstructive jaundice.

Double stone (cystic duct stone causing mucocele and CBD stone causing obstructive jaundice)

Primary CBD stone (non-inflamed gallbladder, may be palpable due to distension)

Spleen (remember 1, 3, 5, 7, 9, 11)

Size 1" x 3" x 5"; 7 ounces (200 gms) in weight and located under 9-11 ribs (left posterior axillary line)

Features of splenic swelling

Located in left hypochondrium, loin or umbilical regions

Intraperitoneal and moves freely with respiration

Grows towards right iliac fossa, crossing the midline (because of the phrenicocolic ligament, which limits downward growth).

Rounded anterior border with a notch

Fingers cannot be insinuated between the swelling and costal margin

Dull on percussion, which is continuous with splenic dullness

No transmitted pulsations felt

If it enters the loin, it may be bimanually palpable

Venous hum may be appreciated over the mass and in the epigastrium

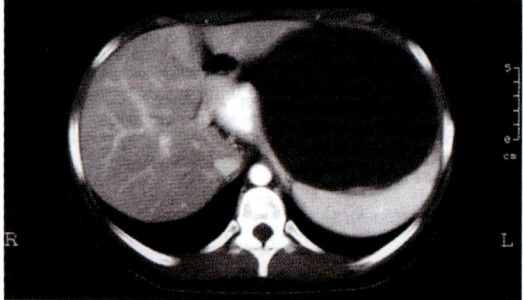

Fig. 103.17. CT scan showing a large cyst arising from the tail of pancreas, displacing the spleen posterioraly

Causes of splenomegaly

Chronic malaria
Tropical splenomegaly
Kala azar (Leishmaniasis)
Blood dyscrasias
Portal hypertension
Infarction
Banti's disease
Felty's syndrome
Amyloidosis
Storage disorders
Autoimmune
An EPIGASTRIC MASS may be arising from
Stomach
Liver
Lesser sac (pseudocyst of pancreas)
Transverse colon
Omentum
Retroperitoneum
Lymph nodes, aorta and body of pancreas
Gastric Swellings
Benign (rare)
Leiomyoma (GIST)
Bezoars
　　Trichobezoar
　　Phytobezoar
Perigastric abscess
Gastrinoma (rare)
Malignant
Carcinoma
Malignant GIST
Lymphoma (NHL)

Features of carcinoma stomach

S　Silent, symptomless
T　Tumor
O　Obstruction, occult bleeding
M　Malena, metastases
A　Anemia, ascites, asthenia, anorexia
C　Cachexia, cervical node, constipation
H　Hepatomegaly, hematemesis, halitosis

Upper G I Symptoms
Dysphagia in tumor at GE junction
GO obstruction in antral tumor
Evidence of upper GI bleeding may be present
Mass epigastrium, hypochondria or umbilical region

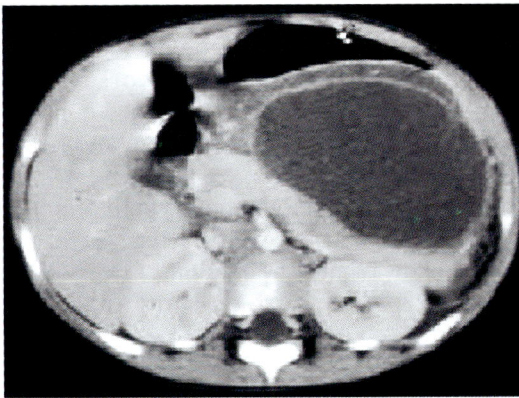

Fig. 103.18. Panreatic pseudocyst, displacing the stomach anteriorly

Moves with respiration, unless fixed
Intraperitoneal
Upper border may be appreciated
Fingers can be insinuated between the mass and the costal margin

Band of resonance between the mass and Liver

Diagnosis: UGI endoscopy and biopsy
Ultrasound scan and CT scan of abdomen to assess nodal and hepatic metastasis.

MRI is superior to CT in identifying the multi-layered cyst wall in clinching the diagnosis

Repeated guided aspirations of the contents and instillation of scolicidal agents have been found to be successful in hydatid disease, thus obviating the need for major (often risky) surgery for them.

Treatment: Radical gastrectomy, Total for

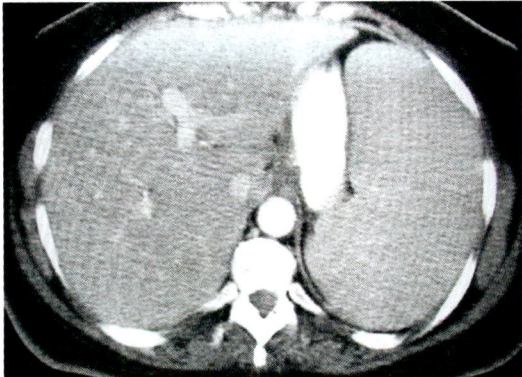

Fig. 103.19. CT scan of abdomen showing massively enlarged spleen

proximal gastric cancer and subtotal for cancer arising from the rest of the stomach. The current recommendation favors a D2 gastrectomy for curative resection, i.e.,nodal stations 1 to 12 along with stomach and lesser and greater omenta.

Postoperative chemotherapy confers some survival advantage. Palliative external radiotherapy is under evaluation.

PANCREATIC PSEUDOCYST

H/O Acute abdomen (pancreatitis)
Epigastric mass
Smooth, cystic, fixed
Some movement with respiration is seen
Upper border not felt
Fluid thrill and transmitted pulse
Resonant (due to overlying stomach)

Constitutional symptoms, only if it gets infected

Pancreatic pseudocyst, displacing the stomach anteriorly.

Diagnosis: CT Scan is the investigation of choice , in terms of anatomic delineation and relation to adjacent structures.

Treatment: If the cyst diameter is greater than 6 cm, the wall thickness is 6 mm and is symptomatic, some form of internal drainage may be done, i.e., endoscopic cystogastrostomy (Juraz), laparoscopic or open cystogastrostomy or cystojejunostomy depending on anatomical position of the pseudocyst. USG-guided aspiration &/or external drainage by a pig-tail catheter, are done only for infection or if the general condition is poor.

Mass in the LOINS (LUMBAR REGIONS)

Kidney
Colon, ascending/ descending
Liver/Gallbladder/Spleen
Pancreas (head/tail)
Appendix (high)
Undescended enlarged testis
Retroperitoneum

    -Ganglioneuroma of adrenal medulla
    -Liposarcoma

Features of a renal mass

Hypochondrium/ loin
Digital insinuation possible
Vertically placed
Rarely crosses midline
Retroperitoneal, doesn't fall forward in knee-elbow position
Limited movement with respiration
Bimanually palpable. Ballotable only if it is relatively small
Can be pushed into renal fossa

Anomalies: Pelvic/horse-shoe kidney and mobile kidney

RENAL MASSES

Cysts (solitary or multiple)
Tumor
Tuberculosis

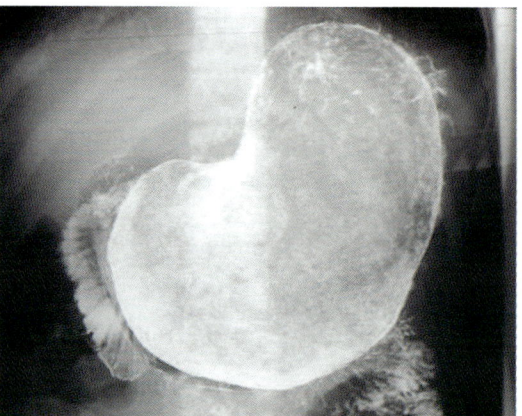

Fig. 103.20. Radiograph of abdomen showing trichobezoar filling the entire stomach

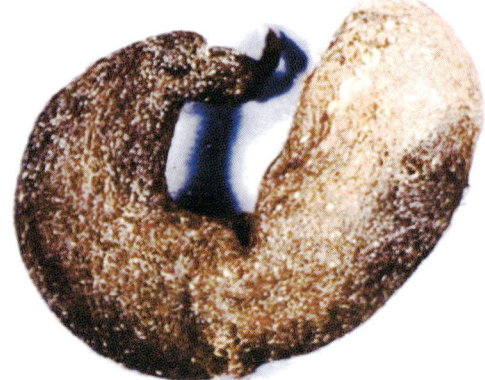

Fig. 103.21. A casted trichobezoar removed by gastrotomy

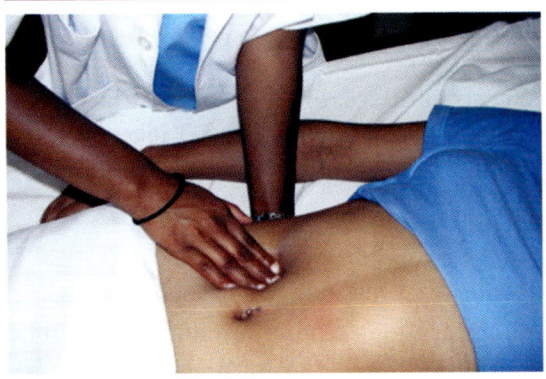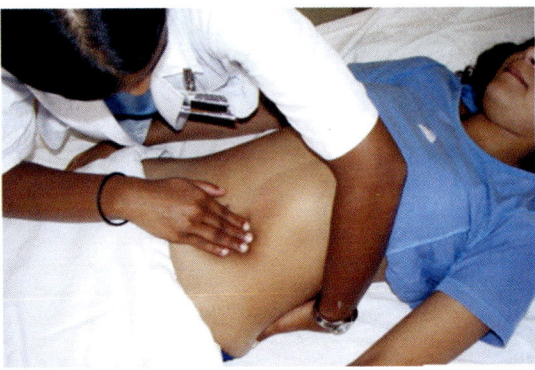

Fig. 103.22. Bimanual palpation of both kidneys

Hydronephrosis

Abscess

Hypertrophy

Congenital polycystic kidney disease (PCKD)

Before the age of 4 or after 40 (infantile is autosomal recessive type, less common and adult is autosomal dominant type, more common)

Bilateral loin masses in most cases, 17% may be initially unilateral

Mobile, irregular, asymmetrical

Recurrent hematuria and anemia

Recurrent fever due to infection

Secondary hypertension

Azotemia/ uremia

Investigations

USG/CT and renal function study

Treatment

Rovsing's operation (deroofing the cysts), earlier described is no longer done.

Watchful expectancy and kidney transplantation

(if the situation warrants) are th only options.

MASSES IN ILIAC FOSSAE

Appendix (on right)

Terminal ileum (on right)

Cecum/ sigmoid colon

Iliac lymph nodes (either side)

Uterine and tubo-ovarian (either side)

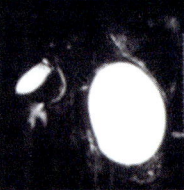

Fig. 103.23. ERCP showing a communicating pseudocyst of pancreas, filled with contrast

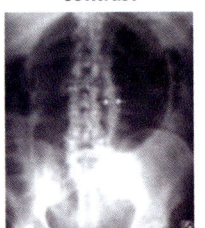

Fig.103.24. Sigmoid volvulus showing typical coffee bean appearance of the gas-filled loops

Psoas abscess (either side)

Less common: vessels, bone, kidney, testis,

retroperitoneum and broad ligament

Features of appendicular mass

History of recent acute pain RIF

Treated nonoperatively

Previous similar pains

Irregular mass, soft/ firm

Without intrinsic mobility

Appears retroperitoneal, due to fixity to the posterior abdominal wall

No bowel symptoms

Usually resolves in 2-3 wks

If not, suspect abscess or review diagnosis

Features of ileocecal tuberculosis

Hyperplastic type young/ middle age

May go into cicatrization later causing obstruction

Vague abdominal pain and constitutional symptoms (anorexia, fever, wight loss)

Alternating diarrhea and constipation, due to subacute small bowel obstruc-tion

Firm mass in RIF

Restricted mobility

Ascites and cold abscess may be present

Para-aortic lymphadenopathy

Hyperperistaltic sounds

Late - intestinal obstruction

Emaciation

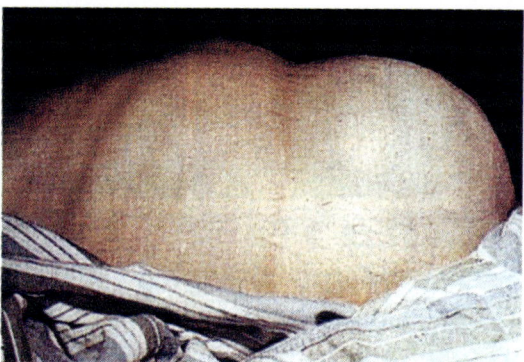

Fig. 103.25. Grossly distended urinary bladder due to benign prostatic hypertrophy

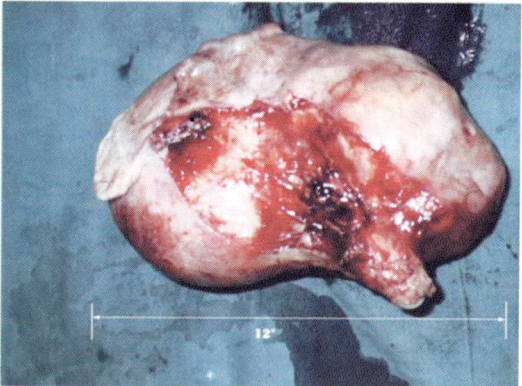

Fig. 103.26. Uterus with multiple large fibroids

Empty RIF (signe de Dance) (as the cecum gets pulled up).

Diagnosis: Ascitic fluid analysis, chest x-ray, ileo-colonoscopy or diagnostic laparoscopy and biopsy.

Treatment:

Anti-Koch's therapy for 9 to 18 months

Indications for surgery:
1. bowel obstruction
2. cold abscess
3. uncertainity about the diagnosis

If obstruction or a large mass, laparoscopic or open 'limited resection' of the terminal ileum, cecum and ascending colon may be done, with ileotransverse colostomy

If the patient's general condition is poor, due to bowel obstruction, a bypass alone may be done. (side-to-side ileotransverse colostomy).

Features of Crohn's disease (regional enteritis)

Recurrent attacks of pain/ fever/ diarrhea
Anemia due to occult or overt GI bleeding
Mass in RIF (usually the terminal ileum)
Perianal disease
Malabsorption
General condition may be well preserved
Acute attack may mimic acute appendicitis

Complications: perforation/abscess/fistula/ obstruction

Diagnosis

1. barium meal series shows the narrow segment (string sign of Cantor).
2. ileo-colonoscopy and biopsy.
3. CT scan

Treatment

1. Primarily medical with salazopyrine, steroids and immunosuppressives like azathioprine. The biological agents like tumor necrosis factor inhibitors (Infliximab) are used for fistulating Crohn's disease.

2. Surgery is indicated mainly for complications like obstruction, perforation, fistula etc. The mainstay of surgery is conservation i.e., stricturoplasty, short segment resections, etc as the disease tends to be recurrent and can involve multiple segments of bowel.

Features of carcinoma cecum

Middle age and above
Painless mass in RIF
Anemia, malena, weight loss, electrolyte problems
Paraaortic nodes/liver
Ascites
Intestinal obstruction (late)
Mass gets fixed (late)
R/O Koch's and NHL

Diagnosis is made by a Colonoscopic biopsy followed by a CT to assess nodal and hepatic metastases.

Treatment is radical right hemicolectomy with ileocolic anastomosis, done open or laparoscopically. Postoperative chemotherapy is generally useful in most cases. In non-resectable cases, palliative bypass may be done, followed by radio/chemotherapy.

MASSES IN HYPOGASTRIUM

Pelvic organs

Uterus, tubo-ovarian
Urinary bladder
Recto-sigmoid

Kidney (pelvic or unascended)
Testis (undescended)
Lymph nodes
Teratoma/ dermoid (presacral)

MASSES IN UMBILICAL REGION

Stomach
Transverse colon/ small bowel
Nodes
Mesentery/ mesocolon
Spleen
Omentum
Pelvic organs
Retroperitoneum

Horse-shoe kidney
Aortic aneurysm
Sympathetic chain

Lumbar vertebra (lordosis)

MESENTERIC CYST

Features of mesenteric cyst

Rounded cystic mass, sometimes with fluid thrill
Location line of mesteric attachment
2" below and right on transpyloric plane to 2" below and left on transtubercular line
Mobility across the line of mesenteric attachment
No bowel symptoms

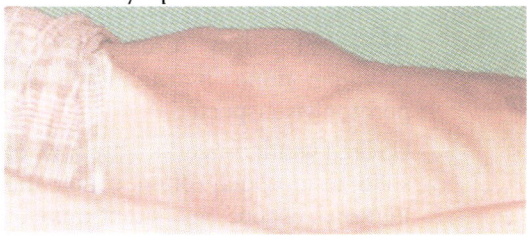

Fig.103.27. Abdominal aortic aneurysm producing a pulsatile epigastric/umbilical mass, better appreciated by tangential inspection

Band of resonance across the mass
No constitutional symptoms, unless infected or in case of a cold abscess

Types of mesenteric cysts

Chylolymphatic (commonest)
Duplication (enteric or urogenital)
Teratomatous
Cold abscess
Parasitic

Diagnosis is made with an ultrasound or a CT scan.

Treatment: Cyst excision is sufficient for the common chylolymphatic variety. Resection of adjacent bowel might become necessary, if it is a duplication cyst as the blood supply to that segment of bowel may be in jeopardy.

Features of lymphoma

Usually NHL
Nodular retroperitoneal swelling in the epigastrium/umbilical region/iliac fossa/ hypogastrium
May be mobile (epiploic/mesenteric/ pericolic/ mesocolic nodes)
Other groups may be involved
Bowel involvement may be present
Constitutional symptoms may be present
Ascites is uncommon
No bowel symptoms, unless bowel is involved

Diagnosis: Chest x-ray, ultrasound and CT scan will identify the disease. Biopsy of any available superficial lymph node will clinch it. Immunohistochemistry is necessary to classify and to select appropriate therapy.

Treatment: Chemotherapy (MOPP, CHOP, COPP, or targeted therapy with Rituximab) is the sheet anchor of treatment.

Abdominal aortic aneurysm (see chapter 81)

INVESTIGATIONS FOR ABDOMINAL MASS

Simple, non-invasive & inexpensive investigations have to be carried out first and only when these do not provide enough information to proceed with treatment, more elaborate, expensive or invasive studies have to be resorted to.

Avoid academic investigations, which do not influence the management; either the diagnosis, treatment or prognostication, e.g. barium study of stomach for an endoscopically proved gastric malignancy (unless some distal disease is suspected)

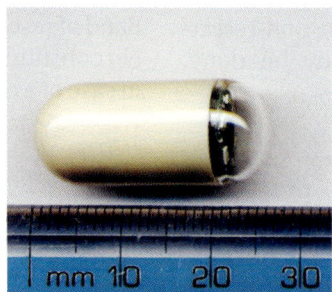

Fig 103.28. A camera-built capsule for enteroscopy

USG is the basic investigation for any abdominal condition, however it is not very sensitive for diseases of hollow viscera, since the gas in the bowel interferes with the sonographic resolution.

CT scan, either contrast-enhanced or multislice has become the gold standard for abdominal diagnosis.

MRI scores over CT in studying vascular or biliary anatomy.

After the advent of fibreoptic endoscopy, barium meal study is rarely done, in view of its low sensitivity in detecting early lesions. Further the all-important tissue diagnosis is possible only with endoscopy. The only place for a contrast study is to ascertain gastric outlet obstruction and to identify distal bowel lesions, beyond the scope of the endoscopes.

Chromoendoscopy has improved the accuracy of detecting early mucosal malignant lesions. It consists of staining the mucosa to delineate pathological areas before endoscopy and is categorized into 3 types:

1. Absorptive (vital) stains (e.g. Lugol's solution and methylene blue) are specifically absorbed through the epithelial membranes

2. Contrast stains (e.g. indigo carmine) highlight the surface topography and mucosal irregularity by permeating into mucosal crevices

3. Reactive stains (e.g. Congo red and phenol red) undergo chemical reaction with specific cellular constituents resulting the color change.

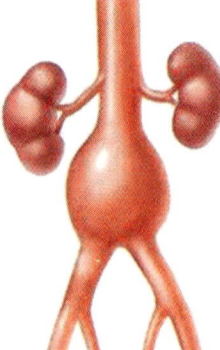

Fig. 103.29. Infrarenal AAA fusiform

These stains are transient in their action, in contrast to more durable tattooing which involves endoscopically injecting a dye through a needle, to mark a site for future identification, e.g. preoperative injection of a polyp through a colonoscope.

For study of distal bowel the colonoscopy has been shown to be superior and more sensitive that barium enema, except in situations where, for technical reasons the endoscope could not be negotiated up to the cecum.

Virtual endoscopy is to study the lumen of the entire bowel (usually colon) using a CT scan employing dedicated software.

Capsule endoscopy

This is used to visualize the areas of GI tract, not in the reach of conventional upper or lower GI endoscopies. A battery operated tiny camera is built in a capsule which is swallowed by the patient. The series of pictures taken or relayed externally through a bluetooth device and the images can be analyzed for any mucosal pathology. The main drawback of this study are:

1. unlike standard endoscopies no biopsy of intervention is possible

2. it is expensive

3. occasional the capsule may get arrested in GI tract, which may have to be removed through endoscopy. Ascitic fluid analysis/Gram stain/cytology (see chapter 18)

Peritoneal biopsy (Cope's needle) may be done if carcinomatosis perotonii is suspected.

USG/CT-guided-needle biopsy of solid lesions may often clinch the matter, except in situations of sampling errors resulting in false negative report. Liver, retroperitoneal lymph nodes/tumors, spleen, pancreas, kidneys, prostate are amenable for this approach and is routinely employed. Though FNAC has become very popular, if the lesion is more than 2-3cm size, it is preferable to use core (Trucut) needle, to improve sensitivity and specificity.

After establishing tissue diagnosis of malignancy, staging investigations have to be done.

IVU/Angio/MRI/Isotope/PET-CT

Immunological studies may be useful in tuberculosis, hydatid disease etc, and are mandatory to immunotype lymphomas.
 Tumor markers (vide infra)
 Laparoscopy/laparotomy.

LIVER BIOPSY

Since many abdominal cancers have a tendency to spread to liver, when the primary inaccessible, tissue diagnosis can often be obtained by a needle biopsy of the liver lesion. The sampling errors of liver biopsy, may be reduced to a great extent by employing the principle of guided biopsy (either USG or CT), 'hitting the target' under vision.

Contraindications for needle biopsy of liver

1. Coagulopathy
2. Vascular lesion
3. Obstructive jaundice
4. Gross ascites
5. In case of doubt whether the lesion is hepatic or extrahepatic
6. Suspected hydatid disease
7. Uncooperative patient

TUMOR MARKERS IN AN ABDOMINAL MASS

Ovary CA 125, β-hCG
HCC   SAlkP, AFP
Prostate   SAcidP, PSA, PSMA (membrane)
Colorectal CA 19-9, CEA
Urinary bladder   BTA (bladder tumor antigen)

Stomach   CA 19-9, Gastrin, pepsinogen 1 & 2
Pancreas   CA 19-9
Testis   AFP, β-hCG, CEA

Chorio Ca β-hCG
Carcinoid 5-HIAA (5-hydroxy indole acetic acid)
Pheochromocytoma   VMA, Catacholamines
Other investigations
Laparoscopy (peeping through key hole?)
Laparotomy

COMMON CONDITIONS IN CHILDREN

Intussusception
Worms
Duplication cysts
Hydronephrosis
Blood dyscrasias
Portal hypertension
Anomalies of Meckel's and Urachus
Choledochal cyst
Polycystic kidney/ liver
Tumors
- Nephroblastoma (Wilm's)
- Neuroblastoma (adrenal)
Tuberculosis

COMMON MISTAKES Checklist for students

Extent of the mass - check costal margins, draw imaginary lines

 Anatomic plane - Carnett's sign
Pulsations - transmitted or expansile
Fecal concretions -   location and moulding sign
Bimanual vs bellotability - for loin and pelvic masses
PV & PR - don't forget in any abdominal case
Groins - missed hernia may be missed exam!
External genitalia - secondaries from testicular tumour may present as an epigastric or umbilical mass
Distended urinary bladder - bladder should be emptied before abdominal examination.

Gravid uterus - menstrual history is very important in child-bearing age

Lumbar lordosis - may accentuate aortic pulsation or feel like a bony hard mass. Hand may be passed under the lumbar spine, if suspected.

Right Hypochondrium	Epigastrium	Left Hypochondrium
Liver/Gallbladder	Stomach	Spleen
Hepatic flexure of colon	Liver	Splenic flexure of colon
Stomach	Transverse colon	Lesser sac
Kidney	Lesser sac	Tail of pancreas
Adrenal	Retroperitoneum	Kidney
Head of pancreas	Lymph nodes	Adrenal
Lesser sac	Aorta	Retroperitoneum
Appendix (subhepatic)	Body of pancreas	
Retroperitoneum	Adrenal	
	Falciform ligament	
Right Lumbar	**Umbilical**	**Left Lumbar**
Right kidney/Adrenal	Stomach	Left kidney/Adrenal
Ascending colon	Transevere colon	Descending colon
Liver/Gallbladder	Mesentery/Mesocolon	Spleen
Head of pancreas	Spleen	Tail of pancreas
Appendix (high)	Omentum	Undescended testis
Retroperitoneum	Pelvic organs	Retroperitoneum
Duodenum	Retroperitoneum	
Undescended testis	Horse-shoe kidney	
	Aorta	
	Lymph nodes	
	Sympathetic chain	
	Psoas sheath	
	Lumbar vertebra (lordosis)	
Right Iliac Fossa	**Hypogastrium**	**Left Iliac Fossa**
Appendix	Pelvic organs	Sigmoid colon
Cecum	Unirary bladder	Unascended kidney
Terminal ileum	Recto-sigmoid	Lymph nodes
Lymph nodes	Kidney (pelvic)	Psoas sheath
Psoas sheath	Undescended testis	Retroperitoneum
Retroperitoneum	Retroperitoneum	Vessels/Bones
Broad ligament	Dermoid/Teratoma	Broad ligament
Unascended kidney	Organ of Zuckerkandl	Undescended testis
Undescended testis	Lymph nodes	Left tube/Ovary
Right tube/Ovary		
Vessels/Bones		

Table-103.3. Origin of abdominal masses in various anatomical zones

104 Portal Hypertension

A vascular system that originates from capillaries and ends in capillaries is called portal system. There are two such systems in the body, namely, hepatic and hypothalamo-hypophysial portal systems.

Hepatic portal venous system

The liver has dual blood supply, $2/3^{rd}$ from the portal vein and the rest from hepatic artery. The portal system includes all the veins which drain the blood from the abdominal part of the digestive tube (with the exception of the lower part of the rectum) and from the spleen, pancreas, and gallbladder. From these viscera the blood is conveyed to the liver by the portal vein. In the liver this vein ramifies like an artery and ends in capillary-like vessels termed sinusoids, from which the blood is conveyed to the inferior vena cava by the hepatic veins. From this it will be seen that the blood of the portal system passes through two sets of minute vessels, viz., (a) the capillaries of the digestive tube, spleen, pancreas, and gallbladder; and (b) the sinusoids of the liver. In the adult the portal vein and its tributaries are devoid of valves; in the fetus and for a short time after birth valves can be demonstrated in the tributaries of the portal vein.

The portal vein is about 8 cm in length, and is formed at the level of the second lumbar vertebra by the junction of the superior

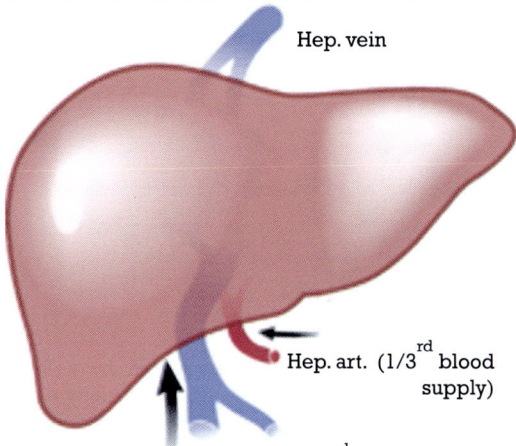

Fig. 104.2. Normal liver blood flow

mesenteric and splenic veins, the union of these veins taking place in front of the inferior vena cava and behind the neck of the pancreas. It passes upward behind the superior part of the duodenum and then ascends in the right border of the lesser omentum to the right extremity of the porta hepatis, where it divides into right and left branches, which accompany the corresponding branches of the hepatic artery

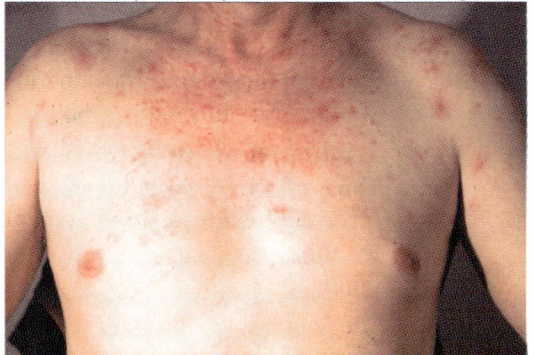

Fig. 104.1. Spider nevi

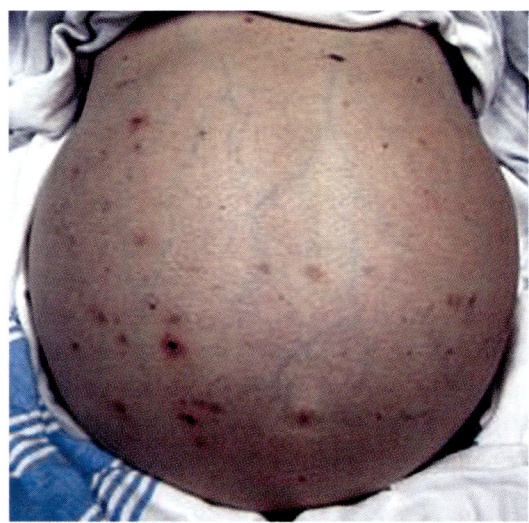

Fig. 104.3. Cirrhosis with ascites

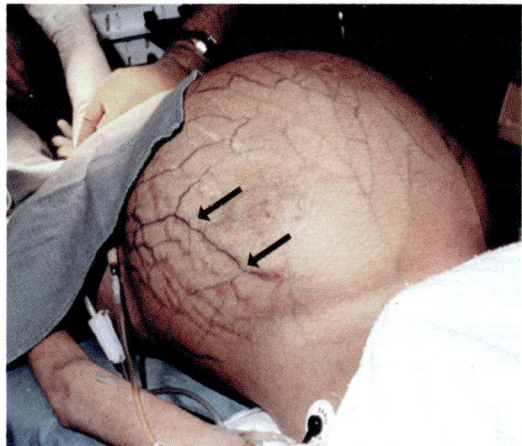

Fig. 104.4. Caput medusae accentuated by a large amount of ascites. A large vein coursing inferiorly along the right flank (arrows) is the superficial epigastric vein

into the substance of the liver. In the lesser omentum it is placed behind and between the common bile duct and the hepatic artery, the former lying to the right of the latter. It is surrounded by the hepatic plexus of nerves, and is accompanied by numerous lymphatic vessels and some lymph glands. The unique feature of the portal vein is, it has unstriated muscle fibres, to regulate the blood flow through it.

The Splenic vein commences by five or six large tributaries which return blood from the spleen. These unite to form a single vessel, which passes from left to right, grooving the upper and back part of the pancreas, below the splenic artery and ends behind the neck of the pancreas by uniting at a right angle with the superior mesenteric to form the portal vein. The splenic vein is of large size, but is not tortuous like the artery.

Tributaries: The splenic vein receives the short gastric veins, the left gastroepiploic vein, the pancreatic veins, and the

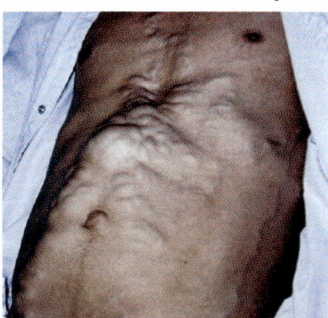

Fig. 104.5. Caput Medusae

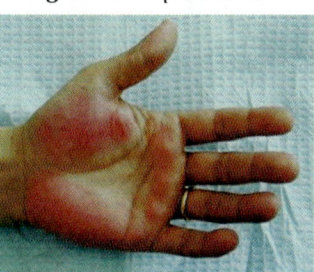

Fig. 104.6. Palmar erythema

inferior mesenteric veins.

The short gastric veins, four or five in number, drain the fundus and left part of the greater curvature of the stomach, and pass between the two layers of the gastrosplenic ligament to end in the splenic vein or in one of its large tributaries.

The left gastroepiploic vein receives blood from the antero-superior and postero-inferior surfaces of the stomach and from the greater omentum; it runs from right to left along the greater curvature of the stomach and ends in the commencement of the splenic vein.

The pancreatic veins consist of several small vessels which drain the body and tail of the pancreas, and open into the trunk of the lienal vein.

The inferior mesenteric vein returns blood from the rectum, sigmoid, and descending colon. It begins in the rectum as the superior rectal (hemorrhoidal) vein, which has its origin in the hemorrhoidal plexus, through which it communicates with the middle and inferior rectal veins. The superior rectal vein leaves the lesser pelvis, crosses the left common iliac vessels with the superior rectal artery, and is continues upward as the inferior mesenteric vein. This vein lies to the left of its artery, and ascends behind the peritoneum and in front of the left psoas major; it then passes behind the body of the pancreas and joins the splenic vein; sometimes it ends in the angle of union of the splenic and superior mesenteric veins.

Tributaries of portal vein

The inferior mesenteric vein receives blood from upper rectum to the distal transverse colon (hindgut).

The superior mesenteric vein received blood from the jejunum, ileum, cecum, ascending and

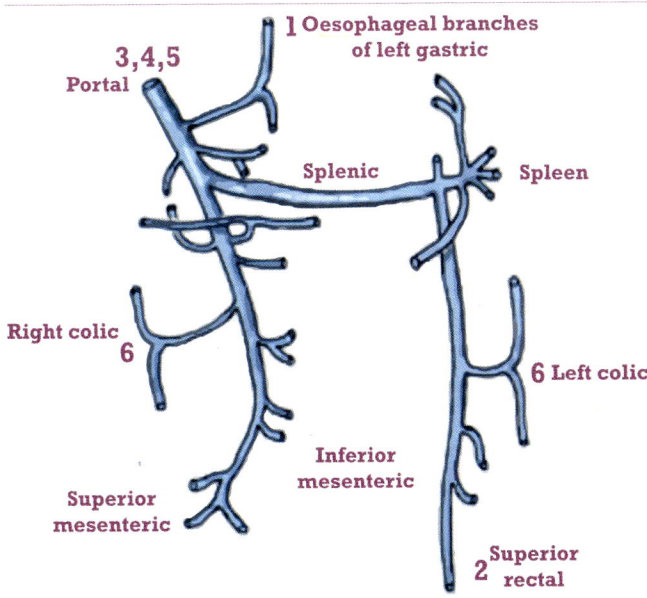

3,4,5
Portal

] Oesophageal branches
of left gastric

Splenic

Spleen

Right colic
6

6 Left colic

Inferior
mesenteric

Superior
mesenteric

Superior
2 rectal

1. **Lower oesophagus**
   Portal: Oesophageal branches of left
   gastric veins
   Systemic: Azygos veins

2. **Upper anal canal**
   Portal: Superior rectal vein
   Systemic: Middle/inferior rectal veins

3. **Umbilical**
   Portal: Veins ofligamentum teres
   Systemic: Superior/inferior epigastric
   veins

4. **Bare area of liver**
   Portal: Hepatic/portal veins
   Systemic: Inferior phrenic veins

5. **Patent ductus venosus (rare)**
   Portal: Left branch of portal vein
   Systemic: Inferior vena cava

6. **Retroperitoneal**
   Portal: Colonic veins
   Systemic: Body wall veins

Fig. 104.7. Portosystemic anastomoses

proximal transverse colon (midgut). It begins in the right iliac fossa by the union of the veins which drain the terminal part of the ileum, the cecum, and vermiform process, and ascends between the two layers of the mesentery on the right side of the superior mesenteric artery. In its upward course it passes in front of the right ureter, the inferior vena cava, 3rd part of the duodenum, and the uncinate process of pancreas. Behind the neck of the pancreas it unites with the splenic vein to form the portal vein.

The coronary (left gastric) vein is the main culprit vein of variceal hemorrhage. It derives tributaries from both surfaces of the stomach; it runs from right to left along the lesser curvature of the stomach, between the two layers of the lesser omentum, to the cardia, where it receives some esophageal veins. It then turns backward and passes from left to right behind the omental bursa and ends in the portal vein.

The other tributaries are the pancreatico duodenal, pyloric and cystic veins.

Periumbilical veins: In the ligamentum teres of the liver and of the medial umbilical ligaments, small veins (paraumbilical) are found which establish an anastomosis between the veins of the anterior abdominal wall and the portal, hypogastric, and iliac veins. The best marked of these small veins is one which commences at the umbilicus and runs backward and upward between the layers of the falciform ligament to end in the left portal vein.

PORTA-AZYGOS COLLATERALS

Collateral venous circulation to relieve portal obstruction in the liver may be effected by communications between

(a) the gastric veins and the esophageal veins which often project as a varicose bunch into the lower esophagus and gastric fundus, emptying themselves into the hemiazygos vein

(b) the veins of the colon and duodenum and the left renal vein

(c) the accessory portal system of Sappey, branches of which pass in the round and falciform ligaments to unite with the epigastric and internal mammary veins, and through the diaphragmatic veins with the azygos system. A single large parumbilical vein, may pass from the hilum of the liver by the round ligament to the umbilicus, producing there a bunch of prominent varicose veins known as the caput medusæ

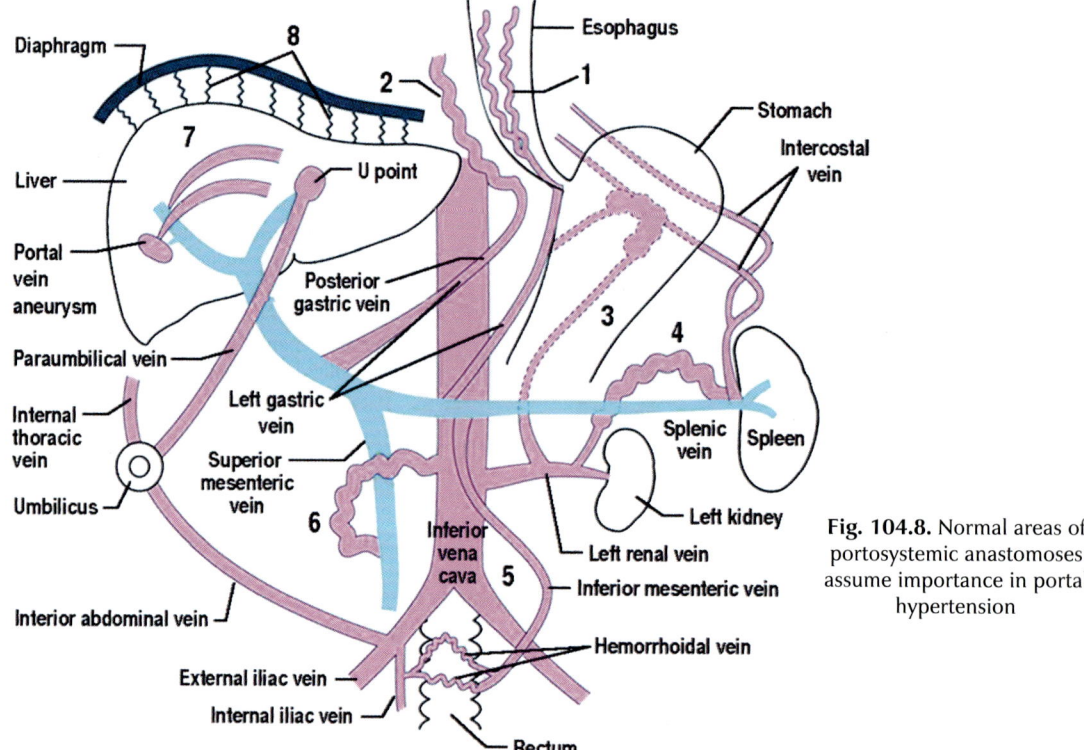

Fig. 104.8. Normal areas of portosystemic anastomoses assume importance in portal hypertension

(d) the veins of Retzius, which connect the intestinal veins with the inferior vena cava and its retroperitoneal tributaries

(e) the inferior mesenteric veins, and the hemorrhoidal veins that drain into the hypogastric veins

(f) very rarely the ductus venosus remains patent, affording a direct connection between the portal vein and the inferior vena cava.

Portal hypertension means the venous pressure is increased in the portal system .

The portal system, which conveys about 60-80% of afferent blood to liver, drains:

(a) from most of GIT (lower third of esophagus to the upper third of rectum)

(b) spleen - 1/5th of portal blood comes from spleen

(c) pancreas

(d) gallbladder

(e) products of digestion

(f) endocrine secretions from stomach, pancreas and small intestines

Normal portal pressure is about 7-8 mmHg and above 10mm is considered portal hypertension. Critical pressure is usually >12mm, below which variceal bleeding does not usally occur. Thus, the idea of chemical or surgical lowering of portal hypertension is to keep the portal pressure below 12mmHg.

Total blood flow through the portal circulation is about 1000-1200ml/minute. The segmental

	EXTRA HEPATIC	INTRA HEPATIC
Presinusoidal	Portal vein thrombosis Splenic vein thrombosis	Congenital hepatic fibrosis Schistosomiasis
Post sinusoidal	Hepatic vein thrombosis IVC thrombosis, web	Cirrhosis

Table-104.1

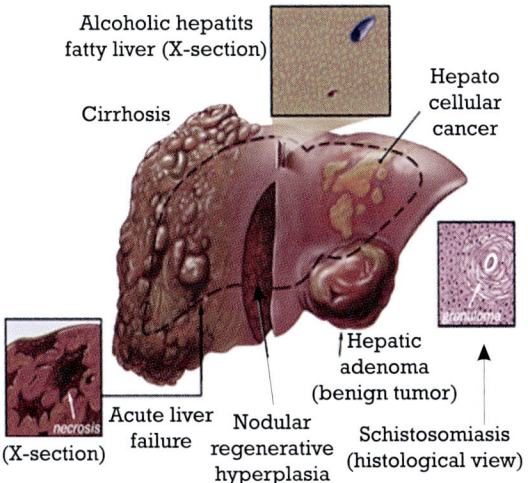

Fig. 104.9. Intrahepatic (sinusoidal) causes

anatomy of the liver is based mainly on the demarcation of hepatic venous branching.

Keeping the hepatic sinusoids as the epicentre, a new nomenclature for portal hypertension has replaced the older one.

Sinusoidal (intrahepatic)
Presinusoidal (prehepatic)
Post-sinusoidal (posthepatic)

CONVENTIONAL CLASSIFICATION
Prehepatic

a) thrombosis/narrowing of portal or: splenic vein

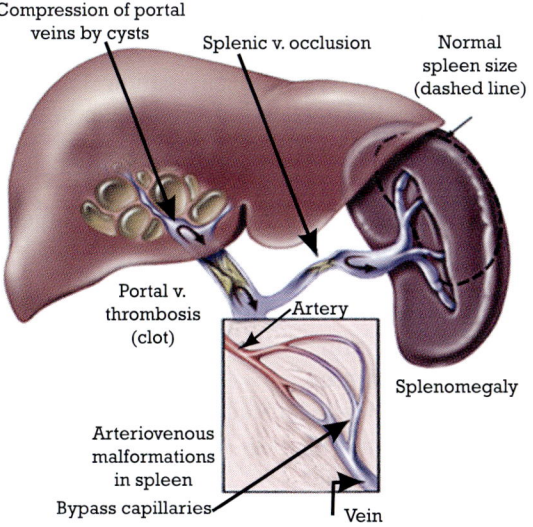

Fig. 104.10. Prehepatic (Pre-sinusoidal) causes

b) tumor around porta hepatis
c) schistosomiasis (most common worldwide, except in India and USA)

Hepatic

a) alcoholic cirrhosis (most common in USA)
b) cirrhosis due to hepatitis
c) nodular regenerative hyperplasia
d) primary biliary cirrhosis
e) primary sclerosing cholangitis

Posthepatic

a) Budd-Chiari syndrome
b) right heart failure (e.g.constrictive pericarditis, cardiomyopathy)
c) hepatic vein thrombosis

NEWER CLASSIFICATION

The importance of the sinusoids is the hepatic lymphatics run into the sinusoids. Ascites in portal hypertension is mainly due to hepatic lymphorrhagia. The more distal the cause of the portal hypertension, the more the ascites, the protein loss and worse the prognosis.

In Budd-Chiari syndrome, which is a post-sinusoidal, extrahepatic disease, there is rapid onset ascites and hepatic failure, whereas in splenic vein thrombosis, which is presinusoidal, extrahepatic, there is neither hepatic dysfunction or ascites.

IMPORTANT POINTS IN HISTORY

1. Nature of hematemesis

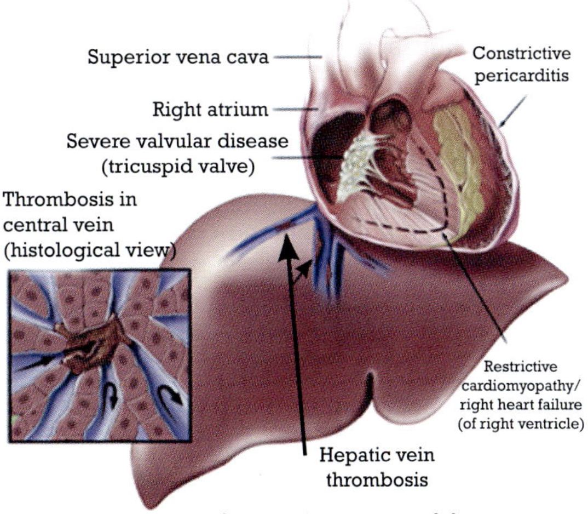

Fig. 104.11. Posthepatic (Post-sinusoidal) causes

a) frank blood - quantity
b) coffee ground vomitus

2. H/o fever
   a) chills and rigors
   b) repeated attacks of fever

3. Pain abdomen
   a) dull ache
   b) biliary colic
   c) burning epigastrium - hyperacidity

4. Features of cirrhosis of liver
   a) ascites
   b) edema of lower limbs
   c) prominent veins over abdominal wall
   d) splenomegaly
   e) shrunken liver
   f) spider nevi
   g) testicular atrophy
   h) palmar erythema
   l) gynecomastia
   j) flapping tremors

5. H/O drug ingestion (e.g. NSAIDs)

6. Anemia

7. Jaundice

8. Personal history
   1. Alcohol ingestion
   a) amount (an alcoholic is one who drinks more than the doctor!)
   b) duration

9. Past history
   a. previous hospitalisation with altered consciousness.
   b. abdominal surgery in the past
   c. hospitalisation for septic appendicular perforation during childhood.
   d. umbilical vein catheterisation.
   e. Tuberculosis, jaundice or any liver problem in the family
   f. α-1 antitrypsin deficiency
   g. Wilson's disease (disease of copper metabolism)
   h. hemochromatosis (disease of iron metabolism).

The commonest causes are:
1. Cryptogenic

2. Viral hepatits (B or C)
3. Alcoholism

PHYSICAL EXAMINATION

1. General
   a) mild icterus
   b) anemia
   c) features of cirrhosis of liver
      hepatosplenomegaly
      spider nevi
      testicular atrophy
      ascites
      palmar erythema
      gynecomastia
      flapping tremors.

2. Abdominal examination may be performed according to the standard protocol detailed in chapter 103.

Left supraclavicular (Virchow) nodes
Vaginal and rectal examination
The sources of hematemesis in portal hypertension:
Esophageal varices
Gastric varices
Congestive gastropathy
Acid-peptic disease

Causes of encephalopathy
a) Bleeding into gastrointestinal tract.
b) Degraded nitrogenous products in the gut, producing ammonia are not detoxified by liver, through the Kreb's urea cycle. Entry of these products into systemic circulation leads to neurological manifestations, including hepatic encephalopathy and coma.
c) Other factors
   I) Following porto-systemic shunt surgery
   ii) Chemicals responsible
      Ammonia
      Gamma aminobutyric acid (GABA)
      Mercaptin
      Methionine
      Short chain fatty acids
d) Precipitating factors
Large protein meal
G I hemorrhage
Hypokalemia

Sepsis

Dehydration

Uremia

Opiate poisoning

Tapping of ascites - large quantities

Diuretic therapy

Alcohol abuse

CLINICAL FEATURES OF ENCEPHALO PATHY

Intellectual deterioration

Personality changes

Disorientation

Slurring speech

Flapping tremors

Cogwheel rigidity of limbs

Ankle clonus

Deep coma

EEG changes slowing of frequency down to delta range

Palmar erythema

cirrhosis with ascitis

caput medusae

spider nevi

Investigations

Routine studies, including liver functions and coagulation profile, INR, serum ammonia.

Stool for occult blood.

Evaluate hypersplenism, if there is pancyto-penia

Serum electrolytes, if the patient is on diuretics

Tumor markers: AFP, CEA, Alk Phosphatase

Viral markers: HBV, HCV, HIV

Barium swallow, USG / CT abdomen

Ascitic fluid analysis and cytology

Upper GI endoscopy

Liver biopsy

Splenoportovenography (SPV), only if shunt surgery is planned. Rarely done now, largely replaced by multislice CT.

Venous phase of celiac axis angiography is found to be safer than SPV and therefore the most preferred.

Cardiac evaluation, if cardiac cirrhosis (congestive hepatopathy) is suspected

Medical treatment

Treatment of underlying disease

Treatment of effects of PH

Beta blockers

Spironolactone

Lactulose and lactitol

Hepatotropic agents

Gut sterilization (metronidazole, rifaximine etc)

Coagulation support

Avoiding hepatotoxic substances

Indications for surgery in PH

1. GI Bleeding
2. Ascites
3. Hypersplenism

Management of bleeding

The therapeutic strategy and ultimate prognosis is largely decided by the state of liver. Child-Pugh's classification is designed to stratify the patients for appropriate regime (Table 104.2).

The bleeding in PH is usually from the esophageal or fundal varices. Occasionally bleeding from a peptic ulcer, which is often associated with PH, may be seen. This is considered to be due to gastrin-like, histamin-like hormones from the gut directly entering into systemic circulation bypassing the liver, to exert their action on the gastric mucosa.

The variceal bleeding may be occult, moderate or massive (life-threatening). The first line of treatment for variceal bleeding is always endos-

Feature	Child's A	Child's B	Child's C
Serum bilirubin (mg%)	<2	2 – 3	>3
Serum albumin (gm%)	>3.5	3 – 3.5	<3
Ascites	None	Minimal	Gross
Encephalopathy	None	Occasional	Advanced
Nutrition	Excellent	Good	Poor

Table - 104.2 - Child's stratification of the state of liver functions
(after Sherlock)

copic therapy, by one of the following methods:

1. Endoscopic peri-variceal injection of sclerosant or endoscopic sclerotherapy (EST)

2. Injection of glue (cyanoacrylate compounds) into and around varices, especially to treat gastric fundal varices.

3. Endoscopic variceal ligation (EVL) or banding.

Since the mortality of first bleed is around 25%, prophylactic endoscopic therapy is advisable for grades 3 & 4 varices. Endoscopic therapy has about 80% success rate in controlling hemorrhage. The question of TIPS or open surgery is considered only if multiple attempts at endoscopic intervention had not arrested bleeding.

TIPS (or TIPSS)

(Trans-jugular intrahepatic porto-systemic shunting) This is done when at least 2-3 attempts of endoscopic therapy failed to arrest bleeding. It involves percutaneous intrahepatic deployment of a self-expanding metal stent from the hepatic vein to the left branch of portal vein. As in any shunt, there is significant incidence of encephalopathy following the procedure, hence should be employed with caution in patients in Child's B & C groups.

Contraindications for TIPS.

Absolute
  Primary prevention of bleeding
  Congestive heart failure
  Severe pulmonary hypertension
  Active biliary obstruction
  Sepsis
  Multiple hepatic cysts or Caroli's disease

Relative
  HCC
  PV or HV thrombosis
  Coagulopathy
  Encephalopathy
  Non-availability of expertise

Complications of TIPS

Procedure-related: hemorrhage from capsular perforation, injury to biliary tree or hepatic artery

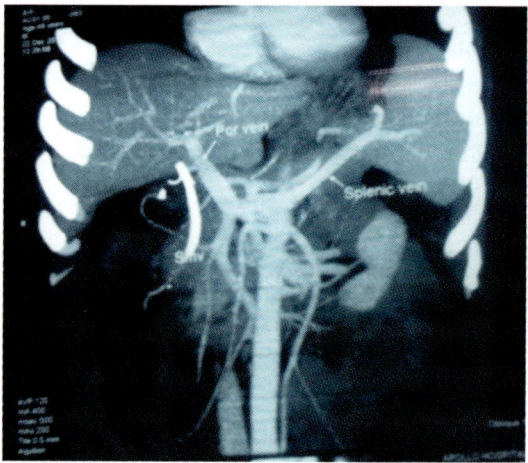

Fig. 104.12. Venous phase of CT angiogram of abdomen showing portal venous system. A biliary stent is also seen

Stent-related: Infection and migration

Contrast-related: anaphylaxis, renal failure, cardiac arrhythmias

Shunt-related: Cardiac overload and congestive failure, pulmonary hypertension, encephalopathy

Open procedures are of two categories: The non-shunt and shunt procedures

Non-shunt procedures

1. Splenic artery ligation &/or splenectomy
2. Gastro-esophageal (porta-azygos) devascularization (Sugiura)
3. Trans-esophageal ligation of varices (Boerema-Crile))
4. Gastro-esophageal dysjunction and reanastamosis
   a) Lower esophageal level (Milnes-Walker)
   b) Proximal gastric level (Tanner)

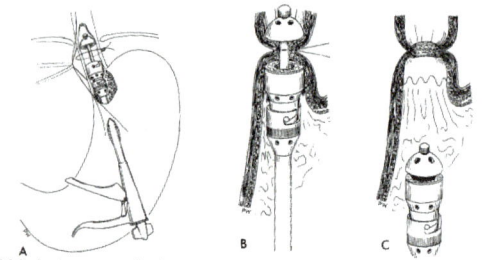

Fig. 104.13. Gastroesophageal disconnection using stapler

c) Only anterior 2/3rd of circumference of fundus (Sadasivan modification)

d) Transluminal stapler (EEA) method at the lower esophagus

5. Transposition of spleen into the chest

Shunt procedures

1. Portacaval shunt

Types of anastomosis

a) Total shunt: end to side (end of portal vein to side of inferior venacava), diverts entire portal flow from the liver

b) Partial shunt (Sarfeh shunt) is side to side portacaval shunt, opening reduced to 8 mm in diameter, there by some amount of portal flow is maintained in about 80% of patients

Criteria for portacaval shunt

Patent portal vein
Serum albumin: >3 g%
Serum bilirubin: <17mmol/L

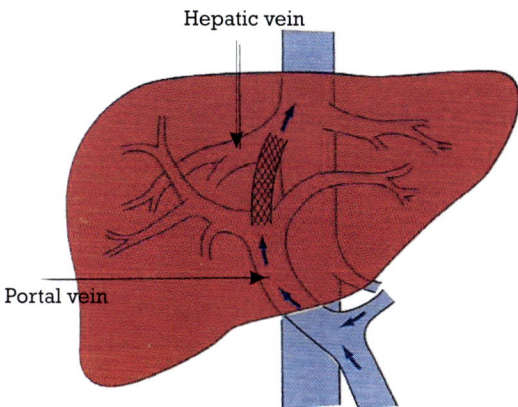

Fig. 104.14. TIPS employing self-expandable metal stent

2. Mesocaval shunt

Jump (H) graft with Dacron or PTFE may be employed, between the superior mesenteric vein and the IVC.

Indications

Portal vein block
Children
Post portocaval shunt block
Advantages
Good graft patency
Risk of encephalopathy minimal

Because of peripheral shunt, blood flow to the liver is maintained

Can be performed as an emergency.

Jewels of Gyan - 104.1

Liver function tests are classified as

a) Those related to carbohydrate metabolism: galactose tolerance test, not very popular

b) Those related to fat metabolism: serum cholesterol, total and esterified fraction

c) Those related to protein metabolism: serum albumin and prothrombin

d) Excretory functions: serum bilirubin, bromsulfophthalein (BSP) retention (normally only <5% of injected dye is retained in 45 min. It is considered to be a highly sensitive test of liver function, in a patient who is not jaundiced)

e) Enzymes: transaminases and alkaline phosphatase. They give an index of sick cells rather than dead cells and may not be useful in acute liver cell necrosis. 5-Nucleotidase estimation is sometimes used when the alkaline phosphatase is elevated, to identify if it is due to biliary or extra-biliary causes.

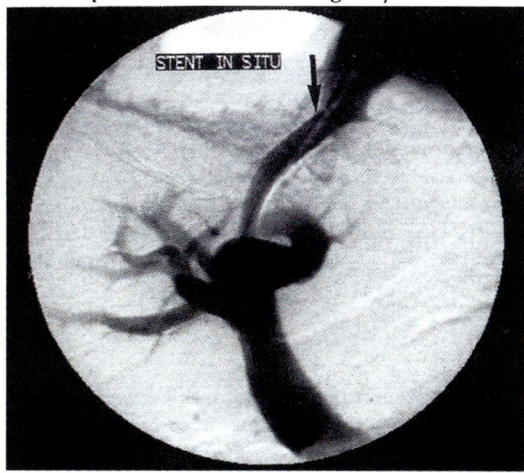

Fig. 104.15. Portal venography demonstrating the stent of TIPS in place

Drawback: portal decompression is not as effective as portocaval shunt

3. **Lienorenal shunt** (proximal splenorenal or Linton- Fisher shunt)

Following splenectomy, the stump of splenic vein is anastomosed to the side of left renal vein

Indications

Thrombosed portal vein
Child's B patients, with moderate risk of encephalopathy
Prerequisite
No thrombosis of splenic vein
Splenic vein size-1 cm in diameter
Left kidney is normal with its vein

Drawback

Splenectomy is inevitable, hence unsuitable for children

Results

Operative mortalility - 10%
Shunt thrombosis - 20%

4. **Selective shunt**

Distal splenorenal (Warren) shunt

Retaining the spleen, the splenic vein is divided behind the pancreas, proximal stump is ligated and the distal splenic vein is anastomosed to renal vein.

Advantages

Maintains normal portal flow
Selective decompression of esophageal and gastric varices
Low incidence of encephalopathy

Disadvantages

Technically difficult, more so in obese and those with massive splenomegaly
Choice of the procedure in a nutshell:
Child's A: Either shunt (including TIPS) or non-shunt procedure
Child's B: Selective shunt or

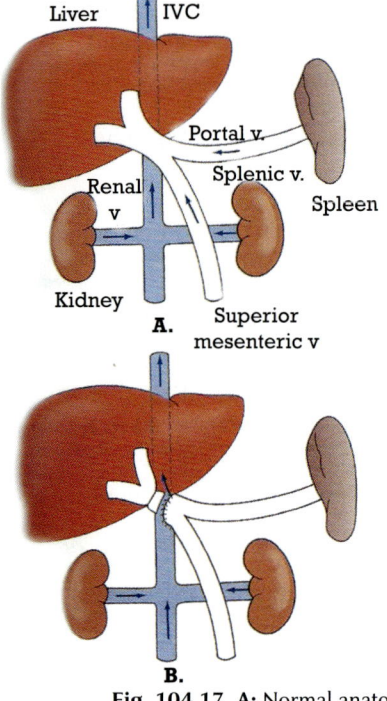

Fig. 104.17. A: Normal anatomy
B: End-to-side portacaval anastomosis

non-shunt preferred
Child's C: Only non-shunt procedures
Acute (massive) upper GI bleeding

Common causes

Portal hypertension and esophageal varices
Peptic ulcer
Erosive gastritis (drug/alcohol induced)

Rare causes

Esophagitis
Gastric carcinoma
Gastric bezoars (phyto and tricho)
Angiodysplasia of gastric mucosa
Post-splenectomy congestive gastropathy
Mallory-Weiss tear
Hemobilia
Hemosuccus pancreaticus
Aorto-enteric fistula

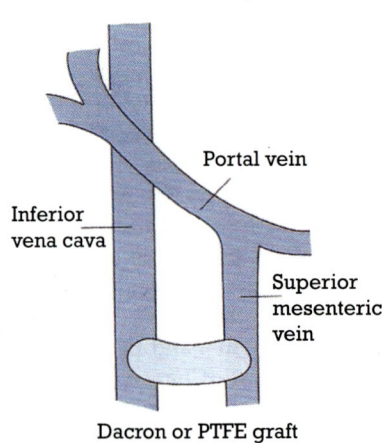

Fig. 104.16. Mesocaval interposition ('H') graft

Management of massive variceal bleeding

Evaluation and monitoring

Resuscitation

Balloon tamponade: Sengstaken-Blakemore tube (Minnisota modification)

Styptics and gastric hypothermia

Non-selective β-blockers (propranolol, nadolol)

Mode of action: β-1 blockade reduces the cardiac output and β-2 blockade induces splanchnic vasoconstriction

Contraindications: COPD, bronchospastic disorder, cardiac A-V block

Vasopressin analogues: Glypressin, or terlipressin. They cause splanchnic vasocons-triction. Problems of their use are impaired coronary flow and rebound bleeding when the infusion is discontinued. Hence they are used to 'tide over the crisis', while getting ready for surgery.

Somatostatin (a hormone released by pancreas, reduces splanchnic blood flow and portal pressure)

Emergency endoscopy and intervention (banding preferred)

Prevention of complications

Hepatorenal syndrome

Systemic infection

Pulmonary aspiration

Encephalopathy

Hepatic failure

Antibiotics

Bowel wash

Gut sterilization

Adequate volume replacement

Hepatoprotective aminoacids

Indication for surgery in massive bleeding

While doing resuscitation, if a patient has to be given blood transfusion equal to half the blood volume in 24 hours, such bleeding is unlikely to stop with other treatment modalities, hence requires immediate surgery.

Other factors that influence the decision: age of the patient, state of liver, coagulation profile, co-morbidities, availability of expertise and infrastructure.

ROLE OF SURGERY

The role of surgery in variceal bleeding is limited to refractory hemorrhage. Most cases are now managed endoscopically, by repeated endoscopic banding and sclerotherapy until the varices are obliterated. However in massive bleeding unresponsive to endoscopic attempts, somatostatin and vasopressin analogues, surgery is considered as a life saving measure. Devascularization of the lower esophageal veins including the coronary vein and the upper gastric veins including the fundic veins, is the mainstay of the procedure, which is usually combined with a splenectomy (Sugiura-Hassab procedure). Transection of the oesophagus using a circular stapler (Johnson) is also added sometimes, to effect complete porta-azygos disconnection.

When liver function is well preserved (Child's A&B) and the portal hypertension is pre-sinusoidal (extrahepatic), e.g. splenic vein or portal vein thrombosis, one of the two shunt procedures may be undertaken, but only in the elective setting. A selective shunt (Warren's DSRS - distal splenorenal shunt) with

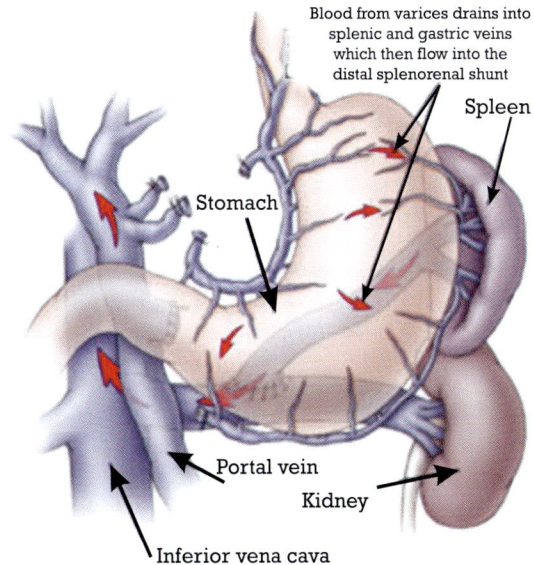

Blood from varices drains into splenic and gastric veins which then flow into the distal splenorenal shunt

Spleen

Stomach

Portal vein

Kidney

Inferior vena cava

Fig. 104.18. Distal splenorenal (Warren) shunt

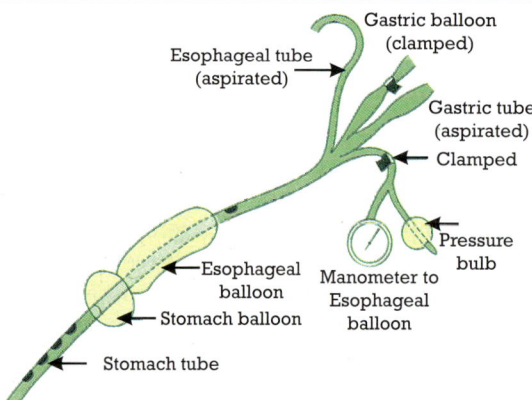

Fig. 104.19. Minnesota modification of Sengstaken-Blakemore tube (with four lumina)

preservation of the spleen or a PSRS (Linton - Fisher shunt) - proximal splenorenal shunt with splenectomy, are the commonest shunts employed.

To summarise

ELECTIVE PROCEDURES

1. Recurrent bleeding with poor hepatic function:

TIPS

Devascularization + transection (Sugiura-Hassab)

2. Recurrent bleeding with good hepatic

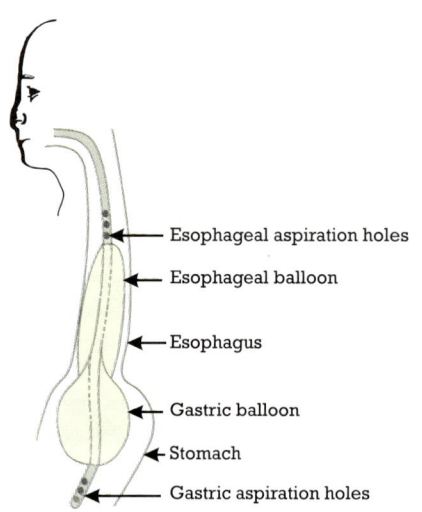

Fig. 104.20. Inflated Sengstaken-Blakemore tube (Minnesota modification) in place

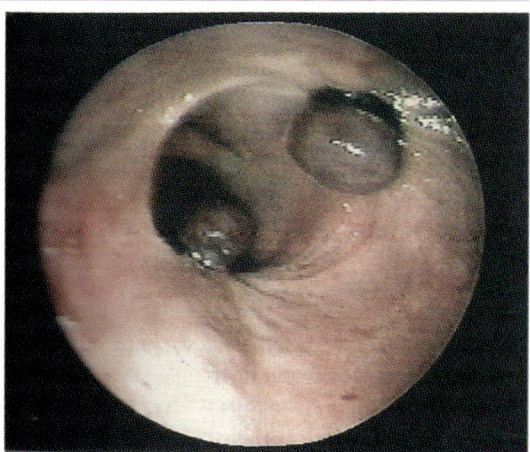

Fig. 104.21. Endoscopic banding (ligation) of esophageal varices
(courtesy: Lifeline Hospital, Chennai)

function:

with hypersplenism - PSRS (splenectomy) - Linton - Fisher shunt.

without hypersplenism - DSRS - Warren shunt.

3. For end-stage liver disease, not responding to conventional therapy, liver transplantation may be the last resort.

Budd-Chiari syndrome (syn: obliterative hepatocavopathy)

This is the result of hepatic venous obstruction, leading to congestive hepatopathy, hemorrhagic hepatic necrosis and its sequella, carrying a very high mortality, if left untreated.

Causes: hepatic vein thrombosis, suprahepatic IVC obstruction (usually due to a web formation) or malignant tumor infiltration. The venacaval web may be congenital or acquired, usually due to infection, under a thrombophilic background. There appears to be some relation to blood dyscrasias (particularly polycythemia), use of oral contraceptives and other thrombophilic disorders to this disease. Some herbal tea used in Jamaica is known to precipitate acute form of this disease.

Acute presentation: severe right hypochondriac pain, nausea, vomiting with rapidly enlarging tender liver and becomes quickly fatal, due to hepatic decompensation. There may be features of portal hypertension with rapidly forming ascites going on to hepatic coma and peripheral failure.

Chronic type: Initial enlarged tender liver leads on to cirrhosis and portal hypertension, with massive refractory ascites, jaundice and pedal edema. Fatality from bleeding esophageal varices or mesenteric venous thrombosis may occur. Markedly enlarged subcutaneous veins over the abdomen are conspicuous. With the advent of noninvasive modalities, more cases are probably being diagnosed in its early stages. If the IVC is occluded, massive pedal edema, engorged flank veins and albuminuria may be seen.

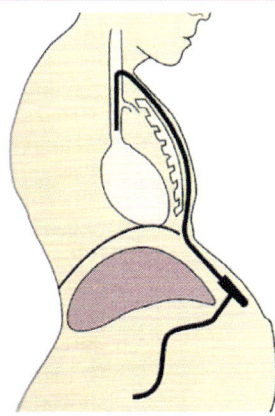

Fig. 104.22. Peritoneo-venous shunt (LeVeen) for intractable ascites

Investigations: Liver function studies, thrombophilia screening, USG, color Doppler, spiral CT abdomen will identify the functional and anatomical nature of the disease. Hepatic venography (functional hepatogram) and inferior venacavography are necessary, to plan surgical strategy. Needle biopsy of liver may be helpful, but not without risk of internal hemorrhage, hence should be done if there is absolute indication.

The caudate lobe of liver, intimately related to the IVC, has its own venous drainage by multiple small veins. In Budd-Chiari syndrome, the other segments of the liver drain blood into the caudate segment. Hence hypertrophy of the caudate lobe is the earliest ultrasonographic sign of this syndrome.

Treatment: If a hematological or coagulative disorder is identified, it should be appropriately treated. If occlusion of hepatic venous outflow (from liver to right atrium) is present, endovascular or open intervention may be required, to relieve the obstruction. If the obstruction is in the hepatic veins, TIPS is the procedure of choice, following which longterm anticoagulation is mandatory. TIPS may also be helpful to 'tide over the crisis' as the patient is being evaluated for liver transplantation. Secondary portal hypertension has to be treated on its merits and its anticipated complications.

Management of ascites in portal hypertension

Medical

Improving nutrition, including serum albumin level. Low sodium intake

Diuretic therapy (spironolactone)

Surgical

Controlled paracentesis

Peritoneo-venous shunting (see Fig. 104.22)

LIVER TRANSPLANTATION

Introduced by Starzl in 1963, liver transplantation has become the standard treatment for end-stage liver disease, for which no alternate therapy is available. The extremely vascular nature of the procedure, especially with portal hypertension and coagulopathy, makes it one of the most difficult operations in surgery, requiring wisdom, skill and endurance. Additional technical difficulties may be encountered in children (below 2), obesity and those undergone previous upper abdominal surgery. Adequate patient counseling is essential, regarding the risk/benefit equation, long term immunosuppression, vulnerability for infections and cancers.

Common technique is orthotopic transplant, removing the liver and placing the graft in the same place. With limited availability of donors, split liver transplant has become necessary, especially for children, though technically demanding. In situations of acute liver damage, with high probability of the patient's liver regenerating, auxiliary liver transplantation is done, retaining the patient's liver. The main advantage of this procedure is to avoid lifelong immunosuppression, if the native liver has a chance to recover.

The recipient surgery has three phases; recipient hepatectomy, anhepatic and post-implantation phases. Anhepatic state can

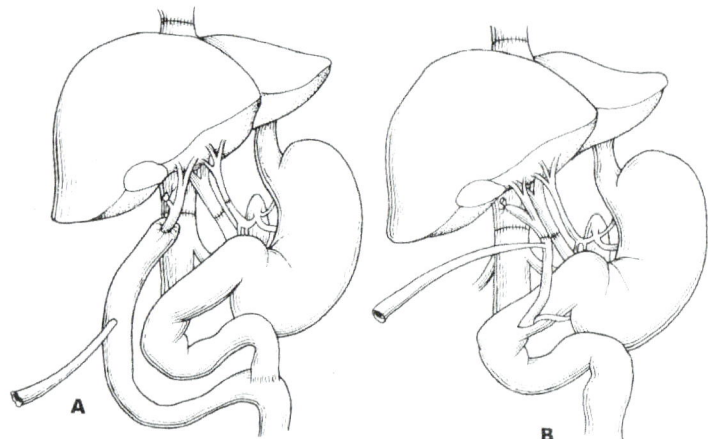

Fig. 104.23. Orthotopic liver transplantation
A. Roux-en-Y biliary anastomosis
B. End-to-end anastomosis of donor and recepient common bile ducts

sustain life only for 24 hrs. High level of postoperative intense care is required with biochemical, hematological, microbiological and immunological monitoring, during the recovery period.

Complications: Besides general complications for any major surgery, specific complications of liver transplantation are:

1. circulatory collapse, due to sudden reduction of venous return to heart via portal circulation and sometimes IVC
2. impaired graft function
3. hemorrhage
4. thrombosis of the anastomosed vessels; portal vein and hepatic artery
5. bile leak
6. sepsis and cholangitis
7. rejection of the graft, which is surprisingly less frequent than the kidney transplantation
8. biliary stricture (late)
9. false aneurysm at the hepatic artery anastomosis (late)
10. 'Vanishing bile duct', due to ischemia or chronic graft-versus-host disease

Early detection and employing appropriate remedial measures are very important in determining the ultimate outcome of surgery and the subsequent quality of life.

Contraindications for liver transplantation have to be strictly observed, in view of the shortage of donors against growing demand, so as not to waste resources on patients, who are not likely to derive optimal benefit from surgery.

Absolute contraindications

Overt sepsis and multiorgan dysfunction syndrome (MODS)
Disseminated malignancy
AIDS
Compromised cardio-pulmonary status

Relative contraindications

Extremes of age: < 2yrs and > 65 yrs
Prior complex hepatobiliary surgery, portocaval shunt or portal vein thrombosis
Multiorgan transplantion
Obesity
Chronic renal insufficiency or severe brain damage

Cholangiocarcinoma: the outcome of liver transplantation is not satisfactory in this condition

Hepatocyte transplantation and stem cell therapy are being currently evaluated, as an alternate to formidable standard surgery, in an attempt to save the patient from considerable risk and expense. As on date, there is no report of successful xenotransplantation, using pig, chimpanzee or baboon liver, due to unmanageable immunological reactions, besides religious and ethical considerations.

105 Stoma

A stoma (from Greek "mouth") is an opening, either natural or surgically created, which connects a portion of the body cavity to the outside environment. Surgical procedures in which stomata are created are ended in the suffix, 'ostomy' and begin with a prefix denoting the viscus being exteriorized.

Any hollow organ can be manipulated into an artificial stoma as necessary. This includes the esophagus, stomach, small bowel, colon, pleural cavity, ureters, urinary bladder and renal pelvis.

The two most common and important types of stoma used in GI surgery are ileostomy and colostomy which involve bringing out of the ileum or colon respectively.

At first sight, one should be able to differentiate the 2 forms based on the fact that an ileostomy appears to sprout with a nipple, while the colostomy appears flush. Although great advances were made with regard to stoma formation and management, both early and late complications are still not uncommon. Understanding enterostomal construction and physiology is essential for providing these patients with optimally functioning stoma and its care. It is important to counsel the patient regarding the stoma, and proper stoma care must be provided by a specialist nurse. Arrange

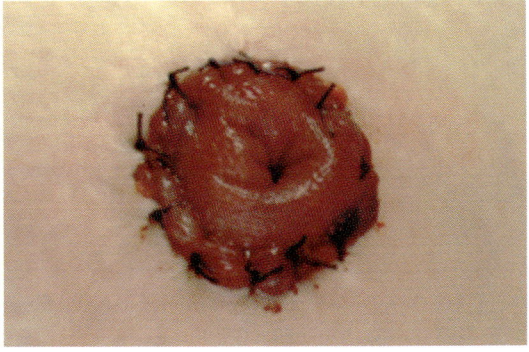

Fig. 105.1. Typical colostomy fashioned

a meeting with a patient who has an ileostomy or colostomy, will boost the morale of the patient, planning for one. Ostomy associations or clubs are established in many countries, to generate confidence in them and to keep them in the main stream of society.

COLOSTOMY

Types

1. End colostomy
2. Loop colostomy
3. Double-barreled colostomy
4. Mucous fistula

END COLOSTOMY

End colostomies are usually created in association with distal colorectal bowel resection. The lateral attachments of the colon are transected along the white line of Toldt until sufficient colon is mobilized to create a colostomy that protrudes from the abdominal wall and can be matured without tension. The premarked stoma site is usually in the left lower quadrant and the cutaneous and fascial openings may need to be slightly larger (admit 2 fingers easily) to facilitate easy passage of the colon through the abdominal wall. Proximal bowel is brought out as an end colostomy and distal bowel is either excised or closed and left in the pelvic cavity. The end of the stump is turned inside out, and the edges sutured to the skin all around, to produce what is known as 'instant maturation'. This prevents exposure of the serosal surface to the exterior, leading to serositis causing diarrhea or intestinal obstruction due to a segmental paralysis of the bowel.

Indications

1. after abdomino-perineal resection (APR) for anorectal cancer
2. Hartmann procedure - following sigmoid resection for cancer or diverticular disease
3. Others - radiation proctopathy, Crohn's disease, sacral decubitus ulcer etc.

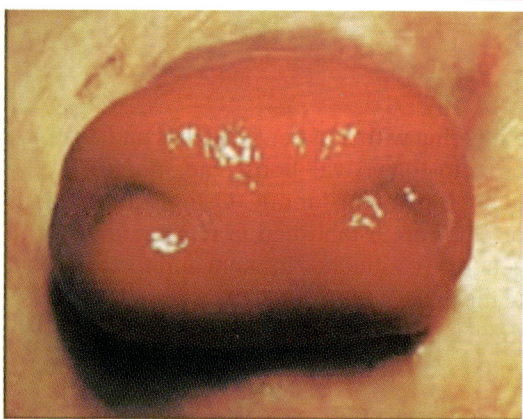

Fig. 105.2. A loop transverse colostomy
(courtesy: Halsted Surgical Clinic, Chennai)

LOOP COLOSTOMY

It may be created to prevent the fecal stream from reaching the rectum and anus in cases of incontinence and severe anorectal infection (diversion), or for proximal protection after complex anal/rectal reconstruction (defunctioning). The stoma is brought out in the left lower quadrant in the form of a loop, opened at the tenia coli, and sutured to the abdominal skin. A disc of skin is excised at the midpoint of the left spino-umbilical line, the loop gently brought out, the serosa sutured to skin all around and then a stoma bag applied over. A plastic rod may be used to hold the loop in position, but this is no longer used in most centres. If the colostomy is done for fecal diversion, it may be opened after 48 hours, using a diathermy (bowel has no pain sensation) and the distal loop is closed with catgut, to prevent fecal spill into the distal segment, defeating the very purpose of the operation.

Indications

1. to cover or defunctionalize a distal anastomosis, e.g. low/ultra low anterior resection, and colo-anal anastomosis (diverting colostomy)

2. Colonic perforation, spontaneous, traumatic or endoscopic (loop brought out at perforated site or proximal to it)

3. RTA- colon injury (especially if the bowel is unprepared!)

4. Rarely in severe ulcerative colitis (fulminating colitis)

5. In some cases of severe refractory pelvic/perianal sepsis, e.g. multiple fistula-in-ano

6. Rectovaginal fistula, usually following difficult labor

DOUBLE-BARREL COLOSTOMY

In this type, the bowel is severed and both ends are brought out onto the abdomen. Only the proximal stoma is functioning and will drain stool. The distal stoma, connected to the rectum and also called a mucous fistula, drains small amounts of mucus material. This is most often a temporary colostomy performed to rest an area of bowel, and to be closed later. This may be closed by Paul-Mikulicz technic, by using Paul's enterotome, without laparotomy

MUCOUS FISTULA

When both ends of a double-barrel type of stoma cannot be brought together, they are brought out through two separate openings, may be few inches apart. The distal opening will only discharge mucosal secretions, hence known as mucous fistula. This will also prevent

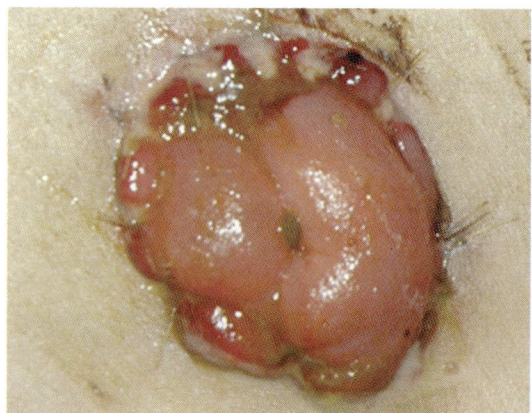

Fig. 105.3. Mature sigmoid colostomy after APR for carcinoma rectum
(courtesy: Lifeline Hospitals, Chennai)

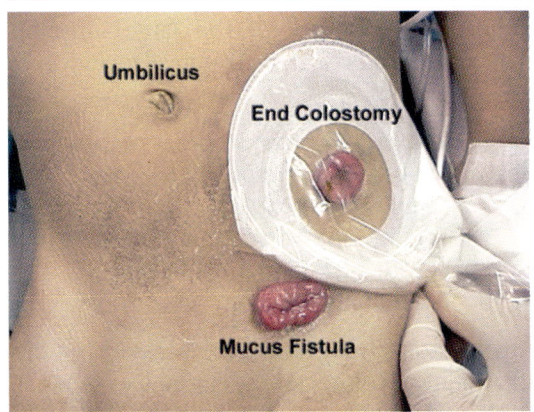

Fig. 105.4. End descending colostomy and mucous fistula of distal sigmoid, following resection of perforated diverticulitis
(courtesy: Halsted Surgical Clinic, Chennai)

retraction of the distal segment, to facilitate reanastomosis, at a later date.

Complications of colostomy

1. Prolapse - it occurs due to improper fixation of the stoma. it is more commonly seen in transverse loop colostomies. Asymptomatic prolapse requires no treatment, especially if the stoma is temporary, but surgical intervention is warranted if the prolapse causes ischemia, obstruction, or pouching problems. The best treatment for a prolapse is to refashion the stoma. If the prolapse is symptomatic, the redundant bowel is amputated and the mucocutaneous border re-established.

2. Retraction - it is a dangerous complication as it leads to the risk of spillage inside the peritoneal cavity, leading to life threatening sepsis.

3. Necrosis - it occurs due to vascular compromise following tight suturing of the blood vessels supplying the stoma. Treated best by refashioning or revision of the stoma and bringing out the proximal healthy colon. The reasons for this complications are:

   a) tension on the bowel segment to be exteriorized
   b) tight fascial opening
   c) tight suturing
   d) pre-existing bowel ischemia or too much of 'skeletonizing' the bowel

4. Parastomal hernia - It occurs due to weakness of the wall surrounding the stoma. It is usually asymptomatic, treated by placing a mesh using an extra peritoneal fascial on-lay technique.It is more common in cases of end colostomy. If the colostomy is temporary, the hernia may be repaired at the time of closing the colostomy.

5. Lateral space herniation - this occurs within the peritoneal cavity, and can happen in 2 ways. Either laterally or under the bowel within the peritoneum. This can sometimes be symptomatic leading to bowel obstruction, and is again treated by mesh placement.

6. Granulation tissue - Sometimes granulation tissue formation can occur over the scar of the sutured line of the stoma. This can often be troublesome for the patient by bleeding from the edges. Treated best by excising the granulation tissue and resuturing.

Bowel training or priming: if the colostomy is regularly irrigated at the same time every day, leading to evacuation, the normal evacuation reflex develops and there may not be a need for using a bag or pouch over the stoma, during the other times.

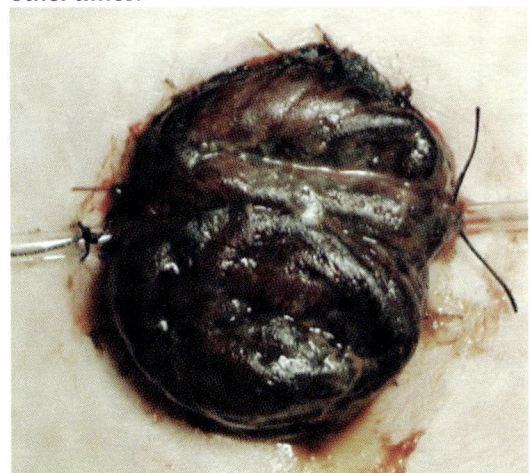

Fig. 105.5. Necrosed loop ileostomy

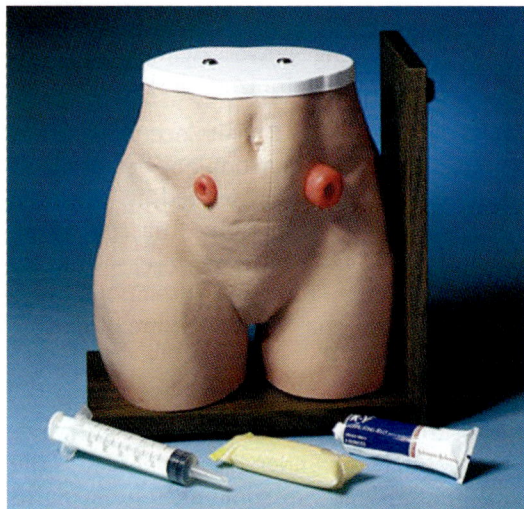

Fig. 105.6. A module to train nurses and prospective ostomy patients

An ileostomy is a surgical opening constructed by bringing the end (more common) or loop of small intestine (the ileum) out onto the surface of the skin. Intestinal waste passes out of the ileostomy and is collected in an external pouching system stuck to the skin. Ileostomies are usually sited above the groin on the right side of the abdomen. Ileostomies are necessary where disease or injury has rendered the large intestine incapable of safely processing intestinal waste, typically because the colon has been partially or wholly removed.

Jewels of Gyan - 105.1

Positioning a Stoma

In a loop ileostomy, the proximal part of the bowel is brought inferior and the distal part brought superior, to avoid necrosis. (remember - PIDS- proximal-inferior, distal-superior).

It is wise to mark the most convenient point of stoma, with the patient standing, especially in obese individuals, in whom surface landmarks can change considerably with posture.

Indications: Diseases of the large intestine which may require surgical removal includes:

1. Crohn's disease
2. Ulcerative colitis: where it precedes an ileal pouch-anal anastomosis
3. Familial adenomatous polyposis
4. Total colonic Hirschprung's disease
5. Severe intra abdominal sepsis
6. Post bowel resection

An ileostomy may also be necessary in the treatment of colorectal cancer; one example is a situation where the tumor is causing a blockage.

Types

1. **End ileostomy:** routinely performed in association with partial or total colorectal resections. Exposure is generally through a midline incision and the stoma is created after performing the indicated bowel resection. An abdominal defect is created, the ileum is prepared, mesentery can be cleared but care must be taken to leave a 1 cm strip with the ileum because it carries a vessel supplying the ileal wall and prevents stomal ischemia.The apex of the ileum is brought out as it has a lesser chance of prolapse.

2. **Standard (Brooke) ileostomy:** this is the most common kind of ileostomy that is done. The end of the ileum is pulled through the abdominal wall, turned inside out and sutured to the skin. The ileostomy is made to evert and sprout outward. This prevents leakage of the digestive secretions on to the skin, leading to digestion and excoriation.

3. **Loop ileostomy:** is generally created in association with distal bowel resection. After a

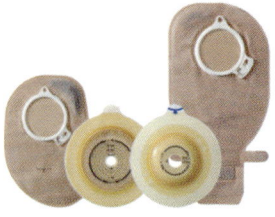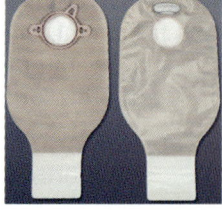

Fig. 105.7. Different types of ostomy pouches available

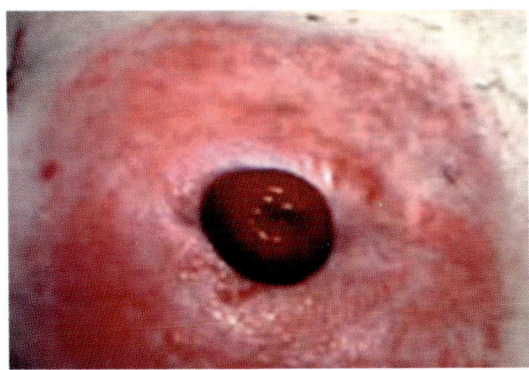

Fig. 105.8. Allergic dermatitis and excoriation around
an ileostomy
(courtesy: Halsted Surgical Clinic, Chennai)

resection-anastomosis is completed, a segment of the terminal ileum that will reach the abdominal wall without any tension is selected and made into a loop which is brought out through the abdominal wall. 3 tripartite sutures are taken similar to loop colostomy between dermis, seromuscular layer of the ileum and a full thickness bite of the open end of the ileum. Maturation is completed with 2 additional sutures between dermis and full thickness of the terminal ileum. The loop stoma should protrude adequately.

4. Kock's continent ileostomy: this is a different but uncommon type of ileostomy. In continent ileostomy, a pouch that collects waste is made from part of the small intestine. This pouch stays inside the body and it connects to the stoma through a valve created. Most people with this kind of ileostomy do not need to wear a pouch on the outside. Waste is drained by putting a catheter through the stoma a few times each day. They can cause many problems that need to be addressed and sometimes may need to be redone.

Complications

The majority of the complications are almost identical to those of a colostomy (i.e., necrosis, obstruction, hernia, retraction, etc.). Other problems include:

1. Ileostomy diarrhea: which is not life threatening but a very troublesome symptom,

best treated by bowel binding agents.

2. Skin irritation and excoriation: occurs due to liquid, caustic effluent from the ileostomy which has a corrosive action on the skin. Patients with a high output stoma are at an increased risk of skin ulceration. Obesity has also been associated with an increased risk of skin irritation. Fungal overgrowth may also be seen in some cases. Peristomal skin irritation may be associated with reactivation of inflammatory bowel disease.

Liberal application of zinc oxide creams may protect skin digestion to some extent.

3. Bowel obstruction: it is seen more with ileostomy than colostomy. Adhesions are suspected to be the most common cause, but small bowel volvulus or internal hernia may occasionally be the culprits! Many patients develop obstruction due to accumulation of partially digested foodstuffs. Bowel irrigations may be repeated using saline carefully till the obstruction is relieved.

Closure of a temporary stoma

a. Timing: by convention, closure is done after six weeks, ensuring that either

    1.   the primary pathology distal to the

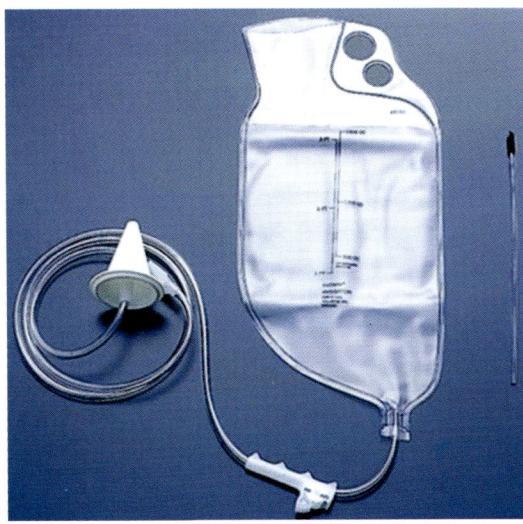

Fig. 105.9. Colostomy irrigation set

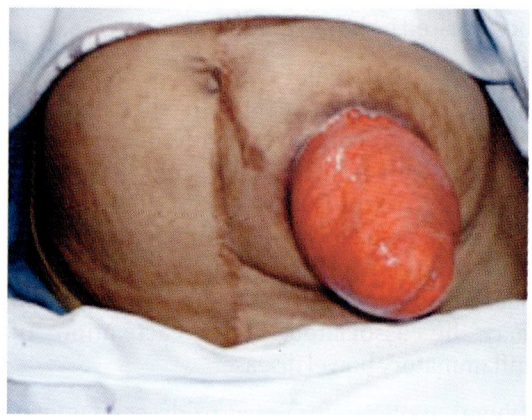

Fig. 105.10. Peristomal ventral hernia and prolapse

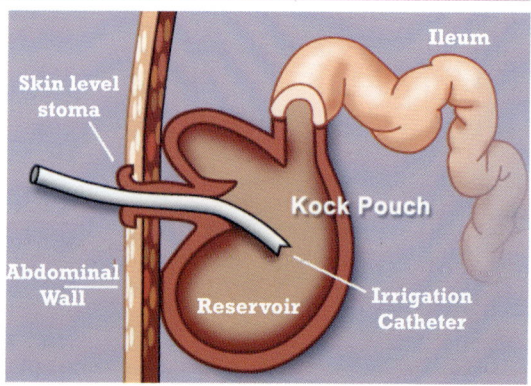

Fig. 105.11. Kock's pouch with continent ileostomy

stoma has settled, e.g. pelvic sepsis, recto-vaginal fistula or peritonitis, or

2. the defunctioned anastomosis is patent and healed, e.g. if a low anterior resection had been done, a contrast study to confirm normalcy.

b. Technique: loop colostomy is closed by a simple interrupted anastomosis of the two lumens of the colon, keeping the intact posterior wall untouched (see Fig. 105.12.)

Loop ileostomy is closed by total resection and anastomosis lest it may result in a stricture.

Jewels of Gyan - 105.1

TIPS in creating a Loop Stoma

When fashioning a sigmoid loop colostomy, choose to open the colon proximal to the apex of the sigmoid. This expedient seems to lower the risk of prolapse.

When forming a loop ileostomy in the right iliac fossa, keep the proximal everted end in the inferior position. This step facilitates better stoma bag handling and decreases skin excoriation.

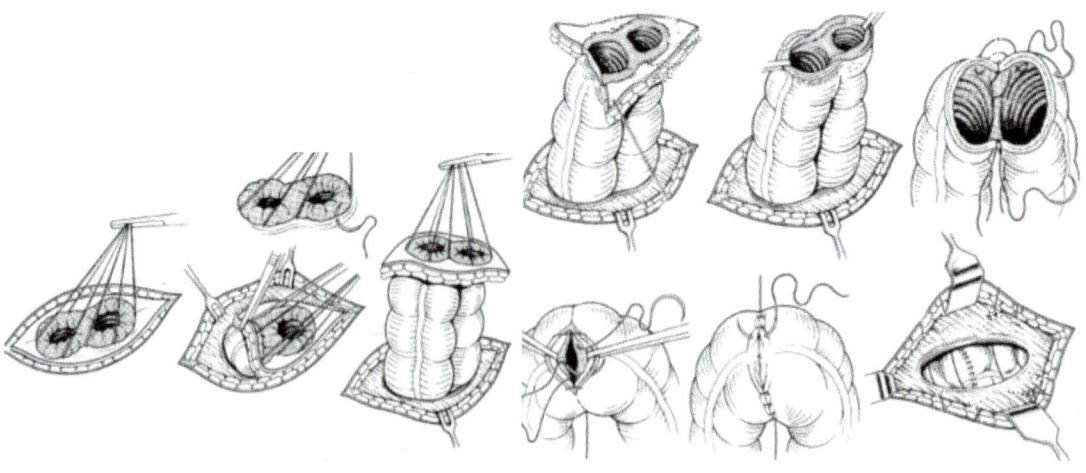

Fig. 105.12. Steps of closure of loop or double-barrelled colostomy

ORTHOPEDICS

(A SYNOPSIS)

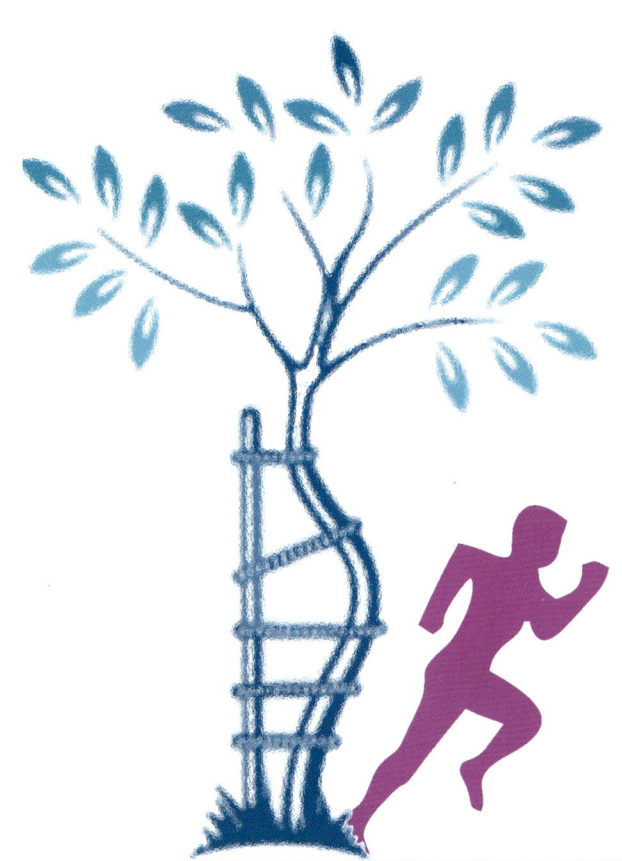

(Ortho: straight; pedios: child)

Orthopedics is the science that deals with diseases of the locomotor system. When Nicolas Andry, a French Surgeon, coined the name in 1741, the subject only dealt with the problem of straightening the deformities in children. In this chapter, only a bird's-eye view of the general principles of orthopedics is given. More detailed information, which may be obtained in standard works on the subject, has been deliberately omitted.

FRACTURE & DISLOCATIONS
Definitions of terms

Fractures: A fracture is present when there is loss of continuity in the substance of a bone. The term covers all bony disruptions, ranging from hairline fractures on one end of the scale to multi-fragmentary (or comminuted) fractures, to the other.

Dislocations: In a dislocation, there is complete loss of contact between the articulating surfaces of a joint.

Subluxations: In a subluxation, the articulating surfaces are no longer congruous, but loss of contact is not complete.

Fracture-dislocations: Certain injuries give rise to specific patterns where a fracture is complicated by a dislocation at the joint in the vicinity.

E.g. Monteggia's fracture - Fracture of proximal ulna with ipsilateral humero-radial dislocation.

Galeazzi's fracture: Fracture of the distal radius shaft with ipsilateral distal radio-ulnar joint.

Types of Fractures

1. Green stick fracture - it is an incomplete fracture seen in children, with one cortex intact. There may or may not be much angulation.

2. Closed fracture - it is a fracture, where the hematoma does not communicate with the exterior.

3. Open or compound fracture - where the hematoma communicates outside through an open wound. This fracture has a high risk of getting infected and is therefore more hazardous.

4. Pathological fracture - it is a fracture occurring in a bone weakened by some disease and the injury is often very trivial or insignificant.

5. Stress or march fracture - it is a fracture occurring at a site subjected to repeated minor stress over a period of time. Sometimes there may not be obvious trauma, but the bone is fractured. This is commonly seen in the neck of 2nd metatarsal bone in soldiers who do a lot of marching and fracture rib in patients having chronic cough.

6. Birth fracture - it is a fracture in the newborn due to obstetric injury.

Types of fracture according to fracture anatomy

1. Simple fracture - which may be transverse, oblique or spiral, depending upon the nature of violence

2. Comminuted fracture - the bone is broken into more than two fragments

3. Avulsion fracture - where a chip of bone is avulsed by sudden violent muscular contraction or pulled by a ligament, e.g. fracture of radial styloid or avulsion fracture of tibial tuberosity

4. Impacted fracture - occurs where a vertical force drives one fragment into other. Here the pain is minimal due to restriction of the mobility of fragments

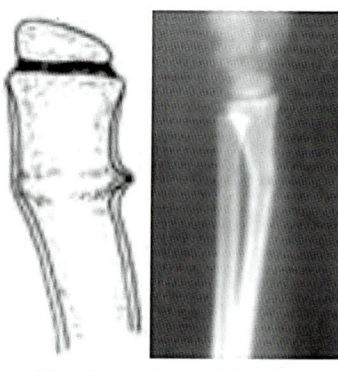

Fig. 106.1. Greenstick fracture.

5. Stellate fracture - this is usually seen in flat bones (e.g. skull bones and patella), where the fracture lines run radially in various directions from one point

6. Depressed fracture- this is also seen in flat bones, where there is a circumferential fracture and the central segment of bone gets depressed

Open fractures

An open or compound fracture refers to the osseous disruption in which a break in the skin and underlying soft tissue communicates directly with the fracture and its hematoma. Any wound occurring in the vicinity of a fracture must be suspected to be an open fracture until proven otherwise.

Soft tissue injuries in an open fracture may have three important consequences:

I) Contamination of the wound and fracture by exposure to the external environment

ii) Crushing, stripping and devascularization that results in soft tissue compromise and increased susceptibility to infection

iii) Destruction or loss of the soft tissue envelop may affect the method of fracture immobilization, compromise the contribution of the overlying soft tissue to fracture healing, and result in loss of function from muscle, tendon, nerve, vascular, ligament, or skin damage

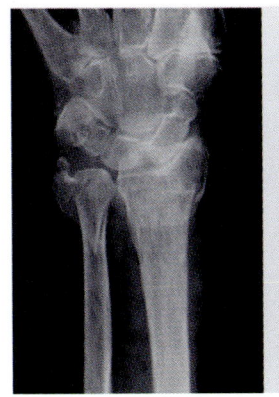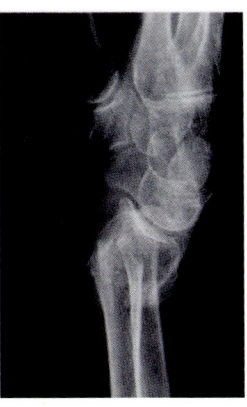

Fig. 106.3. Colles fracture with typical displacement

Gustilo and Anderson classification of open fractures

This was originally designed to classify soft tissue injuries associated with open tibial shaft fractures and was later extended to all fractures. It is useful for communicative purposes despite some variability in inter-observer reproducibility.

Type I: Clean skin opening of <1cm, usually from inside to outside; minimal muscle contusion; simple transverse or short oblique fractures

Type II: Laceration >1cm long, with extensive soft tissue damage; minimal to moderate crushing component; simple transverse or short oblique fractures with minimal communition

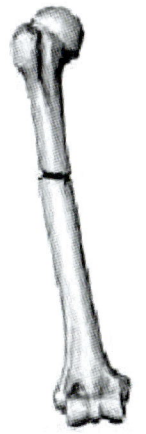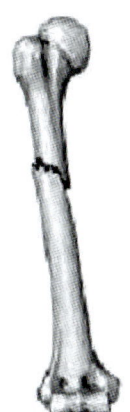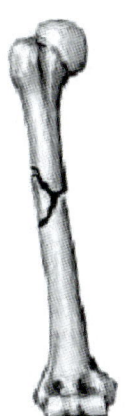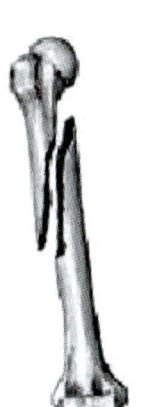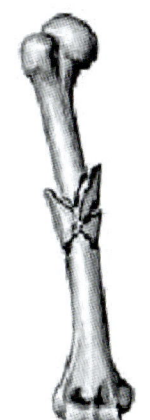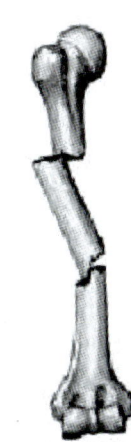

| Transverse Fx | Oblique Fx | Butterfly Fx | Spiral Fx | Communited Fx | Segmental Fx |

Fig.106.2. Anatomical types of fracture

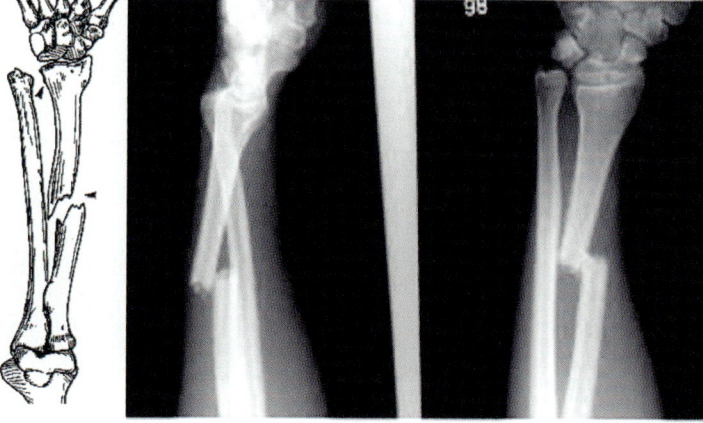

Fig. 106.4. Galeazzi's fracture-dislocation

1.   Displacement: translocation of the two fragments in relation to each other in one or more planes. Traditionally, displacement refers to the position of the distal fragment in relation to the assumed stationary proximal fragment (medial, lateral, anterior and posterior displacement). Specific types of displacement include over-riding in relation to one another and distraction, where essentially the bone ends are pulled apart

Type III: Extensive soft tissue damage, including muscles, skin and neurovascular structures; often a high energy injury with a severe crushing component

III-A: Extensive soft tissue laceration, adequate bone coverage; segmental fractures, gunshot injuries, minimal periosteal stripping

III-B: Extensive soft tissue injury with periosteal stripping and bone exposure, requiring soft tissue flap closure; usually associated with massive contamination

III-C: Vascular injury requiring repair

Closed Fractures

Closed or simple fractures are those in which, either the skin is intact or, if there are any external wounds, they are superficial or unrelated to the fracture.

Fracture Deformities

A fracture can be deformed in any one of three possible planes, i.e. displacement, angulation and rotation.

2. Angulation: this occurs when the two fractured fragments are not aligned and an angular deformity is present. Alignment means that the axes of the proximal and distal fragments are parallel to each other and the joint above and below are in the normal (parallel) relationship. Angulation is typically described by the direction, in which the apex of the angle points, as medial, lateral, dorsal and volar

3. Rotation: Present when there is a torsional relationship between the two fractured fragments

Classification of dislocations

It may be

1. Congenital (as in congental dislocation of hip) or

2. Acquired (traumatic or paralytic)

Traumatic dislocation: the following types are seen in clinical practice

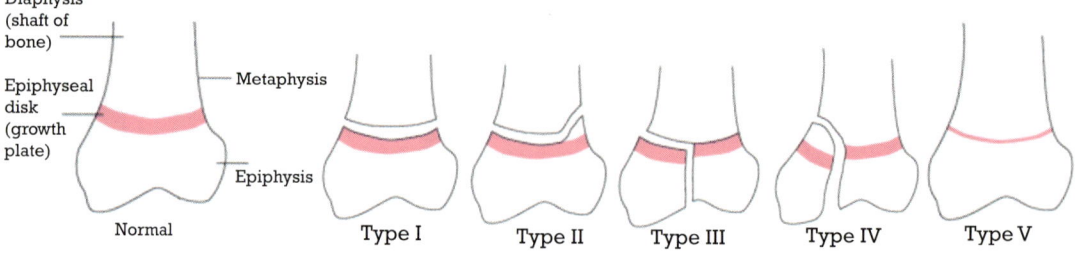

Fig. 106.5. Salter-Harris classification of epiphyseal plate fractures

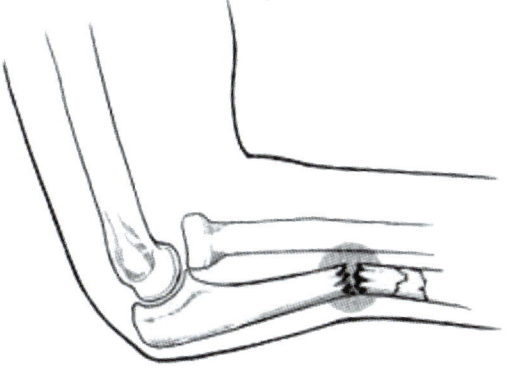 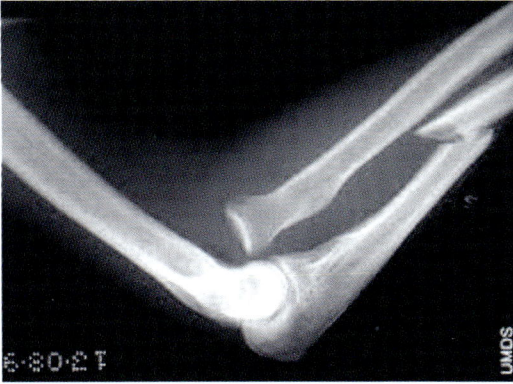

Fig. 106.6. Monteggia fracture-dislocation.

1. Acute traumatic dislocation

2   Old unreduced dislocation, where it is left unreduced for weeks to months

3. Neglected dislocation: where it is neglected (untreated) for months to years

4. Recurrent dislocation: when a traumatic dislocation is followed by repeated dislocations after initial trauma, as seen in shoulder, temporomandibular joint and patella

5   Fracture dislocation: when a fracture of one of the articulating bones is associated with dislocation, e.g. Monteggia fracture dislocation.

Sprain: it is an incomplete tear of a ligament or a complex of ligaments supporting a joint, and is not normally associated with instability (as distinct from a complete ligament tear). The term is also applied to incomplete tears of muscles and tendons.

Healing of a fracture

Healing of a fracture is a complex physiologic process, its striking feature compared to healing in other areas, is that repair is by the original and not by scar tissue.

It involves a combination of intramembranous and endochondral ossification. These two processes participate in the fracture repair sequence by at least four discrete stages of healing:

1. **Hematoma formation (inflammatory) phase:** This phase is characterized by the release of a variety of products, including fibronectin, platelet-derived growth factor (PDGF) and transforming growth factor (TGF), by the activated platelets, triggering the influx of inflammatory cells. This phase peaks within 48 hours of the injury and lasts for a week.

2. **Proliferative (reparative or callus) phase:** This phase is characterized by the formation of connective tissues, including cartilage and formation of new capillaries from preexisting vessels (angiogenesis). During the first 7 to 10 days, the periosteum undergoes an intramembranous bone formation. By the

Jewels of Gyan - 106.1

Stages of bone healing	
Weeks 0-3	Hematoma, macrophages suround fracture site
Weeks 3-6	Osteoclasts remove sharp edges, callus forms within hematoma
Weeks 6-12	Bone forms within the callus, bridging fragments
Months 6-12	Cortical gap is bridged by bone
Years 1-2	Normal architecture is achieved through remodelling

middle of the second week, abundant cartilage overlies the fracture site and this chondroid tissue initiates biochemical preparations to undergo calcification. Thus, the callus becomes a triple-layered structure consisting of an outer proliferating part, a middle cartilaginous layer and an inner portion of new bony trabeculae. The cartilage portion is usually replaced with bone in the course of healing.

3. Maturing (modeling) phase: This phase is characterized by the production of woven bone. The calcification of fracture callus cartilage occurs by a mechanism almost identical to that which takes place in the growth plate. This calcification can occur either directly from mesenchymal tissue (intramembranous) or via an intermediate stage of cartilage (endochondral or chondroid routes). Osteoblasts can form woven bone rapidly, but the result is randomly arranged and mechanically weak. Nonetheless, bridging of a fracture by woven bone constitutes the so-called *clinical union*. Once cartilage is calcified, it becomes a target for the ingrowth of blood vessels.

4. Remodeling phase: By replacing the cartilage with bone and converting the cancellous bone into compact bone, the callus is gradually remodeled. During this phase, the woven bone is converted into stronger lamellar bone by the orchestrated action of osteoclasts (causing bone resorption) and osteoblasts (causing bone formation).

Complications of fractures

A number of complications can occur following fractures and dislocations:

1. Problems of union
   a) Nonunion
   b) Malunion
   c) Delayed union
2. Stiffness and loss of motion
3. Infection and osteomyelitis

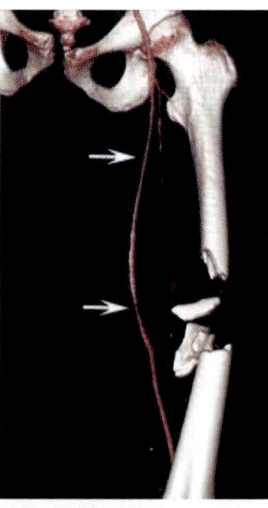

Fig. 106.7. CT femoral angiogram showing displaced femoral vessels due to the fracture hematoma.
(courtesy: Halsted Surgical Clinic, Chennai)

4. Myositis ossificans
5. Avascular necrosis and ischemic contractures
6. Implant failure
7. Chronic regional pain syndrome

1(a).   Nonunion

In nonunion, the fracture has failed to unite and there are radiological changes which indicate that this situation will be permanent i.e. the fracture will never unite unless there is some fundamental alteration in the line of treatment.

Nonunion is also defined as the failure of a fracture to heal in twice the normal period of healing. (at least 6 months after the trauma)

Causes of nonunion

Non- apposition of bone ends
Bone loss at the time of fracture
Interposition of soft tissues
Distraction at fracture site by soft tissues
Reduced blood supply which renders the local tissues non viable
Intact fellow bone in forearm and leg
Untreated delayed union
    Inadequate immobilization
Infection

Clinical features

The most important clinical sign is painless abnormal mobility. There may be shortening deformity and muscle wasting.

Types of nonunion

i). Atrophic nonunion - fracture ends are tapering, rounded, osteoporotic and thin with a distinct gap in the x- rays. Clinically there is obvious abnormal mobility.

ii) Hypertrophic nonunion - there is considerable bone formation at the ends of fractured bone. Radiologically it is termed as 'elephant's foot appearance,' since the bone ends are sclerotic and are flared out so that the diameter of the bone fragments at the level of the fracture is increased. Mobility between the fragments is very limited.

Radiological Features

Sclerosis of the fractured bone ends, sealing and closure of the medullary canal.

Treatment of nonunion

1. Open reduction, internal fixation and bone grafting
2. Ilizarov ring fixation
3. Ortho-fix type external fixation

1(b). Malunion

When the fracture unites in an abnormal position it is called malunion and in practice the term is used in the following circumstances:

Where a fracture has united with angulation or rotation of a degree that gives a displeasing appearance or affects function

Where a fracture has united with a little persistent deformity in situation where even the slightest displacement or angulation is a potential source of trouble. This applies particularly to fractures involving joints

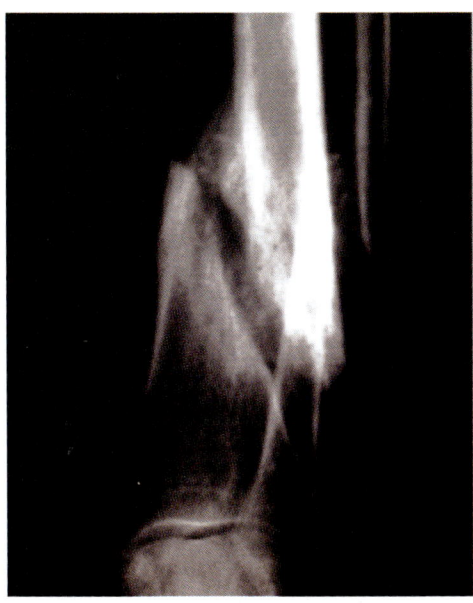

Fig. 106.8. Non-union of fracture lower third of tibia (courtesy: Dr. A N Vivek, Chennai)

Causes of malunion

1. Failure to reduce the fracture properly
2. Failure to immobilize adequately
3 Gradual resorption of fragments in comminuted fractures

Types of malunion according to the cause

i). Primary malunion

When the fracture is initially reduced, immobilized and allowed to unite in a malposition

ii). Secondary malunion

When a fracture is not protected properly after an initial good reduction, leading to displacement or angulation due to muscular contractions or when premature weight bearing was allowed

Types of malnunion according to the displacement

1. Overlapping
2. Angulation
3. Rotation
4. Translocation

Clinical Features

1. Deformity
2. Growth disturbance when malunion occurs at growth plate.
3. Restricted or abnormally increased movements in a few directions.
4. Tendon injury due to friction tear.
5. Abnormal unequal loading of joints which leads on to secondary osteoarthrosis.
6. Tardy ulnar nerve palsy is a complication of long standing cubitus valgus deformity due to malunion of distal humeral or lateral condyle fractures.

Clinically important malunions

1. Cubitus varus (Gun stock deformity) and cubitus valgus in malunion in and around the elbow
2. Manus varus or valgus in fracture around the wrist
3. Genu varum (bow legs) or genu valgum (knock knees) in malunion around the knee
4. Coxa varum in trochanteric fractures

Management

Slight degree of malunion, without much disability, may not require any treatment and in some areas the deformity will get partially corrected by remodeling.

Remodeling depends on

1. Age: better in children, even gross malunions will completely remodel in new borns.

2. Type: translocation (sideway shift) is well corrected.

Angulation upto 10° gets corrected, especially in the plane of movement of the adjacent joints.

Rotation of even minimal degree, will not get corrected

3. Location: Fractures near the growth plate and near joints remodel better

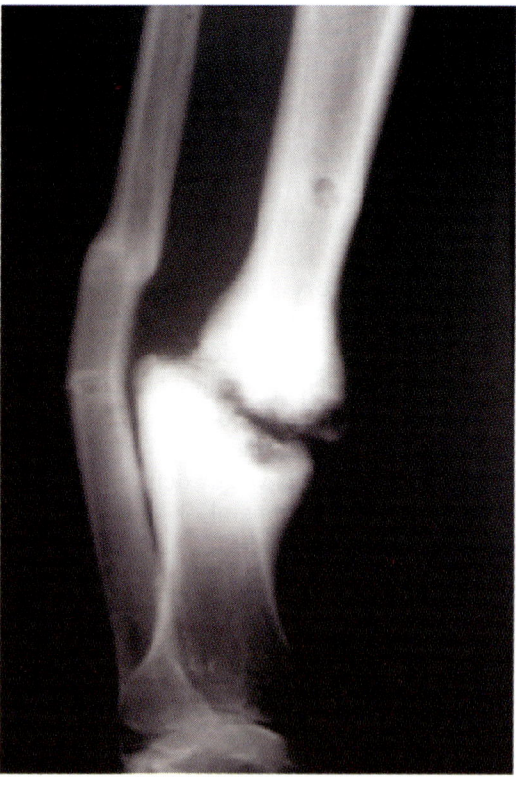

Fig. 106.9. Nonunion of fracture lower third of tibia and malunion of fracture fibula (courtesy: Dr. A N Vivek, Chennai)

Treatment of malunion

a) Osteoclasis (breaking the callus) - closed correction of angulation and immobilization
b) Open reduction and internal fixation
c) Corrective osteotomy
d) Excision of protruding bone

1(c). Delayed union

If a fracture takes more than normal duration to unite, is called delayed union.

Clinical findings

Persistent pain and tenderness
Pain on putting stress at the fracture site

Radiological findings

The fracture line is visible and there is inadequate callus

Management

1. Many of them unite, with additional period of immobilization. Surgical intervention may be required if there is total failure of union, using the following prinicples:

1. Bone grafting only
2. Open reduction, internal fixation and bone grafting
3. Ilizarov/Ortho-fix type of fixator

2. Stiffness and loss of motion

These complications commonly occur in fractures involving articular surfaces, in which arthrofibrosis is known to occur. Additional problems such as bony blocks, loose bodies in the joints, nerve palsies, and posttraumatic arthritis may also be contributory.

Management

Physiotherapy: hot fomentation, wax bath, shortwave diathermy etc. encouraging passive and active movements.

Surgery: Excision of bone blocks, lengthening of contracted muscles or tendon.

3. Infection

Infection in closed fractures, due to hematogenous spread of organisms, is rare and seldom diagnosed in early stages. It is a well-known and feared complication of open fractures or after internal fixation of closed fractures. The presence of a foreign body increases the risk of infection, by interfering with local defense mechanisms. Certain microorganisms have the unique ability to protect themselves under a slime layer called the "glycocalyx," which essentially makes them inaccessible to antimicrobial agents. The presence of necrotic bone, acting as a foreign body, also contributes to infection risk.

4. Myositis ossificans (see chapter 111)

5. Avascular necrosis

This is death of bone due to interference with its blood supply. Because of the tenuous and frequently retrograde blood flow in certain areas, some fractures are more vulnerable for this complication.

a. Femoral head, following intracapsular fracture of the femoral neck or after dislocation of the hip
b. Fracture in the proximal half of scaphoid
c. Fractures neck of talus
d. Dislocation of lunate

6. Implant failure

The use of many metallic implants puts certain fractures at risk, because of their tendency for fatigue, before the bone healing occurs.

7. Chronic regional pain syndrome

syn: reflex sympathetic dystrophy, Sudeck's atrophy or post-traumatic osteodystrophy

This unusual complication is typically seen following trivial trauma in a predisposed patient, who develops abnormal sympathetic response. It may also be due to a partial nerve injury or contusion. In most cases it is not recognized until removal of the plaster. There is swelling of the involved region and the skin is warm, pink and glazed in appearance. There is striking restriction of movements in the involved joints, associated with extreme local pain and tenderness, giving rise to a suspicion of an ununited fracture. However, check radiographs show good union of the fracture, but with diffuse, osteoporotic mottling of the juxta-articular bones. Prognosis depends on early recognition of the symptom and timely intervention.

Management

If general symptomatic therapy fails to give relief, sympathetic blockade of the limb (stellate ganglion block for the upper extremity and epidural or lumbar sympathetic block for the lower extremity) may be helpful. Early aggressive physical therapy and return to normal function are important to the rehabilitation of patients with this troublesome complication.

Scheme of examination of injuries of Bones and Joints

History

In examining a patient suspected to have fracture or dislocation, it is useful to obtain the following details:

1. Age: Fractures may be seen in all ages. Epiphysial separation occurs in children before their fusion, so also the greenstick fracture. Dislocations are common in adults.

2. Nature of the violence, whether direct, indirect or muscular violence

Direct: tapping type: causes transverse fracture, with minimal skin injury

Same injury occurring over a flat bone may lead to a stellate or depressed fracture

Crushing type: multiple fragments, called comminuted fracture

Indirect: Twisting type: leads to spiral fracture and considerable soft tissue damage

Bending or bowing force: transverse or oblique fracture

Combination of these results in butterfly fragments

Muscular: violent muscular contraction may lead to fracture of the bone to which the group of muscle are attached

e.g. patella, olecranon, greater tuberosity of humerus or lesser trochanter of femur.

3. Magnitude of force sustained, if it was not sufficient to break a normal bone, consider a pathological fracture

4. Point of impact and the direction of force

5. Any significance associated with the incident itself (for example, in case of a fall, was it due to any underlying medical cause like syncopal attack or seizure disorder, etc)

6. The site of pain and its severity. Contrary to general belief, sprains are more painful than fractures, where only movements are painful. Pain over a fractured rib may be felt by applying springing pressure over the ends of the involved rib

7. Any loss of functional activity, for example weight bearing is seldom possible following fracture of femur or tibia. Inability to bear weight after an accident is of great significance.

8. Any neurological deficit, to exclude injury to the adjacent nerve.

9. Vascular insufficiency

10. Deformity or swelling is seen if there is a hematoma at a fracture site or a dislocation

11. History of steroid intake which may cause osteoporosis

12. History of diabetes mellitus and smoking which may delay fracture healing

13. Details of any previous treatment taken, especially native treatment

14. History related to other co-morbidities such as ischemic heart disease, hypertension, hypothyrodism etc. which may influence the management, including choice of anesthesia, if required

15. If a pathological factor is suspected, history in relation to possible primary malignancies

PHYSICAL EXAMINATION

The established routine for clinical examination, including general survey and vital signs, is to be followed and the affected side should always be compared with normal side.

Inspection: The area should be carefully inspected for any swelling, shortness, ecchymosis, cyanosis, deformity, attitude, viability and overlying skin. Subcutaneous emphysema may be seen in a rib fracture, due to the breach in the underlying pleura, both visceral and parietal.

Deformity: It is usually due to the displaced fragments of bone, hematoma or edema. Hemorrhage or effusion into the neighboring joint to a major fracture may also produce swelling

Attitude: Certain attitudes are diagnostic of some injuries; e.g. motionless lower limb in abduction in fracture neck of femur. The hip kept in flexion, adduction and internal rotation in posterior dislocation.

Overlying skin: This is important for classification and for the high probability of infection, either nonspecific or specific (clostridial). In gas gangrene, the muscles may protrude through the wound and colored brick red or black, associated with subcutaneous emphysema.

Distal limb: obvious features of loss of viability at the time of admission, either due to crushing or devascularization have to be recorded, for appropriate management and for medico-legal purposes.

Palpation: Feel gently for tenderness (local and remote), swelling, temperature changes, abnormal mobility, and crepitus. Irregularity or gap in the continuity of a bone is pathognomonic of a fracture.

Palpating and recording the peripheral pulses of the affected area is of great significance in terms of management, so also detection of any neurological deficit.

Abnormal movements at the fracture site should be elicited with great caution, since further neurovascular damage may take place

Jewels of Gyan - 106.2

Feeling Crepitus on Palpation

Besides a fracture, crepitus may be observed in surgical emphysema, gas gangrene, osteoarthrosis, rheumatoid arthritis, tenosynovitis and Charcot's joint.

by rough handling. In fact it should be done only to exclude a fracture or if a nonunion is suspected.

Pain elicited by remote manipulation: by rotating the limb in fractures of humerus or femur, by squeezing the both ends of a rib, both bones of forearm or leg, known as springing. Axial pressure produces pain over the fractured carpal or metacarpal bones.

Palpating for the transmitted movements: This proves the continuity of a long bone, such as femur or humerus. The limb is rotated while palpating the greater tuberosity or trochanter with another hand, to see if there is corresponding movement.

Wound exploration: If there is open wound, probing may be done strict aseptic conditions, to identify the bone fragments, foreign body, color of muscles etc.

Measurements (mensuration): measure limb length and girth, using the contralateral limb, kept in the same position as reference.

Movements, both normal and abnormal, of the joint. Move the joint to assess the range of motion, both active and passive.

Stress testing: strain the ligaments to look for abnormal movements

Note: examine the painless areas first to gain confidence of the patient before going to the affected region.

Injuries to other systems, such as neuro, vascular, gastrointestinal, chest, external genitalia etc have to be systematically excluded and if present, properly evaluated. Muscle wasting may be seen only in late stage of nerve injury or prolonged immobilization.

Guidelines for clinical evaluation of an injured

I)   Assess ABCDE - airway, breathing, circulation, disability and exposure
ii) Initiate resuscitation in life-threatening injuries
iii) Evaluate injuries to the head, chest, abdomen, pelvis and spine
iv) Identify all injuries to the extremities

v) Assess the neurovascular status of injured limbs

vi) Assess skin and soft tissue damage (exploration of the wound in the emergency setting is not indicated if operative intervention is planned because it risks further contamination with limited capacity to provide useful information and may precipitate further hemorrhage)

vii) Obvious foreign bodies that are easily accessible may be removed in the emergency room under sterile conditions

viii) Open or compound fractures with bone protrusion through wound should be thoroughly washed and repositioned at the earliest to prevent bone/skin necrosis and infection

ix) Irrigation of wounds with sterile normal saline may be performed in the emergency room if any surgical delay is expected

x) All dislocations should be radiologically documented and reduced at the earliest preferably under anesthesia

xi) Immediate splinting of all obvious fractures with radiolucent materials in the emergency room is of utmost importance since it alleviates pain, prevents further soft tissue damage and arrests bleeding

xii) If there is a possibility of internal malignancy leading to a pathological fracture, it should be appropriately investigated, more so if the magnitude of injury is insufficient to cause fracture of a normal bone.

xiii) Assess co-morbidity such as diabetes, hypertension, ischemic heart disease etc.

INVESTIGATIONS FOR INJURIES TO BONES OR JOINTS

When injuries involve multiple systems, a well coordinated team approach by various specialists, such as thoracic, vascular and abdominal, urological and neurosurgeon etc is very important, giving priority attention to life-threatening injuries. If surgical intervention is anticipated, free interactive counseling regarding the risk/benefit equation has to be arranged, before an 'informed' consent obtained, followed by Anesthesiology evaluation and adequate quantity of blood and other volume expanders are made available.

Routine blood, and urine investigations, a chest x-ray, ECG etc have to be carried out in all cases.

When blood transfusion is anticipated, grouping to be done and the blood bank alerted.

Specific tests if pathologic fracture is suspected

Bence Jones proteins in urine for multiple myeloma and increased serum alkaline phosphatase and urinary excretion of hydroxyprolene in Paget's disease. Assay of tumor markers for some primary malignancies, such as prostate, ovary, thyroid, pheochromocytoma etc. may be indicated. So also serum calcium, phosphorus and parathormone levels for hyperparathyroidism.

A radiographic trauma series consists of the following:

i) Lateral cervical spine: must show all seven vertebrae, including the atlanto-occipital joint and the top of T1

A swimmer's view or CT scan if needed

In the absence of adequate view of all cervical vertebrae, the cervical spine cannot be "cleared" from possible injury, and a rigid cervical collar must be maintained until adequate views or a CT scan can be obtained.

Clinical clearance cannot occur if the patient has a depressed level of consciousness for any reason (e.g. ethanol intoxication or suspected intracranial injury).

ii) AP view of chest

iii) AP view of pelvis

iv) Lateral view of thoracolumbar spine

v) CT of the skull, cervical spine (if not cleared by plain radiographs), thorax, abdomen, or pelvis with or without contrast as dictated by the injury pattern.

vi) Radiograph of the injured region or the limb, minimum of two views (AP and lateral).

vii) Investigations for primary malignancy, if suspected. Common primaries preferentially going to skeletal system are: thyroid, breast, lung, adrenal, kidney and prostate

CT, MRI, isotope scan (^{99m}Tc), arthrography or arthroscopy in appropriate cases.

107 Diseases of Bones and Joints

(syn: Cold orthopedics)

Classification of bony swellings

1. **Traumatic**

a) excess callus formation
b) malunited fracture
c) subperiosteal hematoma
d) myositis ossificans

2. **Inflammatory**

a) acute and chronic osteomyelitis
b) Brodie's abscess
c) specific osteomyelitis due to tuberculosis, syphilis, typhoid, pneumococcal infection.

3. **Developmental disorders**

a) achondroplasia
b) osteogenesis imperfecta
c) mucopolysaccharide disorders such as Hunter's disease and Hurler's disease
d) osteopetrosis (marble bone disease)
e) diaphysial aclasia (multiple exostosis)
f) fibrous dysplasia
g) cleido-cranial dysostosis

4. **Nutritional, metabolic and endocrinal disorders:** rickets, osteomalacia, scurvy, hyper-parathyroidism (osteitis fibrosa cystica or Von Recklinghausen's disease), osteoporosis etc

5. **Malformation syndromes:** Nail-patella syndrome, Marfan's syndrome, Paget's disease of bone (osteitis deformans)

6 **Cysts:** solitary cyst, cysts associated with hyperparathyroidism, hydatid disease, aneurysmal bone cyst

7. **Neoplastic diseases**

a) **Benign:** osteoma, chondroma, osteoid osteoma, periosteal fibroma, hemangioma etc
b) **locally malignant:** osteoclastoma (giant cell tumor)
c) **Malignant**
Primary: osteosarcoma, chondrosarcoma, Ewing's tumor, multiple myeloma, reticulum cell sarcoma, plasmacytoma, fibrosarcoma, liposarcoma, angiosarcoma

Secondary: common primaries are already indicated. Rarely from uterus, GI tract, testis.

Contiguous spread from adjacent soft tissue cancers, such as cheek, tongue etc.

WHO classification of bone tumors - see table 107.1.

Scheme of examination of diseases of bones

Though general principles of examination of a general surgical case apply here, some specific details in the history and physical findings have to be noted. Systematic documentation of the details is important not only for arriving at a diagnosis, assess progress with the ongoing treatment, but also for medicolegal purposes, if such contingency arises. It cannot be overemphasized that many mistakes in clinical practice still occur not because one is not aware of the latest information about the diseases, but because the fundamental principles laid down for good clinical examination are overlooked.

History

It must include patient's occupation, hobbies, history of trauma (obvious or subtle), fever, swelling, previous major illnesses and treatment received. The main presenting symptoms in orthopedics are pain, swelling,

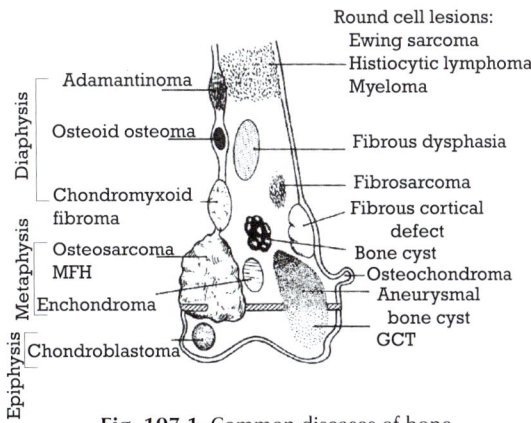

Fig. 107.1. Common diseases of bone

Cartilage forming tumors	Vascular tumors	
Osteochondroma Chondroma Enchondroma Periosteal chondroma Multiple chondromatosis Chondroblastoma Chondromyxoid fibroma Chondrosarcoma	Hemangioma Angiosarcoma	
Osteogenic (bone forming) tumors	**Smooth muscle tumors**	
Osteoma Osteoid osteoma Osteoblastoma Osteosarcoma	Leiomyoma Leiomyosarcoma Lipogenic tumours	
Fibrogenic tumors	**Lipocyte tumors**	
Desmoplastic fibroma Fibrosarcoma	Lipoma Liposarcoma	
Fibrohistiocytic tumors	**Neural tumors**	
Benign fibrous histiocytoma Malignant fibrous histiocytoma	Neurilemmoma Neurofibroma	
Primitive Neuroectodermal tumors	**Miscellaneous tumors**	
Ewing sarcoma Hematopoietic tumors Plasma cell myeloma Malignant lymphoma	Adamantinoma Metastatic malignancy	
Giant Cell tumors	**Miscellaneous lesions**	
Benign giant cell tumor Malignancy in giant cell tumor	Aneurysmal bone cyst Simple cyst Fibrous dysplasia Osteofibrous dysplasia Langerhans cell histiocytosis Erdheim-Chester disease Chest wall hamartoma	
Notochordal tumors	**Articular Lesions**	
Chordoma	Synovial chondromatosis	

Table-107.1. WHO classification of bone tumors

fever, deformity, difficulty in joint movements or locomotion.

Special information is needed regarding site, severity or radiation of pain and its aggravating relieving/factors. The chronological sequence of events is very important to fix the causal relationship of the symptoms to the underlying pathology.

1. Age: osteogenesis imperfecta (brittle bone disease), dwarfism, club foot etc. are seen at birth. Solitary bone cyst and acute osteomyelitis are commoner in children. Monostotic fibrous dysplasia is seen in adolescents, osteosarcoma and osteoclastoma are seen more in young adults. Multiple myeloma and metastatic bone disease are seen in middle aged and elderly.

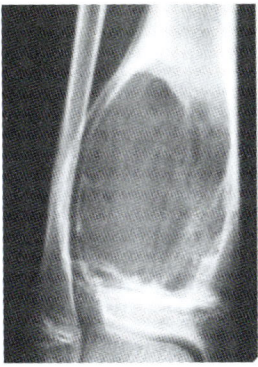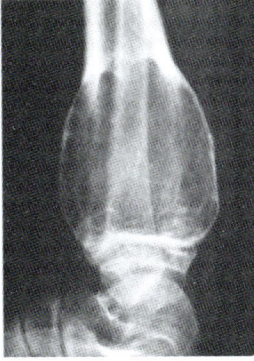

Fig. 107.2. Aneurysmal cyst of lower third of tibia
(courtesy: Dr. A N Vivek, Chennai)

2. Gender: Giant cell tumor has female preponderance. Postmenopausal women are more prone for osteoporosis, with tendency for fractures.

3. Mode of onset and progress

History of trauma may be present in many bone diseases, largely considered incidental, injury serving to bring the matter to light. Spontaneous and insidious onset is typical of neoplastic diseases, but rapid growth may be seen in malignancies. Severe local pain associated with fever and chills, observed in acute osteomyelitis. Fracture developing out of trivial injury should alert the possibility of pathological fracture, due to some underlying osteolytic lesion. Symptoms noted in relation to several bones may indicate some metabolic or metastatic disease.

4. Associated symptoms: symptoms related to primary malignancies, with special predilection to skeletal metastasis, have to be elicited.

5. Pain: Onset of pain before the swelling appeared is in favor of inflammatory disease, typically throbbing in nature, whereas pain is a late feature of tumors and is of dull aching in character. However, in case of osteosarcoma, often the pain may precede the appearance of swelling. Pain may also be due to some underlying pathology, which lead to the fracture.

6. Duration: Rapidly growing swelling of short duration is in favor of malignancy. Acute infections of bone or joint will be of recent onset, whereas chronic inflammations and benign tumors may be of long duration

7. Secondary changes

Presence of erythema, pigmentation, ulceration, sinus formation and the nature of discharge, such as pus or bone chips, the latter being typical of chronic nonspecific osteomyelitis

8. Similar swellings: It is important to know if the swelling is single or multiple. The tumor in early stages may be single, but in diaphysial aclasis, they may be multiple, arising from the metaphysis of several bones.

9. Past history: History of having treated malignancy in other parts in the past, may give a clue to the secondary deposits in a bone. Though not pathognomonic, history of any focus of sepsis, such as middle ear, dental, tonsils, multiple boils of skin may suggest the probability of septic osteomyelitis

10. Family history is relevant in familial diseases, such as osteogenesis imperfecta, achondroplasia, diaphysial aclasia, marble bone disease, Marfan's syndrome etc.

Physical examination
General examination

Full exposure of the body as permissible is essential. General survey to identify any systemic diseases, which may or may not be related to the primary problems, have to be noted, not only to aid diagnosis but also for planning treatment strategies, including choice of anesthesia etc.

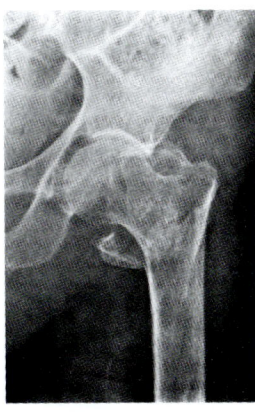

Fig. 107.3. Osteoporosis with severe demineralization (courtesy: Dr. A N Vivek, Chennai)

Routine general survey, including vital signs, should not be omitted.

Local examination

In the loco-regional examination, the normal side should be first examined before the symptomatic side. The standard protocol of inspection, palpation, movements and measurement may be followed. If multiple joints are involved, all of them have to be systematically examined and findings recorded.

Inspection

Physical features, such as changes in size, shape, appearance, have to be noted. Presence of swelling, ulcer, sinus, scar, deformity, muscle wasting and limb shortening have to be recorded, going into more details when they are present. (In unilateral conditions the normal side provides as reference to the abnormal physical findings in the affected site)

Palpation

It must be done with gradually increasing pressure, to ensure it does not cause undue dis-comfort, leading to non-cooperation of the patient. If a mass is present, it has to be examined systematically, as per the standard protocol, including eliciting egg-shell crackling. Deep palpation is done at the end, to identify the bony landmarks, irregularity, fracture and abnormal prominences.

Percussion

Gentle percussion may be done to elicit points of tenderness.

Auscultation

This is done to identify crepitus or bruit in vascular lesion causing pathological fracture.

Movements

The permitted range of movements (ROM) of a joint, both active and passive, have to be observed and measured in terms of degrees, while noting the pain limiting them. *Pain or limitation of any particular movement generally indicates extra-articular disease, whereas in*

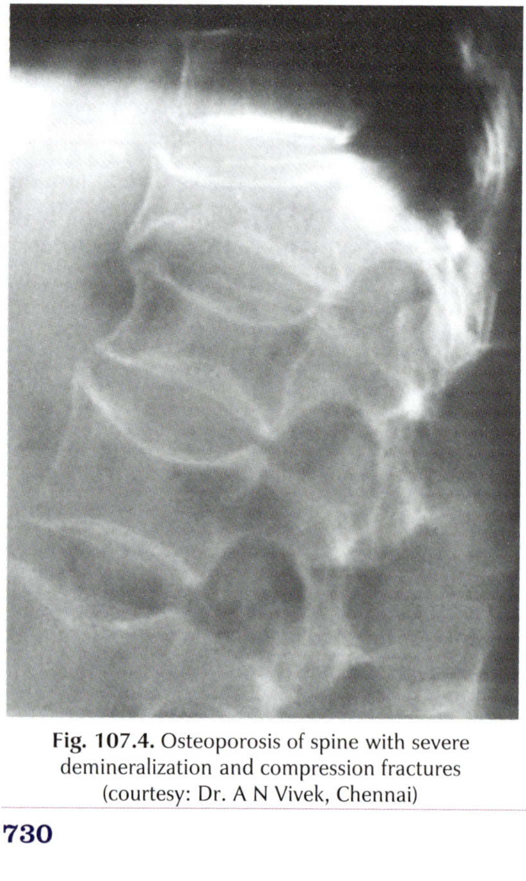

Fig. 107.4. Osteoporosis of spine with severe demineralization and compression fractures
(courtesy: Dr. A N Vivek, Chennai)

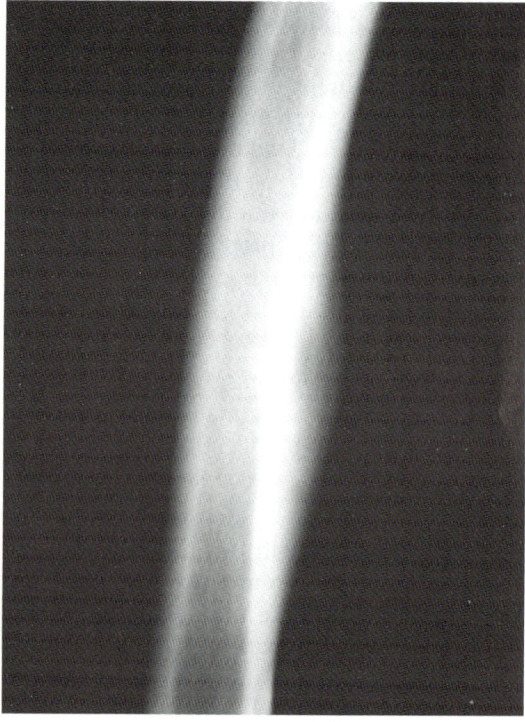

Fig. 107.5. Radiograph of an osteoid osteoma of the shaft of femur
(courtesy: Dr. A N Vivek, Chennai)

joint affection, all movements may be painful and restricted. Any hypermobility or abnormal movements and their range have to be noted.

Pressure effects: Neurovascular deficit has to be evaluated

Measurements (Mensuration)

The length of the entire or a segment of the limb has to be measured, to detect true or apparent shortening or lengthening. The girth of the limb has to be measured at various levels to identify and quantify muscular wasting. (again in unilateral conditions the normal side provides as reference to the extent of deformity and/or discrepancy in length) specific bony land marks are used to perform the measurements

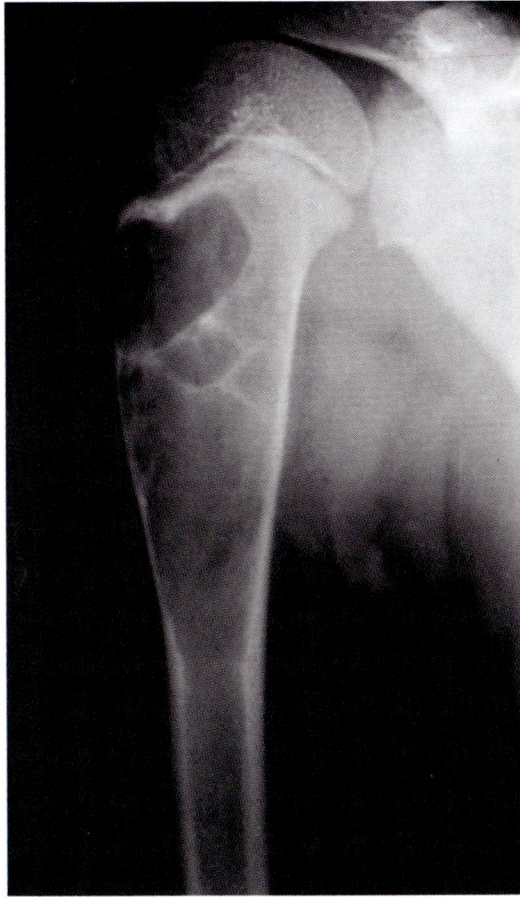

Fig. 107.6. Simple bone cyst of proximal humerus (courtesy: Dr. A N Vivek, Chennai)

Gait

Observation of gait is very important, since many diseases exhibit typical gaits, almost leading to spot diagnoses. (see chapter 130)

Neurological or muscular examination

Both sensory and motor functions of the concerned nerves and grading of muscle power have to be recorded. Superficial and deep reflexes may throw light on the localization of neurological lesions. Autonomic nervous system also has to be evaluated (see chapter 97).

Examination of other systems

a) Tuberculous osteomyelitis: pulmonary tuberculosis, regional lymphadenopathy, weight loss, cough, hemoptysis, fever (more in evening) and night sweats

b) Syphilitis osteitis: history of exposure to STD and presence of syphilitic stigmata

c) Nonspecific (pyogenic) osteomyelitis: primary focus of sepsis

d) Involvement of multiple bones or joints

e) Metastatic bone disease: search for primary malignancy in the areas indicated above

Provisional diagnosis and differential diagnosis: needless to say that this is the basis on which investigations and appropriate therapy can be planned.

DISEASES OF JOINTS

Classification

1) Acute arthritis

   a) Pyogenic
   b) Gonococcal
   c) Rheumatic
   d) Small pox

2) Chronic arthritis

   a) Nonspecific (pyogenic)
   b) Specific
      i) Tuberculous
      ii) Syphilitic (Clutton's)
      iii) Gonococcal
      iv) Dracunculosis (Guinea worm)

3) Degenerative arthropathy

Osteoarthrosis (primary and secondary)

4) Neuropathic arthropathy

A) Charcot's
   b) Diabetes mellitus
   c) Syringomyelia
   d) Hansen's disease

5) Metabolic
   a) Gout (hyperuricemia)
   b) Pseudo gout (chondrocalcinosis)
   c) Alkaptonuria
      i) Stage of simple alkaptonuria
      ii) Stage of ochronosis (colored depo-sits in bones and cartilages)
      iii) Stage of arthritis

6) Arthritis due to systemic diseases
   a) Hemophilia
   b) Reactive arthritis

7) Rheumatoid arthropathy

Rheumatoid arthritis (seropositive and negative)

8) Seronegative spondylarthropathy
   a) Ankylosing spondylitis
   b) Reiter's disease
   c) Psoriatic arthritis
   d) Enteropathic arthritis

Scheme of examination of diseases of Joints

Age and gender: Acute arthritis, tuberculous and rheumatoid arthritis occur in the young, osteoarthrosis in elderly obese, osteoporosis is common in postmenopausal women

Occupation: Osteoarthrosis is common in sedentary workers

Mode of onset: sudden onset in acute arthritis, whereas it is insidious in rheumatoid, tubercu-lous arthritis and typically gout presents as recurrent acute episodes

Pain: Joint disease associated with sensory neuropathy, such as Charcot's joint (tabes dorsalis or syringomyelia) or Clutton's joint (congenital syphilis)

Site: it may be localized over the involved joint or may be referred (e.g. to knee from hip disease). In rheumatoid arthritis, it is typically of fleeting type.

Character: It is throbbing in acute arthritis; it may be dull aching in chronic type.

Relation to movements: Articular pain is felt during all movements of the joint, whereas in extra-articular disease pain is experienced only during some movements, which stretches the inflamed tissue. The pain aggravated at night due to muscle relaxation during sleep allowing joint movements, termed 'night cries' is seen in typically in tuberculous arthritis

Seasonal variation: In rheumatoid arthritis and gout the pain may get worse during new and full moons and also in winter.

Locking: This is due to the presence of loose

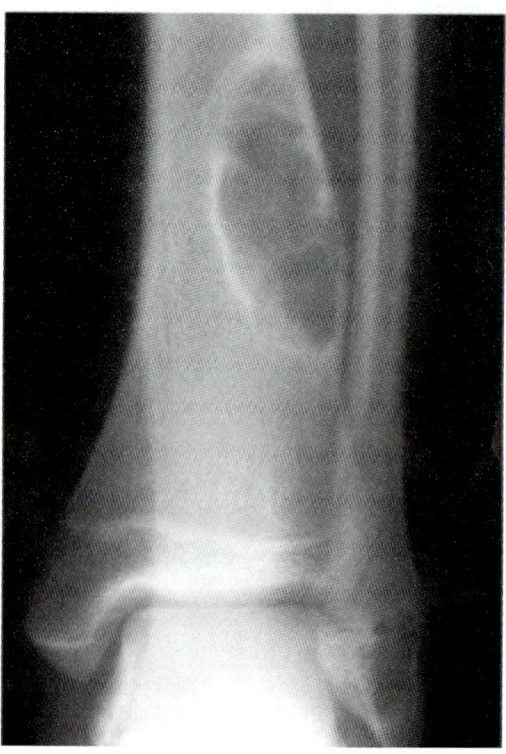

Fig. 107.7. Non-ossifying fibroma of tibia
(courtesy: Dr. A N Vivek, Chennai)

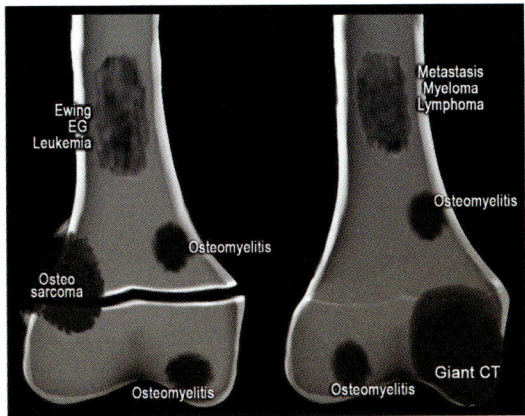

Below 30 years	Above 30 years

Fig. 107. 8. Common bone lesions

bodies in the joint

Deformity: This is seen in late or neglected cases of osteoarthrosis, rheumatoid and tuberculous arthritis

Past history: History of tuberculosis and exposure to STD. Previous injury may predispose to osteoarthrosis

Family history: Hemophilia or gout may be hereditary.

Physical examination

General survey to find out if the patient is in distress due to pain, to assess the nutritional status has to be done, besides the other diseases such as anemia, cyanosis, jaundice, generalized edema, lymphadenopathy etc. Vital signs (pulse, BP, respirations and temperature) have to be recorded. In diseases of lower limbs, any peculiarity in the patient's gait has to be observed.

Local examination

Inspection: The joint has to be inspected in comparison with its normal counterpart

Swelling, which may be diffuse (joint involvement) or on one side (extra articular, such as a bursa, ganglion etc)

Deformity: the concavity of the curvature may be inwards (varus) or outwards (valgus). It may be in relation to hip (coxa), knee (genu), foot (talepes), elbow (cubitus) or wrist (manus). If the effusion is under pressure, the joint assumes the position in which maximum volume of fluid may be accommodated (position of ease). Sometimes the position of the joint depends upon the net product of the strength of various muscles acting on the joint

Skin over the joint: shiny or erythematous appearance is in favor of acute inflammation. Presence of ulcer, (neuropathic joint) sinus (chronic osteomyelitis) or scarring (healed tuberculous ulcer) of the skin

Muscle wasting: The muscles immediately proximal to the involved joint maximally undergo disuse atrophy, e.g. gluteal for hip disease, thigh for knee, calf for ankle etc

Palpation: Points to be noted are, local warmth, tenderness, bony components, swelling and muscle wasting

Fluctuation or cross fluctuation may be elicited if there is considerable quantity of fluid. Patellar tap is specially designed for knee, in which gentle posterior push on the patella (with the knee fully extended and relaxed) will cause a tapping feel or sound, when it touches the femur.

Movements: The permitted range of both passive and active movements of the joint have to be recorded. As always, it is preferable to examine the normal side first, to dispel apprehension and prepare the patient to the similar movement on the affected side. If there is limitation, is it due to pain or mechanical obstruction (ankylosis).

If there crepitus during the movements, it is indicative of degenerative changes of articular cartilage.

Measurements as described in bone diseases, have to be recorded.

Auscultation: The crepitus may be appreciated better by auscultation than by palpation.

Regional lymph nodes: Their number, location and other characteristics have to be noted, including secondary skin changes, such as an ulcer or a sinus.

Examination of other joints: for polyarticular diseases such as rheumatoid, tuberculous arthritis.

Examination of other systems:

CVS for rheumatic arthritis, CNS for Charcot joint or a focus of sepsis in acute arthritis. Skin diseases like psoriasis may cause reactive arthropathy.

INVESTIGATIONS FOR DISEASES OF BONES AND JOINTS

However certain the diagnosis may be, it is prudent to carry out relevant investigations, to support or clinch the diagnosis, before embarking on specific treatment. Besides the routine and specific laboratory investigations, imaging forms the mainstay in orthopedics.

1. Blood: Leukocytosis is seen in acute inflammation. Serum calcium and gamma globulins are raised in multiple myeloma. Calcium is also raised in hyperparathyroidism, multiple skeletal metastases, sarcoidosis, while it is low in hypoparathyroidism, avitaminosis-D, rickets and osteomalacia. Alkaline phosphatase is high in conditions of increased osteoblastic activity (e.g. Paget's disease of bone, osteogenic sarcoma) and in osteomalacia. Elevation of serum acid phosphatase is specific of metastatic prostatic carcinoma, confirmed by raised levels of prostate specific antigen (PSA).

Other tests sometimes necessary: serum uric acid (gout), coagulation profile, including factors VIII and IX (hemophilia), rheumatoid factor - Rose-Waaler (rheumatoid arthritis), HLA-B27 (ankylosing spondylitis), serologic tests for syphilis (STS) etc. Skin has to be carefully examined for any septic focus, psoriasis and leprosy.

2. Urine: Albuminuria may be seen in amyloidosis associated long standing suppurative condition, such as chronic osteomyelitis. Presence of Bence-Jones protein may indicate the diagnosis of multiple myeloma. It is a globulin, detected by heating urine, a floculum develops when it reaches a temperature of 55° C, disappears at 80° C and reappears on cooling.

Urine homogentisic acid for alkaptonuria (on exposure to air, urine turns black, due to oxidation resulting in the formation of a pigment)

3. Radiological investigations:

a) Plain radiography, minimum two views and any special oblique/tangential views, as appropriate, is the initial study done in all cases. In children, it is always safer to compare with the opposite side, in view of the confusion generated by the unfused epiphyseal ends.

b) Contrast radiography, such as myelography, arthrography etc

4. Ultrasonography: It is useful as a simple, inexpensive, non-invasive investigation for conditions such as congenital dislocation of hip, septic arthritis of hip in infancy, (tendo achillis injuries, rotator cuff injuries in adults)

5. Tomography: Conventional tomography has been replaced by computerized axial tomography (CAT or CT), for more accurate 3-dimensional visualization of the pathology

6. Magnetic resonance imaging (MRI) is based on magnetic properties of tissues and considered superior to CT scan, which is density-based imaging, incapable of differentiating two iso-dense tissues or organs.

7. Radionucleide skeletal scan, using ^{99m}Tc, is a

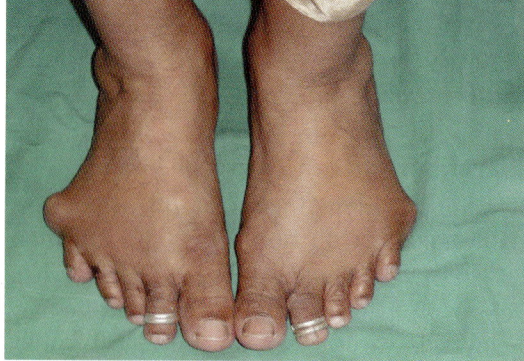

Fig. 107.9. Tophi of gout

very useful and commonly employed study, with high (>95%) sensitivity to detect neoplastic and inflammatory diseases of bone ('hot spots'). However, its specificity is limited to 80%

8. Angiography, if vascular involvement is suspected

9. Biopsy to get histological confirmation of the disease

10. Microbiological examination of pus, blood etc as necessary

ORTHOPEDICS IN EXTREMES OF AGE
PEDIATRIC ORTHOPEDICS

The development and growth of the skeletal system from gestation to skeletal maturity progresses through specific changes, these varied changes of the skeletal system have distinguishing features in terms of, increased susceptibility to injury, and infection, higher capacity of reparative response and remodeling/realignment, as against adult skeletal system.

As a rule, the younger the patient, the greater the remodeling potential; thus, absolute anatomic reduction in a child is less important than in a comparable injury in an adult.

Anatomy of pediatric bone

Pediatric bone has a higher water content and lower mineral content per unit volume than adult bone. Therefore, pediatric bone has a lower modulus of elasticity (less brittle) and a higher ultimate strain-to-failure than adult bone.

The physis (growth plate) is an unique cartilaginous structure that varies in thickness depending on age and location. It is frequently weaker than the adult bone, to torsion, shear, and bending force, predisposing the child to injury through this delicate area.

The periosteum in a child is a thick fibrous structure (up to several mm) that encompasses the entire bone except the articular ends. The periosteum thickens and is continuous with the physis at the perichondral ring (ring of LaCroix),

offering additional resistance to shear force.

As a general rule, ligaments in children are functionally stronger than bone. Therefore, a higher proportion of injuries that produce sprains in adults result in fractures in children.

The blood supply to the growing bone includes a rich metaphyseal circulation with fine capillary loops ending in the physis (in the neonate, small vessels may traverse the physis, ending in the epiphysis).

Mechanism of injury

Because of structural differences, pediatric fractures tend to occur at lower energy than adult fractures. Most are a result of compression, torsion, or bending moments.

Compression fractures are found most commonly at the metaphyseal-diaphysial junction and are referred to as "buckle fractures" or "torus fractures". Torus fractures rarely cause physeal injury, but they may result in acute angular deformity.

Bending moments in the child cause "greenstick fractures" in which the bone is incompletely fractured, resulting in a plastic deformity on the concave side of the fracture.

Bending moments in the child can also result in microscopic fractures that create plastic deformation of the bone with no visible fractures on plain radiographs; however permanent deformity can result.

Clinical evaluation

In pediatric trauma, as with adults, they should undergo full trauma evaluation with attention to airway, breathing, circulation, disability, and exposure (ABCDE).

Children are not good historians; therefore, keen diagnostic skills may be required for even the simplest problems.

It is important to evaluate the entire extremity, because young children cannot always localize the site of injury.

Neurovascular evaluation is mandatory, both before and after manipulation. Periodic evaluation for compartment syndrome should be performed, particularly for nonverbal patient who is irritable and who has an injury due to crush-type mechanism.

Radiographic evaluation

Radiographs must include appropriate views of the involved bones as well as the joint proximal and distal to the suspected area of injury

A thorough understanding of normal ossification patterns is necessary to adequately evaluate plain radiographs. Comparison views of the opposite extremity may aid in appreciating subtle deformities or in localizing a minimally displaced fracture.

"Soft signs" such as the posterior fat pad sign in elbow and pretracheal shadow in cervical spine should be closely evaluated.

Arthrograms are valuable in the intraoperative assessment of intraarticular fractures because radiolucent cartilaginous structures will not be apparent on fluoroscopic or plain radiographic evaluation.

Bone scans may be used in the evaluation of osteomyelitis or tumors.

Ultrasound can be useful for identifying epiphyseal separation in infants and as a screening for developmental dysplasias of the hip in neonates. However, this is not an ideal imaging modality in the diagnosis of bone diseases.

Classification

Five types of pediatric epiphyseal fractures have traditionally been described by Salter-Harris classification:

Type I: separation of epiphysis

Type II: fracture-separation of epiphysis

Type III: fracture of part of epiphysis

Type IV:

(A) fracture of epiphysis and epiphyseal plate
(B) Bony union causing premature closure of plate

Type V:

(C) crushing of epiphyseal plate

(D) Premature closure of plate on one side with resultant angular deformity

Basic principles of treatment

Fracture management in the child differs from that in an adult owing to the presence of a thick periosteum in the case of a diaphysial fracture or open physis in metaphyseal fractures.

A periosteal flap entrapped in the fracture site or buttonholing of a sharp fracture end through the periosteum can prevent an adequate reduction.

Remanipulation of epiphyseal injuries should not be attempted after 5 to 7 days.

Unlike in the adult, considerable fracture deformity may be permitted, because the remodeling potential in a child is significant.

In general, the closer the fracture is to the joint (physis), the better the deformity is tolerated. Rotational deformity does not spontaneously correct or remodel to an acceptable extent even in the young child and should be corrected.

In children, casts or splints should encompass the joint proximal and distal to the site of injury, because post-immobilization stiffness is not a common problem in children.

Indications for open reduction include:
Open fractures
Displaced intraarticular fractures
Fractures with vascular injury
Fractures with an associate compartment syndrome
Unstable fractures that require abnormal positioning to maintain closed reduction.

Complications

1. Complete growth arrest:

This may occur with physeal injuries in Salter-Harris fractures. It may result in limb length inequalities necessitating the use of orthotics, prosthetics, or operative procedures including epiphysiodesis or limb lengthening.

2. Progressive angular or rotational deformities They may result from physeal

Common postop complications in geriatric patients

Stress ulceration and upper GI bleeding

Pulmonary atelectasis and pneumonits

Deep vein thrombosis and pulmonary embolism

Cardiac decompensation due to ischemia, sclerosed valves, myopathy and fluid overload

Nutrition and electrolyte disturbances

Decubitus ulcers

Urinary retention and renal insufficiency

Cerebrovascular events

Constipation and fecal impaction

Postoperative psychosis

injuries with partial growth arrest or malunion. If these result in significant functional or cosmetic deformity, they may require operative intervention, such as osteotomy, for correction.

3. Osteonecrosis:

This may result from disruption of tenuous vascular supply in skeletally immature patients in whom vascular development is not complete (e.g. osteonecrosis of femoral head in case of slipped capital femoral epiphysis).

GERIATRIC ORTHOPEDICS

With improved life expectancy in India, the proportion of geriatric population and their orthopedic problems have increased. The management of orthopedic problems in the elderly (>70) poses special problems due to muscular weakness, senile osteoporosis and joint wear and tear, besides the co-morbidities likely to be present and the risks involved in anesthesia and immobilization. The problem is compounded by the social, economical and emotional factors, with their children living elsewhere, unable to provide them the necessary physical and moral support. Special attention should be paid towards preoperative evaluation, intraoperative care, anticipated postoperative complications, nursing care, early ambulation, physiotherapy and psychological counseling. In the event of requiring amputation, proper motivation to use prosthesis should be done, to restore mobility, productivity and consequent self confidence.

Note: Some subjects relating to orthopedics have been covered in detail in the main text of this book:

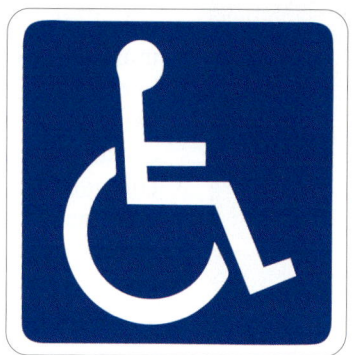

Common Orthopedic Short Cases

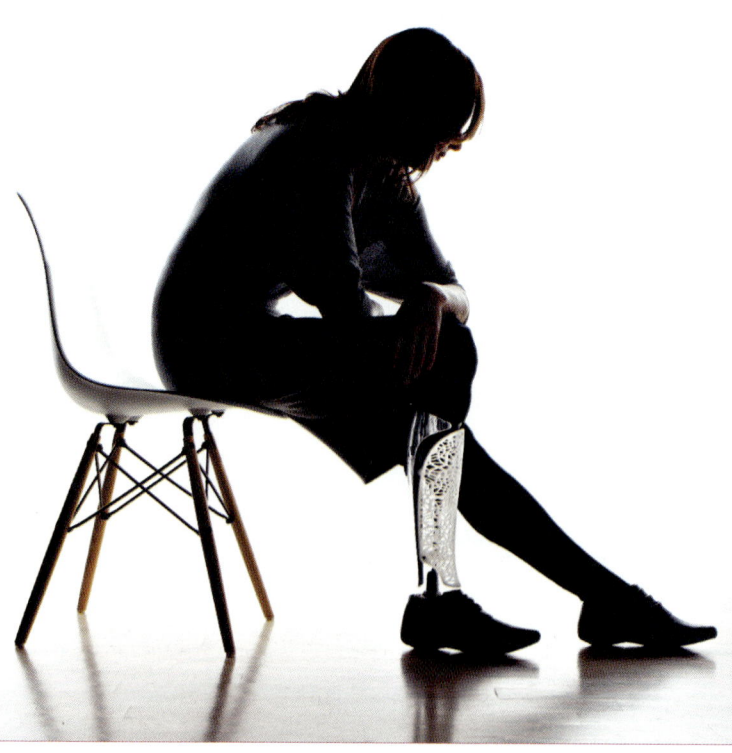

108 Cerebral Palsy

Definition: Cerebral palsy (CP) is a disorder of movement and posture that appears during infancy or early childhood. It is caused by nonprogressive damage to the brain before, during, or shortly after birth.

CP is not a single disease but a name given to a wide variety of static neuromotor impairment syndromes occurring secondary to a lesion in the developing brain. The damage to the brain is permanent and cannot be cured but the consequences can be minimized. Progressive musculoskeletal pathology occurs in most affected children.

The lesion in the brain may occur during the prenatal, perinatal, or postnatal periods. Any nonprogressive central nervous system (CNS) injury occurring during the first 2 years of life is considered to be CP.

In addition to movement and balance disorders, patients might experience other manifestations of cerebral dysfunction.

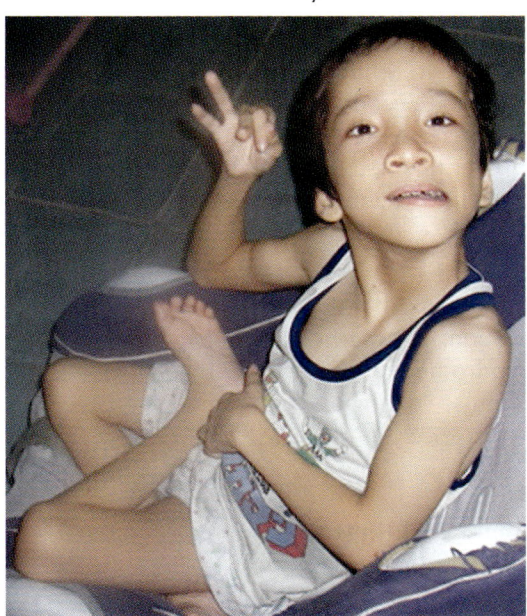

Fig. 108.1. Impaired cerebration and multiple spastic deformites in cerebral palsy

CP was first described by an English physician Sir Francis William Little in 1861 and was known as Little's disease for a long time. Little thought that this condition was caused by neonatal asphyxia. Later, Sigmund Freud and other scientists challenged Little's idea and proposed that a variety of insults during pregnancy could damage the developing brain. Today, it is accepted that only approximately 10% of cases of CP can be attributed to neonatal asphyxia. The majority occurs during the prenatal period, and in most of the cases, a specific cause cannot be identified.

Etiology

The etiology can be identified only in 50% of the cases, however certain risk factors have been identified. The incidence of CP among babies who have one or more of these risk factors is higher than among the normal children. Babies who carry these risk factors should be under close supervision by a pediatric neurologist for signs suggestive of neuromotor developmental delay.

Risk factors

Prenatal period (from the time of conception to the onset of labor)

Prematurity (gestational age <36 weeks)
Low birth weight (<2500 g)
Maternal epilepsy
Infections (TORCH - toxoplasmosis, rebella, cytomegalovirus, herpes simplex)
Bleeding in the third trimester
Incompetent cervix
Severe toxemia, eclampsia
Hyperthyroidism, drug abuse
Trauma
Multiple pregnancies
Placental insufficiency

Perinatal period (28 weeks intrauterine to 7 days postnatal)

Prolonged and difficult labor
Premature rupture of membranes

Manifestations of cerebral palsy	
Neurological	*Associated problems*
Muscle weakness	Intellectual impairment
Abnormal muscle tone	Epilepsy
Balance problems	Visual problems
Loss of selective control	Hearing loss
Pathological reflexes	Speech and communication problems
Loss of sensation	Swallowing difficulty
Musculoskeletal	Feeding difficulty, failure to thrive
Contractures	Respiratory problems
Deformities	Incontinence

Table-108.1

Presentation anomalies
Vaginal bleeding at the time of admission for labor
Bradycardia
Hypoxia

Postnatal period (first two years of life)

CNS infections (encephalitis, meningitis)
Hypoxia
Seizures
Coagulopathies
Neonatal hyperbilirubinemia

Pathology

Specific brain lesions related to CP can be identified in most of the cases. These lesions occur in regions that are particularly sensitive to disturbances in blood supply and are grouped under the term hypoxic ischemic encephalopathy.

Five types of hypoxic ischemic encephalopathy exist; parasagittal cerebral injury, periventricular leukomalacia, focal and multifocal ischemic brain necrosis, status marmoratus and selective neuronal necrosis.

Common sites for deformity	
Spine	Scoliosis, kyphosis
Hip	Subluxation, dislocation
Femur and tibia	Internal or external torsion
Foot	Equinus, valgus, varus

Table-108.2

Clinical findings

Children with CP present with three types of motor problems. The primary impairments of muscle tone, balance, strength and selectivity are directly related to damage in the CNS. Secondary impairments leading to muscle contractures and deformities develop over time in response to the primary problems and musculoskeletal growth. Tertiary impairments are adaptive mechanisms and coping responses that the child develops to adapt to the primary and secondary problems. One typical example is gastrocnemius spasticity as a primary impairment leading to secondary ankle plantar flexion contracture and knee hyperextension in stance as an adaptive mechanism.

Classification

Clinicians classify CP to describe the specific problem, to predict prognosis and to guide treatment, which is based on the change in muscle tone, anatomical region of involvement and severity of the problem and it provides a clearer understanding of the individual patient and directs management.

Spastic CP

Spasticity is defined as an increase in the physiological resistance of muscle to passive motion. It is part of the upper motor neuron syndrome characterized by hyperreflexia, clonus, extensor plantar responses and

Common sites for contracture	
Upper extremity	*Lower extremity*
Wrist and finger flexor	Hip adductor-flexor
Thumb adductor	Knee flexor
	Ankle plantar flexor

Table-108.3

primitive reflexes. Spastic CP is the most common form of CP (70 to 80%) and is anatomically distributed into three types, namely, hemiplegic type, diplegic type, and quadriplegic type.

Dyskinetic CP

Abnormal movements that occur when the patient initiates movement are termed dyskinesia. Dysarthria, dysphagia, and drooling accompany the movement problem. Mental status is generally normal; however severe dysarthria makes communication difficult and leads the observer to think that the child has intellectual impairment.

Ataxic CP

Ataxia is loss of balance, coordination, and fine motor control. Ataxic children are hypotonic during the first 2 years of life. Muscle tone becomes normal and ataxia becomes apparent toward the age of 2 to 3 years. Children who can walk have a wide-based gait and a mild intention tremor (dysmetria) with impaired dexterity and fine motor control. Ataxia is often associated with cerebellar lesions.

Mixed CP

Children with a mixed type of CP commonly have mild spasticity, dystonia, and/or athetoid movement. Ataxia may be a component of the motor dysfunction in patients in this group.

Ataxia and spasticity often occur together. Spastic ataxic diplegia is a common mixed type that often is associated with hydrocephalus.

Exceptions

Some children with CP cannot be fitted into any of these groups because of their varied presentation. Dystonia may be seen in a spastic child, and anatomical classification may not justify because of overlapping clinical findings.

Differential diagnosis

CP has to be distinguished from syndromes of progressive disorders of childhood (shown below), which exhibit more cognitive problems than CP, whereas the motor problems are predominant in CP.

Mental retardation syndromes
Attention deficit disorder
Autism
Non-motor handicaps such as blindness
Emotional disorders

Investigations

Imaging studies enable the physician to define the type and location of the brain lesion and to differentiate progressive neurological syndromes.

Radiology

The indications to perform radiography in cases of CP are:
To monitor hip instability, where baseline hip

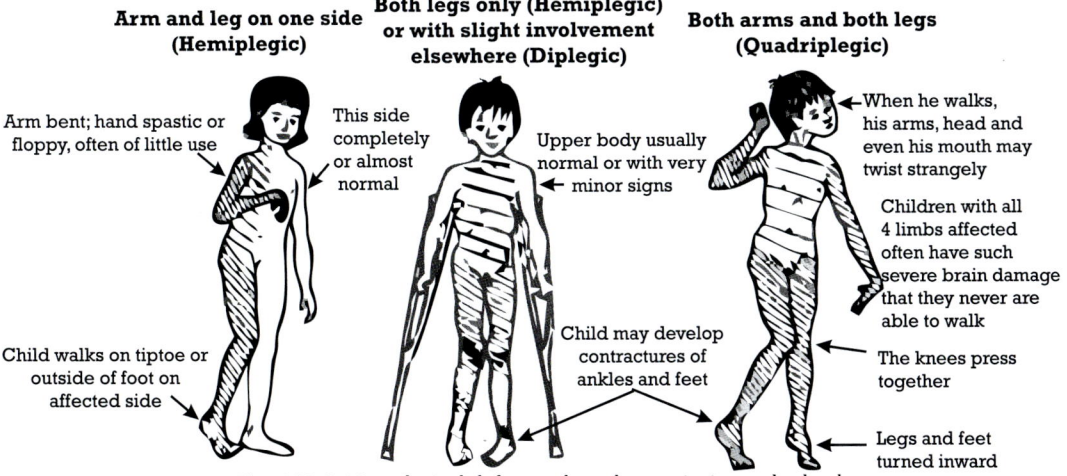

Fig. 108.2. Neurological defect and resultant gaits in cerebral palsy

Arm and leg on one side (Hemiplegic)

Both legs only (Hemiplegic) or with slight involvement elsewhere (Diplegic)

Both arms and both legs (Quadriplegic)

Arm bent; hand spastic or floppy, often of little use

This side completely or almost normal

Upper body usually normal or with very minor signs

When he walks, his arms, head and even his mouth may twist strangely

Children with all 4 limbs affected often have such severe brain damage that they never are able to walk

Child walks on tiptoe or outside of foot on affected side

Child may develop contractures of ankles and feet

The knees press together

Legs and feet turned inward

radiographs are obtained and followed up with interval radiographs for hips 'at risk'. The Reimer's index is the measure of the percentage of femoral head coverage by the acetabulum.

To monitor scoliosis, where interval radiographs are taken to see the progression. Cobb angle is used as a criterion for surgery.

Radiographs of the extremities are necessary for patients planned for osteotomies.

Cranial USG

Cranial USG can help in the differential diagnosis of the infant when the fontanelle is open. It is easy and it does not require sedation as does MRI. Cranial USG evaluates the ventricles, basal ganglia and corpus callosum. Ischemic injury of periventricular white matter and intraventricular hemorrhage are apparent on real-time cranial ultrasonograms.

Cerebral CT

CT is helpful in the diagnosis of intracranial bleeding in the newborn, in evaluating congenital malformations and periventricular leukomalacia (PVL), but this is less helpful compared to MRI.

3 dimensional CT is useful when planning hip reconstruction.

Cerebral MRI

MRI is the best method for diagnosing lesions in the white matter after second week and is at present, most common investigation.

Electroencephalography (EEG)

EEG measures electrical activity on the surface of the brain. It is an essential investigation to diagnose and monitor seizure disorders.

Treatment

The ultimate goal in the management is to minimize disability while promoting independence and full participation in society. All efforts should be directed to gain independence in activities of daily living, ability to go to school, earn a living and a successful integration with the community.

Rehabilitation and physiotherapy

Rehabilitation is the name given to all diagnostic and therapeutic procedures which aim to develop maximum physical, social and vocational function in a diseased or injured person. Physiotherapy begins in early infancy and continues throughout adolescence, with the primary objective of facilitating normal neuromotor development.

Methods of physiotherapy

Conventional exercises

Active and passive range of motion

Stretching

Strengthening

Neurofacilitation techniques (Vojta and Bobath)

These are based on the principle that sensory input to the CNS produces reflex motor output. They aim to normalize muscle tone, to establish advanced postural reactions and to facilitate normal movement patterns.

Occupational therapy, play therapy, sports and recreation

These aim to improve the functions of the exremities through through play and purposeful activities.

Bracing

Braces are devices which hold the extremities in a stable position. The goals of bracing are to increase function, prevent deformity, keep the joint in the functional position, stabilize the trunk and extremities, facilitate selective motor control, decrease spasticity and protect the extremity from injury in the postoperative phase.

Mobility aids, wheeled mobility and assistive devices

Orthopedic Surgery

Orthopedic surgery is widely used in the management of children with CP to prevent or correct certain musculoskeletal problems such as muscle shortening and bony deformities. The goal of orthopedic surgery with walking potential is to improve functional ambulation. For non-ambulatory children, its aim is to facilitate sitting, improve hygiene and prevent pain.

109 Torticollis

(syn: wryneck)

Torticollis is defined as a condition where the head is tilted toward one side and the chin is pointing to the opposite direction (tortus: twisted; collum: neck).

Types:

i) Congenital
   Congenital muscular torticollis
ii) Acquired
   a. Fracture of vertebrae or clavicle
   b. Anomalies of atlantoaxial joint
   c. Posterior fossa tumors
   d. Hysteria
   e. Cervical adenitis, retropharyngeal abscess, or any cervical mass
   f. Ocular abnormalities like strabismus, muscle weakness, and nystagmus
   g. Gastroesophageal reflux disease (GERD)
   h. Drugs- phenothiazines may be associated with abnormal posturing
   i. Grisel's Syndrome- an antecedent inflammatory process in the head of axis bone area may lead to subluxation of the atlantoaxial joint and torticollis.

Congenital muscular torticollis
Etiology

It is usually discovered in the first 2 to 8 weeks of life, with a prediliction to the first-born child, often associated with a difficult delivery or breech presentation, which causes bleeding in to the muscles of the neck, usually the SCM. An associated mass that can be seen or felt within the muscle and usually thought to be a hematoma that is in the process of organization and fibrosis.

Recently, it has been postulated that the shortening of the muscle is a result of scarring due to an intrauterine vascular disturbance.

Clinical features

The condition does not cause pain, but it becomes apparent to the observant mother, as the child persists in holding the head in the tilted position. The right side is more often involved (75%) and the child holds his head tilted to the right, with his face and chin rotated to the left. This is seen within the first 8 weeks of life and may or may not be associated with a SCM mass. When present, the mass, however, tends to resolve spontaneously within 3 months. Congenital muscular torticollis may be associated with hip dysplasia (10 to 20%) so the hips should be carefully examined in children with torticollis. If uncorrected, as the child grows, the face on the affected side may be "flattened", with consequent facial asymmetry. Hence it is important to correct the torticollis before the age of 1, i.e,. before the facial asymmetry develops. Beyond that, some facial asymmetry may remain permanent, which is seen more in congenital torticollis, but rarely those with acquired type and may be useful to distinguish the two types.

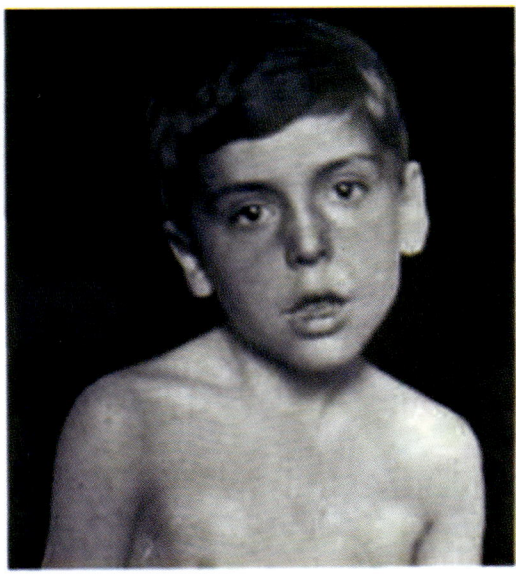

Fig. 109.1. Torticollis
(Right SCM muscle affected)

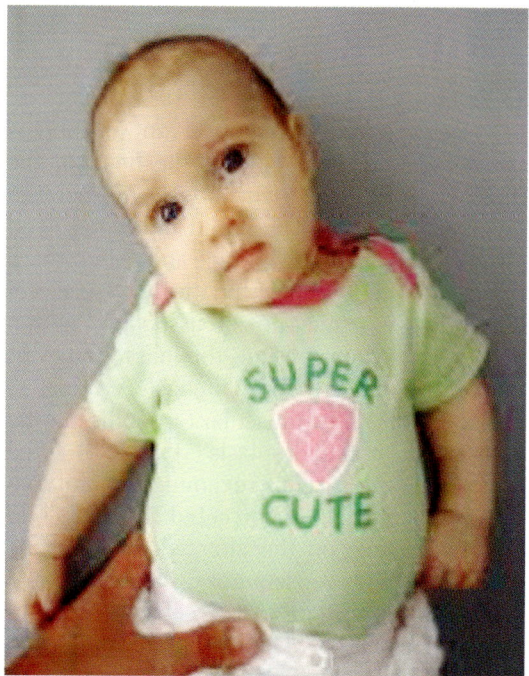

Fig. 109.2. Child with torticollis
(Right SCM muscle affected)

Investigations

Radiological examination of head and neck region is required to rule out atlantoaxial and cervical vertebral anomalies. USG is useful to detect SCM mass, the size of which may be of prognostic significance. It is also useful to rule out associated hip dysplasia. If spinal cord abnormalities are suspected from the sympomatology, a CT scan or MRI may be useful.

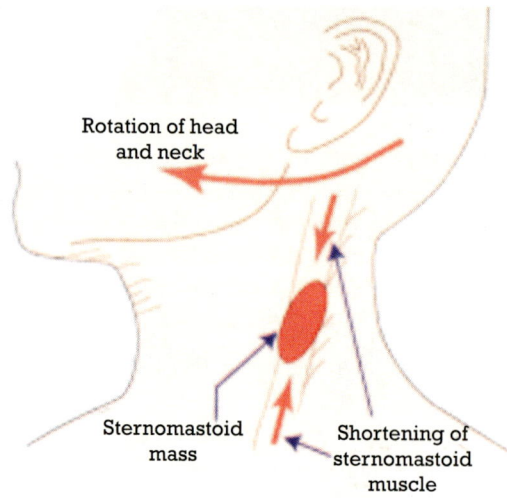

Fig. 109.3. Morbid anatomy of torticollis
(courtesy: Dr. A N Vivek, Chennai)

Treatment

Treatment of congenital torticollis involves stretching exercise program of the shortened neck muscle with 90% success, if started within 3 months of age. In refractory cases, surgical release of the SCM muscle may be required, around the age of 12 months.

Acquired torticollis is treated essentially by treating the underlying cause. Medications used to treat this condition include an anticholinergic drugs e.g. baclofen, skeletal muscle relaxants etc. Injection of botulinum toxin (Botox) into the muscle is shown to give temporary relief, requiring repeat injections at 3 months intervals, reserving surgery to resistant cases.

110 Adhesive Capsulitis
(Frozen Shoulder, Periarthritis Shoulder)

Adhesive capsulitis, or frozen shoulder, is a painful condition in which the synovial lining of the glenohumeral (shoulder joint) is inflamed. It is a clinical diagnosis in which there is loss of both active and passive motion of the joint.

Etiology

The pathophysiology of idiopathic shoulder stiffness remains uncertain, but the disease is commonly limited to contracture of the gleno-humeral capsule. Most prominently involved part of the joint is the coracohumeral ligament. The disease may be idiopathic or posttrauma-tic. Idiopathic types are common in elderly diabetics, especially women between 40 and 60. Other diseases that may predispose to this disorder are:

1. cervical
2. cardiac
3. pulmonary
4. neoplastic
5. neurologic and
6. personality disorders.

Very often the diabetes mellitus is discovered while investigating the patient with the shoulder stiffness. Although all patients may recall some traumatic event that preceded their shoulder stiffness, those with distinct trauma such as a prior fracture, rotator cuff tear, or surgical procedure are grouped under post-traumatic category.

Clinical features

There is insidious onset of shoulder pain felt during rotational movements such as reaching behind the back or putting on a coat. Often the patient may recall a minor trauma that precipitated the condition.

The clinical presentation of idiopathic shoulder stiffness is classically described as having three phases; freezing phase, progressive stiffness phase and thawing phase. It is important, while examining for the range of shoulder move-

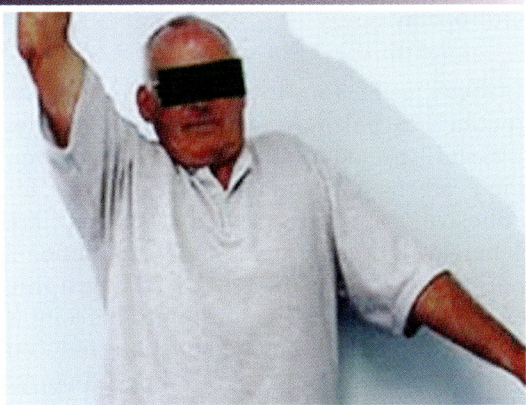

Fig. 110.1. Painful limitation of abduction of left shoulder in periarthritis

ments, to fix the scapula, to eliminate any complementary movements.

Freezing phase: The pain is typically achy, and sudden jolts exacerbate the pain, which may appear more at night, with progressive imitation of shoulder movements. The patients hold the arm in a position of comfort, i.e. adduction, and internal rotation. this phase lasts between 2 and 9 months.

Progressive stiffness phase: Stiffness progresses to the point where shoulder motion is restricted in all planes. Essentially, the shoulder has undergone fibrous ankylosis or arthrodesis. Fortunately, pain progressively decreases from the initial inflammatory phase and in due course patients are able to use the shoulder with little or no pain, within the restricted range of motion, but attempts to exceed this range are accompanied by pain. This phase lasts between 3 and 12 months.

Resolution, or thawing phase: The shoulder progressively becomes supple and the move-ments become pain-free. This phase lasts between 6 months and 3 years.

Differential diagnosis

In early stages, it may mimic impingement. Subtle losses of internal and external rotation in abduction may be in favour of the latter.

Other conditions to be differentiated are, unrecognized trauma (locked posterior shoulder dislocations) and glenohumeral joint arthropathy.

Investigations

Diabetes mellitus and hyperuricemia have to be routinely excluded. A standard shoulder series is useful in excluding other diagnoses; however, there are no plain radiographic findings for adhesive capsulitis. Further studies are generally not indicated unless additional pathology is suspected. Arthrographic evaluation, injecting a contrast into the joint is rarely necessary. It may demonstrate reduced capacity of the joint from 12 ml to 2-3ml. An MRI of the joint confirms the diagnosis.

Treatment

Medical: The treatment of adhesive capsulitis is aimed at resolution of synovial inflammation and restoration of motion. NSAIDs may be used for symptomatic relief, but intraarticular injection of steroid may occasional be necessary. The patient must start on intese pysiotherapy with stretching program to regain motion in all planes. If 3 to 6 months of intense therapy fails to give relief, surgical intervention may be indicated, so also those with posttraumatic adhesive capsulitis.

Surgical: The surgical options are, manipulation under anesthesia, and arthroscopic adhesiolysis. The later is invasive but more effective and involves releasing the shoulder capsule under direct vision with some form of electro frequency device.

Aggressive physical therapy with active-assisted and active range of motion is mandatory to maintain the postoperative range of motion. Shoulder strengthening and resistance therapy is instituted only after restoration of full, active shoulder motion. The overall expected restoration of pain free movements may be around 80%.

111 Myositis Ossificans

This is the commonest type of heterotopic ossification. It is a localized reactive proliferative benign lesion usually confined to muscle, following a fracture or injury in the vicinity, hence it is also called myositis ossificans traumatica.

It is commonly seen in brachialis (following supracondylar fracture of humerus), quadriceps femoris (following supracondylar fracture of femur) and gluteal muscles (following fracture neck of femur). In India it is commonly seen in children after oil massaging of an injured limb.

Pathology: This is essentially ossification in a hematoma, which may follow a fracture and rarely soft tissue injury, involving the periosteum. It is considered to be due to the proliferation of osteogenic cells from the periosteum, however it is not clear why it has special predilection to the region of elbow.

Histologically, it is confirmed by zoning phenomenon, where less mature cells are seen in the center and more mature cells are situated in the periphery of the lesion. This is in contrast to reverse zoning phenomenon of most malignant conditions in which the immature highly neoplastic component of the tumor is at its periphery

Clinical stages

Stage-1:   (0-3 weeks) acute pseudoinflammatory phase, pain, swelling and restricted mobility.

Stage-2:   (3-6 weeks) subacute pseudotumor phase, pain reduces and hard mass starts appearing which may or may not be attached to the bone. In this stage the osteoblasts deposit osteoid in a centripetal fashion (zonal architecture).

Stage-3:   (3-6 months) resolution phase, during which bony mass begins to shrink in size.

Clinical features

History of injury

More rapid development (than malignant tumors)

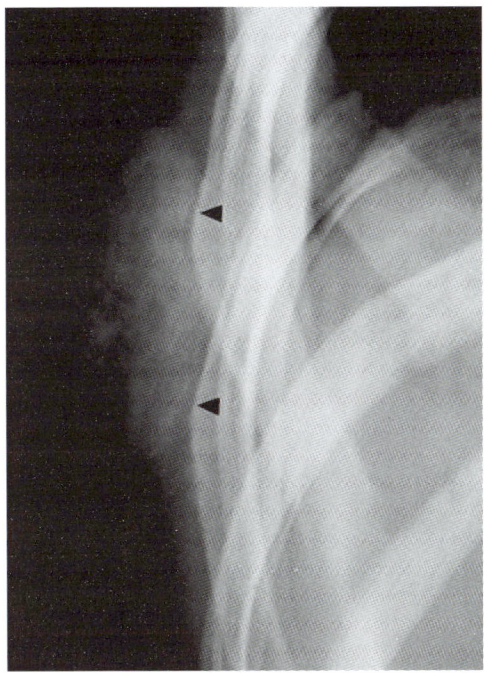

Fig. 111.2. Characteristic appearance of posttraumatic myositis ossificans circumscripta, adjacent to the right ribs. Note the periphery of the lesion is denser than the center. The arrowheads point to the narrow radiolucent cleft that separates the lesion from the cortex of the ribs

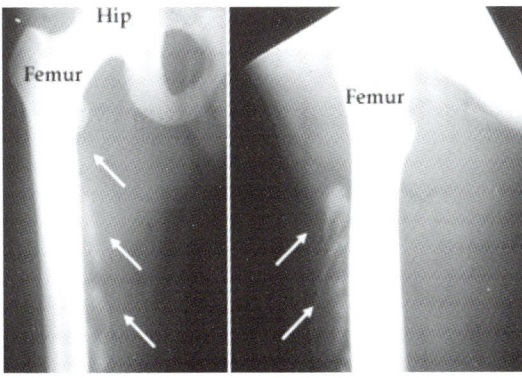

Fig. 111.1. Myositis ossificans of the upper thigh, following blunt injury

Site: brachialis and quadriceps are the common sites

Radiography: radiographically characteristic zonal calcification is seen. The ossific mass matures over a period of 6-18 months. Resorption of the mass occurs over a period of 1-5 years.

Treatment: it is difficult and controversial

In acute phase

Application of a compression dressing, ice, avoidance of additional injury

NSAIDs, e.g. Indomethacin, ibuprofen etc

In established disease

Bisphosphonates

Low dose radiation therapy

Physiotherapy

Surgical resection after myositis mass matures

(if the lesion is excised in acute or subacute stage, prompt recurrence is the rule)

The other types of myositis

Myositis ossificans circumscripta seen in patients with post-traumatic paraplegia or brain injury. There is progressive calcification around several joints, such as shoulders, hips and knees, restricting their movements.

Myositis ossificans progressiva is a disease of unknown etiology, neither associated with injury nor any other identifiable cause. It is seen in children below 10 years, where the heterotropic calcification occurs in trunk and neck muscles, associated with fever and some local signs of inflammation. The disease extends gradually, limiting the movements of spine and thorax, causing respiratory insufficiency. This condition is sometimes associated with congenital short thumbs or big toes.

Treatment: It is only symptomatic, including physiotherapy. Bisphosphonates have been found to be effective in arresting the progression of the disease.

112 Osteomyelitis

Definition: Osteomyelitis is an inflammation of the bone caused by an infecting organism. The infection may be limited to a portion of the bone or may involve a number of regions such as the marrow, cortex, periosteum, and even the surrounding soft tissue.

Classification

Classification of osteomyelitis is based on a number of criteria such as the duration (acute, subacute and chronic), mechanism of infection (exogenous and hematogenous) and based on the host response to the disease (pyogenic and non-pyogenic). Commonly it is based on duration of symptoms, however the time limits defining these categories are somewhat arbitrary.

Acute osteomyelitis

Acute osteomyelitis is a rapidly destructive pyogenic infection, usually hematogenous in origin, occurring most frequently in infants and children. It starts in a metaphysis of an actively growing long bone and runs a fulminant septic course that may terminate fatally.

Etiology

Predisposing causes:

Age: infancy and childhood (bimodal distribution, under 2 years and again between 8 and 12 years)

Sex: males predominate (4:1)

Trauma: history of direct injury to affected region is frequently elicited

Location: metaphysis of a long bone which is the most actively growing region (e.g. upper end of tibia, lower end of femur)

Poor nutrition, unhygienic environment and antecedent focus of infection (e.g. boil, scabies or tonsillitis)

Among the infective agents hemolytic Staphylococcus aureus is the most common organism. Others include Streptococcus, Hemophilus influenza, E.coli, Clostridium perfringens, pneumococcus and salmonelle

Pathogenesis

Acute osteomyelitis is initiated by introduction of bacteria from outside through a wound or a focus of sepsis which leads to septicemia or bacteremia (by hematogenous route). An infective embolus enters the nutrient artery of the bone and is trapped in a small caliber vessel. These small end-arteries are located more in the metaphysis, explaining the predilection of the metaphysis to infection. The infective embolus, which contains the virulent organisms, blocks the small vessels, leading to small area of bone necrosis. There is exudative inflammation with pouring in of polymorphonuclear leucocytes, which follows paths of least resistance, mainly through the Haversian and the cortical Volkmann canals to enter the subperiosteal space, which progressively strips the periosteum to form a subperiosteal abscess. If left untreated, this process eventually results in the formation of extensive sequestrum and goes into a state of chronicity.

Clinical features

Symptoms of acute illness are present, characterized by high fever, chills, rapid pulse, irritability, restlessness, vomiting and convulsions. The extremity affected is held in semiflexion with associated muscular spasm and resistance to passive movements due to pain. Over a period of time soft tissue around the affected region becomes edematous and red, indicating subperiosteal abscess formation. If infection and septicemia proceed unabated, it may threaten the viability of the bone and ultimately life of the child.

Investigations

Radiographs done within the first 10 days may appear normal. Thereafter, a localized area of bone destruction is observed in the metaphysis, later subperiosteal new bone formation is noted. Necrotic bone appears denser with scalloped appearance.

Aspiration of subperiosteal pus reveals the organisms on microscopy and on culture. Blood culture may identify the culprit organism. There may be polymorphonuclear leukocytosis, with elevated ESR and C-reactive proteins (CRP).

^{99m}Technetium phosphate imaging shows increased uptake at the involved area. Gallium citrate and ^{111}Indium-labelled leukocytes have been also used to indentify early stages of acute osteomyelitis. MRI is currently being used to make an expedient diagnosis.

Complications

Spread to surrounding soft tissues may cause suppurative tenosynovitis, suppurative arthritis, and thrombophlebitis. The consequences of septicemia and pyemia, as described above, may supervene.

Treatment

Early administration of wide spectrum antibiotics even before definitive diagnosis is made, should be done. As in any infection in a closed space, immediate provision for drainage and obtaining material for microbiological studies are of paramount importance. This must be done at the earliest possible opportunity, even before signs of subperiosteal abscess formation are evident. Surgical options include, subperiosteal decompression, creation of a bone window, and closed irrigation and suction technique.

Pott's puffy tumor

Subperiosteal infection, caused by osteomyelitis of skull bones, usually the frontal bone. The infection may originate from frontal sinus, infected hematoma following injury or chronic suppurative otitis media

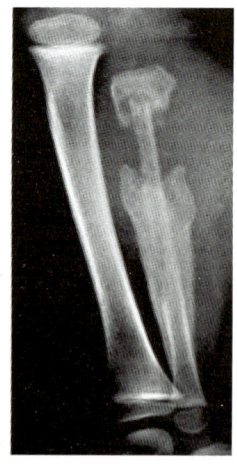

Fig. 112.1. Chronic osteomyelitis of fibula showing extensive sequestrum and surrounding involucrum

(CSOM). Pus collects under the pericraneum and subdural space, often both communicating, forming a dumb-bell abscess.

Constitutional symptoms, such as fever and chills and local signs of boggy swelling over the scalp due to cellulitis, associated with features of an intracranial SOL, like severe headache, vomiting, visual disturbances would provide clue to the diagnosis.

Diagnosis is confirmed by the presence of localizing neurological signs, leukocytosis and a CT scan findings. Diagnostic needling, followed by surgical drainage is the treatment, under cover of high antibiotics. A burr hole may be necessary to drain the intracranial collection, as per the neurosurgical principles. Underlying osteomyelitis has to be treated on its merits and the culprit paranasal sinus or middle ear infection also has to be aggressively treated to prevent recurrence.

Subacute osteomyelitis

Compared with acute osteomyelitis, subacute type has a more insidious onset and lacks the severity of symptoms, which makes the diagnosis more difficult.

Etiology

The indolent course of subacute osteomyelitis is due to better host resistance, low bacterial virulence, or due to the administration of antibiotics early in the course of the disease. Staphylococcus aureus and streptococcus epidermidis are the predominant organisms identified in this condition.

Clinical features

Due to the indolent course and subtle symptomatology, diagnosis is typically delayed for more than 2 weeks. Systemic signs and symptoms, including fever may be minimal. Pain of mild to moderate degree and local muscle spasm are the only consistent signs, to alert the clinician about the possibility of bone infection.

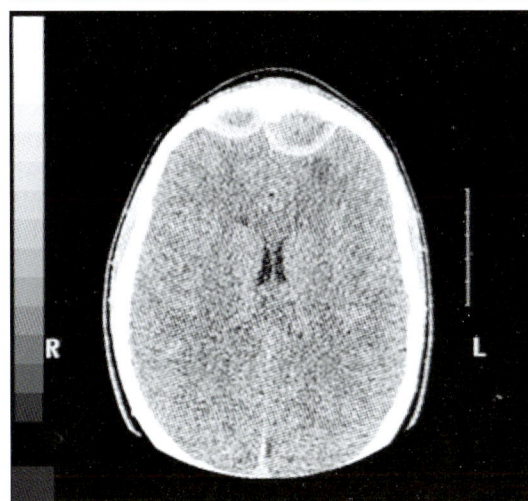

Fig. 112.2. CT scan showing osteomyelitis of the frontal bone.

Investigations

There may not be leukocytosis, but the ESR is elevated in about 50% of patients, and blood cultures are usually negative. Plain radiographs may show solitary localized area of lucency with surrounding new bone formation. Nuclear scans and MRI may indicate the disease, which should be confirmed by an open biopsy and bacteriology.

Treatment

It involves biopsy and curettage, under cover of appropriate antibiotics for about 6 weeks duration.

Primary subacute osteomyelitis

1. Brodie's abscess
2. Garre's osteomyelitis
3. Salmonella osteomyelitis

1.   Brodie's Abscess

A Brodie's abscess is a localized form of subacute osteomyelitis that occurs most often in the metaphysis long bones of lower extremities in young adults, before epiphyseal closure. In adults, the metaphyseal-epiphyseal area is involved, commonest regions being distal femur and proximal tibia. The lesion is caused by organisms of

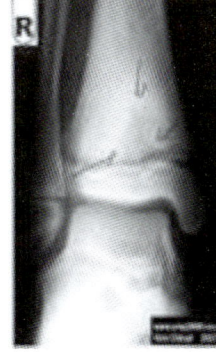

Fig. 112.3. Brodie's abscess of the lower end of tibia.

low virulence commonly staphylococcus aureus

In the adults intermittent pain of long duration is the presenting complaint, along with local tenderness over the affected area. On plain radiographs it generally appears as a lytic lesion with a rim of sclerotic bone and careful evaluation is necessary since it can be easily mistaken for neoplasms. This condition often requires an open biopsy with curettage to make the diagnosis and wound should be closed loosely over a drain. Appropriate antibiotics may be necessary for several weeks, before total resolution occurs. Occasionally it may cause a pathological fracture.

2.   Sclerosing osteomyelitis of Garre

This is a chronic form of disease in which the bone is thickened and distended but abscesses and sequestra are absent. The disease affects children and young adults. Its cause is unknown, but it is thought to be an infection caused by a low-grade, possibly anaerobic bacteria. Patients report intermittent pain of moderate intensity and usually of long duration. Swelling and tenderness over the affected bone may be found. Radiographs show an expanded bone with generalized sclerosis and ESR may be slightly elevated. Biopsy shows chronic, low-grade, nonspecific osteomyelitis, and cultures are usually negative. No treatment has been predictably helpful, but fenestration of the sclerotic bone under cover of antibiotics is recommended. The condition must be distinguished from osteoid osteoma and Pagets' disease.

3.   Salmonella (typhoid) osteo-myelitis

It is a subacute type, commonly occurring in ulna, ribs or vertebra, often several months after the attack of typhoid or paratyphoid fever, presumably from a focus in the gall-bladder. It is also seen as a complication of sickle-cell disease.

Clinically it presents with moderate

signs of inflammation, associated with pain and tenderness over the affected bone. When it occurs in spine, it is often confused with caries spine. Radiograph shows central area of rarefaction with periosteal reaction and new bone formation. The diagnosis is confirmed by Widal test and pus bacteriology (following surgery). Isotope skeletal scan is necessary to detect involvement of other bones. Treatment is by surgery (curettage), under cover of appropriate antibiotics, such as chloramphenicol (not much used nowadays due to the fear of bone marrow depression), ciprofloxacin or 4th generation cephalosporins.

Chronic osteomyelitis

Definition

Chronic osteomyelitis is a sequel of acute osteomyelitis characterized by presence of infected dead bone within a compromised soft tissue envelope.

Pathology

Following an attack of acute osteomyelitis, if the resolution is incomplete, it results in smouldering infection in the form of hyperemia, infected granulation tissue or a sequestrum. The granulation tissue carries osteoclasts and osteoblasts which absorbs necrotic bone and replaces new bone respectively. The absorption of cancellous bone is faster and replaced by new bone, whereas cortical bone is gradually absorbed and is detached from living bone to form a sequestrum in the course of several months. After complete sequestration, there are necrotic bone fragments surrounded by granulation tissue which is encased inside vascular bone. This surrounding living or the vascular bone attempts to wall off the infection by forming a thick, dense wall of periosteal new bone formation called the involucrum. An involucrum usually has multiple openings, called the cloacae, through which exudates, bone debris, and sequestra, which pass through the sinus tracts to the surface. In long standing osteomyelitis multiple cavities and sequestra exist throughout the bone, the shaft becomes thickened, irregular and deformed.

Clinical features

There is persistent local pain, the overlying skin is dusky, thin. scarred and poorly nourished . There may be ulceration which is slow to heal, with multiple nonhealing sinuses, extruding small chips of bone (sequestra) at intervals. The underlying bone is deformed, thickened and adherent to the sinuses. During the periods of inactivity of the infection, the symptoms may be minimal, but if there is a reactivation of infection, increased local pain, swelling, tenderness, warmth and redness may be seen.

Investigations

The diagnosis of chronic osteomyelitis is based on clinical, laboratory, and imaging studies.

Laboratory studies are generally non-specific, CRP and ESR are elevated in most patients, with occasional leukocytosis.

Plain radiographs provide valuable information, with signs of cortical destruction and periosteal reaction. The sequestrum appears denser than the surrounding normal bone (involucrum) due to impaired demineralization, attributable to avascularity, but a CT scan is more sensitive in identifying sequestra, and other bone changes. Sinography can be performed if a sinus tract is present and may be a valuable adjunct to surgical planning. Isotope bone scanning is useful more in acute osteomyelitis than in the chronic form. The gold standard in the diagnosis of chronic osteomyelitis is biopsy and microbiology.

Complications

Complications of chronic osteomyelitis include a reduced rate of growth, pathologic fracture, bone lengthening, muscle contracture, amyloidosis and epithelioma.

Treatment

Chronic osteomyelitis generally cannot be eradicated without surgical treatment. The goal of surgery is elimination of the infection by achieving a viable and vascular environment. Surgery for chronic osteomyelitis consists of sequestrectomy and resection of scarred infected bone and soft tissue. Radical debridement may be required to achieve this goal. Inadequate debridement will result in recurrence.

Surgery for chronic osteomyelitis

a. Sequestrectomy, curettage and saucerization

b. Open bone grafting (Papineau technique)

   i. Stage I - Debridement involves excision of sinus tracts, sequestra and saucerization of the involved region of bone.

   ii. Stage II - Grafting. This is done after granulation tissue has grown on the saucerized area following debridement. Cancellous bone grafts are usually taken from posterior iliac crest and are placed over the granulation bed and dressed (open bone grafting).

   iii. Stage III - Wound coverage one of the several techniques is used; skin grafts, myocutaneous flaps, muscle pedicle flaps, and free flaps.

c. Polymethylmethacrylate (PMMA) antibiotic bead chains after debridement, sequestrectomy and saucerization the dead space is filled by PMMA beads rolled on wires, which are removed after one to three months.

d. Biodegradable antibiotic delivery system: the main advantage of this is that a second procedure is not required to remove the implant.

e. Closed suction drains: in this technique, closed suction antibiotic ingress and egress high-volume irrigation systems are used over a period of 3 to 21 days.

f. Soft tissue transfer

g. Ilizarov technique: this technique has been useful in the treatment of chronic osteomyelitis and infected non-union. The technique allows radical resection of the infected bone. A corticotomy is performed through normal bone proximal and distal to the area of disease and bone is transported until union is achieved.

h. Hyperbaric oxygen therapy: it is recommended only as an adjuvant to traditional methods of treatment.

Specific osteomyelitis

Tuberculous osteomyelitis

Primary source is usually pulmonary disease, it afftects virtually any bone in the body, though it is commonly seen in children and adolescents (up to 30%), while it is very rare in elderly,

Bacteriology and pathology (see chapter 18).

Clinical features: With insidious onset, the constitutional features typically precede the local signs. Adjacent joint may also be involved.

Investigations and chemotherapy (see chapter 18). For skeletal tuberculosis the period of multi-drug chemotherapy is for 12-18 months.

Quiescence of lesion is identified by:

General: Reduction of toxicity, improvement of appetite, weight and overall well-being

Local: Absence of local signs of inflammation, muscle spasm

Laboratory: ESR returning to normal

Radiological: Evidence of clear margins and sclerosis of lesion

Aims of surgery: Drainage of cold abscess, curettage of caseous material, correction of deformities, stabilization the skeletal weakness and preservation of function.

Rarer types of chronic osteomyelitis

Brucellosis
Syphilis
Fungal (nocardiasis)
Parasitic (hydatid)

113 Radial Nerve Palsy

Anatomy: The radial nerve constitutes the termination of the posterior cord of the brachial plexus derived from C-5,6,7,8 and T-1, and descends from the axilla winding posteriorly around the shaft of the humerus (spiral or radial groove). As it passes over the elbow joint, it divides into a terminal motor (posterior interosseous or deep radial) and sensory (superficial radial nerve) branches at the level of the radiocapitellar joint. Motor supply of the radial nerve includes muscles of the posterior compartment of the arm and forearm which are mostly extensors. Before the division it supplies the triceps, anconeus, brachioradialis, extensor carpi radialis longus, and through the posterior interosseous branch, extensor carpi radialis brevis, supinator,

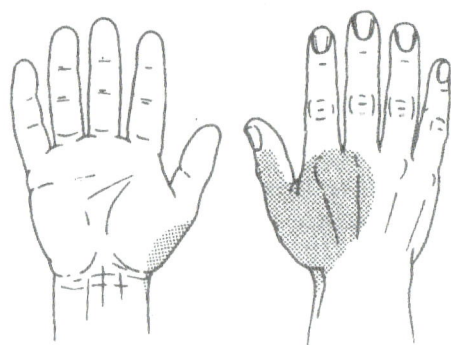

Fig. 113.2. Area of sensory loss in lesion of radial nerve above elbow

extensor digitorum, extensor digiti minimi, extensor carpi ulnaris, the extensor indicis, abductor pollicis longus and two extensors of the thumb, namely extensor pollicis longus and brevis.

Sensory - Inferior lower cutaneous nerve of arm: lower half of the radial aspect of the arm

Posterior cutaneous nerve of forearm: middle of the posterior aspect of the forearm

Superficial branch of radial nerve: the dorsal aspect of the thumb and radial 2nd finger, except nail beds. The distribution to the dorsum of the hand is variable and clinically, sensation should be tested only on the dorsum itself, not over the fingers.

Modes of presentation of radial nerve palsy

'Crutch palsy' - due to compression of the nerve above the spiral groove by crutches as the weight is borne in the axilla.

'Saturday night palsy' - due to compression of the nerve in the upper part of the arm as a result of resting the medial side of the arm against a sharp edge such as the back of a chair for a prolonged period. The person is usually intoxicated. It may also be seen after surgery when the anesthetized patient's limb is allowed to hang over the edge of the operating table.

Humeral fracture - The close relationship of the

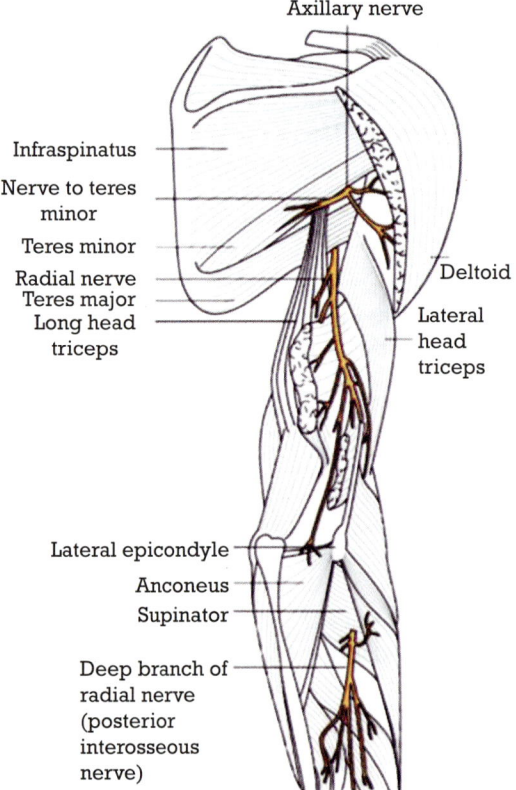

Axillary nerve

Infraspinatus

Nerve to teres minor

Teres minor

Radial nerve
Teres major
Long head triceps

Deltoid

Lateral head triceps

Lateral epicondyle

Anconeus

Supinator

Deep branch of radial nerve (posterior interosseous nerve)

Fig. 113.1. Distribution of radial nerve

radial nerve to the humerus makes it the most common major nerve to be injured by trauma, occurring in about 15% of humeral fractures.

The nerve may be injured:

1. by the traumatic force
2. getting caught in the fracture fragment during reduction
3. under a surgical plate (rare)
4. during dislocation of elbow
5. may be trapped by healing bone.

Clinical features:

The clinical features of radial nerve palsy depend upon the site of the injury.

Lesions in or above the axilla

Results in paralysis and wasting of all the muscles innervated and it is clinically manifested as:

Weakness of elbow extension and flexion (triceps and brachioradialis)

Wrist drop and finger drop - paralysis of the extensors of the wrist and digits

Weakness of the long thumb abductor and extensor muscles

Sensory loss on the dorsum of hand and forearm appropriate to the cutaneous distribution

Lesions around the humerus

These spare triceps, brachioradialis and extensor carpi radialis longus. Therefore these patients will have a wrist and finger drop and the picture more closely resembles posterior interosseous nerve palsy.

Posterior interosseous nerve palsy results from entrapment of the nerve at its point of entry into the supinator muscle. It is often due to a fracture dislocation of the elbow or proximal radial fracture. There is weakness of finger extension and thumb extension and abduction, without wrist drop, or sensory loss.

The extension of the thumb and fingers must be examined carefully since the interossei (ulnar nerve) produce extension of the middle and distal phalanges. However, when the MP joints are kept in acute flexion, the interossei become ineffective in extending the digits.

Investigations:

Radiographs should be obtained if a fracture, dislocation, or foreign body is suspected.

MRI is helpful if a mass is suspected at any level along the course of the radial nerve.

All patients experiencing neural compromise after penetrating injury in the course of the nerves should be explored without the need for preoperative electro diagnostic studies. These will however, help to determine the level of injury or its distribution if the physical examination is unclear, or if the deficit persists beyond 6 to 8 weeks. By 12 weeks, motor unit potentials will be present and will help to differentiate between recoverable injures and those that will require surgery.

Management

It is important while waiting for treatment or recovery to splint the wrist in slight extension and maintain the function with physiotherapy.

Open injuries

In open injuries early exploration is the rule. If the nerve is in continuity at the time of the exploration, it is treated as a closed injury. If the radial nerve has been sharply transected, but there is adequate nerve length and minimal soft tissue injury, it should be repaired primarily. The proximal and distal extent of the transected or injured nerve can be more clearly delineated if the surgery is delayed for 3 weeks. Nevertheless, it may be quite difficult to explore a nerve safely after a delay because of the of the surgical scar. Before 3 weeks, the extent of nerve injury can be determined with intraoperative electro diagnostic studies and by serial frozen section examinations.

Closed injuries

Surgical exploration is indicated only when transection of the radial nerve is suspected, as in the case after a comminuted humeral fracture or if it develops after closed manipulation. Radial palsy following closed intramedullary nailing is often due to a neuropraxia or a 2nd and 3rd degree injury that recovers spontaneously, hence the patient should be observed closely for a period of 3 months. A Tinel sign can be used to follow the progressive recovery of the nerve along its anatomic course in such cases.

Electrodiagnostic studies will help to determine the level and extent of the radial nerve injury and its further management.

Neurorrhaphy and nerve grafting

Nerve grafting is indicated if the nerve defect is large or there is significant tension on the attempted repair. Good results have been noted in 80% of patients following a nerve graft.

Tendon transfer

Tendon transfer is recommended if there is no sign of radial nerve recovery within 1 year.

Nerve transfer

Currently, nerve transfers are indicated under limited circumstances, such as brachial plexus avulsions, when no other options are available.

The median nerve has a limited anatomic variations in the forearm; therefore, it provides a dependable source for nerve transfer to the distal radial nerve. It may provide a useful alternative to tendon transfers in patients with delayed presentation, in high proximal nerve injuries or in situations of complete loss of nerve function. However this needs further evaluation, before it can be recommended for routine application.

Classic Jones transfer for radial nerve palsy	
PT → ECRL and ECRB	To restore wrist extension
FCU → EDL III–V	To restore finger extension
FCR → EI, EDL II & EPL	To restore extension and abduction of the thumb

Table – 113-1.

PT:　pronator teres
ECRL: extensor carpi radialis longus
ECRB: extensor carpi radialis brevis
FCU:　flexor carpi ulnaris
EDL:　extensor digitorum longus
FCR:　flexor carpi radialis
EI:　 extensor indicis
EPL:　extensor pollicis longus

Anatomy: The median nerve receives fibers from C-6,7,8 and T-1 roots, with occasional contribution from C-5. It is formed in the axilla by fusion of the medial and lateral cords of the brachial plexus, where the lateral cord contributes mainly sensory axons from C-6 and C-7 and the medial cord provides main bulk of motor input through C-8 and T-1. The median nerve has no branches above the cubital fossa. The nerve enters the cubital fossa medial to the brachialis tendon and passes between the two heads of the pronator teres, when it gives off the anterior interosseous branch. The nerve continues in the forearm sandwiched between flexor digitorum sublimis and profundus. Just above the wrist, it gives off the palmar cutaneous branch that supplies the skin of the central portion of the palm, it then passes through the carpal tunnel into the hand where it divides into a muscular branch and palmar digital branches. The muscular branch supplies the thenar eminence and the palmar digital branch supplies the lateral two lumbricals and sensation to the palmar aspect of the lateral 3 ½ digits.

Median nerve anomalies

Martin–Gruber anastomosis

It is present in about 10-40% of normal population, in which the fibers that supply the intrinsic muscles of hand are carried in the median nerve to the middle of the forearm where they leave the median nerve to join the ulnar nerve. Functioning intrinsic muscles could be observed with ulnar nerve injury above this anastomosis. This anomaly is bilateral in about 60-70% of cases and is characterized by confluence of branches from median to ulnar nerve in forearm.

Riche-Cannieu anastomosis

Connections between deep ulnar and median nerves in the hand occurs in about 75% of hands, which causes cross innervation between

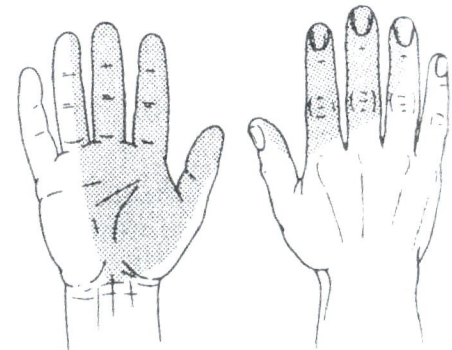

Fig. 114.1. Area of sensory loss in lesion of median nerve

the muscles supplied by the ulnar and median nerves, so much so, even with ulnar nerve injury at the wrist, some intrinsic function is retained.

Etiology

Median nerve palsy may be caused by

1. penetrating injuries to the arm, forearm, or wrist area
2. blunt trauma
3. surgery
4. compression neuropathies
5. mononeuritis multiplex
6. peripheral neuropathies
7. infections like leprosy
8. inflammatory etiology like CIDP (chronic inflammatory demyelinating polyneuropathy)
9. neoplasms, such as neurofibroma and schwannoma
10. ischemic neuropathy (e.g. vasculitis)

Trauma can obviously occur to the nerve anywhere along its course. Types of injury can include penetrating injuries in the axilla and fracture of the shaft of the humerus. Acute compression can occur as a result of bleeding into the forearm or the placement of arteriovenous fistulas for dialysis. Compression of the median nerve at the elbow can result from a supracondylar ligament (ligament of Struthers); and in the forearm it can occur in the proximal arch of the flexor digitorum superficialis or due to presence of lacertus fibrosis.

Entrapment syndromes

There are three well described entrapment syndromes involving the median nerve or its branches, namely, pronator teres, anterior interosseous and carpal tunnel syndromes.

Pronator teres syndrome

This is due to compression of the median nerve as it passes through pronator teres, and classically presents with pain on the volar surface of the forearm following prolonged pronation. Often there are no signs and neurophysiological evaluation may be normal.

Anterior interosseous nerve syndrome

There are a number of causes described for this neuropathy:

1. fractures of the radius mid shaft
2. vigorous exercise
3. penetrating injuries to the forearm
4. presence of Gantzer's muscle, which is an accessory head to flexor pollicis longus
5. brachial neuritis, which presents principally as weakness of the index finger and thumb
6. idiopathic

Carpal tunnel syndrome described in chapter 65

Clinical Features

Clinical features of median nerve palsy depends on the site of involvement of the nerve, accordingly they may be divided into low and high palsies.

Generally in median nerve lesions, there is weak pronation of the forearm, weak flexion and radial deviation of wrist, with thenar atrophy and inability to oppose or flex the thumb. Sensory loss includes radial 3½ fingers, and corresponding portion of palm. With intact nerve, thumb can be pronated, lining up nails of thumb with the rest of the fingers to $180°$, but with median nerve palsy, both these functions are lost.

Low median nerve palsy - the motor deficit primarily involves loss of opposition and

internal rotation of the thumb, with wasting of thenar eminence. Pen touch test is positive and there is sensory loss of the radial 3 ½ fingers.

High median nerve palsy - along with the clinical features seen in low palsies, there is loss of pronation of forearm, wrist flexion, flexion of thumb, index and middle fingers with positive Oschner clasping test.

In lesions **at the wrist,** only the thenar muscles and sensations are affected, long flexors being spared. In long standing palsy, there is thenar wasting and by the unopposed action of adductor pollicis (ulnar nerve) and extensor pollicis longus (radial nerve), the thumb is so rotated that its palmar surface lies in the same plane as the rest of the hand, the so called simian hand or ape-thumb. The straight index, with other fingers flexed, when the palm is held

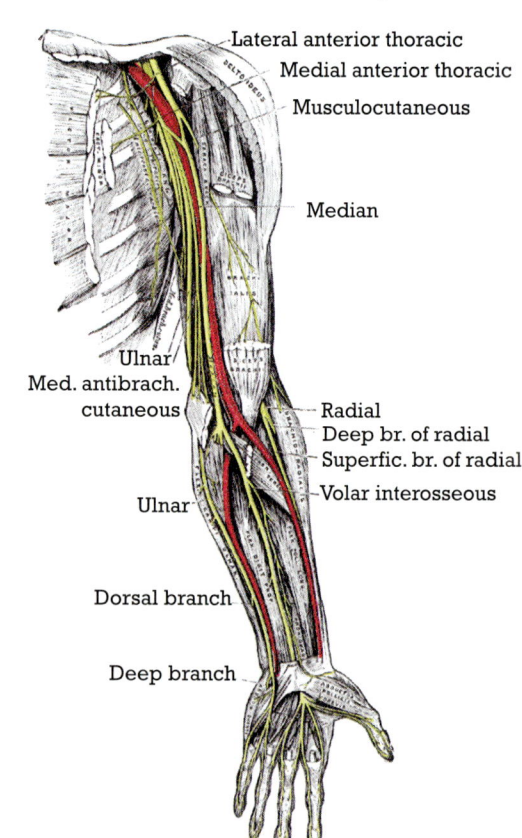

Fig. 114.2. Course and distribution of the median nerve

up, facing forwards, produces an appearance of a priest's hand, known as benediction attitude.

Special clinical tests which aid in diagnosis of carpal tunnel syndrome (see chapter 65).

Tinel's sign: percussion over median nerve region along the volar aspect of wrist; a positive test is identified by eliciting tingling over median nerve sensory area.

Phalen's test: it is positive when tingling or paresthesia is experienced in the distribution of the median nerve when the wrist is held in forced flexion (90°) for 30-60 seconds (Phalen's maneuver). Patients may volunteer that they experience such symptoms when carrying heavy items such as shopping bags, that put the hand in a similar posture.

Reverse Phalen's test: hyperextension of the wrist for 60 seconds produce tingling or paresthesia, experienced in the distribution of the median nerve.

Tourniquet test: sphygmomanometer cuff applied to arm and the pressure is maintained above the systolic pressure for about 2 minutes. The test is positive if tingling or paresthesia is experienced in the distribution of the median nerve.

Luthy's sign: skin fold does not close tightly around a bottle cap; secondary to thumb abduction paresis

Durkan's test: direct pressure over the carpal tunnel produce tingling or paresthesia experienced in the distribution of the median nerve.

Investigations

Electrodiagnostic testing is the mainstay of the diagnosis of median nerve palsy. Electromyography (EMG) shows denervation of median innervated muscles and nerve conduction study (NCS) reveals abnormal median sensory responses. Plain radiographs and CT scan are useful in diagnosing

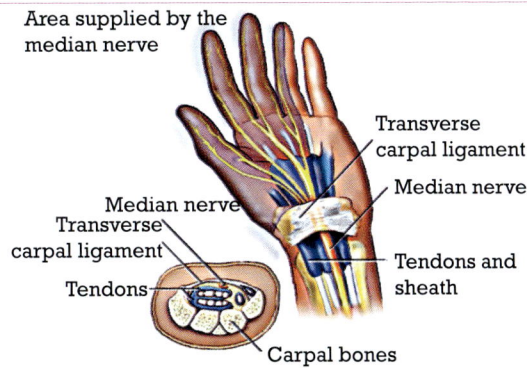
Fig. 114.4. Median nerve compression in the carpal tunnel

conditions due to abnormal bony formations like supracondylar process, elbow dislocation, tumors etc., and MRI is useful in certain compressive neuropathies due to soft tissue structures.

Treatment

Nonsurgical treatment is contemplated when median nerve palsy is expected to resolve, during such course it is necessary to maintain joint flexibility by passive mobilization and to prevent joint contractures by using appropriate splints. In carpal tunnel syndrome conservative modality of management is done by use of corticosteroid injections, splinting especially at night and avoiding activities leading to repeated wrist flexion (chapter 65).

Surgical management depends on the site, extent and the functional demands of the individual with medial nerve palsy. Certain concepts are kept in view while deciding the appropriate surgical modality, such as less recovery of motor function after carpal tunnel release, and of the intrinsics after proximal median nerve repair. Therefore initial transfer to the thumb intrinsics may be undertaken at the time of nerve repair. Various modalities include tendon transfers, nerve repair and/or nerve grafting and arthrodesis.

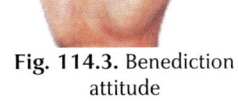
Fig. 114.3. Benediction attitude

115 Ulnar Nerve Palsy

Anatomy: Ulnar nerve is a division of the medial cord of the brachial plexus arising from C-8 and T-1 nerve roots. Initially, it lies medial to the axillary artery and then to the brachial artery at the middle of the arm, where it gives no branches. It pierces the intermuscular septum at this point and follows the medial head of the triceps muscle to the groove between the olecranon process and the medial epicondyle. It then crosses the elbow, giving off articular branches, nerves to the flexor carpi ulnaris and the medial half of the flexor digitorum profundus. It slips between the two heads of the flexor carpi ulnaris and continues into the distal forearm, where it is joined on its lateral side by the ulnar artery. (Refer to Fig. 114.2)

Proximal to the wrist, the nerve gives off a large dorsal branch which supplies sensation to the dorsum of the wrist and the ulnar side of the hand. It enters the hand via the Guyon canal and divides into a superficial or sensory portion and a deep or motor portion. The superficial branch in the Guyon canal supplies the palmaris brevis, the skin of the hypothenar eminence and gives digital branches to the little and ulnar side of the ring finger. The deep branch supplies the 3 small

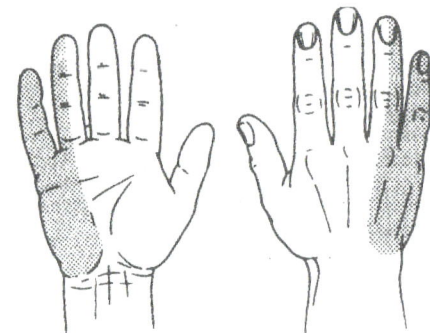

Fig. 115.2. Area of sensory loss in lesion of ulnar nerve

hypothenar muscles, the 3rd and 4th lumbricals, all the volar and dorsal interossei, the adductor pollicis, and the deep head of the flexor pollicis brevis. Anomalous nerve connections must be noted because, in ulnar neuropathy, these anomalies such as the Martin-Gruber anastomosis in the forearm and the Riche-Cannieu anastomosis in palm (see median nerve lesions) may confuse the clinical features.

Gentle tapping of the ulnar nerve over the medial epicondyle elicits an unpleasant tingling sensation over the distribution of the nerve (referred to as 'funny bone', probably called so because it borders on the humerus!).

Etiology

Ulnar nerve palsy is caused by damage, compression or trapping of the ulnar nerve as it makes its way down the length of the arm, at the elbow or at the wrist. It is commonly involved in Hansen's, because of its subcutaneous nature.

Posner has defined 5 areas of potential compression around the elbow as follows:

(1) Intermuscular septum, at two points, at the arcade of Struthers which is a musculofascial band about 8 cm proximal to the medial epicondyle and at the medial intermuscular septum where the nerve pierces to reach the olecranon groove and at the medial head of the

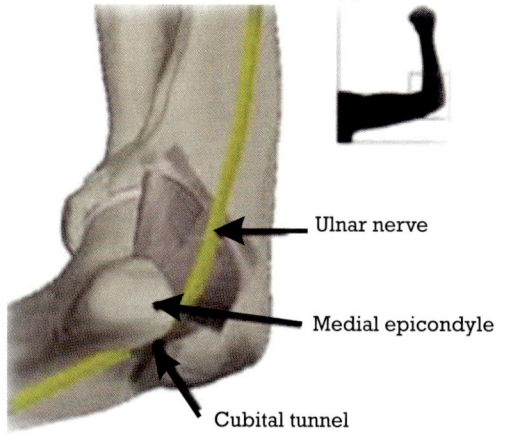

Ulnar nerve

Medial epicondyle

Cubital tunnel

Fig. 115.1. Course of the ulnar nerve behind medial epicondyle of the humerus

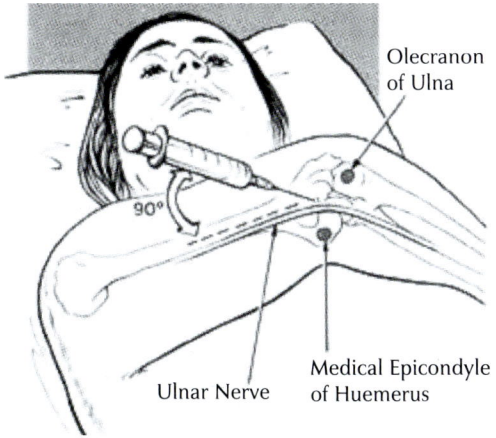

Fig. 115.3. Ulnar nerve block behind the medial epicondyle of humerus

triceps muscle which can be hypertrophied or can chronically snap over the medial epicondyle, causing neuropathy.

(2) At the area of the medial epicondyle, where a cubitus valgus deformity can be caused by malunion or nonunion of a condylar fracture, or an epiphyseal injury to the lateral side of the elbow. These may cause tardy (meaning slow) ulnar palsy secondary to chronic stretching of the ulnar nerve.

(3) The olecranon or epicondylar groove is a fibroosseous tunnel holding the ulnar nerve and its vascular accompaniment. A congenitally shallow groove or a torn fibrous roof can allow the nerve to chronically subluxate or dislocate, causing neuritis and palsy. Fracture fragments and arthritic spurs in or around the groove impinging on the nerve can also cause entrapment and subsequent neuritis. Traumatic hemorrhage, soft tissue tumors, ganglia, infections, osteochondroma, synovitis secondary to rheumatoid diseases, and malposition during work or sleep all may cause entrapment and nerve dysfunction.

(4) The cubital tunnel is the passage between the two heads of the flexor carpi ulnaris, which are connected by a continuation of the fibroaponeurotic covering of the epicondylar groove (Osborne ligament). During elbow flexion, the tunnel flattens as the ligament stretches, causing pressure on the ulnar nerve.

(5) At the flexor-pronator aponeurosis, where the nerve exits the flexor carpi ulnaris, it perforates a fascial layer between the flexor digitorum superficialis and profundus where entrapment can occur.

Claw hand (main-en-griffe) is the result of paralysis of the small muscles of the hand, due to the unopposed action of long flexor and extensor muscles. There is extension at the MP joints and flexion at both IP joints, more of the little and ring fingers; the clawing is made more obvious by the wasting of hand muscles. In lesions at the elbow level, due to the paralysis of flexor profundus component destined for the medial two fingers, there is less flexion of IP joints, i.e. ulnar nerve paradox.

Guyon canal

It is the second most common site of entrapment and is located at the wrist. The ulnar nerve lies on the felxor retinaculum alongside the pisiform bone with the ulnar artery on its radial side. Both are bridged over by a slender ligament between pisiform and hook of hamate, creating a small canal (of Guyon).

Entrapment may cause purely motor, sensory, or a mixed lesion, depending on the site of compression.

Anatomically, the canal is divided into three zones:

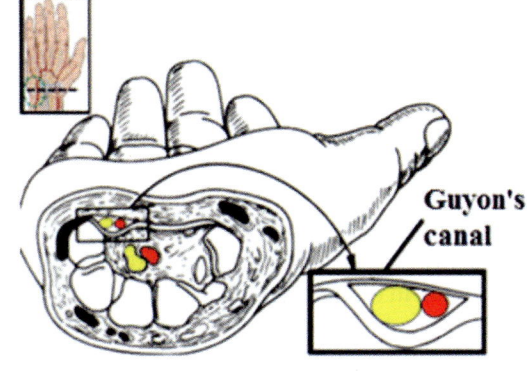

Fig. 115.4. Anatomy of Guyon's canal

Zone-1 is the area proximal to the bifurcation of the ulnar nerve. Compression in this zone causes combined motor and sensory loss. It is most commonly caused by a fracture of the hook of the hamate or a ganglion.

Zone-2 encompasses the motor branch of the nerve after it has bifurcated. Compression causes pure loss of motor function to all of the ulnar-innervated muscles in the hand. Ganglion and fracture of the hook of the hamate are the most common etiological factors.

Zone-3 encompasses the superficial or sensory branch of the bifurcated nerve, where compression causes sensory loss to the hypothenar eminence, the little and part of ring finger, without motor deficit. Common causes are an aneurysm of the ulnar artery, thrombosis and synovial inflammation.

Clinical features

A careful clinical history is imperative, noting the time of occurrence of symptoms and it is important to determine whether symptoms are transient or persistent. The patient may report severe pain at the elbow or wrist with radiation into the hand or up into the shoulder and neck. Presenting symptoms of ulnar nerve entrapment may vary from mild transient paresthesia in the ring and small fingers to clawing of these digits and severe intrinsic muscle atrophy. Fine movements of the hands are affected, usually with patients reporting difficulty in opening jars or turning door knobs.

If ulnar nerve lesion is above mid-forearm, clawing of ulnar two fingers does not occur, because extrinsic muscles producing IP joint flexion are also denervated (see ulnar nerve paradox above).

If ulnar nerve is divided below mid-forearm, ulnar claw hand is produced. In this lesion, 4th and 5th fingers are hyperextended at MP joints by long extensors but flexed at IP joints. This phenomenon of

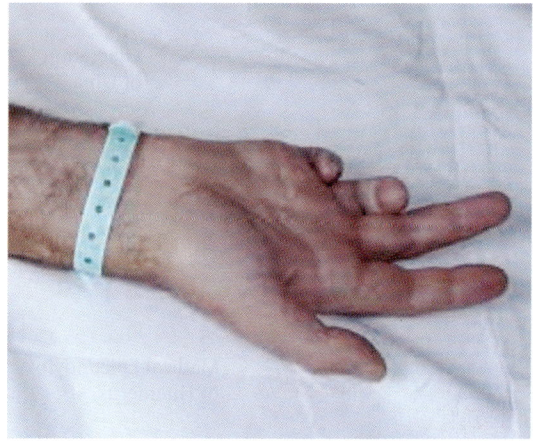

Fig. 115.6. Claw-hand due to ulnar palsy

'higher the lesion, lesser the deformity' is called ulnar nerve paradox.

Division of ulnar nerve at wrist results in paralysis of all small muscles of hand except first and second lumbricles and most of thenar muscles. Paralysis of adductor pollicis produces Froment's sign which is characterized by flexion of the IP joint of the thumb (due to action of flexor pollicis longus supplied by median nerve) when grasping piece of paper between thumb and index finger. It is also known as *Froment's prehensile thumb sign* or the signe de journal. The term is also sometimes used for weakness of little finger adduction, evident when trying to grip a piece of paper between the ring and little finger.

In cases of entrapment of ulnar nerve at wrist, following features may be noted; positive Tinel's sign on percussion over ulnar nerve at Guyon's canal, positive Phalen's test with paresthesia in little and ulnar side of ring finger, increase in two point discrimination and claw hand.

Flexor carpi ulnaris and flexor digitorum profundus strength should be assessed. Intrinsic muscle function is tested by asking the patient to cross the

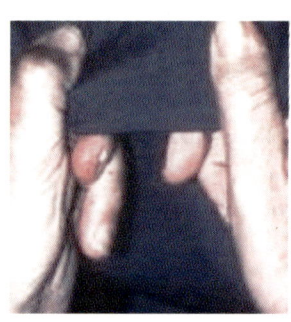

Fig. 115.5. Froment'sign for ulnar palsy

Mechanism of Clawing

1. The interossei cause flexion of MCP joint and lumbricles act to extend the PIP and DIP joints of the fingers.

2. The long finger extensors (extrinsic muscles) can extend the PIP and DIP joints only when the MCP joint is not in hyperextension.

3. In view of the hyperextension of MCP joints the long extensors become ineffective, where as long flexors become more active.

4. The wrist is pulled into flexion by the strong finger flexors which causes a tenodesing effect on the long finger extensors that hyperextends the MCP joints further causing clawing of fingers.

middle finger over the index finger (i.e., crossed finger test). Only two muscles can be tested accurately in the hand, the abductor digiti minimi and the first dorsal interosseous. The tendons or bellies of these muscles can be palpated or visualized. Numbness usually precedes motor loss.

Differential diagnosis

Cervical disc disease

Brachial plexus abnormalities, thoracic outlet syndrome, Pancoast tumor

Elbow abnormalities, epicondylitis

Infections, tumors, diabetes mellitus, hypothyroidism, rheumatoid disease and alcoholism

Wrist fractures

Ulnar artery aneurysms or thrombosis at the wrist.

Hansen's disease

Investigations

Routine laboratory studies for ulnar nerve entrapment are used to rule out anemia, diabetes mellitus, hypothyroidism etc. If rheumatoid disease is suspected, specific investigations should be done to clinch the diagnosis.

Radiographs of the elbow and wrist are mandatory in ulnar nerve compression because 'double crush syndrome', wherein the ulnar nerve may be entrapped at more than one level, may be present. Radiographs of the elbow should be done to diagnose abnormal anatomy, such as a valgus deformity, bone spurs or fragments, a shallow olecranon groove, osteochondroma and other tumors.

Radiographs of the wrist reveal fractures of the hook of the hamate, dislocations of the wrist bones, and to a lesser extent, soft tissue masses and calcifications. MRI is not usually necessary unless delineation of soft tissue masses or visualization of swelling or other abnormalities in the nerve is desired.

Electromyography (EMG) tests and nerve conduction studies are indicated to confirm the area of entrapment, document the extent of the pathology, and to detect or rule out the possibility of double crush syndrome.

Treatment

Conservative treatment

It is most successful when paresthesia is transient and caused by malposition of the elbow or blunt trauma. Patient education, anterior elbow extension splinting (if necessary) and correction of ergonomics at work should help these transient palsies. NSAIDs also are useful adjuncts to relieve nerve irritation. Surgical intervention is indicated if increasing paresthesia occur despite adequate conservative treatment and at the first sign of motor changes.

Surgical treatment

Surgical treatment of ulnar nerve entrapment depends on the site of compression. The most common sites are at the elbow and the wrist. Ulnar nerve compression at the wrist can be decompressed with Guyon's tunnel release surgery. Surgical treatment at the elbow falls

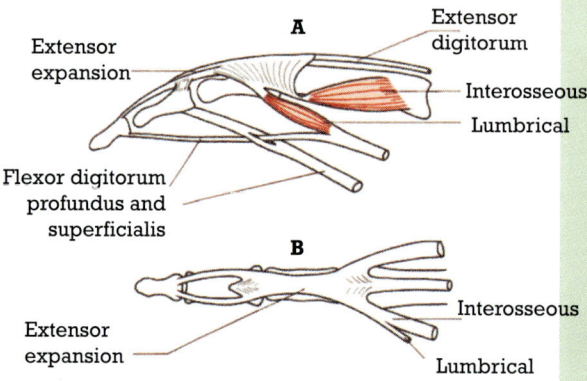

Fig. 115.7. The tendons of a finger; **A:** Lateral view; **B:** Posterior view

into two categories, decompression in situ and decompression with anterior transposition.

Decompression in situ: it is essentially a localized decompression of the nerve, accomplished by incising the Osborne ligament and opening the tunnel beneath the two heads of the flexor carpi ulnaris by dividing the fascia holding them together.

Medial epicondylectomy: although not a true decompression in situ, it is another procedure to release pressure on the ulnar nerve at the elbow, which involves removal of the epicondyle.

Decompression with anterior transposition

Decompression with anterior transposition usually is the operation of choice for tardy ulnar nerve palsy at the elbow because it removes the nerve from its compressive bed and puts it in one that is more suitable, by transferring the nerve anteriorly, it effectively decreases tension on it during elbow flexion. Three types of transposition are possible, subcutaneous, submuscular and intramuscular placements, each with its own set of advocates.

Surgical management for restoration of lost ulnar nerve functions in fixed palsies can be divided into static and dynamic procedures.

The principle that, the long finger extensor can extend IP joints provided that hyperextension of the MCP joints is prevented; is the basis for many of the operations for intrinsic paralysis due to ulnar nerve palsy.

The MCP joint can be stabilized by

a. capsuloplasty (Zancolli)

b. tenodesis (Riordan)

c. bone block (Mikhail)

d. arthrodesis.

Various tendon transfers are also done that actively extend the IP joints as well as flex the MCP joints.

Preferred transfers in ulnar nerve palsy

Thumb Adduction

ECRB → adductor tubercle

FDS (Long) → adductor tubercle

Thumb-index pinch

APL → first dorsal interosseous and arthrodesis of thumb MP joint

EPB → first dorsal interosseous and arthrodesis of thumb MP joint

Clawed fingers

ECRL – four tailed tendon graft

Distal finger flexion (high palsy)

FDP (of long finger) tendodesis to FDP (of ring and little finger)

Radial wrist flexion (high palsy)

FCR → FCU

116 Foot Drop

Anatomy: Common peroneal nerve (CPN) is derived from L-4, 5, S-1 and S-2 roots as a part of the sciatic nerve. The posterior component, supplies short head of biceps femoris in thigh, crosses posterior to lateral head of gastrocnemius, and becomes subcutaneous behind head of fibula. It then divides into superficial and deep peroneal nerves. The CPN also gives off a lateral sural cutaneous branch which joins with the medial sural cutaneous nerve (from tibial nerve) to form the sural nerve.

Superficial peroneal nerve passes in a straight line from the common peroneal nerve along the length of the proximal one third of the fibula where it is on the lateral cortex of the fibula.

Motor: Lateral compartment of the leg (peroneus longus and brevis).

Sensory: Lateral aspect of the lower leg and the dorsum of the foot.

Deep peroneal nerve courses anteriorly taking a sharp turn as it goes around the fibular neck, where it may be readily rolled with a finger, to enter anterior compartment of leg.

Motor: Anterior compartment of the leg (tibialis anterior, extensor hallucis longus, digitorum longus and peroneus tertius)

Sensory: First dorsal webspace.

Etiology

Common cause of foot drop is injury to the CPN at the site where it winds around the neck of fibula. It is encountered following knee dislocation, proximal fracture of both bones of leg, tight casts or bandages causing compression over the nerve at the fibular neck level. It is also seen as a complication following certain surgeries like high tibial osteotomy, total knee replacement, arthroscopic or open lateral meniscal surgery and

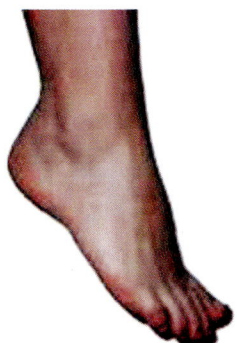

Fig. 116.1. Footdrop due to injury to the common peroneal nerve

resections of proximal fibula. In non-traumatic foot drops, it is important to exclude other causes, such as sciatic nerve injury, lumbosacral root trauma as seen in sacro-iliac joint dislocations and pelvic fractures. Even a herniated lumbar disc compressing the L-5 nerve root can cause foot drop. A combination of neurological assessment and electrophysiological testing excludes the other causes.

Clinical features

Patients have foot extension weakness, as well as numbness or pain on their shin and top of the foot. Gait of the person with foot drop is called as 'high stepping' since one has to raise the thigh to avoid dragging the foot on the floor, as if one is climbing stairs.

Injury to both common and deep peroneal nerves cause foot drop, but CPN injury in addition causes loss of supination of the foot.

Tibialis posterior function should be tested for plantar flexion and inversion against resistance and if it is lost, it would indicate that the lesion is likely from L-5 radiculopathy instead of peroneal nerve palsy, since tibialis posterior is innervated by the tibial nerve.

Investigations

Foot drop is usually diagnosed during a physical examination.

In some cases, additional testing is recommended:

Electromyogram (EMG): This is useful in differentiating between foot drops due to CPN injures and sciatic nerve injuries. For example, in foot drop following hip surgery suspicion of sciatic nerve injury can be confirmed if EMG shows denervation potentials in short head of biceps.

Nerve conduction study (NCS): This helps in differentiating the

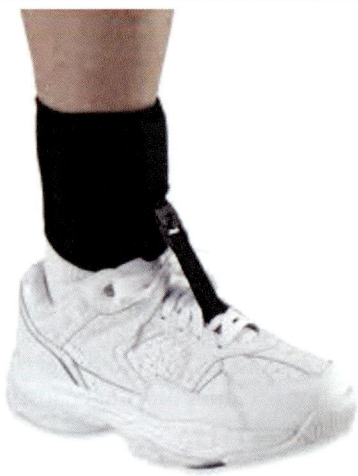

Fig. 116.2. Dynamic footdrop splint

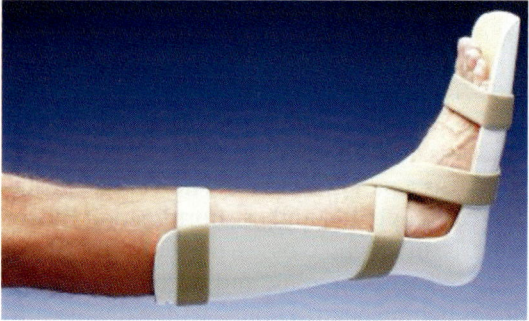

Fig. 116.3. Foot drop splint

level and type of nerve injury and aids in deciding the treatment.

MRI is useful in non-traumatic causes of foot drop as in radiculopathies of lumbar roots.

Treatment
Initial

In acute presentation with limb ischemia compartment compression syndrome has to be excluded and decompression by liberal subcutaneous fasciotomy should be immediately undertaken.

Physiotherapy

Appropriate 'foot-drop' splint has to be used to prevent deformities due to unopposed action of the uninvolved muscles.

Prevention of equinovarus deformity using an ankle-foot orthosis (AFO).

Strengthening any remaining functional muscles and stretching of posterior ankle capsule should be done. Neuromuscular electrical stimulation (NMES) may be useful to prevent atrophy of peroneal supplied muscles.

Peroneal nerve injuries recover very poorly if there is inordinate delay in instituting treatment, therefore in these patients early intervention should be considered, rather than opting for 'wait and see' approach.

Foot drop due to direct trauma to the dorsiflexors generally requires surgical repair. When nerve insult is the cause of foot drop, treatment is directed at restoring nerve continuity, either by direct repair or by removal of the insult.

If foot drop is secondary to lumbar disc herniation consider discectomy. In the early phase of this condition, decreased blood flow due to compression is thought to lead to nerve root ischemia.

Foot drop following hip replacement can also be treated with sciatic nerve decompression. Shortening of the hip prosthesis may be helpful if the limb was lengthened during surgery.

In patients in whom foot drop is due to neurologic and anatomic factors (eg, polio, Charcot joint), arthrodesis may be the preferred option. The goal is to achieve a stable, well-aligned foot and ankle. This may be accomplished via ankle arthrodesis, Lisfranc arthrodesis, and triple or pantalar arthrodesis with or without Achilles tendon lengthening.

Tendon transfer

A common method of tendon transfer moves the posterior tibial tendon, with or without complementary Achilles tendon lengthening. Route of transfer of the posterior tibial tendon may be through the intraosseous membrane or circumtibial (Ober).

Once a transfer route is selected, the point of fixation of the split posterior tibial tendon may be tendon-to-tendon or tendon-to-bone.

117 Rickets

Definition: Rickets is a pediatric disorder characterized by softening and deformity of bones, and growth retardation secondary to defective mineralization of the growth plate, either due to deficiency or defective metabolism of vit-D. Osteomalacia is the adult counterpart of rickets, characterized by defective mineralization of osteoid.

Types

1. Vit-D deficiency - causes classical rickets

2. Congenital disease

A. Vit-D dependent rickets Type 1: due to defective enzyme 1-alpha hydroxylase which converts 25-hydroxycholecalciferol to biologically active 1,25-dihydroxy vit-D (Calcitriol).

B. Vit-D independent rickets Type 2: due to mutations in the vit-D receptor.

C. Familial X-linked hypophosphatemic rickets: autosomal dominant disease which causes vit-D resistant rickets, where there is impaired tubular resorption of phosphate.

3. Vit-D metabolism abnormalities: common causes are renal failure (renal rickets), celiac

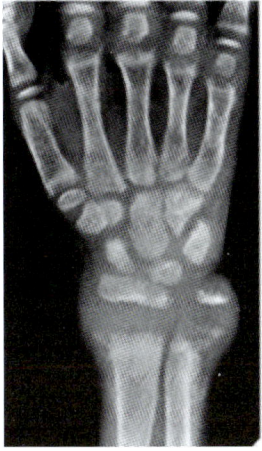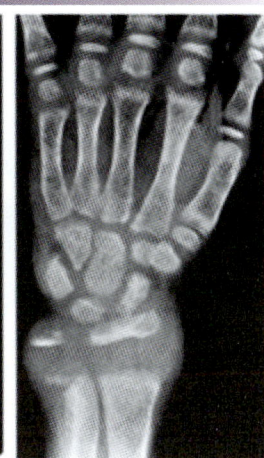

Fig. 117.3. Osteopenia of rickets

disease (celiac rickets) and long term administration of phenytoin, heparin, steroids, INH and tetracycline (drug induced rickets).

Pathology

The histologic feature of rickets is abnormal osteoid tissue which is the protein base in which the calcium and phosphorus salts have failed to deposit. The orderly progression of enchondral ossification is interrupted with widening of the hypertrophic zone of the epiphysis. The most characteristic feature is absence of mineralization of osteoid and absence of the provisional zone of the epiphysis. Women who cover the entire body, including the face for religious reasons (preventing them from exposure to sunlight) may suffer from maternal vit-D deficiency and their children have a tendency for developing the disease.

Clinical features

A history of dietary deficiency may be obtained. The child presents with increased restlessness at night, profuse sweating, skin pallor and is disinterested to play. There is generalized mucous membrane involvement which may manifest as recurrent diarrhea and respiratory infections.

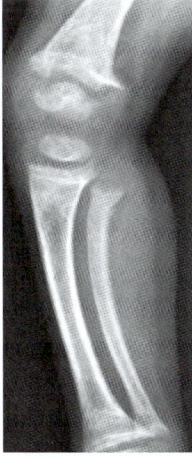

Fig. 117.1
Deformed bones in rickets

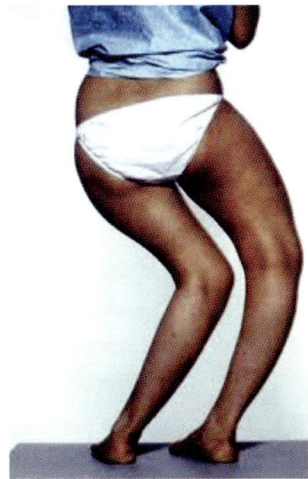

Fig. 117.2. Deformed bones in rickets

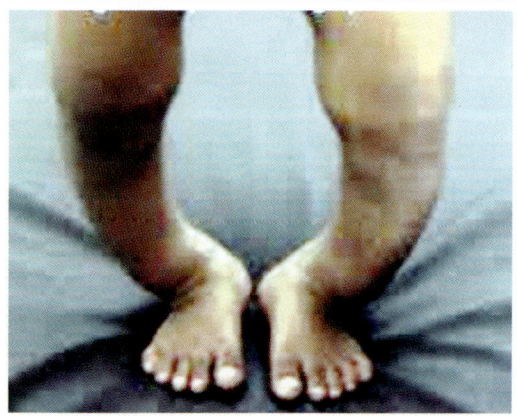

Fig. 117.4. Deformed bones in rickets

Other characteristic features

Head: frontal and parietal bossing, crackling and thinning of bones (craniotabes), enlarged squared appearance due to flattening of occiput and vertex (caput quadratum).

Chest: beaded enlargements at costochondral junctions (rickety rosary), horizontal depression at lower costal margin due to pull of diaphragm (Harrison's groove) and other deformities of chest wall, such as pigeon chest (pectus carinatum) or funnel chest (pectus excavatum).

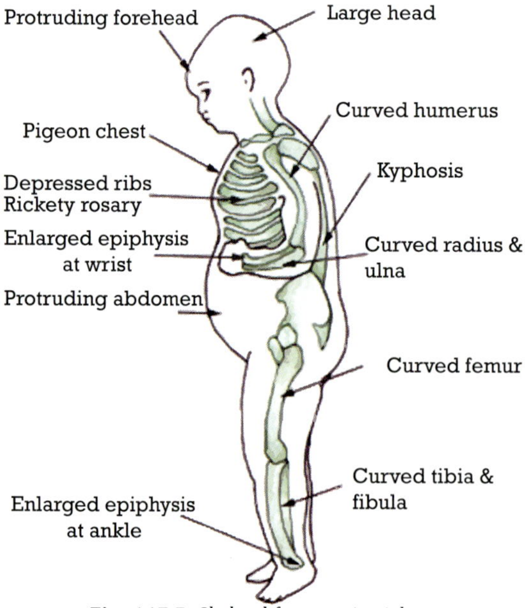

Protruding forehead — Large head
Pigeon chest — Curved humerus
Depressed ribs — Kyphosis
Rickety rosary
Enlarged epiphysis — Curved radius & at wrist ulna
Protruding abdomen
Curved femur
Curved tibia & fibula
Enlarged epiphysis at ankle

Fig. 117.5. Skeletal features in rickets

Abdomen: increased prominence.

Enlarged epiphysis: especially at regions where there is rapid growth, e.g. wrists, knees.

Delayed dentition with defects of the dental enamel and extensive caries are common

Skin pallor: due to secondary anemia may be present.

Poor tone of muscles: may lead to delay in achieving developmental motor milestones.

Deformities: lower extremities are most commonly involved due to weight bearing. Knock knee (genu valgum), bow leg (genu varum), internal torsion of tibia, and coxa varum which causes waddling gait.

Incomplete fractures: commonly seen and are due to trivial trauma.

Growth restriction: usually lasts for a short time and does not affect stature.

Investigations

Radiological findings include widened physeal plate and cupping of the metaphysis which are

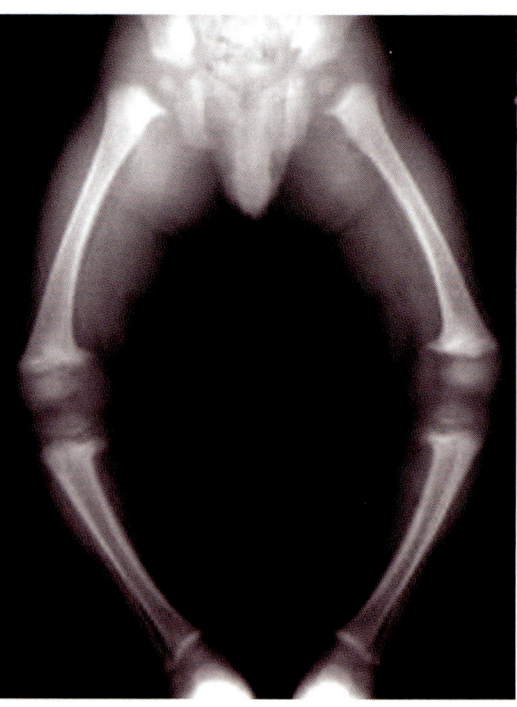

Fig. 117.6. Bowleg deformity in rickets

pathognomonic signs. The classical feature in osteomalacia is the presence of Looser's zones, which are transverse radiolucent lines surrounded by sclerotic bone, not unlike that seen in a stress fracture.

Positive laboratory findings include a typically reduced serum calcium and phosphorus levels and increased alkaline phosphatase levels. Currently direct estimation of vit-D$_3$ levels is used to detect clinical and subclinical deficiency. Urinary calcium output is also reduced. There may be metabolic acidosis.

Treatment

Prophylaxis consists chiefly of administration of vit-D and exposure to sunlight, especially for premature infants and those on artificial milk feedings. Fish (cod and halibut liver) oils and fortified milk are the usual sources of vit-D. Active treatment by vit-D, calcium preparations, and ultraviolet rays will arrest progression of pathology.

Deformity of the lower extremities usually spontaneously regresses to a great degree over a period of months. The application of braces or osteotomy to correct deformity is generally unnecessary.

1,500 to 5,000 IU of vit-D$_3$ per day for about 6-10 weeks is necessary for recovery, though radiological evidence of healing may be seen earlier (after 2-3 weeks). Long term maintenance by supplementation of calcium and vit-D may be necessary, carefully monitoring for any evidence of hypervitaminosis-D.

118 Cubitus Varus (Gunstock Deformity)

Carrying angle is the angle created by the medial borders of the arm and fully extended, supinated forearm with the elbow extended. It is about $10°$ in men and $15°$ in women (to conform to the wider pelvis). Any reduction in this physiological valgus is called cubitus varus.

Etiology

1. The most common cause is malunited supracondylar fracture, as it is a late complication.
2. Medial growth plate suppression (injury or infection) or lateral growth plate stimulation

Displacements of a supracondylar fracture

Medial displacement

Medial tilt

Internal rotation

Posterior displacement

Posterior tilt

Proximal migration

Extension deformity and some medial shift gets corrected over time, other deformities persist.

Clinical features

There are usually no symptoms, except for the deformity. The 3-point relationship (tip of olecranon, medial and lateral epicondyles) is maintained, the arm length may be reduced and thickening of both medial and lateral supracondylar ridges may be present.

Radiology: due to overlapping of capitellum on olecranon 'crescent sign' is seen.

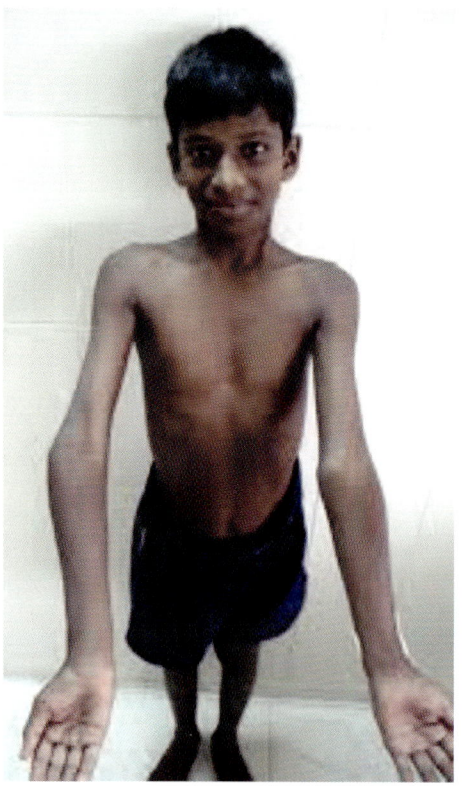

Fig. 118.1. Congenital cubitus varus

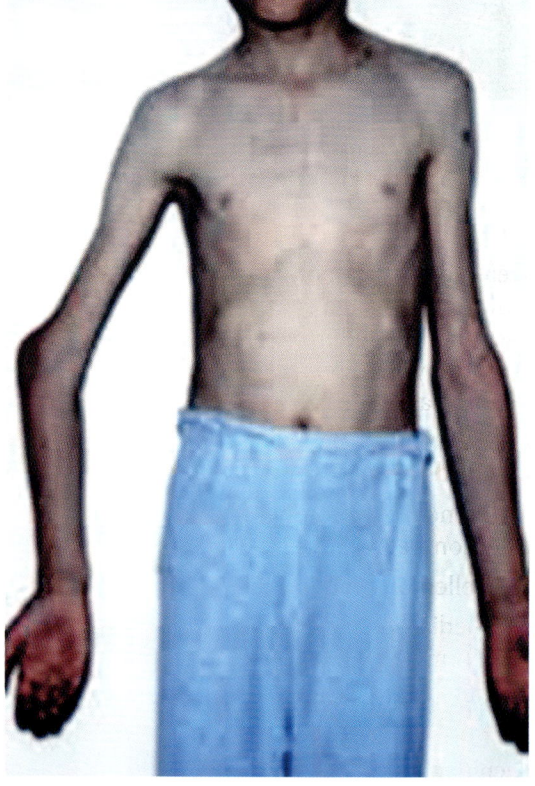

Fig. 118.2. Cubitus varus due to malunited supracondylar fracture

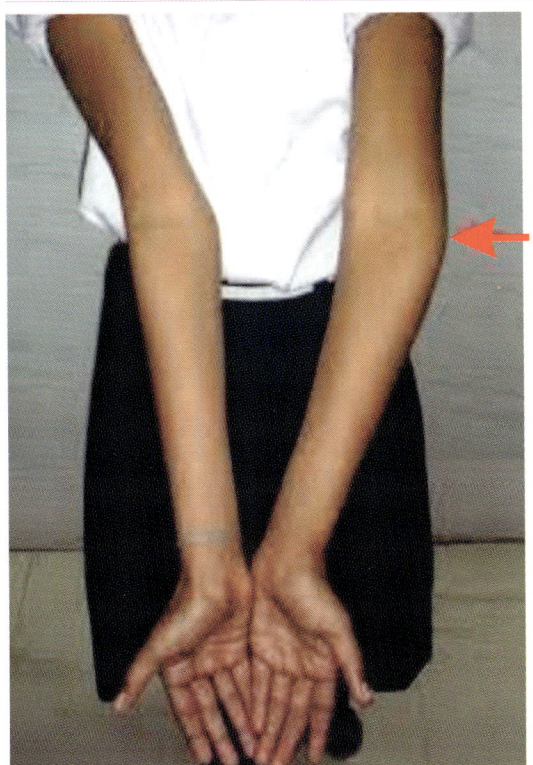

Fig. 118.3. Cubitus varus due to malunited
supracondylar fracture
(courtesy: Prof N D Md Ismail, Chennai)

Treatment

Treatment is mainly for cosmetic reasons,
indicated only in a severe degree of deformity,
and the procedure of choice is corrective
osteotomy. It is preferably done after skeletal
maturity and at least one year after the fracture,
allowing natural remodelling to take place.

Methods of osteotomy

1. French osteotomy - lateral closed wedge
osteotomy at the lower end of humerus

2. Bellemores modified French osteotomy

3. Medial wedge opening osteotomy (King's
osteotomy)

4. Dome osteotomy

5. Oblique osteotomy with derotation
(Uchida)

6. Step cut osteotomy (Desosa and Graziano)

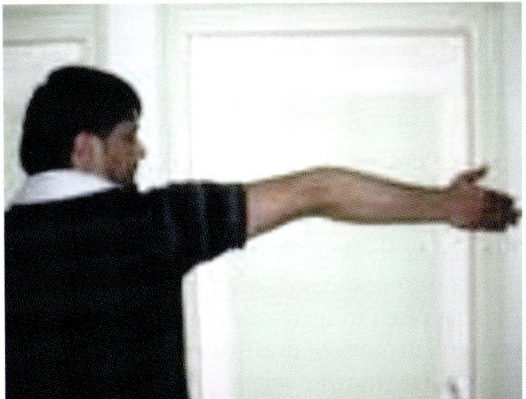

Fig. 118.4. Cubitus varus due to malunited
supracondylar fracture

In contrast to the proximal humeral epiphysis,
the distal epiphysis contributes little (15 - 20%)
to the overall longitudinal growth of the
humerus. Thus, the scope of remodelling and
correction of fracture angulation is limited in
children with supracondylar fractures.

Modern surgical techniques (e.g. closed
reduction with percutaneous pinning) have
reduced the incidence of cubitus varus, which
is mainly of cosmetic significance occurring
years after the original fracture.

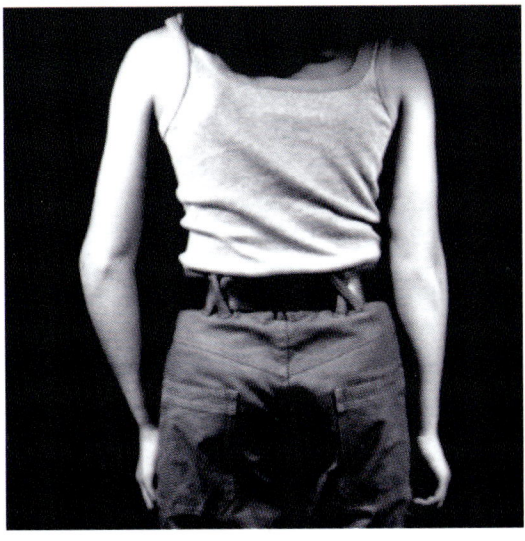

Fig. 118.5. Gun stock deformity left elbow
(courtesy: Dr A N Vivek, Chennai)

119 Genu Varum and Valgum

Genu varum or bowlegs is normally observed in infancy. When a child with genu varum stands with the feet together, there is an increased intercondylar distance at the knees. This may be a result of either one, or both, of the legs curving outward. Walking often exaggerates this bowed appearance and in many of these cases, these children are significantly overweight.

Genu valgum

Genu valgum or 'knock-knee' is a condition where the legs are bowed inwards in the standing position. The bowing usually occurs at or around the knee, so that on standing with the knees together, there is increased intermalleolar distance.

Etiology

Most people have some degree of bowleg or knock-knee and are considered within the limits of normal structure and function.

Physiological

During development in the first few years of life, because of rapid and differential growth around the knees, most children are bowlegged from birth till the age of 3 years, then become knock-kneed till the age of 5, then straighten up by age 6 or 7.

Rickets

Rickets is a pediatric disorder characterized by softening and deformity of bones, and growth retardation secondary to defective mineralization of the growth plate. Classically rickets is

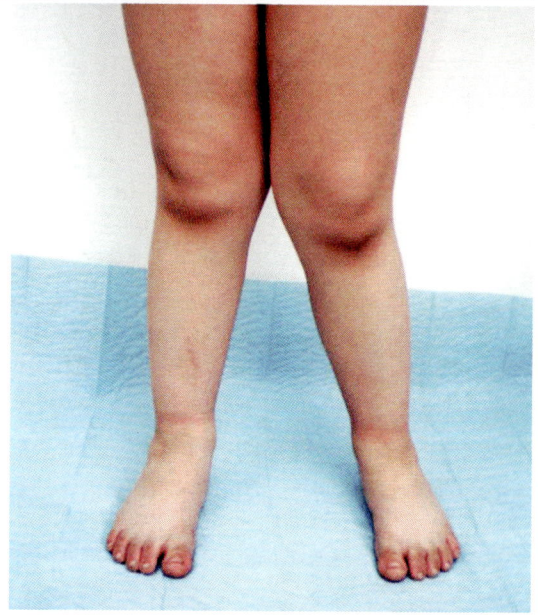

Fig.119.2. Bilateral genu valgum (knock-knee)

caused by vitamin-D deficiency, which can cause both varus and or valgus deformity (see chapter 116).

Growth disturbance

It may be due to epiphyseal dysplasia, either as a part of a generalized bone growth disturbance or due to epiphyseal injuries which may lead to differential growth of the bone, causing either varus or valgus deformities.

Blount's disease is a condition that can occur in infants, as well as in adolescents, results from

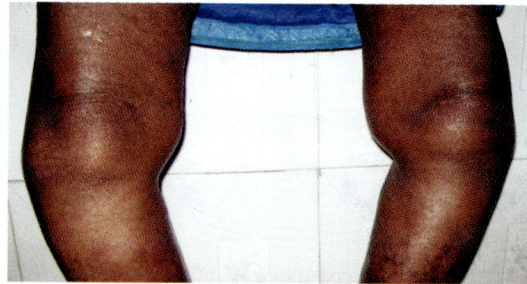

Fig. 119.3. Severe osteoarthrosis causing bilateral genu varum
(courtesy: Prof N D Md Ismail, Chennai)

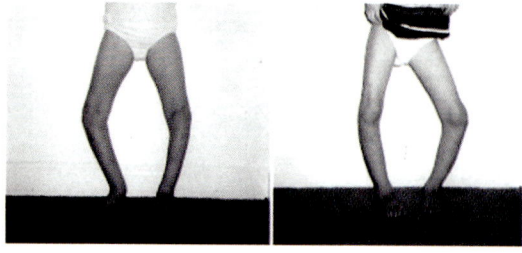

Fig. 119.1. Bilateral genu varum (bow leg)

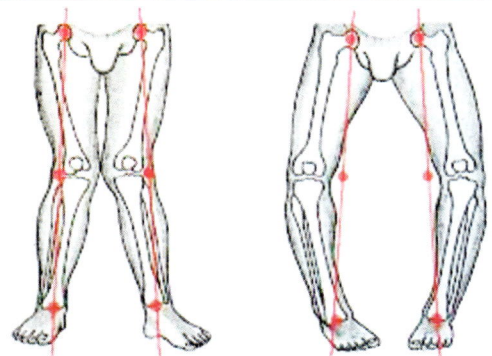

Fig. 119.4. Genu valgus and varus

an abnormality of the growth at the medial proximal epiphysis of tibia. In a child under the age of 2, it may be impossible to distinguish infantile Blount's disease from physiologic genu varum. By the age of 3 years, however, the bowing will worsen and an obvious problem can often be seen in radiographs.

Clinical features

Genu varum or valgus is most evident when a child stands or walks and the most common symptom is an awkward walking pattern. Intoeing of the feet is also commonly associated with genu varum. Both these deformities do not typically cause any pain. During adolescence, however, persistent deformity can lead to discomfort in the hips, knees, and/or ankles due to deviation of the normal axis of weight bearing. The change in the axis of quadriceps pull in genu valgum may result in lateral dislocation of patella.

Investigations

A complete physical examination has to be done in children with knee deformities.

Radiographs of the knee in weight bearing, will show Blount's disease or rickets. In suspected cases estimated of serum vit-D_3 will establish the diagnosis of the rickets.

Treatment

If child is under 2 years, in good health and has minimal symmetrical deformity, only regular follow up at 6 monthly interval is recommended till the age of 6. However if conditions, such as rickets is suspected, it should be promptly treated.

In infantile Blount's disease spontaneous resolution is rare and deformity requires treatment for the bowing to improve. If the disease is diagnosed early, treatment with a brace may be all that is needed, which may be ineffective for adolescents.

Surgical Treatment

In rare instances, physiological genu varum may not completely resolve and during adolescence, the deformity may cause cosmetic concerns. If the deformity is severe enough, an osteotomy to correct the remaining bowing may be needed. In Infantile Blount's disease, if the deformity continues to progress despite the use of a brace, surgery will be needed by the age of 4, which may stop further worsening and prevent permanent damage to the epiphysis.

120 Recurrent Dislocation of Shoulder (RDS)

Definition: the shoulder joint dislocates repeatedly with decreasing injury or effort. It is usually an anterior dislocation.

Pathology: When there is anterior dislocation, anterior capsular tear occurs, which heals in due course, after reduction and immobilization. But if the labrum of the glenoid is injured or detached, it leads to permanent weakness and tendency to dislocate even for trivial reason. This may also follow improper reduction or inadequate immobilization, not allowing the capsular ligaments to heal. There is herniation of the synovial sheath through the defect, forming a ready-made path for the humeral head to sublux. Injury to posterior aspect of humeral head may be another contributory factor.

a) Bankart's lesion: failure of proper healing of the injured anterior capsule and its attachment with labrum

b) Hill Sachs lesion: there is a depression of the posterolateral aspect of the head of humerus due to compression at the time of the first dislocation. During abduction, this depression gets hitched against the posterior margin of glenoid and with further abduction, it levers the head out of the glenoid cavity causing dislocation.

Clinical features: The patient is usually an adult male of athletic nature. The history is

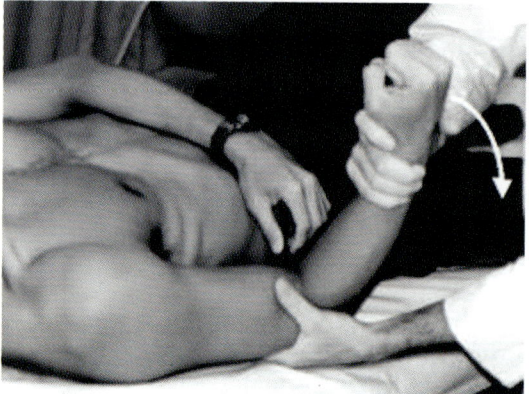

Fig.120.2. Kocher's method of reducing shoulder dislocation

typical and pathognomonic. Initial dislocation following major injury, improper treatment and now the head slips out of its socket and gets 'locked' sometime even on hyperabduction, lateral rotation or after minor violence. Typically patients resist any such passive movement (abduction and external rotation) for fear of dislocation, known as 'apprehension sign'.

Treatment: Initially the dislocation is reduced under general anesthesia, by one of the following methods:

1. Hippocratic method: involves longitudinal traction on the arm and a counterforce to the axilla, usually with the heel of the foot. This

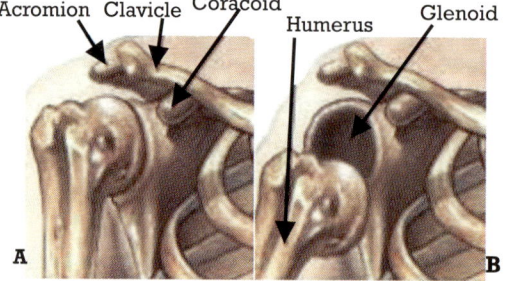

Acromion Clavicle Coracoid Humerus Glenoid

A   **B**

Fig. 120.1. A. Normal shoulder joint
B. Anterior subluxation of the joint

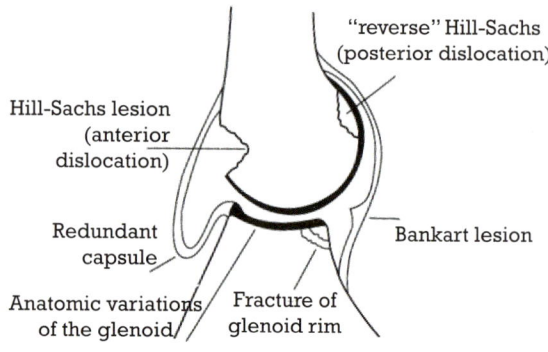

"reverse" Hill-Sachs (posterior dislocation)

Hill-Sachs lesion (anterior dislocation)

Redundant capsule

Anatomic variations of the glenoid

Fracture of glenoid rim

Bankart lesion

Fig. 120.3. Anatomic lesions producing shoulder instability

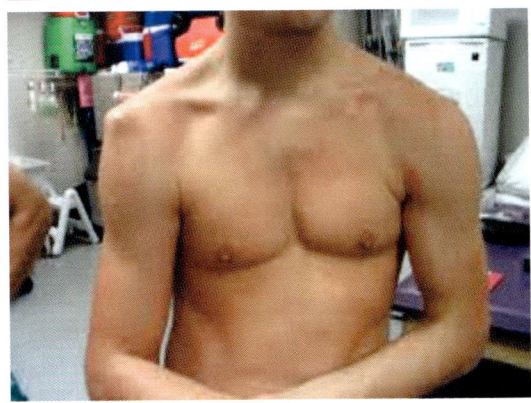

Fig. 120.4 Flattened contour of right shoulder in
dislocation
(courtesy: Dr A N Vivek, Chennai)

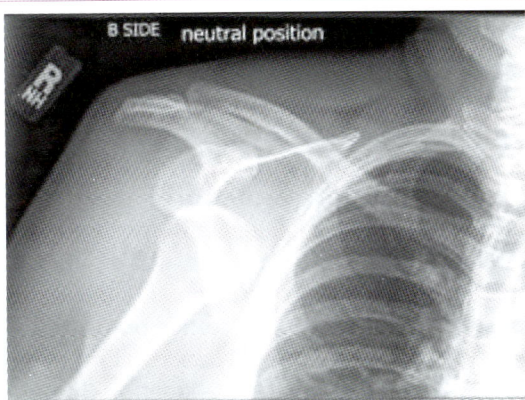

Fig. 120.5. X-ray picture showing anterior dislocation of
shoulder
(courtesy: Dr A N Vivek, Chennai)

method is not currently recommended because of its association with neurovascular complications and proximal humerus fractures.

2. Kocher method: involves traction to the elbow with external rotation of the humerus and adducting the elbow toward the chest. This method is not currently recommended because of its association with neurovascular complications and proximal humerus fractures.

3. External rotation method: which is a modification of the Kocher maneuver, involves flexing the elbow to 90° and slowly adducting the arm to the patient's side. The arm is then carefully externally rotated stopping every few degrees to wait for the muscle spasms to subside.

4. Stimson technique: requires the patient to be positioned prone. The patient's arm is allowed to hang over the edge of the bed with about 10 pounds of weight hanging from the wrist.

5. Milch technique is very successful and relatively atraumatic. It involves the surgeon abducting the patient's arm with one hand while applying pressure to the humeral head with the other hand. When the patient's arm is fully abducted, external rotation and traction are applied.

For RDS in an elderly patient with sedentary occupation, conservative treatment is adopted.

The patient is advised to avoid extreme abduction and external rotation and carry out regular shoulder exercises to strengthen the muscles of internal rotation.

Definitive treatment for RDS is only surgery.

1. Putti-Platt's operation: The aim of surgery is to prevent extreme lateral rotation of shoulder, which can be achieved by plicating or double-breasting the anterior joint capsule and subscapularis muscle, through an anterior approach. The joint is immobilized in internal rotation, for 6 weeks, after which gradual movements were allowed.

2. Bankart's operation: This is essentially aimed at repairing the damaged labrum (Bankart's lesion) and fixing it to the anterior rim of glenoid with nonabsorbable sutures, to prevent recurrence. This procedure is currently done by arthroscopic technique using special bone anchor sutures. If weakness of anterior capsule is detected, that is also repaired and subscapularis is plicated as in Putti-Platt's procedure, for additional protection.

3. Birsto-Helfet operation: In this, the tip of coracoids process with its attached muscles is osteotomized and reattached near the anterior margin of glenoid, to prevent dislocation.

4. Saha operation: This involves changing the direction of the articular surface of the glenoid by osteotomizing the neck of scapula.

121 Recurrent Dislocation of Patella (RDP)

This is characterised by repeated lateral subluxation or dislocation of patella, during flexion of knee. This may follow injury, intial dislocation damaging the bony ridge of the lateral condyle of femur and weakening the quadriceps expansion of the medial side (vastus medialis component). The other predisposing factors are genu valgum and hypermotility of the knee joint, especially hyperabduction. In both these conditions, the traction by the quadriceps will cause lateral force, due to distorted angle of pull. In habitual dislocation, the patella dislocates whenever the knee is flexed and gets spontaneously reduced on extension.

Pathology: In normal knee, the obliquity of the line of quadriceps muscle and its insertion into the tibia, results in an angle (Q angle), which is normally 15-20°. Any condition that exaggerates the Q angle, may predispose to lateral subluxation of patella. It is common in females, where there may be degenerative changes seen in the patella and lateral femoral condyle with flattening of the latter, further increasing the chance of dislocation. Chondromalacia of patella may be another etiological factor or it may be the result of RDP.

Conditions predisposing the RDP:

1. weakness of the quadriceps expansion and capsule of knee joint on the medial side

2. contracture or tightening of the structures on the lateral side of knee

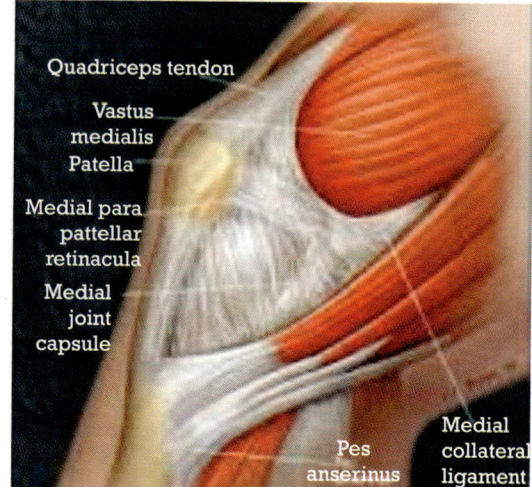

Fig. 121.2. Normal anatomy of the knee - medial view

3. defective development of lateral femoral condyle

4. abnormal (more lateral) insertion of ligamentum patella

5. gross genu valgum

6. anomalies of patella, such as patella alta (high level) or breva (small)

7. in habitual dislocation, there may be abnormal insertion of a part of the iliotibial tract into the superolateral pole of patella

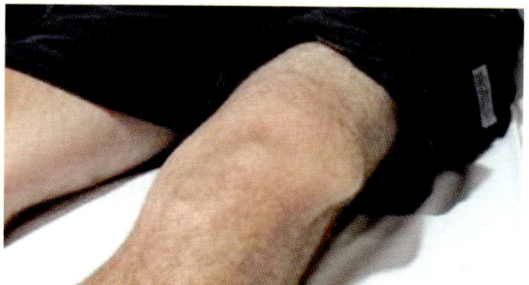

Fig. 121.1. Lateral displacement of patella in dislocation

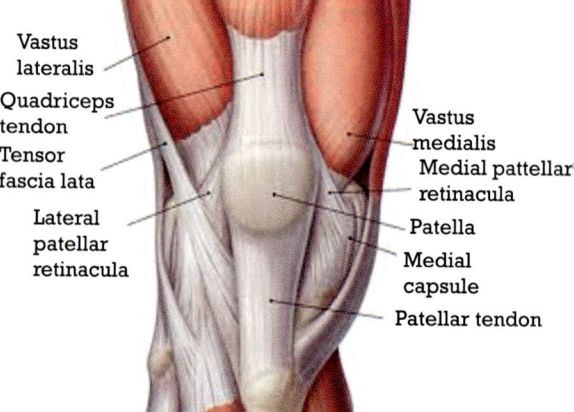

Fig. 121.3. Normal anatomy of the knee - anterior view

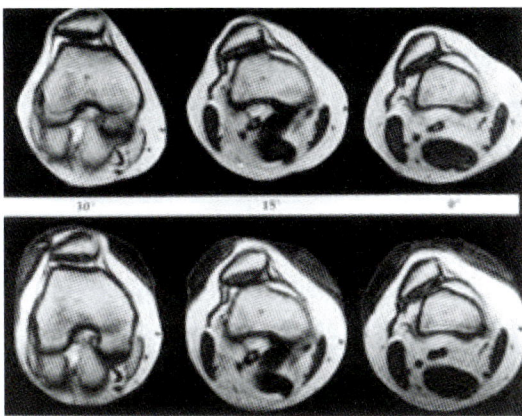

Fig. 121.4. CT scan showing laterally displaced patella

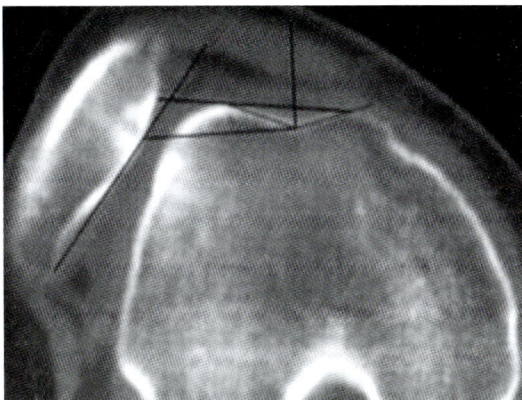

Fig. 121.6. CT scan showing laterally displaced patella

Clinical features: It may be bilateral, sudden 'locking' of the knee in hyperextended position, following minimal effect of knee extension is typical and pathognomonic. The flexed posture of the knee is more than that seen in meniscal injury. The consequent projection of the femur on the medial aspect of knee is mistaken for the patella and gives a false impression of its medial dislocation. The patella may be small in size and its high lateral placement may be seen. As in RDS, here also the patient resists attempts of pushing the patella outwards with knee passively flexed (apprehension sign).

Treatment: Definitive treatment is only surgery; 3 operations are described for this condition:

1. strengthening or plication of the medial capsule, if necessary following a releasing incision on the lateral capsule.

2. shifting the insertion of the ligamentum patella medially, along with a block of bone over the tibial tuberosity.

3. if the chondromalacia of patella is severe, patellectomy may be necessary, along with strengthening of medial capsule.

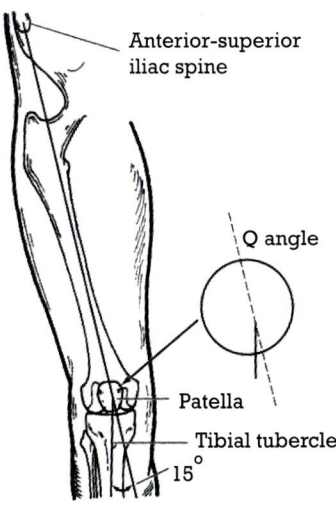

Fig. 121.5. Q angle and valgus angulation

122 Congenital Talipes Equinovarus (Club Foot)

tale: ankle or heel; pes: foot; equinus: horse

Congenital talipes equinovarus (CTEV) or clubfoot is a severe fixed deformity of the foot, characterized by fixed ankle plantar flexion (equinus deformity), inversion and axial internal rotation of the talocalcaneal joint (varus deformity), and medial subluxation of the talonavicular and calcaneocuboid joints (adductus deformity). Severe cavus may be present, with a medial and plantar midfoot crease. Whether unilateral or bilateral, the deformity is more common in males, but when it occurs in females, it tends to be more severe.

The incidence in the newborn population is 1 in 1000. There is considerable evidence that clubfoot is an inherited trait, but the disorder appears to reflect polygenetic expression, and exact inheritance pattern is unclear. Although most are isolated deformities and considered idiopathic, clubfoot may frequently be present in association with a wide variety of syndromes, involving the musculoskeletal system, such as spina bifida and arthrogryphosis multiplexa.

Clinical Features

Clinical diagnosis of clubfoot is uncomplicated. Frequently, the foot is so severely internally rotated and inverted that the sole faces upwards. Occasionally, the plantar flexion of the ankle is not obvious because the posterior tip of the calcaneus is small, high and difficult to palpate. Clubfoot is always associated with a permanent decrease in calf circumference related to fibrosis of the calf musculature. This may not be obvious at birth but becomes more apparent when the child begins to walk. Special attention should be paid to the presence of spine deformity, caudal dimpling, or midline spinal hairy patches, all of which may imply a neurogenic component. Thus, careful search for features of other deformities or syndromes should be made.

Imaging studies

Increasingly, clubfoot is suspected from prenatal ultrasound examination. Radiographs

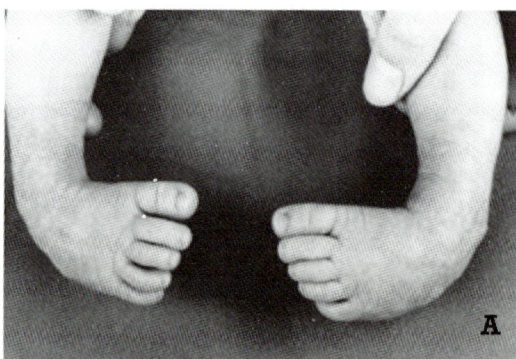
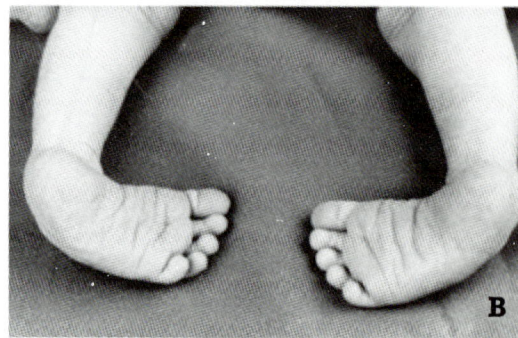

Fig. 122.2. Bilateral congenital talipes equinovarus (CTEV) **A.** Dorsal view **B.** Plantar view

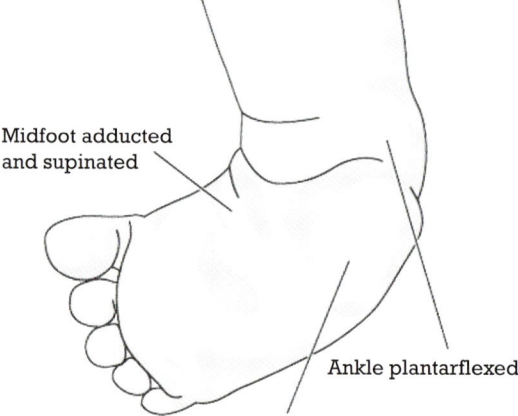

Midfoot adducted and supinated

Ankle plantarflexed

Heel inverted and internally rotated

Fig. 122.1. Congenital talipes equinovarus (CTEV)

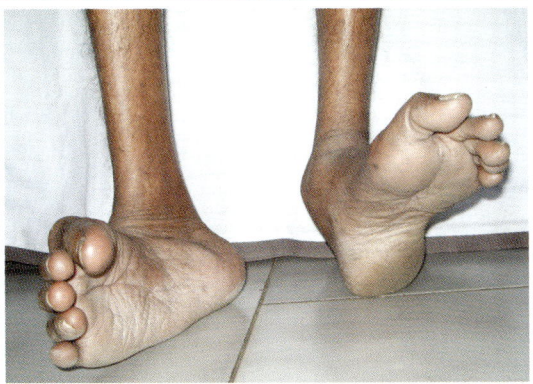

Fig. 122.2. Poliomyelitis affecting both legs, leading to equinovarus on the right and calcanovalgus on the left

are rarely of value in the initial clubfoot evaluation because the bones of the foot are minimally ossified at birth. Radiographs become more important if any surgical intervention is being considered or if the child has reached walking age, when the radiographs can quantify the completeness of correction achieved by casting or surgery. Typical radiographic findings of incompletely treated clubfoot include presence of hindfoot plantar flexion, lack of the normal angular relationship between the talus and calcaneus (parallelism of talus and calcaneus), and residual medial subluxation or displacement of the navicular on the talus and the cuboid on the calcaneus.

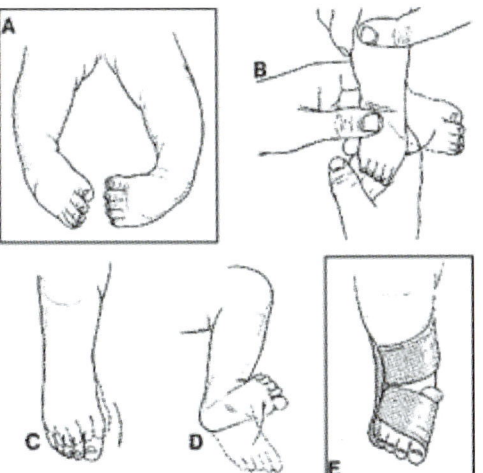

Fig. 122.3. Correction and splinting of CTEV

Treatment

Conservative treatment

Clubfoot always requires treatment, which should begin at birth (when asked by his students, how early it should be corrected after birth, one senior orthopedician, to impress upon them about the urgency, replied in a lighter vain " if it is a breach presentation, the foot deformity should be corrected before the head is delivered !"). The initial approach is passive manipulation and positioning to the corrected position. Serial manipulation and casting, usually at weekly intervals in the first month and at fortnightly intervals thereafter is done. Strapping (with adhesive tape) or splinting with a variety of braces (e.g. foot abduction brace) are also other methods for maintaining the manipulated correction. When casting is performed, there is agreement that specific techniques are more likely to be successful like the Ponseti technique. Even when the deformity responds to casting, there is usually Achilles tendon shortening, so that its lengthening may be needed as early as practical (usually at 4-8 weeks afterbirth) to facilitate cast correction.

The combination of careful casting and limited release allows most clubfeet to be corrected adequately, and long-term bracing for a year or more maintains the correction until the child is walking well. When satisfactory correction is not obtained, more extensive surgery is necessary. Failure of nonoperative treatment is common, particularly in bilateral cases and girls where the deformity tends to be more severe.

Surgical treatment

Surgical correction of all clubfoot deformities is generally performed in one stage. At times, the casting corrects most of the midfoot deformity, and simple posterior release (ankle capsulotomy and Achilles tendon lengthening) are all that is required. Frequently, the surgeon must consider correction of the entire group of deformities through a comprehensive and

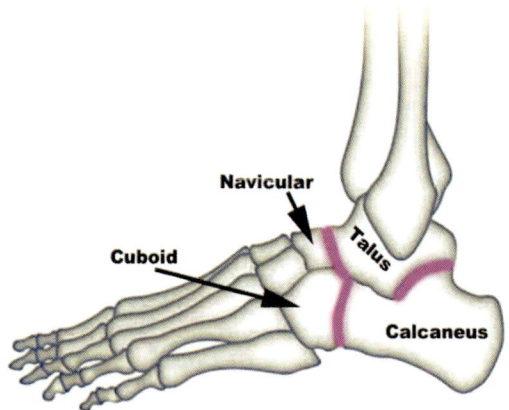

Fig. 122.4. Triple arthrodesis fusion of subtalar, calcaneocuboid and talonavicular joints

often extensive surgical approach.

One common approach uses the so-called Cincinnati incision, which extends from the navicular bone medially, around the superior portion of the heel, to the cuboid bone laterally. During surgery, the medial posterior tibial neurovascular bundle must be identified and protected. The tendons of the tibialis posterior, flexor digitorum longus, hallucis longus, and Achilles tendon are lengthened by z-plasty. The capsules of the talonavicular, subtalar (talocalcaneal) and posterior ankle joints are released to allow repositioning of the bones of the hind and midfoot. In neglected clubfoot, the deformities are rigid and are associated with permanent bony changes. Open

Jewels of Gyan - 122.1

The Ponseti method

It is a complete treatment method that is 97% successful in correcting the clubfoot deformity without major surgery

This program of treatment starts with a series of toe to groin plaster casts starting from birth

Casting continues for 5-12 weeks with weekly change of casts

Achilles tendon tenotomy (Percutaneous) done to correct equinus deformity at about 4 to 8 weeks

Plaster cast reapplied and maintained for 3-4 weeks after tenotomy

Boot and bar orthotic applied and is to be maintained for 23 hours a day for first 12 weeks

Boot and bar orthotic is then worn only at night till child is 4 years old

procedures often fail to correct the deformities to acceptable levels. In these cases JESS (Joshi's external stabilization system) and Ilizarov technique are useful. In very rigid or recalcitrant cases triple arthrodesis is the procedure of choice.

123 Flatfoot (Pes Plannus) and Claw-Foot (Pes Cavus)

Flatfoot is a condition where there is flattening of the arches of foot, especially the medial arch, the foot going into valgus position, during pronation.

Normally the foot has two longitudinal arches, medial and lateral and two transverse arches, one at the midtarsal level and the other at the heads of metatarsals. While standing on the foot, it is important to provide stability and efficient weight transmission. During walking it has to function as a lever and spring, aiding propulsion, adapting to uneven surfaces.

The arches of foot are maintained by

1. the shapes of tarsal bones and their articulation

2. strong ligaments in the foot, such as plantar and spring ligaments

3. resting tone of the intrinsic and extrinsic muscles of foot

Types of flatfoot

1. Congenital type (vertical talus): The feet appear flat in a newborn baby, due to the lack of muscle tone. In some, the sole of the foot is actually convex (rocker bottom foot) and in a valgus or everted position, due to vertical tilt of the talus, with its head pointing the ground.

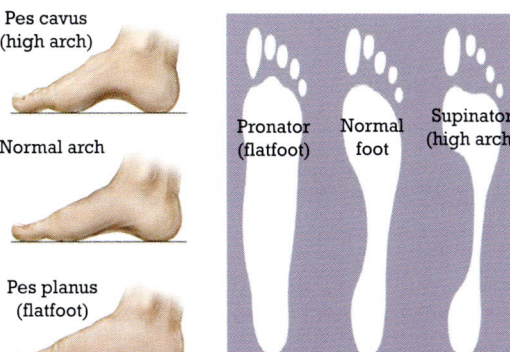

Fig. 123.2. Footprints, flatfoot, normal and claw-foot.

2. Infantile type: This is physiological, before the child starts walking, and disappears in due course.

3. Secondary or compensatory type: This may be associated with genu valgum or paralytic equinus deformity due to poliomyelitis or cerebral palsy.

4. Acquired type: This is due to muscular weakness (neuropathy), obesity or may follow an injury causing fracture of calcaneum or metatarsals, with malunion.

5. Spasmodic type: This is due to spasm of the peroneal muscles, related to some unusual

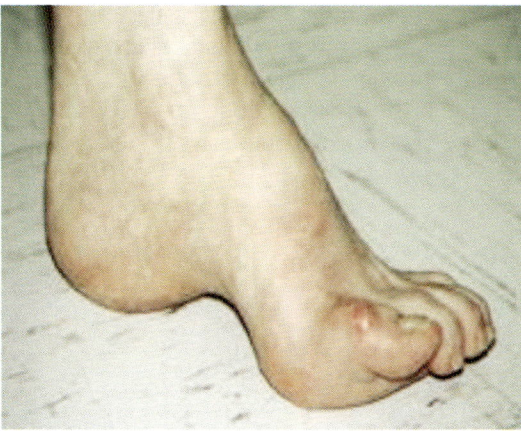

Fig. 123.1. Pes cavus due to poliomyelitis
(courtesy: Prof N D Md Ismail, Chennai)

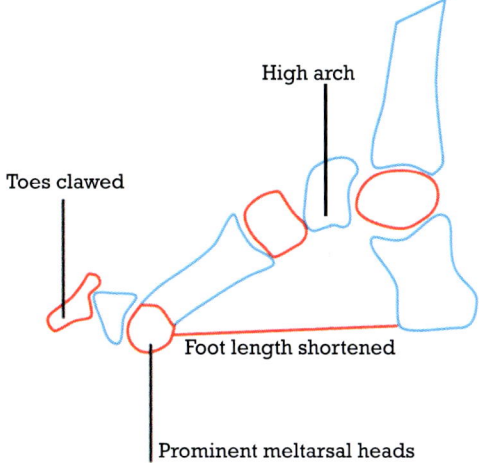

Fig. 123.3. Skeletal structure - pes cavus

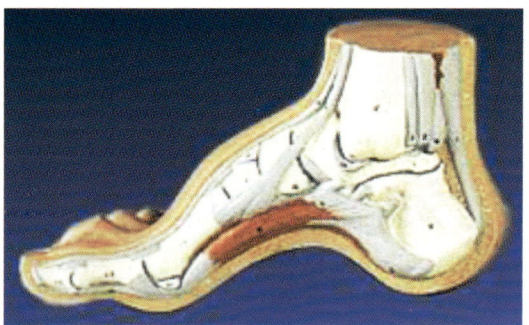

Fig. 123.4. Bony configuration in claw-foot

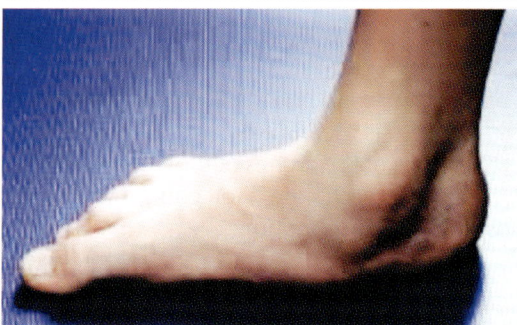

Fig. 123.5. Flatfoot

strain, subtaloid arthritis or anomalies of calceneum or navicular bone

6. Physiological type seen in some children, due to laxity of suspending ligaments, which may get corrected in due course.

Treatment

Intrinsic foot exercises to strengthen the muscles

Footwear modification to elevate the medial foot, to recreate the arch

Treat the primary cause

Gross deformity and disability may need corrective surgery.

PES CAVUS (claw-foot)

It may be caused by a neurological disease, such as poliomyelitis (when unilateral), Charcot-Marie-Tooth disease (peroneal muscular atrophy), Friederich's ataxia or spina bifida, affecting both sides.

Rarely, it may be idiopathic. The basic problem is the imbalance between the muscles of the peroneal and extensor compartments, associated with weakness of intrinsic muscles

of foot, leading to clawing, akin to ulnar nerve palsy resulting in claw hand. The clawed toes may be associated with callosities beneath the MT heads.

Treatment: Conservative treatment with special corrective shoes, physiotherapy and foot exercises, has to be tried if the deformity is minimal.

If the deformity is of moderate degree, Steindler's operation is advisable, which consists of Achilles tendon lengthening and division of tight plantar fascia, to correct the deformity.

In severe cases with eversion of foot (patient waking on the outer border of the foot), Dwyer procedure, which consists of lateral calcaneal osteotomy, may be necessary, to stabilize the foot and replace the heel.

Girdlestone operation: The flexor tendons (f. digitorum profundis and brevis) are transferred to be inserted into dorsal extensor expansion over the proximal phalanges of toes.

A triple arthrodesis, as done for CTEV, may be needed in severe deformities.

124 Deformities of Toes

Hallux valgus: This is a common deformity, where the great toe is deviated laterally to overlap the 2nd toe, and the first metatarsal bone is deviated medially, causing a prominence on the medial aspect of the metatarsophalangeal joint (MTP joint). A bursa forms over the area as a result of the constant pressure, irritation and inflammation, forming a painful swelling called bunion. There may be some degree of foot pronation (flat feet) associated with the condition.

Etiology

1.   Biomechanical instability involving gait cycle

2.   Arthritic conditions: rheumatoid or psoriatic arthritis

3.   Metabolic conditions: gouty arthritis

4.   Connective tissue disorders: Ehlers-Danlos syndrome, Marfan syndrome, Down syndrome, and ligamentous laxity

4.   Neuromuscular diseases: multiple sclerosis, Charcot-Marie-Tooth disease, cerebral palsy

5.   Post-Traumatic conditions: malunions, intra-articular damage, soft-tissue sprains, and dislocations

6.   Structural deformity: malalignment of articular surface or metatarsal shaft, abnormal

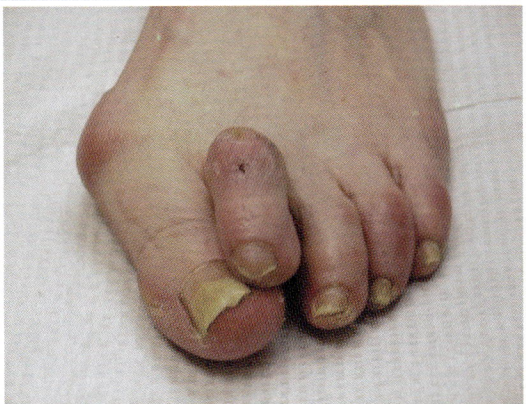

Fig. 124.2. Halux valgus with hammer-toe

metatarsal length, metatarsus primus elevatus

Clinical findings

The physical examination includes an assessment of the vascular, dermatologic, neurologic, and musculoskeletal systems. The musculoskeletal assessment may further be divided into 2 components:

1. determination of the etiology and

2. evaluation of the deformity. Understanding both components is essential in determining the most satisfying and successful treatment plan, whether conservative or surgical. Characteristic findings in hallux valgus are, medial prominence over the first metatarsophalangeal joint (bunion), contracture of extensor hallucis longus, and callus on the dorsum of second digit. The great toe can be overriding, underriding, abutting or without contact depending on the biomechanical abnormality. Lateral deviation of the great toe may result from subluxation of the metatarsophalangeal joint. Bunions are located dorsomedially and erythema or bursa indicates shoe pressure and irritation.

Investigations

Radiographic examination of the forefoot is the most important investigation which helps to identify the degree of deviation, any

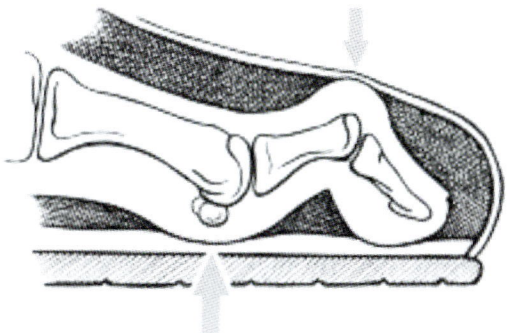

Fig. 124.1. Claw-toe with a tendency for a callosity (vulnerable areas shown with arrows)

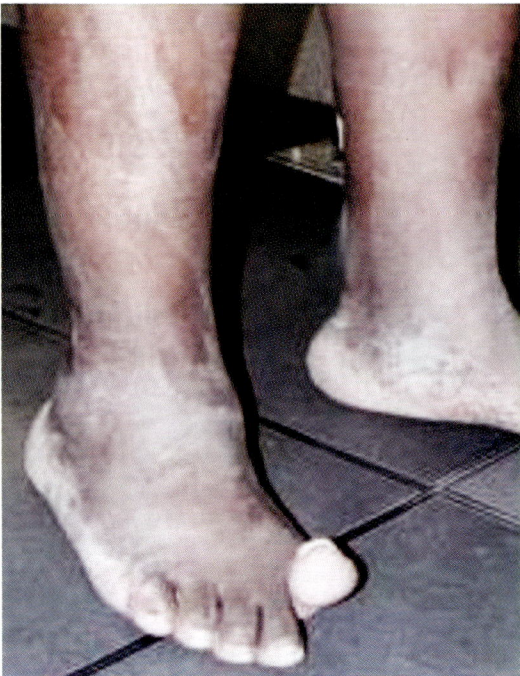

Fig. 124.3. Big toe hyperextended following injury to flexor tendons

subluxation of the metatarsophalangeal joint, position of sesamoids and to assess any arthritic changes in the involved joint. It also provides a template to plan for osteotomies when required. Biochemical or serological investigations to confirm associated conditions like rheumatoid arthritis, gout and other connective tissue disorders should be done.

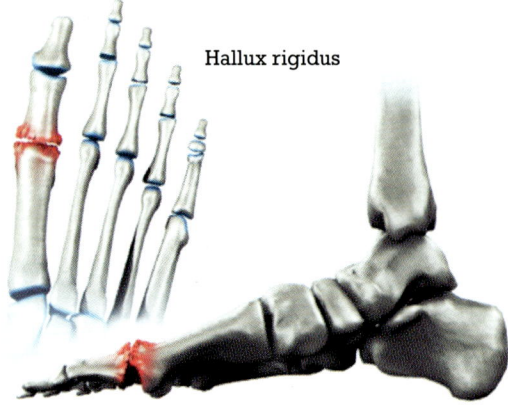

Hallux rigidus

Fig. 124.4. Lesion of first MP joint in hallux rigidus

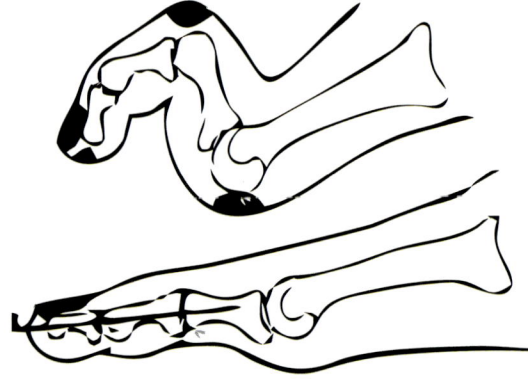

Fig. 124.5. Hammer-toe, stablized with a pin

Treatment

Indications for repair of hallux valgus

1. painful joint Range of Movements (ROM),
2. deformity of the joint complex,
3. pain or difficulty with footwear,
4. interference of activity or lifestyle nce of activity or lifestyle
5. associated secondary foot disorders caused by this condition

Non-operative treatment

Patients without degenerative disease of the metatarsophalangeal joint may benefit from lace up shoes with a wide toe box stiff-soled shoe. Those with equinus contracture may benefit from stretching, which may unload the forefoot and relieve pain.

Operative treatment

1. **Soft tissue procedures:** medial plication with lateral release and capsular repair.
2. **Osteotomies:** proximal phalanx base and/or metatarsal head
3. **Arthrodesis:** of the first metatarsophalangeal joint (in rheumatoid arthritis)
4. **Bunionectomy procedures.**
5. **Partial reduction of the sesamoids**

Hallux rigidus

Hallux rigidus or first metatarsophalangeal joint arthritis is a relatively common problem, often affecting people at a much younger age than arthritis of other joints. Hallux rigidus is seen in patients from their 30s onward. The

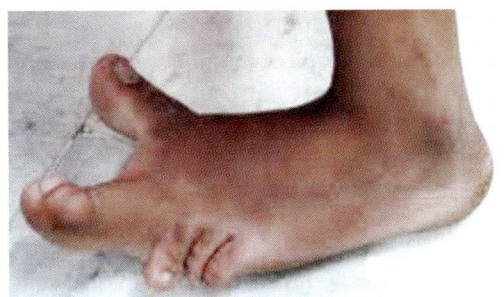

Fig. 124.6. A rare congenital deformity of the toes (courtesy: Halsted Surgical Clinic, Chennai)

reason why arthritis of this joint is seen in younger patients is unclear but may be associated with an unrecognized chondral injury to the metatarsal head. It is also associated with hallux valgus interphalangeus, bilateral involvement in those with a family history and has female preponderance.

Hallux rigidus is not associated with

metatarsus primus elevatus (describes as a structural deformity in which the first ray lies in a dorsiflexed position relative to the lesser toes.

first ray hypermobility,

a long first metatarsal,

Achilles tightness,

abnormal foot posture,

symptomatic hallux valgus,

occupation or faulty shoe wear.

Clinical findings

Patients present with complaints of joint stiffness and pain with dorsiflexion of the joint. The symptoms are worse with increased physical activities. Patients also complain of a painful dorsal prominence over the metatarsal neck that makes shoe wear uncomfortable. Radiographs show varying degrees of joint space narrowing and, invariably, a large osteophyte on the dorsal aspect of the metatarsal neck.

Conservative treatment

Conservative treatment consists of NSAIDs and wearing a stiff-soled shoe with a deep toe box.

In older (more than 60 years), sedentary patients, these measures are usually adequate. In more active individuals, however, surgical treatment is usually indicated.

Surgical treatment

Several surgical treatment methods are available for treating hallux rigidus. Resection of the dorsal bone spur, known as cheilectomy, is efficacious and the least intrusive surgical option. Approximately 25% of the dorsal aspect of the metatarsal head is removed along with the bone spur, and a thorough synovectomy of the joint is performed. This procedure is less likely to have a favorable outcome on joints with advanced arthritis.

A resection arthroplasty (Keller procedure) can be used on older, less active patients, but has a high rate of complications, as previously discussed. Prosthetic replacement of the arthritic first metatarsophalangeal joint can be used in older, lower demand patients but has high rates of failure in younger, more active individuals.

First metatarsophalangeal joint arthrodesis provides predictable pain relief and longevity for advanced arthritis. The drawback is that of lost motion at the joint.

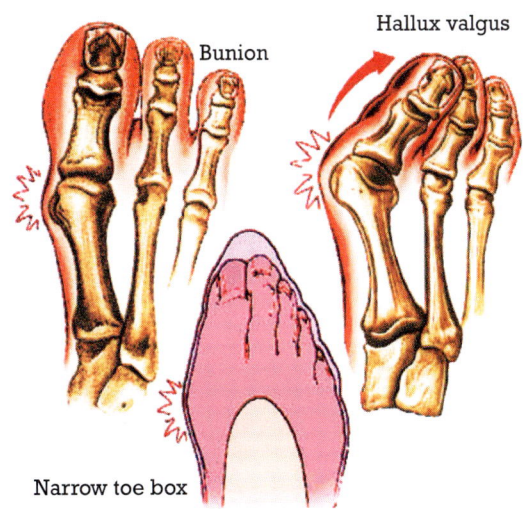

Fig. 124.7. Pathogenesis of hallux valgus

Hammer toe

The deformity occurs at the proximal interphalangeal (PIP) joint. In an infant, it is usually due to hereditary factors. In the older child, it could be due to faulty shoe wear. Most cases are mild, cause no pain, and can be left alone. In the more severe cases, at an older age, surgical correction may be needed.

Mallet toe

The deformity occurs at the distal interphalangeal (DIP) joint. Most cases are mild, and need no treatment. If a corn develops over the deformity, shaving and padding will help. In severe cases, surgical correction can be done.

Claw toe

The deformity involves all joints of the toe - hyperextension of the MTP joints, and flexion at both the PIP and DIP joints. It is a rare condition, but usually occurs in conjunction with a cavus foot, present in neuromuscular diseases like Charcot-Marie-Tooth disease, Volkmann's ischemic contractiure of leg or myelomeningocele.

Curly toe

The affected toe, usually the 4th or 5th is flexed downward and twisted underneath the adjacent toe. It is quite common in infancy and childhood. If it does not cause symptoms, no treatment is needed. If severe, and causes irritation with shoe wear, surgical transfer of the toe flexor may correct the problem.

Supernumerary toes (or Polydactyly)

If the extra toe is not causing problems with walking and shoe wear, no treatment is needed. If the duplication occurs in the little or big toe, and sticks out prominently, surgical excision may be necessary.

Webbed toes (or Syndactyly)

It is a common condition wherein toes are adherernt to each other intervening cleft. Unlike in the fingers it rarely causes problems and may not need surgical separation.

Bunionette (or Tailor's bunion)

The pathology is like that in a bunion, except that it occurs at the 5th MTP joint. The bursa over the lateral aspect of the joint becomes prominent, inflamed and painful. If padding does not help, surgical correction is needed.

125 Tuberculosis of Hip

Tuberculous disease of the hip is very common; the frequency of involvement is next only to spinal tuberculosis. Osteoarticular tuberculosis is caused most often by mycobacterium tuberculosis and by atypical mycobacteria in very few cases.

Etiology

The causative agent is mycobacterium tuberculosis which is a slow growing aerobic organism. In the 'pre-pasteurization' era there was a high incidence of skeletal tuberculosis caused by bovine bacilli. It can also be caused by atypical mycobacteria. Atypical mycobacteria refers to mycobacteria other than M. tuberculosis, e.g. M. kansasi, M. marinum, M. avium complex, M. sacrofulaceum.

Pathology

Any osteoarticular tubercular lesion is the result of a hematogenous dissemination from a primarily infected visceral focus. The primary focus may be active or quiescent, apparent or latent, either in the lungs or in the lymph nodes of the mediastinum, mesentery or cervical region, or kidneys or other viscera. The

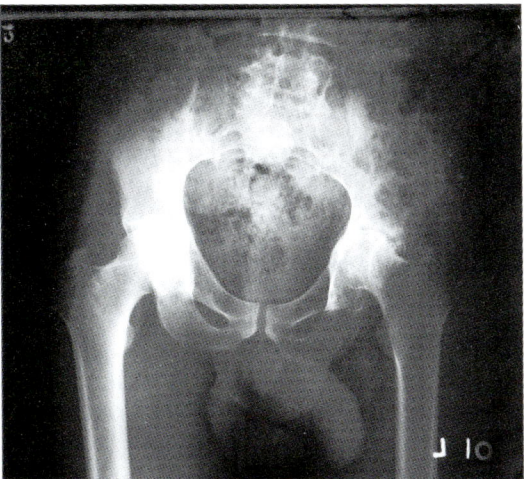

Fig. 125.1. Tuberculosis of hip with destruction of head of left femur
(courtesy: Dr. A N Vivek, Chennai)

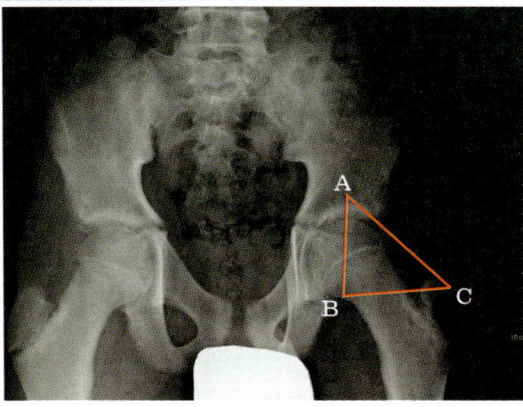

Fig. 125.2. Babcock's Triangle. **A:** upper part of acetabulum, **B:** femoral neck metaphysis, **C:** tip of the greater trochanter.
It represents the common location of osseous origin of tuberculosis of hip joint.
(courtesy: Dr. A N Vivek, Chennai)

infection reaches the skeletal system through vascular channels, generally the arteries as a result of bacillemia or rarely to axial skeleton through Bateson's plexus of veins. Skeletal tuberculosis generally develops 2 to 3 years after the primary focus. In tuberculosis of the hip joint, the initial focus of lesion may start in the acetabular roof, epiphysis, metaphyseal region (Babcock's triangle), or in greater trochanter. Rarely the disease may start in the synovial membrane and many remain as synovitis for a few months. Tuberculosis of the greater trochanter may involve the overlying trochanteric bursa without involving the hip joint for a very long time. As the upper end of femur is entirely intracapsular, the joint gets involved rapidly from any osseous lesion situated within the capsular attachments, the disease becomes 'osteoarticular', and destruction of articular surfaces of femoral head and acetabulum takes place. A cold abscess usually forms within the joint, the inferior weaker part of capsule or rarely the acetabular floor may be perforated and the cold

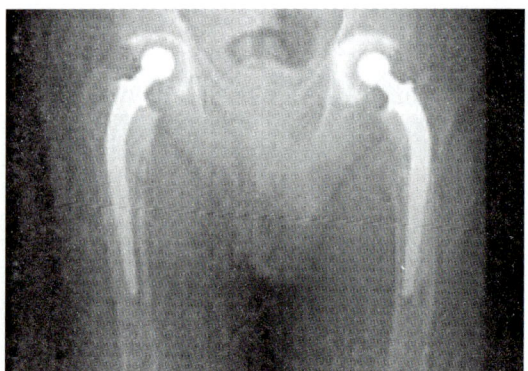

Fig. 125.3. Bilateral total hip replacement for tuberculosis
(courtesy: Dr C R S Reddy, Chennai)

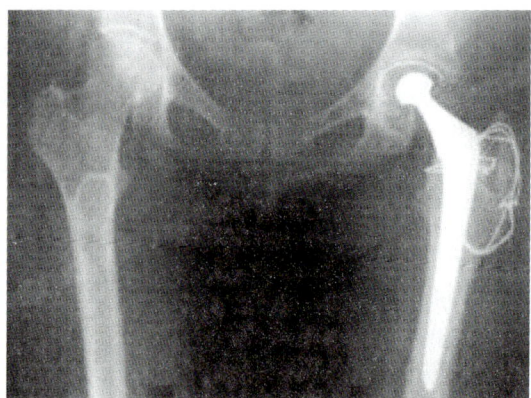

Fig. 125.4. Left total hip replacement for tuberculosis
(courtesy: Dr C R S Reddy, Chennai)

abscess may present anywhere around the hip joint such as femoral triangle, medial lateral or posterior aspects of thigh, ischiorectal fossa, or pelvis. The abscess tracks away from the hip joint mostly along the neighboring vessels and nerves to reach the surface. The intrapelvic abscess above the attachments of the levator ani muscle tracks upwards to point in the inguinal region; whereas those below this muscle track into the ischiorectal fossa.

Clinical features

Like osteoarticular tuberculosis in general, the disease commonly manifests before the 3rd decade, and is associated with pain, limping, deformity and fullness around the hip. Pain is often referred to the medial aspect of the knee and it is maximum during night, the child waking up from sleep due to night cries, from lack of protective muscular spasm. Patients may have clinically palpable cold abscesses with or without sinuses, and may present with varying degrees of pathological subluxation or dislocation of the hip.

The limp is the earliest and commonest symptom. The patient while walking puts as little pressure on the diseased hip joint for a short time as possible (i.e. has shortest possible stance phase) giving rise to the typical antalgic gait. To get relief from the pain of an active hip disease while changing position in the bed, the patient may support or lift the involved limb with the contralateral normal limb, or the patient may "apply traction" on the painful hip by pushing down on the dorsum of foot with the opposite foot while recumbent. Physical examination will reveal tenderness by direct pressure on the hip in the femoral triangle or medial to the greater trochanter posteriorly or indirectly by bitrochanteric pressure or thumping.

Clinical stages of untreated tuberculosis of the hip joint

Stage I – Tubercular synovitis

It is due to juxta-articular osseous lesion which causes an "irritable hip". The joint is held in the position of the maximum capacity i.e. flexion, external rotation and abduction, causing apparent lengthening. There is no true or real shortening. Only extremes of movements are limited and painful. Radiographs may show only soft tissue swelling, with or without rarefaction of the hip bones.

Stage II – Early arthritis

As the disease advances actual destruction or damage to the articular cartilage sets in, the local signs become more prominent and due to the spasm of adductors and flexors, the hip assumes a deformity of flexion, adduction (presenting as apparent shortening) and

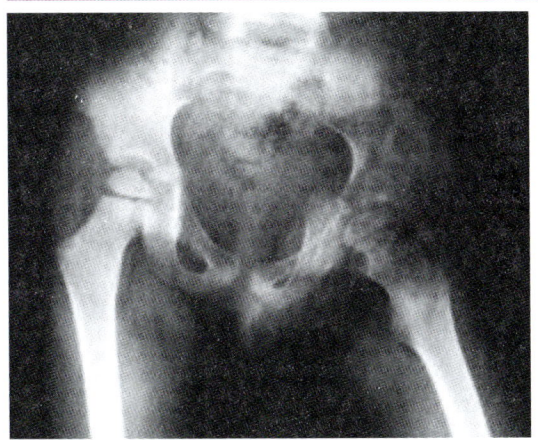

Fig. 125.5. Tuberculosis left hip joint
(courtesy: Dr A N Vivek, Chennai)

internal rotation. There is true shortening of not more than one cm, appreciable muscle spasm and wasting causing painful restriction of movements in all directions. Radiographs show localized osteoporosis, slight diminution of the joint space due to decrease in the vertical height of the articular cartilage and localized erosions at the articular margins.

Stage III – Advanced arthritis

With further advancement of destruction, clinical signs of flexion-adduction-internal rotation deformities, restriction of movements, muscle wasting and true and apparent shortenings are exaggerated. The tendency of the patient to sleep on the side of the uninvolved hip further contributes to the deformity. There is gross destruction of articular cartilage and bones of the femoral head and acetabulum, with capsular thickening and contraction.

Stage IV – Advanced arthritis with subluxation or dislocation

With further destruction of acetabulum, femoral head, capsule and ligaments, the upper end of femur may displace upwards and dorsally in the *wandering or migrating acetabulum* leaving its lower part empty and breaking the Shenton's arc. Rarely the destruction of capsule and acetabulum may be so severe as to lead to frank pathological posterior dislocation of the femoral head. Sometimes the hip may show *protrusio acetabuli*. In some cases the femoral head and neck are grossly destroyed, collapsed and reduced in size contained, in an enlarged acetabulum (mortar and pestle appearance). In general the movements at this stage are grossly restricted; however, in some cases fairly good range of movements may be retained for a long time.

Investigations

General investigations may reveal anemia, elevated ESR and a primary focus in the lung. The Mantoux test is positive only in about 15% of cases.

In early stages i.e., in stages I and II, there may be subtle radiographic changes like soft tissue swelling, localized osteoporosis, slight diminution of the joint space due to decrease in the vertical height of the articular cartilage and localized erosions at the articular margins.

If the disease occurs during childhood, chronic hyperemia leads to enlargement of femoral head epiphysis and metaphysis (coxa magna), thromboembolic phenomenon of selective terminal vasculature may create the changes resembling Perthes' disease or reduction in the size of femoral head and neck (coxa breva). Mismatched growth of capital femoral epiphyseal plate and growth-plate would lead to coxa vara or coxa valga.

Ultrasonography may be a useful investigation to appreciate the swelling of the soft tissues of the hip joint in the early stage of synovitis. MRI at this stage may show synovial effusion and varying degree of bone edema. If the pathological nature is uncertain, a biopsy must be obtained for bacteriology and histo-pathology.

Immunological diagnostics by IgA, IgE and IgM may be corroborative.

Treatment

All patients during active stage are treated by multi-drug therapy (refer chapter 18), and traction to correct the deformity. Bilateral traction is mandatory as traction to the deformed limb alone worsens the abduction deformity. Traction relieves the muscle spasm, prevents or corrects deformity and subluxation, maintains the joint space, minimizes the chances of development of migrating acetabulum and permits close observation of the hip region. Any palpable cold abscess may be aspirated. If there is favorable clinical response, the same treatment is continued. In cases which do not have gross ankylosis, active assisted movements of the hip are started as soon as the pain has subsided. If the response to nonoperative treatment is unfavorable one should perform synovectomy or debridement of the diseased joint as needed. In advanced arthritis the usual outcome is gross fibrous ankylosis. The traction regime and functional exercises in the initial stages help to overcome the deformities and permit assessment regarding the retention or restoration of any useful range of motion.

Surgery

In children with arthritis, the deformity and subluxation or dislocation is corrected or minimized by employing traction, rarely by the application of PoP under general anesthesia with or without adductor tenotomy. Failure to achieve desired results warrants open arthrotomy, synovectomy, debridement of the

---

Jewels of Gyan - 125.1

TB Hip Treatment

All patients during active stage are treated with multi drug therapy

In early stage - bilateral traction

Cold abscess - drainage and streptomycin can be instilled

Non-weight bearing mobilization for 12 weeks

In cases not responding to non-operative treatment - synovectomy or debridement of the joint

In advanced arthritis consider arthrodesis or excisional arthroplasty

---

diseased joint and improvement of displacement. Arthrodesis of the grossly destroyed hip joint or excisional arthroplasty in children should be deferred till the completion of growth potential of the proximal femur.

If the response to conservative treatment is not favorable or the outcome is unacceptable, the following selective operative options may be considered:

Osteotomy
Arthrodesis
Excisional arthroplasty (Girdlestone's excision arthroplasty)

The general management, including attention to nutrition, administration of anabolic steroid,

126 Humeral Supracondylar Fracture in Children

Supracondylar fractures of humerus are typically extraarticular and involve the thin bone between coronoid fossa the olecranon fossa. These fractures occur most often around 6 to 7 years of age.

Classification

Supracondylar fractures are divided into two types depending on the displacement

Extension type (95%)

Flexion type (5%)

Gartland classification for extension fractures recognizes that anterior cortex fails first with resultant posterior displacement of distal fragment

Type I: non-displaced fracture

Type II: displaced with intact posterior cortex

Type III: displaced with no cortical contact

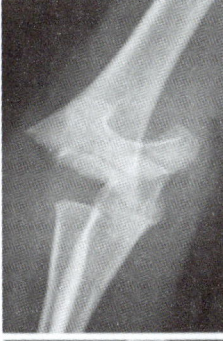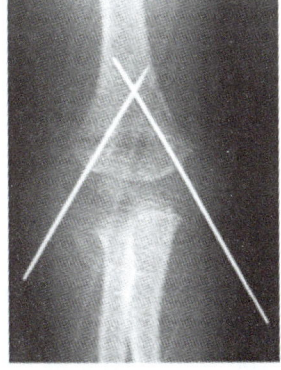
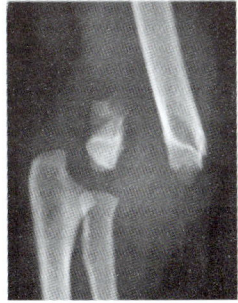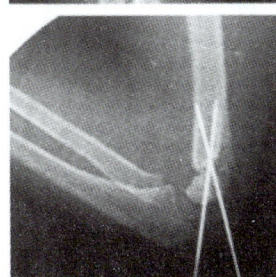

Fig. 126.1. Supracondylar fracture humerus immobilized with pins
(courtesy: Dr. A N Vivek, Chennai)

Mechanism of injury

Extension fractures typically result from a fall on an outstretched hand (FOOSH) mechanism with the elbow hyperextended. The distal condylar complex then shifts in either the posterolateral or posteromedial direction. In contrast to extension injuries, flexion fractures result from a direct blow to the posterior aspect of the flexed elbow. In these cases, the distal condylar complex is displaced in the antero-lateral direction.

Clinical features

The child with a supracondylar fracture typically has elbow pain, swelling, and very limited or no range of motion at the elbow. Open supracondylar fracture often manifests as a puncture wound or laceration in or just above the antecubital region. Displaced fractures may have an "S-shaped" configuration or dimpling in the antecubital fossa associated with marked swelling about the elbow. Ecchymosis over the anteromedial aspect of the forearm suggests brachial artery injury. Undisplaced fractures may have minimal swelling, but observation will show that the child is not using the affected arm normally. Posterior distal humeral palpation is usually painful in such cases.

Examination

Assessment of the injury to identify degree of fracture displacement, neurovascular compromise, and evidence of compartment syndrome should be done expediently.

A complete neurovascular evaluation should be performed which includes an assessment of radial and brachial pulses and the sensory and motor function of the median, radial, and ulnar nerves. Neurovascular assessment has to be repeated after manipulation or splinting.

Investigations

Radiographic assessment of suspected supracondylar fracture requires a true lateral of the elbow with the humerus in anatomic position. Because of the association of supracondylar fractures with forearm fractures, the clinician should also obtain AP and lateral views of the forearm.

Doppler ultrasound should be used to determine the status of distal perfusion if either the brachial or radial pulse is clinically absent. If vascular compromise is suspected, angiogram (conventional or CT) are valuable in assessing nature and extent of the injury and aids in treatment plan.

Pulsoximetry may also provide evidence of pulsatile flow as well as degree of oxygenation distal to the injury and has the advantage of being a dynamic study.

Complications

Early complications

Vascular injury

This constitutes a surgical emergency, which must be promptly identified and immediate intervention should be undertaken. Rarely, these children will require partial closed reduction in the emergency department in an attempt to restore distal circulation. Patients who display a cold, white or cyanotic hand despite reduction attempts require urgent operative exploration and vascular repair.

Acute compartment syndrome

Compartment syndrome may occur prior to or after definitive orthopedic care. Suspected compartment syndrome should prompt measurement of compartment pressure and emergent measures to decompress the compartments by removing all external pressure and if necessary by performing fasciotomies. Ischemia and primary swelling from the injury can lead to the development of compartment syndrome within 12-24 hours. Without timely intervention, the associated ischemia and infarction may progress to Volkmann's ischemic contracture.

Neurologic deficit

The frequency of neurologic deficit after supracondylar fractures varies from 10-50% depending on the type of fracture. Posterolaterally displaced fracture puts the median nerve and its anterior interosseous branch at the greatest risk of injury. Posteromedial fracture displacement increases the chance of radial nerve impingement. Ulnar nerve injuries are most commonly associated with flexion type of supracondylar fractures. Although nerve injuries may be associated with long-term sequel, the majority are neurapraxias that will resolve within two to three months. Surgical exploration should be considered for nerve deficits that persist beyond three months. An MRI scan may differentiate various types of nerve injuries, in making a decision for surgical intervention.

Late complications

Myositis ossificans

Cubitus varus deformity

Physeal growth arrest/growth disturbance

Tardy ulnar nerve palsy

Treatment

Initial treatment varies for each type of fracture:

Type I fracture must be immobilized for three weeks using posterior splint and sling which should extend from the wrist to the axilla, with the elbow at 90° flexion and the forearm in neutral position.

Type II and Type III fractures require closed reduction and percutaneous pin fixation.

Surgical intervention is mandatory in any of the following circumstances:

Open fracture

Fracture with neurovascular compromise

Type II or type III fracture

Evidence of compartment syndrome.

127 Giant Cell Tumor (Osteoclastoma)

Giant cell tumors constitute about 20% of all bone tumors. They may be benign, locally malignant or malignant.

1. BENIGN GIANT CELL TUMORS (95%) are osteolytic lesions arising from epiphysis. They typically occur between the ages of 20 and 40 years, with a slight female predominance. Although these tumors are typically benign, they are locally malignant and pulmonary metastasis occurs in approximately 3% of the cases. Histologic hallmark of this disease is the presence of tumor giant cells.

Common sites

Lower end of femur
Upper end of tibia and fibula
Distal end of radius

Gross pathology

Ragged, friable, bleeding tissue filled with old or fresh blood clots with various sized cysts and cavities. Colored bluish grey to reddish brown, the epiphyseal end of the bone is distorted and expanded. Tumor does not breach articular cartilage in early stages and no periosteal reaction is seen in cases without pathological fracture.

Histopathology

Fibrous capsule is present at periphery. Presence of abundant giant cells which are

characteristic with large and multiple nuclei (more than 150 in number) distributed throughout the cell. There is no correlation between histologic appearance and biological behavior of this tumor.

Clinical features

Most patients with giant cell tumors have progressive pain, often related to activity initially and only later becomes persistent. There is swelling at the epiphyseal end of bone, skin over the swelling is stretched and dilated veins are conspicuously absent. There may be minimal tenderness unless a pathological fracture has occurred, which is a late feature. *Eggshell crackling sensation may be appreciated.*

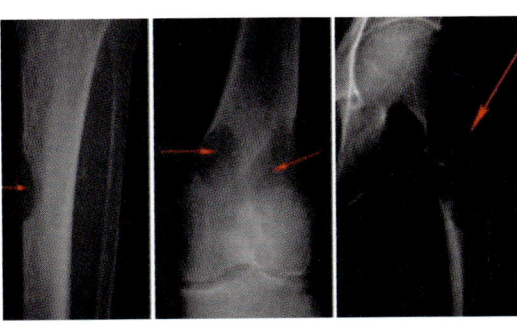

Fig. 127.2. Multiple myeloma (plasmacytoma). X-rays showing typical lesions in various areas of the leg. (Left) A lesion in the shinbone (tibia). (Center) Two lesions in the thighbone (femur) near the knee. (Right) A large lesion in the upper thighbone near the hip
(courtesy: Dr. A N Vivek, Chennai)

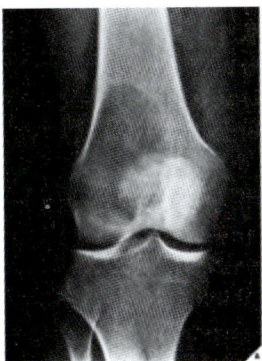
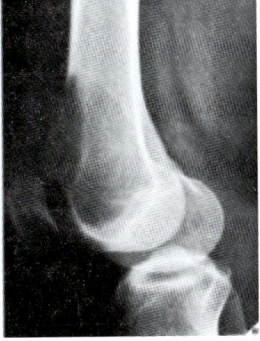

Fig. 127.1. Osteoclastoma of lower end of femur
(courtesy: Dr. A N Vivek, Chennai)

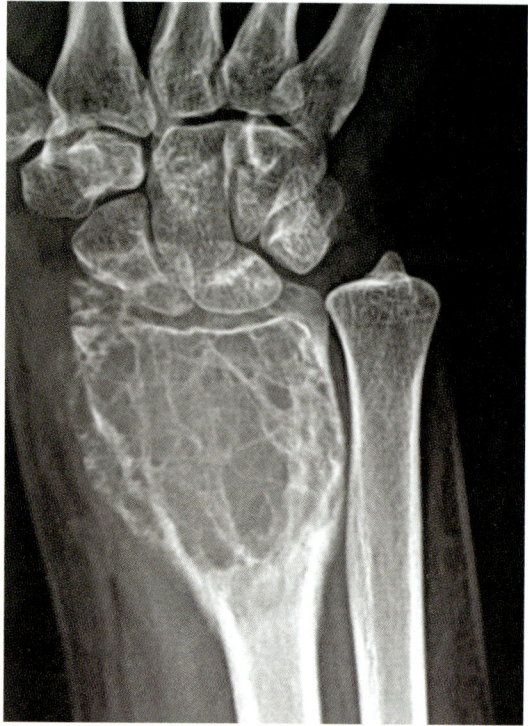

Fig. 127.3. Typical soap bubble appearance in osteoclastoma, distal radius (courtesy: Dr A N Vivek, Chennai)

2. MALIGNANT GIANT CELL TUMOUR

Malignant giant cell tumors represent less than 5% of the cases and are classified as primary or secondary. Primary malignant giant cell tumors are extremely rare and are defined as sarcomas that occur within lesions that otherwise are typical of benign giant cell tumors. Secondary malignant giant cell tumors are sarcomas that occur at the sites of giant cell tumors that have been treated, usually with radiation.

Investigations

Radiographic findings often are diagnostic. The lesions appear osteolytic, are eccentrically located in the epiphysis of long bones and abut the subchondral bone. There is thinning and expansion of the cortex. Thin septa of bone traverse the interior of the lesion and produce a *soapbubble appearance*. There is no periosteal new bone formation unless a pathological fracture is present and the cortex may be disrupted in late stages. Joint extension is rare.

MRI allows more accurate assessment of intramedullary and extraosseous extension of the lesion and a liberal bone biopsy will establish the true nature of the lesion.

Arteriography shows a very great increase in the number of arterioles and venules both inside and outside the bone in malignant disease, which does not happen in any other bone disease. In osteoclastoma though there is increased vascularity, there is never the picture of increased arterioles and venules as in osteosarcoma. It will also differentiate osteoclastoma from an aneurysmal bone cyst

Differential diagnosis

Plasmacytoma
Adamantinoma (ameloblastoma)
Giant cell reparative granuloma
Osteitis fibrosa of focal and generalized types

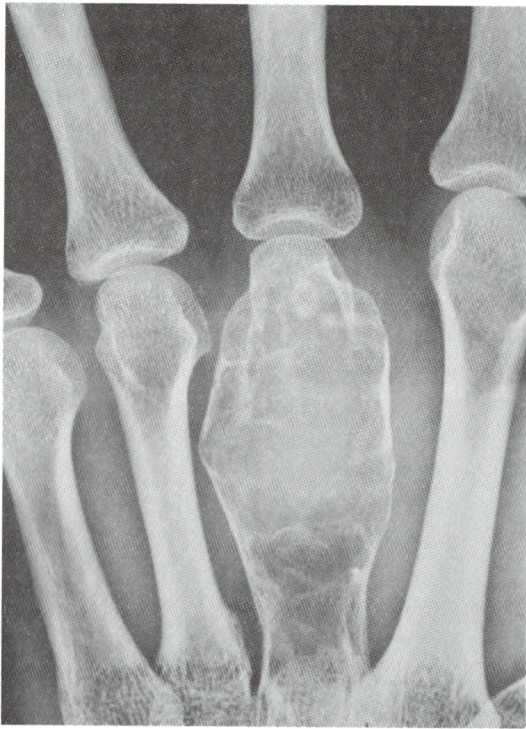

Fig. 127.4. Osteoclastoma of metacarpal bone (courtesy: Dr C R S Reddy, Chennai)

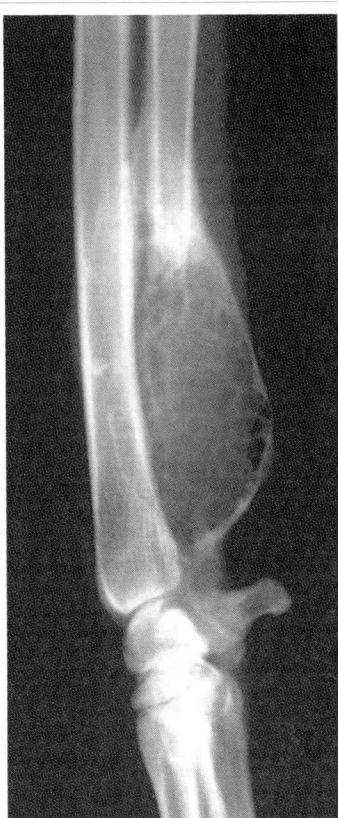

Fig. 127.5. Aneurysmal bone cyst, presenting like osteoclastoma

Chondromata

Bone cysts, including aneurysmal bone cyst

Osteolytic sarcoma

Metastatic carcinoma

Cystic type of tuberculosis

Plasmacytoma: The solitary type is to be differentiated. The trabeculae are few, well-defined and coarse; urine may show Bence-jones protein and sternal puncture, plasma cells.

Adamantinoma (in the jaw): The line of demarcation from the normal bone is sharp, the trabeculae are coarse and sometimes the tumor gives a honeycombed appearance. It is not radiosensitive.

Focal osteitis fibrosa: Though usually solitary other bones may show similar lesions, trabeculae are few and course, outline is sharp and progress is slow.

Generalized osteitis fibrosa cystica (von Recklinghausen): There is generalized osteoporosis; blood chemistry shows changes and deposition of calcium in urinary tract may occur.

Chondroma: It may be anywhere in the shaft, has a well-defined and clear cut boundary and on radiographic examination of the skeleton similar lesions may be found in other bones.

Bone cyst: It has a clear cut sclerosed margin and may be situated anywhere in the shaft.

Osteolytic sarcoma: There is no definite line of demarcation from normal bone; periosteal reaction and invasion of the tumor into the shaft occur.

Metastatic carcinoma: The secondary deposits from thyroid have a soapbubble appearance and this has to be borne in mind. Age and site as also the history or presence of primary lesion

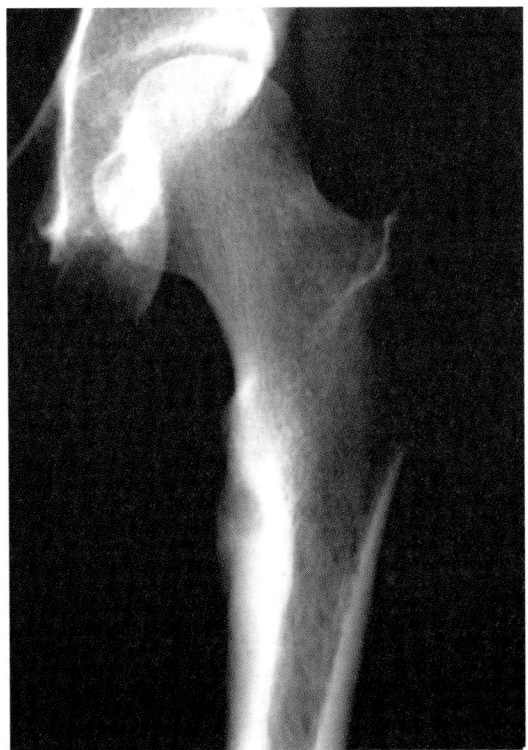

Fig. 127.6. Osteoid osteoma

help in differentiation. Urine may show Bence-Jones protein. These lesions have invasive and destructive properties.

Cystic type of tuberculosis: Repeated examination at short intervals shows the cysts to coalesce; the articular surface later breaks down and ultimately the joint may be destroyed.

Treatment

Surgery

Curettage and bone grafting: for lesions which are clinically benign without pathological fracture.

Enbloc excision: for aggressive type of lesions and in those lesions where there is a pathological fracture.

Curettage and acrylic bone cementation: for juxta-articular lesions which are unstable following conventional curettage.

Curettage and cryosurgery: liquid nitrogen is used to achieve tumor free field following curettage.

Excision and reconstruction: this is performed for aggressive tumors, lesions with pathological fractures and in cases of recurrence which can be contained. Reconstruction can be performed with allogenic banked bone.

Amputation: performed in malignant GCT, aggressive lesions with soft tissue involvement and in recurrence.

Radiation therapy

It is a radiosensitive tumor and RT is employed in several situations:

1. as a primary modality for inaccessible lesions like in spine or pelvis
2. neoadjuvant therapy
3. postoperative adjuvant therapy
4. palliative therapy

128 Osteogenic Sarcoma (Osteosarcoma)

Osteosarcoma is a highly malignant primary bone tumor characterized by production of osteoid by malignant cells. It is the second most common primary malignancy of bone next to multiple myeloma.

Etiology

There is no racial predilection, but genetic factors have occasionally been demonstrated to play a role; it is seen in association with hereditary form of retinoblastoma, Rothmund-Thomson syndrome, and Li-Fraumeni syndrome. It is also associated with certain viral infections (polyoma and SV 40 virus), with exposure to radiation of more than 2000 rads to osteoprogenitor cells in areas of active growth at metaphysis, and with exposure to chemicals like 20-methyl cholanthrene benzyllium. It is common in second decade of life with a male preponderance (3:1). All skeletal locations can be affected; however, most primary osteosarcomas occur at the sites of the most rapid bone growth, namely the distal femur, the proximal tibia, and the proximal humerus.

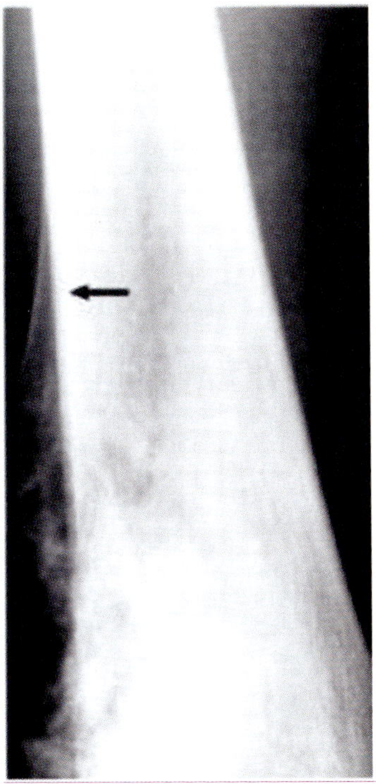

Pathology

Osteosarcomas are categorized as primary or secondary. Primary osteosarcomas are subcategorized as follows:

1. Central (medullary)
· Conventional central (classic) (75% of all osteosarcoma)
· Telangiectatic
· Intraosseous/intramedullary well differentiated (low grade)

Fig. 128.1. Osteosarcoma of lower end of femur with Codman's triangle (courtesy: Dr. A N Vivek, Chennai)

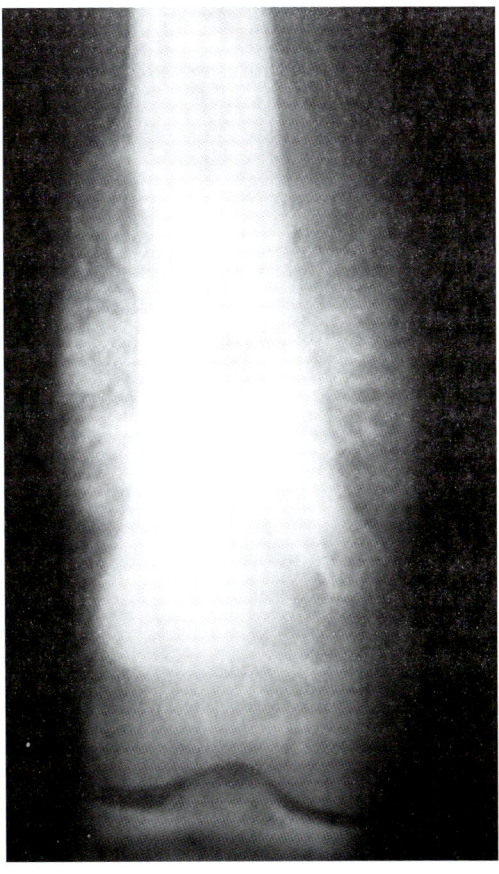

Fig. 128.2. Osteosarcoma of lower end of femur with typical sun ray appearance (courtesy: Dr. A N Vivek, Chennai)

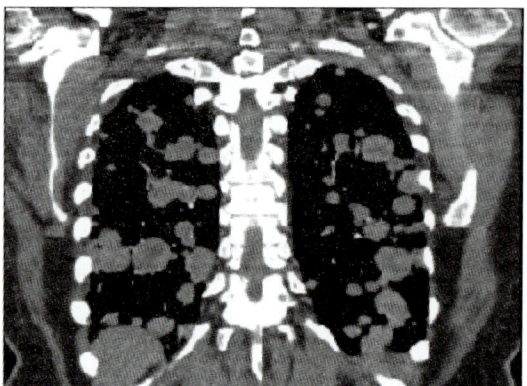

Fig. 128.3. Mlultiple pulmonary secondaries (cannon balls) from osteosarcoma
(courtesy: Dr. A N Vivek, Chennai)

· Small cell
2. Surface (peripheral)
· Parosteal (low grade)
· Periosteal (low to intermediate grade)
· High grade surface

Based on histology, they may be primarily:
- Osteoblastic
- Chondroblastic
- Fibroblastic

On gross examination the tumor is situated in the metaphysis of large long bone with areas of destruction giving an appearance of leg of mutton. Consistency may be variable ranging from stony hard to soft. Color of the specimen may be bluish white (if the tumor is cartilaginous), fish flesh appearance (in fibroblastic type) and yellowish white (in osteoblastic type). In telangiectatic type there are necrotic foci, cavitations and hemorrhages may be present and is in reddish brown in color..

Clinical features

Usually a history of trauma is present drawing the attention of the patient to the swelling. Pain is the first symptom and is later followed by the appearance of the swelling. Pain is persistent and night pain is an important clue to the diagnosis and it is not specifically related to activity. Pain is due to the microinfarctions of the involved bone which occurs due to the invasion of the tumor cells, weakening the

bone. General condition of the patient is good till the late stages, but the patient is usually anemic. There may be pyrexia with increased leukocytosis. Skin over the tumor is stretched, shiny and mobile (until infiltrated), with erythema and dilated veins. The swelling is tender, with local rise of temperature and the margins of the swelling are not well defined. Tumor souffle may be appreciated in highly vascular osteosarcomas. Pathological fracture is an unusual presentation.

Differential diagnosis

1. Myositis ossificans
2. Sessile osteochondroma
3. Ossifying soft tissue sarcoma
4. Ossifying fibromyxoid tumor

Investigations

Plain radiographs are valuable tools for making diagnosis. Common appearance is that of an

Jewels of Gyan - 128.1

Guidelines for Surgical Resection

1. The major neurovascular bundle must be free of tumor.

2. Wide resection of the affected bone with a normal muscle cuff in all directions should be done.

3. All previous biopsy sites and all potentially contaminated tissues should be removed en bloc.

4. Bone should be resected 3 to 4 cm beyond abnormal uptake as determined by bone scan.

5. The adjacent joint and joint capsule should be resected.

6. Adequate motor reconstruction must be accomplished by regional muscle transfers.

7. Adequate soft tissue coverage is needed to decrease the risk of skin flap necrosis and secondary infection.

Overall Treatment Strategy

The patient with a primary tumor of the extremity without evidence of metastases requires surgery to control the primary tumor and chemotherapy to control micrometastatic disease.

The choice between amputation and limb-sparing resection must be made taking into account tumor location, size or extramedullary extent, the presence or absence of distant metastatic disease, and patient factors such as age, skeletal development, and lifestyle preference that might dictate the suitability of limb salvage or amputation.

Routine amputations are no longer performed; all patients should be evaluated for limb-sparing options.

Patients who are judged unsuitable for limb-sparing options may be candidates for presurgical (neo-adjuvant) chemotherapy; those with a good response may then become suitable candidates for limb-sparing operations.

aggressive lesion in the metaphysis of a long bone, which is permeative with ill defined borders and areas of bone production and destruction. Periosteal reaction may take the form of a 'Codman's triangle,' or it may have a 'sunburst' or 'hair on end' appearance. MRI is the best study to measure the extent of the tumor both within the bone and in the soft tissue and to determine the relationship of the tumor to nearby anatomical structures. Bone scan is done to look for skeletal metastasis and CT scan of the chest for pulmonary secondaries since the lungs are the most common sites of metastases.

Biopsy of the specimen is confirmatory. Increased serum alkaline phosphatase and serum lactate dehydrogenase are noted in laboratory investigations.

Treatment

The main treatments for osteosarcoma are chemotherapy and surgery.

Chemotherapy protocols have typically included various combinations and dosage schedules of high-dose methotrexate (HDMTX), doxorubicin hydrochloride (adriamycin), Ifosfamide and cisplatin. Multiagent chemotherapy, using various dosing schedules, is now considered standard treatment for osteosarcoma.

The aim of this course of chemotherapy is to shrink the primary tumor, facilitating surgical excision and subsequent limb salvage, and to kill any cells that have spread to other parts of the body.

Chemotherapy given after the surgery is known as adjuvant chemotherapy.

Radiotherapy: Osteosarcoma is not very radiosensitive, but may be employed as neoadjuvant therapy (Stanford) or palliative measure for advanced nonresectable tumors.

Limb-sparing resection

The majority of OS can be treated safely by a limb-sparing resection combined with effective neo-adjuvant and adjuvant treatments. Successful limb-sparing surgery consists of three phases:

1. Resection of tumor. Resection strictly follows the principles of oncologic surgery. Avoiding local recurrence is the criterion of success and the main determinant of the amount of bone and soft tissue to be removed.

2. Skeletal reconstruction. The average skeletal defect following adequate bone tumor resection measures 15 to 20 cm. Techniques of reconstruction (prosthetic replacement,

arthrodesis, allograft, or combination) vary and are independent of the resection, although the degree of resection may favor one technique over the other.

3. Soft tissue and muscle transfers. Muscle transfers are performed to cover and close the resection site and to restore lost motor power. Adequate skin and muscle coverage is mandatory to decrease postoperative morbidity.

Resection of large solitary pulmonary metastasis, if necessary criteria are met.

SECONDARY OSTEOSARCOMA

Secondary osteosarcomas occur at the site of another disease process. They rarely occur in young patients but constitute almost half of the osteosarcomas in patients over 50 years of age, Paget's disease and previous radiation are the most common pre-existing conditions.

Paget's osteosarcoma most commonly occurs in patients between the sixth and the eighth decades of life, and pelvis is the most common location.

Other diseases predisposing to secondary osteosarcoma:

1. Rothmund-Thomson syndrome
2. Werner's syndrome
3. Osteogenesis imperfecta
4. McCune Albright syndrome
5. Retinoblastoma
6. Neuroblastoma
7. Bone infarct
8. Chronic osteomyelitis
9. Osteochondromas

Investigation and treatment: Same as above.

Li-Fraumeni syndrome

It is a rare disorder that greatly increases the risk of developing several types of cancer, particularly in children and young adults.

The CHEK2 and TP53 genes (tumor suppressor genes) are associated with Li-Fraumeni syndrome.

The cancers most often associated with are breast cancer, osteosarcoma, soft tissue sarcomas, brain tumors, leukemias, and adrenocortical carcinoma.

Rothmund-Thomson syndrome

It is a rare condition that affects particularly the skin. People with this condition develop telangiectasia which persist for life, and are collectively known as poikiloderma.

It is also characterized by sparse hair, slow growth and small stature; abnormalities of the teeth and nails; and gastrointestinal problems in infancy, such as chronic diarrhea and vomiting. Some affected children develop cataract, skeletal abnormalities including absent or malformed bones, delayed bone formation, and low bone density (osteopenia). Some of these abnormalities affect the development of bones in the forearms and the thumbs, and are known as radial ray malformations. People with this syndrome have an increased risk of developing osteosarcoma. These bone tumors most often develop during childhood or adolescence. Several types of skin cancer are also more common in people with this disorder.

Recent advances

Targeted radiotherapy with an isotope [153]Sm-EDTMP, for locally advanced or disseminated osteosarcoma is under evaluation.

129 Diaphyseal Aclasis

syn: Hereditary multiple exostoses (HME), External chondromatosis syndrome, Multiple cartilaginous exostoses, Multiple exostoses, Multiple exostoses syndrome, Multiple osteochondromatosis.

Diaphyseal aclasis is an autosomal dominant, rare skeletal disorder, characterized by multiple bony growths or exostoses, often on the epiphysis of the long bones of extremities. These bony growths may cause deformities, are covered by cartilage or adventitious bursa and usually continue to grow until after puberty.

Pathology

Though it is mostly inherited, 10% may have no family history. The two genes most strongly associated with this condition are EXT1 on 8q24.1 and EXT2 on 11p13. The mutation of these genes causes lack of production of two specific proteins called exostosin 1 and 2 and leads to deficiency of heparan sulfate, which is necessary for normal bone metabolism. However, the precise mechanism of the development of multiple exostosis is not clear. Cartilaginous exostoses arise from the metaphysis, point away from epiphysis, and appear to extend down the diaphysis during growth; they increase in size and number in course of time, but become latent at maturity. In over 90% of cases both ends of tibia, proximal femur, and proximal humerus are involved. Other areas include iliac crests, scapulae and ribs. Sarcomatous degeneration, in the form of chondrosarcoma may develop in 1-2% of patients with this condition.

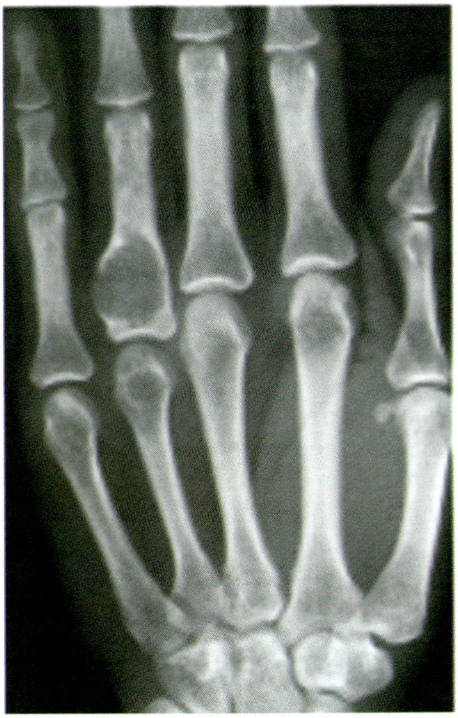

Fig. 129.1. Enchondroma of proximal phalanx of ring finger
(courtesy: Dr A N Vivek, Chennai)

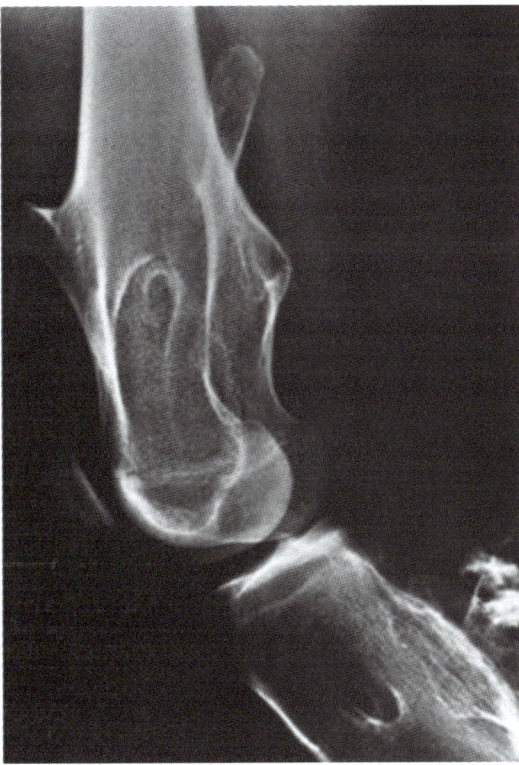

Fig. 129.2. Diaphyseal aclasis of femur

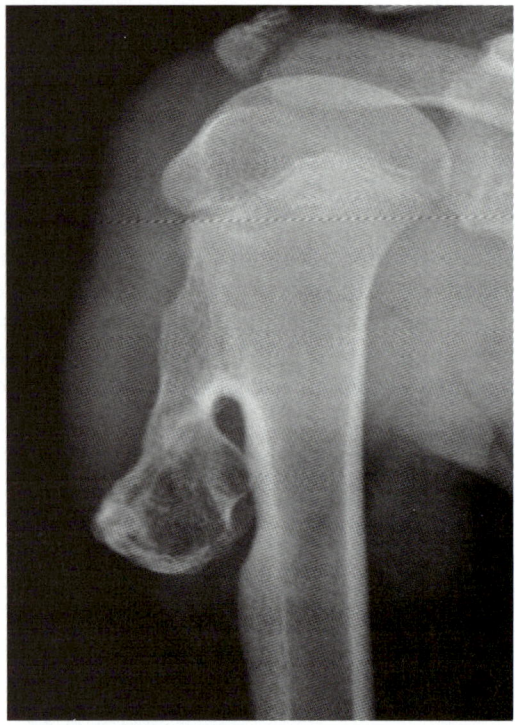

Fig. 129.3. Diaphyseal aclasis of humerus

Clinical features

Majority of the bony outgrowths are asymptomatic. Symptoms from a lesion are usually due to fracture, pressure on surrounding soft tissues, neurovascular compromise or **causing** mechanical hindrance for joint function. 40% of patients will demonstrate short stature, but not to the extent of causing dwarfism. Inequality of leg length may be severe enough to cause a disturbance in gait, often requiring special foot-wear or surgical correction.

Differential diagnosis

Other benign lesions of bone

Investigations

Radiography is characteristic with isodense bony outgrowths which arise from metaphyses, and appear to extend down the diaphysis. Due to the widespread nature of the disease, a limited skeletal survey may be needed with additional modalities like CT of areas with severe symptoms.

Treatment

Majority of patients do not require any treatment. They learn to compensate for the deformity or decreased range of motion, to maintain normal function. When the patient is disabled to carry normal daily activities, intervention may be necessary.

Indications for surgery

1. Disability to carry on normal functions
2. Painful or causing pressure symptoms
3. Cosmetic considerations
4. Early surgery may prevent boney deformity by allowing remodelling.

Surgery: Besides excision of the exostosis, other corrective procedures employed:

1. osteotomy
2. epiphysiodesis
3. Ilizarov technique by distraction osteogenesis.

Non-ossifying fibroma

Nonossifying fibroma or fibrous cortical defect is a common benign fibrous tumor, which is usually incidentally found on radiographs taken for other purposes. Most occur in children and adolescents between the ages of 10 and 20 years. Radiogaphically they appear as oval, osteolytic areas which are located eccentrically. Unless they are large (more than 50% of the diameter of the native bone), they can be left alone. surgery involves excision and curettage, often done to prevent the pathological fracture.

Unicameral bone cyst

Unicameral or solitary bone cyst occurs anywhere in the skeleton, but commonly in the proximal humerus and proximal femur, presenting in the first two decades of life with male predominance. There is an elevated level of prostaglandin (PGE2) in the fluid within the cyst. It has a characteristic appearance on radiographs, and does not require any treatment if small. It causes symptoms only if it gets large enough to cause weakness in the bone, resulting in a fracture, when the treatment is usually directed towards the fracture.

Frequently, with the bleeding from the fracture occurring in to the cyst, the fracture healing obliterates the cyst. If the cyst persists even after the fracture heals, it is advisable to excise the cyst and fill it up with bone graft to prevent future problems.

Treatment

Methylprednisolone injection into the cyst reduces the PGE2 and is used as a treatment modality.

Aneurysmal bone cyst

Aneurysmal bone cyst can occur anywhere in the body, but commonly in the posterior part of the spine, and the long bones, seen between first and second decades of life. Biopsy is indicated since radiologically aneurysmal bone cysts, giant cell tumors and osteosarcomas may appear similar. It exhibits expansile pulsation with a characteristic honeycomb appearance on radiographs. It may cause pain, pathological fracture and diagnostic difficulties with neoplastic conditions, hence surgery consisting of excision and bone grafting, is indicated. there is a high incidence of recurrence following simple curettage.

Enchondroma is a cartilage tumor that occurs within the long bones of the limbs and fingers. Sometimes it occurs in multiple sites, and is called Ollier's disease.

Osteoid osteoma

Osteoid osteoma is a small painful lesion, typically causing discomfort at night relieved by aspirin. It can occur anywhere in the body, but commonly in the long bones and the spine. Diagnosis is by its typical appearance of a small dense lesion on radiography. CT scan may be needed to delineate the lesion. Treatment is usually excision.

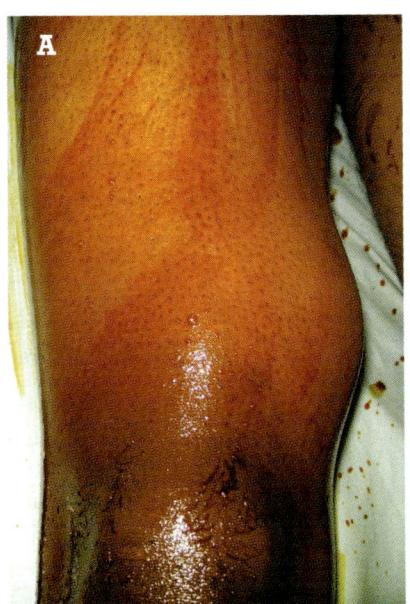
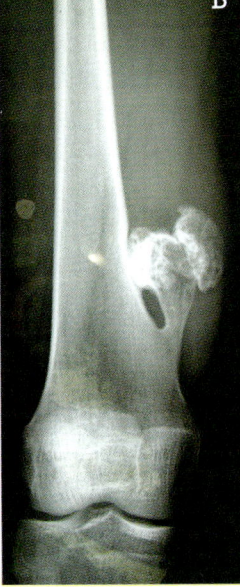
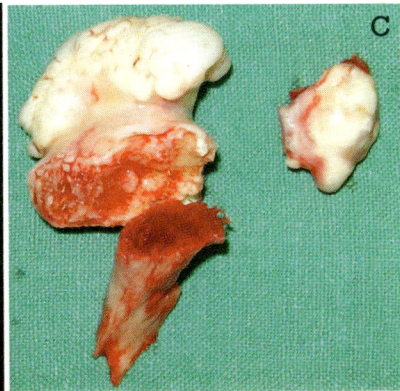

Fig. 129.4. Diaphyseal aclasis of lower end of femur
A: Clinical appearance
B: Radiograph of the lesion
C: Excised surgical specimen
(courtesy: Dr C J Reddy, Gudur)

DEFORMITIES: it is an alteration in the shape of a limb, spine or any part of the body, causing esthetic or functional disability. They may be congenital or acquired.

1. Congenital

As in any congenital defect, a combination of genetic and environmental factors influence the development and the ultimate outcome in a deformity. The atomic bombing on Hiroshima and Nagasaki during Second World War, not only resulted in enormous number of congenital deformities in children, but provided a unique opportunity to understand their pathogenesis and natural course of radiation induced deformities. Some of the common congenital deformities are shown in Table-130.1.

2. Acquired

Common causes of acquired deformities are trauma, infection, neurogenic, metabolic and postural.

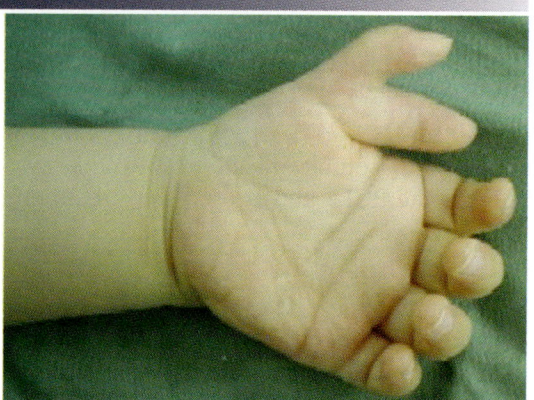

Fig. 130.1. Polydactyly and syndactyly of thumb

a) Traumatic conditions may be injuries to bones (malunited fractures), joints (unreduced dislocations), nerves (e.g. claw hand in ulnar nerve palsy or foot drop in lateral popliteal nerve injury), blood vessels (e.g. Volkmann's ischemic contracture), soft tissue (e.g. contractures following burns or badly placed incisions across joints)

Stage	Etiology	Deformity
Cellular stage	Genetic	Achondroplasia Polydactyly Club foot Arthrogryphosis
Embryonic stage	Chromosomal (trisomy-21) Folic acid deficiency	Down's syndrome Anencephaly and neural tube defects
Early fetel stage	a) Drugs (thalidomide, steroids, alchohol) b) Radiation (diagnostic, therapeutic) c) Maternal diseases (diabetes, rubella)	Cong. limb deficiency Club foot Spina bifida
Late fetal stage	Combination of factors	Structural deformities
Peripartum stage	Mechanical & postural factors Trauma, cerebral hypoxia	Club foot (easy type) Cerebral palsy Genu recurvatum

Table-130.1. Some causes of congenital deformities

b) Infections, such as tuberculosis or nonspecific pyogenic infections of bones &/or joints are the leading causes of deformities in India, whereas rheumatoid arthritis is the main reason in the West.

c) Neurogenic deformities may be lesions of upper motor neurone (e.g. cerebral palsy, infantile hemiplegia etc. causing spastic paralysis), lower motor neurone (e.g. anterior poliomyelitis causing flaccid paralysis) or peripheral nerves (e.g. Leprosy or peripheral nerve injury)

d) Metabolic diseases, such as rickets, osteomalacia, hyperparathyroidism and generalized bone diseases like osteoporosis, Paget's disease

e) Diseases of soft tissue, such as myopathies (pseudohypertrophic muscular dystrophy) causing equinus deformity and Dupuytren's contracture causing finger deformities. Before the routine immunization, anterior poliomyelitis (APM) was a leading cause of lower limb deformities.

f) Postural deformities: These are due to habitual assumption of bad postures and are mostly correctable by voluntary efforts and by exercises aimed to over correct the deformity, e.g. postural kyphosis, scoliosis or flat foot.

g) Functional or hysterical and rarely malingering

i) Idiopathic: e.g. idiopathic scoliosis occurring in adolescence

Management

Evaluation of deformity

It is important to identify if a deformity is primary or secondary to some other condition, e.g. an equinus deformity may be a result of imbalance of muscular activity due to limb shortening, caused by knee or hip disease, or it may be due to venous disease of leg, in which plantar flexion of ankle gives comfort. Next is to find out if the deformity is mobile (or flexible), which can be passively corrected or fixed. Lastly the extent of disability or disfigurement

caused by the deformity has to be assessed. Naturally, more the magnitude of defect, more difficult it is to correct, but once accomplished, greater the patient's satisfaction.

Methods of correction

1. Conservative (non-operative) methods
   a) Physiotherapy
   b) Splinting or use of an appliance
   c) Traction
   d) Plaster casts and wedging
   e) Manipulation under anesthesia

2. Surgical methods

This is resorted to when the deformity cannot be corrected by other means and is causing

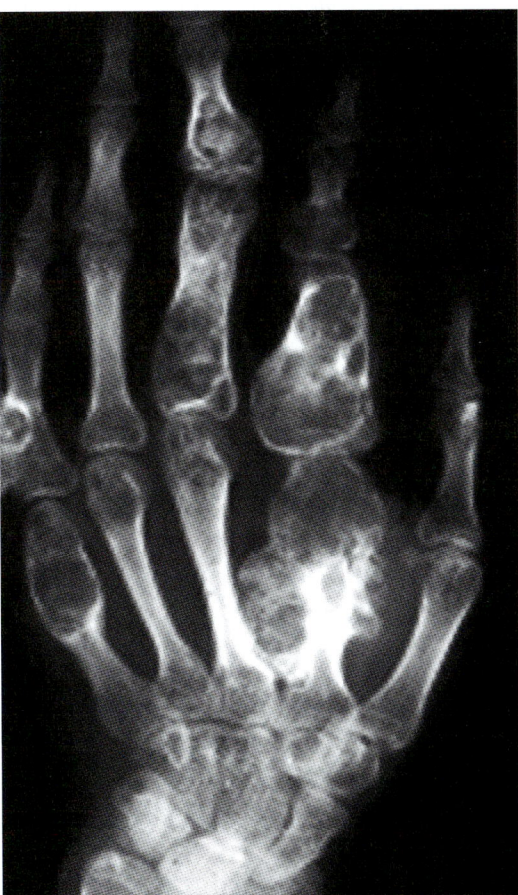

Fig. 130.2. Ollier disease. Large, lobulated cartilaginous masses markedly deform the bones of the hand (courtesy: Dr. A N Vivek, Chennai)

significant disability or disfigurement. This may be by means of operations on:

a) Soft tissues: this may be possible in younger age groups when permanent bone changes have not yet occurred. e.g. soft tissue release for club foot, tendo Achilles lengthening for equinus deformity. It is also possible in adults, if the pathology is confined to soft tissues

b) Bones: this may be necessary in long standing deformities, often in conjunction with release of soft tissue. e.g. osteotomy, orthodesis or Ilizarov's operation

GAIT

As the patient enters the consultation chamber, observation of gait may provide a valuable clue to the diagnosis, which is according to altered biomechanics of muscles, joints and the necessary sensory (proprioceptive) feedback. The visual and labirinthine sensory inputs are very essential for the normal smooth, graceful, coordinated human gait.

Definition of normal gait

Human gait is bipedal, biphasic, forward propulsion of centre of gravity, in which there is alternate sinuous movement of head and body, with least expenditure of energy.

Phases

During every 'walking cycle', there is a stance phase (70%) and a swing phase phase (30%) for each leg.

During stance phase, the foot is on the ground, whereas in swing phase that same foot is no longer in contact with the ground and the leg is swinging through in preparation for the next foot strike.

The stance phase may be subdivided into three separate phases.

1. First double support, when both feet are in contact with the ground

2. Single limb stance, when one foot is swinging through, while the other foot is in ground contact.

3. Second double support, when both feet are again in ground contact.

The first double support for the right side is second double support for the left side, and vice versa. In normal gait there is a natural symmetry between the left and right sides, but in pathological gait an asymmetrical pattern very often exists.

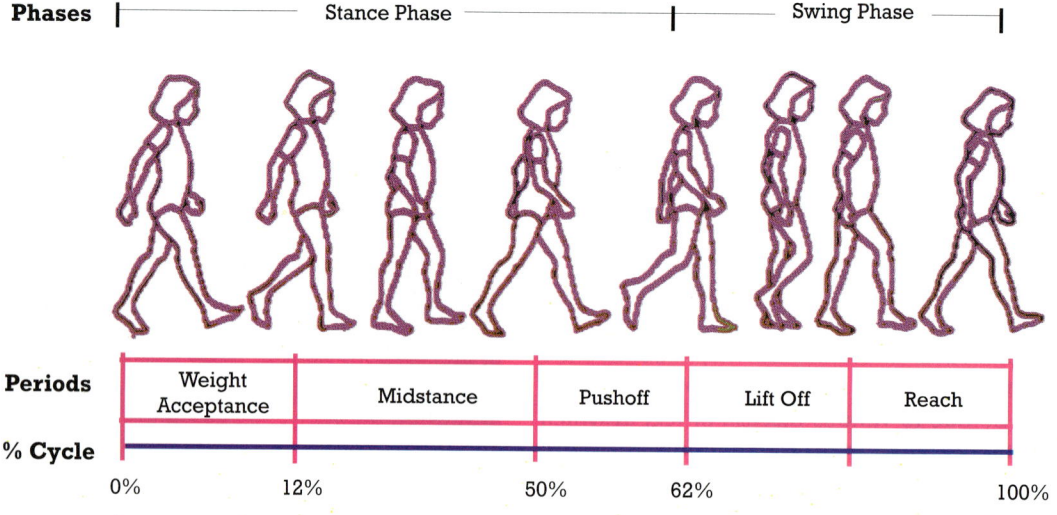

Phases	Stance Phase			Swing Phase	
Periods	Weight Acceptance	Midstance	Pushoff	Lift Off	Reach
% Cycle	0%	12%	50%	62%	100%

Fig. 130.3. Components of normal walking

Events

Traditionally the gait cycle has been divided into eight events or periods, five during stance phase and three during swing. The names of these events are self-descriptive and are based on the movement of the foot.

In the traditional nomenclature, the *stance phase* events are as follows:

1. Heel strike initiates the gait cycle and represents the point at which the body's centre of gravity is at its lowest position.
2. Foot-flat is the time when the plantar surface of the foot touches the ground.
3. Midstance occurs when the swinging (contralateral) foot passes the stance foot and the body's centre of gravity is at its highest position.
4. Heel-off occurs as the heel loses contact with the ground and the pushoff is initiated by the plantar flexors of the ankle.
5. Toe-off terminates the stance phase as the foot leaves the ground.

The *swing phase* events are as follows:

6. Acceleration begins as soon as the foot leaves the ground and the subject activates the hip flexor muscles to accelerate the leg forward.
7. Midswing occurs when the foot passes directly beneath the body, coincidental with midstance for the other foot.
8. Deceleration describes the action of the muscles as they slow the leg and stabilize the foot in preparation for the next heel strike.

This traditional nomenclature best describes the gait of normal subjects. However, there are a number of patients with pathologies, such as ankle equinus secondary to spastic cerebral palsy, whose gait cannot be described using this approach.

An alternative nomenclature, developed by Perry and her associates, has also eight events, but these are sufficiently general to be applied to any type of gait:

1. Initial contact (0%)
2. Loading response (0-10%)
3. Midstance (10-30%)
4. Terminal stance (30-50%)
5. Preswing (50-60%)
6. Initial Swing (60-70%)
7. Midswing (70-85%)
8. Terminal swing (85-100%)

Normal walk of an adult has a speed of 5 kmph, with about 50-60 steps per minute and at no point of time, the body losses the ground support through the one foot or the other. While running however, there will be a period during the walk cycle, when both the feet are off the ground and the body moves forwards at a greater speed.

Types of gait

Trendelenburg gait (unstable hip gait or gluteus medius gait):

It may be unilateral or bilateral. When unilateral, the patient lurches on the affected side (to move the center of gravity to the weight bearing limb) and the pelvis drops on the opposite side of the hip. Any condition, in which there is deficit in abduction mechanism of the hp joint, medial deviation of the lower limb and gross costo-pelvic impingement, will cause this type of gait. Bilateral *Trendelenburg* gait is like waddling gait.

Antalgic gait

Due to pain anywhere from foot to hip, the patient avoids bearing of weight on the affected limb (reduced stance phase, shortened step length, stride length and reciprocal arm swing with increased velocity of steps).

Short limb gait

Initially if the shortening is less than 1.5 cm it can be compensated by pelvic tilt while walking; if shortening increases upto 5 cm it can be made up by equinus at the ankle. With more shortening (>5 cm) the patient dips his body on that side due to marked pelvic tilt and increased equinus.

High stepping gait (foot drop gait)

During the heal strike attempt, the toes drop on ground first, hence to clear the ground, the patient flexes the hip and knee excessively,

807

raises the foot and slap it on the ground forcibly.

Stamping gait

The patient raises his feet abnormally high and jerks them forward to strike the ground slowly with a 'stamp' due to lack of kinesthetic. It is seen in sensory ataxia like tabes dorsalis, syringomyelia, hansen's disease and diabetes mellitus.

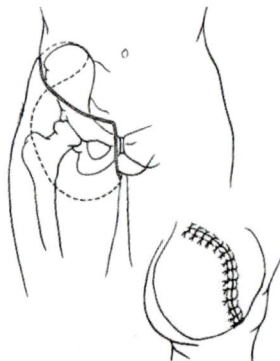

Fig. 130.4. Hind quarter amputation

Ataxic gait (broad based gait)

A gait in which foot is raised higher than necessary and brought down suddenly in a flapping manner, seen in cerebellar disease or alcoholic intoxication.

Quadriceps gait (hand to knee gait)

In quadriceps palsy seen in poliomyelitis the locking maneuver of the knee at the last stage of stance phase is lost and is compensated by the hand pres-sure over the thigh, to prevent the knee giving way to flexion. In due course, the patient may develop genu recurvatum deformity.

Gluteus maximus gait (rocking horse gait)

In gluteus maximus weakness during mid-stance phase, while the body propels forward, the trunk lurches posteriorly to effect the posterior pelvic tilting and shifting the center of gravity in line with the leg.

Stiff hip gait

When the movements of hip joints are restricted due to ankylosis, it is not possible to flex it to clear the ground in the swing phase and the patient improvises circumduction of the hip to bring the limb forward.

Scissoring gait

This is the characteristics of a spastic child of cerebral palsy, due to marked bilateral adductor spasm, legs crossing each other (like scissors) during walking.

Waddling gait (duck gait)

When there is disturbance in abduction mechanism of both hips, there is increased lordosis. While walking, the body sways from side to side on a wide base. Therefore, the patient lurches on both sides like a duck. It is seen in bilateral DDH, coxa varum, paralysis of abductors of both hips and myopathies.

In-toeing gait

It is usually due to metatarsus adductus, tibial bowing with torsion and persistent femoral anteversion. It usually resists correction by any orthotics. Hence, exact cause should be localized and treated.

Out-toeing gait

It is usually associated with lateral tibial torsion which needs surgical correction.

Festinant gait (short shuffling gait or toe-heel gait)

As a result of rigidity of muscles, the patient with stooping body, is propelled forward quickly in successions as if trying to catch up with the center of gravity, hence there will be short steps, lack of heel strike, and toe off, loss of arm swing and lack of pelvic rotation. Since the heel strike is absent, toe strike first, hence it is also called toe-heel gait. It is seen in Parkinsonism and Wilson's disease.

AMPUTATIONS

It is defined as surgical removal of a protruding functional unit of body. The ablation of a limb is such an extreme step resulting in profound physical and emotional consequences, utmost care should be exercised before deciding to perform an amputation. It is generally done

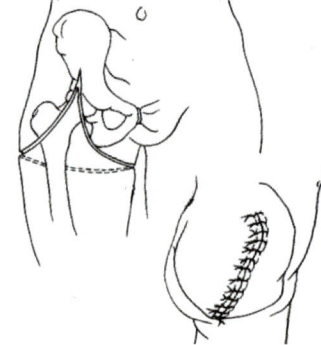

Fig. 130.5. Hip disarticulation

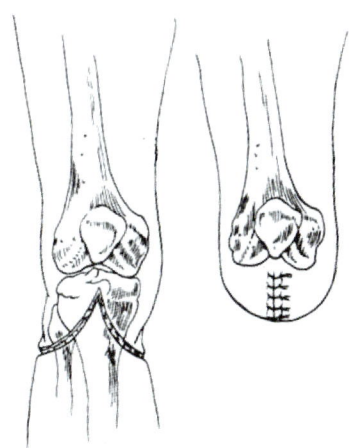

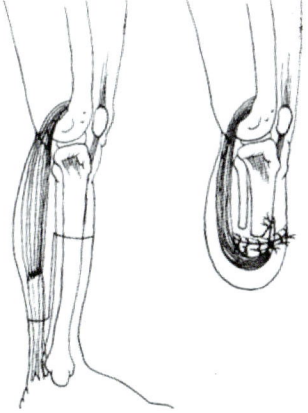

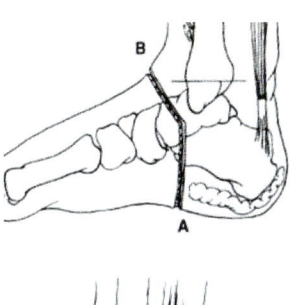

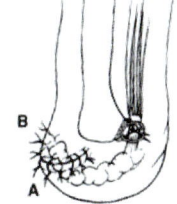

Fig. 130.6. Knee disarticulation

Fig.130.7. Below-knee amputation with a long posterior flap

Fig. 130.8. Syme's amputation

as a last resort, when all attempts of limb salvage had failed. It should be considered as a reconstructive procedure rather than an ablative procedure.

Removal of a limb through one or more bones is called amputation, whereas removal through a joint is called disarticulation.

Indications

1. Traumatic conditions: crush injuries with devitalized tissues

2. Vascular diseases: ischemia leading to gangrene

3. Malignancies of skin, soft tissue or bone

4. Infections: gas gangrene, actinomycosis, leprosy, filarial elephantiasis

5. Congenital deformity, so gross that makes the limb functionally useless

Types of amputations

1. Standard or classical amputation using fish-mouth or racquet incision

2. Guillotine amputation, using circular incision, cutting all tissues at the same level. This is done in emergencies to dismember grossly devitalized, potentially infected wound, as in gas gangrene to save life. The wound is left open for free drainage of infected fluid and closed secondarily, or converted to classical amputation after the infection is resolved.

3. Revision amputation

Selection of level (sites of election) of amputation

In the lower limb

1. Toe amputation or disarticulation

2. Ray amputation through the neck of the metatarsal bone

3. Forefoot (trans-metatarsal) amputation

4. Lisfranc amputation(through the tarso-metatarsal joints)

5. Chopart amputation (disarticulation through the talonavicular and calcaneocuboid joints)

6. Boyd amputation (arthrodesis between distal tibia and the tuber of calcaneus)

7. Pyragoff (trans-calcaneal) amputation

8. Syme's (trans-ankle) amputation

9. Below-knee (BK) amputation

10. Gritti-Stokes (trans-knee) amputation

11. Above-knee (AK) amputation

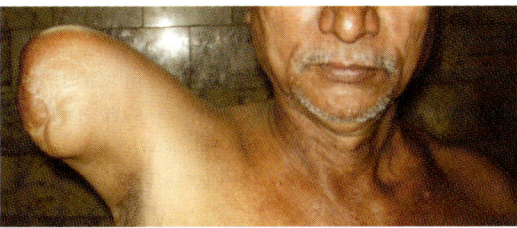

Fig. 130.9. Proximal arm amputation for crush injury

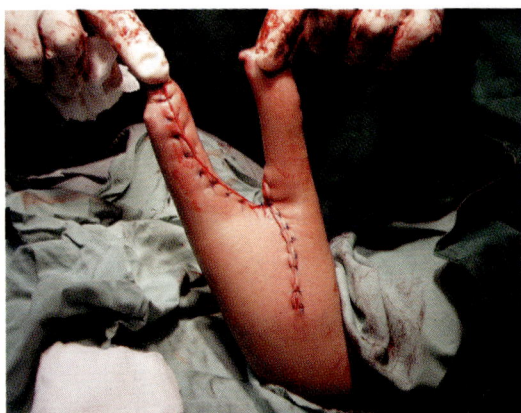

Fig. 130.10. Krukenberg reconstruction of distal forearm amputation
(courtesy: Prof G Balakrishnan, Chennai)

12. Mid-thigh amputation
13. Hip disarticulation
14. Hindquarter amputation

In the upper limb

1. Finger amputation
2. Mid-palm (trans-metacarpal) amputation
3. Above-wrist (AW) amputation
4. Krukenberg operation
5. Below-elbow (BE) amputation
6. Elbow disarticulation
7. Above-elbow (AE) amputation
8. Mid-arm amputation
9. Shoulder disarticulation
10. Forequarter amputation

Procedure

Mark out the level of amputation and by raising appropriate skin flaps, usually fish-mouth or racquet incision, the fascia and muscles are divided about 2cm proximal to skin. The main blood vessels and their major branches are identified and ligated. The nerves should not be crushed nor cut with scissors, but cut only with a sharp knife, after applying traction and allowed to retract. The bone is cut at about 5cm above the skin incision, with a saw and the sharp end is filed. If a tourniquet was applied, it should be removed or deflated at this stage, to look for and control bleeding points. Muscle loses its contractile function when the skeletal attachments are divided during amputation. Stabilizing the distal insertion of muscle can improve residual limb function by preventing muscle atrophy, providing counterbalance to the deforming forces resulting from amputation, and providing stable padding over the end of the bone. The muscles are sutured in 2 techniques.

Myodesis – Myodesis is the direct suturing of muscle or tendon to the bone or the periosteum. Myodesis techniques are most effective in stabilizing strong muscles needed to counteract strong antagonistic muscle forces, such as in cases involving transfemoral or transhumeral amputation and in cases involving knee or elbow disarticulation.

Myoplasty - Myoplasty involves the suturing of muscle to muscle over the end of the bone. The distal stabilization of the muscle is more secure with myodesis than with myoplasty. Care must be taken to prevent a mobile sling of muscle over the distal end of the bone, which usually results in a painful bursa.

A drain may be placed if the hemostasis is considered suboptimal or if the patient has been on anticoagulant/antiplatelet therapy. Compression dressings are applied and the stump is immobilized in a splint, as soon as possible. If the indication for amputation is ischemia, it is preferable not to use a tourniquet, especially in elderly with athero-sclerotic vessels whenever a torniquet is applied, as a matter of abundant precaution the end of the tape is tied to the operation table, so that a rare accident of not releasing the tourniquet after the procedure, may be prevented. While doing amputation in children, the skin flaps should be tailored loose and redundant, so as to accommodate the growing bone in future.

Krukenberg reconstruction

It is employed for an above-wrist amputation, to make the forearm stump functional, by dividing it vertically between the two bones and providing them skin cover. This essentially converts the stump into a fork, with which the patient can hold objects, including a pen for writing.

Ideal stump

1. it should be of optimal length
2. it should have a smooth, rounded or conical shape, without the surgical scar over the weight bearing surface, especially in the lower limb
3. it should be firm, with the bone end cushioned by muscles
4. it should have good vascularity
5. opposing groups of muscles should be sutured over the bone, to maintain neutral position
6. the skin over the stump should neither be too tight nor redundant.

Complications of amputations

Immediate

1. Hematoma
2. Infection
3. Hemorrhage
4. Flap necrosis
5. Deep vein thrombosis and embolism
6. Bone eroding through the suture line or skin flap

Late

1. Stump neuroma
2. Causalgia
3. Phantom-limb pain (page 218)

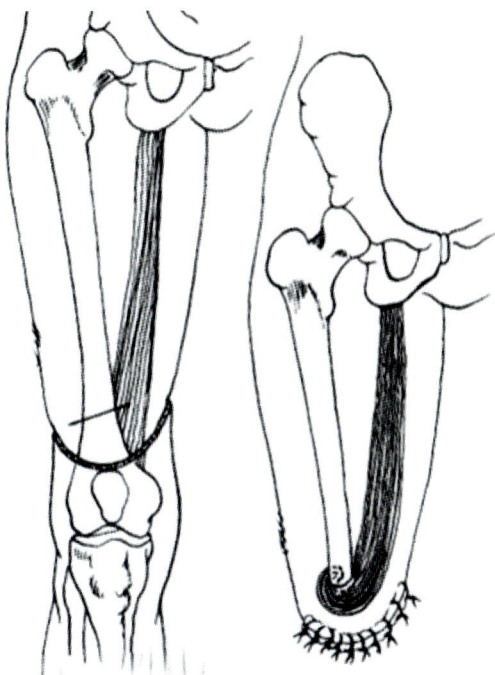

Fig. 130.11. Above-knee amputation with adductor myodesis

4. Pressure sores of stump, due to ill-fitting prosthesis
5. Osteomyelitis and ring sequestrum of the bone stump
6. Non-healing sinus
7. Contractures.

Index

A

Index...

Index...

Index...

Index...

Index...

Index...

Index...

Index...

Index...

Index...

Index...

Index...

Index...

P

Index...

Index...

Index...

Index...

Index...

Index...

Index...

Index...

Reader's Note